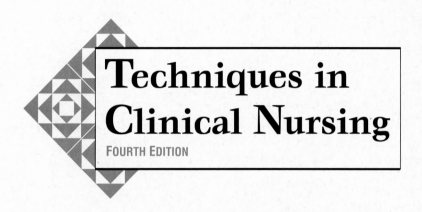

Techniques in Clinical Nursing

FOURTH EDITION

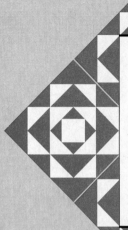

Techniques in Clinical Nursing

FOURTH EDITION

Barbara Kozier, RN, MN

Glenora Erb, RN, BSN

Kathleen Blais, RN, EdD
FLORIDA INTERNATIONAL UNIVERSITY

Joyce Young Johnson, RN, PhD, CCRN
GEORGIA STATE UNIVERSITY

Jean Smith Temple, RN, MSN
UNIVERSITY OF SOUTH ALABAMA

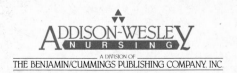
ADDISON-WESLEY NURSING
A DIVISION OF
THE BENJAMIN/CUMMINGS PUBLISHING COMPANY, INC.

Redwood City, California • Menlo Park, California
Reading, Massachusetts • New York • Don Mills, Ontario
Wokingham, U.K. • Amsterdam • Bonn • Sydney • Tokyo • Madrid • San Juan

SPONSORING EDITOR: Patricia L. Cleary
PROJECT EDITOR: Wendy Earl
PRODUCTION EDITOR: Wendy Earl
ASSISTANT EDITOR: Bradley Burch
TEXT DESIGNER: Paula Schlosser
COVER DESIGNER: Yvo Reizebos Design
MANUSCRIPT EDITOR: Sally Peyrefitte
PRINCIPAL PHOTOGRAPHER: Richard Tauber
ILLUSTRATOR: Jack Tandy
PRODUCTION ASSISTANT/ART COORDINATOR: Robert Kearns
PROOFREADER: Holly Wunder
INDEXER: Elinor Lindheimer
COMPOSITOR: Jonathan Peck Typographers
PRINTER AND BINDER: Banta Company

Library of Congress Cataloging-in-Publication Data
Techniques in clinical nursing / Barbara Kozier . . . [et al.].—4th ed.
      p.   cm.
      Rev. ed. of: Techniques in clinical nursing / Barbara Kozier,
Glenora Erb. 3rd ed. © 1989.
      Includes index.
      ISBN 0-8053-5950-8
      1. Nursing.   I. Kozier, Barbara.   II. Kozier, Barbara.
Techniques in clinical nursing.
      [DNLM: 1. Nursing Process.   WY 100 T2545]
RT41.K723   1993
610.73—dc20
DNLM/DLC
for Library of Congress   92-48922
                                                                         CIP

ISBN 0-8053-5950-8

1 2 3 4 5 6 7 8 9 10-BA-96 95 94 93 92

The cover illustration is from a quilt entitled "Pinnacle" by Setsuko Segawa.

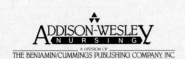
ADDISON-WESLEY
NURSING
A DIVISION OF
THE BENJAMIN/CUMMINGS PUBLISHING COMPANY, INC.

390 Bridge Parkway, Redwood City, CA 94065

The authors and publisher thank the following institutions for their kind permission to photograph in their facilities:

California Pacific Medical Center, San Francisco, California

East Bay Pediatrics, Berkeley, California

Hillhaven Convalescent Center, San Francisco, California

Jewish Home for the Aged, San Francisco, California

Kaiser Permanente Medical Center, Oakland Campus, Oakland, California

Joseph M. Long Hospital, University of California, San Francisco, California

San Francisco General Hospital, San Francisco, California

Stanford University Medical Center, Palo Alto, California

In addition, the authors and publisher thank Bette Ann Greene, Patricia Larson, RN, DNSc, Mary Matejov, RN, Karen Rago, RN, and Patricia Wong, RN for their valuable assistance in providing client and nurse models and access to their facilities.

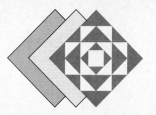

Preface

Technical expertise—a vital part of quality nursing care and an integral part of the intervention phase of the nursing process—must be synthesized with knowledge, interpersonal expertise, critical thinking and humanistic caring. In the words of Patricia Benner and Judith Wrubel:

". . . Nursing can never be reduced to mere technique. The way medicines are given and the way patients are taught all have different effects when they are done in a context of care."*

The fourth edition of *Techniques in Clinical Nursing* includes

- A total of 237 techniques. In some instances, separate techniques from earlier editions have been combined, e.g., measuring body temperature by mouth, axilla, and rectum; and administering oxygen by cannula, face mask, and face tent.

- A total of 500 illustrations and 355 photographs. Where appropriate, illustrations and photographs have been revised to reflect the Centers for Disease Control's universal precautions.

Techniques in Clinical Nursing may be used as a primary text in all nursing education programs, as a supplemental text in a skills course, by nurses needing reorientation when returning to clinical practice, or by beginning practitioners who need to refamiliarize themselves with specific skills required for various clinical settings. The text may be used effectively in a laboratory or a clinical setting, as well as in independent or instructor-led learning situations.

The content for this edition was selected on the basis of market surveys by the publisher, valuable suggestions from users and reviewers of previous editions, and an evaluation of changing nursing practices.

*From *The Primacy of Caring: Stress and Coping in Health and Illness* by Patricia Benner and Judith Wrubel, Addison-Wesley Publishing Company, 1989 and AJN, August 1988, p. 1073.

Goals of the Fourth Edition

The goals of this edition are:

- To provide information that complements fundamentals, medical-surgical, pediatric, and obstetrical nursing textbooks.

- To help students learn and perform the most commonly used techniques in nursing practice.

- To provide an understanding of not only *how* to perform a particular technique but *why* it is performed and why certain actions must be implemented throughout its performance.

- To help learners implement techniques within a nursing process framework.

- To assist learners to accurately document all nursing assessments and interventions.

- To encourage students to consider potential clinical problems that may arise while performing the technique.

New Features

Eleven New Chapters

- Introduction to Nursing
- Nursing Process and Critical Thinking
- Recording and Reporting
- Helping and Communicating
- Teaching
- Assessing Adult Health
- Assessing Infant and Child Health
- Assessing Maternal Health During the Perinatal Period
- Stress Management
- Pain Management
- Therapeutic Beds

38 New Techniques

These additions are indicated by an asterisk on the list of techniques beginning on page xi.

40 Assessment Techniques

New 3-column formats are used in Chapters 11 (Assessing Adult Health), 12 (Assessing Infant and Child Health), and 13 (Assessing Maternal Health During the Perinatal Period).

Special Learning Aids

- Safety alert logos (S) indicate when safety precautions are essential.
- Blood and body fluid alert logos reinforce awareness of CDC universal precautions.
- Pediatric logos (P) alert the learner to information within techniques that is pertinent to infants and children.
- Boxes that highlight special considerations for care of the elderly.
- A full-color introduction to the nursing process.
- A full-color overview of physical health assessment.
- A full-color guide to skin disorders.

Nursing Process Guides

Most chapters begin with a nursing process guide that includes comprehensive data for the techniques in the chapter, nursing diagnostic categories relating to the chapter content, and a planning section outlining client goals and outcome criteria that may be used to evaluate the effectiveness of nursing interventions.

New Technique Format

Each technique contains purposes, an assessment focus, a list of equipment, a list of step-by-step interventions describing how to perform the technique, an evaluation focus, a sample recording, and a summary of key elements. In addition, critical steps of the technique are supported by a *rationale*. Many techniques have a variation section that describes an alternative method of performing the technique or information essential for pediatric application.

Guide to Required Nursing Actions

Specific nursing actions that are common to most techniques have been omitted from each technique to avoid repetition. These actions are summarized on the inside front cover, providing easy access for the student.

Key Elements Boxes

At the end of each technique involving a client, a summary of key elements helps students learn and evaluate their performance. We consider a key element a nursing activity that meets any or all of the following criteria:

- Prevents injury to the client
- Safeguards the client's and the nurse's current health status, and
- Is essential for the effectiveness of the technique.

Although elements that protect the client from emotional jeopardy—such as explaining the procedure and using therapeutic communication—are also considered essential, these elements have not always been repeated in each technique because they apply to all techniques.

Critical Thinking Challenges

Each chapter contains a potential clinical problem that may arise when providing care. These exercises are designed to help the student apply knowledge gained from the chapter and to stimulate critical thinking. Responses to these items, as well as additional critical thinking challenges and responses, are provided in the Instructor's Guide that accompanies the text. They may be used as a basis for post-clinical conference discussions or in a classroom setting.

Related Research References

Each chapter concludes with a brief list of nursing research articles that relate to the chapter content and emphasize the role that research plays in changing nursing practice.

Universal Precautions

A summary of the Centers for Disease Control recommendations regarding universal blood and body fluid precautions appears on the back cover of the book.

Organization

The fourth edition of *Techniques in Clinical Nursing* contains 45 chapters that may be used independently and in any sequence. The first five chapters provide a broad introduction to concepts essential for synthesizing technical and interpersonal competencies and selected nursing knowledge. The remaining chapters are listed in the table of contents. The glossary at the end of the text facilitates flexibility in using this text.

Each chapter contains behavioral objectives, a chapter outline, a nursing process guide (where appropriate), and a theory base for the techniques. Included in the theory section of some chapters are relevant developmental changes and common health problems.

Supplemental Teaching and Learning Package

Instructor's Manual

To help instructors enhance the use of this new edition, an instructor's manual, prepared by Kathleen Blais and Judith Wilkinson, includes:

- An article entitled "Promoting Critical Thinking" by Judith Wilkinson

- An article entitled "A Curricular Basic for Our Multiethnic Future" by Carlos E. Cortéz

- Responses to the Critical Thinking Challenges in each chapter of the basic text

- An additional Critical Thinking Challenge (situation) for each chapter, with responses

- Suggested learning activities for each chapter

Acknowledgments

The participation of many persons of diverse talent and expertise is required to prepare a textbook of this magnitude. We extend our warmest appreciation and sincere thanks to all who participated.

- Users of the previous editions, who sent us many useful suggestions and who always help us focus on their needs.

- The nursing educators who shared their knowledge and experience in reviewing selected portions of this edition to ensure accuracy, clarity, and currency. They are listed on page viii.

- Patti Cleary, the sponsoring editor, whose guidance in this project provided stimulation and motivation for this work. She has the ability to instill confidence, understanding, and support when it is most needed. Her inspiration, advice, and feedback have been invaluable and our association with her has been a most enriching experience.

- Wendy Earl, the project editor and production editor, who provided ongoing momentum for the developing manuscript, and performed the indispensable task of coordinating the production of this book. We are grateful for her special qualities of commitment, involvement, diligence, unremitting attention to detail, and high standards. We value her continued support.

- Bradley Burch, assistant editor, for his continued goodwill, seemingly effortless help whenever it was needed, and dedicated efforts in developing the instructor's manual and obtaining reviews for this edition.

- Paula Schlosser, for the aesthetic page and book design, cover design, and page layouts that are so creative, visually appealing, and streamlined.

- Sally Peyrefitte, copy editor, who transposed so many passive to active sentences and provided many other helpful suggestions for clarity, style, and syntax.

- Jack Tandy of St. Louis, whose artistic talents produced new line drawings that make explicit what words alone cannot and, as usual, are models of clarity.

- Richard Tauber, whose talents as a photographer are obvious in the clarity, sensitivity, and authentic realism of the many new photographs.

- Robbi Kearns, who competently organized and managed the art program.

- Elinor Lindheimer, for her skill, speed, and judgment in creating a comprehensive index.

- Holly Wunder, for her careful attention to detail when reading the galleys.

- Mary Tobin, our typist, for her accommodating nature, expertise, and speed, which enabled us to meet many deadlines.

- Joan Andrews, Carol MacFarlane, and Linda Edge at the Registered Nurses' Association of British Columbia, for their continued support in obtaining reference materials for this manuscript.

- Marjorie E. Wilson, Head Nurse, ICU, Beth Israel Hospital North, New York, for her advice regarding intensive care equipment and practices.

- The administrators, staff, and clients at many hospitals in the California community for their generosity and cooperation in conducting photography in the clinical setting.

- Finally, our families and friends, who provided balance to our lives and much encouragement, understanding, and support throughout another demanding schedule.

We invite users of the fourth edition to send their reactions and suggestions to the publisher so that subsequent editions of this book can be improved.

Barbara Kozier

Glenora Erb

Kathleen Blais

Joyce Johnson

Jean Temple

Reviewers

Sandra Cesario, BSN, MS
USPHS Indian Hospital, Claremore, OK

Rosario T. DeGracia, MS, RNC
Seattle University School of Nursing, Seattle, WA

Hubert M. D'Entremont, BA, BSN
Yarmouth Regional Hospital, Yarmouth,
Nova Scotia

Margaret Fried, BSN, MSN
Pima Community College, Tucson, AZ

Ruby F. Graber, BSN, MSN
Hesston College, Hesston, KS

Marguerite Jackson, MS, CIC, FAAN
University of California Medical Center,
San Diego, CA

Carol Kilmon, BSN, MSN, PhD
The University of Texas School of Nursing at
Galveston, Galveston, TX

Linda L. Larson, BSN, MS, PhD
Regis University, Denver, CO

Kate McClure, BSN, MS, CCRN
Samuel Merritt College, Oakland, CA

Frieda A. Muwakkil, BSN, MS, MEd
Gate Way Community College, Phoenix, AZ

Julie Novak, MA, CPNP, DNSc
San Diego State University, San Diego, CA

Lynne Peterson, BSN, MSN
Hocking College, Nelsonville, OH

Jennifer Reilly, BSN, MEd, MSN
Hocking College, Nelsonville, OH

Judith M. Wilkinson, MA, MS, RNC
Johnson County Community College,
Overland Park, KS

Carol Zack, BSN, MSN, DEd
Wilkes University, Wilkes Barre, PA

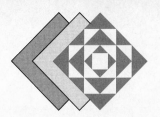

Contents

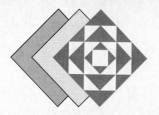

Techniques

*Asterisked techniques are new to this edition.

continued

continued

continued

Clinical Guidelines Boxes

The following logos are used throughout the text:

 Blood and Body Fluid Precautions

This logo draws attention to the need for blood and body fluid precautions. These precautions are intended to protect the nurse and others from infection. See also the Universal Precautions on the back cover, and check with your instructor regarding agency protocol to determine which precautionary measures to implement.

 Safety Precautions

This logo highlights nursing actions that are of particular significance for maintaining client and nurse safety. If you require clarification, consult your instructor or check agency protocol to ensure safe practice.

 Pediatric Considerations

This logo highlights information that pertains to the care of infants and children.

1

Introduction to Nursing

OBJECTIVES

- Identify essential aspects of nursing or the practice of nursing, according to Florence Nightingale, Virginia Henderson, the ANA, and the CNA

- Differentiate independent, dependent, and collaborative nursing actions

- Identify four cognitive skills nurses use when implementing nursing care

- Discuss essential aspects of the nurse's roles

- Explain how nurse practice acts legally help the nurse practitioner

- Describe essential elements of the legal concepts of privileged communication, privacy, battery, and informed consent

- Identify the nurse's legal responsibilities in relation to record keeping, carrying out physician's orders, and implementing nursing actions

- Describe the purposes of codes of ethics

- Outline the essentials of the Patient's Bill of Rights established by the American Hospital Association

CONTENTS

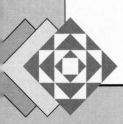

Nursing Practice

Florence Nightingale defined nursing over 100 years ago as "the act of utilizing the environment of the patient to assist him in his recovery" (Nightingale 1860). Nightingale considered a clean, well-ventilated, and quiet environment essential for recovery. Often considered the first nurse theorist, Nightingale raised the status of nursing through education. Nurses were no longer untrained housekeepers but people trained in the care of the sick.

Virginia Henderson was one of the first modern nurses to define nursing. In 1960, she wrote, "The unique function of the nurse is to assist the individual, sick or well, in the performance of those activities contributing to health or its recovery (or to peaceful death) that he would perform unaided if he had the necessary strength, will, or knowledge, and to do this in such a way as to help him gain independence as rapidly as possible" (Henderson 1966, p. 3). Like Nightingale, Henderson described nursing in relation to the client and the client's environment. Unlike Nightingale, however, Henderson saw the nurse as concerned with both well and ill individuals, acknowledged that nurses interact with clients even when recovery may not be feasible, and mentioned the teaching and advocacy roles of the nurse.

The American Nurses' Association (ANA) describes nursing practice as "direct, goal oriented, and adaptable to the needs of the individual, the family, and community during health and illness" (ANA 1973, p. 2). In its 1987 House of Delegates, the ANA adopted a statement on the scope of nursing practice: "There is one scope of clinical nursing practice. The core, or essence, of that practice is the nursing diagnosis and treatment of human responses to health and to illness" (ANA 1987, p. 76). The Canadian Nurses' Association (CNA) published a definition in 1984 that serves as a practice standard for nurses in Canada. In this definition, *nursing* or *the practice of nursing* means the identification and treatment of human responses to actual or potential health problems; it includes the practice of and supervision of functions and services that, directly or indirectly, in collaboration with a client or providers of health care other than nurses, have as their objectives the promotion of health, prevention of illness, alleviation of suffering, restoration of health, and optimum development of health potential; and it encompasses all aspects of the nursing process (CNA 1984, p. 8).

The recipients of nursing are sometimes called *consumers*, sometimes *patients*, and sometimes *cli-*

ents. A **consumer** is an individual, a group of people, or a community that uses a service or commodity. A family that uses electricity in their home is a consumer of electricity. People who use health care products or services are consumers of health care. A **patient** is a person who is waiting for or undergoing medical treatment and care. The word *patient* comes from a Latin word meaning "to suffer" or "to bear." Traditionally, the person receiving health care has been called a patient. Usually, people become patients when they seek assistance because of illness or for surgery.

Some nurses believe that the word *patient* implies passive acceptance of the decisions and care of health professionals. Additionally, as a result of the emphasis on health promotion and prevention of illness, many recipients of nursing care are not ill. Moreover, nurses interact with family members and significant others in addition to the persons actually receiving nursing care. For these reasons, nurses are increasingly referring to recipients of health care as clients. A **client** is a person who engages the advice or services of another who is qualified to provide this service. The term *client* presents the receivers of health care less as passive recipients and more as collaborators in the care, i.e., as persons who are also responsible for their health. Thus, the health status of a client is the responsibility of the individual in collaboration with health professionals.

Types of Nursing Actions

The terms *independent*, *dependent*, and *collaborative* (*interdependent*) are often used to describe nursing actions. An *action*, in this context, is an activity appropriate to a person's role. It is also called a *nursing strategy*. An **independent nursing action** is an activity that the nurse initiates as a result of the nurse's own knowledge and skills. Examples of independent nursing actions include providing self-care assistance and providing client teaching.

Dependent nursing actions are those activities carried out on the order of the physician, under the physician's supervision, or according to specified routines. An example of a dependent action is giving an antibiotic by injection to a client as a result of a physician's written order. The dependent activity in nursing practice is usually directly related to the client's disease, and its importance should not be minimized. In addition to the task of carrying out the physician's order, the nurse who performs a dependent nursing action also conducts the appropriate nursing activities associated with the order. In the example above, for instance, the nurse would also monitor the client for signs of improvement, worsening infection, or toxic effects of the antibiotic.

Collaborative nursing actions are those activities performed either jointly with another member of the health care team or as a result of a joint decision by the nurse and another health care team member. For example, a nurse and a respiratory therapist together may decide on a schedule of breathing exercises for a client. The therapist may initially teach the exercises to the client, and the nurse reinforces the learned behavior and assists the client in the therapist's absence.

Protocols and Standing Orders

A **protocol** is a written plan specifying the procedure to be followed in a particular situation. For example, agencies often have protocols regarding a client's admission and discharge. Nurse practitioners in a community clinic often have protocols about which clients to refer to the physician and which clients to treat directly. Nurses in a home setting usually have protocols about the procedure to follow when a client dies. Nurses in hospitals often have protocols regarding the steps to follow when a postoperative client returns to the unit.

A **standing order** is a written document about policies, rules, regulations, or orders regarding client care. Standing orders give nurses the authority to carry out specific actions under certain circumstances, often when a physician is not immediately available. In a hospital critical care unit, a common example is the administration of emergency antiarrhythmic medications when a client's cardiac monitoring pattern changes. In a home care setting, a physician may write a standing order for the administration of epinephrine for a client who becomes excessively dyspneic.

Categories of Nursing Skills

There are three categories of actions or skills needed in nursing practice: cognitive, interpersonal, and technical skills.

Cognitive Skills
Cognitive skills are intellectual skills. The cognitive skills needed in nursing practice are problem solving, decision making, critical thinking, and creative thinking. They are crucial to safe, intelligent nursing care.

Problem Solving There are various approaches to problem solving. Four of the most commonly used

are trial and error, intuition, experimentation, and the scientific method.

In solving a problem by *trial and error*, the nurse tries a number of approaches until a solution is found. However, by failing to consider the alternatives systematically, the nurse cannot determine *why* the solution works. Trial-and-error methods in nursing care can be dangerous, because the client might suffer harm from an inappropriate approach.

Intuition as a problem-solving method has not been considered either sound or legitimate. Rather, it has been viewed as a form of guessing and, as such, an inappropriate basis for nursing decisions. However, according to recent investigations, intuition appears to be an essential and legitimate aspect of clinical judgment acquired through knowledge and experience (Benner and Tanner 1987). Nurses develop intuitive judgment through clinical experience with similar types of situations. In other words, nurses develop expertise in a specialty area, such as cardiovascular nursing, from continuous and meaningful exposure to clients who have experienced cardiovascular problems.

Experimentation is more controlled than trial and error. It is based on knowledge and research and is therefore a more valid method than trial-and-error or intuitive problem solving. Experimentation is used in pilot projects and limited trials to solve problems. For example, a nurse caring for a client with intractable pain may try one specific nursing intervention for 3 days to reduce the pain. If the pain is not reduced, the nurse may then implement a second plan for another 3 days.

The **scientific method** is a logical, systematic approach to solving problems. The classic scientific method is most useful in a laboratory, where the scientist works in a controlled situation. The steps of the scientific method are outlined in Table 1–1.

Health professionals require a modified approach of the scientific method for solving problems. This modified scientific problem-solving method is used in the nursing process as well as the medical process. Like the scientific process, it has seven steps. See Table 1–1 on the following page for a comparsion of the problem-solving process, the nursing process, and the scientific method.

Decision Making **Decision making** is the process of choosing the best action to meet a desired goal. Three conditions must prevail: freedom, rationality, and voluntary (Schaefer 1974, p. 1852). Freedom means that the individual has the authority to make the decision without pressure from others. Rationality, in the context of decision making, means that the individual makes the best or optimal decision consistent with personal values and preferences.

TABLE 1–1 COMPARISON OF STEPS IN THE PROBLEM-SOLVING PROCESS,
THE NURSING PROCESS, AND THE SCIENTIFIC METHOD

Problem-Solving Process	Nursing Process	Scientific Method
1. Encounter the problem.	1. Assessing	1. Recognize and define the problem.
2. Collect data.		2. Collect data from observation and experimentation.
3. Analyze information and identify exact nature of the problem.	2. Diagnosing	3. Formulate hypothesis (an assumption made to test the logic of a proposition).
4. Determine a plan of action.	3. Planning	4. Select plan to test the hypothesis.
5. Carry out the plan.	4. Implementing	5. Test the hypothesis.
6. Evaluate the plan and its outcomes.	5. Evaluating	6. Interpret test results (evaluate whether the hypothesis is correct).
7. Terminate or modify the plan.		7. Conclude or modify hypothesis.

Rationality involves both deliberation and judgment. Voluntarity means that the person makes the choice voluntarily.

Critical Thinking **Critical thinking** is a pattern of thinking based on knowledge, experience, and the abilities to conceptualize and analyze relationships. To conceptualize means to form a concept. A *concept* is an abstract idea generalized from particular instances. Critical thinking involves organizing information, picking out relevant information, relating, conceptualizing, and making judgments. Critical thinking enables nurses to make decisions quickly without bias.

The ability to think critically is learned. It requires knowledge, experience, and mature, healthy nervous systems. As people grow and develop, they attempt to deal with new experiences largely through trial and error. As a result, individuals build up a repertoire of thinking skills. With increasing knowledge and experience, individuals enlarge their repertoire, test and modify their skills, and learn to think critically. For more information about critical thinking, see Chapter 2, page 17.

Creative Thinking **Creative thinking** is a form of directed thinking that involves establishing new relationships and new concepts, thereby solving problems innovatively. When thinking creatively, the individual cannot always weigh alternatives or establish the logic behind all actions. For nurses, planning nursing strategies and changing nursing actions provide opportunities for creative thinking. Creative thinking helps nurses change a nursing activity efficiently.

Interpersonal Skills
Interpersonal skills are all the activities people use when communicating directly with one another, both verbally and nonverbally. The effectiveness of a nursing action often depends largely on the nurse's ability to communicate with others. Even when giving a medication to a client, the nurse needs to understand the client and in turn to be understood. A nurse delegating a nursing action also needs to be understood.

Interpersonal skills are necessary for all nursing activities: caring, comforting, referring, counseling, and supporting are just a few. Interpersonal skills are crucial to the nurse's ability to convey knowledge, attitudes, feelings, interest, and appreciation of the client's cultural values and life-style. Before nurses can be highly skilled in interpersonal relations, they must be self-aware and sensitive to others. See Chapter 4 for more detailed discussions about interpersonal skills.

Technical Skills
Technical skills are "hands-on" skills, such as manipulating equipment, giving injections, and bandaging, moving, lifting, and repositioning clients. To master technical skills, nurses need to acquire considerable knowledge about the principles behind the steps of the procedure, about equipment and supplies, and, in some instances, about when the procedure is required. Knowledge of underlying principles is particularly important because it enables the nurse to adapt a procedure to the individual client safely. For example, if a client cannot turn on the left side for an enema, the nurse can adjust the client's position and still administer the enema effectively, provided that the nurse understands the position of the rectum and large intestine in the body and the gravitational flow of fluids.

It is important that the nurse make significant assessments of the client *before, during,* and *after* carrying out procedures requiring technical skills. Before initiating any procedure, nurses must relate their own knowledge and competence to the client's needs. Sometimes they need assistance to prevent undue stress on the client and to ensure that the procedure is both safe and effective. Evaluating the effectiveness of the procedure is equally important.

Technical skills require knowledge and, frequently, manual dexterity. The number of technical skills expected of nurses has increased greatly in recent years. Because of the increased use of technology, especially in acute care hospitals, the importance of humanizing health care and communicating effectively with clients has received increased recognition.

Roles of the Nurse

The following nurse roles are ways of describing the nurse's activities in practice. Each role is described as a separate entity for the sake of clarity. The roles are not, however, exclusive of one another; in practice, several roles often coincide. For example, the nurse may be acting as a client advocate while also caring, communicating, teaching or counseling, and acting as a change agent and a leader.

Carer

The role of the nurse as carer and comforter is difficult to define specifically. It has traditionally included those activities that preserve the dignity of the individual and those often referred to as the "mothering actions" in nursing. However, caring also involves knowledge of and sensitivity to what matters and what is important to clients. The chief goal of the nurse in this role is to convey understanding and to provide support. The nurse supports the client by attitudes and actions that show concern for client welfare and acceptance of the client as a person, not merely a mechanical being.

Communicator/Helper

Effective communication is an essential element of all helping professions, including nursing. Communication shapes relationships between nurses and clients, nurses and support persons, and nurses and colleagues. It plays a role in every action the nurse undertakes. The communication process, listening and responding skills, and ways to establish helping relationships are discussed in detail in Chapter 4.

Communication facilitates all nursing actions. The nurse communicates to other health care personnel the nursing interventions planned and implemented for each client. The nurse writes planned nursing interventions on the client's care plan and, once they are implemented, documents them on the client's record. Assessment findings, procedures implemented, and the client's responses are recorded. Nurses also communicate pertinent information verbally at change of shift reports, on a client's transfer to another unit, at client rounds, and on a client's discharge to another health care agency. This type of communication needs to be concise, clear, and relevant. See Chapter 3 for details of reporting and recording.

Teacher

Teaching refers to activities by which one person helps another to learn. It is an interactive process between a teacher and one or more learners in which specific learning objectives or desired behavior changes are achieved (Redman 1988, pp. 9 and 15). The focus of the behavior change is usually the acquiring of new knowledge or technical skills. The teaching process has four components—assessing, planning, implementing, and evaluating—which can be viewed as parallel to the parts of the nursing process. In the assessment phase, the nurse determines the client's learning needs and readiness to learn; during planning, sets specific learning goals and teaching strategies; during implementation, enacts teaching strategies; and, during evaluation, measures learning. See Chapter 5 for detailed information about the teaching/learning process.

Counselor

Counseling is the process of helping a client to recognize and cope with stressful psychologic or social problems, to improve interpersonal relationships, and to promote personal growth. Counseling involves providing emotional, intellectual, and psychologic support. In contrast to the psychotherapist, who counsels individuals with identified problems, the nurse counsels primarily healthy individuals with normal adjustment difficulties. The focus is on helping the person develop new attitudes, feelings, and behaviors rather than on promoting intellectual growth. The nurse encourages the client to look at alternative behaviors, recognize the choices, and develop a sense of control.

Obviously, counseling requires therapeutic communication skills. In addition, the nurse must be a skilled leader, able to analyze a situation, synthesize information and experiences, and evaluate the progress and productivity of the individual or group. The nurse must also be willing to model and teach desired behaviors, to be sincere when dealing with people, and to demonstrate interest and caring in the welfare of others.

Client Advocate

An **advocate** pleads the cause of another or argues or pleads for a cause or proposal. Advocacy involves concern for and defined actions in behalf of another person or organization to bring about a change. A **client advocate** is an advocate of clients' rights. According to Disparti (1988, p. 140), advocacy involves promoting what is best for the client, ensuring that the client's needs are met, and protecting the client's rights. Some nurses believe client advocacy is an essential nursing function. Others believe that a client advocate need not be a nurse. All, however, recognize that many clients need an advocate to protect their rights and to help them speak up for themselves.

Some people believe that the client advocate should be accountable to the client and be the client's representative. The client advocate should be able to call in qualified consultants, participate actively in hospital committees monitoring the quality of client care, present complaints directly to the hospital director and hospital executive committee, delay discharges, and participate at the client's request and direction in discussions of the client's case (Annas 1975, pp. 209, 211). An advocate can represent a client by presenting the client's point of view and by interpreting and explaining the client's rights. The box below outlines the characteristics of responsible advocacy.

Change Agent

A **change agent** is a person or group who initiates changes or who assists others in making modifications in themselves or in the system (Kemp 1986). When assuming the role of change agent, nurses must recognize that they serve as an important link between various components of the change project or people participating in the change project. The change agent should hold a variety of expectations and expect the final outcome to be different from the original plan. The change agent must also be accessible to all people involved in the change process and be honest and straightforward about goals and problems.

A key element is trust. The change agent must trust the participants in the change, and they in turn must trust the change agent. One of the greatest risks is that the system can become disrupted, even nonfunctional. For example, changing the method of assigning nurses could result in gaps and missed care for some clients. To avoid this problem, the change agent must closely observe the situation during the change process.

Mauksch and Miller (1981) list three key characteristics of a change agent:

1. The ability to take risks. This involves the ability to calculate potential risks associated with the change and then to decide whether the risks are worth taking.

2. A commitment to the efficacy of the change. The change agent should investigate the change and be convinced of its value and effectiveness.

3. Comprehensive nursing knowledge that combines research findings and basic science data; competence in nursing practice, interpersonal relations, and communication skills.

Leader

The leadership role can be applied at many different levels: individual, family, groups of clients, professional colleagues, or the larger society. At the client level, **nursing leadership** is defined as a process of interpersonal influence through which the nurse helps the client establish and achieve goals to improve well-being (Leddy and Pepper 1989, p. 336). Effective leadership is a learned process requiring an understanding of the needs and goals that motivate people, the knowledge to apply the leadership skills, and the interpersonal skills to influence others.

Manager

Management and leadership are often confused, because in much of the literature, leadership is associated with group interaction within an organizational setting. **Management** is defined as "the use of delegated authority within the formal organization to organize, direct, or control responsible subordinates ... so that all service contributions are coordinated

---

Characteristics of Responsible Advocacy

- Conveying concern for the client's total situation

- Recognizing that what the client really wants may not be what the client verbalizes under stress

- Recognizing the effect a change in a client's situation may have on others

- Balancing the client's needs against others' needs and recognizing that change must come slowly

- Recognizing the importance of good working relationships and communication with others

Source: J. Zusman, Want some good advice? Think twice about being a patient advocate, *Nursing Life*, November/December 1982, 6:49.

to attain a goal" (Yura, Ozimek, and Walsh 1981, p. 5). Leadership, by contrast, may or may not involve delegation of authority within a formal organization.

The nurse manages the nursing care of individuals, families, and communities. The nurse-manager also delegates nursing activities to ancillary workers and other nurses and supervises and evaluates their performance. Managing requires knowledge about organizational structure and dynamics, authority and accountability, leadership, change theory, advocacy, delegation, and supervision and evaluation.

Researcher

Increasingly, nurses are expected to participate in research activity. Many constraints in clinical settings must be reckoned with before research can become a legitimate and comfortable activity. However, if nursing is to develop as a research-based practice, it is not unreasonable to expect the nurse in the clinical area to (a) have some awareness of the process and language of research, (b) be sensitive to issues relating to protecting the rights of human subjects, (c) participate in the identification of significant researchable problems, and (d) be a discriminating consumer of research findings.

Legal Aspects of Nursing

Because nurses are accountable for their professional judgments and actions, they must be familiar with the basic legal concepts that govern nursing practice. **Accountability** means being responsible for one's actions and accepting the consequences of one's behavior.

Nurse Practice Acts

Each state in the United States has nurse practice acts, and each province in Canada has a nurse practice act or an act for professional nursing practice. Nurse practice acts protect the nurse's professional capacity and legally control nursing practice through licensing. Nurse practice acts legally define and describe the scope of nursing practice, which the law seeks to regulate, thereby protecting the public as well. Because of the number of acts there are many definitions and descriptions of nursing. In 1981, the ANA described nursing practice as including but not limited to "administration, teaching, counseling, supervison, delegation, and evaluation of practice and execution of the medical regimen, including the administration of medications and treatments prescribed by any person authorized by state law to prescribe" (ANA 1981, p. 6).

Privileged Communication

A *privileged communication* is information given to a professional who is forbidden by law from disclosing the information in a court without the consent of the person who provided it.

Legislation regarding privileged communications is highly complicated. A nurse would be unwise to encourage disclosures or advise a client about the subject. The privileged communication law is for the benefit of the client; a nurse who is given confidential information should be prepared to answer questions fully and honestly if required to testify in a court of law. Many states with statutes granting privileged communications between the client and various health care providers do not extend the privilege to nurse-client communication.

Privacy

When a client enters a hospital or nursing facility, the loss of privacy is instantly obvious. *Privacy* has been described as a comfortable feeling reflecting a deserved degree of social retreat. Its dimensions and duration are controlled by the individual seeking the privacy.

People need varying degrees of privacy and establish boundaries for privacy; when these boundaries are crossed, they feel invaded. Hospital personnel sometimes show little concern for clients' privacy. Clients are asked to provide information that many consider private; they may share a room with strangers; and their health is frequently discussed among many health professionals.

The boundaries of privacy are highly individual. The adult who lives alone may be used to privacy while eating, sleeping, and reading. A child from a large family may be accustomed to sharing these activities with others. It is important for nurses to ascertain what privacy means to the individual and try to support accustomed practices whenever possible. A nurse has a qualified privilege to make statements that could be considered invasions of a client's privacy, both orally and in writing, but only as a part of nursing practice and only to a physician or another health team member caring directly for the client.

Informed Consent

Informed consent is a client's agreement to accept a course of treatment or a procedure after receiving complete information, including the risks of treatment and facts relating to it, from the physician. Informed consent, then, is an exchange between a client and a physician. Usually the client signs a form provided by the agency. The form is a record of the informed consent, not the informed consent itself.

Obtaining informed consent is the responsibility of a physician. Although this responsibility is delegated to nurses in some agencies, the practice is highly undesirable. The nurse's responsibility is often to witness the giving of informed consent. This involves the following:

- Witnessing the exchange between the client and the physician

- Witnessing the client's signature

- Establishing that the client really did understand, i.e., was really informed

If a nurse witnesses only the client's signature and not the exchange between the client and the physician, the nurse should write "witnessing signature only" on the form (Northrop 1988, p. 218). If the nurse finds that the client really does not understand the physician's explanation, then the physician must be notified.

To give informed consent voluntarily, the client must *not* feel coerced. Sometimes fear of disapproval by a health professional can be the motivation for giving consent; such consent is not voluntarily given.

To give informed consent, the client must receive sufficient information to make a decision; otherwise, the client's right to decide has been usurped. Information needs to include benefits, risks, and alternative procedures. It is also important that the client understand. Technical words and language barriers can inhibit understanding. If a client cannot read, the consent form must be read to the client before it is signed. If the client does not speak the same language as the health professional who is providing the information, an interpreter must be acquired.

If given sufficient information, the client can make decisions regarding health. To do so, the client must be competent and an adult. A competent adult is a person over 18 years of age who is conscious and oriented. A person under 18 years who is considered "an emancipated minor," i.e., self-supporting or married, can also give consent. A client who is confused, disoriented, or sedated is not considered functionally competent at that time.

Battery and False Imprisonment

Battery is the willful touching of a person (or the person's clothes or even something the person is carrying), which may or may not cause harm. To be actionable at law, however, the touching must be wrong in some way, e.g., done without permission, embarrassing, or causing injury. For example, the nurse who administers a hypodermic injection to a client or ambulates a client without the client's con-

sent could be held liable for battery. Liability applies even though the physician ordered the medication or the activity and even if the client benefits from the nurse's action.

In Canada, the term *battery* is not used. Instead, assault is classified into three categories: assault with intention to injure (for example, threatening someone by making a menacing gesture with a knife), assault causing bodily injury, and sexual assault.

Although nurses may suggest under certain circumstances that a client remain in the room or in bed, they must not detain the client against the client's will. To do so may be considered false imprisonment. **False imprisonment** is unjustifiable detention that deprives a person of personal liberty for any length of time. For example, a nurse who locks a client in a room unjustifiably is guilty of false imprisonment. Nurses must also be careful not to commit false imprisonment when applying restraints to a client. For information about restraints, see Chapter 6.

The client has a right to leave even though it may be detrimental to health. In this instance, the client may leave by signing an AMA (against medical authority) form. For further information, see Chapter 8.

Record Keeping

The client's medical record is a legal document and can be produced in court as evidence. Often the record is used to remind a witness of events surrounding a lawsuit, events that may have taken place several months or years before the suit came to trial. The effectiveness of a witness's testimony can depend on the accuracy of such records. Nurses therefore need to keep accurate and complete records of nursing care provided to clients. Failure to keep proper records can constitute negligence and be the basis for tort liability. Insufficient or inaccurate assessments and documentation can hinder proper diagnosis and treatment and result in injury to the client. Types of records and essential facts about recording are discussed in Chapter 3.

Carrying Out Physician's Orders

Many techniques are carried out as a result of a physician's order. Nurses are expected to know basic information about these procedures and medications.

Becker (1983, pp. 21–23) outlines five orders that nurses must question to protect themselves legally:

1. *Question any ambiguous order.* It is the nurse's responsibility to seek clarification of ambiguous or seemingly erroneous orders from the prescribing physician. Clarification from any other source is

unacceptable and regarded as a departure from competent nursing practice.

2. *Question any order a client questions.* For example, if a client who has been receiving an intramuscular injection tells the nurse that the doctor changed the order from an injectable to an oral medication, the nurse should recheck the order before giving the medication.

3. *Question any order if the client's condition has changed.* The nurse is considered responsible for notifying the physician of any significant changes in the client's condition, whether the physician requests notification or not. For example, if a client who is receiving an intravenous infusion suddenly develops a rapid pulse, chest pain, and a cough, the nurse must notify the physician immediately and question continuance of the ordered rate of infusion. If a client who is receiving morphine for pain develops severely depressed respirations, the nurse must withhold the medication and notify the physician.

4. *Question and record verbal orders to avoid miscommunications.* In addition to recording the time, the date, the physician's name, and the orders, the nurse documents the circumstances that prompted the call to the physician, reads the orders back to the physician, and documents that the physician confirmed the orders as the nurse read them back.

5. *Question standing orders, especially if the nurse is inexperienced.* Standing orders give the nurse added responsibility to exercise appropriate judgment when implementing them. The nurse is delegated the authority to, for example, adjust the amount of a medication or other substances and make decisions about when a medication is needed. Nurses need to take the same precautions when implementing these orders as when implementing any other orders. In addition, the nurse who does not feel confident about exercising discretionary judgment should request specific guidelines from the physician or assistance from a more experienced nurse. In some states, standing orders are not allowed except in intensive care or coronary care units.

If the order is neither ambiguous nor apparently erroneous, the nurse is responsible for carrying it out. For example, if the physician orders oxygen to be administered at 4 liters per minute, the nurse must administer oxygen at that rate, and not at 2 or 6 liters per minute. If the orders state that the client is not to have solid food after a bowel resection, the nurse must ensure that no solid food is given to the client. Nurses also have a responsibility to check for changes in orders from previous shifts of duty.

Implementing Nursing Actions

Nurses implementing care need to take the following precautions (Grane 1983, pp. 17–20; Rhodes and Miller 1984, pp. 153–60):

- Know your own job description. This enables nurses to function within the scope of the description and know what is and what is not expected. Job descriptions vary from agency to agency.

- Follow the policies and procedures of the agency in which you are working.

- Always identify clients, particularly before initiating major interventions, e.g., surgical or other invasive procedures, or when administering blood transfusions.

- Make sure the correct medications are given in the correct dose, by the right route, at the scheduled time, and to the right client. See Chapters 35 and 36 for more detailed information about the administration of medications.

- Perform procedures appropriately. Incidents of negligence that take place during procedures generally relate to equipment failure, improper technique, and improper performance of the procedure. For instance, the nurse must know how to safeguard the client in the event that a respirator or other equipment fails.

- Promptly and accurately document all assessments and care given. Records must show that the nurse provided and supervised the client's care daily.

- Report all incidents involving clients. Prompt reports enable those responsible to attend to the client's well-being, to analyze why the incident occurred, and to prevent recurrences.

- Build and maintain good rapport with clients. Keeping clients informed about diagnostic and treatment plans, giving feedback on their progress, and showing concern for the outcome of their care prevent a sense of powerlessness and a buildup of hostility in the client.

- Maintain clinical competence in your area of practice. For students, this demands study and practice before caring for clients. For graduate nurses, it means continued study, including maintaining and updating clinical knowledge and skills.

- Know your own strengths and weaknesses. For example, nurses who recognize that they have

Legal Precautions for Nurses

- Function within the scope of your education, job description, and area nurse practice act.
- Follow the procedures and policies of the employing agency.
- Observe and monitor the client accurately.
- Communicate and record significant changes in the client's condition to the physician.
- Check any orders that a client questions.
- Identify clients before initiating any interventions.
- Protect clients from falls and preventable injuries.
- Document all nursing assessments and interventions accurately.
- Ask for assistance and supervision in situations for which you feel inadequately prepared.
- Delegate tasks to persons with the knowledge and skill to carry them out.
- Build and maintain good rapport with clients.

difficulty calculating medication dosages should always ask someone to check the calculations before proceeding.

- When delegating nursing responsibilities, make sure that the person who is delegated a task understands what to do and has the required knowledge and skill to do it. The delegating nurse can be held liable for harm caused by the person to whom the care was delegated.

- Be alert when implementing nursing interventions and give each task your full attention and skill.

Ways nurses can protect themselves legally are summarized in the box above.

Legal Responsibilities of Students

Nursing students are responsible for their own actions and are liable for their own acts of negligence committed during the course of clinical experiences. When they perform duties that are within the scope of professional nursing, such as administering an injection, they are legally held to the same standard of skill and competence as a registered professional nurse (Rhodes and Miller 1984, p. 163). Lower standards are *not* applied to the actions of nursing students.

In cases arising from acts of negligence, the nursing student has traditionally been treated as an employee of the hospital, which was held liable under the doctrine of *respondeat superior*. Today, associate degree and baccalaureate nursing students are not usually considered employees of the agencies in which they receive clinical experience, since these nursing programs contract with agencies to provide clinical experiences for students. In future cases of negligence involving such students, the hospital or agency (e.g., public health agency) and the educational institution will be held potentially liable for negligent actions by students (Rhodes and Miller 1984, p. 164).

Students in clinical situations must be assigned activity within their capabilities and be given reasonable guidance and supervision. Nursing instructors are responsible for assigning students to the care of clients and for providing reasonable supervision. Failure to provide reasonable supervision and/or the assignment of a client to a student who is not prepared and competent can be a basis for liability.

To fulfill responsibilities to clients and to minimize chances for liability, nursing students need to

- Make sure they are prepared to carry out the necessary care for assigned clients.

- Ask for additional help or supervision in situations for which they feel inadequately prepared.

- Comply with the policies of the agency in which they obtain their clinical experience.

- Comply with the policies and definitions of responsibility supplied by the school of nursing.

Students who work as part-time or temporary nursing assistants or aides must also remember that *legally* they can perform only those tasks that appear in the job description of a nurse's aide or assistant. Even though a student may have received instruction and acquired competence in administering injections or suctioning a tracheostomy tube, the student cannot legally perform these tasks while employed as an aide or assistant.

Ethical Aspects of Nursing

Values

Values, beliefs, and attitudes differ from one another but are often interconnected. A **value** can be defined as something of worth, a belief held dear by a person. A value is an affective disposition toward a person, object, or idea (Steele and Harmon 1983, p. 1). Values common to many people are peace, truth, and freedom, for example. Values form a basis for behavior; a person's real values are shown by consistent patterns of behavior. Once one is aware of one's values, the values become an internal control for behavior. Values thus underlie people's purposive behavior, i.e., behavior performed "on purpose" or intentionally.

Beliefs

A **belief** (opinion) is something people judge to be true on the basis of probability rather than actuality. A belief is a special type of attitude whose cognitive (intellectual) component is based more on faith than on fact. People hold beliefs that may be true or that can, with reliable evidence, be proved true. Family traditions and folklore are beliefs passed from one generation to another.

Beliefs may or may not involve values. For example, a client may believe that all nurses are honest. The client has accepted that a relationship exists between "nurse" and "honesty," nurse being the object and honesty the value. The client considers this relationship self-evident. A belief of this type is sometimes called a value judgment.

Attitudes

An **attitude** is a feeling tone directed toward a person, object, or idea. Attitudes are made up of many beliefs (Steele and Harmon 1983, p. 3). For example, a child may learn such attitudes as cooperation and kindness from parents and in turn exhibit these in behavior.

Ethics

Ethics is the rules or principles that govern right conduct. The word *ethics* is derived from the Greek *ethos*, meaning "custom" or "character." The term *bio-*

ethics is being used increasingly in the health field. **Bioethics** is the ethics concerning life.

Since ethics govern right conduct, it deals with what "should" or "ought to" be done. Ethics is not unlike the law in that each deals with rules of conduct that reflect underlying principles of right and wrong and codes of morality. Protecting the rights of human beings is the primary underlying principle of ethics. In nursing, ethics provides professional standards for nursing activities; these standards protect both the nurse and the client. Ethical practice refers to a nurse's moral decisions regarding ethical dilemmas (Ketefian 1989, p. 509).

Nursing Codes of Ethics

A **code of ethics** provides a means by which professional standards of practice are established, maintained, and improved. It is essential to a profession. Codes of ethics are formal guidelines for professional action. They are shared by the persons within the profession and should be generally compatible with a professional member's personal values.

A code of ethics gives the members of the profession a frame of reference for making judgments in complex nursing situations. No two situations are identical, and nurses are frequently in situations that require them to choose which course of action to take. A code of ethics serves as a guide in many of these situations. It identifies the values and beliefs behind ethical standards (Thompson and Thompson 1985, p. 12).

The American Nurses' Association (ANA) first adopted a code of ethics in 1950, which was revised in 1968, 1976, and 1985. See Table 1–2. This code is

---

TABLE 1–2 AMERICAN NURSES' ASSOCIATION CODE FOR NURSES

1. The nurse provides services with respect for human dignity and the uniqueness of the client unrestricted by considerations of social or economic status, personal attributes, or the nature of health problems.

2. The nurse safeguards the client's right to privacy by judiciously protecting information of a confidential nature.

3. The nurse acts to safeguard the client and the public when health care and safety are affected by the incompetent, unethical, or illegal practice of any person.

4. The nurse assumes responsibility and accountability for individual nursing judgments and actions.

5. The nurse maintains competence in nursing.

6. The nurse exercises informed judgment and uses individual competence and qualifications as criteria in seeking consultation, accepting responsibilities, and delegating nursing activities to others.

7. The nurse participates in activities that contribute to the ongoing development of the profession's body of knowledge.

8. The nurse participates in the profession's efforts to implement and improve standards of nursing.

9. The nurse participates in the profession's effort to establish and maintain conditions of employment conducive to high-quality nursing care.

10. The nurse participates in the profession's effort to protect the public from misinformation and misrepresentation and to maintain the integrity of nursing.

11. The nurse collaborates with members of the health professions and other citizens in promoting community and national efforts to meet the health needs of the public.

Source: Reprinted with permission from *Code for Nurses with Interpretive Statements,* © 1985, American Nurses' Association, Washington, DC.

designed to provide guidance for nurses by stating principles of ethical concern. In 1988, the ANA published *Ethics in Nursing*, which addresses a wide range of nursing situations that involve ethical action. In 1980, the Canadian Nurses' Association adopted a code of ethics. It was revised in 1985. Nurses have a responsibility to be familiar with the code that governs their nursing practice.

International, national, state, and provincial nursing associations have established codes of ethics. If a nurse violates the code, the association may expel the nurse from membership.

Health Care System

A **health care system** is the totality of services offered by all health disciplines. Traditionally, the health care delivery system in North America provides two general types of services: illness care services (restorative) and health care services (preventive). Illness care services help the ill or injured. Health care services promote better health and help prevent disease and accidents. Although most facili-

ties within the system—for example, hospitals, clinics, and physicians' offices—provide both types of services, illness care services predominate. In recent years, however, the awareness of the need to promote health and to prevent disease has increased. Considerable emphasis has been placed on the role of the nurse in these areas.

The providers of health care, also referred to as the **health care team**, are health personnel from different disciplines who coordinate their skills to assist a client and/or support persons. The choice of personnel for a particular client depends on the needs of the client. In the present system of health care in North America, health care teams commonly include nurses, physicians, pharmacists, dietitians, physiotherapists, respiratory therapists, occupational therapists, paramedical technologists, social workers, and chaplains.

Rights to Health Care

The movement for clients' rights in health care arose in the late 1960s. At that time, the broad goals of the

---

TABLE 1–3   A PATIENT'S BILL OF RIGHTS

1. The patient has the right to considerate and respectful care.

2. The patient has the right to obtain from his physician complete current information concerning his diagnosis, treatment, and prognosis, in terms the patient can be reasonably expected to understand. When it is not medically advisable to give such information to the patient, the information should be made available to an appropriate person in his behalf. He has the right to know by name the physician responsible for coordinating his care.

3. The patient has the right to receive from his physician information necessary to give informed consent prior to the start of any procedure and/or treatment. Except in emergencies, such information for informed consent should include but not necessarily be limited to the specific procedure and/or treatment, the medically significant risks involved, and the probable duration of incapacitation. Where medically significant alternatives for care or treatment exist, or when the patient requests information concerning medical alternatives, the patient has the right to such information. The patient also has the right to know the name of the person responsible for the procedures and/or treatment.

4. The patient has the right to refuse treatment to the extent permitted by law and to be informed of the medical consequences of his action.

5. The patient has the right to every consideration of his privacy concerning his own medical care program. Case discussion, consultation, examination, and treatment are confidential and should be conducted discreetly. Those not directly involved in this care must have the permission of the patient to be present.

6. The patient has the right to expect that all communications and records pertaining to his care should be treated as confidential.

7. The patient has the right to expect that within its capacity a hospital must make reasonable response to the request of a patient for services. The hospital must provide evaluation, service, and/or referral as indicated by the urgency of the case. When medically permissible, a patient may be transferred to another facility only after he has received complete information and explanation concerning the needs for and alternatives to such a transfer. The institution to which the patient is transferred must first have accepted the patient for transfer.

8. The patient has the right to obtain information as to any relationship of his hospital to other health care and educational institutions insofar as his care is concerned. The patient has the right to obtain information as to the existence of any professional relationships among individuals, by name, who are treating him.

9. The patient has the right to be advised if the hospital proposes to engage in or perform human experimentation affecting his care or treatment. The patient has the right to refuse to participate in such research projects.

10. The patient has the right to expect reasonable continuity of care. He has the right to know in advance what appointment times and physicians are available and where. The patient has the right to expect that the hospital will provide a mechanism whereby he is informed by his physician or a delegate of the physician of the patient's continuing health.

11. The patient has the right to examine and receive an explanation of his bill regardless of source of payment.

12. The patient has the right to know what hospital rules and regulations apply to his conduct as a patient.

Source: American Hospital Association, A patient's bill of rights, *Nursing Outlook*, February 1973, 21:82, and January 1976, 24:29. Reprinted with the permission of the American Hospital Association.

movement were to improve the quality of health care and to make the health care system more responsive to clients' needs. Today, clients are also seeking more self-determination and control over their own bodies when they are ill. Informed consent, confidentiality, and the right of the client to refuse treatment are all aspects of this self-determination. The need for clients' rights is largely the result of two circumstances: the client's vulnerability due to illness and the complexity of the relationships in the health care setting.

When people are ill, they are frequently unable to assert their rights as they would if they were healthy. Asserting rights requires energy and an underlying awareness of one's rights in the situation.

The complexity and variety of health care relationships also increase the need for clients' rights. In this day of specialization, a client is often helped by a variety of health professionals. The client becomes one person among many health professionals. Thus, the client's needs or priorities, for example, can become lost in the communications among health professionals.

A new pattern of health care relationships is emerging as a result of several forces in society, including an increase in the consumer's knowledge of health issues and recognition of the role of lifestyle in disease. Today, the goals of health include the client's return to autonomy and independence and the acceptance of good health as a responsibility of the care provider, the client, and society. These goals cannot be met unless clients accept active responsibility for their health and health care and unless clients and care providers have mutual respect.

In 1973, the American Hospital Association published "A Patient's Bill of Rights" in an effort to promote the rights of hospitalized clients. See Table 1–3. Clients frequently do not know their rights, although many hospitals today give clients on admission a statement of their rights while in hospital.

CRITICAL THINKING CHALLENGE

As a nursing student, you are assigned to provide nursing care to Anita Evans, a 64-year-old female admitted to the nursing unit with a fractured hip. The primary nurse has just received a telephone order from Ms Evans' physician for Demerol 75 mg IM for pain, stat. The nurse asks you to administer the medication. You have not given an IM injection to a client before. Your instructor is busy assisting another student with a treatment. How will you reply to the nurse? What principles guide your reply? What sources provide you with assistance in your actions?

RELATED RESEARCH

Benner, P., and Tanner, C. January 1987. Clinical judgment: How expert nurses use intuition. *American Journal of Nursing* 87:23–31.

Berger, M. C.; Seversen, A.; and Chvatal, R. August 1991. Ethical issues in nursing. *Western Journal of Nursing Research* 13:514–21.

Curran, M., and Curran, K. January 1991. The ethics of information. *Journal of Nursing Administration* 21:47–49.

Kruger, S. February 1991. The patient educator role in nursing. *Applied Nursing Research* 4:19–24.

REFERENCES

American Hospital Association. January 1976. A patient's bill of rights. *Nursing Outlook* 24:29 (also February 1973, *Nursing Outlook* 21:82).

American Nurses' Association. 1973. *Standards of nursing practice.* Kansas City, Mo.: ANA.
_____. 1981. *Facts about nursing 80–81.* New York: American Journal of Nursing Co.
_____. 1985. *Code for nurses.* Kansas City, Mo.: ANA.
_____. 1987. *Facts about nursing. 86–87.* Kansas City, Mo.: ANA.
_____. 1988. *Ethics in nursing: Position statements and guidelines.* Kansas City, Mo.: ANA.

Annas, G. J. 1975. *The rights of hospital patients: The basic ACLU guide to a hospital patient's rights.* New York: Avon Books.

Bandman, E. L., and Bandman, B. 1990. *Nursing ethics through the life span.* 2d ed. Norwalk, Conn.: Appleton & Lange.

Becker, M. January/February 1983. Five orders you must question to protect yourself legally. *Nursing Life* 3:21–23.

Benner, P., and Tanner, C. January 1987. How expert nurses use intuition. *American Journal of Nursing* 87:23–31.

Cameron, M. July/August 1991. Justice, caring, and virtue. *Journal of Professional Nursing* 7:206.

Canadian Nurses' Association. April 1984. CNA connection: Canada Health Act. *Canadian Nurse* 80:8–9.
_____. 1987. *A definition of nursing practice: Standards for nursing practice.* Ottawa: CNA.

Cassidy, V. R. March/April 1991. Ethical responsibilities in nursing: Research findings and issues. *Journal of Professional Nursing* 7:112–18.

De Tornyay, R. May 1991. Reshaping the nation's health care. *Journal of Nursing Education* 30:195–96.

Disparti, J. 1988. Nutrition and self care. In Caliandro, G., and Judkins, B. L., editors. *Primary nursing practice*. Glenview Ill.: Scott, Foresman & Co.

Dunn, B. January 1991. Who should be doing the research in nursing? *Professional Nurse* 6:190, 192–94.

Gordin, P. January/February 1991. Launching a leadership role. *American Journal of Maternal Child Nursing* 16:24–26.

Grane, N. B. January/February 1983. How to reduce your risk of a lawsuit. *Nursing Life* 3:17–20.

Green, M., and Jones, F. January 1991. WHO code? Who cares? *Canadian Nurse* 87:26–28.

Harris, M. D. November/December 1990. The ethical dilemmas. *Home Health Care Nurse* 8:47–48.

Henderson, V. 1966. *The nature of nursing: A definition and its implications for practice, research, and education*. New York: Macmillan Co.

Ivy, S. S. January/March 1991. Ethics in practice. *Journal of Urological Nursing* 10:1133–35.

Jarczewski, P. H. May/June 1990. What is an ethical decision? Ethics for contemporary nursing practice. *Advancing Clinical Care* 5:28.

Kaplan, S. M. November/December 1990. The nurse as a change agent. *Pediatric Nursing* 16:603–5.

Kemerer, A. A. March/April 1989. Nurse practice acts. *A D Nurse* 4:29–33.

Kemp, V. H. 1986. An overview of change and leadership. In Hein, E. C., and Nicholson, M. J., editors. *Contemporary leadership behavior: Selected readings*. 2d ed. Boston: Little, Brown and Co.

Ketefian, S. June 1989. Moral reasoning and ethical practice in nursing. *Nursing Clinics of North America* 24:509–21.

Kohnke, M. F. 1990. *The nurse as advocate . . . 1980*. In Pence, T., and Cantrall, J. pp. 56–58. *Ethics in nursing: An anthology*. NLN Pub. no. 20–2294. New York: National League for Nursing.

Kurtz, R. J., and Wang, J. 1991. The caring ethic: More than kindness, the core of nursing science. *Nursing Forum* 26(1):4–8.

Leddy, S., and Pepper, J. M. 1989. *Conceptual bases of professional nursing*. 2d ed. Philadelphia: J. B. Lippincott Co.

Murphy, E. K. March 1991. Patient's rights vs. court orders. *AORN Journal* 53:794–95, 798–99.

Nightingale, F. 1860. *Notes on nursing: What it is, and what it is not*. London: Harrison. Reprinted in Bishop, F. L. A., and Goldie, S. 1962. *A bio-bibliography of Florence Nightingale*. London: Dawsons of Pall Mall.

Northrop, C. 1988. Legal aspects of nursing. In McCann Flynn, J. B., and Heffron, P. B. *Nursing: From concept to practice*. 2d ed. East Norwalk, Conn.: Appleton & Lange.

Omery, A. June 1989. Values, moral reasoning, and ethics. *Nursing Clinics of North America* 24:499–508.

Pence, T., and Cantrall, J. 1990. *Ethics in nursing: An anthology*. NLN Pub. no. 20–2294. New York: National League for Nursing.

Redman, B. K. 1988. *The process of patient education*. 6th ed. St. Louis: C. V. Mosby Co.

Rhodes, A. M., and Miller, R. D. 1984. *Nursing and the law*. 4th ed. Rockville, Md.: Aspen Systems Corporation.

Schaefer, J. October 1974. The interrelatedness of decision making and the nursing process. *American Journal of Nursing* 74:1852–55.

Smith, J. 1990. Privileged communication: Psychiatric/mental health nurses and the law. *Perspectives in Psychiatric Care* 26(4):26–29.

Steele, S. M., and Harmon, V. M. 1983. *Values clarification in nursing*. 2d ed. Norwalk, Conn.: Appleton-Century-Crofts.

Sweeney, M. L. August 1991. Your role in informed consent. *RN* 54:55–60.

Thompson, J. B., and Thompson, H. O. 1985. *Bioethical decision making for nurses*. Norwalk, Conn.: Appleton-Century-Crofts.

White, G. February 1991. Ethical, rights issues abound. *American Nurse* 23:25.

Yura, H., Ozimet, D., and Walsh, M. B. 1981. *Nursing leadership: Theory and process*. New York: Appleton & Lange.

Zusman, J. November/December 1982. Want some good advice? Think twice about being a patient advocate. *Nursing Life* 6:49.

2

The Nursing Process and Critical Thinking

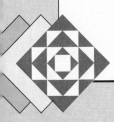

CONTENTS

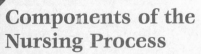

Components of the Nursing Process

The **nursing process** is a systematic rational method of planning and providing nursing care. Its goals are to identify a client's health status and actual or potential health care problems, to establish plans to meet the identified needs, and to deliver specific nursing interventions to meet those needs. To carry out the nursing process effectively and individualize approaches to each person's particular needs, the nurse must collaborate with the client and other members of the health care team.

The nursing process consists of a series of five problem-solving steps: assessing, diagnosing, planning, implementing, and evaluating. These five steps are interrelated and cyclical and build on each other. Accuracy in each step is crucial to ensuring that the client receives the maximum benefit of nursing care.

Assessing is the process of collecting, verifying, and organizing data (information) about a client's health status. In the assessment phase, nurses and clients establish the database from which they derive individualized client care plans. During this phase of the process, the nurse strategically collects from a variety of sources the data needed to care for the client.

Diagnosing is the process that results in a diagnostic statement or nursing diagnosis that provides the basis for the selection of nursing interventions for the client.

Diagnosis is a process of analysis and synthesis. **Analysis** is the separation into components; i.e., breaking down the whole into its parts. **Synthesis** is the opposite; i.e., putting together the parts into the whole. The cognitive skills required for analysis and synthesis are objectivity, critical thinking, decision making, and inductive and deductive reasoning.

Planning is a process in which the nurse and the client set priorities, write goals or expected outcomes, and establish a written care plan designed to resolve or minimize the identified problems of the client and to coordinate the care provided by all health team members. In collaboration with the client, the nurse develops specific interventions required to prevent, reduce, or eliminate those client health problems identified and validated during the diagnostic phase.

Through the written nursing care plan, nurses communicate to one another significant assessment findings, nursing diagnoses, client goals, and progress in solving problems. By using the care plan, the nurse can individualize client care and at the same time ensure that care remains consistent from nurse to nurse and shift to shift.

Implementing is the carrying out of the planned nursing interventions to help the client attain the goals, that is, putting the plan into action. During the implementation phase, the nurse continues to collect data, carries out the prescribed nursing activities or delegates the care to an appropriate person, and validates the nursing care plan. Continued data collec-

TABLE 2–1 OVERVIEW OF THE PURPOSES AND ACTIVITIES OF THE NURSING PROCESS

Component and Purpose(s)	Activities
ASSESSING To establish a database	Obtain health history. Perform physical assessment. Review records, e.g., laboratory records, other health care records. Interview support persons. Review literature. Validate assessment data.
DIAGNOSING To identify the client's health care needs and to prepare diagnostic statements	Organize data. Compare data against standards. Cluster or group data (generate tentative hypotheses). Identify gaps and inconsistencies. Determine the client's health problems, risks, and strengths. Formulate nursing diagnoses/diagnostic statements.
PLANNING To identify the client's goals and appropriate nursing interventions	Set priorities in collaboration with client. Write evaluation goals and outcome criteria in collaboration with client. Select nursing strategies. Consult other health care personnel. Write nursing orders. Write nursing care plan.
IMPLEMENTING To carry out planned nursing interventions and to help the client attain goals	Reassess client. Update database. Review and revise care plan. Perform or delegate planned nursing interventions.
EVALUATING To determine the extent to which goals of nursing care have been achieved	Collect data about the client's response. Compare the client's response to evaluation (outcome) criteria. Analyze the reasons for the outcomes. Modify the care plan.

The Nursing Process

Assessing

- Collect data
- Validate data
- Classify (organize) data

The nursing process is a systematic, rational method of planning and providing nursing care. Its goal is to identify a client's health status, actual or potential health care problems, to establish plans to meet the identified needs, and to deliver specific nursing interventions to meet those needs. The nursing process is cyclical; that is, its components follow a logical sequence, but more than one component may be involved at any one time. At the end of the first cycle, care may be terminated if goals are achieved, or the cycle may begin again with reassessment.

Diagnosing

- Analyze data
- Formulate a diagnosis
- Validate the diagnosis

Evaluating

- Evaluate goal achievement
- Terminate care for goals achieved
- Reassess, and revise care plan if goals were not achieved

Planning

- Establish short-term and long-term goals
- Develop outcome criteria
- Write the care plan

Implementing

- Carry out the care plan
- Communicate care plan to members of care team
- Document assessments and interventions

The nursing process in practice . . .

Luisa Westley, a 28-year-old married attorney, was admitted to the hospital with an elevated temperature, a nonproductive cough, and rapid, labored respirations. In taking a nursing history, Mary Medina, RN, finds that Ms. Westley has had a "chest cold" for two weeks, and has been experiencing shortness of breath upon exertion. Yesterday she developed an elevated temperature and began to experience "pain" in her "lungs."

Assessing: Nurse Medina's physical assessment reveals that Ms. Westley's vital signs are: Temperature, 39.4 C (103 F); pulse, 92 BPM; respirations, 28; and blood pressure, 122/80 mm Hg. Nurse Medina observes that Ms. Westley's skin is dry, her cheeks are flushed, and she is experiencing chills. Auscultation reveals inspiratory crackles with diminished breath sounds in the right lung.

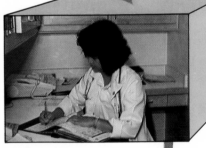

Diagnosing: After analysis, Nurse Medina formulates a nursing diagnosis:
Ineffective airway clearance
related to thick sputum obstructing airways.

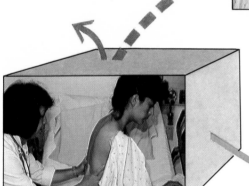

Evaluating: Upon assessment of respiratory excursion, Nurse Medina detects failure of the client to achieve maximum ventilation. She and Ms. Westley reevaluate the care plan and modify it to increase coughing and deep breathing exercises to q2h.

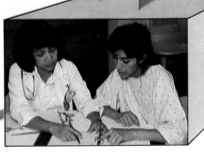

Planning: Nurse Medina and Ms. Westley collaborate to establish goals (e.g., restore effective breathing pattern and lung ventilation); set outcome criteria (e.g., have a symmetrical respiratory excursion of at least 4 cm and so on); and develop a care plan that includes, but is not limited to, coughing and deep breathing exercises q3h, fluid intake of 3000 mL daily, and daily postural drainage.

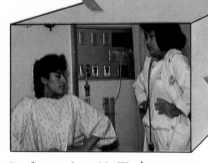

Implementing: Ms. Westley agrees to practice deep breathing exercises q3h during the day. In addition, she understands the need to increase her fluid intake and to plan her morning activities to accommodate postural drainage.

tion is essential not only to keep track of changes in the client's condition but also to obtain evidence for evaluating goal achievement, which is the next phase of the nursing process.

Evaluating is determining the client's response to nursing interventions and then comparing the response to predetermined standards. These standards are often referred to as *outcome criteria*. The nurse determines the extent to which the goals or predetermined outcomes of care have been achieved, partially achieved, or not met. If goals have not been met, the nurse needs to reassess the care plan. Reassessment may involve changes in any or all of the previous phases of the nursing process.

Table 2–1 contains an overview of the purposes and activities of the nursing process.

Characteristics of the Nursing Process

The five steps of the nursing process are not discrete entities but overlapping, continuing subprocesses. For example, assessing, the first step of the nursing process, may also be carried out during implementing and evaluating. The nurse must continually update each step as the situation changes. Just as a client's health is never static but constantly changing, the nursing process, because it is responsive to the client's health, is also dynamic.

Each step or phase of the nursing process affects the others; they are closely interrelated. For example, if the nurse uses an inadequate database during assessment, the nursing diagnoses will be incomplete or incorrect; this will be reflected in the planning, implementing, and evaluating phases. Incomplete or incorrect assessment necessarily means equivocal evaluation because the nurse will have incomplete or incorrect criteria against which to evaluate changes in the client and the effectiveness of intervention.

The success of the nursing process depends on open and meaningful communication and the development of rapport between the client and the nurse. See the accompanying box for a summary of the characteristics of the nursing process.

Characteristics of the Nursing Process

- The system is open, flexible, and dynamic.
- It individualizes the approach to each client's particular needs.
- It is planned.
- It is goal directed.
- It is flexible to meet the unique needs of client, family, or community.
- It permits creativity for the nurse and client in devising ways to solve the stated health problem.
- It is interpersonal. It requires the nurse to communicate directly and consistently with clients to meet their needs.
- It is cyclical. Since all steps are interrelated, there is no absolute beginning or end.
- It emphasizes feedback, which leads either to reassessment of the problem or to revision of the care plan.
- It is universally applicable. The nursing process is used as a framework for nursing care in all types of health care settings, with clients of all age groups.

Critical Thinking

Critical thinking is both an attitude and a reasoning process involving a number of intellectual skills—a purposeful mental activity in which ideas are produced and evaluated and judgments are made. (Wilkinson 1992, p. 24). Critical thinking is disciplined, self-directed, rational thinking that "certifies what we know and makes clear wherein we are ignorant. . . ." It is "the art of thinking about your thinking while you're thinking so as to make your thinking more clear, precise, accurate, relevant, consistent, and fair" (Paul 1988b, pp. 2–3).

Characteristics

Wilkinson (1992, pp.25–26) outlines the characteristics of critical thinking as follows.

Critical thinking involves conceptualization. Conceptualization is the intellectual process of forming a concept. A **concept** is a mental image of reality. In conceptualization, an abstract idea is generalized from particular instances, and exists as a symbol in the mind. Concepts are ideas about events, objects, and properties, as well as the relationships between them.

Critical thinking is rational and reasonable. This is the most obvious feature of critical thinking. Reason and **rationality** refer to the fact that the thinking is based on reasons rather than prejudice, preferences, self-interest, or fears.

Critical thinking is reflective. This means that the person who thinks critically does not jump to conclusions or make a hurried decision, but takes the time to collect data and then think the matter through in a disciplined manner, weighing facts and evidence.

Critical thinking is, in part, an attitude. It is an attitude of inquiry. A critical thinker examines existing claims and statements to see if they are true or valid rather than blindly accepting them. In response to a claim like, "Fords are better than Chevrolets," a critical thinker might ask: (1) What do you mean by "better than"; better in what ways? and (2) What information do you have that this is so? Critical thinkers are skeptical, but constructively so. They ask, "Why?" and "How?"

Critical thinking is autonomous thinking. A critical thinker thinks for himself. He does not passively accept the beliefs of others, but analyzes the issues and decides which authorities are credible.

Critical thinking includes creative thinking. **Creative thinking** is a productive intellectual skill that creates original ideas by establishing relationships among thoughts and concepts. It involves the ability to break up and transfer a concept to new settings or uses. For example, the concept of *brick* could be thought of along the lines of its molecular structure, its dimensions, its color, its effect on the economy, its hardness, its ability to transfer heat, and so on. Whatever the idea is, the creative thinker is able to transfer it—to find it again in other settings (e.g., a remembered smell, a relationship, a psychomotor procedure). Creative thinkers do not simply memorize and evaluate existing knowledge; they create alternative courses of action, make reasonable hypotheses and find new solutions to problems.

Creative thinking involves more or less random thought and occurs at different levels of consciousness. It may not establish logical explanations for actions, especially when the problem is unusual; nor does it necessarily consider possible outcomes in forming the new idea. Creative thinking, however, is directed, even though it is more random than systematic. **Directed thinking** is purposeful and goal-directed, unlike **associative thinking**, which involves random, unstructured thoughts (for example, daydreaming).

Critical thinking is fair thinking. Critical thinkers attempt to remove bias and one-sidedness from their own thinking and to recognize it in others. This requires them to examine the reasons for their choices and decisions. It also requires an awareness of one's own values and feelings and a willingness to examine the basis for them.

Critical thinking focuses on deciding what to believe or do. Critical thinking is used to evaluate arguments and conclusions, create new ideas or alternative courses of action, decide upon a course of action, produce reliable observations, draw sound conclusions, and solve problems. Critical thinkers use

accepted standards to examine their own views as well as the views of others; they do the following (Paul, 1988a):

1. Explore the thinking that underlies their emotions and feelings.

2. Suspend judgments when they lack sufficient evidence.

3. Develop criteria for evaluation and apply them fairly and accurately.

4. Evaluate the credibility of sources used to justify beliefs.

5. Make interdisciplinary connections and use insights from one subject to illuminate and correct other subjects.

6. Distinguish facts from ideals and what they would like to be from what they are.

7. Examine assumptions that underlie thoughts and behavior.

8. Distinguish the relevant from the irrelevant, and the important from the trivial.

9. Make plausible inferences and distinguish conclusions from the reasoning that supports them.

10. Seek out evidence and give evidence when questioned.

Relationship to the Nursing Process

Critical thinking is an essential part of problem solving and decision making and is, therefore, an essential skill for all aspects of the nursing process. See Table 2–2.

Assessing

Assessing involves the collection and validation of the data the nurse uses to make the nursing diagnosis. In effect, assessing is a continuous process carried out during all phases of the nursing process. It may be used during the diagnosis phase to validate a diagnosis. During the planning and implementing stages, the nurse may collect data to determine the proper nursing intervention or obtain information about a client's response to the nursing strategies. In the evaluation phase, assessment is done to determine the outcomes of the nursing strategies and to evaluate goal achievement.

In *Nursing: A Social Policy Statement* (ANA 1980, p. 9), the American Nurses' Assocation states that nursing is "the diagnosis and treatment of human responses to actual or potential health problems." Thus the focus of assessment is to establish a data-

TABLE 2–2 CRITICAL THINKING THROUGHOUT THE
NURSING PROCESS

The Nursing Process	Critical-Thinking Skills
ASSESSING	Observing Distinguishing relevant from irrelevant data Distinguishing important from unimportant data Validating data Organizing data Categorizing data
DIAGNOSING	Finding patterns and relationships Making inferences Stating the problem Suspending judgment
PLANNING	Generalizing Transferring knowledge from one situation to another Developing evaluative criteria Hypothesizing
IMPLEMENTING	Applying knowledge Testing hypotheses
EVALUATING	Deciding whether hypotheses are correct Making criterion-based evaluations

Source: J. M. Wilkinson, *Nursing process in action: A critical thinking approach.*
(Redwood City, Calif.: Addison-Wesley Nursing), p. 29. Reprinted with
permission.

base about a client's *response* to health concerns or
illness in order to determine the client's nursing care
needs. Clients' responses include areas of daily living,
health, and biophysical, emotional, socioeconomic,
cultural, and religious concerns. In contrast to other
health professionals, the nurse is concerned with
human needs that affect the total person rather than
one problem or segment of need fulfillment (Yura and
Walsh 1988, p. 110).

Establishing the database begins with obtaining
the client's health history and culminates with validation of the assessment data. The nurse obtains data
by interviewing the client and family or support persons, by consulting other health care personnel, and
by performing a physical assessment on the client.
In addition, the nurse reviews the client's health care
records, along with literature that validates the
assessment data.

Types of Data

All phases of the nursing process depend on the accurate and complete collection of data. Data can be
objective or subjective. **Objective data** are detectable
by an observer or can be tested against an accepted
standard. They can be seen, heard, felt, or smelled.
For example, a discoloration of the skin, a blood pressure reading, the act of crying, or a hand tremor are
objective data. **Subjective data** are apparent only to

the person affected and can be described or verified
only by that person. Itching, pain, and feeling worried
are examples of subjective data. Subjective data are
collected during the nursing health history and
include the client's perception of personal health
status and life situation. Information supplied by family members, significant others, or other health professionals is also considered subjective, if it is based
on opinion rather than fact.

Objective data are sometimes called **signs** or
overt data, and subjective data are sometimes called
symptoms or **covert data**. Data can also be
described as **variable** or **constant**. Blood pressure
is variable; it changes from day to day or even hour
to hour and needs updating. Constant data, for example, a date of birth, are unchanging.

Sources of Data

Sources or data are *primary* or *secondary*. The client
is the primary source of data. Secondary, or indirect,
sources include significant others, other health personnel, records and reports, and relevant literature.

Client
The chief source of data is usually the client unless
the client is too ill, young, or confused to communicate clearly. The client can usually provide subjective data that no one else can offer.

Significant Others
Significant others or support persons know the client
well and often can provide data. They may supplement information or verify information provided by
the client. They might convey information about the
stresses the client was experiencing before the illness,
family attitudes to illness and health, and the client's
home environment. Significant others are an important source of data, particularly when the client is
very young, unconscious, or confused.

Health Personnel
Health personnel are sources of information about a
client's health. Nurses, social workers, physicians,
and physiotherapists, for example, may have information from either previous or current contact with
the client. A physician who knows the client's home
setting may provide valuable data about the family
and environmental stressors.

Medical Records
Medical records are a source of a client's present and
past patterns of health and illness. These records can
provide nurses with information about a client's coping behaviors, health practices, previous illnesses,
and allergies.

Other Records and Reports

Other records and reports can also provide pertinent health information. Laboratory tests are frequently ordered as part of the physician's initial examination to aid in a medical diagnosis. Laboratory tests are also used to monitor medical treatment, e.g., determination of blood glucose level to monitor the administration of oral hypoglycemic medications.

Other records and reports—for example, a social agency's report on a client's living conditions or a home health care agency's report on a client's coping at home—can also be helpful to the nurse conducting an assessment.

Literature

The review of nursing and related literature, such as professional journals and reference texts, can provide additional information for a database. A literature review includes but is not limited to the following information:

- Standards or norms against which to compare findings, e.g., height and weight tables, normal developmental tasks for an age group

- Cultural and social health practices

- Spiritual beliefs

- Additional required assessment data

- Nursing interventions and evaluation criteria relative to a client's health problems

- Information about medical diagnoses, treatment, and prognoses

Methods of Data Collection

The major methods of collecting data are observing, interviewing, and examining.

Observing

To **observe** is to gather data by using the five senses. Although nurses observe mainly through sight, all of the senses are engaged during careful observations. Observation has two aspects: (a) noticing the stimuli and (b) selecting, organizing, and interpreting the data, i.e., perceiving them. A nurse who observes that a client's face is flushed must relate that observation to, for example, body temperature, activity, environmental temperature, and blood pressure. Because observation involves selecting, organizing, and interpreting data, there is a possibility of error. For example, a nurse might not notice certain signs simply because they are unexpected in a certain client or situation or because they do not conform to preconceptions about a client's illness.

Interviewing

An **interview** is a planned communication or a conversation with a purpose, e.g., to gather data, to give information, to identify problems of mutual concern, to evaluate change, to teach, to provide support, and to provide counseling or therapy. Interviewing can be applied in most phases of the nursing process. One type of interview is the nursing health history, which is the primary tool for data collection during the assessment phase of the nursing process. See Nursing Health History in Chapter 11.

There are two approaches to interviewing: directive and nondirective. The **directive interview** is highly structured and elicits specific information. The nurse establishes the purpose of the interview and controls the interview, at least at the outset, by asking *closed* questions (see Table 2–3) that call for a specific amount of data. The client responds to questions but may not have an opportunity to ask questions or discuss concerns. Directive interviews are frequently used to gather and to give information in a limited amount of time. During a **nondirective**, or rapport-building, **interview**, the nurse allows the client to control the purpose, subject matter, and pacing. The nurse encourages communication by using *open-ended* questions (see Table 2–3) and empathetic responses. Nondirective interviewing is used for problem solving and counseling. A combination of directive and nondirective approaches is usually appropriate for information-gathering interviews.

Technique 2–1 explains the steps involved in interviewing a client.

Examining

A **physical examination** or **physical assessment** is the means by which the nurse obtains the objective data needed to complete the assessment phase of the nursing process. Developing the skills needed to conduct a physical assessment requires knowledge, practice, and time. The physical assessment is carried out systematically. It may be organized according to the examiner's preference, in a head-to-toe approach or as a body systems approach. Findings are measured against norms or standards, such as ideal height and weight standards or norms for body temperature or blood pressure levels.

To conduct the examination, the nurse uses techniques of inspection, auscultation, palpation, and percussion. These techniques are discussed in Chapter 11.

TABLE 2–3   KINDS OF INTERVIEW QUESTIONS

Type	Description	Indications for Use	Examples
Closed questions	Are restrictive and generally require only short answers. Often begin with *when*, *where*, *who*, *what*, *do* (*did*, *does*), *is* (*are*, *was*) and sometimes *how*.	Used (a) in directive interview; (b) for clients who are highly stressed and who have difficulty communicating; and (c) in an emergency or other acute situation when information must be obtained quickly.	"What medications did you take?" "Are you having pain now? Show me where it is." "How long has it been since you had your last physical examination?" "When did you fall?" "What were you doing before the fall?"
Open-ended questions	Are questions that lead or invite clients to explore (elaborate, clarify, or illustrate) their thoughts or feelings and allow them the freedom to talk about what they wish. They are broad questions that invite answers longer than one or two words and require more than a yes or no or other short response, such as "Yesterday," or "I don't know." Usually begin with *what* or *how*.	Used (a) in nondirective interview; (b) at the beginning of an interview or to change topics; and (c) to enable clients to divulge only the information they are ready to disclose.	"How have you been feeling lately?" "What brought you to the hospital?" "How did you feel about coming to the hospital?" "How did you feel in that situation?"

2-1   Interviewing the Client

PURPOSES
- To gather data
- To identify problems of mutual concern
- To begin to establish rapport
- To evaluate change
- To teach, provide support, or provide counseling

ASSESSMENT FOCUS

Health status and ability to provide information and participate in the interview; immediate concerns; age and educational level; sociocultural background; barriers to communication; family or significant others from whom information may be needed; home environment.

EQUIPMENT
- ☐ Pen or pencil
- ☐ Information form

Technique 2–1 Interviewing a Client CONTINUED

INTERVENTION

1. Prepare for the interview.

- Review the chart to find out information about the client that may already be documented. *This provides a base of personal data that may help the nurse begin to establish a relationship with the client.*

- Familiarize yourself with the data-collection form to be used or the information to be obtained. *This reduces reliance on forms and papers and facilitates a more successful interview in which communication skills will be more effective.*

- Identify any special needs to be addressed before proceeding with the interview. *If the client is critically ill, experiencing pain, disoriented, or unable to communicate clearly, the information obtained may not be valid.*

2. Establish an appropriate environment for the interview.

- Arrange the environment as needed. Ensure that there is adequate privacy, lighting, and ventilation and minimal or no noise or other distractions, such as televisions or radios. *An appropriate setting enhances client cooperation and communication.*

- Establish an appropriate seating arrangement that places client and nurse on equal terms. Avoid sitting at the head of the table or in any other superior positon. *This creates a less formal atmosphere.*

- Establish an appropriate distance, i.e., about 3 to 4 ft apart. *Most people feel uncomfortable when talking to someone who is too close or too far away.*

3. Open the interview.

- Establish rapport—a sense of goodwill and trust—by beginning with a greeting ("Good morning, Mr. Henderson") or a self-introduction ("Good morning. I'm Becky James, a nursing student"), accompanied by nonverbal gestures such as a smile, a handshake, and a friendly manner. Ask questions about the person and proceed with some small talk about the weather, sports, families, and the like. *This sets the tone for the remainder of the interview and clearly elicits client participation.* Avoid overdoing this stage. *Too much superficial talk can arouse anxiety about what is to follow and may appear insincere.*

- Explain the purpose and nature of the interview, how long it will take, and what is expected of the client.

4. Continue the interview, using the following guidelines.

- Begin with an open-ended question or questions, e.g., "What brought you to the hospital today?" *An open-ended question facilitates the transition from the opening stage to this stage and allows clients to express their concerns first. In this way, the nurse indicates that the client's concerns will be a priority in planning care.*

- Plan questions to follow a logical sequence. Refer as necessary to the data-collection form to avoid omissions and appearing disorganized.

- Ask only one question at a time. *Double questions limit the client to answering only one of the two and may confuse both the nurse and the client.*

- Obtain the most important information first, such as the client's main problem, allergies, emergency contact numbers, and so on. If the client is uncomfortable (in pain, nauseated, or dizzy, for example), defer less important information to a later time.

- Ask personal or delicate questions later in the interview, when a degree of rapport and trust is established.

- Use open-ended and closed questions throughout the interview as needed.

- Use communication techniques that make the client feel comfortable and serve the purpose of the interview. (see Table 4–1 on page 71).

- Listen attentively, using all of the senses, and speak slowly and clearly.

- Use language the client understands, and clarify any vague or confusing responses, for instance, by asking what a certain word means to the client: "What do you mean by a 'normal' amount of exercise, Mr. Henderson?"

- Note verbal and nonverbal gestures, such as grimacing, wringing of hands, crossing of arms, or change in voice tone. *This may give an indication that some information needs to be further investigated.*

- Allow clients the opportunity to look at things the way they appear to them and not the way they appear to the nurse or to someone else.

- Do not impose values on the client. Avoid using personal examples, such as saying, "If I were you. . . . "

► **Technique 2–1** *CONTINUED*

- Nonverbally convey respect, concern, interest, and acceptance.

- Use and accept silence to help the client search for and organize thoughts.

- Use eye contact, and be calm, unhurried and sympathetic.

5. Close the interview in a manner that maintains rapport and trust with the client.

- Signal that the interview is coming to a close by offering to answer any questions the client may have.

- Declare completion of the purpose or task by a statement such as, "Well, that's about all I need to know for now." Preceding a remark with the word "well" generally signals that the end of the interaction is near.

- Express concern for the person's welfare and future: "Take care of yourself. I'll see you on Thursday." "I hope all goes well for you. If you run into any additional problems, be sure to get in touch with me."

- Plan for the next meeting, if there is to be one. Include the day, time, place, topic, and purpose.

- Reveal what will happen next for the client in relation to the nursing care regimen, such as the number of times per day dressings will be changed, and so on.

- Signal that the time is up, if a time limit was agreed upon, or explain why the interview must now close: "Well, I see our time is up. We'll have to continue this discussion this afternoon."

- Provide a summary to verify accuracy. *Summarizing helps terminate the interview, reassures the client that the nurse has listened, checks the accuracy of the nurse's perceptions, and helps the client to note progress and forward direction.*

- State appreciation or satisfaction about what was accomplished: "I really enjoyed meeting you, and I think we accomplished a great deal." "Those are all the questions I have. Thank you for your time and help." "The questions you have answered will be helpful in planning your nursing care."

EVALUATION FOCUS	Chief complaints; perceptions of illness; untoward responses to being interviewed; potential risk factors for illness; status of family resources and support.

SAMPLE RECORDING

Date	Time	Notes
9/7/93	1400	53-year-old male admitted with complaint of sharp abdominal pain in right upper quadrant for last 4 hours. Tearful and guarding abdomen during data collection. Encouraged to ventilate concerns. States is afraid he has cancer. Additional data as per admission nursing assessment sheet. ———————————————————— Becky L. James, RN

KEY ELEMENTS OF INTERVIEWING A CLIENT

- Identify any special client needs before proceeding with the interview.
- Establish a comfortable informal interview environment.
- Open the interview with a sense of goodwill and trust and an explanation of the purpose of the interview.
- Begin with open-ended questions.

- Obtain the most important information first.
- Listen attentively to the client and use and accept periods of silence.
- Use language the client understands.
- Close the interview by offering to answer questions, providing a summary, and stating what activities will follow the interview.

Structuring Data Collection

To obtain data systematically during the nursing health history, the nurse needs to use an organized assessment framework or structure.

Gordon (1987b, p. 93) established a framework of 11 functional health patterns. See the box below. Gordon uses the word *pattern* to signify a sequence of behavior. The nurse collects data about dysfunctional as well as functional behavior. Thus, using Gordon's framework to analyze data, nurses are able to discern emerging patterns. There are many other frameworks associated with nursing models available to structure data collection.

Gordon's Typology of 11 Functional Health Patterns

- *Health-perception–health-management pattern.* Describes client's perceived pattern of health and well-being and how health is managed.
- *Nutritional-metabolic pattern.* Describes pattern of food and fluid consumption relative to metabolic need and pattern indicators of local nutrient supply.
- *Elimination pattern.* Describes patterns of excretory function (bowel, bladder, and skin).
- *Activity-exercise pattern.* Describes pattern of exercise, activity, leisure, and recreation.
- *Cognitive-perceptual pattern.* Describes sensory-perceptual and cognitive pattern.
- *Sleep-rest pattern.* Describes patterns of sleep, rest, and relaxation.
- *Self-perception–self-concept pattern.* Describes self-concept pattern and perceptions of self (e.g., body comfort, body image, feeling state).
- *Role-relationship pattern.* Describes pattern of role-engagements and relationships.
- *Sexuality-reproductive pattern.* Describes client's patterns of satisfaction and dissatisfaction with sexuality; describes reproductive patterns.
- *Coping–stress-tolerance pattern.* Describes general coping pattern and effectiveness of the pattern in terms of stress tolerance.
- *Value-belief pattern.* Describes patterns of values, beliefs (including spiritual), or goals that guide choices or decisions.

Source: M. Gordon, *Nursing diagnosis: Process and application*, 2d ed. (New York: McGraw-Hill, 1987), p. 93.

Diagnosing

Nursing diagnosis emerged in the 1970s and provided the profession with an appropriate focus on the content and the diagnostic categories that were in the domain of nursing. Since that time, over 100 nursing diagnoses have been developed. See the box on page 25.

In March 1990, the Ninth Conference on the Classification of Nursing Diagnoses in Orlando, Florida, accepted the following working definition of **nursing diagnosis**: "Nursing diagnosis is a clinical judgment about individual, family, or community responses to actual and potential health problems/life processes. Nursing diagnoses provide the basis for selection of nursing interventions to achieve outcomes for which the nurse is accountable" (Carroll-Johnson 1990, p. 50).

Implied in this definition are the following characteristics:

- Professional nurses (registered nurses) are the persons responsible for making nursing diagnoses. Even though other nursing personnel may contribute data to the process of diagnosing and may implement specified nursing care, the formulation of a diagnostic statement lies within the realm of the professional nurse.
- A **health problem** is any condition or situation in which a client requires help to promote, maintain, or regain a state of health or to achieve a peaceful death. It does not always refer to an undesirable state but does refer to a situation for which the client needs nursing assistance.
- **Life processes** are normal life events.
- Nursing diagnoses describe (a) **actual health problems** (deviations from health), (b) **potential health problems** (risk factors that predispose persons and families to health problems), and (c) areas of enriched personal growth. Examples of diagnoses that describe actual health problems are **Ineffective airway clearance**, **Fluid volume deficit**, and **Knowledge deficit**. Examples describing potential health problems are **High risk for Infection** and **High risk for Injury**. Examples of diagnoses that identify life processes or areas of enriched personal growth are **Family coping: Potential for growth**, **Altered parenting**, and **Anticipatory grieving**.
- The domain of nursing diagnosis includes only those health states that nurses are able and licensed to treat. For example, nurses are not educated to diagnose or treat diseases such as diabetes mellitus; this task is defined legally as

Approved Nursing Diagnoses

North American Nursing Diagnosis Association (NANDA)
April 1992

Activity intolerance
Activity intolerance: High risk for
Adjustment, Impaired
Airway clearance, Ineffective
Anxiety
Aspiration: High risk for
Body image disturbance
Body temperature, Altered: High risk for
Breast-feeding, Effective (potential for enhanced)
Breast-feeding, Ineffective
Breast-feeding, Interrupted
Breathing pattern, Ineffective
Cardiac output, Decreased
Caregiver role strain: Actual or High risk for
Communication, Impaired verbal
Constipation
Constipation, Colonic
Constipation, Perceived
Coping, Defensive
Coping (family), ineffective: Compromised
Coping (family), ineffective: Disabling
Coping (family), potential for growth
Coping (individual), ineffective
Decisional conflict (specify)
Denial, Ineffective
Diarrhea
Disuse syndrome: High risk for
Diversional activity deficit
Dysreflexia
Family processes, Altered
Fatigue
Fear
Fluid volume deficit
Fluid volume deficit: High risk for
Fluid volume excess
Gas exchange, Impaired
Grieving, Anticipatory
Grieving, Dysfunctional
Growth and development, Altered
Health maintenance, Altered
Health-seeking behaviors (specify)
Home maintenance management, Impaired
Hopelessness
Hyperthermia
Hypothermia
Incontinence, Bowel
Incontinence, Functional (urinary)
Incontinence, Reflex (urinary)
Incontinence, Stress (urinary)
Incontinence, Total (urinary)
Incontinence, Urge (urinary)
Infant feeding pattern, Ineffective
Infection: High risk for
Injury: High risk for
Knowledge deficit (specify)

Management of therapeutic regimen, Ineffective individual
Mobility, Impaired physical
Noncompliance (specify)
Nutrition, Altered: Less than body requirements
Nutrition, Altered: More than body requirements
Nutrition, Altered: High risk for more than body requirements
Oral mucous membrane, altered
Pain [Acute]
Pain, Chronic
Parental role conflict
Parenting, Altered
Parenting, Altered: High risk for
Peripheral Neurovascular Dysfunction: High risk for
Personal identity disturbance
Poisoning: High risk for
Post-trauma response
Powerlessness
Protection, Altered
Rape-trauma syndrome
Rape-trauma syndrome: Compound reaction
Rape-trauma syndrome: Silent reaction
Relocation stress syndrome
Role performance, Altered
Self-care deficit: Bathing/hygiene
Self-care deficit: Dressing/grooming
Self-care deficit: Feeding
Self-care deficit: Toileting
Self-esteem disturbance
Self-esteem, Low: Chronic
Self-esteem, Low: Situational
Self-mutilation: High risk for
Sensory/perceptual alterations: Visual, auditory, kinesthetic, gustatory, tactile, olfactory (specify)
Sexual dysfunction
Sexuality patterns, Altered
Skin integrity, Impaired
Skin integrity, Impaired: High risk for
Sleep pattern disturbance
Social interaction, Impaired
Social isolation
Spiritual distress
Spontaneous ventilation, Inability to sustain
Suffocation: High risk for
Swallowing, Impaired
Thermoregulation, Impaired
Thought processes, Altered
Tissue integrity, Impaired
Tissue perfusion, altered: Renal, cerebral, cardiopulmonary, gastrointestinal, peripheral (specify type)
Trauma: High risk for
Unilateral neglect
Urinary elimination, Altered
Urinary retention
Ventilary Weaning Response, Dysfunctional
Violence, High risk for: Self-directed or directed at others

within the practice of medicine. Yet they can diagnose a **Knowledge deficit, Ineffective individual coping, Altered nutrition,** and **High risk for Injury**, all of which may accompany diabetes mellitus. These problems are within the nurse's capabilities, the nurse's *independent* functions, and the scope of the nurse's licensing laws; thus, the nurse is responsible and accountable for the treatment provided in response to these nursing diagnoses. Nursing diagnoses are differentiated from medical diagnoses in Table 2–4.

• A nursing diagnosis is a judgment made only after a thorough, systematic process of data collection.

Nursing diagnoses accepted by NANDA (North American Nursing Diagnosis Association) have generally focused on altered health patterns. To date, four wellness-oriented nursing diagnoses are listed in the NANDA Taxonomy I: **Anticipatory grieving; Effective breastfeeding; Family coping: Potential for growth;** and **Health-seeking behaviors** (Popkess-Vawter 1991, p. 19). Efforts are underway to generate others. In the meantime, nurses caring for basically healthy individuals may find it necessary to use **potential nursing diagnoses**, such as

• **Potential diversional activity deficit** related to post-retirement status

• **Potential ineffective individual coping** related to new parenting role

TABLE 2–4 COMPARISON OF NURSING AND MEDICAL DIAGNOSES

Nursing Diagnosis	Medical Diagnosis
Describes an individual's response to a disease process, condition, or situation.	Describes a specific disease process.
Is oriented to the individual.	Is oriented to pathology.
Changes as the client's responses change.	Remains constant throughout the duration of illness.
Guides independent nursing activities: planning, intervening, and evaluating.	Guides medical management, some of which may be carried out by the nurse.
Is complementary to the medical diagnosis.	Is complementary to the nursing diagnosis.
Has no universally accepted classification system; such systems are in the process of development.	Has a well-developed classification system accepted by the medical profession.
Consists of a two-part statement with etiology when known.	Consists of two or three words.

• **Potential impaired adjustment** related to divorce and inadequate support from family members

• **Potential activity intolerance** related to lack of motivation

• **Potential ineffective airway clearance** related to smoking

Nursing Diagnosis Format

There are three essential components of nursing diagnostic statements; they are referred to as the **PES format** (Gordon 1976, p. 1299):

1. *The terms describing the problem (P).* This component, referred to as the *diagnostic category label* or *title*, is a description of the client's (individual, family, community) health problem (actual or potential) for which nursing therapy is given. The state of the client is described clearly and concisely in a few words. See the box on page 25 for a list of nursing diagnostic categories adopted by the North American Nursing Diagnosis Association's Tenth National Conference on Classification of Nursing Diagnoses in 1992. To be clinically useful, category labels need to be specific. When the word *specify* follows a category label in the list, the nurse states the area in which the problem occurs. For example, a knowledge deficit may be in the area of medication prescription, dietary adjustments, or disease process and therapy.

2. *The etiology of the problem (E)* or contributing factors. This component identifies one or more probable causes of the health problem and gives direction to the required nursing therapy. Etiology may include behaviors of the client, environmental factors, or interactions of the two. For example, the probable causes of **Altered health maintenance** include perceptual or cognitive impairment, lack of gross or fine motor skills, lack of material resources, and ineffective individual coping. See Table 2–5. Differentiating among possible causes in the nursing diagnosis is essential because each may require different nursing therapies.

3. *The defining characteristics or cluster of signs and symptoms (S).* The defining characteristics provide information necessary to arrive at the diagnostic category label (component 1). Each nursing diagnostic category is associated with signs and symptoms that occur as a clinical entity. *Major* signs and symptoms are those that must be present to make the diagnosis valid. *Minor* characteristics may or may not be present. Nursing diagnostic categories are similar to medical diagnostic categories. For example, the medical diagnostic category myocardial infarction (heart

TABLE 2–5   COMPONENTS OF A NURSING DIAGNOSTIC CATEGORY

Diagnosis	Definition	Etiology	Defining Characteristics
Altered health maintenance	Inability to identify, manage, and/or seek out help to maintain health	Lack of or significant alteration in communication skills (written, verbal, and/or gestural)	Demonstrated lack of knowledge regarding basic health practices
		Lack of ability to make deliberate and thoughtful judgments	Demonstrated lack of adaptive behaviors to internal or external environmental changes
		Perceptual or cognitive impairment	Reported or observed inability to take the responsibility for meeting basic health practices in any or all functional pattern areas
		Complete or partial lack of gross and/or fine motor skills	
			History of lack of health-seeking behavior
		Ineffective individual coping; dysfunctional grieving	Expressed interest in improving health behaviors
		Lack of material resources	
		Unachieved developmental tasks	Reported or observed lack of equipment, financial, and/or other resources
		Ineffective family coping: disabling spiritual distress	Reported or observed impairment of personal support system

Source: M. J. Kim, G. K. McFarland, and A. M. McLane, *Pocket guide to nursing diagnoses*, 4th ed. (St. Louis: C. V. Mosby Co., 1991). Used by permission.

attack) is associated with a standard set of signs and symptoms that are universally understood and accepted. Likewise, the nursing diagnostic category **Altered health maintenance** is associated with a standard cluster of signs and symptoms. See Table 2–5. For most nursing diagnoses, the list of defining characteristics is still being developed and refined. Partial listings have been published to assist nurses in developing and validating nursing diagnoses.

The Diagnostic Process

The diagnostic process has the following steps:

1. Data processing (interpreting collected data)

2. Determining the client's health problems, health risks, and strengths

3. Formulating nursing diagnoses

Step 1: Data Processing
Data processing, the act of interpreting collected data, involves the following steps: (a) Organize data, (b) Compare data against standards, (c) Cluster data (generate tentative hypotheses), and (d) Identify gaps and inconsistencies. These activities occur continuously rather than sequentially.

Organizing the Data   Once the data are collected, they need to be organized into a usable framework for the nurse and others who may need access to them. Theoretical frameworks and conceptual models often guide the format of the assessment tool, thus facilitating the organization of data.

To illustrate data organization, a summary of the nursing assessment data for a client, Mr. Frederick Smith, is shown in the box on page 28. In this instance, a functional health pattern assessment format is used.

Comparing Data against Standards   The nurse compares the client's data to a wide range of standards, such as normal health patterns, normal vital signs, laboratory values, basic food groups, growth, and development. The nurse also uses personal knowledge—e.g., of physiology, psychology, and sociology—as well as past experience when comparing the data.

Standards used for comparison include the Daily Food Guides, Erikson's stages of development, and the Metropolitan Life Insurance charts for normal ranges of height and weight. The nurse compares the client data against standards and norms in order to identify significant and relevant cues. A **cue** is a piece of information or data that influences decisions (Gordon 1987b, p. 182).

Clustering Data   Clustering or grouping data is a process of determining the relatedness of facts and finding patterns in the facts. Data are examined to determine whether any patterns are present, whether the data represent isolated incidents, and whether the data are significant.

To relate and group data, the nurse must consider nursing diagnostic categories (see the box on page 25) or areas of nursing responsibility. Gordon (1987b, p. 20) states that clustering information involves a search in the nurse's memory stores for previously learned meaningful groups of clinical cues that are associated with a diagnostic category. Gordon believes that clustering occurs in conjunction with data collection and interpretation, as evidenced in such remarks or thoughts as "I'm getting a picture of" or "This cue doesn't fit the picture."

During data clustering, the nurse interprets the possible meaning of the cues and labels the cue clusters with tentative diagnostic hypotheses. Data clustering or grouping for Mr. Frederick Smith is illustrated in Table 2–6. The data are clustered according to nursing diagnostic categories.

Identifying Gaps and Inconsistencies in Data
Gaps are missing information the nurse needs to determine a data pattern. For example, during the assessment phase, the nurse needs data about a client's definition of health to interpret his statement "I am sick all the time." Data may be completely missing or incomplete.

Inconsistencies are conflicting data. Possible sources of conflicting data include measurement error, expectations, and conflicting or unreliable reports (Gordon 1987b, p. 259). For example, if the client reports a history of high blood pressure but the nurse obtains a low reading, the nurse should check the equipment and procedure for possible error. All inconsistencies must be clarified before a valid pattern can be established.

Organization of Data for Mr. Frederick Smith

Health Perception/Health Management
- No energy
- Shortness of breath
- Had left hip replacement 2 years ago
- Eats a good diet
- Does not smoke
- Does not drink

Nutritional/Metabolic
- Has diabetes
- Does not eat sugar
- Lost 5 pounds over past year

Elimination
- Urinates frequently

Activity/Exercise
- Lacks energy to do daily ranch chores
- Moves more slowly since hip surgery

Cognitive/Perceptual
- Slightly hard of hearing
- Wears glasses
- Doesn't read much, prefers to be told how to do things

Roles/Relationships
- Lives with wife and 6 of 13 children
- Family "scared" about his illness
- Cattle rancher and farmer

Self-Perception/Self-Concept
- Too weak to do day work on the farm

Coping/Stress
- Usually too busy to worry about things
- Perceives his son Tom as helpful in talking things over
- Wants family to visit

Value/Belief
- Religion/spirituality is important to him
- Wants to see hospital chaplain

Medication/History
- Tolazamide (Tolinase) 250 mg daily
- Furosemide (Lasix) 20 mg daily
- Slow K 20 mEq daily
- Nitroglycerin 1/150 gr prn for angina

Nursing Physical Assessment
- 81 years old
- Height 171 cm
- Weight 95.3 kg
- TPR 36.5, 80, 16
- Blood pressure 124/80 mm Hg
- Large, slightly obese
- Joint stiffness
- Slight limp
- No pedal edema
- Femoral pulses very strong (R) and bounding (L)
- Popliteal, dorsalis pedis, posterior tibial pulses absent in left leg
- Left leg cooler than right leg
- Heart rhythm is regular
- Loud heart murmur in aortic area
- History of angina (6 months)
- Rales in bases of both lungs cleared by coughing
- Urinary frequency due to Lasix
- No allergies

TABLE 2–6   FORMULATING NURSING DIAGNOSES FOR MR. FREDERICK SMITH

Diagnostic Category	Data Clustering/ Grouping Data	Determining Strengths and Health Problems	Formulating Nursing Diagnostic Statements
Activity intolerance	Shortness of breath Lacks energy to do daily chores Does not smoke	Does not smoke (strength) Activity intolerance (problem)	**Activity intolerance** related to shortness of breath and lack of energy secondary to decreased strength of cardiac contraction
Ineffective airway clearance	Rales in bases of both lungs relieved by coughing	Able to expel secretions by coughing (strength) Secretions in lung bases (problem)	**Potential ineffective airway clearance** postoperatively related to chest incision
High risk for Injury	Left hip replacement Movement slightly limited Joint stiffness Slight limp	Carries out daily activities independently (strength) Movement slightly limited (problem)	**High risk for injury** (trauma) related to joint stiffness and limp from hip replacement surgery
Altered nutrition: More than body requirements	Is diabetic Takes tolazamide (Tolinase) daily "No sugar" in diet "Eats a good diet" Overweight for height Weight loss of 5 pounds in past year	Controls diabetes with Tolinase and "no sugar" (strength) Weight loss of 5 pounds in past year (strength) Overweight (problem)	**Altered nutrition: More than body requirements** related to imbalance of intake versus activity expenditure
Knowledge deficit	Takes furosemide (Lasix) daily Takes Slow K daily Urinates frequently	Complies with medical regimen (strength) Does not relate urinary frequency to diuretic (problem)	**Knowledge deficit:** side-effects of diuretic therapy
Altered peripheral tissue perfusion	Vital signs normal Heart rhythm regular Loud heart murmur (aortic area) Femoral pulses stronger than normal Absent pulses (popliteal, dorsalis pedis, posterior tibial) in left leg Left leg cooler than right leg Integument pink and intact	Vital signs within normal range (strength) Skin intact and of good color (strength) Impaired circulation in left leg (problem)	**Altered peripheral tissue perfusion** (left leg) related to impaired arterial circulation
Fear	Hospitalized for cardiac catheterization and possible aortic valve replacement States family "scared" about illness Wants to see chaplain Wants family to visit Perceives son Tom as helpful Says is usually too busy to worry about things	Perceives family as supportive (strength) Says family anxious about illness. Did not indicate own feelings (problem)	**Fear** related to cardiac catheterization, possible surgery, and its outcome
Pain	History of angina (6 months) Takes nitroglycerin for angina	Has not needed nitroglycerin for 2 months (strength)	**Potential pain (angina)** related to excessive activity or stress

Step 2: Determining the Client's Health Problems, Health Risks, and Strengths

After data are clustered, the nurse and the client can together identify strengths and problems. This second phase of the diagnostic process is primarily a decision-making process. The nurse determines which groups of data identify actual or potential health problems or risks for the client and which problems require nursing intervention. The client must accept the existence of the problem. The nurse, by contrast, determines whether the client needs help dealing with the problem. See Table 2–6 for examples of Mr. Frederick Smith's problems.

At this stage, the nurse and client also establish the client's strengths, resources, and abilities to cope. Generally, people have a clearer perception of their problems or weaknesses than of their strengths and assets, which they often take for granted. By taking an inventory of strengths, the client can develop a more well-rounded self-concept and self-image. Awareness of one's strengths can be an aid to mobilizing health and regenerative processes.

One client's strength might be that his weight is within the normal range for his age and height, thus enabling him to cope better with surgery. Another client's strengths might be that she is allergy-free and a nonsmoker. The same client's resources could be a supportive family and an ability to cope.

A client's strengths can be found in the nursing assessment record (health, home life, education, recreation, exercise, work, family and friends, religious beliefs, and sense of humor, for example), the health examination, and the client's records. See Table 2–6 for examples of Mr. Frederick Smith's strengths.

Step 3: Formulating Nursing Diagnoses

At this final stage, the nurse formulates causal relationships between the health problems and the factors related to them. These factors may be, for example, environmental, sociologic, psychologic, physiologic, or spiritual. More than one factor may be related to one health problem. It is also important to determine at this time whether the problem can be resolved by independent nursing interventions. If it cannot, the nurse should refer the client to the appropriate health team member. By including the causal factors in diagnostic statements, the nurse can tailor a plan of care for the client. For example, the diagnosis **Impaired physical mobility** tells the nurse the problem but does not suggest the direction the nursing intervention should take, whereas **Impaired physical mobility related to neuromuscular impairment** suggests a direction for plans and interventions to deal with the problem. Obviously, the causative factor *neuromuscular impairment* suggests a different direction than the factor *fear of falling* would.

Nurses can refer to a list of accepted nursing diagnoses, shown on page 25, to select a diagnostic category. The causal factors are obtained from the data. If no causal factor appears in the data, the nurse may wish to make a tentative diagnosis based on scientific nursing knowledge and experience. The nurse should then review the database for inconsistencies and gaps. Once the causal relationships have been established, the nurse is ready to write the diagnostic statements.

See Table 2–6 for Mr. Frederick Smith's nursing diagnostic statements.

Writing a Diagnostic Statement

Nurses may write diagnoses as either two-part or three-part statements. The two-part nursing diagnostic statement includes

1. Problem (P)—Statement of the client's response

2. Etiology (E)—Factors contributing to or probable causes of the responses

The two parts are joined by the words *related to* or *associated with* rather than *due to*. The phrase *due to* implies a cause-and-effect relationship; one clause causes or is responsible for the other clause. By contrast, the phrases *related to* and *associated with* merely imply a relationship. The phrase *related to* is most commonly used. If one part of the diagnostic statement changes, the other part may change as well. Here are some examples of two-part nursing diagnoses:

- **Self-esteem disturbance** (problem) related to *altered body image (loss of arm)* (etiology)

- **Anticipatory grieving** (problem) related to *anticipated loss* (etiology) secondary to *husband's illness* (etiology)

A three-part nursing diagnosis statement includes

1. Problem (P)—Statement of the client's response

2. Etiology (E)—Factors contributing to or probable causes of the responses

3. Signs and symptoms (S)—Defining characteristics manifested by the client

The three-part diagnostic statement includes the problem, the etiology, and the observed signs and symptoms (PES). Actual nursing diagnoses can be documented by using the three-part statement (using *related to* and *manifested by*), since the signs and symptoms have been identified. Here are some examples of three-part statements:

- **Self-esteem disturbance** (problem) related to *altered body image (loss of arm)* (etiology) manifested by *crying and hostility* (signs and symptoms)

- **Anticipatory grieving** (problem) related to *husband's terminal illness* (etiology) manifested by *anorexia and withdrawn behavior* (signs and symptoms)

Possible nursing diagnoses are used when evidence about a response is unclear or when the related factors are unknown. The nurse writes the possible nursing diagnosis and collects more data either to support or refute the possible response. For example, an elderly widow who lives alone is admitted to hospital. The nurse notices that she has no visitors and is pleased with attention and conversation from the nursing staff. Until more data are collected, the nurse may write a possible nursing diagnosis of **Social isolation** related to *unknown etiology*.

The accuracy of nursing diagnostic statements also depends on a complete database and appropriate data processing. If data are omitted, a diagnosis can be missed. If data are not processed properly, e.g., are not clustered appropriately, a diagnosis can be made prematurely or incorrectly or be missed.

Table 2–7 presents guidelines to writing clear, concise, client-centered nursing diagnoses.

Planning

Although the planning process is basically the responsibility of the nurse, the plan can be effective only if the client and support persons provide input. It is no

---

TABLE 2–7   GUIDELINES FOR WRITING A NURSING DIAGNOSTIC STATEMENT

Guideline	Correct Statement	Incorrect and/or Ambiguous Statement
1. State in terms of a problem, not a need.	**Fluid volume deficit** (problem) related to fever	**Fluid replacement** (need) related to fever
2. State so that it is legally advisable.	**Impaired skin integrity** related to immobility (legally acceptable)	**Impaired skin integrity** related to improper positioning (implies legal liability)
3. Use nonjudgmental statements.	**Spiritual distress** related to inability to attend church services secondary to immobility (nonjudgmental)	**Spiritual distress** related to strict rules necessitating church attendance (judgmental)
4. Make sure that both elements of the statement do *not* say the same thing.	**High risk for Impaired skin integrity** related to immobility	**Impaired skin integrity** related to ulceration of sacral area (response and probable cause are the same)
5. Make sure that the client's response precedes the contributing or causal factor.	**Noncompliance with diet** (response) related to lack of knowledge (contributing factor)	**Knowledge deficit** (contributing factor) related to noncompliance with diet (response)
6. Use statements that provide guidance for planning independent nursing interventions.	**Social isolation** related to loss of speech (loss of speech provides direction for planning alternative communication methods)	**Social isolation** related to laryngectomy (the nurse can do nothing about the laryngectomy)
7. Word diagnosis specifically and precisely to provide direction for planning nursing intervention.	**Altered oral mucous membrane** related to decreased salivation secondary to radiation of neck (specific)	**Altered oral mucous membrane** related to noxious agent (vague)
8. Use nursing terminology rather than medical terminology to describe the client's response.	**Potential ineffective airway clearance** (nursing terminology)	**Potential pneumonia** (medical terminology)
9. Use nursing terminology rather than medical terminology to describe the probable cause of the client's response.	**Potential ineffective airway clearance** related to accumulation of secretions in lungs (nursing terminology)	**Potential ineffective airway clearance** related to emphysema (medical terminology)
10. Do not start the nursing diagnosis with a nursing intervention.	**Altered nutrition: Less than body requirements** related to inadequate intake of protein (directs but does not state nursing intervention)	Provide high-protein diet because of **Potential altered nutrition** (starts with nursing intervention)
11. Avoid using a symptom, such as nausea, as the client's response. A symptom does not reflect a pattern and requires additional data collection.	Insufficient data for a diagnosis	**Nausea** related to medication

longer sufficient that nurses plan *for* the client; whenever possible, the client must participate actively.

Planning is a deliberative, systematic process that is critical to providing quality nursing care. It is a process in which decision making and problem solving are carried out. The planning process uses (a) data obtained during assessing and (b) the diagnostic statements that present the client's health problems (potential and actual). Accurate nursing diagnoses provide direction for determining client goals and developing a plan of care.

Planning has five components: (a) Setting priorities; (b) Establishing client goals and outcome criteria; (c) Planning nursing strategies; (d) Writing nursing orders; and (e) Writing the nursing care plan.

Setting Priorities

Priority setting is the process of establishing a preferential order for nursing strategies. To set priorities, the nurse and the client first order the nursing diagnoses preferentially, i.e., they decide which deserves attention first, which second, and so on. Diagnoses can be grouped as having high, medium, or low priority. This priority setting, however, does not mean that all the high-priority diagnoses must be resolved before any others are considered. A high-priority diagnosis may be dealt with partially, and then a diagnosis of lesser priority may be dealt with. In addition, the nurse may address more than one diagnosis at a time. Because client problems are usually multiple, this is often the case.

The priorities assigned to problems should not remain fixed. Nursing priorities must change as a client's health problems and therapy change. The nurse can determine the relative value or priority level of the client's problem by noting the following factors:

- *Urgency of the health problem.* Life-threatening situations, such as loss of cardiac or respiratory function, have high priority. Health-threatening problems, either actual or potential, that may result in delayed development or impaired functioning usually have medium priority. For example, growth needs, such as self-esteem, are not necessary for sustaining life. Thus, in planning care for a client with unmet physiologic needs and unmet growth needs, the nurse gives first priority to the basic or physiologic needs.

- *The client's health values, beliefs, and priorities.* For example, one nursing diagnosis may relate to smoking and another to nutrition. The nurse may give the smoking problem a higher priority than the problem of obesity, but the client may see the problem of obesity as more important. When there is such a difference of opinion, the client

and nurse should discuss it openly to resolve the conflict. However, in a life-threatening situation, the nurse needs to take the initiative.

- *Resources available to the nurse and client.* If necessary resources (e.g., money, equipment, or personnel) are not readily accessible, the problem may be assigned a lower priority and addressed after the resources become available. For example, a client who is unemployed may defer dental treatment.

- *Medical treatment plan.* The priorities for treating health problems must be congruent with treatment by other health professionals. For example, a high priority for the client might be to become ambulatory; however, if the physician's therapeutic regimen calls for extended bed rest, then ambulation must assume a lower priority or deferment in the nursing strategy plan.

See Table 2–8 for the assignment of priorities to the diagnostic statements for Mr. Frederick Smith.

Establishing Client Goals and Outcome Criteria

Goals A **client goal** is a desired outcome or change in client behavior in the direction of health. Goal attainment reflects the resolution of the client concern or health problem specified in the nursing diagnosis. The nursing diagnosis guides the type of goal statement: goals may reflect health restoration, health maintenance, or health promotion (Christensen 1986, p. 173).

A client goal is a broad statement about the expected or desired change in the status of the client after the client receives nursing interventions. Since goals are broad indicators of performance, the use of such verbs as *increase, decrease, maintain, improve, develop,* and *restore* is appropriate. See examples of client goals in the box below.

Examples of Client Goals

The client/clients will

- Increase activity tolerance.
- Maintain urinary elimination pattern.
- Restore fluid volume.
- Decrease potential for injury.
- Develop coping abilities.
- Improve nutritional pattern.
- Increase parenting knowledge.
- Establish change in family roles.

TABLE 2–8 ASSIGNING PRIORITIES TO DIAGNOSTIC STATEMENTS FOR MR. FREDERICK SMITH (BEFORE CARDIAC CATHETERIZATION)

Diagnostic Statement List	Priority Rating	Rationale
Activity intolerance related to shortness of breath and lack of energy secondary to decreased strength of cardiac contractions	Medium priority	Lack of energy is the client's stated major concern. Too much activity can create excessive cardiac demands, resulting in further decreased cardiac output with lowered blood pressure and inadequate circulation. However, because Mr. Smith is able to handle basic activities of daily living, strategies to deal with this diagnostic statement can be deferred until after cardiac catheterization and/or cardiac surgery.
Potential ineffective airway clearance postoperatively related to chest incision	Low priority	Until surgery is performed, ineffective airway clearance is not likely, because he is currently able to clear his airways by coughing.
High risk for Trauma related to joint stiffness and limp from hip replacement surgery	High priority	The client is independent and moves slowly to accommodate his limitations. However, new surroundings and a sedative given before cardiac catheterization increase his risk of injury.
Knowledge deficit: side-effects of diuretic therapy	Medium priority	Although the client complies with his medical regimen, he does not seem to understand the side-effects of the prescribed diuretic, e.g., its relation to increased urination.
Altered peripheral tissue perfusion (left leg) related to impaired arterial circulation	High priority	Decreased circulation and tissue perfusion to the client's left leg can result in damage to the tissues of the limb.
Fear related to cardiac catheterization, possible heart surgery, and its outcome	High priority	Extreme fear could impair his coping capacity.
Potential pain (angina) related to excessive activity or stress	Medium priority	Angina has not been a problem for 2 months, but it could recur with the stress of hospitalization and planned treatments.

The purpose of client goals is to

• Provide direction for planning nursing interventions that will achieve the anticipated changes in the client.

• Provide direction for establishing evaluation criteria to measure the effectiveness of the interventions.

The nurse derives client goals from the first clause of the nursing diagnosis, i.e., from the identified client response. For example, if the first clause of the nursing diagnosis or problem (P) is **Self-care deficit: Feeding**, the goal might be stated as follows: "Client will demonstrate increased ability to feed self." See establishing goals from nursing diagnosis, in the accompanying box. Then, from this goal, the nurse determines more specific client outcomes (criteria); these criteria form the basis of evaluation. For example, if the goal is "The client will demonstrate increased ability to feed self," two criteria might be,

---

Establishing Goals from Nursing Diagnosis

Client goals are derived from the first clause of the nursing diagnosis, which is the client problem (P).

Nursing diagnosis	**Impaired physical mobility** related to pain
Client response or problem	Impaired physical mobility
Client goal	Client will demonstrate increase in physical mobility.
Nursing diagnosis	**Self-care deficit: Feeding** related to depression
Client response or problem	Self-care-deficit: Inability to feed self
Client goal	Client will perform self-feeding.

"Will drink from a glass through a straw" and "Will feed self using utensils with sponge-wrapped handles." See the section on outcome criteria in this chapter.

Goals may be short term or long term. A short-term goal might be, "Client will raise right arm to shoulder height by Friday." In the same context, a long-term goal might be, "Client will regain full use of right arm in 6 weeks." Because a great deal of the nurse's time is focused on the immediate needs of the client, most goals are short term. In addition, the nurse is better able to evaluate the client's progress or lack of it with short-term goals.

Long-term goals are often appropriate for clients who live at home and have chronic health problems or clients in nursing homes, extended care facilities, and rehabilitation centers. Short-term goals are useful (a) for clients who require health care for only a short time and (b) for persons who are frustrated by long-term goals that seem difficult to attain and who need the satisfaction of achieving a short-term goal.

Outcome Criteria Outcome criteria add specificity to the broad goal statements. **Outcome criteria** are statements that describe specific, observable, and measurable responses of the client. They determine whether the stated goals have been achieved and are therefore essential to the evaluation phase of the nursing process.

Generally, three to six outcome criteria are needed for each goal. Some nurses consider outcome criteria to be part of goals and add criteria directly to the goal statement, as follows: "Client's hydration status will be maintained (goal) as evidenced by (outcome criteria): (a) fluid intake of at least 2500 ml daily, (b) urinary output in balance with fluid intake, (c) normal skin turgor, (d) moist mucous membranes." Other nurses find this method cumbersome and separate the goal statement from the criteria statements.

Whichever method is used, the process of developing outcome criteria is the same. The nurse needs to ask two questions:

1. How will the client look or behave if the desired goal is achieved?

2. What must the client do and how well must the client do it to attain the goal?

Outcome criteria generally have all or some of the following components:

• *Subject.* The subject, a noun, is the client, any part of the client, or some attribute of the client, such as the client's pulse or urinary output. Often, the subject is omitted in nursing care plan goals; it is assumed that the subject is the client unless indicated otherwise.

• *Verb.* The verb denotes an action the client is to perform, e.g., what the client is to do, learn, or experience. The nurse selects verbs that denote directly observable behaviors, such as *administer, demonstrate, show, walk, drink, tell, list, state,* and so on.

• *Conditions or modifiers.* Conditions or modifiers may be added to the verb to explain the circumstances under which the behavior is to be performed. They explain what, where, when, or how. For example:

Walks *with the help of a walker* (how)
After attending two group diabetes classes, lists signs and symptoms of diabetes (when)
When at home, maintains weight at existing level (where)
Discusses *four food groups and recommended daily servings* (what)
Conditions need not be included if the standard of performance clearly indicates what is expected.

• *Criterion of desired performance.* The criterion indicates the standard by which the nurse evaluates a performance or the level at which the client performs the specified behavior. A criterion may specify time or speed, accuracy, distance, and quality. To establish a time-achievement criterion, the nurse needs to ask, "How long?" To establish an accuracy criterion, the nurse asks, "How well?" Similarly, the nurse asks, "How far?" and "What is the expected standard?" to establish distance and quality criteria, respectively. Examples are:

Weighs 75 kg *by April* (time)
Lists *five out of six* signs of diabetes (accuracy)
Walks *one block per day* (time and distance)
Administers insulin *using aseptic technique* (quality)

Table 2–9 shows examples of client goals and outcome criteria associated with the diagnostic statements for Mr. Frederick Smith. Note that the diagnostic statements have been reordered according to established priorities.

Planning Nursing Strategies

Nursing strategies, or interventions, are nursing actions that address a specific nursing diagnosis to achieve client goals. The nurse chooses specific strategies that focus on eliminating or reducing the *cause* (etiology) of the nursing diagnosis, which is the second clause of the diagnostic statement. When nurses determine strategies for *potential* nursing diagnoses, the interventions should focus on measures to reduce the client's contributing factors, i.e., signs and symptoms.

TABLE 2–9 GOALS AND OUTCOME CRITERIA FOR MR. FREDERICK SMITH (BEFORE CARDIAC CATHETERIZATION)

Diagnostic Statement*	Client Goals	Outcome Criteria
1. **Fear** related to cardiac catheterization, possible heart surgery, and its outcome	Experience increased emotional comfort and feelings of control.	Verbalizes specific concerns. Communicates thoughts clearly and logically. Facial expressions, voice tone, and body posture correspond to verbal expressions of increased emotional comfort or feelings of control. After instruction, describes the cardiac catheterization procedure and what is expected of him before and after the procedure.
2. **Altered peripheral tissue perfusion (left leg)** related to impaired arterial circulation	Improve circulation to left leg and foot.	Skin intact, pink, and moist. Skin temperature warm (as other foot). Left dorsalis pedis, posterior tibial, and popliteal pulses palpable and of same strength as corresponding right pulses. Verbalizes factors that improve and inhibit peripheral circulation. Capillary refill of left toenails within 1 to 3 seconds.
3. **High risk for Trauma** related to joint stiffness and limp from hip replacement surgery	Prevent injury.	Moves in and out of bed and ambulates without falling or injuring self.
4. **Activity intolerance** related to shortness of breath and lack of energy secondary to decreased strength of cardiac contraction	Avoid performance of activities causing shortness of breath and excessive cardiac workload.	Rests after meals. No shortness of breath during activities. Pulse and blood pressure remain stable at 80 beats per minute and 124/80 mm Hg.

*Note new order of diagnostic statements to reflect highest priorities.

The correct identification of the etiology during the nursing assessment provides the framework for choosing successful nursing interventions. For example, **Activity intolerance** may have several etiologies—pain, weakness, sedentary life-style, anxiety, or heart palpitations. The interventions vary according to the cause of the problem.

Selecting nursing strategies is a decision-making process. Planning nursing strategies involves generating a number of alternative nursing actions likely to solve the client's problem, considering the consequences of each alternative action, and choosing one or more nursing strategies. See Table 2–10 for examples of possible nursing strategies that address the diagnosis **Sleep pattern disturbance**.

The following criteria can help the nurse choose the best nursing strategy for a particular client. The planned action must be

- Safe and appropriate for the individual's age, health, and so on.
- Achievable with the resources available (e.g., if the nurse chooses the first strategy in Table 2–10, food and milk must be available).
- Congruent with the client's values and beliefs.

TABLE 2–10 DEVELOPING ALTERNATIVE NURSING STRATEGIES

Diagnostic Statement	Client Goal	Alternative Nursing Strategies
Sleep pattern disturbance related to anxiety	Obtain 6 to 9 hours of sleep.	Provide warm milk and a snack in the evening. Provide more activity during daytime. Encourage client to decrease activity 2 hours before bedtime. Assess diet for stimulants, i.e., caffeine. Provide soft music. Encourage verbalization of worries.

- Congruent with other therapies (e.g., if the client is not permitted food, the nurse must defer the strategy of an evening snack until health permits).
- Based on nursing knowledge and experience or knowledge from relevant sciences.

- Within established standards of care as determined by state laws, professional associations (American Nurses' Association, Canadian Nurses' Association), and the policies of the institution.

Writing Nursing Orders

Nursing orders are the specific actions the nurse takes to help the client meet established health care goals. Nursing orders should include the following five components (Carnevali 1983, p. 222):

1. *Date.* The nurse dates the nursing order at the time of writing and reviews it regularly at intervals appropriate to the client's needs.

2. *Action verb.* The verb starts the order and needs to be precise. For example, "Explain (to the client) the actions of insulin" is a more precise statement than "Teach (the client) about insulin." "Measure and record ankle circumference daily at 0900 hr" is more precise than "Assess edema of left ankle daily." Sometimes a modifier for the verb can make the nursing order more precise. For example, "Apply spiral bandage to left lower leg *firmly*" is more precise than "Apply spiral bandage to left leg."

3. *Content area.* The content is the where and the what of the order. In the above order, "spiral bandage" and "left leg" state the what and the where of the order. The nurse can also clarify in this example whether the foot or toes are to be left exposed.

4. *Time element.* The time element answers when, how long, or how often the nursing action is to occur. Examples are: "Assist client with tub bath at 0700 daily"; "Immerse client's left arm in sterile saline soak for 20 minutes"; or "Assist client to change position every 2 hr between 0700 and 2100 hr."

5. *Signature.* The signature of the nurse prescribing the order shows the nurse's accountability and has legal significance.

Writing the Nursing Care Plan

The **nursing care plan** is a written guide that organizes information about a client's health into a meaningful whole; it focuses on the actions nurses must take to address the client's identified nursing diagnoses and meet the stated goals. It is also referred to as the *client care plan*, since its focus is the client.

The nurse in charge (head nurse, primary nurse, or team leader) starts the care plan as soon as a client is admitted to the health care agency. It is constantly updated and revised throughout the client's stay, in response to changes in the client's condition and evaluations of goal achievement.

The purposes of a written care plan are

- To provide direction for *individualized care* of the client. The nurse organizes the plan according to each client's unique nursing care needs.

- To provide for *continuity of care.* The written plan is a means of communicating and organizing the actions of a constantly changing nursing staff.

- To provide *direction about what needs to be documented* on the client's progress notes. The care plan specifically outlines which observations to make, what nursing actions to carry out, and what instructions the client or family members require. In this way, recording is facilitated.

- To serve as a *guide for assigning staff* to care for the client. Certain aspects of the client's care may need to be delegated to someone who can make necessary judgments about the client's responses.

- To serve as a *guide for reimbursement* from medical insurance companies, often called third-party reimbursement. The medical record is used by the insurance companies to determine what they will pay in relation to the hospital care received by the client.

Format Although formats differ from agency to agency, the plan is generally organized into four columns or categories: (a) nursing diagnoses or problem list, (b) goals, (c) nursing strategies/interventions/nursing orders, and (d) outcome or evaluation criteria. Many agencies use a nursing Kardex or Rand system for organizing and storing nursing care plans.

See Table 2–11 for a sample care plan for Mr. Frederick Smith.

Guidelines for Writing Nursing Care Plans In addition to following the earlier suggestions for writing nursing orders, the nurse can use the guidelines in the box on page 38 when writing nursing care plans.

Implementing

In the implementation phase, also called the intervention phase, the nurse puts the nursing strategies listed in the nursing care plan into action to attain the desired outcome or the client's goals.

To implement nursing care, the nurse generally performs the following activities: caring, communicating, helping, teaching, counseling, acting as a client advocate and change agent, leading, and managing. These activities are associated with nursing roles (see Chapter 1) and include (a) assigning and delegating care to other nursing personnel and (b) supervising and evaluating the nursing activities of others. Guidelines for implementing nursing strat-

TABLE 2–11   NURSING CARE PLAN FOR MR. FREDERICK SMITH

Diagnostic Statement	Goals	Nursing Orders	Outcome Criteria
1. **Fear** related to cardiac catheterization, possible heart surgery, and its outcome	Experience increased emotional comfort and feelings of control.	Establish a trusting relationship with the client and family. Encourage client and family to express feelings and concerns. Discuss the cardiac catheterization procedure and what is expected of him before and after the procedure. Encourage conversation with another client who has recuperated from similar surgery.	Verbalizes specific concerns. Communicates thoughts clearly and logically. Facial expressions, voice tone, and body posture correspond to verbal expressions of increased emotional comfort or feelings of control. After instruction, describes the cardiac catheterization procedure and what is expected of him before and after the procedure.
2. **Altered peripheral tissue perfusion (left leg)** related to impaired arterial circulation	Improve circulation to left leg and foot.	Consult with physician about exercise program such as walking and ROM exercises to hip, knee, and ankle. Keep the extremity in a *dependent* position (i.e., lower than the heart). Use Doppler ultrasound stethoscope (DUS) to assess blood flow in left dorsal pedis, posterior tibial, and popliteal arteries q2h. Instruct client to keep his leg warm, e.g., wear warm socks but discourage use of external heat sources.	Skin intact, pink, and moist. Skin temperature warm (as other foot). Left dorsalis, posterior tibial, and popliteal pulses palpable and of same strength as corresponding right pulses. Capillary refill of left toenail within 1 to 3 seconds.
3. **High risk for Trauma** related to joint stiffness and limp from hip replacement surgery	Prevent injury.	Closely assess ambulation and transfers during first few days. Keep bed at lowest level. Encourage client to request assistance to ambulate during the night. Closely attend or put side rails up when client is sedated.	Moves in and out of bed and ambulates without falling or injuring self.
4. **Activity intolerance** related to shortness of breath and lack of energy secondary to decreased strength of cardiac contraction	Avoid performance of activities causing shortness of breath and excessive cardiac workload.	Organize client care and provide undisturbed rest periods. Discuss energy conservation methods, such as taking periodic rest periods. Tell the client to reduce the intensity, duration, and frequency of activity if he experiences chest pain, shortness of breath, dizziness, or abnormal pulse and blood pressure after activity. Monitor vital signs q2h, and report decreasing blood pressure, increasing heart rate, or increasing respiratory rate.	Rests after meals. No shortness of breath during activities. Pulse and blood pressure remain stable at 80 beats per minute and 124/80 mm Hg.

Guidelines for Writing Nursing Care Plans

- Date and sign the plan. The date the plan is written is essential for evaluation, review, and future planning. The signature of the nurse who writes the plan demonstrates accountability to the client and to the nursing profession, since the effectiveness of nursing actions can be evaluated.

- Use the category headings "Nursing Diagnoses," "Goals," "Nursing Orders/Interventions," and "Evaluation," and include a date for the evaluation of each goal.

- Indicate that goals are met or revised by a signature or some other method specified by the agency.

- List the nursing orders for each goal in order of priority. For example, the nursing orders for a client with a decubitis ulcer might include "Apply an occlusive dressing for 24 hours" and "Clean the ulcer with Betadine solution daily." The appropriate sequence is to clean the ulcer before applying the dressing, and the orders should be listed in that sequence.

- Use standardized medical or English symbols and key words rather than complete sentences to communicate your ideas. For example, write "Turn and reposition q2h" rather than "Turn and reposition the client every two hours."

- Refer to procedure books or other sources of information rather than including all the steps on a written plan. For example, write: "See unit procedure book for tracheostomy care," or attach a standard nursing plan about such procedures as radiation-implantation care and preoperative or postoperative care.

- Tailor the plan to the unique characteristics of the client by ensuring that the client's choices, such as preferences about the times of care and the methods used, are included. This reinforces the client's individuality and sense of control. For example, the written nursing order "Provide prune juice at breakfast rather than orange juice" indicates that the client was given the choice between beverages.

- Ensure that the nursing plan incorporates *preventive* and health maintenance aspects as well as restorative. For example, carrying out the order "Provide active-assistance ROM exercises to affected limbs q2h" prevents joint contractures and maintains muscle strength and joint mobility.

- Include collaborative and coordination activities in the plan. For example, write orders to ask a nutritionist or physical therapist about specific aspects of the client's care.

- Include plans for the client's discharge and home care needs. It is often necessary to consult and make arrangements with the community health nurse, social worker, and specific agencies that supply client information and needed equipment.

egies, shown in the box on page 39, serve as a blueprint.

The process of implementing normally includes five components: (a) Reassessing the client; (b) Validating the nursing care plan; (c) Determining the need for nursing assistance; (d) Implementing the nursing strategies; and (e) Communicating the nursing actions. Reassessing the client and validating the nursing care plan are subprocesses that operate continuously throughout the implementing phase.

Reasssessing the Client

Assessing or reassessing is carried out throughout the nursing process—in fact, whenever the nurse has contact with the client. While providing care, nurses must continue to collect data about changes (subtle or acute) in the client's level of wellness, i.e., health problems as well as reactions, feelings, and strengths. Whereas the nurse performs an extensive assessment during the first phase of the nursing process, reassessing in later phases usually focuses on more specific needs or responses of the client, i.e., fluid intake, pain, pulse rate, and urine output. Through this mechanism, nurses are able to determine whether planned nursing strategies are currently appropriate for the client.

Validating the Nursing Care Plan

A nursing care plan cannot be fixed; it must be a flexible tool. The nurse should compare new data with the database. Sometimes, the new data are incongruent with baseline data. The nurse must judge the value of the new data and determine whether the nursing care plan is still valid. When a client's health status changes, i.e., when physical or psychosocial responses change, the nurse needs to adjust the nursing care plan. If the data regarding the client's health status are unchanged, the nurse proceeds with the implementing process.

Determining the Need for Assistance

When implementing some nursing strategies, the nurse may require assistance for one of the following reasons: The nurse alone is unable to implement the

Guidelines for Implementing Nursing Strategies

- Nursing actions are based on scientific knowledge and nursing research. Be aware of the scientific rationale for all interventions and any possible side-effects or complications of the activities.

- Nursing actions resulting from a physician's order must be understood by the nurse. The nurse is responsible for intelligent implementation of these orders. This requires a knowledge of the activity, procedure, or medication; its purpose in the client's plan of care; and any contraindications (e.g., allergies) or changes in the client's condition that may be applicable. If there is any question regarding prescribed nursing actions, consult the nurse-manager or supervisor and/or physician.

- Nursing actions are adapted to the individual. A client's beliefs, values, age, health status, and environment can affect a nursing action.

- Nursing actions should always be safe. Nurses and clients need to take precautions to prevent injury. For example, when changing a sterile dressing, practice sterile technique to prevent infection; when turning a client, protect the client's skin from abrasions, which could also lead to infection.

- Nursing actions often require teaching, supportive, and comfort components. These independent nursing activities can often enhance the effectiveness of a specific nursing action.

- Nursing actions should always be holistic. Always view the client as a whole and consider the client's responses in that light.

- Nursing actions should respect the dignity of the client and enhance the client's self-esteem. Providing privacy and encouraging clients to make their own decisions are ways of respecting dignity and enhancing self-esteem.

- Encourage the client's active participation in implementing nursing actions as health permits. Active participation enhances the client's sense of independence and control. Clients vary in the degree of participation they desire. Some clients want total involvement in their care, whereas others prefer little involvement. The amount of involvement desired is often related to the severity of the illness and the number of stressors, as well as the client's energy, fear, understanding of the illness, and understanding of the intervention.

nursing strategies safely (e.g., turning an obese client in bed) or to reduce stress on a client (e.g., turning a person who has acute pain when moved). In addition, nurses should obtain assistance if they lack the knowledge or skills to implement a particular nursing activity. For example, nurses who are not familiar with a particular model of oxygen mask need assistance the first time they apply it.

Implementing Nursing Strategies
Nursing strategies help the client meet established health goals. When implementing these strategies, the nurse considers the following factors:

- The client's individuality
- The client's need for involvement
- Prevention of complications
- Preservation of the body's defenses
- Provision of comfort and support to the client
- Accurate and careful implementation of all nursing activities

Communicating Nursing Actions
Nursing actions are communicated in writing and often verbally, but only *after* they have been carried out. Nursing actions must not be recorded in advance

because the nurse may determine on reassessing the client that the action should not or cannot be implemented.

In some instances, it is important to record a nursing action immediately after it is implemented—particularly the administration of medications, treatments, and so on—because recorded data about a client must be up to date, accurate, and available to other nurses and health care professionals. Immediate recording helps safeguard the client, for example, from receiving a second dose of medication.

The nurse may record such nursing actions as providing mouth care every 2 hours or turning a client at the end of a shift; in the meantime, the nurse maintains a personal record of these interventions so that they can be accurately recorded later. The method of documentation is guided by the policies of the health care agency. See Chapter 3 for information on recording.

Nursing actions are often communicated verbally as well as in writing. When a client's health is changing rapidly, the charge nurse and/or the physician may want to be kept up to date with verbal reports. Verbal reports are given to another nurse or other health professionals. Nurses also give verbal reports at a change of shift and on a client's discharge to another unit or health agency. Some hospitals use tape recorders to facilitate change-of-shift reports.

Evaluating

To evaluate is to judge or to appraise. In the evaluation phase, the nurse identifies whether or to what degree the client's goals have been met. Evaluation is an exceedingly important aspect of the nursing process because conclusions drawn from the evaluation determine whether the nursing interventions can be terminated or must be reviewed or changed.

Evaluating is both a concurrent and a terminal process: It is concurrent in that the nurse normally evaluates during the implementing phase of the process. How is the client reacting to this nursing action? Is the reaction expected or unexpected? At this stage, the nurse may change a nursing action to help the client meet the planned goals. Evaluating is also a terminal process in that after completing the nursing activity, the nurse evaluates whether the client's goals have been met. Often the nurse uses the time frame stated in the outcome criteria to gauge the client's progress.

The evaluation process has four components: (a) Collecting data related to the identified criteria; (b) Comparing the data collected with the identified criteria and judging whether the goals have been attained; (c) Reexamining the client's care plan; and (d) Modifying the care plan.

Collecting Data

The nurse collects data, either by observation, direct communication, and purposeful listening or from reports of other health professionals, to determine whether the goals have been met. The data must relate to the specified criteria, and both objective and subjective data may be necessary. The nurse records the data concisely and accurately to facilitate the third part of the evaluating process. Recording aids include flowsheets and problem-oriented medical records in the SOAP format (discussed in Chapter 3).

Judging Goal Achievement

After collecting the data, the nurse determines whether

- The goal was met; i.e., the client responded as expected.

- The goal was partially met; i.e., a short-term goal was achieved, but the long-term goal was not; or, some, but not all, of the outcome criteria were attained.

- The goal was not at all met.

If goals are fully met, the nurse states "Problem resolved" on the care plan and dates and signs the entry.

Reexamining the Client's Care Plan

If problems are partially met or not met at all, the nurse determines whether the diagnosis may be incorrect, whether the goals and outcome criteria are unrealistic, and whether all or some of the nursing strategies need to be reevaluated and restructured.

Modifying the Care Plan

When it is determined that the care plan needs revising, the nurse follows five steps:

1. Change the data in the assessment column to reflect the more recent findings. Date and flag the new data in some way to indicate they are new. Follow agency practice: Some nurses use ink of a different color; others put a colored tab at the edge of the paper.

2. Revise the nursing diagnoses to reflect the new data. Also date the new nursing diagnoses.

3. Revise the client's priorities, goals, and outcome criteria to reflect the new nursing diagnoses. Date these also.

4. Establish new nursing strategies to correspond to the new nursing diagnoses. New nursing strategies may reflect the client's increased or decreased need for nursing care, scheduling changes, and rearrangement of nursing activities to group similar activities or to permit longer rest or activity periods for the client.

5. Change the outcome criteria to reflect the other changes in the plan. These changes should project the client's desired level of wellness. Delete criteria that apply to outdated nursing diagnoses.

CRITICAL THINKING CHALLENGE

Deborah Maples is a 78-year-old female who has been admitted to the nursing unit for evaluation of arthritis. She has severe deformity of her hands, which impairs her ability to grasp objects. She states she has difficulty dressing and preparing meals. She complains of joint stiffness, which interferes with her ability to move about, especially when awakening. She states that at times she experiences severe pain in her joints that is somewhat relieved by heat and aspirin. She is fearful of falling and breaking a bone. On observation you note that the distal and proximal joints of her fingers are deformed with reddened and inflamed nodules that are tender to palpation. What client-specific nursing diagnoses would you develop for Ms Maples? Support your diagnoses with data from the situation.

RELATED RESEARCH

Brunckhorst, L.; Placzek, L.; Payne, J.; McInerney, J.; and Parzuchowski, J. February 1989. Who's using nursing diagnoses? *American Journal of Nursing* 89:267–68.

Byrne-Coker, E.; Fradley, T.; Harris, J.; et al. July/September 1990. Implementing nursing diagnoses within the context of King's conceptual framework. *Nursing Diagnosis* 1:107–14.

Hardy, M., Maas, M., and Akins, J. 1989. The prevalence of nursing diagnoses among the elderly and long-term care residents: A descriptive study. In R. M. Carroll-Johnson, editor. *Classification of nursing diagnoses, Proceedings of the eighth national conference.* Philadelphia: J. B. Lippincott Co.

Johnson, J. E. October 1987. Selecting nursing activities for hospitalized clients. *Journal of Gerontological Nursing* 13:29–33, 44–45.

Lenihan, A. A. July/August 1988. Identification of self-care behaviors in the elderly: A nursing assessment tool. *Journal of Professional Nursing* 4:285–88.

REFERENCES

American Nurses' Association. 1980. *Nursing: A social policy statement.* ANA Pub. no. NP–63 35M 12/80. Kansas City, Mo.: ANA.

Baretich, D. M., and Anderson, L. B. September 1987. Diagnostics. Should we diagnose strengths? No—stick to the problem. *American Journal of Nursing* 87:1211–12.

Brider, P. May 1991. Who killed the nursing care plan? *American Journal of Nursing* 91:34–38.

Brigdon, P., and Todd, M. January 1990. In search of the perfect assessment. *Professional Nurse* 5:181–84.

Carpenito, L. J. 1987. *Nursing diagnosis: Application to clinical practice.* 3d ed. Philadelphia: J. B. Lippincott Co.

———. 1989. *Handbook of nursing diagnosis 1989–1990.* Philadelphia: J. B. Lippincott Co.

Carroll-Johnson, R. M. (editor). April/June 1990. Reflections on the ninth biennial conference. *Nursing Diagnosis* 1:49–50.

Christensen, P. J. 1986. Planning: Priorities, goals and objectives. In Griffith, J. W., and Christensen, P. J., editors. pp. 169–82. *Nursing process: Application of theories, frameworks, and models.* St. Louis: C. V. Mosby Co.

Derdiarian, A. March 1988. A valid profession needs valid diagnoses. *Nursing and Health Care* 9:136–40.

Dolan, M. B. November 1990. Why nurses and doctors should be partners in diagnosis. *Nursing* 20:41.

Flynn, J. B., and Heffron, P. B. 1988. *Nursing: From concept to practice.* 2d ed. San Mateo: Appleton & Lange.

Gordon, M. August 1976. Nursing diagnosis and the diagnostic process. *American Journal of Nursing.* 76:1298–300.

———. 1987a. *Manual of nursing diagnosis.* New York: McGraw Hill.

———. 1987b. *Nursing diagnosis: Process and application.* 2d ed. New York: McGraw-Hill.

Guzzetta, C. 1988. Nursing diagnosis. In McCann Flynn, J. B., and Burroughs Heffron, P. *Nursing: From concept to practice.* 2d ed. Norwalk, Conn: Appleton & Lange.

Guzzetta, C.; Bunton, S.; Prinkey, L.; Sherer, A.; and Seifert, P. 1989. *Clinical assessment tools for use with nursing diagnosis.* St. Louis: C. V. Mosby Co.

James, S., and Mott, S. 1988. *Child health nursing.* Menlo Park, Calif.: Addison-Wesley Publishing Co.

Kim, M. J.; McFarland, G. K.; and McLane, A. M. 1989. *Pocket guide to nursing diagnoses.* 3d ed. St. Louis: C. V. Mosby Co.

Leddy, S., and Pepper, J. M. 1989. *Conceptual bases of professional nursing.* 2d ed. Philadelphia: J. B. Lippincott Co.

Lederer, J. R.; Marculescu, G.; Mocnik, B., and Seaby, N. 1990. *Care planning pocket guide: A nursing diagnosis approach.* 3d ed. Redwood City, Calif.: Addison-Wesley Nursing.

Maas, M., and Hardy, M. March 1988. Focus: Nursing diagnosis. A challenge for the future. *Journal of Gerontological Nursing* 14:8–13.

MacLeod, E., and MacTavish, M. Spring 1988. Solving the nursing care plan dilemma: Nursing diagnosis makes the difference. *Journal of Nursing Staff Development* 4:70–73.

McElroy, D., and Herbelin, K. February 1988. Writing a better patient care plan. *Nursing 88* 18:50–51.

McHugh, M. K. April 1991. Does the nursing process reflect quality care? *Holistic Nursing Practice* 5:22–28.

Merry, J. A. January 1988. Take your assessment all the way down to the toes. *RN* 51:60–63.

Miers, L. J. January/March 1991. NANDA's definition of nursing diagnosis: A plea for conceptual clarity. *Nursing Diagnosis* 2:9–18.

Mills, W. C. January/March 1991. Nursing diagnosis: The importance of a definition. *Nursing Diagnosis* 2:3–8.

Niziolek, C., and Shaw, S. M. May/June 1991. Whose plan—whose care? *Journal of Professional Nursing* 7:145.

Paul, R. 1988a. *The critical student and person.* From The Eighth Annual and Sixth International Conference on Critical Thinking and Educational Reform. The Center for Critical Thinking and Moral Critique, Sonoma State University, Rohnert Park, CA 94928.

———. 1988b. *What, then, is critical thinking?* From The Eighth Annual and Sixth International Conference on Critical Thinking and Educational Reform. The Center for Critical Thinking and Moral Critique, Sonoma State University, Rohnert Park, CA 94928.

Popkess-Vawter, S. January/March 1991. Wellness nursing diagnoses: To be or not to be? *Nursing Diagnosis* 2:19–25.

Rundell, S. April 17–23, 1991. Care about care plans! *Nursing Times* 87:32.

Tribulski, J. December 1988. Nursing diagnosis: Waste of time or valued tool? *RN* 51:30–34.

Turkoski, B. May/June 1988. Nursing diagnosis in print, 1950–1985. *Nursing Outlook* 36:142–44.

Wilkinson, J. M. 1992. *Nursing process in action: A critical thinking approach.* Redwood City, Calif.: Addison-Wesley Nursing.

Yura, H., and Walsh, M. B. 1988. *The nursing process: Assessing, planning, implementing, evaluating.* 5th ed. Norwalk, Conn.: Appleton & Lange.

3

Recording and Reporting

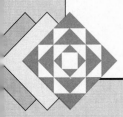

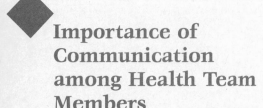

Importance of Communication among Health Team Members

Written and verbal communication among health team members is vital to the quality of client care. Generally, health team members communicate through discussions, reports, and records. A *discussion* is an informal oral consideration of a subject by two or more members of the health team, often leading to a decision. A *report* is an oral or written account by one member to others in the health team; for instance, nurses always report on clients at the end of a hospital work shift. A *record* is always written; it is a formal, legal documentation of a client's progress and treatment.

The client's record is protected legally as a private record of the client's care. Thus, access to the record is restricted to health workers involved in giving care to the client. Insurance companies, for example, have no legal right to demand access to medical records, even though they may be determining compensation to the client. However, a client who is making a claim for compensation may ask to have the medical history used as evidence. In this instance, the client must sign an authorization for review, copying, or release of information from the record. This form clearly indicates what information is to be released and to whom. In no instance may a nurse allow family members or any person other than a caregiver access to a client's record.

For purposes of education and research, most agencies allow student and graduate health professionals access to client records. The records are used in client conferences, clinics, rounds, and written papers or client studies. The student or graduate is bound by a strict ethical code to hold all information in confidence. Some agencies code medical records when they are filed, removing the names of clients. This allows records to be used without identifying individuals. When this is not the practice, it is the responsibility of the student or health care professional to protect the client's privacy by *not* using a name or any statements in the notations that identify the client. Many agencies also require documentation from the student or health professional wishing to use medical records of discharged clients. A permission note from the student's instructor confirms the person's status as a student at a particular school.

Purposes of Client Records

A client's **medical record**, or **chart**, is an account of the client's health history, current health status, treatment, and progress. It is a highly confidential, legal document by means of which physicians, nurses, social workers, and other health team members communicate about that client. When a client goes to a physician's office or enters a hospital, a record is usually started. Records are generally kept in folders, in binders, or on clipboards and are updated continually while clients attend the health care facility. When clients are discharged, their records are stored for future reference in the medical records department of the agency.

Although the forms of client records may vary considerably from agency to agency, nurses are universally required to make entries about clients' health, including, for example, all assessments and interventions. The process of making entries on client records is called **recording** or **charting**.

Client records are kept for a number of purposes: communication, legal documentation, research, statistics, education, audit, and planning client care.

Communication

The record serves as the vehicle by which different members of the health team communicate with each other. Although these members also communicate verbally, the record is an efficient and effective method of sharing information. It also allows health team members on different shifts to convey to one another meaningful data about the client.

Legal Documentation

The client's record is a legal document and is admissible in court as evidence. In some jurisdictions, however, the record is considered inadmissible as evidence when the client objects, because information the client gives to the physician is confidential. A record is usually considered the property of the agency, although there is increasing belief that the client has a right to the information in the record upon request. Legal decisions have recognized this right (Creighton 1986, p. 104).

Research

The information in a record can be a valuable source of data for research. The treatment plans for a number of clients with the same illness can yield information helpful in treating a particular client. A record made years earlier may also assist members of the health team with a current problem. A client's memory of an illness may provide limited data, but a record of that illness generally reveals additional and more accurate data.

Statistics
Statistical information from client records can help an agency anticipate and plan for people's future needs. For example, the number of births or kinds of illnesses can be obtained from records. Some statistics, such as records of births and deaths, are required by law. They are filed with a government agency and become a part of the local, national, and international statistics.

Education
Students in health disciplines often use client records as educational tools. A record can frequently provide a comprehensive view of the client, the illness, and the kinds of assistance given. In this context, records are used by nursing students, medical students, dietitians, and other health team members.

Audit
The client's record is used to monitor the care the client is receiving and the competence of the people giving that care. A nursing **audit**, for example, is a process in which the nursing interventions are monitored and measured against established standards. Often the audit is a retrospective audit of care that has already been given.

A nursing audit carried out by other nurses is sometimes referred to as a *peer review*. Many agencies have audit committees that monitor the practice of individual nurses. Audits are also carried out by outside groups for approval and accreditation purposes.

Planning Client Care
The entire health team uses data from the client's record to plan care for that client. A physician, for example, may order a specific antibiotic after establishing that the client's temperature is steadily rising and that laboratory tests reveal the presence of a certain microorganism. Nurses use data from the history they took on the client's admission to establish an individual nursing care plan. The social worker's data about the client's home environment can assist the nurse in developing an appropriate discharge teaching plan. Data from the physical therapist help the nurse to implement specific physical exercises for the client.

Types of Records

Source-Oriented Medical Records

In the traditional client record, or **source-oriented medical record**, each health care worker or department makes notations in a separate section or sections of the client's chart. For example, the admission department has an admission sheet; the physician has a doctor's order sheet, a doctor's history sheet, and progress notes; nurses use the nurse's notes; and other departments or personnel have their own records. In this type of record, information about a particular problem is distributed throughout the record. For example, for a client with left hemiplegia (paralysis of the left side of the body), data about this problem might be found in the doctor's history sheet, on the doctor's order sheet, in the nurse's notes, in the physical therapist's record, and in the social service record.

Source-oriented client records generally have five components: 1. Admission sheet; 2. Physician's order sheet; 3. Medical history sheet; 4. Nurse's notes; and 5. Special records and reports.

The *admission sheet* is a part of the record in most agencies. It generally contains demographic data about the client, such as name, address, date of birth, marital status, and admitting diagnosis.

The *physician's order sheet* is a written record of orders. The physician is expected to write the date of the order and sign each order (or sign for several orders written at once). Various agencies have different methods (e.g., using red "flags" on the front or extending out from the chart and/or placing the chart in a designated area of the nursing station) of indicating to the nurse or clerk that there is a new order. When the doctor phones in orders about a client, these are written on the physician's sheet by the recipient of the call and signed by that person, indicating a telephone order. Often the physician is expected to countersign the telephone order within 24 or 48 hours of the call. Before a nurse can accept a verbal order from a physician, however, agency policies and procedures must be checked. Usually, nursing students are not allowed to accept verbal orders.

The *medical history sheet* is a record of the client's health history, written by the physician. The physician may also use this sheet to record progress notes on the client and future plans, although most agencies have separate records for progress notes. At some facilities, the record of the client's admitting physical examination may also be on the history sheet, which is then usually called the *history and physical* sheet.

The *nurse's notes* are a record of the nursing assessments of the client, identified nursing diagnoses, interventions carried out, and evaluations of the effectiveness of the interventions. See the section Nurse's Notes, later in this chapter.

Special records and reports also become part of the client's permanent record. These may include consultations from medical specialists, roentgenographic reports, laboratory findings, reports of surgery, anesthesia records, physical therapy records, occupational therapy records, and social service records. In addition, special flowsheets are often used to record certain data about the client. These include graphic records for vital signs, fluid intake and output, and medications. See page 49, later in this chapter, for details.

Problem-Oriented Medical Records

In a **problem-oriented medical record** (**POMR** or **POR**), data about the client are recorded and arranged according to the client's problems, rather than according to the source of the information. The record integrates all data about a problem, whether gathered by physicians, nurses, or others involved in the client's care. Plans for each active problem are drawn up, and progress notes are recorded for each problem. Unlike the traditional record, which separates the medical data on a problem from the nursing data and other data into different sections of the record, the POR coordinates the care given by all health team members and focuses on clients and their health problems.

The POR has four basic components: 1. Defined database; 2. Problem list; 3. Initial list of orders or care plans; and 4. Progress notes.

Defined Database
The defined database consists of all information known about the client when the client first entered the health care agency. It includes the nursing assessment, the physician's history, and the physical health examination. To these are added social and family data from other sources, such as the social worker, and baseline laboratory and roentgenographic data. Most agencies use a standardized form to help team members obtain a complete database.

Problem List
The problem list (Figure 3–1) is carefully compiled once the databases have been collected and analyzed. Some problems are obvious on initial contact with the client; others are established as additional data are gathered. In this context, a *problem* is essentially a need that the client is unable to meet without assistance from members of the health care team.

The initial problem list is usually made either by the first health care worker to encounter the client or by the person who assumes primary responsibility for the client's care. Subsequent contributions are made by other members of the health team.

To be complete, the problem list should include socioeconomic, demographic, psychologic, and physiologic problems. The list is usually found at the front of the client's record. Each problem is labeled and numbered so that it can be identified throughout the record. This list has been likened to an index or table of contents. Problems are usually categorized as active or inactive.

A problem that is potential rather than actual is generally entered on the progress notes rather than the problem list. Only when a problem actually becomes active is it added to the list.

Signs, symptoms, and abnormal diagnostic measures, if used, are considered temporary labels until diagnosis is established. With the development of nursing diagnoses, many nurses are now using the NANDA taxonomy of nursing diagnoses to state nursing problems. Problem statements should refer to one problem only, be written unambiguously (so that no interpretation is required) in behavioral terms, and provide direction for client care. (See Chapter 2.)

When several problems have a common etiology or cause, nurses use two methods to relate the problems: sublisting and cross-referencing. A *sublist* is a group of all manifestations of a major problem that require separate management. Manifestations may be either behavioral or clinical indicators of the same problem. For example, consider the following segment of Figure 3–1:

No.	Client Problem
1	Several CVAs resulting in Rt hemiplegia and left-sided weakness
1A	Self-care deficit (hygiene, toileting, grooming, feeding)
1B	Impaired physical mobility
1C	Total incontinence
ID	Progressive dysphasia

The *cross referencing method* lists all problems separately, using consecutive numbers. A "Related to" column to the right of the "Client Problem" column lists the number of the major problem to which the manifestations are related. For example, Figure 3–1 could also include the following:

No.	Date Entered	Date Inactive	Client Problem	Related to
#1	Mar 9/92		Several CVAs resulting in Rt hemiplegia and left-sided weakness. Redefined Feb 7/94	
#1A	Mar 9/92		Self-care deficit (hygiene, toileting, grooming, feeding).	
#1B	Mar 9/92		Impaired physical mobility. Redefined Feb 7/94	
#1C	Mar 9/92		Total incontinence. Redefined Nov 17/93	
#1D	Mar 9/92		Progressive dysphasia.	
#2	Mar 9/92		Colonic constipation. Redefined Nov 10/92	
#3	Mar 9/92		History of depression.	
#4	Mar 9/92		Essential hypertension.	
#5	June 6/92	Nov 92	PRURITIS.	
#2	Nov 10/92		Potential for constipation.	
#1C	Nov 17/93		Nocturnal urinary incontinence.	
#1	Feb 7/94		Cerebral vascular disease (multiple CVAs) resulting in bilateral hemiplegia	
#1B	Feb 7/94		Needs major assistance to transfer/ unable to walk	

FIGURE 3–1 A client's problem list using the sublisting method to relate problems. Note that problems 1, 1B, 1C, and 2 were redefined on the dates indicated and listed subsequently. *Source* Courtesy of the Nursing Department, University Hospital—UBC site, Vancouver, British Columbia.

No.	Client Problem	Related to
1	Multiple CVAs resulting in Rt hemiplegia and left-sided weakness	
2	Self-care deficit (hygiene, toileting, grooming, feeding)	#1
3	Impaired physical mobility	#1
4	Total incontinence	#1
5	Progressive dysphasia	#1

Major problems can also be cross-referenced to other major problems:

No.	Client Problem	Related to
1	Cerebral vascular disease	#4
4	Essential hypertension	#1

Often, the nurse needs to "redefine" problems to reflect a change in the client's problem or to increase understanding of the problem. Redefining does *not* involve changing the stated nature of the problem; it involves changing the wording of the problem to reflect a change in its frequency or intensity, or increased knowledge. The problem retains the same number (e.g., see Figure 3–1):

No.	Client Problem
1C	Total incontinence Redefined Nov 17/93
1C	Nocturnal urinary incontinence

Initial List of Orders or Care Plans

The initial list of orders or care plans is developed with reference to the active problems. Care plans or orders are generated by the person who lists the problems. Physicians write physician's orders or medical care plans; nurses write nursing orders or nursing care plans. The written plan in the record is listed under each problem in the progress notes (discussed next) and is not isolated as a separate list of orders.

Progress Notes

Progress notes in the POMR are made by all members of the health team involved in a client's care: nurse, occupational therapist, dietitian, physician, social worker, and others. All members of the health team add progress notes on the same type of sheet. Progress notes are numbered to correspond to the problems on the problem list. See the section Types of Progress Records, later in this chapter.

Kardex and Nursing Care Plan

The **Kardex** is a widely used, concise method of organizing and recording data about a client, making information quickly accessible to all members of the health team. The system consists of a series of cards kept in a portable index file. The card for a particular client can be quickly turned up to reveal specific data. Often Kardex data are recorded in pencil so that they can be changed and kept up-to-date. The information on Kardexes may be organized into sections, for example:

- Pertinent information about the client.

- List of medications.

- List of daily treatments and procedures.

Although much of the information on the Kardex may be recorded by the nurse in charge or a delegate (e.g., the ward clerk), any nurse who cares for the client plays a key role in initiating the record and keeping the data current. When caring for the client, a nurse has the best opportunity to assess and reassess with the client the accuracy of the information and the effectiveness of treatment.

Computer Records

Initially, hospital computers were installed primarily in business offices for such applications as client billing, maintaining financial records, and long-term planning. However, increasing numbers of computers are being used in health care planning and delivery, as well as in laboratories and physicians' clinics. By the turn of the century, most nurses will use computers in many aspects of their practice. Already, "user-friendly" machines, often operated with a light-pen and simple keyboard or by touching the screen (Figure 3–2), are of great help to the nurse in assessing, planning, implementing, recording, and evaluating nursing care. Computer skills and knowledge will soon be expected and perhaps required in a great many nursing positions.

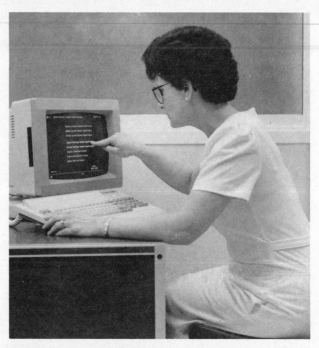

FIGURE 3–2 User-friendly computers with touch screens are used by many agencies.

By using computerized systems, nursing staffs create care plans easily, customize them for each client, type in additions as needed, evaluate and update information at any time, and retrieve data appropriate to a specific nursing diagnosis. Such systems can be programmed to provide work lists, as needed, directly from the computer. In this way, lists generated for treatments, procedures, and medications can always be kept up-to-date. Such an application eliminates the need for multiple flowsheets, since all of the same information is available both in the computer and on computer-printed update forms. To record nursing actions, the nurse either enters data directly into the computerized records or completes the computer-generated flowsheet in the client's chart.

A well-designed database system can make the entry and retrieval of information a relatively easy task for the nurses who use it. Figure 3–3 shows how a portion of a client's record might appear on the computer screen. The nurse enters the appropriate information into the form by typing it on the computer's keyboard. Changes can be made easily to update this record. Later, as the needs of the nurse dictate, information about a particular client, diagnosis, or physician can be recalled to the screen.

Specific ways in which an *automated client care plan* can facilitate the role of the nurse include the following:

- Entry of nursing assessments is simplified; e.g., the nurse can touch a computer screen display of possibilities.

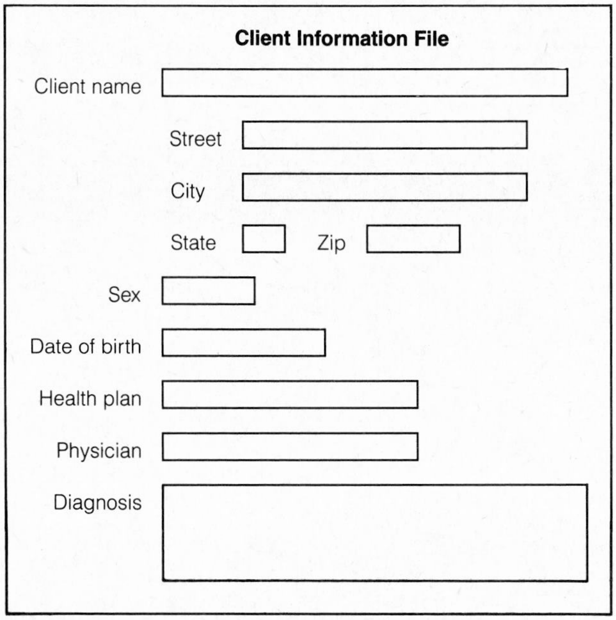

Client Information File

Client name

Street

City

State   Zip

Sex

Date of birth

Health plan

Physician

Diagnosis

FIGURE 3–3   Segment of a client's database.

- The nurse can order laboratory data by entering a request at a terminal in the nurse's station and retrieve results over the same terminal in a shorter time with less paperwork.

- The system facilitates complete and legible medication orders.

- The nursing implications of a doctor's order can be sent to the nurse. Client preparation needs for a particular test can be listed automatically in the client's nursing care plan.

- The use of a common format facilitates nursing diagnosis.

- Current information can be updated easily. Discontinued medication orders can be deleted easily, making all information timely, legible, and complete.

With access to a completely automated care plan, the nurse can prepare client discharge summaries that include information from the time of admission. These reports can include all current unresolved nursing diagnoses and the relevant interventions. Computer-generated reports can include relevant information for teaching the client, including instructions about the use of drugs, details of a required diet, activity restrictions, and the date of the next visit to the physician's office.

Nurses are bound by their professional ethics to maintain a client's privacy. This means that information about a client cannot be disseminated outside of the realm of the caregivers. The use of computer-based information systems to store client data has increased the risk of an accidental or intentional vio-

lation of a client's rights. Just as computers are becoming easier to use, they are becoming easier to abuse. Clients have a right to privacy and confidentiality even where computer-based information systems are used. Nurses should not give their signature codes to anyone or let anyone without an access code use the computer.

Types of Progress Records

Three kinds of progress notes are generally recognized; nurse's, or narrative, notes; flowsheets; and discharge notes, or referral summaries. These are used in both source-oriented and problem-oriented medical records.

Nurse's Notes

Nurse's notes record the client's progress descriptively. In some hospitals, because of the prospective payment system based on diagnostic related groups (DRGs), a note *must* be written every 24 hours. In general, the nurse's notes record the following kinds of information:

- Assessments of the client by various nursing personnel, e.g., pale or flushed skin color or dark or cloudy urine

- Independent nursing interventions, such as special skin care or health teaching, carried out on the nurse's initiative

- Dependent nursing interventions, such as medications or treatments ordered by a physician

- Evaluation of the effectiveness of each nursing intervention

- Measures carried out by the physician (e.g., shortening a postoperative drainage tube) that affect subsequent nursing measures

- Visits by members of the health team, such as a consulting physician, social worker, or chaplain

Nurse's notes and the manner of recording vary, depending on whether a source-oriented medical record or POR is used. See the section Formats for Writing Progress Notes, later in this chapter.

Flowsheets

When specific client variables, such as pulse, blood pressure, medications, and progress in learning a new skill, need to be recorded accurately, narrative notes are often too long. Instead, the **flowsheet**, a graphic record, is used as a quick way to reflect the client's condition. The time parameters for flowsheets can vary from minutes to months. In a hospital

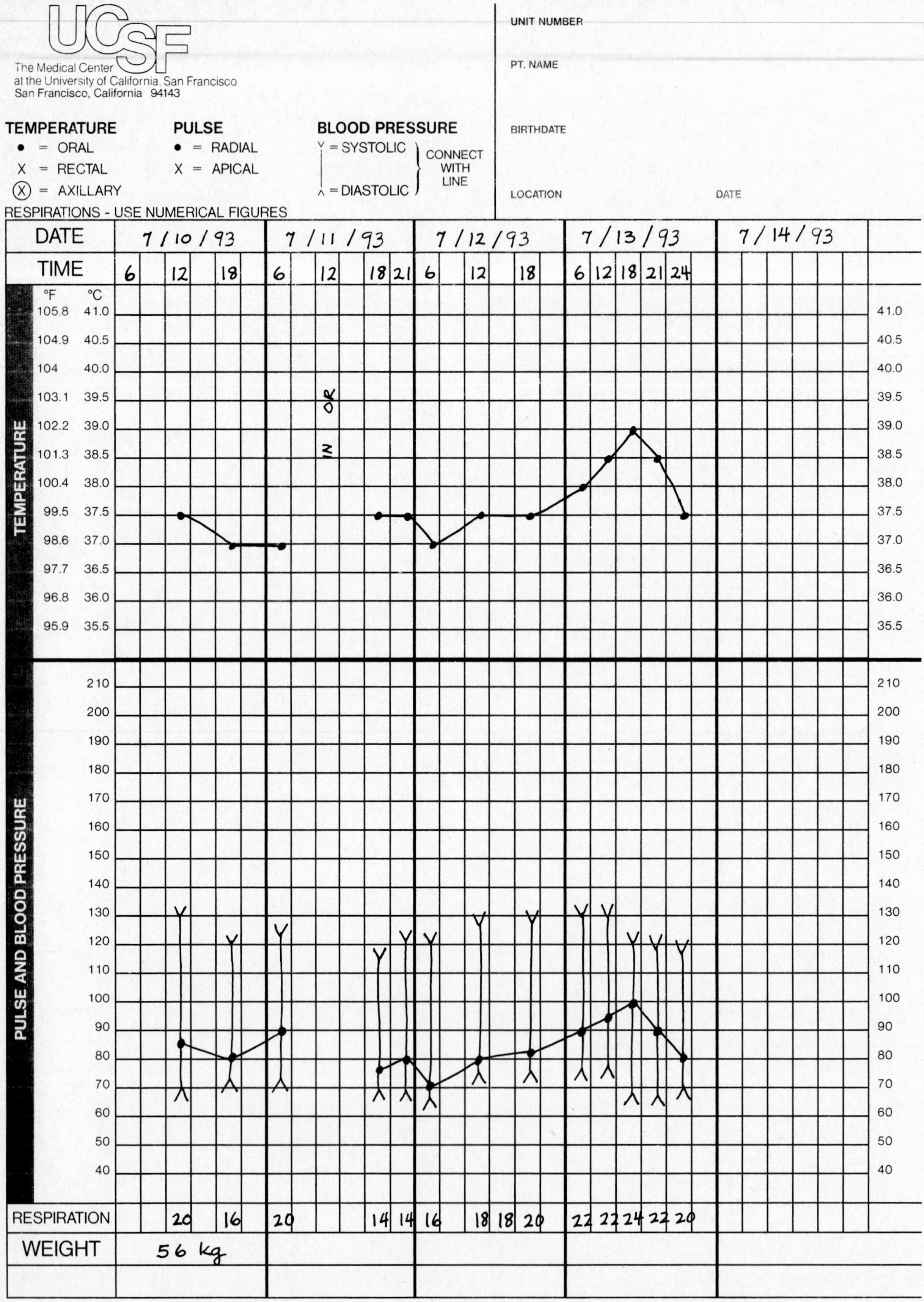

UCSF

The Medical Center
at the University of California, San Francisco
San Francisco, California 94143

UNIT NUMBER

PT. NAME

BIRTHDATE

LOCATION   DATE

TEMPERATURE	PULSE	BLOOD PRESSURE
● = ORAL	● = RADIAL	ᵛ = SYSTOLIC
X = RECTAL	X = APICAL	CONNECT WITH LINE
Ⓧ = AXILLARY		ᴧ = DIASTOLIC

RESPIRATIONS - USE NUMERICAL FIGURES

DATE	7 / 10 / 93	7 / 11 / 93	7 / 12 / 93	7 / 13 / 93	7 / 14 / 93
TIME	6 12 18	6 12 18 21	6 12 18	6 12 18 21 24	

TEMPERATURE scale:
°F / °C
105.8 / 41.0
104.9 / 40.5
104 / 40.0
103.1 / 39.5
102.2 / 39.0
101.3 / 38.5
100.4 / 38.0
99.5 / 37.5
98.6 / 37.0
97.7 / 36.5
96.8 / 36.0
95.9 / 35.5

(notation on chart: OR / IN)

PULSE AND BLOOD PRESSURE scale:
210 200 190 180 170 160 150 140 130 120 110 100 90 80 70 60 50 40

| RESPIRATION | 20 16 | 20 | 14 14 16 | 18 18 20 | 22 22 24 22 20 | |
| WEIGHT | 5 6 kg | | | | |

FIGURE 3–4 A clinical graph record. *Source* Courtesy of the Department of Nursing, The Medical Center at the University of California, San Francisco.

intensive care unit, a client's blood pressure may be monitored by the minute, whereas in an ambulatory clinic, a client's blood glucose level may be recorded once a month.

Flowsheets commonly used are the clinical record (also called the graphic chart or graphic observation record), the fluid intake and output record, the medication record, and daily nursing care records.

Clinical Record

The *clinical record* (Figure 3–4) indicates body temperature, pulse rate, respiratory rate, blood pressure readings, and weight. Some agencies also show special medications (such as dicumarol), central venous pressure (CVP), 24-hour fluid intake and output, bowel movement, glucose and acetone in the urine, and so on.

24-Hour Fluid Balance Record

Before making notations on a *24-hour fluid balance record* (Figure 3–5), the nurse records the amount of the client's fluid intake and output on a form kept at the client's bedside. The client and support persons should be taught to use this record. It documents intake and output for the duration of one shift only (8 or 12 hours). The totals for each shift are then recorded on the 24-hour fluid balance record. In the sample shown in Figure 3–5, the totals for each 8-hour shift (days, evenings, and nights) are recorded, and then the 24-hour totals are calculated. All routes of fluid intake and all routes of fluid loss or output must be measured and recorded (see Chapter 24).

Medication Record

Medication flow sheets usually include designated areas for the date of the medication order, the expiration date, the medication name and dose, the frequency of administration and route, and the nurse's signature. Some records also include a place to document the client's allergies.

Daily Nursing Care Record

In POMRs the daily nursing care is often recorded on a flowsheet See Figure 3–6 on page 52.

Discharge Note and Referral Summary

The nurse completes a discharge note and referral summary (Figure 3–7 on page 53) when the client is discharged and transferred to another institution or

EL CAMINO HOSPITAL

INTAKE AND OUTPUT RECORD

PATIENT LABEL

PATIENT NAME ____________________

PATIENT # ____________________

PHYSICIAN ____________________

INTAKE						OUTPUT					
TOTAL IV	INTRAVENOUS			TUBE FEED	ORAL	TIME	URINE	NG	EMESIS	BM	MISC.
					DATE:						
						6-2					
						2-10					
						10-6					
						24°					
					DATE:						
						6-2					
						2-10					
						10-6					
						24°					

FIGURE 3–5 A sample 24-hour fluid intake and output record. *Source* Courtesy of El Camino Hospital, Mountain View, California.

UBC HEALTH SCIENCES CENTRE HOSPITAL

NURSING CARE FLOW SHEET

Legend:
I — Independent
S — Supervised
(A) — Assisted

T — Total Care
NN — Refer to Nurses' Notes

	Date	10/2								
	Time Period	0730 1930								
	Initials of nurse assigned to patient	BKE								
EXCRE-TORY CT – Catheter CM – Condom I – Incontinent	Urine	CT 750ml								
	Stool (#)	1								
INGESTIVE N – Normal B – Blenderized MS – Mechanical Soft FF – Fluid CF – Clear Fluid P – Pureed NPO	Diet (T – Therapeutic)	NPO								
	Eating Poorly									
	Eating Well									
	Weight (kg.)									
PROTECTIVE HYGIENE	Sponge Bath	✓								
	Tub Bath									
	Shower									
	Mouth Care	q 6h								
SKIN INTEGRITY	Intact									
	Turns	q 2h								
SAFETY P – Posey W – Wrist M – Mitts LT – Lap Tray LR – Lap Restraint	Restraint	M								
	Bed Rails Up (x1) (x2)	x 2								
REPARATIVE MOBILITY AIDS C – Cane CR – Crutches W – Walker WC – Wheelchair	Bedrest (+D = Dangle)	✓ + D								
	B.R.P.									
	Chair									
	Walking									
REST DURING NIGHT	Slept Poorly	✓								
	Slept Well									
Catheter Care		x 1								
I. V. Intact		✓								

KN 109-1-85 Rev. 1

FIGURE 3–6 A nursing care flowsheet used in conjunction with the problem-oriented record. *Source* Courtesy of the Nursing Department, University Hospital—UBC site, Vancouver, British Columbia.

THE UNIVERSITY OF BRITISH COLUMBIA
HEALTH SCIENCES CENTRE
EXTENDED CARE UNIT

NURSING
SUMMARY

MISS ANN SMITH
Age 82 years BD: 1 Aug. 06
Admitted: March 5, 1993

DISCHARGE SUMMARY – June 10, 1993

Admitted March 5, 1993 from Victoria General Hospital in Victoria, B.C.

Problems

1. Multiple CVAs with bilateral hemiplegia resulting in need for assistance with ADLs and mobility/ transfers—needs 2 person assist to transfer, needs maximum assist with ADLs; dressing, washing and bathing done by staff. She is concerned about her appearance.

2. Continent of urine if routinely toileted during the day—occasionally incontinent of urine at night.

3. Prone to constipation—has soft formed BM q 2–3 days when toileted—needs occasional glycerine suppository and receives Metamucil 15cc daily.

4. Essential hypertension—B.P. ranges from 150/90 to 184/108—monitored 2 days weekly (Tues & Fri.). Receives Nadolol 80 mg daily

5. Has a history of depression—has become lethargic, withdrawn and weepy at times. Minimal response to antidepressant drugs (Amitriptyline 25 mg ghs - was D/C May 19/81). Involved in numerous social groups and 1-1 interaction—responded well to both. Family visited frequently and very supportive.

6. Diet—minced—has occasional difficulty swallowing and tongue mobility due to dysarthria.

7. Progressive dysphasia—speech slurred—difficult to understand; very slow to respond; appreciates help from staff.

Next of Kin

Ray Smith—phone 123-4567 (brother)

Sue Brown—phone 261-0941 (niece)

Medical regime

Metamucil 15 cc daily

Nadolol 80 mg daily

Brandy 30 cc q h.s. prn

Allergies

—elastoplast—suffered period of general pruritis but was unable to relate to specific drugs or food—spontaneously resolved.

Safety Needs

Vision—good/able to read clock on wall and small print

Hearing—able to hear normal conversation

Mechanical aids—side rails and support in chair with pillows and belt restraints

        —trunk balance poor

Orientation—well oriented to time, place, person despite deterioration in physical condition

Strengths and Resources

Miss Smith has a very supportive family. She is concerned about her appearance and feels comfortable letting staff know what her needs are.

Resident and family wish Miss Smith to move to LTC facility (X-E.C.U) in South Vancouver as it is much closer for family to visit—family visits 2-3 x weekly.

                                    J. Doe, R.N.

June 10, 1993
Date

J. Doe, RN
Signature

FIGURE 3–7 A nursing discharge summary. *Source* Courtesy of the Nursing Department, University Hospital—UBC site, Vancouver, British Columbia.

to a home setting where a visit by a public health nurse is required. Referral summaries usually include the following:

- Any active health problems
- Current medications
- Current treatments that are to be continued
- Eating and sleeping habits
- Self-care abilities
- Support networks
- Life-style patterns
- Religious preferences

This exchange of information ensures continuity of health care for the client.

Formats for Writing Progress Notes

Nurses use four methods to write progress notes: narrative charting, the SOAP format, focus charting, and charting by exception.

Narrative Charting

Narrative charting (Figure 3–8) is a description (narration) of information, and **chronologic charting** records data in sequence as time moves forward. Chronologic charting is commonly associated with source-oriented medical records. The forms used for the nurse's notes vary from place to place. Some agencies have separate columns for treatments, nursing observations, and comments. The major disadvantage of narrative charting is that it is difficult for a reader to find all the data about a specific problem without examining all of the recorded information. For this reason, certain information is documented on specific flow records (discussed earlier).

SOAP Format

SOAP is an acronym for subjective data, objective data, assessment, and planning. The SOAP format originated with the POMR but is used increasingly in many different types of records. The acronyms SOAPIE and SOAPIER refer to formats that add implementation, evaluation, and revision. Many agencies use only the SOAP format. A more recent format is the **APIE** (assessment, plan, implementation, and

	NURSING NOTES	

Date	Time	
2/13/93	1400	Passive R O M exercises provided for R arm and leg. Active assistive exercises to L arm and leg. Has scratch marks on L and R forearms. States, "My skin on my back and arms has been itchy for a week." Rash not evident. No previous history of pruritis. Is allergic to elastoplast but has not been in contact. Dr. J. Wong notified. —————————————— Tom Ritchie, R. N.
	1430	Applied calamine lotion to back and arms. Incontinent of urine. Is restless.———Tom Ritchie, R. N.

FIGURE 3–8 An example of narrative nurse's notes.

evaluation), which condenses the client data into fewer statements (Groah and Reed 1983, p. 1184). In APIE, the assessment combines the subjective and objective data with the nursing diagnosis; the plan combines the nursing actions with the expected outcomes; and the implementation and evaluation are the same. Figure 3–9 shows a nurse's progress notes in the SOAP, SOAPIER, and APIE formats.

Subjective data report what the client perceives and the way the client expresses it. *Objective data* include such measurements as vital signs, observations of health team members, laboratory and roentgenographic findings, and client responses to diagnostic and therapeutic measures (see Chapter 2, page 19).

In the *assessment stage,* the observer interprets and draws conclusions from the subjective and objective data. Again, all team members have made assessments, using the knowledge in their possession. At this point, the nurse writes a nursing diagnostic statement in accordance with the guidelines discussed in Chapter 2. The *plan* is a plan for action based on the above data. The initial plan is written by the person who enters the problem into the record. All subsequent plans, considered revisions, also are entered into the progress notes. Plans may include termination of certain activities if the problem is resolved, initiation of new actions if the problem is unchanged, and activities being done to resolve a particular problem.

Implementation, or *intervention,* is documentation of activities in the plan that were actually done for the client. These entries specify which plans were actually carried out. *Evaluation* is documentation of the client's response to the plan, stated in terms of client behavior (e.g., what the client did or said). The question asked at this stage is "Does the client's behavior indicate that the plan was unsuccessful in lessening or alleviating the identified problem?" *Revision,* or *reassessment,* refers to changes that must be made in the initial or original plan. From the evaluation notes and decision, the nurse may determine that the client's condition may have improved or deteriorated. New data may now be available.

SOAP Format

2/13/93 #5 Generalized pruritus

1400 S —"My skin is itchy on my back and arms and it's been like this for a week."

O —Skin appears clear—no rash or irritations noted. Marks where client has scratched noted on left and right forearms. Allergic to elastoplast but has not been in contact.

A —No previous history of pruritus. Altered comfort (pruritus): cause unknown

P —Instructed to not scratch skin
—Applied calamine lotion to back and arms at 1430 hrs.
—Cut fingernails
—Assess further to determine if recurrence associated with specific drugs or foods
—Refer to physician and pharmacist for assessment
Tom Ritchie, R.N.

SOAPIER Format

2/13/93 #5 Generalized pruritus

1400 S —"My skin is itchy on my back and arms and it's been like this for a week."

O —Skin appears clear—no rash or irritation noted. Marks where client has scratched noted on left and right forearms. Allergic to elastoplast but has not been in contact.
No previous history of pruritus.

A —Altered comfort

P —Instruct not to scratch skin
—Apply calamine lotion as necessary
—Cut nails to avoid scratches
—Assess further to determine if recurrence associated with specific drugs or foods
—Refer to physicians and pharmacist for assessment

I —Instructed not to scratch skin
Applied calamine lotion to back and arms at 1430 hrs.
Assisted to cut fingernails
Notified physician and pharmacist of problem

1600 E —States "I'm still itchy. That lotion didn't help."

R —Remove calamine lotion and apply hydrocortisone ungt. as ordered.
Tom Ritchie, R.N.

APIE Format

2/13/93 #5 Generalized pruritus

1400 A —Altered comfort; cause unknown. States "My skin is itchy on my back and arms and it's been like this for a week." Skin appears clear
—No rash or irritations noted. Marks where client has scratched noted on left and right forearms. Allergic to elastoplast but has not been in contact. No previous history of pruritus.

P —Instruct not to scratch skin
—Apply calamine lotion as necessary
—Cut nails to avoid scratches
—Assess further to determine if recurrence associated with specific drugs or foods
—Refer to doctor and pharmacist for assessment

I —Instructed not to scratch skin
Applied calamine lotion to back and arms at 1430 hrs.
Assisted to cut fingernails
Notified physician and pharmacist of problem

E —States "I'm still itchy. That lotion didn't help."
Tom Ritchie, R.N.

FIGURE 3–9 Examples of nursing progress notes using the SOAP, SOAPIER, and APIE formats.

Focus Charting

Focus charting uses key words that describe what is happening to the client. Unlike problem-oriented charting, focus charting is *not* limited to clinical problems. The term "focus" was developed to encourage nurses to view the client's status from a positive perspective rather than the negative one that "problem" suggested. The term "focus" has a broad definition. It can denote (Lampe 1985, p. 43)

- A current client concern or behavior (e.g., decreased fluid intake)

- A significant change in the client status or behavior (e.g., sudden loss of sensation in one extremity)

- A significant event in the client's therapy (e.g., return from surgery)

In summary, a nursing focus outlines the occasions for and the activities of the *nursing care* the client is receiving. A focus is *not* a medical diagnosis, but it sometimes describes what is happening to the client as a result of the medical diagnoses. For example, some of the foci for a client with a medical diagnosis of myocardial infarction may include admission information, chest pain, anxiety about medical diagnosis, and education about cardiac medications.

The focus charting system uses three columns in the nurse's notes:

Date/Hour	Focus	Notes
2/11/93 0900	Neuro status	DATA. Unresponsive to verbal stimuli; responsive to painful stimuli. Pupils pinpoint and equal. Dr. Ward visited. ACTION. Neuro assessment and vital signs q2h. RESPONSE. See flowsheets.

Compared with a narrative documentation, this list facilities (a) more rapid scanning to find the desired entries and (b) better communication. In the nurse's notes column, the SOAP format is replaced by DAR (data, action, response). *Data* include client behaviors, client status, and nursing observations. *Action* includes plans for action and immediate nursing actions. *Response* includes the client response to nursing and/or medical care. This system is therefore compatible with use of the nursing process: data equates with assessment, action with planning and implementation, and response with evaluation.

Focus charting relies on an adequate database or assessment forms and the use of flowsheets, such as vital signs records, neurologic checklists, intake and output flowsheets, and hygiene checklists. Agencies that use focus charting often provide a simple assessment checklist of key words that pertain to the special needs of clients in specific nursing units. For each key word, the checklist shows both normal and abnormal characteristics. Those applicable to the client can be circled. Normal characteristics may be underlined.

Charting by Exception

Charting by exception (CBE), developed in 1983 by staff nurses at St. Luke's Hospital in Milwaukee, is a documentation system in which only significant findings or exceptions to norms are recorded. CBE incorporates three key components (Burke and Murphy 1988, p. 7):

1. Unique *flowsheets* that highlight significant findings and define assessment parameters and findings. These include the nursing/physician order flowsheet, the graphic record, the client teaching record, and the discharge note.

2. Documentation by reference to agency-developed *Standards of Practice*, which eliminates much of the repetitive charting of routine care. An example of a standard related to hygiene patterns is "The nurse shall ensure that the client has a complete linen change every three days and as needed." Documentation of care according to these specified standards involves only a check mark in the routine standards box on the graphic record.

3. Bedside accessibility of documentation forms. In the CBE system, all flowsheets are kept at the client's bedside to allow immediate recording and to eliminate the need for transcribing data from the nurse's worksheet to the permanent record.

Guidelines about Recording

Because the client's record is a legal document and may be used to provide evidence in court, the nurse must consider many factors in recording. Health care personnel not only maintain the confidentiality of the client's record but also meet legal standards in the process of recording. Some of these factors are restricted access, use of ink, signature, errors, blanks, accuracy, appropriateness, completeness, use of standard terminology, and brevity.

For *each* notation, documentation of the *date* and *time* is essential not only for legal reasons but also for safe care. For example, the time at which a narcotic was administered to a client needs to be determined before the next one can safely be given. Time

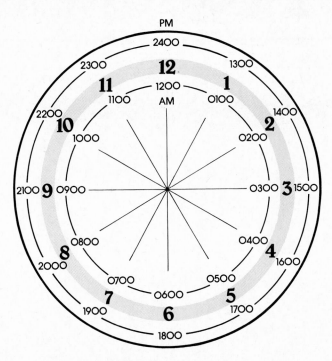

PM

FIGURE 3–10 The 24-hour clock.

can be recorded in the conventional manner (i.e., 9:00 A.M. or 3:20 P.M.) or according to the 24-hour clock, or military clock (Figure 3–10), which avoids confusion about whether a time was A.M. or P.M.

Use of Ink
All entries on the client's record are made in dark-colored ink so that the record is permanent and changes can be identified. Dark-colored ink is generally required because it reproduces well on microfilm and in duplication processes. Entries need to be legible. Hand printing or easily understood handwriting is permissible.

Signature
Each recording on the nursing notes is signed by the nurse making it. The signature includes the *name* and *title*, for example, "Susan J. Green, R.N." The following title abbreviations are often used, but nurses are advised to check the practice in their agencies.

RN   registered nurse
LVN   licensed vocational nurse
LPN   licensed practical nurse
NA   nursing assistant
NS   nursing student
SN   student nurse

Errors
When an error is made in charting, a line is drawn through it, and the word "error" is written above it, with the nurse's initials or name (depending on

agency policy). Errors should not be erased or blotted out, so that there is no doubt about the nursing care given or the charting error made.

SAMPLE RECORDING

Date: Dec 10/93	Time: 0100
error A.J.R.	
Pulse ~~100 beats/minute~~ 108 beats/minute	
——— Abby J. Roberts, NS	

If the nature of the error is not clear, many attorneys feel it is helpful and legally acceptable to indicate what the error was, in order to protect the client and the nurse. An example might be, "Charted for wrong client." The nurse must check the policy of the agency, however.

Blanks
If a blank appears in a notation, the nurse draws a line through the blank space so that no additional information can be recorded at any other time or by any other person, and signs the notation.

SAMPLE RECORDING

Date: Nov 7/93	Time: 0730
Urine appears cloudy, light brown with dark flecks. No odor. ——— Lin I. Ma, NS	
C/o burning pain in pubic region prior to voiding. ——— Lin I. Ma, NS	

Accuracy
It is essential that notations on records be accurate and correct. Accurate notations consist of facts or exact observations, rather than opinions or interpretations of an observation. It is more accurate, for example, to write that the client "refused medication" (fact) than to write that the client "was uncooperative" (opinion); to write that a client "was crying" (observation) is preferable to noting that the client "was depressed" (interpretation). Opinions or interpretations may or may not be accurate. Similarly, when a client expresses worry about the diagnosis or problem, this should be quoted directly on the record: "Stated: 'I'm worried about my leg.' " Nurses should record what they hear as well as what they observe.

Correct spelling is essential for accuracy in recording. If unsure how to spell a word, the nurse looks it up in a dictionary. Most agency units have one available for this purpose. Two decidedly different medications may have similar spellings—for example, digitoxin and digoxin.

Appropriateness
The nurse records only information that pertains to the client's health problems and care. Any other personal information that the client conveys to the nurse

is inappropriate for the record. If irrelevant information is recorded, it can be considered an invasion of the client's privacy and/or libelous. A client's disclosure that she was a prostitute and has smoked marijuana, for example, *would not* be recorded on the client's medical record unless it had a direct bearing on the client's health problem.

Completeness

Not all data a nurse obtains about a client can be recorded. However, the information that is recorded needs to be complete and helpful to the client, physicians, other nurses, and participating health care workers. Incomplete records could be used as evidence in court to show that the client did not receive the quality of care considered to meet generally accepted standards. For example, if a diabetic client's record does not indicate that insulin was given and that the urine was tested, the record could be used as evidence of negligence on the part of the nurse responsible for providing care. Of course, other examples and evidence are needed to support a finding of negligence by the nurse. However, the client's record can be used to indicate the kind of care given. A complete notation for a client who has vomited, for example, includes the time, the amount, the color, the odor of the vomit, and any other data about the client (e.g., pain).

SAMPLE RECORDING

Date: Aug 12/93	Time: 1410

Vomited approx 500 ml of black liquid with foul fecal odor. C/o cramplike pain in epigastric region immediately prior to vomiting.
— Nancy R. Long, NS

The following guide may assist nurses in selecting essential and complete information to record about clients. Note that the emphasis is on facts that denote a change in the client's health status or behavior that indicate a deviation from what is usually expected. Essential information for recording includes the following:

1. Any behavior changes, for example
 • Indications of strong emotions, such as anxiety or fear
 • Marked changes in mood
 • A change in level of consciousness, such as stupor
 • Regression in relationships with family or friends

2. Any changes in physical function, such as
 • Loss of balance
 • Loss of strength
 • Difficulty hearing or seeing

3. Any physical sign or symptom that
 • Is severe, such as severe pain
 • Tends to recur or persist
 • Is not normal, such as elevated body temperature
 • Gets worse, such as gradual weight loss
 • Indicates a complication, such as inability to void following surgery
 • Is not relieved by prescribed measures, such as continued failure to defecate or to sleep
 • Indicates faulty health habits, such as lice on the scalp
 • Is a known danger signal, such as a lump in the breast

4. Any nursing interventions provided, such as
 • Medications administered
 • Therapies
 • Activities of daily living, if agency policy dictates
 • Teaching clients self-care

5. Visits by a physician or other members of the health team

Use of Standard Terminology

The nurse needs to use only commonly accepted *abbreviations, symbols,* and *terms* that are specified by the agency. Then, if the record is used in court as evidence, other professionals responsible for interpreting the data can do so correctly. Many abbreviations are standard and used universally; others are used only in certain geographic areas. Some agencies supply a list of the abbreviations they accept. When in doubt about whether to use an abbreviation, the nurse writes the term out in full, until certain about the abbreviation. Table 3–1 lists some commonly used abbreviations (except those used for medications, which are described in Chapter 35). Table 3–2 contains commonly accepted symbols.

Medical terminology is generally made up of root words, prefixes, and suffixes. A root word may be derived from Latin or Greek. A prefix is a sequence of letters that comes before the word and often describes a variation of the normal. A suffix is a sequence of letters that occurs at the end of the word; it often describes a condition of or act performed on the root word. Root words, suffixes, and prefixes are provided in Appendix A. Additional terms are given in the glossary at the end of the book.

Brevity

Recordings need to be brief as well as complete, to save time in communication. The client's name and word *client* are omitted. For example, the nurse may write "Perspiring profusely. Respirations shallow, wet, 28/min." Each thought or sentence is terminated with a period.

TABLE 3–1 COMMONLY USED ABBREVIATIONS

Abbreviation	Term	Abbreviation	Term
abd	abdomen	neg	negative
ABO	the main blood group system	nil (ō)	none
ac	before meals (*ante cibum*)	no. (#)	number
ADL	activities of daily living	NPO (NBM)	nothing by mouth (*per ora*)
ad lib	as desired (*ad libitum*)	NS (N/S)	normal saline
adm	admitted or admission	O₂	oxygen
A.M.	morning (*ante meridiem*)	od	daily (*omni die*)
amb	ambulatory	OD	right eye (*oculus dexter*); overdose
amt	amount	OOB	out of bed
approx	approximately (about)	os	mouth
bid	twice daily (*bis in die*)	OS	left eye (*oculus sinister*)
BM (bm)	bowel movement	pc	after meals (*post cibum*)
BP	blood pressure	PE (PX)	physical examination
BR	bed rest	per	by or through
BRP	bathroom privileges	P.M.	afternoon (*post meridiem*)
c̄ (C)	with	po	by mouth (*per os*)
C	Celsius (centigrade)	postop	postoperative(ly)
CBC	complete blood count	preop	preoperative(ly)
CBR	complete bed rest	prep	preparation
Cl	client	prn	when necessary (*pro re nata*)
c/o	complains of	pt	patient
DAT	diet as tolerated	q	every (*quaque*)
dc (disc)	discontinue	qd	every day (*quaque die*)
drsg	dressing	qh (q1h)	every hour (*quaque hora*)
Dx	diagnosis	q2h, q3h, and so on	every two hours, three hours, and so on
ECG (EKG)	electrocardiogram	qhs	every night at bedtime (*quaque hora somni*)
F	Fahrenheit	qid	four times a day (*quater in die*)
fld	fluid	req	requisition
GI	gastrointestinal	Rt (rt, R)	right
GP	general practitioner	S (s̄)	without (*sine*)
gtt	drops (*guttae*)	SI	seriously ill
h (hr)	hour (*hora*)	spec	specimen
H₂O	water	stat	at once, immediately (*statim*)
hs	at bedtime (*hora somni*)	tid	three times a day (*ter in die*)
I & O	intake and output	TL	team leader
IV	intravenous	TLC	tender loving care
Lab	laboratory	TPR	temperature, pulse, respirations
liq	liquid	Tr.	tincture
LMP	last menstrual period	VO	verbal order
LT (L)	left	VS (vs)	vital signs
meds	medications	WNL	within normal limits
ml (mL)	milliliter	wt	weight
mod	moderate		

TABLE 3–2 COMMONLY USED SYMBOLS

Symbol	Term	Symbol	Number
>	greater than	ō	0
<	less than	s̄s̄	½
=	equal to	ī	1
↑	increased	īī	2
↓	decreased	īīī	3
♀	female	īv̄	4
♂	male	v̄	5
°	degree	v̄ī	6
#	number; fracture	v̄īī	7
ℨ	dram	v̄īīī	8
℥	ounce	īx̄	9
×	times	x̄	10
@	at		

Reporting

Reports can be either oral or written. The purpose of reporting, in general, is to communicate specific information to a person or group of people. A report should be concise. A good report includes pertinent information, but no extraneous detail. Two common types of reports are the change-of-shift report and the incident report.

A *change-of-shift report* is an oral report usually given by the on-duty charge nurse to all nursing personnel coming on duty. Variations occur, however. In units where primary nursing is employed, the report may be given from one RN to another; in units where team nursing is practiced, the report may be given from one team leader to another. Change-of-shift reports may be given either in a face-to-face exchange or by audiotape recording. The face-to-face report allows the listener to ask questions during the report,

---

Information to Include in an Incident Report

- Identify the client by name, initials, and hospital or identification number.
- Give the date, time, and place of the incident.
- Describe the facts of the incident. Avoid any conclusions or blame. Describe the incident as you saw it even if your impressions differ from those of others.
- Identify all witnesses to the incident.
- Identify any equipment by number and any medication by name and number.
- Document any circumstance surrounding the incident, e.g., another client (Mrs. Losas) was experiencing cardiac arrest.

Guidelines for Giving Reports About Clients

- Follow a particular order when reporting about a series of clients. For example, follow room numbers in a hospital or times of appointments in a community clinic.
- Identify the client by name, room number, and bed designation. For example, Ms Jessie Jones, 702, Bed D. This enables the listeners, especially float nurses or those returning from days off or vacation, to relate subsequent information immediately to this client's case.
- Depending on the type of unit, provide the reason for admission, that is, the client's medical diagnosis or original complaint. This information may not be necessary in long-term geriatric units or newborn nurseries; in acute-care settings, however, it is often necessary because of multiple tests, consultations, and transfers.
- Include diagnostic tests and/or results and other therapies performed in the past 24 hours, such as blood transfusions, surgery, initiation of intravenous therapy, narcotics administered, blood gas levels, and group therapy data.
- Note any significant changes in the client's condition. Oncoming nurses must know about changes for the worse to monitor the client's condition appropriately. Significant improvements toward goal attainment

should also be noted so that the nurse can provide positive feedback to the client.
- When reporting about changes, present the pertinent information in this order: assessment, nursing diagnoses (if appropriate), planning, intervention, and evaluation. For example, "Mr. Ronald Oakes said he had an aching pain in his left calf at 1400 hours. Inspection revealed no other signs. Calf pain is related to altered blood circulation. Rest and elevation of his legs on a footstool for 30 minutes provided relief."
- Provide exact information, such as "Ms Jessie Jones received Demerol 100 mg intramuscularly at 2000 hours (8 P.M.)," not "Ms Jessie Jones received some Demerol during the evening."
- Do not include unremarkable measurements, such as normal temperature, pulse, and blood pressure, unless a desired change is involved. For example, a normal body temperature for a client who has had an elevated temperature should be reported.
- Report the client's emotional responses that need attention before other interventions can be implemented. For example, a client who has just learned his biopsy results revealed malignancy and who is now scheduled for a laryngectomy needs time to discuss his feelings before the nurse commences preoperative teaching.

Sources: G. Hesse, A better shift report means better nursing care, *Nursing 83,* February 1983, 13:65 (Canadian edition 13:17); C. E. Smith, Upgrade your shift reports with the three R's, *Nursing 86,* February 1986, 16:63–64.

although if given to all on-coming nurses it can be time-consuming. On-coming nurses are required, for example, to listen to the report on all clients, including many not under their care. The tape-recorded report is often briefer and less time-consuming. Some agencies or units combine these methods of giving the change-of-shift report, following the taped report or a brief report to all on-coming staff with a more extensive individual report given by the nurse going off duty to the nurse who will be providing client care during the coming shift. This more detailed report is often given at the bedside, and clients as well as nurses may participate in the exchange of information.

The *incident report* is an agency record of an accident or incident. This report is used to make all the facts about an accident available to agency personnel, to contribute to statistical data about accidents or incidents, and to help health personnel prevent future accidents. All accidents are usually reported on incident forms. Some agencies also report other inci-

dents, e.g., the occurrence of client infection or the loss of personal effects. The box at the top of page 60 lists the information to be included in an incident report. The report should be completed as soon as possible, always within 24 hours of the incident.

When an accident occurs, the nurse should first assess the client and intervene to prevent injury. If a client is injured, nurses must take steps to protect the client, themselves, and their employer. Most agencies have policies regarding accidents. It is important to follow these policies and not to assume one is negligent. Although this may be the case, accidents do happen even when every precaution has been taken to prevent them.

The guidelines shown in the box at the bottom of page 60 can help nurses prepare and present reports about clients. Nursing students may want to practice giving reports in clinical postcare conferences or by taping themselves giving a simulated report of the current status of their assigned clients.

CRITICAL THINKING CHALLENGE

On several occasions the head nurse tells you she has difficulty reading your handwritten charting and asks you to correct the problem. What potential problems may result from illegible handwriting? What actions can you take to correct the problem?

RELATED RESEARCH

Edelstein, J. November 1990. A study of nursing documentation. *Nursing Management* 21:40–43.

Lucatorto, M.; Petras, D. M.; Drew, L. A.; et al. March 1991. Documentation: A focus for cost savings. *Journal of Nursing Administration* 21:32–36.

Richard, J. A. Spring 1988. Congruence between intershift report and patients' actual conditions. *Image: Journal of Nursing Scholarship* 20:4–6.

REFERENCES

Afferbach, D. January 1986. A flow sheet that saves time and trouble. *RN* 49:42–44.

Bailey-Allen, A. M. January/February 1986. Avoid legal pitfalls in charting. *Orthopedic Nursing* 5:21–23.
———. April 1988. More about charting with a jury in mind. *Nursing 88* 18:50–58.

Blount, M.; Green, S. S.; Hamory, A.; Kinney, A. B.; and Sanborn, C. W. September 1978. Documenting with the problem-oriented record system. *American Journal of Nursing* 78:1539–42.

Buckley-Womack, C., and Gidney, B. October 1987. A new dimension in documentation: The PIE method. *Journal of Neuroscience Nursing* 19:256–60.

Burke, L. J., and Murphy, J. 1988. *Charting by exception: A cost-effective, quality approach.* New York: John Wiley and Sons.

Creighton, H. 1986. *Law every nurse should know.* 5th ed. Philadelphia: W. B. Saunders Co.

Cushing, M. December 1982. The legal side: Gaps in documentation. *American Journal of Nursing* 82:1899–1900.

Exstrom, S., and Gollner, M. L. October 1990. There is more than one use of SOAP. *Nursing Management* 21:12.

Fairless, P. R. September 1986. Nine ways a computer can make your work easier. *Nursing 86* 16:54–56.

Fiesta, J. August 1991. If it wasn't charted, it was done! *Nursing Management* 22:17.

Fox, L., and Woods, P. January 1991. Nursing process—evaluation of documentation. *Nursing Management* 22:57–58.

Groah, L., and Reed, E. A. May 1983. Your responsibility in documenting care. *Association of Operating Room Nurses Journal* 37:1174, 1176–77, 1180–85.

Gruber, M., Gruber, J. M. Spring 1990. Nursing malpractice: The importance of documentation, or saved by the pen! *Gastroenterological Nursing* 12:255–59.

Gryfinski, J. J., and Lampe, S. S. Winter 1990. Implementing focus charting: Process and critique. *Clinical Nurse Specialist* 4:201–5.

Harkins, B. December 1986. Keep your eye on the patient's problems. *RN* 49:30–32.

Hesse, G. February 1983. A better shift report means better nursing care. *Nursing 83* 13:65. Canadian edition 13:17.

Killian, W. H. March 1991. Keep medical records accurate, timely. *American Nurse* 23:22–23.

Kilpack, V., and Dobson-Brassard, S. October 1987. Intershift report: Oral communication using the nursing process. *Journal of Neuroscience Nursing* 19:266–70.

Laing, M. December 1981. Flow sheets: Meeting the charting challenge. *The Canadian Nurse* 77:40–42.

Lampe, S. S. 1984. *Focus charting.* Minneapolis, Minn.: Creative Nursing Management.

———. July 1985. Focus charting: Streamlining documentation. *Nursing Management* 16:43–46.

Miller, P., and Pastorino, C. November 1990. Daily nursing documentation can be quick and thorough. *Nursing Management* 21:47–49.

Murphy, J., Burke, L. J. May 1990. Charting by exception: A more efficient way to document. *Nursing 90* 20:65, 68–69.

Neubauer, M. P. November 1990. Careful charting—your best defense. *RN* 53:77–78.

Philpott, M. August 1986. Twenty rules for good charting. *Nursing 86* 10:63.

Rich, P. L. July 1985. With this flow sheet less is more. *Nursing 85* 15:25–29.

Simpson, K. June 1985. Using Kardex cards to improve the quality of patient care. *The Canadian Nurse* 81:37–40.

Smith, C. E. February 1986. Upgrade your shift reports with the three R's. *Nursing 86* 16:63–64.

Svanda, C. December 1986. Key words show what's important . . . focus charting. *RN* 49:32–33.

Weed, L. L. 1971. *Medical records, medical education and patient care: The problem-oriented record as a basic tool.* Cleveland: Case Western Reserve University Press.

4

Helping and Communicating

OBJECTIVES

- Describe essential aspects of communication and the communication process

- Explain four elements of the communication process

- Identify ways in which selected factors influence the communication process

- Differentiate verbal from nonverbal communication

- Describe effective and ineffective methods nurses use to communicate with clients

CONTENTS

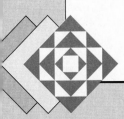

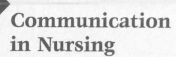

Communication in Nursing

The term **communication** has various meanings, depending on the context in which it is used. To some, communication is the interchange of information between two or more people—in other words, the exchange of ideas or thoughts. This kind of communication uses methods such as talking and listening or writing and reading. However, painting, dancing, and storytelling are also methods of communication. People convey thoughts to others not only by spoken or written words but also by gestures or body actions.

Communication may have a more personal connotation than the interchange of ideas or thoughts. It can be a transmission of feelings. In this context, communication often is synonymous with relating. Frequently one member of a couple comments that the other is not communicating. Some teenagers complain about a generation gap—being unable to communicate with understanding or feeling to a parent or authority figure. Sometimes a nurse is said to be efficient but lacking in something called *bedside manner*. For the purpose of this text, *communication* is any means of exchanging information or feelings between two or more people. It is a basic component of human relationships.

The intent of any communication is to elicit a response. Thus, communication is a process. It includes all the techniques by which an individual affects another. It has two main purposes: to influence others and to obtain information. Communication can be described as helpful or unhelpful. The former encourages a sharing of information, thoughts, or feelings between two or more people. The latter hinders or blocks the transfer of information and feelings.

Communication is a significant aspect of nursing practice. Nurses who communicate effectively are better able to initiate change that promotes health, establish a trusting relationship with a client and support persons, and prevent legal problems associated with nursing practice. Effective communication is essential for the establishment of the nurse-client relationship.

Nursing practice involves three kinds of communication: social, structured, and therapeutic. **Social communication** is unplanned communication, often carried out in an informal setting and usually at a leisurely pace. It is usually satisfying to all parties participating. **Structured communication** refers to definite planned content (Sundeen, Stuart, Rankin, and Cohen 1989, p. 129). An example of struc-

tured communication is teaching a client to give an injection or discussing postoperative care with a person anticipating surgery. **Therapeutic communication** is a process that helps "overcome temporary stress, to get along with other people, to adjust to the unalterable, and to overcome psychological blocks which stand in the way of self-realization" (Ruesch 1961, p. 7). Nurses use therapeutic communication in many settings and in many circumstances, for example, to support the anxious preoperative client or to help the person who has cancer accept and cope with this diagnosis.

Nurse-client relationships are referred to by some as *interpersonal relationships*, by others as *therapeutic relationships* and by still others as *helping relationships*. Helping is a growth-facilitating process in which one person assists another to solve problems and to face crises in the direction the assisted person chooses (Brammer 1988, p. 5). Several terms are used to describe the persons involved in a helping relationship: *helper* and *helpee*; *giver* and *receiver*; and *counselor* and *client*. For purposes of consistency, in this text the term *nurse* or *helper* refers to the person who gives the help, and the term *client* denotes the person receiving the help. However, we recognize that various people in all walks of life act as helpers and receivers of help.

In many nurse practice settings, such as critical care, where the nurse has time to only attend to physiologic variables that are life-threatening, interpersonal relationships may be difficult to establish. In these situations the nurse and client focus on goal-oriented interactions, i.e., they mutually identify goals and the means to achieve them (King 1981, p. 61).

Modes of Communication

Communication is generally carried out in two different modes: verbal and nonverbal. **Verbal communication** uses the spoken or written word; **nonverbal communication** uses other forms, such as gestures or facial expressions. Although both kinds of communication occur concurrently, the majority of communication (some say 80% to 90%) is nonverbal.

Verbal Communication

Verbal communication is largely conscious, because people choose the words they use. The words vary among individuals according to culture, socioeconomic background, age, and education. As a result, ideas are exchanged in countless ways. An abundance of words can be used to form messages. In addition, speech can convey a wide variety of feelings. The intonation of the voice can express animation, enthusiasm, sadness, annoyance, or amusement. The number of different intonations heard when people say, "Hello," or "Good morning," illustrates the variety that is possible. The pacing or rhythm of a person's communication is another variable. Monotonous rhythms or very rapid rhythms can be products of lack of energy or interest, anxiety, or fear.

When choosing words to say or to write, nurses need to consider several criteria of effective communication. These include (a) simplicity, (b) clarity, (c) timing and relevance, (d) adaptability, and (e) credibility.

Simplicity
Simplicity includes the use of commonly understood words, brevity, and completeness. Many people have a tendency to overcommunicate. Their messages are wordy, contain too many extraneous explanations, or use words that are highly academic, technical, or slangy. In the world of nursing, many complex technical terms become natural to nurses. However, these terms can often be misunderstood even by informed laypeople. Nurses need to learn to select simple words intentionally even though effort is required to do so. For example, instead of saying to a client, "The nurse will be catheterizing you tomorrow for a urine specimen," it is better to say, "Tomorrow we need a sample of urine, and we will collect it by putting a tube into your bladder." The latter statement is likely to produce a response from the client about why it is needed and whether it will hurt or be uncomfortable. The former statement may simply make the client wonder what the nurse means.

Another aspect of simplicity is brevity. Most people have heard others give lengthy explanations of events, to which they respond, "Get to the point." Using short sentences and avoiding unnecessary material are particularly important in writing, e.g., nurse's notes (see Chapter 3). Reports or memos need to be concise and should be condensed into a single paragraph or page, if possible.

The opposite of overcommunicating is undercommunicating. For example, initials or abbreviations such as b.i.d. (twice a day) or ICU (intensive care unit) should be avoided unless the nurse is certain that the client understands them. At the first use, terms should be expressed in full; later they can be shortened when the nurse is sure that the client or reader knows the meanings.

Clarity
Clarity means saying exactly what is meant. It also is aligned with meaning what is said. The speaker achieves the latter by matching behavior (nonverbal communication) with the words that are spoken.

When the words and the behavior blend together or are unified, the communication is regarded as consistent or congruent.

Clarity ensures that people know the what, how, why (if necessary), when, who, and where of any specific event. Without knowing these facts, people are left to make assumptions. To ensure clarity in communication, the nurse also needs to speak slowly and enunciate words well. It may be helpful to repeat the message and to reduce distractions such as surrounding noises. Some common pitfalls that can produce unclear communications are ambiguous statements, generalizations, and opinions.

Timing and Relevance
No matter how clearly or simply words are stated or written, the timing needs to be appropriate to ensure that words are heard. Keeping communication relevant involves being sensitive to the client's needs and concerns. For example, if a female client is enmeshed in fear of cancer, she may not hear the nurse's explanations about the expected procedures before and after her gallbladder surgery. In this situation it is better for the nurse first to encourage her to express her concerns, and to then deal with those concerns. The necessary explanations can be provided at another time. Other pitfalls include asking several questions at once and asking a question without waiting for an answer before making another comment.

Adaptability
The speaker needs to alter messages in accordance with behavioral cues from the listener. This adjustment is referred to as *adaptability*. Moods and behavior may change minute by minute, hour by hour, or from day to day. In this sense, nurses need to avoid routine or automatic speech, individualizing and carefully considering what they say and how they say it. This requires astute assessment and sensitivity. For example, a nurse who usually smiles, appears cheerful, and greets her client every afternoon with an enthusiastic "Hi, Mr. Brown!" notices that he is not smiling and appears distressed when she appears. In response to the client's cues, the nurse adapts her usual greeting and tones down her cheery manner. She may say "Hi" in a much softer and caring manner and express concern in her facial expression while she moves toward him.

Credibility
Credibility means worthiness of belief, trustworthiness, reliability. Credibility may be the most important criterion of effective communication. A nurse's credibility to clients depends in part on the opinion of others. If other health professionals and clients regard the nurse as trustworthy, then the client also is likely to.

To become credible, the nurse needs to be knowledgeable about the subject matter being discussed and to have accurate information. Nurses also need to convey confidence and certainty in what they are saying. This is often referred to as *positivism*. People tend to perceive confidence, which is dynamic and emphatic, as more credible than hesitance or uncertainty, which is less forceful and less active. However, the nurse should not sound overconfident or authoritarian. To avoid this, the nurse states messages in a constructive way and focuses on being helpful to clients.

Nurses develop reliability by being consistent, dependable, and honest. People value the nurse who acknowledges limitations and can say, "I don't know the answer to that, but I'll find someone who does."

Nonverbal Communication

Nonverbal communication is sometimes called *body language*. It includes gestures, body movements, and physical appearance, including adornment. Nonverbal communication often tells others more about what a person is feeling than actually saying, because nonverbal behavior is controlled less consciously than verbal behavior. Nonverbal communication either reinforces or contradicts the speaker's words. For example, a nurse may say to a client, "I'd be happy to sit here and talk to you for a while," yet if she glances nervously at her watch every few seconds, the actions contradict the verbal message. The client is more likely to believe the nonverbal behavior, which conveys "I am very busy."

To observe nonverbal behavior efficiently requires a systematic approach. As part of an initial assessment, the nurse observes the person's overall physical appearance, manner of dress, (including adornments), posture, and gait, and then assesses specific parts of the body, such as the face and the hands, for nonverbal cues.

Posture and Gait

The ways people walk and carry themselves are often reliable indicators of self-concept, current mood, and health. Erect posture and an active, purposeful stride suggest a feeling of well-being. Slouched posture and a slow, shuffling gait suggest dejection or physical discomfort. Tense posture and a rapid, determined gait suggest anxiety or anger. Likewise, the sitting or lying postures of clients can communicate feelings.

Facial Expression

No part of the body is as expressive as the face (Figure 4–1). Facial expressions can convey feelings of joy, sadness, fear, surprise, anger, and disgust. The muscles around the eyes and the mouth are particularly expressive. Although actors learn to control these

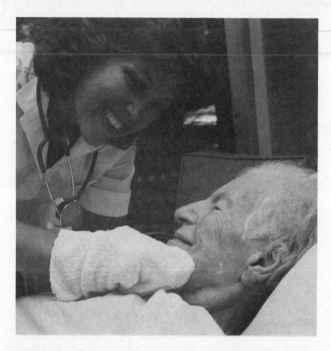

FIGURE 4–1 The nurse's facial expression communicates warmth and caring.

muscles to convey emotions to audiences, most other people generally do not consciously control their facial expressions.

Hand Movements and Gestures

Like faces, hands are expressive. They can communicate feelings at any given moment. An anxious person, for instance a man awaiting word about his daughter in surgery, may wring his hands or pick his nails; relaxed persons may interlock their fingers over their laps or allow their hands to fall over the ends of armrests. Hands also communicate by touch: slapping someone's face or caressing another's head communicates obvious feelings.

The Communication Process

A communication model has two main parts: people and messages. Face-to-face communication involves a sender, a message, a receiver, and a response, or feedback (Figure 4–2). In its simplest form, communication is a two-way process involving the sending and receiving of a message. Since the intent of communication is to elicit a response, the process is ongoing; the receiver of the message then becomes the sender of a response, and the original sender then becomes the receiver.

Sender

The sender, a person or group who wishes to convey a message to another, is sometimes called the *source-encoder*. This term suggests that the person or group sending the message must have an idea or reason for

Sender   Receiver

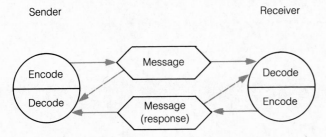

FIGURE 4–2 The communication process. The dashed arrows indicate internal feedback from the sender of the message (or response).

communicating (source) and must put the idea or feeling into a form that can be transmitted. **Encoding** involves the selection of specific signs or symbols (codes) to transmit the message, such as which language and words to use, how to arrange the words, and what tone of voice and gestures to use. For example, if the receiver speaks English, English words will usually be selected. If the message is "No, Johnny, you may not have any more cookies before dinner!" the tone of voice selected will be one firmness, and a shake of the head or a pointing index finger can reinforce it. The nurse must not only deal with dialects and foreign languages but also must cope with two language levels—the layperson's and the health professional's.

Message

The second component of the communication process is the message itself—what is actually said or written, the body language that accompanies the words, and how the message is transmitted. Various channels can be used to convey messages, and frequently combinations are used. It is important that the channel be appropriate for the message and make the intent of the message clear.

Talking face-to-face with a person may be more effective in some instances than telephone or writing a message. Recording messages on tape or communicating by radio or television may be more appropriate for larger audiences. Written communication is often appropriate for long explanations or for a communication that needs to be preserved. The nonverbal channel of touch is often highly effective.

Receiver

The receiver, the third component of the communication process, is the listener, who must listen, observe, and attend. This person, sometimes called the *decoder*, must perceive what the sender intended (sensation) and then analyze the information received (interpretation). Perception involves use of all the senses to receive all verbal and nonverbal messages. To **decode** means to relate the message per-

ceived to the receiver's storehouse of knowledge and experience and to sort out the meaning of the message. Whether the message is decoded accurately by the receiver, according to the sender's intent, depends largely on their similarities in knowledge and experience. For example, Johnny may perceive the message accurately—"No more cookies for me right now." However, if experience has taught him that he can help himself to the cookie jar without punishment, he will interpret the intent of the message differently.

Response

The fourth component of the communication process, the response, is the message that the receiver returns to the sender. It is also called **feedback**. Feedback can be either positive or negative. Nonverbal examples are a nod of the head or a yawn. Either way, feedback allows the sender to correct or reword a message. In the case of Johnny, the receiver may cry or move away from the cookie jar or say, "Well, Judy had three cookies and I only had two." The sender then knows the message was interpreted accurately. However, now the original sender becomes the receiver, who is required to decode and respond.

The receiver is not the sole source of feedback. Communicators constantly receive *internal feedback* from themselves. Internal feedback is often used for written messages. For example, after composing a letter, a person will read it silently or out loud to see how it sounds; or a person who makes a social blunder (*faux pas*) may instantly realize the mistake and say, "That isn't what I really meant," or "I didn't mean it that way."

Factors Influencing the Communication Process

In addition to the person's sociocultural background, language, age, and education and the limitations and attributes of nonverbal communication, the following factors affect the communication process.

Ability of the Communicator The person's abilities to speak, hear, see, and comprehend stimuli influence the communication process. People who are hard of hearing may require messages that are short, loud, and clear. Those who are unable to read will be unable to comprehend written information. Some, because of disease processes, are unable to see or to speak, and individual methods for communication need to be devised with them.

The receiver of a message also needs to be able to interpret the message. Mental faculties can be impaired for such reasons as brain damage or use of sedative drugs or alcohol. Even if a client is free of physical impairments, the nurse needs to determine how many stimuli the client is capable of receiving in a given time frame. Frequently the receiver is expected to assimilate too much information. The nurse may be talking too quickly or presenting too many ideas at once, particularly when offering health instruction.

Perceptions Because each person has unique personality traits, values, and life experiences, each will perceive and interpret messages differently. For example, the nurse may draw the curtains around a crying woman and leave her alone. The woman may interpret this as "The nurse thinks that I will upset others in the room and that I shouldn't cry" or "The nurse doesn't like crying" or "The nurse respects my need to be alone." It is important in many situations to validate or correct the perceptions of the receiver.

Personal Space **Personal space** is the distance people prefer to maintain when interacting with others. Middle-class North Americans use definite distances in various interpersonal relationships, along with specific voice tones and body language. Hall (1969, p. 45) has identified four distances, each with a close and a far phase, that characterize different levels of communication:

1. Intimate: Physical contact to 1½ feet.

2. Personal: 1½–4 feet

3. Social: 4–12 feet

4. Public: 12 feet and beyond

Roles and Relationships The roles and the relationship between sender and receiver affect the communication process. Roles, such as nursing student and instructor, client and physician, or parent and child, affect the content and responses in the communication process. Choice of words, sentence structure, and tone of voice vary considerably from role to role. In addition, the specific relationship between the communicators is significant. The nurse who meets with a client for the first time will communicate differently from the nurse who has previously developed a relationship with that client.

Time The time factor in communication includes the events that precede and follow the interaction. The hospitalized client who is anticipating surgery or who has just received news that a spouse has lost a job will not be very receptive to information. A client who has had to wait for some time to express needs may respond quite differently from one who has endured no waiting period.

Environment People usually communicate most effectively in a comfortable environment. Temperature extremes, excessive noise, and poor ventilation can all interfere with communication. Also, lack of privacy may interfere with a client's communication about matters the client considers private.

Attitudes Attitudes convey beliefs, thoughts, and feelings about people and events convincingly and rapidly. Such attitudes as caring, warmth, respect, and acceptance facilitate communication, whereas condescension, lack of interest, and coldness inhibit communication.

Emotions and Self-Esteem Most people have experienced overwhelming joy or sorrow that is difficult to express in words. Anger may produce loud, profane vocalizations or controlled speechlessness. Fright may produce screams of terror or paralyzed silence.

Emotions also affect a person's ability to interpret messages. A receiver experiencing strong emotion may misinterpret a message or simply not hear parts of it. This situation occurs frequently in nursing. For example, the client feeling great fear may not remember all the preoperative instructions offered by a nurse.

Developing Helping Relationships

Whatever the practice setting, the nurse establishes some sort of helping relationship in which mutual goals are set with the client, or with support persons if the client is unable to participate. Although *special* training in counseling techniques is advantageous, there are many ways of helping clients that do not require special training. Shanken and Shanken (1976, pp. 24–27) have outlined ten of these:

1. *Listen actively.* (See Figure 4–3, and the discussion of attentive listening, later in this chapter.)

2. *Help to identify what the person is feeling.* Often clients who are troubled are unable to identify or to label their feelings and consequently have difficulty working them out or talking about them. A response by the nurse such as "You sound as if you've been lonely since your wife died" can help clients recognize what they are feeling and talk about it.

3. *Put yourself in the other person's shoes.* The ability to do this is referred to as **empathy**. According to Egan (1975, p. 76), empathy involves the ability to discriminate what the other's world is like and to communicate to the other this understanding in a way that shows the other that the helper has picked up both the client's *feelings* and the *behavior* and *experience* underlying these feelings. Empathetic nurses respond in ways that indicate they have listened to what was said and understand how the client feels. The nurse's nonverbal behaviors are also important.

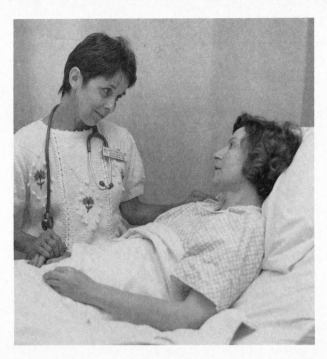

FIGURE 4–3 The nurse conveys attentive listening through a posture of involvement.

High-empathy nurses employ moderate head nodding, a steady gaze, moderate gesturing, and little activity or body movement. *Low-empathy nurses* nod the head and gesture more frequently, laugh more than the high-empathy nurse, display more eye movement, leg movement, and torso movement and sit with crossed arms and legs (Hardin and Halaris 1983, p. 15).

4. *Be honest.* In effective relationships, nurses honestly recognize any lack of knowledge by saying, "I don't know the answer to that right now"; openly discuss their own discomfort by saying, for example, "I feel uncomfortable about this discussion"; and admit tactfully that problems do exist, for instance, when a client says "I'm a mess, aren't I?"

5. *Do not tell a person not to feel.* Feelings expressed by clients often make nurses uncomfortable. Common examples are a client's expressions of anger or worry or a client's crying. When a nurse feels this discomfort, common responses are "Don't worry about it, everything will be fine" or "Please don't cry." Such responses inhibit the client's expression of feelings. Unless feelings are extremely inappropriate, it is best to encourage the client to ventilate (voice) them. Ventilation allows the client to express feelings in words and examine them objectively. Indirectly, such an attitude conveys this message: "Your feelings are not that awful, since I am not bothered by them."

6. *Do not tell a person what to feel.* Statements that indicate to clients how they should feel, rather than how they actually do feel, in essence deny clients' true feelings and suggest that they are inappropriate. Examples are "You shouldn't complain about pain; many others have gone through this same experience stoically" and "You should be glad that you are alive and not worry about the loss of your arm."

7. *Do not make excuses for the other person.* When a person reacts with an intense feeling such as anger or grief and seems to have lost control of behavior to the astonishment or discomfort of others, a common error is to explain the behavior by offering excuses. Examples are: "Well, Mr. Brown, you're upset about not finishing your lunch, but the dietitian and I gave you too much" and "I guess you've had a tough session in physical therapy." These responses discourage and divert the person from discussing feelings of anger or inadequacy. The nurse has made assumptions about the reasons for the client's behavior and therefore inhibits exploration of what the client is really experiencing and feeling.

8. *Be genuine.* Personal statements can be helpful in solidifying the rapport between the nurse and the client. The nurse might offer such comments as "I recall when I was in (a similar situation), and I felt angry about being put down." Egan (1982, p. 128) states that the helper "must be spontaneous, open. He can't hide behind the role of counselor. He must be a human being to the human being before him." Egan refers to this quality as *genuineness* and outlines five behaviors that constitute it. See the box below. Nurses need to exercise caution when making references about themselves. Matching each of the

---

Behaviors/Components of Genuineness

- The genuine helper does not take refuge in or over-emphasize the role of counselor.
- The genuine person is spontaneous.
- The genuine person is nondefensive.
- The genuine person displays few discrepancies—that is, the person is consistent and does not think or feel one thing but say another.
- The genuine person is capable of deep self-disclosure (self-sharing) when it is appropriate.

Source: G. Egan, *The skilled helper. Model, skills, and methods for effective helping*, 2d ed. (Monterey, Calif.: Brooks/Cole Publishing Co., 1982), pp. 127–31.

client's problems with a better story of the nurse's own is of little value to the client.

9. *Use your ingenuity.* There are always many courses of action to consider in handling problems. Whatever course is chosen must lead to further achievement of the client's goals, be compatible with the client's value system, and offer the probability of success. The client needs to choose the ways to achieve goals; however, the nurse can assist in identifying options. For example, a client has asked for help because he is depressed and anxious about retirement. The nurse knows he loves animals, young children, and storytelling. In this case, the nurse might direct his thoughts toward acquiring a puppy, writing children's stories, and volunteering at the public library.

10. *Know your role and your limitations.* Every person has unique strengths and problems. When the nurse feels unable to handle some problems, the client should be informed and referred to the appropriate health professional.

Techniques for Therapeutic Communication

Therapeutic communication promotes understanding on the part of both the sender and the receiver. A number of techniques can help establish a constructive relationship between the nurse and the client, although the use of the techniques is no guarantee of effective communication. So many factors are involved in communication that the nurse is ill-advised to rely on any one technique or even several techniques. Not all people feel comfortable with all techniques, and skill in using them appropriately is essential. The nurse must be comfortable with the technique used and convey sincerity to the client. A phony or false response is usually quickly identified by clients and hinders the development of an effective relationship.

Nurses need to respond not only to the content of a client's verbal message but also to the feelings expressed. It is important to understand how the client views the situation and feels about it before responding. The content of the client's communication is the words or thoughts, as distinct from the feelings. Sometimes people can convey a thought in words while their emotions contradict the words; i.e., words and feelings are incongruent. For example, a client says, "I am glad he has left me; he was very cruel." However, the nurse observes that the client has tears in her eyes as she says this. To respond to the client's *words*, the nurse might simply rephrase, saying "You are pleased that he has left you." To

respond to the client's *feelings*, the nurse would need to acknowledge the tears in the client's eyes, saying, for example, "You seem saddened by all this." Such a response helps the client to focus on her feelings. In some instances, the nurse may need to know more about the client and her resources for coping with these feelings.

Sometimes clients need time to deal with their feelings. Strong emotions are often draining. People usually need to deal with feelings before they can cope with other matters, such as learning new skills or planning for the future. This is most evident in hospitals when clients learn that they have a terminal illness. Some require hours, days, or even weeks before they are ready to start other tasks. Some need only time to themselves, others need someone to listen, others need assistance identifying and verbalizing feelings, and others need assistance making decisions about future courses of action.

Nurses can learn much by examining and becoming aware of their own reactions (feelings) and responses. Although it is difficult for nurses to see their own nonverbal communication other than by videotape feedback, much can be learned by reflecting on what the nurse heard, what the nurse said, and when and how the nurse said it. Methods such as role playing, process recordings, and audiotapes can be useful.

Attentive Listening

Attentive listening is listening actively, using all the senses, as opposed to listening passively with just the ear. It is probably the most important technique in nursing and is basic to all other techniques. Attentive listening is an active process that requires energy and concentration. It involves paying attention to the total message, both verbal messages and nonverbal messages, and noting whether these communications are congruent. Attentive listening means absorbing both the content and the feeling the person is conveying, without selectivity. The listener does not select or listen solely to what the listener wants to hear; the nurse focuses not on the nurse's own needs but rather on the client's needs. Attentive listening conveys an attitude of caring and interest, thereby encouraging the client to talk. In summary, attentive listening is a highly developed skill, but fortunately it can be learned with practice.

A nurse can convey attentiveness in listening to clients in various ways. Common responses are nodding the head, uttering "uh huh" or "mmm," repeating the words that the client has used, or saying, "I see what you mean." Each nurse has characteristic ways of responding, and the nurse must take care not to sound insincere or phony.

Actions of Physical Attending

- *Face the other person squarely.* This position says, "I am available to you." Moving to the side lessens the degree of involvement.

- *Maintain good eye contact.* Mutual eye contact, preferably at the same level, recognizes the other person and denotes a willingness to maintain communication. Eye contact neither glares at nor stares down another but is natural.

- *Lean toward the other.* People move naturally toward one another when they want to say or hear something—by moving to the front of a class, by moving a chair nearer a friend, or by leaning across a table with arms propped in front. The nurse conveys involvement by leaning forward, closer to the client.

- *Maintain an open posture.* The nondefensive position is one in which neither arms nor legs are crossed. It conveys that the person wishes to encourage the passage of communication, as the open door of a home or an office does.

- *Remain relatively relaxed.* Total relaxation is not feasible when the nurse is listening with intensity, but the nurse can show relaxation by taking time in responding, allowing pauses as needed, balancing periods of tension with relaxation, and using gestures that are natural.

These five attending postures need to be adapted to the specific needs of clients in a given situation. For example, leaning forward may not be appropriate at the beginning of an interview. It may be reserved until a closer relationship grows between the nurse and the client. The same applies to eye contact, which is generally uninterrupted when the communicators are very involved in the interaction.

Egan (1982, pp. 60–61) has outlined five specific ways to convey physical attending. He defines physical attending as the manner of being present to another or being with another. Listening, in his frame of reference, is what a person does while attending. The five actions of physical attending, which convey a "posture of involvement," are shown in the box above.

Table 4–1 provides descriptions and examples of the major techniques that facilitate communication and focus on the client's concerns.

Nontherapeutic Responses

Nurses need to recognize nontherapeutic techniques that interfere with effective communication. See Table 4–2. Failure to listen, improperly decoding the client's intended message, and placing the nurse's needs above the client's needs are major barriers to communication.

TABLE 4–1 THERAPEUTIC COMMUNICATION TECHNIQUES

Technique	Description	Examples
Offering self	Suggesting one's presence, interest, or wish to understand the client without making any demands or attaching conditions that would make the client comply to the suggestion to receive the nurse's attention.	"I'll stay with you until your daughter arrives." "We can sit here quietly for a while; we don't need to talk unless you would like to." "I'll help you to dress to go home."
Giving information	Providing, in a simple and direct manner, specific factual information the client may or may not request. When information is not known, the nurse states this and indicates who has it or when the nurse will obtain it.	"Your surgery is scheduled for 11 A.M. tomorrow." "You will feel a 'pulling' sensation when the tube is removed from your abdomen." "I do not know the answer to that, but I will find out from Mrs. King, the nurse in charge."
Acknowledging	Giving recognition, in a nonjudgmental way, of a change in behavior, an effort the client has made, or a contribution to a communication. Acknowledgement may be with or without understanding, verbal or nonverbal.	"You trimmed your beard and mustache and washed your hair." "I notice you keep squinting your eyes. Are you having difficulty seeing?" "You walked twice as far today with your walker."

▶

▶ TABLE 4–1 **Therapeutic Communication Techniques** *CONTINUED*

Technique	Description	Examples
Using silence	Accepting pauses or silences that may extend for several seconds or minutes without interjecting any verbal response.	Sitting quietly (or walking with the client) and waiting attentively until the client is able to put thoughts and feelings into words.
Providing general leads	Using statements or questions that (a) encourage the client to verbalize; (b) choose a topic of conversation; and (c) facilitate continued verbalization.	"Perhaps you would like to talk about . . ." "Would it help to discuss your feelings?" "Where would you like to begin?" "And then . . . what?" "I follow what you are saying."
Being specific and tentative	Making statements that are specific rather than general, and tentative rather than absolute.	"You scratched my arm." (specific statement) "You are as clumsy as an ox." (general statement) "You seem unconcerned about Mary." (tentative statement) "You don't give a damn about Mary and you never will." (absolute statement)
Using open-ended questions	Asking broad questions that lead or invite the client to explore (elaborate, clarify, describe, compare, or illustrate) thoughts or feelings. Open-ended questions specify only the topic to be discussed and invite answers that are longer than one or two words.	"I'd like to hear more about that." "Tell me about . . ." "How have you been feeling lately?" "What brought you to the hospital?" "What is your opinion?" "You said you were frightened yesterday. How do you feel now?"
Using touch	Providing appropriate forms of touch to reinforce caring feelings. Because tactile contacts vary considerably among individuals, families, and cultures, the nurse must be sensitive to the differences in attitudes and practices of clients and self.	Putting an arm over the client's shoulder. Placing the hand over the client's hand.
Restating or paraphrasing	Actively listening for the client's basic message and then repeating those thoughts and/or feelings in similar words. This conveys that the nurse has listened and understood the client's basic message and also offers clients a clearer idea of what they have said.	Client: "I couldn't manage to eat any dinner last night—not even the dessert." Nurse: "You had difficulty eating yesterday." Client: "Yes, I was very upset after my family left." Client: "I have a lot of trouble talking to strangers." Nurse: "You find it difficult talking to people you do not know?"
Seeking clarification	A method of making the client's *broad overall* meaning of the message more understandable. It is used when paraphrasing is difficult or when the communication is rambling or garbled. To clarify the message, the nurse can restate the basic message or confess confusion and ask the client to repeat or restate the message.	"I'm puzzled." "I'm not sure I understand that." "Would you please say that again?" "Would you tell me more?"
	Nurses can also clarify their own message with statements.	"I meant this rather than that." "I guess I didn't make that clear—I'll go over it again."
Perception checking or seeking consensual validation	A method similar to clarifying that verifies the meaning of *specific words* rather than the overall meaning of a message.	Client: "My husband *never* gives me any presents." Nurse: "You mean he has *never* given you a present for your birthday or Christmas?" Client: "Well—not *never*. He does get me something for my birthday and Christmas, but he never thinks of giving me anything at any other time."

▶

► **TABLE 4–1** *CONTINUED*

Technique	Description	Examples
Clarifying time or sequence	Helping the client clarify an event, situation, or happening in relationship to time.	Client: "I vomited this morning." Nurse: "Was that after breakfast?" Client: "I feel that I have been asleep for weeks." Nurse: "You had your operation Monday, and today is Tuesday."
Presenting reality	Helping the client to differentiate the real from the unreal.	"That telephone ring came from the program on television." "That's not a dead mouse in the corner; it is a discarded washcloth." "Your magazine is here in the drawer. It has not been stolen."
Focusing	Helping the client expand on and develop a topic of importance. It is important for the nurse to wait until the clients think they have talked about the main concerns before attempting to focus. The focus may be an idea or a feeling; however, the nurse often emphasizes a feeling to help the client recognize an emotion disguised behind words.	Client: "My wife says she will look after me, but I don't think she can, what with the children to take care of, and they're always after her about something—clothes, homework, what's for dinner that night." Nurse: "You are worried about how well she can manage."
Reflecting	Directing ideas, feelings, questions, or content back to clients to enable them to explore their own ideas and feelings about a situation.	Client: "What can I do?" Nurse: "What do you think would be helpful?" Client: "Do you think I should tell my husband?" Nurse: "You seem unsure about telling your husband."
Summarizing and planning	Stating the main points of a discussion to clarify the relevant points discussed. This technique is useful at the end of an interview or to review a health-teaching session. It often acts as an introduction to future care planning.	"During the past half hour we have talked about . . ." "Tomorrow afternoon we may explore this further." "In a few days I'll review what you have learned about the actions and effects of your insulin."

TABLE 4–2   NONTHERAPEUTIC RESPONSES

Response	Description	Examples
Unwarranted reassurance	Using cliches or comforting statements of advice as a means to reassure the client. These responses block the fears, feelings, and other thoughts of the client.	"You'll feel better soon." "I'm sure everything will turn out all right." "Don't worry."
Passing judgment	Giving opinions and approving or disapproving responses, moralizing, or implying one's own values. These responses imply that the client *must* think as the nurse thinks, fostering client dependence.	"That's good (bad)." "You shouldn't do that." "That's not good enough." "What you did was wrong (right)."
Giving common advice	Telling the client what to do. These responses deny the client's right to be an equal partner. Note that giving *expert* rather than common advice is therapeutic.	Client: "Should I move from my home to a nursing home?" Nurse: "If I were you, I'd go to a nursing home, where you'll get your meals cooked for you."

►

▶ TABLE 4–2 **Nontherapeutic Responses** *CONTINUED*

Technique	Description	Examples
Stereotyping	Offering generalized and oversimplified beliefs about groups of people that are based upon experiences too limited to be valid. These responses categorize clients and negate their uniqueness as individuals.	"Two-year olds are brats." "Women are complainers." "Men don't cry." "Most people don't have any pain after this type of surgery."
Agreeing and disagreeing	Akin to judgmental responses, agreeing and disagreeing imply that the client is either right or wrong and that the nurse is in a position to judge this. These responses deter clients from thinking through their position and may cause a client to become defensive.	Client: "I don't think Dr. Broad is a very good doctor. He doesn't seem interested in his patients." Nurse: "Dr. Broad is head of the Department of Surgery and is an excellent surgeon."
Being defensive	Attempting to protect a person or health care services from negative comments. These responses prevent the client from expressing true concerns. The nurse is saying, "You have no right to complain." Defensive responses protect the nurse from admitting weaknesses in the health care services, including personal weaknesses.	Client: "Those night nurses must just sit around and talk all night. They didn't answer my light for over an hour." Nurse: "I'll have you know we literally run around on nights. You're not the only client, you know."
Challenging	Giving a response that makes clients prove their statement or point of view. These responses indicate that the nurse is failing to consider the client's feelings, making the client feel it necessary to defend a position.	Client: "I felt nauseated after that red pill." Nurse: "Surely you don't think I gave you the wrong pill?" Client: "I feel as if I am dying." Nurse: "How can you feel that way when your pulse is 60?" Client: "I believe my husband doesn't love me." Nurse: "You can't say that; why, he visits you every day."
Probing	Asking for information chiefly out of curiosity rather than with the intent to assist the client. These responses are considered prying and violate the client's privacy. Often asking "why" is probing and places the client in a defensive position.	Client: "I was speeding along the street and didn't see the stop sign." Nurse: "Why were you speeding?" Client: "I didn't ask the doctor when he was here." Nurse: "Why didn't you?"
Testing	Asking questions that make the client admit to something. These responses permit the client only limited answers and often meet the nurse's need rather than the client's.	"Who do you think you are?" (enforces people to admit their status is only that of client) "Do you think I am not busy?" (forces the client to admit that the nurse really *is* busy)
Rejecting	Refusing to discuss certain topics with the client. These responses often make clients feel that the nurse is rejecting not only their communication but also the clients themselves.	"I don't want to discuss that. Let's talk about . . ." "Let's discuss other areas of interest to you rather than the two problems you keep mentioning." "I can't talk now. I'm on my way for coffee break."
Changing topics and subjects	Directing the communication into areas of self-interest rather than considering the client's concerns. It often arises as a self-protective response to anxiety-causing topics. These responses imply that what the nurse considers important will be discussed and that clients are not capable of helping themselves.	Client: "I'm separated from my wife. Do you think I should have sexual relations with another woman?" Nurse: "I see that you're thirty-six and that you like gardening. This sunshine is good for my roses. I have a beautiful rose garden."

CRITICAL THINKING CHALLENGE

Maxwell Rowland, a 64-year-old male, has been admitted to the nursing unit for treatment of peptic ulcer disease. When receiving report from the previous shift, you are told that he has been uncooperative with the physician's treatment orders, and has told the nursing staff to leave him alone. When you visit him to assess his status at the beginning of your shift, he states, "I don't need your help; you probably don't know what you're doing, either. No one around here does! Leave me alone." What might be causing Mr. Rowland's behavior? How do you feel about Mr. Rowland's behavior? What do you think he might be feeling? What would you say to Mr. Rowland to enable you to assess the reason for his behavior? What communication techniques will you use?

RELATED RESEARCH

Apse, A. December 1985. Avoiding terms of bewilderment. *Nursing 85* 15:42–43.

Harrison, T. M.; Pistolessi, T. V.; and Stephen, T. D. February 1989. Assessing nurses' communication: A cross-sectional study. *Western Journal of Nursing Research* 11:75–91.

Rosendahl, P. B., and Ross, V. October 1982. Does your behavior affect your patient's response? *Journal of Gerontological Nursing* 8:572–75.

REFERENCES

Brammer, L. M. 1988. *The helping relationship: Process and skills.* 4th ed. Englewood Cliffs, N.J.: Prentice-Hall.

Carkhuff, R. R., and Anthony, W. A. 1979. *The skills of helping.* Amherst, Mass.: Human Resource Development Press.

Davis, A. J. 1984. *Listening and responding.* St. Louis: C. V. Mosby Co.

Egan, G. 1975. *The skilled helper: A model for systematic helping and interpersonal relating.* Monterey, Calif.: Brooks/Cole Publishing, Co.

———. 1982. *The skilled helper: Model, skills, and methods for effective helping.* 2d ed. Monterey, Calif.: Brooks/Cole Publishing Co.

Hardin, S. B., and Halaris, A. L. January 1983. Nonverbal communication of patients and high- and low-empathy nurses. *Journal of Psychosocial Nursing and Mental Health Sciences* 21:15–20.

Kaul, T., and Schmidt, L. 1971. Dimensions of interviewer trustworthiness. *Journal of Counseling Psychology* 34:134–39.

King, I. M. 1981. *A theory for nursing. Systems, concepts, process.* New York: John Wiley and Sons.

Peplau, H. E. July 1960. Talking with patients. *American Journal of Nursing* 60:964–66.

Raudsepp, E. April 1990. Seven ways to cure communication breakdowns. *Nursing 90* 20:132, 134, 137–38.

Ruesch, J. 1961. *Therapeutic communication.* New York: W. W. Norton and Co.

Scott, A. L. August 1988. Human interaction and personal boundaries. *Journal of Psychosocial Nursing and Mental Health Services* 26:23–27.

Seaman, L. May/June 1982. Affective nursing touch. *Geriatric Nursing* 3:162–64.

Shanken, J., and Shanken, P. February 1976. How to be a helping person. *Journal of Psychiatric Nursing and Mental Health Services* 14:24–28.

Stewart, C. J., and Cash, W. B. 1988. *Interviewing principles and practices.* 5th ed. Dubuque, Iowa: Wm. C. Brown Publishers.

Sundeen, S. J.; Stuart G. W.; Rankin, E. A. D.; and Cohen, S. A. 1989. *Nurse-client interaction.* 4th ed. St. Louis: C. V. Mosby Co.

Thomas, M. 1970. Trust in the nurse-patient relationship. In Carlson, C. E., editor. *Behavioral concepts and nursing intervention.* Philadelphia: J. B. Lippincott Co.

Travelbee, J. February 1963. What do we mean by rapport? *American Journal of Nursing* 63:70–72.

5

Teaching

OBJECTIVES

- Identify factors that facilitate client learning

- Identify factors that inhibit learning

- Outline five principles of teaching

- Describe the essential steps in preparing a teaching plan

- Explain essential factors in assessing for learning needs

- Identify nine guidelines to implementing a teaching plan

CONTENTS

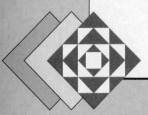

NURSING PROCESS GUIDE

TEACHING

ASSESSMENT

Determine

- Client learning needs and need for specific teaching program. Three sources for identifying learning needs are the client, the client's behavior, and other health care professionals.

- Age of client. Age provides information on the person's developmental status, such as the motor and intellectual development of children and possible psychomotor and learning difficulties of older adults.

- Education of client. This may influence present knowledge as well as the teaching method that is most effective; e.g., the client's abilities to read or write affect teaching style.

- Cultural beliefs and practices. Cultural beliefs and practices related to diet, health, illness, and life-style and folk medical practices influence teaching content and in some instances may impinge on learning.

- Economic considerations. Some clients may not be able to afford certain equipment, such as a new sterile syringe for each injection or certain ostomy appliances or oxygen equipment.

- Client readiness and openness to learning. Clients who are ready to learn often behave differently from those who are not. A client who is ready may search out information, for instance, by asking questions, reading books or articles, talking to others, and generally showing interest. The person unready to learn is more likely to avoid the subject or situation and hope or believe that someone else will take care of the problem (Smitherman 1981, pp. 126–27). In addition, somatic symptoms (such as headaches, upset stomach, or gas pains) may make it difficult for clients to pay attention.

- Client motivation. Motivation is usually greatest when the client is ready and the content is meaningful to the client.

- Client learning style. Does the person learn best by visual or auditory methods? Is the person a thinking or feeling person? A thinking person uses logical decision making to arrive at a conclusion, whereas a feeling person is more likely to arrive at conclusions using subjective personal values. A nurse should stress logic and knowledge when teaching a thinking person but should stress interpersonal skills when teaching a feeling person.

RELATED DIAGNOSTIC CATEGORIES

Nursing diagnoses pertinent to a client's learning needs are all grouped under the diagnostic category of **Knowledge deficit**. It is extremely important that the nurse specify which exact deficits individual clients manifest. Examples include the following:

- Knowledge deficit: low-calorie diet related to newly ordered therapy

- Knowledge deficit: diabetic diet related to prescribed treatment

- Knowledge deficit: preoperative care related to impending surgical procedure

- Knowledge deficit: medications related to language differences

- Knowledge deficit: home safety hazards related to denial of declining health

- Knowledge deficit: substance abuse related to lack of motivation to acquire information

PLANNING

Client Goals

The client will

- Increase knowledge or decrease knowledge deficit in such areas as self-care; activities related to health care regimens; decision-making regarding health; enhancement of life processes, such as birth, human development, and death; health maintenance and coping.

- Use and obtain health care information.

Outcome Criteria

The client

- Makes health care decisions based on information provided.

- Explains how and why to take a specified health care action.

- Demonstrates adequate knowledge/skill to perform health care regimen (specify) or to carry out activities necessary for well-being.

- Monitors self for signs and symptoms of illness.

- Experiences a decrease in manifestations of disease state and an increase in indicators of health.

- Verbalizes when to seek health care service.

- Verbalizes where to obtain specific health care information.

- Uses appropriate community resources.

Facilitating Learning

Teaching can occur without any learning taking place, and learning can occur in the absence of teaching. Client education is a major aspect of nursing practice and an important independent nursing function. Legislation relating to nursing frequently has included client teaching as a function of nursing, thereby making teaching a legal and professional responsibility (Phillips and Hekelman 1983, pp. 42–46).

Clients have a variety of learning needs. A **learning need** is a need to change behavior or "a gap between the information an individual knows and the information necessary to perform a function or care for self" (Gessner 1989, p. 593). **Learning** is a change in human disposition or capability that persists over a period of time and that cannot be solely accounted for by growth. Learning is represented by a change in behavior. An important aspect of learning is the individual's desire to learn and to act on the learning. This is referred to as **compliance**.

Factors Facilitating Learning

Genuine Motivation

Motivation to learn is the desire to learn. It is a term that describes forces acting on or from within the person to initiate, direct, and maintain behavior and to explain differences in the intensity and direction of behavior (Redman 1988, p. 21). Such motivation is generally greatest when a person recognizes a need and believes the need will be met through learning. It is not enough for the need to be identified and verbalized by the nurse; it must be experienced by the client. Often the nurse's task is to help the client personally work through the problem and identify the need.

Nurses can positively influence a client's motivation in three ways:

1. By relating the learning to something the client values and helping the client see the relevance of the learning

2. By helping the client to make the learning situation pleasant

3. By encouraging self-direction

To influence the externally motivated learner, a nurse can use *positive reinforcement*, which involves rewarding the learner for achievements, e.g., giving praise or reading a bedtime story to a child. Reinforcement is most effective when given immediately after the desired response. **Negative reinforcement**, or punishment for undesirable responses, is considered less motivating than positive reinforcement. However, negative reinforcement can be motivating if it is accompanied by encouragement and an explanation of how to correct the response (for instance: "I agree that looks right, but if you place the tube like this the urine should flow more readily").

Physical and Emotional Readiness

Readiness to learn is the behavior that reflects motivation at a specific time. Readiness sometimes comes with time, and the nurses role is often to encourage its development (Redman 1988, p. 36). Readiness involves two facets: emotional, or motivational, and experiential. *Emotional readiness* determines the person's willingness to put forth the effort needed to learn. Emotional factors affecting readiness include anxiety. A high level of anxiety narrows the person's perceptions and thus interferes with learning. *Experiential readiness* involves the person's background of experiences, skills, attitudes, and ability to learn. Experiential factors include occupational status, client capabilities, and educational level. In health, physical readiness is also important to consider. Clients may be too ill or weak to attend to learning.

Nurses can sometimes facilitate a client's readiness by tactfully calling attention to a learning need (for example, "Have you thought about learning to change your dressing?"). Two other ways to facilitate readiness are to give the client information to read and to point out an opportunity to learn (for instance: "There is a baby bath demonstration at 3 P.M. today in the next room").

Active Involvement

Active involvement in the learning process makes learning more meaningful. For example, the person who actively participates in planning and discussion learns faster and retains more (Figure 5–1). Passive learning, such as listening to a lecture or watching a film, does not foster optimal learning.

Successful Learning

Once learners have succeeded in accomplishing a task or understanding a concept, they gain self-confidence in their ability to learn. This reduces their anxiety about failure and can motivate greater learning. Successful learners have increased confidence with which to accept failure.

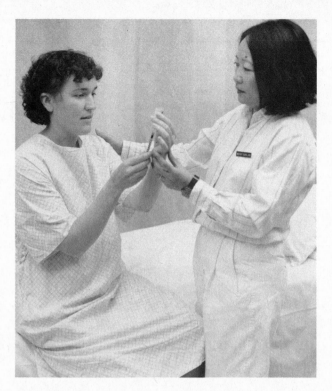

FIGURE 5–1 The client's interest and active involvement facilitate learning.

Accepting, Nonjudgmental Environment

People learn best when they believe they are accepted and will not be judged. The person who expects to be judged as a "poor" or "good" client will not learn as well as the person who feels no such threat.

Feedback

Feedback is information relating a person's performance to a desired goal. It has to be meaningful to the learner. Feedback that accompanies practice of psychomotor skills helps the person to learn those skills. Support or desired behavior through praise, positively worded corrections, and suggestions of alternative methods are ways of providing positive feedback. Negative feedback such as ridicule, anger, or sarcasm can lead people to withdraw from learning. Such feedback, viewed as a type of punishment, may cause the client to avoid the teacher in order to avoid punishment.

Progression from Simple to Complex

Learning is facilitated by material that is logically organized and proceeds from the simple to the complex. Such organization enables the learner to comprehend new information, assimilate it with previous learning, and form new understandings. Of course, simple and complex are relative terms, depending on the level at which the person is learning. What is simple for one person may be complex for another.

Repetition

Repetition of key concepts and facts facilitates retention of newly learned material. Practice of psychomotor skills improves performance of those skills and facilitates their transfer to another setting.

Relevance

When a person appreciates the relevance of specific material, learning is facilitated. For example, the man who understands the relevance to his health of a special diet is better able to learn about the diet than a person who sees no such connection.

Time between Learning and Use

People retain information and psychomotor skills when the time between learning and use is short; the longer the time interval, the more is forgotten. For example, a woman who is taught how to administer her own insulin but is not permitted to do so until discharge from hospital is unlikely to remember much of what she learned. However, if she is allowed to give her own injections while in hospital, her learning will be enhanced.

Optimal Learning Environment

An optimal learning environment has adequate lighting that is free from glare, a comfortable room temperature, good ventilation, and freedom from noise. Privacy is essential for some learning. For example, when a client is learning to irrigate a colostomy, the presence of others can be embarrassing and thus interfere with learning.

Barriers to Learning

Table 5–1 on page 80 outlines specific barriers to learning and their implications for the nurse.

Teaching

Teaching is a system of activities intended to produce learning. The teaching process is intentionally designed to produce specific learning. Teaching also involves a type of communication for which there are specific goals. For example, clients who need to administer their own eye drops or to change an incision dressing share these goals with the nurse. Another aspect of teaching is the relationship between the teacher and the learner. It is essentially one of trust and respect. The learner trusts that the teacher has the knowledge and skill to teach, and the teacher respects the learner's ability to attain the recognized goals. Once a nurse starts to instruct a client and/or support persons, it is important that the teaching process continue until the participants reach the goals, change the goals, or decide that the goals will not help meet the learning objectives.

TABLE 5–1 BARRIERS TO LEARNING

Barrier	Explanation	Nursing Implications
Acute illness	Client requires all resources to cope with illness.	Defer teaching until client is less ill.
Pain	Pain decreases ability to concentrate.	Deal with pain before teaching.
Age	Vision, hearing, and motor control can be impaired in the elderly.	Allow for sensory and motor defects in teaching.
Prognosis	Client can be preoccupied with illness and unable to concentrate on new information.	Defer teaching to a better time.
Biorhythms	Mental and physical performances have a circadian rhythm.	Change time of teaching to suit client.
Emotion (e.g., anxiety, denial, depression)	Emotions require energy and distract from learning.	Deal with emotions first and possible misinformation.
Language and ethnic background	Client may not be fluent in the nurse's language.	Obtain services of an interpreter or nurse with appropriate language skills.
Iatrogenic barriers	The nurse may set up barriers by appearing condescending or hurried or by ignoring client cues.	Establish a helping relationship and be sensitive to client's needs.

Principles of Teaching

The following five principles of teaching may be helpful to nursing students:

1. *Teaching activities should help the learner meet individual learning objectives.* Teacher and learner should mutually determine these objectives. If certain activities do not assist the learner, these need to be reassessed; perhaps other activities can replace them. For example, explanation alone may not be able to teach a client to handle a syringe. Actually handling the syringe may be more effective.

2. *Rapport between teacher and learner is essential.* A relationship that is both accepting and constructive will best assist learning.

3. *The teacher who can use the client's previous learning in the present situation encourages the client and facilitates the learning of new skills.* For example, a person who already knows how to cook can use this knowledge when learning about a special diet.

4. *A teacher must be able to communicate clearly and concisely with words that have the same meaning to the learner as to the teacher.* For example, a client who is taught not to put water on an area of the skin may think a wet washcloth is permissible for washing the area. In effect, the nurse needs to explain that no water or moisture should touch the area.

5. *The teaching activities need to be oriented around the learning objectives.* Information and skills not related to the learner's objectives need to be eliminated from the teaching process because they may confuse or distract the learner.

Developing a Teaching Plan

The nurse develops a teaching plan by following a series of steps. Involving the client at this time promotes the formation of a meaningful plan and stimulates client motivation. The client who participates in the formulation of the teaching plan is more likely to achieve the desired outcomes.

Determining Teaching Priorities
The client and nurse together must rank the client's learning needs according to priority. For pediatric clients, the nurse consults both the parent and child to determine priorities and proper timing for teaching.

Setting Learning Objectives
The terms *goals* and *objectives* are used interchangeably by some educators and distinguished by others. Used interchangeably, they can be considered as both immediate and long-term aims to be accomplished in a learning situation. However, *goal* is often the more general term, describing a general, long-range intended outcome of learning, whereas *objective* is used to mean a specific, immediate, short-range intended outcome of a learning situation.

The client (or support persons) and the nurse set the goals and objectives. Objectives relate to immediate client needs, such as perineal care after the birth of a baby. Goals relate to long-term needs, such as an obese new mother's need to lose weight (in which case the goal may be a specific weight loss through diet and exercise).

The objectives for learning should be both specific and observable in terms of behavior. A specific objective might be "to take 60 mg furosemide (Lasix) upon identifying ankle edema." An objective needs to be stated in terms of client behavior, not nurse behavior: for example, "Will write his own diets as instructed" (client behavior), not "To teach the client about his diet" (nurse behavior). See the box below for a list of behavioral (observable) verbs and nonbehavioral verbs.

The nurse may need to modify objectives according to the client's age and developmental capacity. For young children with short attention spans, the nurse should set objectives that can be achieved within a short period of time. For elderly persons, who generally require more time to digest smaller amounts of material, the nurse may need to develop several objectives to help the clients meet goals in stages.

Objectives should contain these three types of information:

1. *Performance, or behavior, that the learner will exhibit after mastering the objective.* The objective must reflect an observable activity. The performance may be visible, e.g., walking, or invisible, e.g., adding a column of figures. However, it is necessary to be able to deduce whether an unobservable activity has been mastered from some performance that represents the activity. Therefore, the performance of an objective might be written: "Writes the total for a column of figures in the indicated space" (observable), not "Adds a column of figures" (unobservable).

2. *Conditions under which the client is to carry out a performance, so that the objective is clear.* For example, "Walks to the end of the hall and back without crutches" describes a performance clearly; "without crutches" is a condition of the objective. Nurses always need to determine the conditions in which an activity will be carried out. Then, the objectives for the learning plan can reflect those conditions. For example, if Mr. Jones lives alone and must irrigate his own colostomy, then "Irrigates his colostomy *independently* as taught" is the correct objective.

3. *Criteria, or the standards of performance that are considered acceptable.* Each objective should specify a standard against which the performance can be measured. Examples include speed, quality, and accuracy. Learners need to understand the criteria so that they can evaluate their performance validly.

Choosing Content

The objectives determine the content to be taught. For instance, "Identify appropriate sites for insulin injections" means the nurse must include content about the body sites suitable for insulin injections. Any content that does not address the objectives should be omitted.

There are many sources of content information. Nurses will have some knowledge as a result of their own education. Pamphlets, books, and journals can also assist nurses and clients.

Selecting Teaching Strategies

The method of teaching the nurse chooses should be suited to the individual, to the material to be learned, and to the teacher. For example, the person who cannot read needs material presented in other ways; a discussion is usually not the best strategy for teaching a client to give an injection; and a teacher using group discussion for teaching should be a competent group leader. Some people are visually oriented and learn best through seeing; others learn best through hearing and having the skill explained. These attributes should be considered during the planning phase.

Audio-visual aids (film strips, films, posters, pamphlets, line drawings) are often helpful for client learning. It is important, however, that the nurse review these aids before presenting them to clients to ensure that information is consistent; these materials can be out of date or differ in content from other materials (even minimal differences can be confusing to clients) and hinder the learning process.

Peer groups or representatives from support organizations can also be helpful. For example, the client who has recently had a colostomy often can learn a great deal from a person who has had a colostomy for several years. Self-help groups function on this premise.

The nurse may use multiple teaching strategies in one teaching session, and consider alternative strategies when the client has problems in comprehension. See Table 5–2 on page 82 for selected teaching strategies.

The use of puppetry or dolls for teaching young pediatric clients is beneficial. The nurse can demonstrate the procedures by using the doll or puppet. The child can then handle the equipment and pretend to perform the procedure on the doll or puppet. Older children can be encouraged to draw pictures or write

---

Selected Verbs for Objectives

Behavioral Verbs	Nonbehavioral Verbs
Defines	Knows
Identifies	Understands
Chooses	Appreciates
Demonstrates	Feels
Differentiates	
Applies	
Compares	

TABLE 5–2 SELECTED TEACHING STRATEGIES

Strategy	Major Type of Learning	Characteristics
Explanation or description (e.g., lecture)	Cognitive	Teacher controls content and pace. Feedback is determined by teacher. May be given to individual or group. Encourages retention of facts.
One-to-one discussion	Affective, cognitive	Encourages participation by learner. Permits reinforcement and repetition at learner's level. Permits introduction of sensitive subjects.
Answering questions	Cognitive	Teacher controls most of content and pace. Teacher must understand question and what it means to learner. Can be used with individuals and groups. Teacher sometimes needs to confirm whether question has been answered by asking learner, e.g., "Does that answer your question?"
Demonstration	Psychomotor	Often used with explanation. Can be used with individuals, small or large groups. Does not permit use of equipment by learners.
Group discussion	Affective, cognitive	Learner can obtain assistance from supportive group. Group members learn from one another.
Practice	Psychomotor	Allows repetition and immediate feedback. Permits "hands-on" experience.
Printed and audio-visual materials	Cognitive	Forms include books, pamphlets, films, programmed instruction, and computer learning. Learners can proceed at their own speed. Nurse can act as resource person, need not be present during learning.
Role playing	Affective, cognitive	Permits expression of attitudes, values, and emotions. Can assist in development of communication skills. Involves active participation by learner.
Modeling	Affective, psychomotor	Nurse sets example by attitude, psychomotor skill.

about feelings and reactions related to the impending procedure. Expression of concerns through play, art, or writing helps the child to work through anxiety and may decrease fear.

Clients who require greater explanations or time for learning, particularly young children, adolescents, or the elderly, may benefit from group discussions that follow brief individualized teaching sessions.

Ordering Learning Experiences

Some health agencies have developed teaching guides and materials for lessons that nurses commonly give. The nurse often needs to adapt these guides to suit the individual client or client group. Whether the nurse is implementing a plan devised by another or developing an individualized teaching plan, these guidelines can help the nurse order the learning experience:

- *Start with something the learner is concerned about.* For example, before learning how to administer insulin to himself, an adolescent wants to know how he can adjust his life-style and still play football.

- *Begin with what the learner knows, and proceed to the unknown.* This gives the learner confidence.

- *Address any area of learning that is anxiety provoking first.* A high level of anxiety can impair concentration in other areas. For example, a woman highly anxious about turning her husband in bed might not be able to learn about bathing him until she has successfully learned to turn him.

- *Teach the basics first, then proceed to the variations or adjustments.* For example, when teaching a female client how to insert a retention catheter, it is best to teach the basic procedure before teaching any adjustments that might be needed if the catheter stops draining after insertion.

Implementing the Teaching Plan

The nurse needs to be flexible in implementing any teaching plan, since the plan may need revising, e.g., because the client tires sooner than anticipated, the client is faced with too much information too quickly, the client's needs change, or external factors intervene. For instance, the nurse and the client, Mr. Brown, may have planned for him to learn to administer his own insulin at a particular time, but when the time comes the nurse finds that he wants additional information before actually giving himself the insulin. In this case, the nurse alters the teaching plan and discusses the desired information, provides written information, and defers teaching the psychomotor skill until the next day.

Technique 5–1 explains the essential steps involved in implementing a teaching plan.

5-1 Implementing a Teaching Plan

PURPOSES
- To inform clients about health risk factors
- To provide information about specific health measures
- To increase compliance to health restoration and maintenance procedures
- To reduce anxiety

ASSESSMENT FOCUS

> Cognitive level/ability to comprehend; current knowledge related to the content; readiness to learn (motivation, health beliefs, and so on); barriers to learning (environmental, physical, emotional, language); parental suggestions regarding timing, content, and methodology for teaching of young children.

EQUIPMENT

- Audio-visual aids, charts, illustrations
- Pen and paper
- Pamphlets or other written material
- Hand puppet or doll
- Equipment for demonstration and return demonstration (e.g., syringe and medication if injection is being explained)

INTERVENTION

1. Determine any modifications required for the teaching plan.

- Determine the client's physiologic readiness by noting the degree of physical discomfort, mental alertness, and acuity of illness.
- Determine psychologic readiness by noting the client's emotional state and level of comprehension.
- Ensure that the time planned is appropriate for the client.
- Review goals for this specific teaching session with the client. *Ensuring that the goals are realistic enhances learner satisfaction.*

2. Assemble the teaching materials, and prepare the environment.

- Ensure that the room or setting where the teaching is to occur is comfortable and quiet. Consider environmental characteristics such as lighting, temperature, ventilation, sound, visibility, and a chair or support for the learner. *Noise or other interruptions usually interfere with concentration, whereas a comfortable environment enhances learning.*
- Assemble all teaching materials required for the client's learning needs and teaching strategies selected.

3. Teach the planned content, using the following guidelines.

- Use a layperson's vocabulary to enhance communication. Words such as *urine* or *feces* may be unfamiliar to clients, and abbreviations such as "RR" (recovery room) or "PAR" (postanesthesia room) are often misunderstood.
- Use the type of supplies or equipment that the client will eventually use. *This facilitates the transfer of learning.*
- Be sensitive to any signs that the pace is too fast or too slow. A client who appears confused or does not comprehend material when questioned may be finding

▶

▶ **Technique 5–1 Implementing a Teaching Plan** *CONTINUED*

the pace too fast. When the client appears bored and loses interest, the pace may be too slow, the learning period may be too long, or the client may be tired.

- Use "organizers" to introduce material to be learned. *These provide a means of relating unknown material to known material and generating logical relationships. For example:* "You understand how urine flows down a catheter from the bladder. Now I will show you how to inject fluid so that it flows up the catheter into the bladder." *The details that follow such an introduction are then seen within its framework, and the details have added meaning.*

- Obtain evaluative feedback from the client throughout the session, e.g., ask, "Do you have any questions?" *Feedback enables the nurse to make necessary modifications in the teaching process.*

- Use techniques of repetition, rephrasing (using other words), and approaching the material from another point of view. For instance, after discussing the kinds of foods that can be included in a diet, the nurse describes the foods again, but in the context of the three meals eaten during one day. *These techniques reinforce learning.*

- Provide positive feedback for the client's accomplishments as war-

ranted. *Positive feedback enhances motivation and learning.*

- At the end of the session, summarize the content taught. *A summary reinforces the learning and may provide a sense of accomplishment.*

- At closure, plan for the next teaching session as indicated. Include day, time, place, topic, and purpose.

4. Document the teaching on the client's record.

- Record the kind of teaching provided, the client's achievements, and the client's reaction to the teaching.

EVALUATION FOCUS	Behaviors indicating knowledge and understanding of material covered; measurable changes in behavior; compliance to health restoration and health maintenance routines.

SAMPLE RECORDING

Date	Time	Notes
01/11/93	0800	Client teaching provided regarding impending surgery for tonsilectomy. Mother in room, discussed the use of oxygen mask for anesthesia using the doll. Allowed client to place mask over doll's face. Observed client telling doll "not to be afraid, the doctor would fix her throat and she will be all better". Minimal anxiety noted. ———————— Joyce Y. Johnson, RN

KEY ELEMENTS OF IMPLEMENTING A TEACHING PLAN

- Determine client readiness and comfort.
- Assess and eliminate barriers to learning.
- Use terms the client understands and equipment the client will eventually use.
- Obtain evaluative feedback throughout the session, and be sensitive to any signs that the pace is too fast or too slow.
- Provide positive feedback for the client's accomplishments.
- Use techniques of repetition, rephrasing, and summarizing to facilitate learning.

CRITICAL THINKING CHALLENGE

Steven Brown, a 29-year-old male with a history of seizure disorder, has been admitted to your nursing unit for the second time in 2 months with seizures. He is well known to the nursing staff because of his repeated hospital admissions for seizures. He is being treated with antiepileptic medication, which he is required to take daily. He has monthly outpatient clinic appointments for follow-up care. The clinic staff tells you that he has not kept his clinic appointments. You suspect that he might not be taking his medication. The staff has labeled him as "noncompliant." How do you feel about Mr. Brown's noncompliant behavior? What information do you need to decide what to do? Would teaching interventions be effective in changing Mr. Brown's behavior? Why or why not?

RELATED RESEARCH

Streiff, L. D. Summer 1986. Can clients understand our instructions? *Image: Journal of Nursing Scholarship* 18:48–52.

Vessey, J. A. September/October 1988. Comparison of two teaching methods on children's knowledge of their internal bodies. *Nursing Research* 38:262–87.

REFERENCES

Armstrong, M. L. September 1989. Orchestrating the process of patient education: Methods and approaches. *Nursing Clinics of North America* 24:597–604.

Cross, K. P. 1988. *Adults as learners.* San Francisco: Jossey-Bass.

Gessner, B. A. September 1989. Adult education: The cornerstone of patient teaching. *Nursing Clinics of North America* 24:589–95.

Kick, E. September 1989. Patient teaching for elders. *Nursing Clinics of North America* 24:681–86.

Lawrence, G. 1982. *People types and tiger stripes: A practical guide to learning styles.* Gainesville, Fla.: Center for Applications of Psychological Type, Inc.

Phillips, J. A., and Hekelman, F. P. September/October 1983. The role of the nurse as a teacher: A position paper. *Nephrology Nurse* 5:42–46.

Redman, B. K. 1988. *The process of patient education.* 6th ed. St. Louis: C. V. Mosby Co.

Robinson, Y. K. January 1986. Teaching adults: Some issues in adult education for health education. *Physiotherapy* 72:49–52.

Rorden, J. W. 1987. *Nurses as health teachers: A practical guide.* Philadelphia: W. B. Saunders Co.

Smith, C. E., editor. 1987. *Patient education: Nurses in partnership with other health professionals.* Orlando, Fla.: Grune & Stratton.

Smitherman, C. 1981. *Nursing actions for health promotion.* Philadelphia: F. A. Davis Co.

Thurlow, J. G. Spring 1990. Tools for patient education. *Gastroenterological Nursing* 12:286–88.

Tripp-Reimer, T. September 1989. Cross-cultural perspectives on patient teaching. *Nursing Clinics of North America* 24:613–19.

Ward, D. B. January 1986. Why patient teaching fails. *RN* 49:45–47.

6

Client Comfort and Safety

OBJECTIVES

- Identify six psychosocial aspects of a client's environment

- Describe the characteristics of a safe and comfortable physical environment

- State three nursing diagnoses that apply to the safety of a client's environment

- List five types of fire extinguishers and when each should be used

- Explain six measures to prevent falls in hospitals

- Describe various kinds of restraints and situations in which each may be used

- Apply the restraints discussed in this chapter

- Identify appropriate assessments and care to clients with restraints

CONTENTS

A Client's Environment

Strategies in Response to Environmental Hazards

TECHNIQUE 6–1   Using an Ambularm Safety Monitoring Device

Restraining Clients

TECHNIQUE 6–2   Applying Restraints

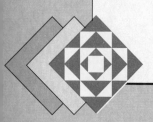

NURSING PROCESS GUIDE
CLIENT SAFETY

ASSESSMENT

Determine

- Age of client for ability to protect self.

- Client's level of awareness or consciousness, specifically, orientation to time, place, and person; ability to concentrate and make judgments; ability to assimilate many kinds of information at one time; ability to perceive reality accurately and act on those perceptions. Consider clients whose judgment is altered by medications, such as narcotics, tranquilizers, hypnotics, and sedatives.

- Life-style factors, such as risk-taking behavior and use of safety equipment.

- Sensory alterations, such as impaired vision, hearing, smell, tactile perception, and taste.

- Mobility status. Note in particular individuals who have muscle weakness, poor balance or coordination, or paralysis; those weakened by illness or surgery; and those who use ambulatory aids.

- Emotional state, which can alter the ability to perceive environmental hazards. Persons who are acutely anxious, angry, or depressed may have reduced perceptual awareness or may think and react to environmental stimuli more slowly.

- Ability to communicate. Individuals with diminished ability to receive and convey information (e.g., aphasic clients) and those with language barriers may not be able to read such safety signs as "No Smoking— Oxygen in Use."

- Previous accidents and frequency or predisposition to accidents.

- Safety knowledge about use of potentially dangerous equipment and precautions to take to prevent injury (e.g., fire safety, water safety, oxygen precautions, radiation protection, accident prevention).

RELATED DIAGNOSTIC CATEGORIES

- High risk for Injury
- High risk for Trauma
- High risk for Suffocation
- High risk for Poisoning

PLANNING

Client Goal
The client will experience no physical, mechanical, thermal, chemical, or radiation injury.

Outcome Criteria
The client

- Relates factors (e.g., physiologic) that increase the potential for injury.

- Identifies potentially hazardous factors in the environment.

- Identifies preventive measures for specific hazards (e.g., fire, falls, poisoning, burns).

- Reports an intent to carry out selected preventive measures.

- Identifies information about safety precautions and safety habits for children.

- Demonstrates appropriate use of countermeasures to protect self form injury.

- Alters physical environment to reduce risk of injury.

- Seeks instruction to (a) handle new equipment (e.g., household, occupational, or recreational) or (b) implement safe child-rearing practices.

A Client's Environment

Nurses care for clients in many environments. An **environment** is the aggregate of surrounding things, conditions, or influences, with particular reference to those aspects that affect the existence or development of people and other living things. Environments should be safe, comfortable, and therapeutic; that is, the environment should support the client's health (*Therapeutic* refers to therapy or cure.)

Psychosocial Environment

Two major aspects of the environment are the psychosocial and physical. The psychosocial environ-ment encompasses past and present influences from people and the culture or society. Aspects of the psychosocial environment that have a particular impact on clients are autonomy, life-style, and territoriality.

Autonomy
Autonomy is the state of being independent and self-directed without outside control. People vary in their sense of autonomy; some are accustomed to functioning independently in most of their life activities, whereas others are more accustomed to direction from others.

Hospitalized people frequently give up much of their autonomy. Decisions about meals, hygienic practices, and sleeping are frequently made for them. This loss of individuality is often difficult to accept, and the client may feel dehumanized into "just a piece of machinery."

 For the hospitalized child, autonomy has additional importance. Children at various stages of development require different degrees of autonomy to accomplish developmental tasks. Hospitalization may limit development if the child is restricted in activity or other needed stimulation. To perform the developmental tasks of infancy and early childhood, the child needs opportunities to develop self-control and control over the environment and to learn to live within set rules or restrictions.

Life-Style

Nurses can help clients adapt to life in a hospital in several ways:

- Providing explanations about hospital routines

- Making arrangements wherever possible to accommodate the client's life-style, such as providing a bath in the evening rather than in the morning.

- Encouraging other health professionals to become aware of the person's life-style and to support healthy aspects of that life-style.

- Reinforcing desirable changes in practices to help make them a permanent part of the client's lifestyle.

Territoriality

Territoriality is a concept of the space and things that individuals consider their own. Territories may be visible to others. For example, clients in a hospital often consider their territory the area bounded by the curtains around the bed unit or by the walls of a private room. All health care workers must recognize this human tendency to claim territory. Clients often feel the need to defend their territory when others invade it; for example, a visitor who removes a chair to use at another bed inadvertently violates the territoriality of the client whose chair is moved.

Physical Environment

A safe physical environment is one in which people can function without injury and feel a sense of security. A comfortable environment is one that is free from unpleasant stimuli to the senses of sight, smell, hearing, touch, and temperature.

Temperature and Humidity

Nurses may need to help clients adjust to uncomfortable temperatures. Warm socks, additional bedding, and shawls can provide added warmth, while a sponge bath may refresh and cool a client who is perspiring excessively on a hot day.

Generally, a humidity range of 30% to 60% is comfortable to most people. A very low humidity, such as 10%, is drying to the skin and mucous membranes of the air passages, and it accelerates the evaporation of perspiration. A high humidity, such as 90%, impedes the evaporation of perspiration and thus interferes with one of the body's major cooling mechanisms.

A highly humid environment is sometimes provided as a therapeutic measure. For example, cool air vaporizers or humidifiers may be used for clients with respiratory infections, since increasing the humidity of the inhaled air facilitates breathing. In other situations dehumidifiers are necessary, especially if the individual has an allergy to mold or mildew, since these frequently grow in humid environments. Many air conditioners regulate both temperature and humidity.

Lighting

Most health care facilities are designed to provide adequate natural and artificial light. Although many clients do not require or use night lights, children and the elderly often find them helpful for orienting themselves to strange surroundings at night and for getting to a bathroom. Nurses also use night-lights for observing critically ill clients throughout the night. For clients who have eye problems or have had eye surgery, nurses may need to dim overhead lights and natural light from the windows in the daytime, since the eyes may be photosensitive.

Noise

People who are ill are frequently sensitive to noises that normally would not disturb them. Nurses need to make a concerted effort to maintain a quiet, restful environment for all clients. Ways to control noise levels include the following:

- Reduce talking and laughing to a minimum, especially in long corridors, which tend to conduct sound.

- Wear shoes with rubber or soundless soles.

- Handle equipment and trays of dishes carefully.

- Help clients to keep television and radio volumes low. Most agencies supply earphones to prevent disturbance to adjacent clients.

- Monitor visiting hours and, when necessary, tactfully remind visitors of the need for quiet.

- Keep all conversations at low volumes.

Odors

Mild odors that normally are innocuous or even pleasant can be unpleasant to the ill person. Many people find that the smell of food cooking produces a feeling of nausea when they have the flu. Unpleasant scents may arise from refuse, such as dressings and body discharges. Ways to reduce odors include the following:

- Discard waste and refuse promptly.

- Empty bedpans, urinals, and emesis basins immediately after use, and clean them effectively.

- Change soiled linen promptly.

- Provide adequate ventilation.

Strategies in Response to Environmental Hazards

Fire

Fire is a constant danger in homes and hospitals. Common causes of fires are smoking in bed and faulty electrical equipment. Hospital fires are particularly hazardous to clients who are incapacitated and unable to leave the building without assistance. Many health care agencies have instituted no-smoking policies both to decrease the chances of fire and to promote employee and client health.

A fire can burn only if three elements are present: sufficient heat to start the fire, a combustible material, and sufficient oxygen to support the fire. To prevent fires, the nurse controls the environment to ensure that the three essential elements are not simultaneously present.

Health care agencies usually follow established procedures in an emergency or during a fire. Nurses need to become familiar with the practices of their employing agency. When a fire occurs, the nurse has two major goals:

1. To protect clients from injury

2. To contain and put out the fire

General protective practices to meet these goals include the following:

- Making sure the telephone numbers of emergency services are displayed on all telephones

- Knowing the location of fire exits

- Knowing the location and types of fire extinguishers and learning to operate them

- Learning the agency's fire drill or fire evacuation procedure

- Keeping access to firehoses clear at all times

- Keeping hallways free of unnecessary furniture and equipment

- Posting signs on elevator doors so that people will know to use the stairs in the event of fire

- Making sure the location of fire exits is clearly marked

In the event of fire, nurses follow the guidelines in the box below.

Carrying Clients from Fires

There are a number of methods of carrying persons from the scene of a fire. Generally, nurses use these carries when they cannot wheel out clients confined to their beds or transfer them out on stretchers. Non-nursing hospital personnel (e.g., maintenance, housekeeping, and dietary staff) may assist with evacuating clients and should receive inservice education on using these carries.

- *Swing carry.* The swing is a two-person carry used for heavy clients. The client, in a sitting position, places the arms around each nurse's shoulders. Each nurse holds the client's wrists, which are

---

Steps to Follow in the Event of Fire

- Evacuate clients who are in immediate danger. First, direct ambulatory clients to a safe area, or enlist their help in moving clients in wheelchairs. This clears the area for the evacuation of nonambulatory clients, who can be moved in a stretcher or bed, carried, or dragged on sheets and blankets.

- Activate the fire alarm if one is nearby.

- Notify the hospital switchboard of the location of the fire.

- If the fire is small, use the fire extinguisher on the fire.

- Close windows and doors in the area of the fire to reduce ventilation.

- Turn off oxygen and any electrical appliances in the vicinity of the fire.

- Clear fire exits, if necessary.

- Contain smoke as necessary by placing damp cloths or blankets around the outside edges of doors.

- Protect clients from smoke inhalation by giving them wet washcloths through which to breathe.

over each nurse's shoulders, to support the client. The nurses then reach behind the client and grasp each other's shoulder or upper arm. The nurses then release the client's wrists, reach under the client's thighs, and grasp each other's wrists. They lift and carry the client in this sitting position (Figure 6–1). This carry is sometimes referred to as the two-handed seat, in which a hand-forearm interlock is used. A variation is the four-handed seat (Figure 6–2), used for clients who are able to sit up with less support.

• *Pack strap carry.* The packstrap is a one-person carry. The nurse faces the seated client and grasps the wrists. The nurse's right hand grasps the client's left wrist; the left hand grasps the client's right wrist. The nurse then pivots and slips under one of the client's arms so that the nurse's back is to the client and the client's arms are crossed in front of the nurse. The nurse assumes a broad stance, one leg in front of the other, and rolls the client onto the nurse's back (Figure 6–3).

• *Piggy-back carry.* This carry is used for clients who are conscious and have some strength to help. The client sits at the edge of the bed. The nurse stands in front of the client with the back toward the client. The client reaches over the nurse's shoulders, and clasps the hands in front of the nurse while the nurse grasps the backs of the client's legs above the knees. With this carry,

the nurse can support the client's weight more easily than with the pack strap carry.

• *Cradle carry.* The cradle carry is used for children or adults who are light in weight. The nurse lifts the client by placing one arm beneath the person's knees and the other around the back.

Containing the Fire

Fires are categorized into four classes according to the type of material burning. Several types of fire

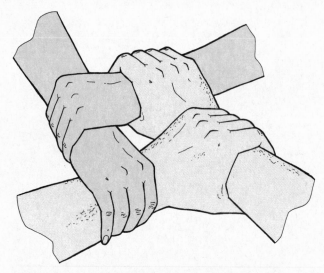

FIGURE 6–2 Position of hands for a four-handed seat.

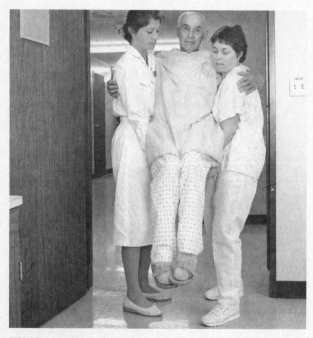

FIGURE 6–1 The swing carry.

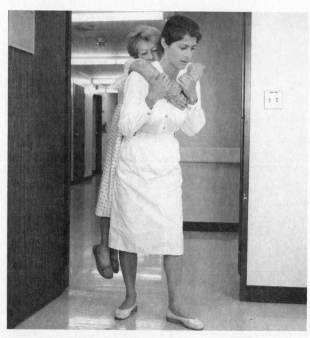

FIGURE 6–3 The pack strap carry.

extinguishers are in use today. The right type of extinguisher must be used to fight a fire. Fire extinguishers are now commonly labeled with picture symbols showing on which fires they should and should not be used. Directions for use are also attached to the extinguisher.

Scalds and Burns

A **scald** is a burn from a hot liquid or vapor, such as steam. A **burn** results from excessive exposure to thermal, chemical, electrical, or radioactive agents.

 In health care agencies, the risk of scalds and burns is greater for clients whose skin sensitivity to temperature is impaired. Scalds can occur from overly hot bath water or from overly hot moist dressings. Heat lamps can cause burns. It is important for the nurse to assess how well clients can protect themselves and what special precautions, if any, need to be taken.

Falls

Falls are common among the elderly ill or injured, who are weak. To prevent falls and subsequent injury of hospitalized clients, the nurse should consider the guidelines in the accompanying box.

Some agencies have a protocol to prevent client falls. Technique 6–1 shows how to use the Ambularm safety monitoring device.

Preventing Falls in Hospitals

- On admission, orient clients to their surroundings, and explain the call system.
- Carefully assess the client's ability to ambulate and transfer; provide walking aids and assistance as required.
- Closely supervise the clients at risk for falls during the first few days, especially at night.
- Encourage the client to use call bell to request assistance; ensure that the bell is within easy reach.
- Place beside tables and overbed tables near the bed or chair so that clients do not overreach and consequently lose their balance.
- Always keep hospital beds in the low position when not providing care so that clients can move in or out of bed easily.
- Encourage clients to use grab bars mounted in toilet and bathing areas and railings along corridors.
- Make sure nonskid bath mats are available in tubs and showers.
- Encourage the client to wear nonskid footwear.
- Keep the environment tidy, especially keep light cords from underfoot and furniture out of the way.
- Attach side rails to the beds of confused, sedated, restless, and unconscious clients, and keep the rails in place when the client is unattended.

 6-1 ## Using an Ambularm Safety Monitoring Device

The Ambularm is an electronic device with a position-sensitive switch that triggers an audio alarm when the client attempts to get out of bed unassisted. When activated, the alarm alerts the nurse and provides an opportunity for the nurse to intervene.

PURPOSES
- To alert the nurse that the client is attempting to get out of bed
- To help decrease the risk of client falls

ASSESSMENT FOCUS

Mobility status; judgment about ability to get out of bed safely; skin integrity of leg to which band is applied; vascular status of leg; proximity of client's room to nurses' station; position of side rails and functioning status of call light.

EQUIPMENT
- Alarm device
- Leg band of appropriate size
- Ambularm sticker

▸ Technique 6–1 Using an Ambularm *CONTINUED*

INTERVENTION

1. Explain to client and support persons the purpose and procedure of using safety monitoring device.

- Explain that the device does not limit mobility in any manner; rather, it alerts the staff when the client is about to get out of bed.

- Explain that the nurse must be called when the client needs to get out of bed.

2. Measure for proper size of leg band. Measure thigh circumference just above the knee with the tape measure:

- For a thigh circumference of up to 18 inches, use a regular size band.

- For a thigh circumference of 18 inches or larger, use a large size band.

3. Test the battery device and alarm sound. Touch alarm snaps on the Ambularm device to the corresponding snaps on the leg band (Figure 6–4). *This ensures that the device is functioning properly prior to use.*

4. Apply the Ambularm.

- Place the leg band just above the knee (Figure 6–5).

- Securely snap the Ambularm onto the leg band at the corresponding snap junctions (Figure 6–6). *This activates the position-sensitive alarm device.*

- Place the client's leg in a straight horizontal position. *The alarm device is position-sensitive; i.e., when it approaches a near-vertical position (such as in walking, crawling, or kneeling as the client attempts to get out of bed), the audio alarm is triggered, causing a sharp, shrill sound* (Figure 6–7).

5. Instruct the client to call the nurse when the client wants or needs to get up, and assist as required.

- When assisting the client up, deactivate the alarm by unsnapping the alarm device from the elastic band (Figure 6–8).

- Assist the client back to bed, and reattach the alarm device to the leg band.

6. Ensure client safety with additional safety precautions.

- Place call light within client reach, lift all side rails, and lower the bed to its lowest position. *The alarm device is not a substitute for other precautionary measures.*

- Periodically assess the skin and vascular status of leg being used.

- Place ambulation monitoring stickers on the client's door, chart, and Kardex.

7. Document relevant data.

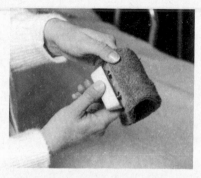

FIGURE 6–4 Testing an Ambularm by contacting corresponding snaps on the leg band.

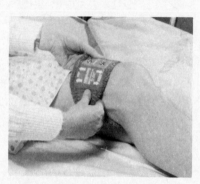

FIGURE 6–5 Placing the leg band around the leg just above the knee.

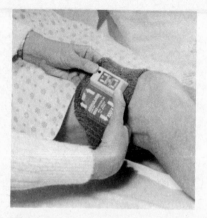

FIGURE 6–6 Attaching the Ambularm to the leg band.

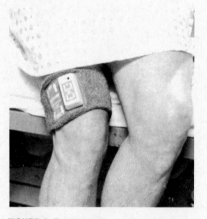

FIGURE 6–7 Triggering of the alarm when the leg is in a near-vertical position.

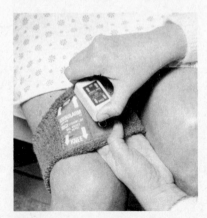

FIGURE 6–8 Detaching the Ambularm from the leg band.

- Record that ambulation device is intact when applied.

- Record all assessments.

- Record all safety precautions and interventions discussed and employed.

▶ **Technique 6–1** *CONTINUED*

<table>
<tr><td>**EVALUATION
FOCUS**</td><td colspan="3">Status of the Ambularm device; effectiveness of safety precautions.</td></tr>
</table>

SAMPLE RECORDING

Date	Time	Notes
5/2/93	1515	Returned to room following TUPR. Irrigation system and retention catheter patent. Urine bright red. BP 118/78 P 88. Disoriented to time and place. States "I must go milk the cows." Trying to get out of bed. Side rails up. Explained x 2 about need to stay in bed. Wife present during both explanations. ———— Laurie R. Ens, RN
	1530	Wife unable to stay. Remains disoriented. Ambularm applied to L leg. Skin intact and pedal pulse strong (88). Side rails up and call light within reach. ———— Laurie R. Ens, RN

KEY ELEMENTS OF USING AN AMBULARM SAFETY MONITORING DEVICE

- Test the device for function.
- Measure the leg band correctly.
- Snap the Ambularm on the leg band correctly.

- Evaluate the skin and vascular status of leg.
- Use additional safety precautions (side rails, call light, correct bed position).

Poisoning

A **poison** is any substance that injures or kills through its chemical action when inhaled, injected, applied, or absorbed in relatively small amounts. For certain poisons, specific antidotes or treatments are available; for many, there is no specific therapy.

The major reasons for poisoning in children are inadequate supervision and improper storage of many household toxic substances. Adolescent and adult poisonings are usually caused by insect or snake bites and drugs used for recreation or in suicide attempts. Poisoning in elderly people usually is a result of accidental ingestion of a toxic substance due to failing eyesight or an overdose of a prescribed medication due to impaired memory.

The box on page 94 provides guidelines in teaching clients to prevent poisoning.

Electric Shock

Nurses need to use electrical equipment that is properly **grounded** (that transmits an electric current from an object or surface to the ground). The electrical plug of grounded equipment has three prongs. The two short prongs transmit the power to the equipment. The third, longer prong is the grounding device, which carries short circuits or stray electric current to the ground (Figure 6–9). Grounding prongs offer a path of least resistance to stray electric currents.

Faulty equipment, e.g., a frayed cord, presents a danger of electric shock. Also, faulty electrical equipment can start fires. For example, an electric spark near certain anesthetic gases or a high concentration of oxygen may cause a serious fire.

Radiation

Radiation as a health hazard is a recent source of concern. Nurses are concerned specifically with those radioactive materials used in diagnostic and therapeutic practices. Radiation injury can occur from overexposure or from exposure to radiation that treats specific tissues and at the same time injures other tissues.

Radioactive materials are used in such diagnostic procedures as radiography, fluoroscopy, and nuclear medicine. In nuclear medicine, radioactive isotopes

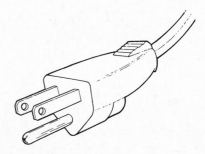

FIGURE 6–9 Three-pronged ground plug.

CLIENT TEACHING

Preventing Poisoning

- Place potentially toxic agents, including drugs and cleaning agents, out of reach of crawling infants.

- Lock cleaning agents in a cupboard, or attach special plastic hooks to the inside of cabinet doors to keep them securely closed. Unlatching these hooks requires firmer thumb pressure than small children can usually exert.

- Avoid storing toxic liquids or solids in food containers, such as soft drink bottles, peanut butter jars, or milk cartons.

- Do not remove container labels or reuse empty containers to store different substances. Laws mandate that the labels of all poisons specify antidotes.

- Keep poisonous house plants out of reach of young children. Be able to identify the poisonous plants in your neighborhood.

- Do not rely on cooking to destroy toxic chemicals in plants. Never use anything prepared from nature as a medicine or "tea."

- Teach children never to eat any part of an unknown plant or mushroom and not to put leaves, stems, bark, seeds, nuts, or berries from any plant into their mouths.

- Do not take medications in front of children. They may imitate you.

- Never call medicine "candy" when giving it to children.

- Read and follow label directions on all products before using them.

- Keep syrup of ipecac on hand at all times. Syrup of ipecac is a nonprescription emetic available in single-dose 15 ml vials in all drugstores. Use it only after advice from the local poison control center or the family physician.

- Display the phone number of the poison control center near or on all telephones in the home so that it is available to baby-sitters, family, and friends.

that have an affinity for specific tissues are given orally or intravenously.

Radioactive materials are provided in sealed sources and unsealed liquid sources. For example, cobalt implants are sealed; iodine 131 and phosphorus 32 are unsealed liquids. Principles governing the degree of exposure to radiation are as follows:

- The longer the time in the presence of radiation, the greater the exposure.

- The closer a person is to the radioactive source, the greater the exposure.

- The more extensive the use of lead and other radiation shields, the greater the protection against radiation.

Nurses often care for clients treated or diagnosed with radioactive substances. The client diagnosed through radiography or fluoroscopy generally receives minimal exposure, and few precautions are necessary. The nurse restraining a small child during radiography needs to wear a lead apron. Clients with radioactive implants are a source of radiation to the immediate environment. The nurse who is in close contact with such clients also needs to wear a lead apron.

Nurses must deal safely with radioactive body discharges by wearing gloves and in some instances placing excreta in containers for special disposal. The nurse must wash gloved hands well before and after

removing the gloves and place contaminated materials in a special container for disposal.

One important aspect of caring for clients receiving radiation treatment is making sure they understand the treatment and the precautions they need to take. Often such clients are restricted to bed or to a confined area to protect others. These clients need emotional support to deal with the precautions and will likely accept treatments and precautions better when they know what will happen, when, and why.

Restraining Clients

Restraints are protective devices used to limit the physical activity of the client or a part of the body. Restraints can be classified as physical or chemical. *Physical restraints* are any manual method or physical or mechanical device, material, or equipment attached to the client's body; they cannot be removed easily and they restrict the client's movement. *Chemical restraints* are medications such as neuroleptics, anxiolytics, sedatives, and psychotropic agents used to control socially disruptive behavior.

Because restraints restrict the individual's ability to move freely, their use has legal implications. In some settings, the nurse makes the decision to use a restraint; in others, a physician must make the decision. Often a nurse can apply a restraint as a temporary emergency measure. Nurses need to know their agency's policies and the state or provincial laws about restraining clients. Increasingly, determining the need for safety measures is viewed as an independent nursing function.

Restrained clients often become restless and anxious as a result of the loss of self-control. Nurses may need to remain with the restrained client and speak quietly to give reassurance and allay distress. Understanding why the body part has to be kept relatively still helps the client to view the restraint as a protective measure.

The nurse must document the type of restraint used, the exact times the restraint was applied and removed, the client's behavior before and with the restraint, care given while the restraint was applied, and notification of the physician. Nurses must explain the need for the restraint, both to the client and to support persons, and document the substance of these explanations.

Selecting a Restraint

Before selecting a restraint, nurses need to understand its purpose clearly and measure it against the following five criteria:

1. It restricts the client's movement as little as possible. If a client needs to have one arm restrained, do not restrain the entire body.

2. It is the least obvious to others. Both clients and visitors are often embarrassed by a restraint, even though they understand why it is being used. The less obvious the restraint, the more comfortable people feel.

3. It does not interfere with the client's treatment or health problem. If a client has poor blood circulation to the hands, apply a restraint that will not aggravate that circulatory problem.

4. It is readily changeable. Restraints need to be changed frequently, especially if they become soiled. Keeping other guidelines in mind, choose a restraint that can be changed with minimal disturbance to the client.

5. It is safe for the particular client. Choose a restraint with which the client cannot self-inflict injury. For example, a physically active child could incur injury trying to climb out of a crib if one wrist is tied to the side of the crib. A jacket restraint would restrain the child more safely.

Kinds of Restraints

There are several kinds of restraints. Among the most common are the jacket restraint, the belt restraint, the mitt or hand restraint, limb restraints, elbow restraints, mummy restraints, and crib nets. Geri chairs, wheelchairs, and bedsheets used to confine client activity can also be considered restraints. There are several types of *jacket restraints*, but all are essentially sleeveless jackets (vests) with straps (tails) that can be tied to the bed frame under the mattress or to the legs of a chair (Figure 6–10). The jacket may be put on with the ties at the front or at the back, depending on the type. Jackets intended to open at the front must be applied in this manner. These body restraints are used to ensure the safety of confused or sedated clients in bed or wheelchairs.

Belt or safety strap body restraints (Figure 6–11) are used to ensure the safety of all clients who are being moved on stretchers or in wheelchairs. Some

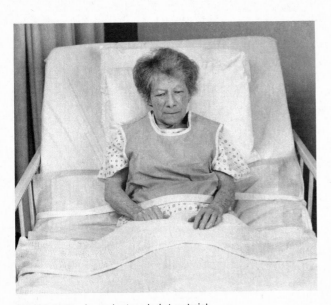

FIGURE 6–10 A poncho-type jacket restraint.

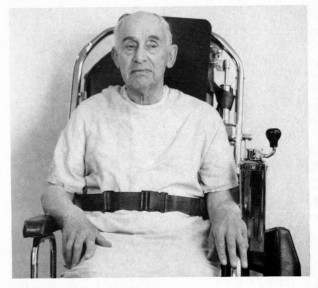

FIGURE 6–11 A belt restraint.

wheelchairs have a soft padded safety bar that attaches to side brackets that are installed under the arm rests. To prevent the person from slumping forward, the nurse then attaches a shoulder "Y" strap to the bar and over the client's shoulders to the rear handles. Other safety belt models have a three-loop design. One loop surrounds the person's waist and attaches to the rear kick spurs; a second loop connects the first loop to the third loop, which crosses over the shoulders and attaches to the rear handles. If such restraints are unattainable, the nurse can place a folded towel or small sheet around the client's waist and fasten it at the back of the wheelchair. Belt restraints may also be used for certain clients confined to bed or to chairs.

A *mitt or hand restraint* (Figure 6–12) is used to prevent confused clients from using their hands or fingers to scratch and injure themselves. For example, a confused client may need to be prevented from pulling at intravenous tubing or a head bandage following brain surgery. Hand or mitt restraints allow the client to be ambulatory and/or to move the arm freely rather than be confined to a bed or a chair. Mitt restraints are commercially available. Also, nurses can make hand restraints using large dressings and stockinette. See Technique 6–2. Mittens need to be removed at least every two hours to permit the client to wash and exercise the hands. The nurse also needs to take off the mitten regularly to check the circulation to the hand.

Limb restraints (Figure 6–13), which are generally made of cloth, may be used to immobilize a limb, primarily for therapeutic reasons (e.g., to maintain an intravenous infusion). Some commercially prepared restraints are available. Nurses can also improvise a clove hitch limb restraint using padded dressing and gauze.

Elbow restraints (Figure 6–14) are used to prevent infants or small children from flexing their elbows to touch or scratch a skin lesion or to reach the head when a scalp vein infusion is in place. This restraint consists of a piece of material with pockets into which plastic or wooden tongue depressors are inserted to provide rigidity.

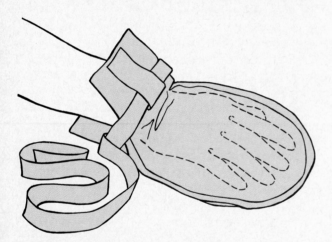

FIGURE 6–12   A commercially made mitt restraint.

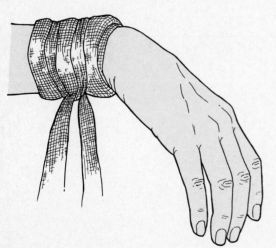

FIGURE 6–13   A limb restraint.

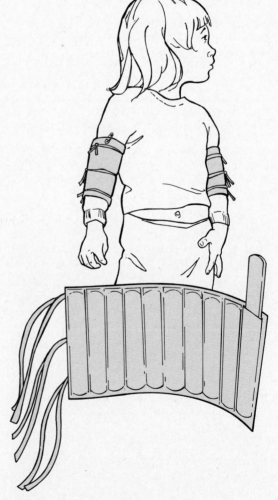

FIGURE 6–14   An elbow restraint for a young child.

The *mummy restraint* (Figure 6–15) is a special folding of a blanket or sheet around the child to prevent movement during a procedure such as gastric washing, eye irrigation, or collection of a blood specimen. A *crib net* or *dome* (Figure 6–16) is simply a device placed over the top of a crib to prevent active young children from climbing out of the crib. At the same time, it allows them freedom to move about in the crib. The crib net or dome is not attached to the movable parts of the crib so that the caregiver can have access to the child without removing the dome or net.

When using restraints, the nurse may find the guidelines in the box below helpful.

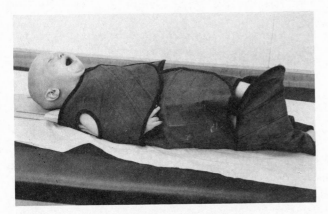

FIGURE 6–15   A commercially made mummy restraint.

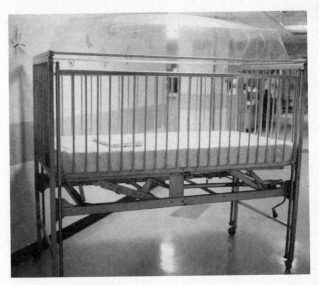

FIGURE 6–16   A crib dome.

CLINICAL GUIDELINES

Applying Restraints

- Assure the client and the client's support persons that the restraint is temporary and protective. A restraint must never be applied as punishment for any behavior or merely for the nurse's convenience.

- Apply the restraint in such a way that the client can move as freely as possible without defeating the purpose of the restraint.

- Ensure that limb restraints are applied securely but not so tightly that they impede blood circulation to any body area or extremity.

- Pad bony prominences (e.g., wrists and ankles) before applying a restraint over them. The movement of a restraint without padding over such prominences can quickly abrade the skin.

- Always tie a limb restraint with a knot, e.g., a clove hitch, that will not tighten when pulled.

- Tie the ends of a body restraint to the part of the bed that moves when the head is elevated. Never tie the ends to a side rail or to the fixed frame of the bed if the bed position is to be changed.

- Assess the restraint every 30 minutes. Some facilities have specific forms to be used to record ongoing assessment.

- Release all restraints at least every 2 to 4 hours, and provide range-of-motion (ROM) exercises (see Chapter 21) and skin care (see Chapter 15).

- Reassess the continued need for the restraint every 8 hours. Include an assessment of the underlying cause of the behavior necessitating use of the restraints.

- When a restraint is temporarily removed, do not leave the client unattended.

- Immediately report to the nurse in charge and record on the client's chart any persistent reddened or broken skin areas under the restraint.

- At the first indication of cyanosis or pallor, coldness of a skin area, or a client's complaint of a tingling sensation, pain, or numbness, loosen the restraint and exercise the limb.

- Apply a restraint so that it can be released quickly in case of an emergency and with the body part in a normal anatomic position.

- Provide emotional support verbally and through touch.

6-2 **Applying Restraints**

PURPOSE To enable the reception of treatment and to allow the treatment to proceed without client interference, e.g., to prevent movements that would disrupt therapy to a limb connected to tubes or appliance.

ASSESSMENT FOCUS Behavior indicating the possible need for a restraint; underlying cause for assessed behavior (to ascertain what other protective measures may be implemented before applying a restraint); status of skin to which restraint is to be applied; circulatory status of extremities; effectiveness of other available safety precautions.

EQUIPMENT

Select the kind and size of restraint required by the client. See "Selecting a Restraint," earlier in this chapter. If a commercial hand, wrist, or ankle restraint is not available, the supplies that follow are needed.

Mitt Restraint
- Four large padded dressings, e.g., ABD pads
- Pieces of thick gauze
- Stockinette dressing or elastic bandage
- Adhesive tape

Wrist or Ankle Restraint
- Padded or thick gauze dressing, e.g., an ABD pad
- Strip of gauze bandage or cloth tie 5 to 8 cm (2 to 3 in) wide and 90 to 120 cm (3 to 4 ft) long

---

INTERVENTION

1. Explain to client and support persons the purpose and procedure of using restraint.

2. Apply the selected restraint.

Belt Restraint (Safety Belt)

- Determine that the safety belt is in good order. If a Velcro safety belt is to be used, make sure that both pieces of Velcro are intact.

- If the belt has a long portion and a shorter portion, place the long portion of the belt behind (under) the bedridden client and secure it to the movable part of the bed frame. *The long attached portion will then move up when the head of the bed is elevated and will not tighten around the client.* Place the shorter portion of the belt around the client's waist, over the gown. There should be a finger's width between the belt and the client.

or

Attach the belt around the client's waist, and fasten it at the back of the chair.

or

If the belt is attached to a stretcher, secure the belt firmly over the client's hips or abdomen. Belt restraints need to be applied to all clients on stretchers even when the side rails are up.

Jacket Restraint

- Place vest on client, with opening at the front or the back, depending on the type.

- Pull the tie on the end of the vest flap across the chest, and place it through the slit in the opposite side of the chest.

- Repeat for the other tie.

- Use a half-bow knot to secure each tie around the movable bed frame or behind the chair to a chair leg (Figure 6–17). *A half-*

bow knot does not tighten or slip when the attached end is pulled but unties easily when the loose end is pulled.

or

Fasten the ties together behind the chair using a square (reef) knot (Figure 6–18). *This knot does not tighten with pulling and does not slip when pressure is released.*

- Ensure that the client is positioned appropriately to enable maximum chest expansion for breathing.

Mitt Restraint

- Apply the commercial thumbless mitt (Figure 6–12, earlier) to the hand to be restrained. Make sure the fingers can be slightly flexed and are not caught under the hand.

- Follow the manufacturer's directions for securing the mitt.

Technique 6–2 Applying Restraints *CONTINUED*

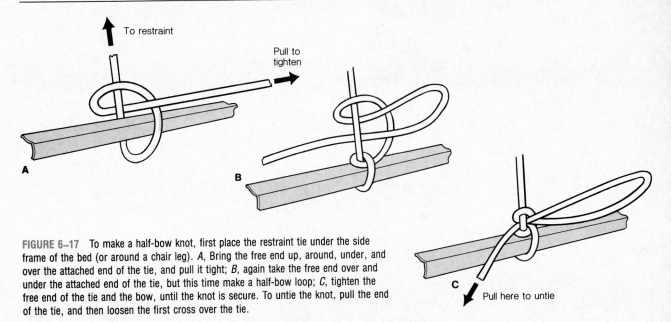

FIGURE 6–17   To make a half-bow knot, first place the restraint tie under the side frame of the bed (or around a chair leg). *A*, Bring the free end up, around, under, and over the attached end of the tie, and pull it tight; *B*, again take the free end over and under the attached end of the tie, but this time make a half-bow loop; *C*, tighten the free end of the tie and the bow, until the knot is secure. To untie the knot, pull the end of the tie, and then loosen the first cross over the tie.

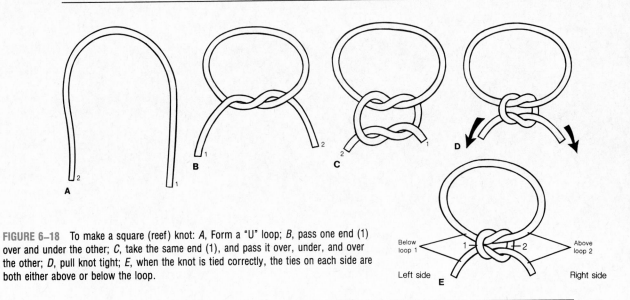

FIGURE 6–18   To make a square (reef) knot: *A*, Form a "U" loop; *B*, pass one end (1) over and under the other; *C*, take the same end (1), and pass it over, under, and over the other; *D*, pull knot tight; *E*, when the knot is tied correctly, the ties on each side are both either above or below the loop.

- If there is no commercial mitt, make a mitt as follows:

  a. Place a large folded dressing, such as an abdominal (ABD) pad, in the client's palm. Ensure that the hand is in a natural position with the fingers slightly flexed.

  b. Separate the fingers with pieces of large dressing or thick gauze. *This prevents skin abrasion.*

c. Put a padded dressing around the client's wrist. *This prevents pressure and skin abrasion.*

d. Place two large dressings (ABD pads) over the hand. Place the first one from the back of the hand over the fingers to the palm; then wrap the other from side to side around the hand.

e. Cover these dressings by placing a stockinette dressing over the hand or wrapping them with an elastic bandage, using a recurrent pattern. See Figure 40–5, on page 000. See also Chapter 40 for basic turns used in bandaging.

f. Secure the stockinette or elastic bandage with adhesive tape.

► Technique 6–2 Applying Restraints CONTINUED

• If a mitt is to be worn for several days, remove it at least every 2 to 4 hours. Wash and exercise the client's hand, then reapply the mitt. Check agency practices about recommended intervals for removal.

• Assess the client's circulation to the hands shortly after the mitt is applied and at regular intervals. *Feelings of numbness or discomfort or inability to move the fingers could indicate impaired circulation to the hand.*

Wrist or Ankle Restraint

• Apply the padded portion of a commercially prepared restraint around the ankle or wrist.
or
Improvise a restraint as follows:

a. Cushion the wrist or ankle with a padded or thick gauze dressing, e.g., an ABD pad.

b. Wrap a long, narrow strip of gauze bandage or a cloth tie around the padding.

• Pull the tie of the commercially made restraint through the slit in the wrist portion or through the buckle.
or
Use a clove hitch to secure the gauze strip or cloth tie of the improvised restraint (Figure 6–19). *The clove hitch knot does not tighten with pulling and is readily released.*

• Using a half-bow knot or a square knot as appropriate, attach the other end of the commercial restraint (or the two ends of the improvised restraint)

to the movable portion of the bed frame. *If the ties are attached to the movable portion, the wrist or ankle will not be pulled when the bed position is changed.*

Elbow Restraint

• Examine the restraint to make sure that the tongue depressors are intact, i.e., all in place and not broken.

• Place the infant's elbow in the center of the restraint. Make sure that the ends of the tongue depressors are covered by the padded material. *This prevents them from irritating the skin.*

• Wrap the restraint smoothly around the arm.

• Secure the restraint, using safety pins, ties, or tape. Ensure that it is not so tight that it obstructs blood circulation.

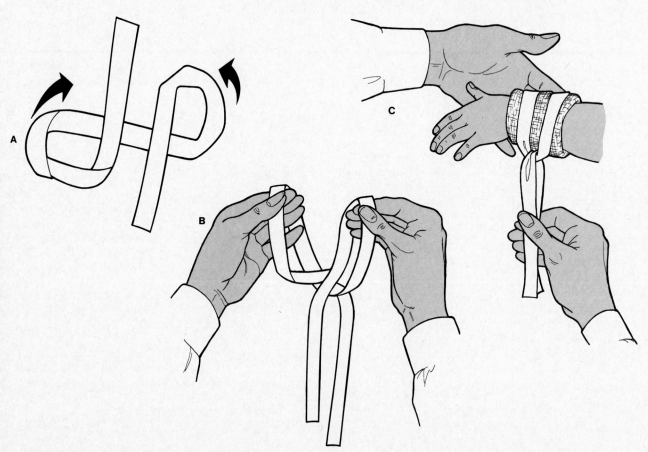

FIGURE 6–19 To make a clove hitch: *A*, make a figure-eight; *B*, pick up the loops; *C*, put the limb through the loops, and secure it.

▶ **Technique 6–2** *CONTINUED*

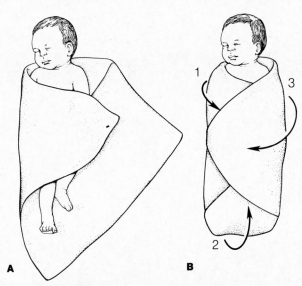

FIGURE 6–20 Making a mummy restraint.

• (Optional) After the restraint is applied, pin it to the child's shirt. *This prevents it from sliding down the arm.*

▶ **Mummy Restraint**

• Obtain a blanket or sheet large enough so that the distance between opposite corners is about twice the length of the infant's body. Lay the blanket or sheet on a flat dry surface.

• Fold down one corner, and place the baby on it in the supine position.

• Fold the right side of the blanket over the infant's body, leaving the left arm free (Figure 6–20, A). The right arm is in a natural position at the side.

• Fold the excess blanket at the bottom up under the infant (Figure 6–20, B[2]).

• With the left arm in a natural position at the baby's side, fold the left side of the blanket over the infant, including the arm, and tuck the blanket under the body (Figure 6–20, B[3]).

• Remain with the infant who is in a mummy restraint until the specific procedure is completed.

▶ **Crib Net**

• Place the net over the sides and ends of the crib.

• Secure the ties to the springs or frame of the crib. *The crib sides can then be freely lowered without removing the net.*

• Test with your hand that the net will stretch if the child stands in the crib against it.

3. Document relevant information for all kinds of restraints.

• Record on the client's chart the time the physician was notified, the type of restraint applied, the time it was applied, the reason for its application, the client's response to the restraint, and the times that the restraints are removed and skin care given.

• Record any other interventions, assessments, and explanations to client and significant others. See sample recording below.

• Adjust the nursing care plan as required, e.g., to include releasing the restraint q2h, providing skin care, and providing ROM exercises.

EVALUATION FOCUS

Client response to restraint; circulatory status of restrained limbs; skin status beneath restraints.

SAMPLE RECORDING

Date	Time	Notes
9/29/93	0320	Found climbing over side rails. Explained possibility of falling and injury. Sat with client for 10 minutes. She continued to try to climb over side rails. Stated "Don't know where I am." ———————————————— Edward R. King, NS
	0330	Dr. Singh notified. Jacket restraint applied. ————————Edward R. King, NS
	0345	Daughter with client. Resting more comfortably. Restraint removed. ————
	0400	130 ml clear fluid taken. Voided. ————————————Edward R. King, NS

▶ **Technique 6–2 Applying Restraints** *CONTINUED*

KEY ELEMENTS OF APPLYING RESTRAINTS

- Use means other than restraints as much as possible, and stay with the client.
- When restraints are used, explain the reasons for and the protective nature of the restraints to clients and support persons.
- Obtain a physician's order for the restraint.
- Pad bony prominences, such as wrists and ankles, before applying a restraint over them.
- Tie restraints with knots that will not tighten when pulled and to parts of the bed that move when the bed is elevated.
- Remove limb restraints at least every 4 hours, and provide ROM exercises and skin care. Remove mitt restraints at least every 2 hours.

- Assess restrained limbs for signs of impaired blood circulation.
- Always stay with a client whose restraint is temporarily removed.
- Document notification of the physician, the type of restraint used, other protective measures tried and found ineffective, exact times the restraint was applied and removed, the client's behavior before and with the restraint, care given while the restraint was applied, and information given to the client and support persons.

CRITICAL THINKING CHALLENGE

Gladys Henderson is an 82-year-old female who has been admitted to an extended care facility because she is no longer able to live on her own. She has impaired coordination and is occasionally confused. What information do you need when planning interventions to protect her safety? How might you ensure her safety while still considering her basic needs for privacy, autonomy, and self-esteem?

RELATED RESEARCH

Craven, R., and Bruno, P. August 1986. Teach the elderly to prevent falls. *Journal of Gerontological Nursing* 12:27–33.
Johnston, J. E. November 1988. The elderly and fall prevention. *Applied Nursing Research* 1:140.
Wolf-Klein, G. B.; Silverstone, F. A.; Basavaraju, N.; et al. September 1988. Prevention of falls in the elderly population. *Archives of Physical Medicine and Rehabilitation* 69:689–91.

SELECTED REFERENCES

Berger, M. E., and Hubner, K. F. August 1983. Hospital hazards: Diagnostic radiation. *American Journal of Nursing.* 83:1155–59.
Brammer, L. M. 1988. *The helping relationship: Process and skills,* 4th ed. Englewood Cliffs, N. J.: Prentice-Hall.
Campbell, E. B.; Williams, M. A.; and Mlynarczyk, S. M. February 1986. After the fall: Confusion. *American Journal of Nursing* 86:151–53.
Carpenito, L. J. 1989. *Nursing diagnosis: Application to clinical practice.* 3d ed. Philadelphia: J. B. Lippincott Co.
Dallaire, L. B., and Burke, E. V. January 1989. A new program for reducing patient falls. *Nursing 89* 19:65.
Denomy, E. B. April 1990. Accidental killers. *Canadian Nurse* 86:22–24.
Easterling, M. L. January 1990. Which of your patients is headed for a fall? *RN* 53:56–59.
Fitzgibbon, M., and Roberts, F. M. 1988. Prevention of accidents to hospital patients. *Recent Advances in Nursing* (22): 33–48.
Friedman, F. B. January 1983. Restraints: When all else fails, there still are alternatives. *RN* 46:79–80, 82, 84.
Hall, E. T. 1969. *The hidden dimension.* Garden City, N. Y.: Doubleday and Co.
Hernandez, M., and Miller, J. March/April 1986. How to reduce falls. *Geriatric Nursing* 7:97–102.
Houston, K. A., and Lach, H. W. September/October 1990. Restraints: How do you score? *Geriatric Nursing* 11:231–32.
Innes, E. M., and Thurman, W. G. February 1983. Evaluation of patient falls. *Quality Review Bulletin* 9:30–35.
Kim, M. J.; McFarland, G. K.; and McLane, A. M. 1989. *Pocket guide to nursing diagnoses.* 3d ed. St. Louis: C. V. Mosby Co.

McHutchion, E., and Morse, J. M. February 1989. Releasing restraints: A nursing dilemma. *Journal of Gerontological Nursing* 15:16–21.

Schuster, E. A. October 1976. Privacy: The patient and hospitalization. *Social science medicine* 10:245.

Smith, D. P., editor. 1991. *Comprehensive child and family nursing skills.* St. Louis: Mosby-Year Book, Inc.

Tideiksaar, R. July 1989. Restraint use declines as fall prevention options rise. *Provider* 15:35–36.

————. November/December 1989. Home safe home: Practical tips for fall-proofing. *Geriatric Nursing* 10:280–84.

Whaley, L. F., and Wong, D. 1991. *Nursing care of infants and children,* 4th ed. St. Louis: Mosby-Year Book, Inc.

Widder, B. September/October 1985. A new device to decrease falls. *Geriatric Nursing* 6:287–88.

Wyatt, D. M. February 1985. Are you prepared for a hospital fire? *Nursing 85* 15:51.

Admissions

7

OBJECTIVES

• Identify preliminary admission procedures

• Describe the essential activities in preparing a client's room prior to admission

• List information needed to orient a client to the agency

• Describe policies related to handling of clothes, valuables, and medications

• Explain rationales for routine admission tests

• Discuss the importance of determining the client's allergies

CONTENTS

Admission Practices and Trends

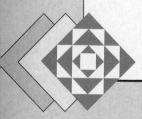

NURSING PROCESS GUIDE
ADMISSIONS

ASSESSMENT

Observe general appearance and responses

- Sex, race
- Posture and gait
- General condition (e.g., alert, oriented, lethargic, cachectic)
- Respiratory status (e.g., wheezing, coughing, shortness of breath)
- Skin condition: color, temperature, turgor, lesions, abrasions, decubitus ulcers, scars
- Mobility
- Affect/mood/self-perception
  - Revealed through verbal responses to explanation and greetings
  - Revealed through nonverbal behaviors
- Behaviors indicative of stress (e.g., increased muscle tension, clammy hands and skin, false cheerfulness)
 For children observe
  - Age and apparent as well as anticipated developmental stage
  - Temperament—usual adjustment to new people, places, and routines

Measure

- Height and weight
- Vital signs
  - Temperature, pulse, respirations
  - Blood pressure

Determine

- Current health status and past health history
  - Reason for admission
  - Past illness and previous agency admissions
  - Current medications, their dosages and frequency
  - Allergies to food, medications, and substances that may cause contact dermatitis (soaps, creams, lotions, ointments)
  - Immunization status (for children and elderly)
  - Substance use/abuse (e.g., tobacco, alcohol, coffee, tea, colas, sleeping or mood-altering medications, mind-altering drugs such as marijuana)

- Activities of daily living
  - Eating pattern (usual times of eating, food preferences, special diets)
  - Sleep/rest pattern (difficulties sleeping, use of aids to facilitate sleep, rest patterns)
  - Elimination pattern (problems with urinary or fecal elimination and how managed; use of laxatives)
  - Activity/exercise pattern (mobility or activity limitations; usual exercise, activity, leisure, and recreation)
  - Use of prostheses (presence and management of dentures; eyeglasses; contact lenses; hearing aids; wigs; mastectomy or limb prostheses; colostomy, ileostomy, or ureterostomy appliance)
- Social and family data
  - Ability or desire of family member to remain with pediatric client throughout hospital stay, or during the night or daytime hours
  - Languages spoken (document the fact that English is a second language or not well spoken and understood)
  - Occupation or school (note feelings about how illness will affect employment or education)
  - Family/home situation (family members and effect of client's illness on them)
  - Religious practices and how these can be supported throughout hospitalization
  - Financial concerns about health care

RELATED DIAGNOSTIC CATEGORIES

- Anxiety
- Activity intolerance
- Fatigue
- Potential altered growth and development
- Potential ineffective family coping: Compromised
- High risk for infection
- High risk for injury
- Knowledge deficit (specify)
- Impaired physical mobility
- Pain
- Self-care deficits: Bathing/hygiene, dressing/grooming, feeding, toileting
- Sensory/perceptual alterations: Visual, auditory, kinesthetic, gustatory, tactile, olfactory (specify)
- Impaired skin integrity
- Altered thought processes

Continued on page 106

Nursing Process Guide *CONTINUED*

PLANNING

Client Goal
The client will experience minimal anxiety while adapting to the nursing unit (hospitalization).

Outcome Criteria
The client

- Manifests minimal signs of anxiety or fear, e.g., absence of (a) excessive sympathetic stimulation such as increased pulse rate, blood pressure, res-

piratory rate, muscle tension; (b) insomnia; (c) feelings of restlessness.

- Manifests minimal disruption of developmental advancement during hospitalization.

- Communicates appropriately with other clients and staff.

- Participates in plan of care.

- Reports feelings of psychologic and physiologic comfort.

Admission Practices and Trends

Entering a health care facility is a stressful experience for clients. They may or may not be in discomfort, but most—if not all—feel anxious. Relatives and friends are also worried. Thus, the first contact of the client and the support persons with personnel in the facility is extremely important. Admitting and health care personnel need to convey kindness, concern, and competence in what they do.

Each health care agency has established policies and procedures for the admission of clients, the transfer of clients within the agency and to outside agencies, and the discharge of clients. This chapter focuses on the admission procedures common to many agencies. Chapter 8 presents transfer and discharge procedures.

Recent admission nursing practices in North American agencies include preadmission clinics or screening programs and home visits. These practices are implemented for clients requiring elective surgery and for elderly clients entering nursing homes.

Preadmission Clinics

Preadmissions are usually scheduled 6 to 14 days before the client's surgery. All support persons are encouraged to attend. Overall goals of preadmission clinics for elective surgery clients are to facilitate client recoveries, decrease client stays, and generally improve the use of beds and outpatient services.

Care at the clinics includes (a) preoperative diagnostic testing, (b) screening of test results, (c) nursing assessments, and (d) client teaching. The entire process takes approximately 4 to 5 hours. The objectives of the preadmission screening are the following (Haines and Viellion 1990, p. 54):

- To prepare the client physically and emotionally for surgery and subsequent effects

- To assist the client and support persons in identifying appropriate discharge arrangements

- To obtain the nursing history and physical and laboratory tests

- To prevent last minute surgical cancellations for medical reasons

Before preadmission clinics existed, diagnostic laboratory tests, X-ray studies, electrocardiograms, and respiratory tests were performed the night before surgery. This night-before testing left no time to deal with abnormalities and resulted in surgical cancellations, longer client stays, and ineffective use of beds. At preadmission clinics, the clinic nurse screens diagnostic test results within 72 hours and reports abnormalities to the client's surgeon and documents them as part of the client's permanent record.

The nurse performs assessments either before or after diagnostic testing and, to promote continuity of care, sends them to the appropriate nursing unit on the client's admission. Seigel (1988, p. 38) recommends a risk assessment model so that interventions can be applied early to *prevent* a health problem and facilitate early discharge planning. Four categories of risk are outlined: Social-emotional factors, health condition, functional status, and educational needs (Figure 7–1).

Preoperative client-teaching sessions, in which the nurses from specific units participate, may include slide presentations and discussions by the nurse, equipment displays, guest speakers, and question-and-answer periods. Pamphlets and other reading materials may also be provided. Both preadmission assessments and client-teaching ses-

Social-Emotional Factors	Health Condition	Functional Status	Educational Needs
Age 70 years or older, under 18 years with no known guardian. Admission from another institution, readmission after recent discharge, recurrent admissions Single parent with minor children Financial need Known to several community agencies Sporadic use of needed healthcare Living arrangements prior to admission include: living alone, homebound, unable to return to pre-admission address, no known address Lack and/or limitation of support system Caretakers' failing health, finances, coping Environmental barriers in home— stairs, safety Socially isolated; depressed; recently bereaved; suspicion neglect/abuse victim	Prognosis poor or deteriorating Newly diagnosed disease Catastrophic illness Substance abuser Psychiatric history Scheduled for mutilating surgery Multiple diagnoses Ongoing respiratory needs Dehydration and/or malnutrition High-risk diagnoses such as: Hip fracture, CVA, MI, burns, brain failure, gunshot wounds, arthritis, hypertension, chronic renal failure, diabetes mellitus, CHF, cancer Certain stages of disease, e.g., terminal, pre-terminal Premature infant Newborn with major birth defects	Dependent in activities of daily living, eating, dressing, bathing, etc. Impaired mobility Incontinent Mental status changes; confusion, agitation Sensory losses Communication disorder	Lack of knowledge of preadmission treatments and medications Request by client and/or family for follow-up care New medications, treatments, diet, prosthesis Complex medication regimen, treatments, diet, wound care, ostomies, tubes

Potential Community Resources

Family Friends	Neighbors	Church Employer	Volunteers	

Other recovered patients
Community mental health centers
Family counseling agencies
Home health agencies
Community health nurse
Legal assistance
		Support groups related to:
		  disease/problem
		  e.g., battered women
		  diabetes, cerebrovascular,
		  accident, alcoholism, etc.
		Government agencies/programs
		Day programs
		Respite care
			Telephone reassurance
			Friendly visiting
			Transportation
			Shopping
				Nutrition programs
				  Home delivered meals
				  Nutrition centers
				Multiple service home care
				  Aides, PT, OT programs
				  Equipment, etc.

Smooth Transition to Home Recovery—Maintenance— Comfortable Death

FIGURE 7–1 Risk factor assessment for planning community discharge at hospital admission.
Source: H. Seigel, Nurses improve hospital efficiency through a risk assessment model at admission, *Nursing Management*, October 1988, 19(10):42.

sions provide major advantages. First, they decrease the amount of time required for preventive interventions on admission for surgery. Second, they enable the nurse to prepare surgical clients better, because their anxiety levels are less intense than at the time of admission. In addition, the preadmission assessments and teaching sessions facilitate earlier client referrals to home and auxiliary hospital personnel, such as dietitians and family counselors, and increased coordination of care and workload plans.

 Preadmission Processes for the Pediatric Client
Preadmission is recommended for the pediatric client whenever hospitalization or an outpatient clinical procedure is anticipated. The timing of preadmission for the pediatric client depends on the age of the child.

The younger the child, the closer to the actual date of hospitalization the preadmission process is performed—the 2-year-old may be preadmitted 2 days prior to admission, the 10-year-old one week prior to the admission date. Parents play an essential role in the preparation of the young to preadolescent child, and they themselves must be prepared if the child is to be properly prepared. Along with the nurse, parents must plan the appropriate timing, the amount and type of information, and the way the information should be presented to the child. Films, pamphlets, and dolls or puppetry may be used for teaching, depending on the age of the child. Adolescents are often treated with the same consideration as the young adult; however, their level of maturity varies, and each individual must be considered separately and support provided as indicated.

Home Visits

Preadmission home visits for elective admissions to hospitals or nursing homes facilitate discharge planning, improve client relations, enhance continuity of care, and reduce admission times. Members of the nursing staff visit a client's home 2 to 3 days before agency admission and generally, if they do so on off-duty hours, are compensated at an hourly rate of pay. Such visits provide opportunities (a) to implement the admission process in an environment where both the client and family members feel comfortable and therefore retain more of the information provided; (b) to evaluate the client's available support system; and (c) to begin client teaching. Advantages of preadmission home visits include the following (Werdal 1989, p. 50):

- A smooth, nonthreatening admission process in the client's own environment

- Reduction of client and family anxiety about hospitalization

- Reduced agency admission time

- Better and earlier data collection about the client's health status, which can initiate a preventive plan of action

- Enhanced continuity of care, especially if the client is cared for by the same nurse who made the preadmission visit

- Implementation of early discharge planning

- Improvement in the image of the role of nurses, since the client and family can recognize and therefore value the nurse's assessment expertise

- Positive influence on the public's perception of nurses and the nursing profession

- Creation of a positive image for the agency

Preliminary Admission Practices

The admission of clients to a health care agency involves (a) routine admitting office procedures, (b) preparation of the client's room, and (c) admission procedures conducted by the nurse when the client arrives at the room.

Clients who are not critically ill generally report first to the admitting office. In some agencies, nurses carry out the initial admission functions; in other agencies, admitting receptionists do so. Clients who are critically ill or injured are admitted directly to the emergency unit or, in some agencies, the intensive care unit (ICU).

Preliminary admitting office procedures generally include

- *Obtaining essential personal and identifying data for the admission record.* Such data include the client's full name, age, birth date, address, next of kin and/or support person, physician, religion, and dates of past admissions.

- *Acquiring a signed general consent for care.* A signed general consent for care legally permits the health care agency to provide routine care.

- *Legal consent for procedures on minor children.* This must be obtained from a custodial parent or legal guardian. If the child is adolescent and of sound mind, the adolescent *and* the custodial parent or legal guardian should read and sign the consent form.

- *Putting an identification bracelet (Identaband) on the client.* These bracelets are usually made of clear, waterproof plastic and cannot be removed except by cutting. Information on the bracelet may include the client's name and admission number, the attending physician, and the client's room number. Bands listing the client's allergies can also be applied at this time.

- *Notifying the nursing unit that a new client is being admitted.* The room and bed the client will occupy, the client's diagnosis, the attending physician, and other information relevant to the admission (such as "requires continuous oxygen")—must be specified. Notification alerts the nursing staff to possible immediate intervention required and enables them to make necessary arrangements.

- *Transporting the client to the room.* For safety reasons the client is always accompanied to the nursing unit by a person designated or assigned by the agency. Many agencies have volunteer staff or porters for this purpose. Depending upon the client's condition, a wheelchair or stretcher may be necessary. Most clients, however, can walk to the unit. The unit clerk or nurse there then assists the client to the room.

Before admitting a client, the nurse needs to know the following:

- The agency's policies and practices for admitting clients, particularly those regarding the client's medications, personal property, and security for valuables

- The bed and/or room to which the client will be admitted

- For a small child, what type of bed is used at home—if a crib has not been used and hospital

policy allows, a regular bed with side rails may be substituted when appropriate

- The client's general condition and/or medical diagnosis

- Whether on admission the client needs any special equipment, such as an oxygen device

- Whether the physician has written special orders to be implemented immediately upon the client's arrival

Techniques 7–1 and 7–2 explain the steps in admitting the adult and pediatric client, respectively, to the nursing unit.

7-1 Admitting the Adult Client to the Nursing Unit

PURPOSES
- To minimize the client's anxiety and facilitate adaptation to the agency environment
- To ensure the client's comfort and safety
- To ensure the protection of the client's personal property
- To encourage verbalization of client concerns and participation in care planning
- To obtain baseline data for subsequent care planning

ASSESSMENT FOCUS
Physical, emotional, and intellectual status; level of comfort; mobility; activity tolerance; affect and mood; behaviors indicative of stress.

EQUIPMENT

- Hospital gown (and pajama bottoms for males) as necessary
- Clothes list or clothing responsibility form
- Envelope to enclose valuables for safekeeping
- Appropriate hospital forms, e.g., a responsibility release for personal possessions

- Labels to attach to client's personal articles at bedside
- Thermometer, if not provided at bedside
- Watch with second hand
- Stethoscope and sphygmomanometer with cuff

- Portable scale
- Bedpan or urinal in which to acquire urine specimen, if ordered
- Clearly labeled urine specimen container and laboratory urinalysis requisition
- Client's chart, Kardex card, and care plan

INTERVENTION

1. Prepare the client's room.

- Open a closed bed for the client's convenience. (The bed unit is described in Chapter 18).

- In most cases, place the bed in a low position or place a footstool by a bed that is not adjustable, to make it easier and safer for the client to get into bed. If the client

is being transported by stretcher, however, place the bed in a high position to facilitate transfer from stretcher to bed.

- Check that all necessary unit supplies are provided: a full water jug if not contraindicated, bedpan or urinal, bath basin, kidney basin, and call signal.

- Provide equipment essential to the client's specific needs, e.g., intravenous pole, footboard, overhead frame with trapeze, and oxygen equipment.

- Verify that bedside equipment (e.g., call signal, light control, TV and remote control, bed controls) is functional.

► **Technique 7–1 Admitting the Adult Client** CONTINUED

2. Greet the client in a manner that conveys interest and concern.

- Introduce yourself, ask by what name the client wishes to be called, and inquire about any immediate problems the client may have. If the client is feeling distraught or upset, take time to listen and talk, to allay these concerns. If the client is in acute pain, attend to this at once, contacting the physician for medication orders and/or providing other nursing interventions. *By attending to the client's immediate problems, the nurse indicates a primary concern for the client's welfare. This makes the client feel that problems will be attended to and does much to initiate a sense of security and a trusting relationship.*

- Obtain other essential information about the client's physical and emotional status from the client's record or from health team members. *Knowledge of the client's health status assists the nurse in attending to the client's immediate problems.*

3. Orient the client to the unit.

- Introduce the client to the other clients in the room and to any other staff members encountered, even though the client cannot be expected to remember all their names. *Introduction to roommates facilitates the client's adjustment to the agency; introduction to staff members helps the client recognize caregivers.*

- Tell the client the name of the nurse in charge of the unit and that person's role. *Knowing the name of the nurse in charge and that person's problem-solving role helps the client feel more secure and provides a means for the client to communicate problems.*

- Explain and demonstrate use of equipment. *Knowledge about the location and appropriate use of equipment ensures the client's safety and sense of security in being able to obtain assistance if needed.*

  a. Explain how the call system works.

  b. Explain equipment in the bedside table and location of the client's locker.

  c. Show location of the bathroom and showers.

  d. Demonstrate overhead room lighting and night lighting.

  e. If applicable, demonstrate use of bedside television.

- Provide information about the agency to the client and support persons. *Knowledge of the agency's policies promotes the client's and support persons' feelings of security and minimizes anxiety.* Many agencies provide information pamphlets that cover most of this information. Check available materials.

  a. Inform the client about meal hours and nourishment times. If the client is placed on a special diet, stress the importance of restricting the diet to that supplied by the hospital unless otherwise ordered by the physician.

  b. Explain visiting hours and policies.

  c. Describe other areas in the hospital that the client or support persons may use, such as lounges, the cafeteria, the chapel, the canteen or snack area, and public restrooms.

  d. Discuss restrictions, requirements, and liability related

to electrical equipment supplied to the client from outside the hospital. Most facilities require that all equipment be inspected and approved by the hospital engineering department. Explain how the client may obtain a television or radio.

  e. Inform the client of smoking regulations.

  f. Describe facilities and services available, such as gift shop, library, newspaper delivery, cafeteria, chapel, and chaplain visitation.

  g. Inform the client of the location of the public telephone and operation of the portable or bedside telephone.

- Describe the staff's expectations of the client. For example, tell the client what to wear, to remain in the room until the doctor has visited, or to inform the nursing staff of the client's whereabouts.

4. Inform the client about the admission procedure, and begin the procedure.

- Explain that the admission procedure includes a physical examination and a nursing assessment. *Although the admission procedure often becomes routine for health personnel, it is unfamiliar to clients.*

- Direct support persons to the lounge area unless they can assist the client to undress. Reassure them that they will be called when it is best for them to return.

- Provide privacy, and assist the client to change into hospital gown or, if agency policy allows, into personal sleeping garments. Some agencies or specific units even allow clients to wear lounging garments or daytime dress.

▶ **Technique 7–1** CONTINUED

Some psychiatric units, for example, encourage full daytime dress. Many medical-surgical units, however, require hospital gowns. Many clients do not require assistance undressing but need to be informed how to put on a hospital gown, i.e., with the ties at the back. *Because the physical examination is an essential part of the admission procedure, the client's body parts are more readily exposed if a gown or pajamas are worn.*

- Assist the client as needed to a comfortable position in bed or in a chair. *Client comfort reduces anxiety and tension, which can elevate cardiac and respiratory rates and blood pressure. Accuracy of assessment findings is essential for baseline data used to compare subsequent findings.*

- Place the clothes in the bedside locker, and either list the clothes or have the client sign a form assuming responsibility for them, following the policy of the agency. Some agencies have support persons take the client's clothing home.

- Inform the client of agency policy regarding valuables. When possible, valuables should be taken home by family members. When this is not possible, special envelopes are usually provided by the agency to store valuables, such as money, jewelry, and keys, in a locked safe in the business office. Supply an envelope, if this is agency policy. Assure the client that the valuables will be safely handled and returned at discharge. Have the client sign a statement absolving the hospital of responsibility for valuables kept at the bedside. Agency policies generally state the amount of money the client should keep

at the bedside. Clients undergoing prolonged hospitalization sign special release forms to be able to withdraw small amounts of money from safekeeping as needs arise. Label large items, such as radios, with the client's full name.

- Arrange for proper storage of prostheses (dentures, artificial limbs, contact lenses) as needed or desired by clients. *A proper storage place for prostheses reduces the chance of damage.*

- Ask whether the client has brought medications. If so, request that they be taken home, or send them to the hospital pharmacy or designated area for safekeeping. It is usual for only certain medications, such as nitroglycerin, to be kept at the bedside. Check agency policy. *While the client is in the hospital, medications must be carefully regulated to be therapeutic, to avoid incompatibilities, and to avoid duplication of medication administration by the client and nurse.*

- Take the client's temperature, pulse, respirations, and blood pressure (see Chapter 10.) *These vital signs provide baseline data for subsequent assessments during hospitalization, indicate the client's general condition, and may be used to assess the effect of specific therapies.* Also take height and weight, if agency requires. In many agencies, these are recorded as the client states them. See Chapter 11.

5. Instruct the client about any specimens required and tests or treatments ordered by the physician.

- Obtain a urine specimen if ordered (see Chapter 28). Explain to the client the reason for it, e.g., to detect an infection of the uri-

nary tract. Direct ambulatory clients to the bathroom to provide a specimen. Provide a bedpan or urinal for bed clients to use. *A urine specimen is ordered if there is a reason to suspect a urinary problem. Because it is not cost-effective, urinalysis is no longer a routine screening procedure in many agencies.*

- Inform the client that a blood specimen and chest X-ray film will be taken by a technician, if applicable. *A blood specimen is routinely taken from many or all clients for hemoglobin assessment and blood typing and crossmatching for clients having surgery. Some agencies are also doing routine AIDs screening. Chest X-ray films may be taken to ascertain the presence of any lung disease, such as tuberculosis.*

- Inform the client of any treatment to be administered in the near future, e.g., during the next shift or day. For example, clients who are having surgery need to know what preoperative preparations (such as surgical shave) are required. See Chapter 42. *Knowledge of what to expect reduces anxiety.*

6. Ensure client comfort and safety.

- Place the call signal within easy reach of the client, and ensure that the bed is in the low position and that side rails are raised if indicated.

- Inform support persons when they can return, and inform them about visiting hours. *Consideration of support persons conveys your understanding of their concern and needs.*

- Place allergy alerts, if necessary, on the client and the chart, according to agency policy. Record

▶

▶ **Technique 7–1** *CONTINUED*

allergies in red ink, both on the front of the client's chart and on the nursing Kardex. A sign indicating specific allergies may also be placed on the foot of the client's bed or on the wall above the head of the bed. If the client has food allergies, notify the dietary department. *Allergy alerts prevent constant questioning of the client when therapies are administered, serve as reminders to all caregivers, and safeguard the client.*

• Place the client on "risk management" or other such precautions as indicated by assessment data suggesting possible risk for falls and accidental injury, and as dictated by hospital policy. Label the client's chart, Kardex, and hospital door appropriately. Obtain special safety equipment (e.g., bed alert, additional side rails) as indicated. *Risk alert serves as a reminder to the care provider to take special precautions with this client to avoid injury.*

7. Obtain a nursing assessment if not previously performed during preadmission programs.

• See assessment guide on page 105 and the nursing health history in Chapter 11.
 or
 Use the agency assessment form. *The nursing assessment provides baseline data for subsequent care planning.*

8. Send specimens to the laboratory with appropriate labels and requisitions. *Inappropriate* *identification of the specimen can lead to errors of diagnosis or therapy for the client.*

9. Document relevant information on the client's records.

• Record assessment data on the appropriate forms of the client's record, in accordance with agency procedure. For example, some agencies record the vital signs on both the nurse's notes and the graphic record. Selected data from the nursing assessment form are generally transferred to the nurse's notes as well as the client's Kardex.

• Record on the nurse's notes and on the valuables envelope the disposition of the valuables.

• Initiate the client's care plan.

EVALUATION FOCUS

Behaviors indicating initial adaptation to the nursing unit (see Outcome Criteria on page 106).

SAMPLE RECORDING

Date	Time	Notes
12/5/93	1140	Admitted walking. T 97, P 82, R 14, BP on "L" arm 130/70. Is alert. States is in to have gallbladder removed, has no discomfort at present. States has no known allergies. States takes thyroid pills twice a day before breakfast and at bedtime. Clean voided urine specimen sent to lab. Gave watch and ring to wife to take home. $50.00 cash placed in valuables envelope and given to hospital Business Office to place in safe. Oriented to hospital routines and equipment. Given information pamphlet about preop prep. ————— Sheila S. Murphy, NS
	1150	Dr. L. Stein notified of admission. ————— Sheila S. Murphy, NS
	1230	Blood sample for CBC, Hb, blood typing and cross-matching taken by lab technician. ————— Sheila S. Murphy, NS

KEY ELEMENTS OF ADMITTING THE ADULT CLIENT

• Assess the client's physical, emotional, and intellectual ability.

• Determine the client's allergies and place allergy alerts according to agency policy.

• Promptly implement any nursing interventions required to maintain the client's safety and comfort.

• Acquire baseline data for monitoring the client's condition and for planning care.

• Ensure that the client knows how to use the call system for assistance and what assistance the nurse will provide.

• Promptly implement physician's orders that should be initiated on arrival.

7-2 Admitting the Pediatric Client to the Nursing Unit

PURPOSES
- To minimize anxiety in the client, parent, and support persons
- To prevent significant disruption of the client's growth and development during hospitalization
- To avoid disruption of parent-child relationship during hospitalization
- To ensure the client's comfort and safety
- To facilitate the client's adaptation to the agency environment
- To ensure the protection of the client's personal property
- To obtain baseline data for subsequent care planning

ASSESSMENT FOCUS

Age; developmental status (actual and standard for age); temperament or usual adjustment to new people, places, and routines; level of comfort; behaviors indicative of stress; activity tolerance; mobility.

EQUIPMENT

- Hand puppet
- One or two favorite toys from home, or other age-appropriate items for diversional sedentary activity (game, book, coloring book, or hospital-approved electrical device such as radio or tape player)
- Pediatric gown or favorite pajamas, if allowed

- Stethoscope and sphygmomanometer with pediatric or appropriate-sized cuff
- Thermometer
- Portable scale
- Bedpan or urinal, if specimen of urine is ordered
- Specimen containers, with labels

- Appropriate hospital forms for clothes, valuables, and other personal belongings
- Admission kit with pitcher, cup, and other items of appropriate size
- Pad and pencil for bedside, if record keeping is needed

INTERVENTION

1. Prepare the client's room.

- Obtain the appropriate type of bed for the client's age and stage of development (crib, bed with four side rails, or regular bed for adolescent), and open a closed bed for the client's convenience.

- In most cases, place the bed in low position, and if needed, place a footstool by the bed for the child's use when getting into the bed. If the client is being transported by stretcher, place the bed in a high position to facilitate transfer from the stretcher.

- Check that bedside supplies are in the client's reach; confirm that bedside controls (light, call sig-

nal, television control, and so on) are functional.

- Partially fill the water pitcher, if not contraindicated.

- Obtain bedside equipment as appropriate for the child's age and needs. Such equipment may include an IV pole, a footboard, or oxygen equipment.

2. Meet the client and family.

- Whenever possible, have the primary nurse who participated in the preadmission process available when the client is admitted.

- Introduce yourself, and ask by what name the client prefers to be called. *Using a familiar and*

preferred name facilitates the development of a therapeutic nurse-client relationship.

- Follow Technique 7–1, Step 2, for inquiring about any immediate concerns or discomfort, addressing these concerns, and obtaining other essential information about the client's physical and emotional status from the client's record or from health team members.

3. Orient the client to the unit.

- See Step 3 in Technique 7–1. In addition:

- Explain and demonstrate the use of equipment at the bedside, and encourage the child, if develop-

▶ **Technique 7–2 Admitting the Pediatric Client** CONTINUED

mentally able, to demonstrate in return the use of equipment, e.g., call system, lighting, bed control, bedside telephone, television, and bedside table.

- Provide information about the agency to the client, parents, and support persons (see Step 3 in Technique 7–1). Include meal hours and nourishment times; visiting hours and related policies; smoking regulations; restrictions regarding medications at the bedside; location of lounges, cafeteria, chapel, cafeteria/snack area; gift shop; library; public telephones and restrooms; how to obtain a newspaper, television, or radio; restrictions regarding electrical equipment brought from the home; chaplain services.

- Whenever possible, arrange for rooming-in of parent or family member, and ask who will stay with the child and what assistance will be needed (e.g., guest tray, cot).

- Inform parents of client care measures in which they may participate—if the parent wishes and is comfortable doing so—and explain care measures, such as recording intake and output.

- Inform client and family of the required clothing, dietary, and activity restrictions, the need to remain in the hospital room during particular time periods (e.g., until shift assessment has been performed, medications administered, and the doctor has visited) and to inform the nursing staff of the client's whereabouts.

4. Inform the client about the admission procedure, and begin the procedure.

- Explain that the procedure includes a physical examination

and nursing assessment, using easy-to-understand words. Use a doll or puppet to explain the examination procedure to young children.

- Encourage a parent or support person to remain with a young child whenever possible. *The presence of a parent or familiar support person will decrease anxiety related to separation, the unfamiliar environment, and the procedures being performed.*

- For preadolescents or adolescents, direct support persons to the waiting area when the nursing history and physical examination are being performed. Reassure them that they will be called when it is best for them to return. *Privacy and modesty is important and should be preserved with older children and adolescents. Older youths may be reluctant to reveal some kinds of information (e.g., dietary intake of snacks, alcohol/drug experimentation) when parents are present.*

- Follow Step 4 in Technique 7–1 for assisting the client to change into a hospital gown or personal sleeping garments, assisting the client to a comfortable position, and appropriate handling of the client's clothing, valuables, prostheses, and medications brought from home.

- Take the client's temperature, pulse, blood pressure, respiratory rate, weight, and height (see Chapters 10 and 12). *In addition to providing baseline data, height and weight are also used to determine the growth of children and the dosages of medication appropriate for them.*

5. Instruct the client and parents regarding any specimens required and tests or treatments ordered by the physician.

- Obtain a urine specimen or specimens of other bodily fluids, if ordered; inform the child and parents of treatments planned for the immediate future; and place allergy alerts, if indicated, on the client's chart, Kardex, and at the bedside in accordance with agency policy (see Technique 7–1, Step 5).

- If X-ray studies or blood work has been ordered, notify the appropriate department that the client has been admitted, and transport the client (accompanied by the parent, if the child is young) to the appropriate department. If blood specimens are to be drawn or other painful procedures are to be performed, transport the child to the treatment room. *The child's bedside should be preserved as a safe place; painful procedures should therefore be performed elsewhere to preserve the child's sense of security while in the hospital room.*

- Avoid having parents restrain infants or young children during painful procedures. *This could negatively affect the child's trust in the parent.*

6. Ensure the client's comfort and safety.

- Place the call signal within easy reach of the client, or parent of a young child.

- Place the bed in low position with side rails or crib rails raised.

- Obtain cot for parent or support person, or inform support persons when they may return to the bedside. *Consideration of family or support persons conveys the nurse's understanding of their concern and needs.*

7. Obtain a nursing assessment, if not previously performed during the preadmission program.

▶ **Technique 7–2** *CONTINUED*

- Record data using the assessment guide on page 105 or in Chapter 12, or use the agency assessment form. *The nursing assessment provides baseline data for subsequent care planning.*
- Document the name of the person providing information about the client.

8. Document relevant information on the client's records (see Technique 7–1, Step 9).

- Record in the nurse's notes the client's physical and emotional state on admission, the relationship of support persons with the client and rooming-in arrangements, disposition of the client's

property and valuables, diagnostic procedures performed, and specimens obtained and sent to the laboratory. Fully document any client teaching performed and verbalizations indicating that the information was understood.

- Initiate the client's care plan.

EVALUATION FOCUS

Client and parental behaviors indicative of initial adaptation to the nursing unit (see Outcome Criteria on page 106).

SAMPLE RECORDING

Date	Time	Notes
12/6/93	1400	Four-year-old male admitted to unit for T & A in AM. Prefers to be called "Bry." Mother in attendance and verbalizes intent to remain at the hospital with the client. Cot and linen obtained. Oriented to room and bedside equipment; mother verbalized understanding. Preassessment data obtained. No diagnostic tests pending. Mother states understanding of preoperative preparations needed and states has begun teaching with child. Minimum anxiety noted from client or mother. Child sitting on the bed in pajamas, and is dressing doll in hospital gown. Supportive parent-child interaction noted. — James Dee, RN, CCRN

KEY ELEMENTS OF ADMITTING THE PEDIATRIC CLIENT

- Preadmit pediatric clients whenever possible; the younger the child, the closer to the time of admission the preparations should begin.
- Assign a primary nurse for each hospital shift to decrease the anxiety of the client and family members.
- Perform all painful procedures in areas away from the bedside.
- Allow parent to accompany the young child during procedures.

- Do not have a parent restrain the infant or young child during a painful procedure.
- Provide privacy for children, particularly older children or adolescents, during the assessment to allow modesty.
- Interview older children and adolescents separately from their parents.
- Use appropriate forms for documentation.
- Identify the person who has provided information about the child.

CRITICAL THINKING CHALLENGE

Eleanor Lambert is admitted to the nursing unit for evaluation of a cardiac arrhythmia. During the admission procedures, Mrs. Lambert expresses concern that physician specialists other than her private physician will be examining and treating her. She states that she doesn't know them and expects that she must trust the judgment of her personal physician but that she feels unsure about the specialists. She asks your opinion. What do you think Mrs. Lambert is thinking and feeling? Give two examples of responses that might help Mrs. Lambert, and give reasons for your choices.

RELATED RESEARCH

Gavey, J. December 7–13, 1988. Baby admissions. *Nursing Times* 84(49):43–45.

MacDowell, N. M. Winter 1989. Willingness to provide care to AIDS patients in Ohio nursing homes. *Journal of Community Health Nursing* 14(4):205–13.

Marriner, J.; Brown, S.; McPherson, L.; LeBail, J.; and Allen, A. October 5–11, 1988. A children's tour . . . a pre-admission visit. *Nursing Times* 84(40):38–40.

Mulhearn, S. October 1989. The nursing process: Improving psychiatric admission assessment? *Journal of Advanced Nursing* 14:808–14.

Schepp, K. G. January/February 1991. Factors influencing the coping effort of mothers of hospitalized children. *Nursing Research* 40(1):42–46.

REFERENCES

Adams, J.; Gill, S.; and McDonald, M. January 2–8, 1991. Child health: Reducing fear in hospital. *Nursing Times* 87(1):62–64.

Haines, N., and Viellion, G. March/April 1990. A successful combination: Pre-admission testing and pre-operative education. *Orthopedic Nursing* 9(2):53–57.

Harrington, A. M., and Waltman, R. E. May 1989. Eight steps for evaluating a new longterm care patient. *Nursing* 19:74–76, 78.

Kennedy, C. M.; Gyr, P. M.; and Garst, K. F. March/April 1991. A nursing tool to assess children upon hospital admission *MCN* 16(2):78–82.

Knight, S. July 1989. Assessment to discharge, this form does it all. *RN* 52:36–40.

Lathrop, L.; Corcoran, S.; and Ryden, M. March 1989. Description and analysis of pre-admission screening. *Public Health Nursing* 6(1):23–27.

LeNoble, E. February 1991. Pre-admission possible . . . pre-admission clinics have shown benefits in promoting patient recoveries, decreasing patient stays and generally improving bed utilization. *Canadian Nurse* 87:18–20.

McConnell, E. A. December 1988. Seeing your patient as a mosaic. *Nursing* 18:50–51.

Prescott, T. August 1990. We get an early start on a.m. admits . . . preop testing and teaching before the day of surgery. *RN* 53:21, 23–24.

Price, S. February 27–March 5, 1991. Preparing children for admission to hospital. *Nursing Times* 87(9):46–49.

Seigel, H. October 1988. Nurses improve hospital efficiency through a risk assessment model at admission. *Nursing Management* 19:38–40, 42, 44.

Werdal, L. May 1989. Pre-admission home visits: From concept to implementation. *Nursing Management* 20:49–50, 52–54.

Transfer, Discharge, and Postmortem Care

CONTENTS

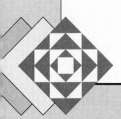

Nursing Process Guide

Discharge

ASSESSMENT

Determine

- Abilities to perform activities of daily living (ADL)
  - Bathing (shower, tub, or sponge bath)
  - Dressing (obtaining needed clothing from closet or drawers, getting dressed, closing fasteners)
  - Toileting (going to bathroom, cleaning self after elimination, arranging clothing)
  - Transferring (moving from bed to chair; in and out of bath, in and out of car)
  - Continence (controlling bowel and bladder elimination)
  - Eating (getting food from dishes into mouth)
  - Ambulating (with or without aids such as cane, crutches, walker, wheelchair)
  - Transportation and shopping
  - Meal preparation
- Disabilities or limitations
  - Sensory losses (auditory, visual, gustatory, kinesthetic)
  - Energy limitation
  - Motor losses (paralysis)
  - Communication disorder
  - Mental status changes (confusion)
  - Social isolation and/or depression
- Adequacy of support network
  - Financial needs
  - Family, friends, neighbors, volunteers
  - Caretaker's health or coping abilities
  - Availability of community resources (health centers, community health nurse, legal assistance, day programs, respite care, nutrition programs, home care)
- Environmental hazards or barriers in the home
  - Safety precautions (stairs with or without hand rails; lighting in rooms, hallways, stairways; night-lights in hallways or bathroom; grab bars near toilet and tub; firmly attached carpets and rugs)
  - Self-care barriers (lack of running water, lack of wheelchair access to bathroom or home, lack of space for required equipment, lack of elevator)
- Educational needs
  - Knowledge of illness

- Self-administration of medications
- New treatments, such as wound care, ostomy care, tracheostomy care, indwelling catheter care, or other tube maintenance
- Diet management
- Prosthesis application and care
- Health status restrictions (e.g., exercise limitations)
- Signs and symptoms of complications
- Preventive measures (life-style or environmental changes)
- Health care assistance in the home
  - Home-delivered meals
  - Volunteers for telephone reassurance, friendly visiting, transportation, shopping
  - Assistance with bathing
  - Assistance with housekeeping
  - Assistance with wound care, ostomies, tubes, intravenous medications, and so on

RELATED DIAGNOSTIC CATEGORIES

- Self-care deficits: Bathing/hygiene, dressing/grooming, feeding, toileting
- Knowledge deficit (specify)
- Activity intolerance
- Altered health maintenance
- Impaired home maintenance management
- Social isolation

PLANNING

Client Goal

The client will perform self-care activities with or without assistance and will manage health care requirements in the home.

Outcome Criteria

The client

- Verbalizes feelings about discharge.
- Identifies life-style changes required as a result of illness.
- Identifies required environmental changes due to disabilities or limitations.
- Explains reasons for all information provided in health care instruction.
- Demonstrates skills required to manage prescribed self-care treatments in the home.
- Arranges necessary nursing and self-care assistance in the home.

Transfers

Clients may be transferred to another bed within the unit, to another unit within the agency, or to another agency. Some transfers are required because of the client's health; others are undertaken at the client's request.

In-unit transfers are usually made to place a client closer to the nursing station for more frequent observation, to provide a requested private or semiprivate room, or to provide the client with a roommate more compatible in age or interests. This type of transfer involves minimal change. The nurse records the new room number on the client's chart and other documents (the medication record, the nursing care plan, Kardex, and so on). The nurse should also notify the business office, the information desk, the dietary department, and other departments as appropriate to ensure continuity of services. All the client's personal belongings and equipment are moved with the client.

Interunit or interagency transfers may be made to provide special care for the client (e.g., in an intensive care unit) or to provide a different level of care, such as long-term, rehabilitative, or hospice care. These transfers require considerable coordination of activities between the sending and receiving units or agencies. To ensure continuity of care, complete information about the client's medical and nursing needs must be provided.

Transfers are usually stressful for clients. People worry about the move to a new setting, the care they will receive in that setting, and the loss of their belongings. It is important that transfers be safe and comfortable for clients. Technique 8–1 describes essential steps in transferring a client.

8-1 Transferring a Client

PURPOSES
- To provide care to suit the client's needs
- To provide privacy or a compatible roommate and thus psychologic comfort

ASSESSMENT FOCUS

> Health status; level of comfort; mobility; activity tolerance; any concerns of client.

EQUIPMENT
- ☐ All personal belongings
- ☐ Equipment used at bedside
- ☐ Client's record and related supplies and medications
- ☐ Wheelchair or stretcher

INTERVENTION

Nurse in Current Unit

1. Explain the transfer to the client and/or family members.

- Include the purpose of transfer, the type of nursing unit receiving the client, the time the transfer will occur, and assurance that the hospital's information desk will be given the new room number so that visitors can be told.

Clients may experience fear or anxiety about moving to a different area with unfamiliar nursing personnel and worry that family members and friends will not locate them.

2. Assess the client's current physical health status.

- Note respirations, blood pressure, and pulse. *The client's*

health status may change during transport.

- Determine the need for supportive equipment during the move. *Special equipment, such as oxygen tanks, suction devices, intravenous therapy apparatus, or cardiac monitoring equipment, may need to be maintained during transport.*

▶

► Technique 8–1 Transferring a Client *CONTINUED*

3. Gather all the client's personal belongings.

- Check all closets and drawers for the client's personal items to ensure that all belongings are assembled.

- Include any clothing, footwear, suitcase, cosmetic items, cards, flowers, books, magazines, eyeglasses, dentures, and hearing aid.

- Check agency policy about moving reusable bedside equipment and supplies, such as a bedpan or urinal, washbasin, towels, kidney or emesis basin, denture cup, and water pitcher. In some agencies, clients are billed for this equipment.

4. Assemble all the client's records and medications.

- Ensure that all documentation in the client's record and Kardex is current and complete. *Accurate information is essential for the receiving nurses to implement and maintain the client's care.*

- Assemble all medications, medication forms, or tickets.

5. Document the transfer.

- Record in the chart the time of the transfer, the unit to which the client is moving, the mode of transport, and any significant assessments, including the condition of the client. Complete this recording just prior to moving the client (see the sample recording for this technique.)

6. Ensure the client's safety and comfort during the move.

- Establish the method by which the client can move, e.g., by wheelchair or stretcher. This may be indicated in the client's record or by the nurse. Clients normally are transferred by wheelchair unless they are too ill to sit up.

- Lock the wheels on the stretcher or wheelchair when the client moves on and off it. *Locking prevents the wheels from moving and thus protects the client's safety.*

- Assist the client to the wheelchair or stretcher. Provide warm coverings as needed. *Assistance prevents undue exertion. Coverings prevent chilling and maintain the client's sense of modesty.*

7. Transport the client to the new unit.

- Take the client and the supplies to the other unit, or arrange for transport service.

- Stop at the nurses' station on arriving at the receiving unit, and introduce the nurse in charge to the client.

- Review the client's record or discharge summary with a nursing staff member (receiving nurse) on the new unit.

- Leave the chart, nursing care plan, and any medications at the nurses' station.

- Take the client to the new room, and assist the client into bed. Have the receiving nurse go along.

- Ensure that the client is comfortable.

8. Return to your nursing unit, and ensure that all required hospital departments are notified of the transfer.

- Notify the information desk, admitting, dietary, housekeeping, pharmacy, and business department. Most agencies have a list of the departments that need to be notified. Often this is done in writing, and a unit clerk may perform this function. *Notification ensures continuity of care for the client and facilitates communication of the client's location to family and friends.*

Nurse in Receiving Unit

- With the transferring nurse, review the client's chart or discharge summary (if written) and the assessments, nursing diagnoses, and so on. This is particularly important when interventions are carried out just prior to the transfer, e.g., administration of an analgesic.

- Assess the client's immediate health and provide any interventions immediately needed. Record data in the client's record.

- Welcome the client and any accompanying support persons. Introduce other clients in the room. Orient the client to any practices that are different on this unit from those of the previous unit.

- Confirm that other departments, such as the dietary department, know the client's new location.

- Record on the client's chart the time of arrival, method of transport, assessment data, and any care provided. See sample recordings below.

EVALUATION FOCUS	See Assessment Focus.

▶ **Technique 8–1** *CONTINUED*

SAMPLE RECORDING: Transferring Nurse

Date	Time	Notes
6/12/93	1100	Transferred by wheelchair to A6. P 96, BP 160/120/90. All personal items, including dentures, moved with client. Meds given to L. Jones, HN ————— ————————————————————————————————— Eliza L. Begbie, NS

SAMPLE RECORDING: Receiving Nurse

Date	Time	Notes
6/12/93	1115	Received by wheelchair. Color pale. P 106, BP 165/90. C/o fatigue. Oriented to unit practices. Dr. Bedow notified. ————— Karen S. Stockley, NS

KEY ELEMENTS OF TRANSFERRING A CLIENT

- Use method of transfer appropriate for client's health status.
- Implement safety precautions during transfer.

- Communicate pertinent data regarding the client's condition and the transfer to others.

Discharge

Planning for a client's discharge involves the collaborative efforts of the client, support persons, and many health care professionals: physician, unit nurse, community health nurse, social worker, dietitian, and so on. The physician authorizes the discharge by a written order, such as "May go home tomorrow," and specifies all medications and medical therapies to be continued at home. The unit nurse's continuous communication with the client's physician during the course of the client's hospitalization is essential to identifying the client's changing needs. If the unit nurse determines that the client requires skilled home nursing care, that nurse makes a referral to a community health nurse for home visits. Skilled nursing services may include providing wound care and dressing changes, administering intravenous fluids or injections, and providing ongoing health teaching for ostomy care.

In many agencies, the client's risk factors for discharge planning are assessed by the unit nurse and a social worker at the time of admission to the agency. See Figure 7–1 on page 107. Social problems, such as finances and living arrangements, must also be considered. More suitable living arrangements may be necessary for the client who has no support network in place or who cannot, for example, manage stairs to a third floor apartment.

By the day of discharge, clients should feel comfortable about their abilities to (a) resume normal activities at home and (b) manage any medication administration or other required health care skills.

Discharge Holding Units

A recent trend to expedite the availability of beds of discharged clients and maximize bed usage is the development of a discharge holding unit (Ashley 1989, p. 32). These units are areas set aside for discharged clients who have an unintentional discharge delay that hinders the admission of new clients. Reasons for delays include (a) lack of transportation for the client; (b) inability of support persons to pick the client up until late evening; (c) inability of pharmacy to expedite discharge medications; and (d) no written physician's orders for an anticipated discharge (Ashley 1989, p. 33).

Clients waiting in a discharge holding area are self-care clients who require no nursing intervention other than instructions for administering their take-home medications and treatments. Usually, clients accepted to the area must have a definite place to go by 1900 hours. While waiting, clients are allowed to choose a bed or a chair. Diversional activities, food, and safety are provided for them.

Discharging a Client AMA

Occasionally, clients leave an agency without the permission of the physician. These are *unauthorized discharges*, often referred to as *discharge against medical authority (AMA)*. The client is asked to sign a special form releasing the hospital from any responsibility after the departure (Figure 8–1 on page 122).

It is important the client understands that refusing a particular treatment or medication is not the

EL CAMINO HOSPITAL

LEAVING HOSPITAL AGAINST ADVICE

Date...

This is to certify that..,
a patient in the above named hospital, is leaving the hospital against the advice of the attending physician
and the hospital administration. I acknowledge that I have been informed of the risk involved and hereby
release the attending physician, and the hospital, from all responsibility and any ill effects which may result
from this action.

....
Patient

....
Other Person Responsible

....
Relationship

Witness...

Witness...

Form 224

FIGURE 8–1 A discharge form for a client who is being released against medical authority.
Source: El Camino Hospital, Mountain View, California. Reprinted with permission.

same as refusing all treatments and desiring to leave the hospital. The AMA form is used in the latter instance, whereas refusing a particular aspect of care is the client's right and needs to be documented on the chart and reported to the nurse in charge.

When a client decides to leave a health care facility AMA, the following activities are indicated:

1. Ascertain why the person wants to leave the agency. Sometimes clients misunderstand information or have fears the nurse can resolve. As a result, the client may decide to stay in the agency.

2. Notify the physician of the client's decision.

3. Offer the client the appropriate form to complete (Figure 8–1).

4. If the client refuses to sign the form, document the fact on the form and have another health professional witness this.

5. Provide the client with the original of the signed form and place a copy in the record.

6. When the client leaves the agency, notify the physician, nurse in charge, and agency administration as appropriate.

7. Assist the client to leave as if this were a usual discharge from the agency. The agency is still responsible while the client is on the premises.

Technique 8–2 explains essential steps in discharging a client.

8-2 Discharging a Client

PURPOSES
- To ensure that the client has the proper knowledge and skill to perform self-care after discharge
- To ensure appropriate preparation of the client's home environment at discharge
- To ensure adequate home health care support
- To minimize the client's anxiety at discharge

ASSESSMENT FOCUS

See Assessment in Nursing Process Guide on page 118.

EQUIPMENT

- Any equipment the client requires, e.g., walker, wheelchair, commode, crutches, oxygen, antiemboli stockings
- Medications
- Dressing materials
- Educational booklets and/or written instructions

INTERVENTION

Before Day of Discharge

1. Determine home care needs, required teaching, and available community resources.

- Collaborate with the client, support persons, and/or the home care nurse regarding needs required in the home. *Adaptations in the home environment can often contribute to independent functioning and to a client's safety.*

- Establish a teaching program for the client and support persons as soon as convenient during hospitalization. The program may include how to give injections, colostomy care, and diet. Provide written information when possible. *People usually need time to practice new skills and ask questions. Written information can be referred to after discharge.*

- Provide the client and/or support person with information about any community health resources that may be helpful. *Most communities have a variety of services that can support clients and help meet their continued health needs, e.g., meals-on-wheels, day-care centers for the elderly.*

- Complete a referral form. *Nurses make referrals for health care services in collaboration with the physician. The nurse may be the first person to recognize the client's need for a dietitian, home care nurse, nutritionist, or social worker.*

Day of Discharge

2. Verify and implement the physician's discharge orders.

- Check that the physician's orders for discharge have been written. *Discharge is authorized only by the physician.*

- Verify orders for prescriptions, change in therapies, or need for special appliances. *Checking orders early enables the nurse to implement any procedures required in advance of discharge.*

- Ensure that all laboratory tests, X-ray studies, and procedures are completed before discharge.

3. Review health care instructions and needs with the client.

- Instruct the client and/or support person about the dosage and frequency of administration, precautions, and any other relevant information of all prescriptions or medications ordered by the physician. *Proper instruction about medications ensures correct drug administration and achieves the intended benefit for the client.*

- Allow the client and support persons to ask questions about medications, physical care, and supplies. *This relieves anxiety about self-care and facilitates final clarification of information and compliance with required care.*

- Provide the client with necessary written instructions, pertinent pamphlets (if available), and supplies. Some agencies provide at discharge limited supplies of syringes, dressing materials, crutches, or canes.

4. Determine whether the client's transportion home has been arranged.

- Note the time arranged for transport and the method of transport. The client's condition will determine the method of transportion.

- Usually clients and/or support persons are responsible for making arrangements for their own transportation. If an ambulance is required, at some agencies the nurse may telephone to make the arrangements.

5. Assist the client as required to perform any hygiene measures,

▶

► **Technique 8–2 Discharging a Client** CONTINUED

dress, and pack all personal belongings.

- Check whether the client being discharged to a nursing home may wear bed clothing.

- Check all closets and drawers to ensure that all belongings are packed.

- If there are valuables in safe-keeping, obtain the client's signature on the release form, and return all valuables listed.

- Inspect and change all surgical dressings as required.

6. Ensure that all required hospital departments are notified of the discharge.

- Notify admitting, dietary, housekeeping, business office, and/or cashier. Usually the unit clerk performs this function. *Notification enables these departments to prepare for the next admission.*

- Confirm that the business office has completed its procedures. If it has not, make arrangements for the client to visit the office or for an office representative to visit the client. Arrangements for

paying are usually made at the time of admission.

7. Escort the client from the nursing unit to the arranged mode of transport.

- Contact the transport service, or obtain a wheelchair if required, unless an ambulance will be used. Obtain a utility cart to transport personal effects if the client cannot hold them. Because of the danger of overexertion, some hospitals require that a wheelchair be used even though the client feels able to walk. *This ensures a safe exit from the agency.* The ambulance crew will have a stretcher for the person who needs an ambulance.

- Ⓢ Lock the wheels of the chair. Raise the foot supports. Then, assist the client into the wheelchair, and support the feet appropriately. *Locking the wheels prevents the chair from moving and thus protects the client's safety.*

- Take the client and the personal belongings to meet the arranged transportation.

- Ⓢ Lock the wheels of the chair and raise the foot supports before assisting the client to move to the mode of transport.

8. Report and document the client's discharge.

- Report to the nurse in charge and/or the unit clerk that the client has been discharged.

- Document on the client's chart the discharge, the time, the method of transport to the agency door, and assessment data. Some agencies also suggest that the client's destination, e.g., a nursing home, be included in the discharge notes.

9. Write a discharge profile or referral summary for specified institution or community health nurse.

- Include any active health problems, current medications, current treatments that are to be continued, eating and sleeping habits, self-care abilities, support networks, life-style patterns, and religious preference (optional). See Figure 3–7 on page 53.

EVALUATION FOCUS	Ability to perform ADL; disabilities or limitations; knowledge and understanding of required life-style changes and environmental changes; ability to perform skills required to manage prescribed self-care treatments.

SAMPLE RECORDING

Date	Time	Notes
12/5/93	1400	Discharged by wheelchair to Sunnyvale Lodge. Eye drops and oral medications taken by wife. Written instructions provided to client and wife about eye drop insertion; medication dosage, schedule, and precautions; and leg exercises. — Maria L. Chevez, NS

KEY ELEMENTS OF DISCHARGING A CLIENT

- Assess the client's and/or support person's ability to carry out required care.

- Help the client and support persons plan support services and make any necessary home adjustments.

- Instruct the client and/or support persons regarding follow-up care.

Postmortem Care

Postmortem care is an unpleasant subject for most people and a technique that nurses carry out from necessity, often with considerable feelings. Because so many people in the United States and Canada die in hospitals, nurses encounter death more often than most people.

Care of the dying and the dead has cultural, social, religious, and legal implications. It is important for nurses to understand how these apply in their own communities. Nurses also need to understand the stages of clients' emotional reactions to their own death in order to offer emotional support and necessary care.

Clinical Signs of Death

Various consciousness levels occur just before death. Some clients are alert, whereas others are drowsy, stuporous, or comatose. Hearing is thought to be the last sense lost.

The traditional *clinical signs of death* were cessation of the apical pulse, respirations, and blood pressure. However, since the advent of artificial means to maintain respirations and blood circulation, identifying death is more difficult. In 1968, the World Medical Assembly adopted the following guidelines for physicians as indications of death (Benton 1978, p. 18):

- Total lack of response to external stimuli
- No muscular movement, especially breathing
- No reflexes
- Flat encephalogram

In instances of artificial support, absence of electric currents from the brain (measured by an electroencephalogram) for at least 24 hours is an indication of death. Only a physician can pronounce death, and only after this pronouncement can life-support systems be shut off.

Another definition of death is **cerebral death**, which occurs when the higher brain center, the cerebral cortex, is irreversibly destroyed. The client may still be able to breathe but is irreversibly unconscious. People who support this definition of death believe the cerebral cortex, which holds the capacity for thought, voluntary action, and movement, *is* the individual (Schulz 1978, p. 92).

Changes in the Body after Death

Rigor mortis is the stiffening of the body that occurs about 2 to 4 hours after death. It results from a lack of adenosine triphosphate (ATP), which is not synthesized because of a lack of glycogen in the body.

ATP is necessary for muscle fiber relaxation. Its lack causes the muscles to contract, which in turn immobilizes the joints. Rigor mortis starts in the involuntary muscles (heart, bladder, and so on), then progresses to the head, neck, and trunk, and finally reaches the extremities.

Because the deceased's family members often want to view the body, it is important that the deceased appear natural and comfortable. Positioning the body, placing the dentures in the mouth, and closing the eyes and mouth must take place before rigor mortis occurs. Rigor mortis usually leaves the body about 96 hours after death.

Algor mortis is the gradual decrease of the body's temperature after death. When blood circulation terminates and the hypothalamus ceases to function, body temperature falls about 1 C (1.8 F) per hour until it reaches room temperature. Simultaneously, the skin loses its elasticity and can easily be broken when removing dressings and adhesive tape.

After blood circulation has ceased, the skin becomes discolored. The red blood cells break down, releasing hemoglobin, which discolors the surrounding tissues. This discoloration, referred to as **livor mortis**, appears in the lowermost or dependent areas of the body.

Tissues after death become soft and eventually liquefied by bacterial fermentation. The hotter the temperature, the more rapid the change. Therefore, bodies are often stored in cool places to delay this process. Embalming reverses the process through injection of chemicals into the body to destroy the bacteria.

Legal Aspects of Death

Legal issues surrounding death include the death certificate, labeling of the deceased, autopsy, organ donation, and inquest.

Death Certificate

By law, a death certificate must be made out when a person dies. It is usually signed by the attending physician and filed with a local health or other government office. The family is usually given a copy to use for legal matters, such as insurance claims.

Labeling of the Deceased

Nurses have a duty to handle the deceased with dignity and label the corpse appropriately. Mishandling can cause emotional distress to survivors. Mislabeling can create legal problems if the body is inappropriately identified and prepared incorrectly for burial or a funeral. Usually, the deceased's wrist identification tag is left on, and another tag is tied to the client's ankle or big toe, in case one of the tags becomes detached. Tags tied to the ankle or toe are preferred, since any tissue damage they cause will be concealed by bed linen or clothing. A third tag is attached to the shroud. All identification tags should include the client's name, hospital number, and physician's name.

Autopsy

An **autopsy**, or **postmortem examination**, is an examination of the body after death. It is performed only in certain cases. The law describes under what circumstances an autopsy must be performed, e.g., when death is sudden or when it occurs within 48 hours of admission to a hospital. The organs and tissues of the body are examined to establish the exact cause of death, to learn more about a disease, and to assist in the accumulation of statistical data.

It is the responsibility of the physician or, in some instances, of a designated person in the hospital to obtain consent for autopsy. Consent must be given by the decedent (before death) or by the next of kin. Laws in many states and provinces prioritize the family members who can provide consent as follows: surviving spouse, adult children, parents, siblings. After autopsy, hospitals cannot retain any tissues or organs without the permission of the person who consented to the autopsy.

Organ Donation

Under the Uniform Anatomical Gift Act in the United States or the Human Tissue Act in Canada, any person 18 years or older and of sound mind may make a gift of all or any part of the body for the following purposes: for medical or dental education, research, advancement of medical or dental science, therapy, or transplantation. The donation can be made by a provision in a will or by signing a cardlike form in the presence of two witnesses. This card is usually carried at all times by the person who signed it. In most states and provinces, the gift can be revoked either by destroying the card or by an oral revocation in the presence of two witnesses. Nurses may serve as witnesses for persons consenting to donate organs. In some states (e.g., California) health care workers are required to ask survivors for consent to donate the deceased's organs.

Inquest

An **inquest** is a legal inquiry into the cause or manner of a death. When a death is the result of an accident, for example, an inquest is held into the circumstances of the accident to determine any blame. The inquest is conducted under the jurisdiction of a coroner or medical examiner. A **coroner** is a public official, not necessarily a physician, appointed or elected to inquire into the causes of death, when appropriate. A **medical examiner** is a physician who usually has advanced education in pathology or forensic medicine. Agency policy dictates who is responsible for reporting deaths to the coroner or medical examiner.

Technique 8–3 explains the steps involved in caring for a body after death.

8-3   Caring for a Body after Death

Generally a nurse is responsible for preparing the body after death and making arrangements for the client's property. Postmortem care begins after the physician has confirmed death. Although procedures differ among agencies, there are certain common elements.

PURPOSES

- To maintain the best possible appearance of the body by preventing skin damage and discoloration.
- To maintain the dignity of the deceased by safeguarding belongings and handling the body with respect and care

EQUIPMENT

- ☐ Clean gown
- ☐ Valuables list and envelopes for valuables
- ☐ Paper bags or other containers provided by the agency for the client's clothing
- ☐ Moistened cotton fluffs for eyelids (optional)
- ☐ Shroud or sheets
- ☐ Dressing materials if a wound is present
- ☐ Two identification tags
- ☐ Absorbent pads or a diaper
- ☐ Masking tape

▶ **Technique 8–3** *CONTINUED*

INTERVENTION

1. Determine the agency's policies about the following:

- Identification of the body.

- Removal of equipment from the body.

- Tissue and organ removal and donation.

- Autopsy requirements and permission.

- The death certificate.

- Practices for positioning the client's body; handling dentures, hairpieces, and so on; and wrapping the body.

- If death occurred following an infectious disease, the precautions to be taken to prevent the spread of the disease to others. Practices depend on the causative organism and its mode of transmission.

2. Provide privacy.

- Close the room door and/or pull the bed curtains around the bed. *Screening provides privacy for the deceased and the family and is less disturbing to other clients.*

- If there are other clients in the room, give them an honest explanation.

3. Position the client appropriately.

- Place the body in straight alignment in the supine position, with the arms laid palm down at the sides or according to agency policy. Some agencies prefer the arms to be laid across the abdomen. If this is the case, avoid placing one hand on top of the other. *The underlying hand will become discolored.*

- Place one pillow under the head and shoulders. *This prevents the settling of blood in the face and subsequent discoloration.*

- Close the eyelids by gently holding your fingertips over each eyelid for a few seconds. Do not use Scotch tape or adhesive tape to close the eyelids. *These are difficult to remove without damaging the tissues.* If the eyelids do not remain closed, place a moistened cotton fluff on each eyelid for a few moments. *Closed eyelids give the face a natural appearance for viewing.*

- Put the client's dentures, if any, in the client's mouth. If this is not possible, label and store them properly for the mortician to insert.

- If the mouth does not remain closed, place a small rolled towel under the chin.

4. Detach and remove equipment from the body in accordance with agency policy.

- Detach bottles, bags, and receptacles from intravenous tubes, nasogastric tubes, urinary catheters, and so on.

- Follow agency policies about whether the tubes are to be removed or clamped and left in place. In some agencies, the policy is to clamp all tubes and leave them in place if an autopsy is to be performed. In other agencies, tubes are cut 2.5 cm (1 in) from the body and taped to the skin. In still others, tracheostomy or endotracheal tubes are removed, but other tubes, such as intravenous and nasogastric tubes, are left in place and clamped. And in some agencies, all tubes are removed and discarded.

5. Clean the body as needed.

- Using plain water, wash soiled areas of the body. A complete bath is unnecessary, since the body is washed by the mortician.

However, excessive soil, such as feces, emesis, or blood, needs to be removed to prevent odor caused by microorganisms.

- Place absorbent pads under the buttocks if soiling occurs, or apply a diaper according to agency practice. *Sphincter muscles relax after death and may release urine or feces.*

- Remove soiled dressings if necessary, and replace them with light gauze dressings.

- Put a clean gown on the client if agency policy recommends this. *A clean gown is generally put on if the family wishes to view the deceased.*

- If the support persons are to view the decreased, adjust the top linen as necessary, and cover the client to the shoulders. *A clean and neat appearance is important to the family.*

- Brush and comb the hair. Remove hairpins. *The client should appear nicely groomed for viewing by the family. Hairpins are removed to prevent damage to the scalp or face of the deceased.*

6. Assemble the client's clothing, valuables, and other personal effects.

- Remove all jewelry, with the possible exception of a wedding band. Family members may request that a wedding band be left on. If a wedding band is not to be removed, check agency policies about whether it is to be taped on or tied with gauze.

- List all the client's valuables, label them, and give them to the next of kin or put them in a secure place at the nursing station. *The nurse is responsible for preventing the loss of personal items, such as eyeglasses, keys, and re-*

► **Technique 8–3 Caring for a Body after Death** CONTINUED

ligious medals. Generally, eyeglasses, dentures, and hair that was shaved for surgery are labeled and sent with the body to the mortician.

- Place the client's clothing and other personal effects in a labeled container for the next of kin.

7. Label the body.

- Attach identification tags to the body. Leave the wrist identification band in place, and tie another identification tag to the client's ankle or big toe. If the wrist band is restrictive, however, remove it. All identification tags should include the client's name, hospital number, and physician's name. *Appropriate identification cannot be overemphasized. More than one tag is applied in case one becomes detached. Tags tied to the ankles or toes are preferred, since any tissue damage they cause will be concealed by bed linen or clothing.*

8. Assist support persons as needed to view the deceased.

- Provide soft lighting and chairs for family members. *Lowered lighting softens the stark features of the deceased.*

- Stay with the support persons at first, then leave them with the body. *Some people may at first want the comfort of the nurse's presence and then privacy with the deceased.*

9. After the family leaves, wrap the body, and ensure appropriate labeling.

- After the family leaves, apply a shroud or wrap the body in a sheet (Figure 8–2). In some agencies, the ankles are first tied together. *Wrapping prevents damage to the extremities, avoids unnecessary exposure, and maintains the dignity of the deceased.*

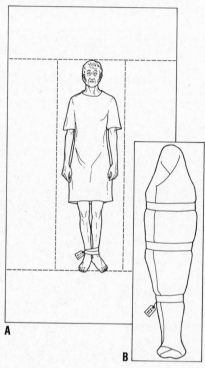

FIGURE 8–2 *A,* Position of body on sheet or shroud. Note identification tag. *B,* Body wrapped in shroud with another identification tag attached.

- Securely attach the sheet or shroud in accordance with agency policy. *Because safety pins can create pressure and damage the deceased's skin, masking tape is generally preferred to fasten the shroud.*

- Attach a second identification tag to the outside of the shroud.

- If the client had an infectious disease, attach a special tag with that information.

10. Transfer the client's body to the morgue.

- Arrange for the body to be transported to the morgue for cooling, if arrangements have not been made for the mortician to take the body from the client's room.

- Move the body gently when transferring it to a stretcher. Ensure that the alignment of the body is maintained. *Rough movements could damage the body tissues.*

- Transport the body as inconspicuously as possible. In some agencies, other clients' room doors are closed before transporting the deceased through the corridors, and service elevators are used. *The sight of a body is often disturbing to clients and hospital visitors.*

11. Document all relevant information.

- Record the events leading to the actual death, the date and time of death (i.e., termination of vital signs), the time the physician was notified, who pronounced the death, how valuables and personal belongings were handled, care given the body, any forms signed by the family, visits by any family or clergy, identification attached to the body, disposition of the body, and information given to support persons and their responses.

SAMPLE RECORDING

Date	Time	Notes
1/4/93	0630	Pronounced dead by Dr. Darcy. Family members notified by physician. Signed permission for autopsy obtained by Dr. Darcy. Gold-colored wedding band taped to finger on body; other valuables given to Mrs. Robert Brown (daughter). Body viewed by family. Family's clergyman present. Body transported with I.D. according to agency policy and death certificate to hospital morgue. —————————————— Matthew S. Lewis, RN

▶ **Technique 8–3** *CONTINUED*

KEY ELEMENTS OF CARING FOR A BODY AFTER DEATH

- Provide privacy.
- Handle the body with respect and care; clean the body as needed to remove excessive secretions and excretions.
- Apply a clean gown on the client if the family wishes to view the deceased.
- Avoid movements or actions that could cause skin damage and discoloration of the body.
- Label the body appropriately.
- Follow agency policies about positioning the body; handling dentures, hairpieces, and so on; detaching and removing equipment from the

body; wrapping the body; tissue and organ donation and removal; autopsy requirements and permission; and the death certificate.
- Support family members and friends as needed to view the body.
- Ensure that appropriate infection control precautions are implemented if death occurred following an infectious disease.
- Safeguard the client's personal effects.
- Arrange for transport of the body to the morgue.

CRITICAL THINKING CHALLENGE

Maria Rodriguez was admitted to the special care unit in congestive heart failure 3 days ago. She has been progressing well, and the physician has ordered her transfer to a general medical nursing unit. Since she was informed of the proposed transfer, she has been complaining of chest pain and shortness of breath. What factors (physiologic or psychologic) might be causing Ms Rodriguez's symptoms? What nursing actions should you take?

RELATED RESEARCH

Edelstein, J. November 1990. A study of nursing documentation. *Nursing Management* 21:40–43, 46.

Jackson, M. F. February 1990. Use of community support services by elderly patients discharged from general medical and geriatric medical wards. *Journal of Advanced Nursing* 15:167–75.

Oktag, J. S., and Volland, P. J. January 1990. Post-hospital support program for the frail elderly and their care-givers: A quasi-experimental evaluation. *American Journal of Public Health* 80:39–46.

Schaefer, A. L.; Anderson, J. A.; and Simms, L. M. October 1990. Are they ready? Discharge planning for older surgical patients. *Journal of Gerontological Nursing* 16:16–19, 36–37.

Sharer, K.; Reich, M.; Evoy, K.; et al. August 1990. Evaluating written discharge instructions in a pediatric setting. *Journal of Nursing Quality Assurance* 4(4):63–71.

REFERENCES
Ashley, M. H. December 1989. Discharge holding area: Using inpatient beds more efficiently. *Journal of Nursing Administration* 19:32–38.

Benton, R. E. 1978. *Death and dying: Principles and practices in patient care.* New York: D. Van Nostrand Co.

Gerardi, R. 1989. Western spirituality and health care. In Carson, V., editor. *Spiritual dimensions of nursing practice.* Philadelphia: W. B. Saunders Co.

Penticuff, J. H. February 1990. Ethical issues in redefining death. *Journal of Neuroscience Nursing* 22:48–49.

Schulz, R. 1978. *The psychology of death, dying and bereavement.* Reading, Mass.: Addison-Wesley Publishing Co.

Smith, J. B. January/February 1990. Effective discharge planning and home health care: How-tos for the staff nurse. *Advancing Clinical Care* 5(1):6–8.

Wolf, Z. R. January/February 1991. Care of dying patients and patients after death: Patterns of care in nursing history. *Death Studies* 15(1):81–93.

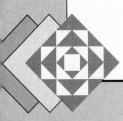

9

Preventing the Transfer of Microorganisms

CONTENTS

NURSING PROCESS GUIDE
PREVENTING INFECTION

ASSESSMENT

Determine

- Risk for acquiring an infection:

  - Last immunization dates for diphtheria, tetanus, poliomyelitis, rubella, measles, influenza, and pneumococcal pneumonia, and hepatitis B

  - Current administration of antineoplastic, anti-inflammatory, and antibiotic medications

  - Recent diagnostic procedure or treatment that penetrated the skin or a body cavity

  - Current nutritional status

- Signs and symptoms indicating the presence of an infection:

  - Localized signs (swelling, redness, pain or tenderness with palpation or movement, palpable heat at infected site, loss of function of affected body part, presence of exudate)

  - Systemic indications (fever, increased pulse and respiratory rates, lassitude, malaise, lack of energy, anorexia, enlarged lymph nodes)

  - Laboratory data: elevated leukocyte (white blood cell) count (i.e., over 11,000/mm³); elevated erythrocyte sedimentation rate (ERS); urine, blood, sputum, or other drainage cultures

- Signs associated with specific body systems (difficulty urinating, urinary frequency, sore throat, productive cough, nausea, vomiting, diarrhea)

RELATED DIAGNOSTIC CATEGORIES

- High risk for Infection

PLANNING

Client Goals
The client will

- Avoid infection or extension of present infection during hospitalization.

- Avoid transmission of infectious agents to others.

Outcome Criteria
The client

- Verbalizes understanding of individual risk factors.

- Identifies measures to prevent or reduce the risk of infection.

- Practices appropriate precautions to reduce the risk of infection.

- Obtains recommended immunization(s).

- Experiences no signs of infection in surgical wound.

- Has normal flora in cultures of body secretions, excretions, and exudates.

- Has a leukocyte count within normal limits.

Chain of Infection

There are six links in the chain of infection: the etiologic agent, or microorganism; the place where the organism naturally resides (reservoir); a portal of exit from the reservoir; a method (mode) of transmission; a portal of entry into a host; and the susceptibility of the host. See Figure 9–1. It is important for nurses to understand this chain so as to reduce the risk of transmission at portals of exit and entry.

Etiologic Agent (Microorganism)

A **parasite** is a microorganism that lives in or on another and obtains its nourishment from it. All viruses are parasites. The extent to which any microorganism or parasite is capable of producing an infectious process depends on the number of organisms

present, the virulence and potency of the organisms (pathogenicity), the ability of the organisms to enter the body, the susceptibility of the host, and the ability of the organisms to live in the host's body.

Some microorganisms, such as the smallpox virus, have the ability to infect almost all susceptible people after exposure. By contrast, microorganisms such as the tuberculosis bacillus infect a relatively small number of the population who are susceptible and exposed, usually people who are poorly nourished and living in unsanitary conditions. The presence of organisms in body secretions or excretions that does not cause illness is called **colonization**. A **carrier** is a person or animal that harbors a specific infectious agent and serves as a potential source of infection yet does not manifest any clinical signs of disease.

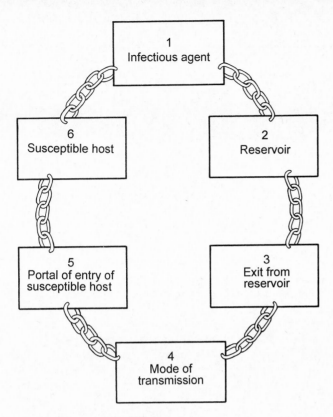

FIGURE 9–1 The chain of infection.

TABLE 9–1 HUMAN RESERVOIRS AND PORTALS OF EXIT

Reservoir	Portals of Exit
1. Respiratory tract	Nose/mouth through sneezing, coughing, breathing, or talking; endotracheal tubes or tracheostomies
2. Gastrointestinal tract	Mouth: through saliva, vomitus; anus/ostomies: feces; drainage tubes: e.g., nasogastric or T-tubes
3. Urinary tract	Urethral meatus and urinary diversion ostomies
4. Reproductive tract	Vagina: vaginal discharge; may be further transported by urine; urinary meatus: semen, urine
5. Blood	Open wound, needle puncture site, any disruption of intact skin or mucous membrane surfaces

The carrier state may also exist in the incubation period, convalescence, and postconvalescence of an individual with a clinically recognizable disease. This type of carrier is referred to as an *incubatory* or *convalescent carrier*. Under either circumstance, the carrier state may be of short duration (*temporary* or *transient carrier*) or long duration (*chronic carrier*) (Beneson 1990, p. 497).

Reservoir

There are many **reservoirs**, or sources of microorganisms. Common sources are other humans, the client's own microorganisms, plants, animals, or the general environment. People are the most common source of infection for others and for themselves. The person with, for example, an influenza virus frequently spreads it to others. When resistance is lowered by fatigue and other factors, an infection emerges.

Portal of Exit

Before an infection can establish itself in a host, the microorganisms must leave the reservoir. If the reservoir is within a human, the microorganisms have a number of exits, depending on the site of the reservoir. Common human reservoirs and their associated portals of exit are summarized in Table 9–1.

Method of Transmission

After a microorganism leaves its source or reservoir, it requires a means of transmission to reach another person or host through a *receptive portal of entry*. There are three mechanisms:

1. *Direct transmission*. Direct transmission involves immediate and direct transfer of microorganisms from person to person through touching, biting, kissing, or sexual intercourse. Droplet spread is also a form of direct contact but can occur only if the source and the host are within 3 feet of each other. Sneezing, coughing, spitting, singing, or talking can project droplet spray into the conjunctiva or onto the mucous membranes of the eye, nose, or mouth of another person.

2. *Indirect transmission*. Indirect transmission may be either vehicle-borne or vector-borne.
 a. *Vehicle-borne*. A *vehicle* is any substance that serves as an intermediate means to transport and introduce an infectious agent into a susceptible host through a suitable portal of entry. *Fomites* (inanimate materials or objects), such as handkerchiefs, toys, soiled clothes, cooking or eating utensils, and surgical instruments or dressings, can act as vehicles. For example, an intravenous needle can be a vehicle for transmission of microorganisms from the reservoir to the host. Water, food, milk, blood, serum, and plasma are other vehicles. For example, food or water may become contaminated by a food handler who transports the hepatitis A virus. The food is then ingested by a susceptible host.

b. *Vector-borne.* A *vector* is an animal or flying or crawling insect that serves as an intermediate means of transporting the infectious agent. Transmission may occur by injecting salivary fluid during biting or by depositing feces or other materials on the skin through the bite wound or a traumatized skin area.

3. *Airborne transmission.* Airborne transmission occurs when **droplet nuclei** (residue of evaporated droplets that may remain in the air for long periods of time) emitted by an infected host (e.g., one with tuberculosis) or dust particles containing the infectious agent (e.g., *Clostridium difficile* spores from the soil) are transmitted by air currents to a suitable portal of entry, usually the respiratory tract, of another person.

Portal of Entry

Before a person can become infected, microorganisms must enter the body. The skin is a barrier to infectious agents; however, any break in the skin can also readily serve as a portal of entry. Microorganisms can enter the body through the same routes they use to leave the body. Often, microorganisms enter the body by the same route they used to leave the source.

Susceptible Host

A **susceptible host** is any person who is at risk for infection. **Compromised hosts** are persons "at increased risk," individuals who for one or more reasons are more likely than others to acquire an infection. Impairment of the body's natural defenses and a number of other factors can affect susceptibility to infection.

Breaking the Chain of Infection

Various practices break the chain of infection or interrupt the infectious disease process. For example, the first link in the chain, the etiologic agent, is interrupted by the use of **antiseptics** (agents that inhibit the growth of some microorganisms) and **disinfectants** (agents that destroy microorganisms other than spores), and by **sterilization**. Nurses carry out practices that break other links in the chain. The aim of most hospital precautions is breaking the chain during the mode of transmission phase of the cycle.

Reducing Risks for Infection

Planned nursing strategies to reduce the risk of transmission of organisms from one person to another include the use of meticulous medical and surgical asepsis. **Asepsis** is the freedom from infection or infectious material. There are two basic types of asepsis: medical and surgical. **Medical asepsis** includes all practices intended to confine a specific microorganism to a specific area, limiting the number, growth, and spread of microorganisms. **Surgical asepsis**, or sterile technique, refers to those practices that keep an area or objects free of all microorgan-

TABLE 9–2   CATEGORY-SPECIFIC ISOLATION PRECAUTIONS

Isolation Category	Purpose	Private Room	Gowns
1. *Strict isolation*, e.g., for diphtheria, pneumonic plague, smallpox, varicella (chickenpox), zoster.	To prevent airborne or contact transmission of highly contagious or virulent microorganisms.	Necessary; door must be kept closed.	Must be worn by all persons entering room; for smallpox, coverings for cap and shoes are also recommended.
2. *Contact isolation*, e.g., for acute respiratory infections and influenza in children, pediculosis, wound infections, herpes simplex, impetigo, rubella, scabies.	To prevent highly transmissible infections not requiring strict isolation but spread by close or direct contact.	Necessary.	Must be worn if soiling is likely.
3. *Respiratory isolation*, e.g., for epiglottitis, measles, meningitis, mumps, pertussis, pneumonia in children.	To prevent infections spread by contaminated articles (e.g., tissues) and respiratory droplets that are coughed, sneezed, or exhaled.	Necessary.	Not necessary.

isms; it includes practices that destroy all microorganisms and spores. A **spore** is a round or oval structure enclosed in a tough capsule. Some microorganisms assume this structure in response to adverse conditions; in this form, they are highly resistant to destruction. Sterile technique is required for invasive procedures, such as injections, intravenous therapy, or urinary catheterization.

Isolation Precautions in Hospital

CDC Guidelines

Isolation practices are indicated when a client has an infection that can be transmitted to others. In 1983, the Centers for Disease Control (CDC) published recommendations regarding isolation practices in hospitals. The CDC recommended that hospitals either choose *one* of the following alternative systems for isolation or design their own system (Garner and Simmons 1983, p. 245).

- *Category-specific isolation system* based on seven categories: strict isolation, contact isolation, respiratory isolation, tuberculosis isolation, enteric precautions, drainage/secretions precautions, and blood/body fluid precautions (see Table 9–2)

- *Disease-specific isolation precautions*

In 1987, the CDC also presented recommendations for *universal precautions* (*UP*) on all clients to decrease the risk of transmitting unidentified pathogens (U.S. Department of Health and Human Services pp. 35–85). The CDC guidelines for universal precautions are shown on the back cover. They apply primarily to reducing the transmission of blood-borne pathogens.

The Body Substance Isolation System (BSIS)

The *body substance isolation system* is a more recent system based on three premises (Jackson and Lynch 1991, p. 448):

1. All people have an increased risk for infection from microorganisms placed on their mucous membranes and nonintact skin.

2. All people are likely to have potentially infectious microorganisms in all of their moist body sites and substances.

3. An unknown portion of clients and health care workers will always be colonized or infected with potentially infectious microorganisms in their blood and other moist body sites and substances.

The purposes of the BSIS are similar to those of all precaution systems: (a) to prevent cross-transmission of microorganisms from the hands of health care workers to clients and (b) to protect the health

Masks	Gloves	Hand Washing	Disposal of Contaminated Articles
Must be worn by all persons entering room.	Must be worn by all persons entering room.	Necessary after touching client or potentially contaminated articles and before caring for another client.	Discard in plastic-lined container or bag and label before sending for decontamination and reprocessing.
Must be worn if person comes near the client.	Worn if touching infected material.	Same as for strict isolation.	Same as for strict isolation.
Must be worn by all persons in close contact.	Not necessary.	Same as for strict isolation.	Same as for strict isolation.

▶ **TABLE 9–2** CATEGORY-SPECIFIC ISOLATION PRECAUTIONS *CONTINUED*

Isolation Category	Purpose	Private Room	Gowns
4. *Tuberculosis isolation* (AFB isolation) for pulmonary tuberculosis when clients have positive sputum smear or suggestive chest X-ray film.	To prevent spread of acid-fast bacilli (AFB).	Necessary, with special ventilation.	Necessary only if clothing may become contaminated.
5. *Enteric precautions*, e.g., for hepatitis A, some gastroenteritis, typhoid fever, cholera, diarrhea with suspected infectious etiology, encephalitis, meningitis.	To prevent infections spread through direct or indirect contact with feces.	Necessary if client hygiene is poor, e.g., client is incontinent.	Same as for tuberculosis isolation.
6. *Drainage/secretion precautions*, e.g., for any draining lesion, abscess, infected burn, infected skin, decubitis ulcer, conjunctivitis.	To prevent infections spread through direct or indirect contact with material or drainage from body site.	Not necessary unless client hygiene is poor.	Same as for tuberculosis isolation.
7. *Blood/body fluid precautions*, e.g., for hepatitis B, syphilis, AIDS, malaria.	To prevent infections spread through direct or indirect contact with infected blood or body fluids.	Necessary if client hygiene is poor.	Same as for tuberculosis isolation.

care worker from microorganisms harbored by clients. See the accompanying box for use of appropriate precautions in the BSIS.

Maintaining Surgical Asepsis

An object is sterile only when it is free of all microorganisms. It is well known that surgical asepsis is practiced in operating rooms, labor and delivery rooms, and special diagnostic areas. Less known, perhaps, is that surgical asepsis is also employed for many procedures in general care areas (i.e., procedures such as administering injections, changing wound dressings, performing urinary catheterizations, and administering intravenous therapy). In these situations, all of the principles of surgical asepsis are applied as in the operating or delivery room; however, not all of the sterile techniques that follow are always required. For example, before an operating room procedure, the nurse generally puts on a mask and cap, performs a surgical hand scrub, and then dons a sterile gown and gloves. In a general care area, the nurse may only perform a hand wash and don sterile gloves. The nine basic principles of surgical

---

Body Substance Isolation System*

Use appropriate barriers as follows:

- *Gloves.* Put on clean gloves immediately before contact with a client's mucous membranes or non-intact skin. Wear gloves before contact with any moist body substance. Use sterile gloves when in contact with sterile areas.

- *Gowns and plastic aprons.* Wear a gown or plastic apron if soiling of clothing is likely. There is little evidence that clothing can serve to transmit infectious organisms.

- *Masks and eyewear.* Wear a mask and/or eye protection only if there is a likelihood of being splashed in the nose, mouth, or eyes. They are not indicated most of the time.

- *Private room.* Place the client in a private room if the client's hygienic practices are poor or if the client has an airborne communicable disease.

*Care providers for clients with airborne communicable diseases (e.g., chickenpox) should be immune to those diseases. Susceptible hosts should not be assigned to care for these clients. Care providers of clients who have pulmonary tuberculosis should follow agency protocol regarding use of masks.

Masks	Gloves	Hand Washing	Disposal of Contaminated Articles
Necessary if client is coughing and does not always cover mouth.	Not necessary.	Same as for strict isolation.	Clean and disinfect, although these articles rarely transmit disease.
Not necessary.	Necessary if touching infected material.	Same as for strict isolation.	Same as for strict isolation.
Not necessary.	Same as for enteric precautions.	Same as for strict isolation.	Same as for strict isolation.
Not necessary. Goggles are used if spatter is considered likely.	Necessary if touching infected blood or body fluid with visible blood.	Necessary if hands can become contaminated and before caring for another client.	Same as for strict isolation; used needles must be placed in puncture-proof container for disposal.

Source: Adapted from J. S. Garner and B. P. Simmons, CDC guidelines for isolation precautions in hospitals, *Infection Control*, July/August 1983. 4:258–60.

asepsis and practices that relate to each principle appear in Table 9–3 on page 138.

Hand Washing

Hand washing is important in every setting where people are ill, including hospitals. It is considered one of the most effective infection control measures. The goal of hand washing is to remove transient microorganisms that might be transmitted to the nurse, clients, visitors, or other health care personnel.

Any client may harbor microorganisms that are currently harmless to the client yet potentially harmful to another person or to the same client *if they find a portal of entry.* It is important that hands be washed at the following times to prevent the spread of these microorganisms: before eating, after using the bedpan or toilet, and after the hands have come in contact with any body substances, such as sputum or drainage from a wound. In addition, health care workers should wash their hands before and after any direct client contact.

For routine client care, the CDC recommends a vigorous hand washing under a stream of water for

at least 10 seconds using bar soap, granule soap, soap-filled tissues, or antimicrobial liquid soap (Garner and Favero 1985, p. 7). Liquid soaps are frequently supplied in dispensers at the sink. Antimicrobial soaps are usually provided in high-risk areas, e.g., the newborn nursery. In the following situations, the CDC recommends antimicrobial hand-washing agents with any chemical germicides listed with the Environmental Protection Agency:

- When there are known multiple resistant bacteria

- Before invasive procedures

- In special care units, such as nurseries and ICUs

This book recommends that the hands be held down (below the elbows) when they are soiled with body substances and during routine hand washing so that the microorganisms are washed directly into the sink. For surgical asepsis, the hands should be held above the elbows so that the water runs from the cleanest to the least clean area. Nurses usually dry their hands with paper towels, discarding them in an appropriate container immediately after use. Technique 9–1 on page 139 provides more detailed instructions for hand washing.

TABLE 9–3   PRINCIPLES AND PRACTICES OF SURGICAL ASEPSIS

Principles	Practices
All objects used in a sterile field must be sterile.	All articles are sterilized appropriately by dry or moist heat, chemicals, or radiation before use.
	Sterile articles can be stored for only a prescribed time; after that, they are considered unsterile.
	Always check a package containing a sterile object for intactness, dryness, and expiration date. Any package that appears already open, torn, punctured, or wet is considered unsterile. Never assume an item is sterile.
	Storage areas should be clean, dry, off the floor, and away from sinks.
	Always check the sterilization dates and periods on the labels of wrapped items before using the items.
	Always check chemical indicators of sterilization before using a package. The indicator is often a tape used to fasten the package or contained inside the package. The indicator changes color during sterilization, indicating that the contents have undergone a sterilization procedure. If the color change is not evident, the package is considered unsterile. Commercially prepared sterile packages may not have indicators but are marked with the word *sterile*.
Sterile objects become unsterile when touched by unsterile objects.	Handle sterile objects that will touch open wounds or enter body cavities only with sterile forceps or sterile gloved hands.
	Discard or resterilize objects that come into contact with unsterile objects.
	Whenever the sterility of an object is questionable, assume the article is unsterile.
Sterile items that are out of vision or below the waist level of the nurse are considered unsterile.	Once left unattended, a sterile field is considered unsterile.
	Sterile objects are always kept in view. Nurses do not turn their backs on a sterile field.
	Only the front part of a sterile gown (from the waist to the shoulder) and 2 inches above the elbows to the cuff of the sleeves are considered sterile.
	Always keep sterile gloved hands in sight and above waist level; touch only objects that are sterile.
	Sterile draped tables in the operating room or elsewhere are considered sterile only at surface level.
	Once a sterile field becomes unsterile, it must be set up again before proceeding.
Sterile objects can become unsterile by prolonged exposure to airborne microorganisms.	Doors are closed, and traffic is kept to a minimum in areas where a sterile procedure is being performed because moving air can carry dust and microorganisms.
	Areas in which sterile procedures are carried out are kept as clean as possible by frequent damp cleaning with detergent germicides to minimize contaminants in the area.
	Keep hair clean and short or enclose it in a net to prevent hair from falling on sterile objects. Microorganisms on the hair can make a sterile field unsterile.
	Surgical caps are worn in operating rooms, delivery rooms, and burn units.
	Sneezing or coughing over a sterile field can make it unsterile because droplets containing microorganisms from the respiratory tract can travel 3 feet. Some nurses recommend that masks covering the mouth and the nose should be worn by anyone working over a sterile field or an open wound.
	Nurses with mild upper respiratory tract infections refrain from carrying out sterile procedures or wear masks.
	Anyone working over a sterile field keeps talking to a minimum. Avert the head from the field if talking is necessary.
	Refrain from reaching over a sterile field unless sterile gloves are worn and from moving unsterile objects over a sterile field because microorganisms can fall onto it. Always reach around a sterile field or carefully turn it by reaching under the wrapper or by touching the wrapper edges.
Fluids flow in the direction of gravity.	Unless gloves are worn, always hold wet forceps with the tips below the handles. When the tips are held higher than the handles, fluid can flow onto the handle and become contaminated by the hands. When the forceps are again pointed downward, the fluid flows back down and contaminates the tips.
	During a surgical hand wash, hold the hands higher than the elbows to prevent contaminants from the forearms from reaching the hands.
Moisture that passes through a sterile object draws microorganisms from unsterile surfaces above or below to the sterile surface by capillary action.	Sterile waterproof barriers are used beneath sterile objects. Liquids (sterile saline or antiseptics) are frequently poured into containers on a sterile field. If they are spilled onto the sterile field, the barrier keeps the liquid from seeping beneath it.
	The sterile covers on sterile equipment are kept dry. Damp surfaces can attract microorganisms in the air.
	When pouring sterile solutions into sterile containers, take care to avoid dampening the sterile field.
	Replace sterile drapes that do not have a sterile barrier underneath when they become moist.

TABLE 9–3 *CONTINUED*

Principles	Practices
The edges of a sterile field are considered unsterile.	A 2.5 cm (1 in) margin at each edge of an opened drape is considered unsterile, since the edges are in contact with unsterile surfaces.
	All sterile objects are placed more than 2.5 cm (1 in) inside the edges of a sterile field.
	Any article that falls outside the edges of a sterile field is considered unsterile.
The skin cannot be sterilized and is unsterile.	Wear sterile gloves and/or use sterile forceps to handle sterile items.
	Prior to a surgical aseptic procedure, wash the hands to reduce the number of microorganisms on them.
Conscientiousness, alertness, and honesty are essential qualities in maintaining surgical asepsis.	When a sterile object becomes unsterile, it does not necessarily change in appearance.
	The person who sees a sterile object become contaminated must correct or report the situation.
	Do not set up a sterile field ahead of time for future use.

9-1   Hand Washing

PURPOSES
- To reduce the number of microorganisms on the hands
- To reduce the risk of transmission of microorganisms to clients
- To reduce the risk of cross-contamination among clients
- To reduce the risk of infection among other health care workers
- To reduce the risk of transmission of infectious organisms to oneself

EQUIPMENT
- ☐ Soap
- ☐ Warm running water
- ☐ Towels

INTERVENTION

1. Prepare and assess the hands.

- File the nails short. *Short nails are less likely to harbor microorganisms, scratch a client, or puncture gloves. Long nails are hard to clean.*

- Remove all jewelry. Some nurses prefer to slide their watches up above their elbows. Others pin the watch to the uniform. *Microorganisms can lodge in the settings of jewelry and under rings (Larson 1989, p. 936). Removal facilitates proper cleaning of the hands and arms.*

- Check hands for breaks in the skin, such as hangnails or cuts. Report cuts to the instructor or nurse in charge before beginning work, or check agency policy about cuts. Use lotions to prevent hangnails and cracked, dry skin. A nurse who has open sores may have to change work assignments or wear gloves to avoid contact with infectious material.

2. Turn on the water, and adjust the flow.

- There are four common types of faucet controls:

  a. Hand-operated handles.

  b. Knee levers. Move these with the knee to regulate flow and temperature. (Figure 9–2).

  c. Foot pedals. Press these with the foot to regulate flow and temperature. (Figure 9–3 on page 140).

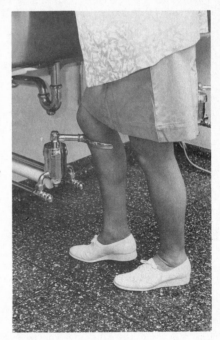

FIGURE 9–2   A knee-lever faucet control.

▶ **Technique 9–1 Hand Washing** *CONTINUED*

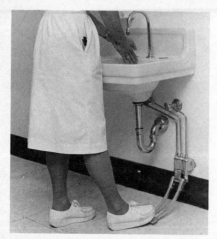

FIGURE 9–3   A foot-pedal faucet control.

d. Elbow controls. Move these with the elbows instead of the hands.

- Adjust the flow so that the water is warm. *Warm water removes less of the protective oil of the skin than hot water.*

3. Wet the hands thoroughly by holding them under the running water, and apply soap to the hands.

- Hold the hands lower than the elbows so that the water flows from the arms to the fingertips. *The water should flow from the least contaminated to the most contaminated area; the hands are generally considered more contaminated than the lower arms.*

- If the soap is liquid, apply 2 to 4 ml (1 tsp). If it is bar soap, rub it firmly between the hands.

4. Thoroughly wash and rinse the hands.

- Use firm, rubbing, and circular movements to wash the palm, back, and wrist of each hand. Interlace the fingers and thumbs, and move the hands back and forth (Figure 9–4). Then continue this motion for 10 seconds. *The circular action helps remove microorganisms mechanically. Interlacing the fingers and thumbs cleans the interdigital spaces.*

- Rinse the hands.

- Wash hands for a minimum of 10 seconds. For a more thorough washing, extend the time for wetting, washing, and rinsing.

5. Thoroughly dry the hands and arms.

- Dry hands and arms thoroughly with a paper towel. *Moist skin becomes chapped readily; chapping produces lesions.*

- Discard the paper towel in the appropriate container.

6. Turn off the water.

- Use paper towels to grasp a hand-operated control (Figure 9–5). *This prevents the nurse from picking up microorganisms from the faucet handles.*

VARIATION: Hand Washing before Sterile Techniques

- Hold the hands higher than the elbows during this hand wash. Wet the hands and forearms under the running water, letting it run from the fingertips to the el-

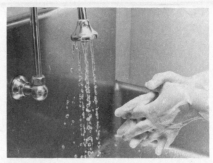

FIGURE 9–4   Interlacing the fingers during hand washing.

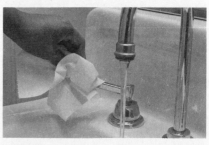

FIGURE 9–5   Using a paper towel to grasp the handle of a hand-operated faucet.

bows so that the hands become cleaner than the elbows (Figure 9–11, later in this chapter). *In this way, the water runs from the area with the fewest microorganisms to areas with a relatively greater number.*

- Apply the soap and wash as described earlier in Step 4, maintaining the hands uppermost.

- After washing and rinsing, use a towel to dry one hand thoroughly in a rotating motion from the fingers to the elbow. Use a clean towel to dry the other hand and arm. *A clean towel prevents the transfer of microorganisms from one elbow (least clean area) to the other hand (cleanest area).*

KEY ELEMENTS OF HAND WASHING

- Ensure that the hands and arms are free of lesions and jewelry.
- Ensure that the nails are short.
- Use tepid water.
- Hold the hands lower than the elbows.

- Wash the hands thoroughly, using firm, rubbing, circular movements and interlacing thumbs and fingers.
- Wash the hands for a minimum of 10 seconds.
- Thoroughly rinse and dry the hands.
- Use paper towels to turn off hand-operated tap handles.

Face Masks

Masks are worn to prevent the spread of organisms by the droplet contact and airborne routes. The CDC recommends that masks be worn (Garner and Simmons 1983, p. 254):

1. Only by those close to the client if the infection (e.g., acute respiratory diseases in children, measles, or mumps) is transmitted by large-particle aerosols (droplets). Large-particle aerosols are transmitted by close contact and generally travel short distances (about 1 m, or 3 ft).

2. By all persons entering the room if the infection (e.g., diphtheria) is transmitted by small-particle aerosols (droplet nuclei). Small-particle aerosols remain suspended in the air and thus travel greater distances by air.

Masks are worn by all persons entering the rooms of clients who require strict isolation. They are also worn during certain techniques requiring surgical asepsis. During a procedure requiring sterile technique, masks are worn to prevent the airborne or droplet contact transmission of exhaled microorganisms to the sterile field or to a client's open wound. Nurses should wear masks when they are in close contact with clients who require contact isolation, respiratory isolation, and tuberculosis isolation when the client does not cover the mouth when coughing.

Technique 9–2 describes how to don and remove a face mask.

 ## 9-2   Donning and Removing a Face Mask

PURPOSES

- To prevent the inhalation of infective airborne microorganisms
- To prevent the spread of airborne microorganisms from the nurse's respiratory tract to clients at risk (e.g., a person who has an exposed open wound) or to a sterile area

---

EQUIPMENT

☐ Clean mask

INTERVENTION

1. Don the face mask.

- High-efficiency disposable masks are more effective than cotton gauze or paper tissue masks (Garner and Simmons 1983, p. 254).

- Locate the top edge of the mask. The mask usually has a narrow metal strip along the edge.

- Hold the mask by the top two strings or loops.

- Place the upper edge of the mask over the bridge of the nose, and tie the upper ties at the back of the head or secure the loops around the ears. If glasses are worn, fit the upper edge of the mask under the glasses. *With the edge of the mask under the glasses, clouding of the glasses is less likely to occur.*

- Secure the lower edge of the mask under the chin, and tie the lower ties at the nape of the neck (Figure 9–6). *To be effective, a mask must cover both the nose and the mouth, because air moves in and out of both.*

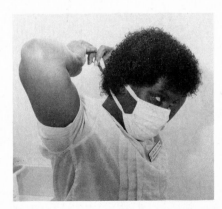

FIGURE 9–6   Tying a mask snugly over the mouth and nose.

- If the mask has a metal strip, adjust this firmly over the bridge of the nose. *A secure fit prevents both the escape and the inhalation of microorganisms around the edges of the mask and the fogging of eyeglasses.*

- Avoid unnecessary talking and, if possible, sneezing or coughing when caring for an at-risk client (e.g., when exposing an open wound).

- Wear the mask only once, and do not wear any mask longer than the manufacturer recommends or once it becomes wet. Do not leave a used face mask hanging around the neck. *A mask should be used only once because it becomes ineffective when moist.*

2. Remove the mask.

▶ **Technique 9–2 Donning and Removing a Face Mask** CONTINUED

- Remove gloves, if used, or wash hands if they are soiled.

- If using a mask with strings, first untie the *lower* strings of the mask. *This prevents the top part of the mask from falling onto the chest.*

- Untie the top strings, and while holding the ties securely, remove the mask from the face. *This prevents hand contact with the moistened, contaminated portion of the mask.*
  or
  If side loops are present, lift the side loops up and away from the ears and face.

- Discard a disposable mask in the waste container.

- Wash the hands if they have become contaminated by accidentally touching the soiled part of the mask.

KEY ELEMENTS OF DONNING AND REMOVING A FACE MASK

When donning a mask:
- Fit the mask securely over the bridge of the nose and under the chin.
- Use a mask only once, and wear it no longer than the manufacturer recommends.

When removing a mask:
- Avoid hand or other contact with the moistened, contaminated portion of the mask.
- Wash hands.

Gowning

Clean or disposable gowns or plastic aprons are worn for isolation precautions when the nurse's uniform is likely to become soiled. Gowns are also required when persons enter the room of a client who has an infection, for example, varicella (chickenpox), that could cause serious illness if spread to others, even though soiling of the clothing is not likely (Garner and Simmons 1983, p. 254). Sterile gowns may be indicated when the nurse is changing the dressings of a client with extensive wounds, e.g., burns.

Technique 9–3 describes the steps in gowning.

9-3 Gowning for Isolation Precautions

PURPOSES
- To prevent soiling of the nurse's clothing
- To prevent transmission of microorganisms from the nurse to the client at risk (barrier technique)

EQUIPMENT
☐ Clean gown

INTERVENTION

1. Prepare to don the gown.
- Wash hands thoroughly to prevent the transmission of microorganisms to the client. *Infected clients may have a lowered resistance to microorganisms that do not usually cause infection.*

- Don a face mask, if required.

2. Don a clean gown.
- Pick up a clean gown, and allow it to unfold in front of you without allowing it to touch any area soiled with body substances.

- Slide the arms and the hands through the sleeves.

- Fasten the ties at the neck to keep the gown in place.

- Overlap the gown at the back as much as possible, and fasten the waist ties or belt (Figure 9–7). *Overlapping securely covers the uniform at the back. Waist ties keep the gown from falling away from the body and prevent inadvertent soiling of the uniform.*

▶ **Technique 9–3 Gowning for Isolation Precautions** *CONTINUED*

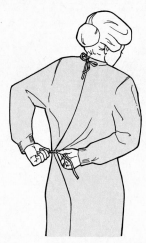

FIGURE 9–7 Overlapping the gown at the back to cover the nurse's uniform.

3. Don disposable gloves, if required. See Technique 9–4.

4. Remove the gown when preparing to leave the room. Unless a gown is grossly soiled with body substances, no special precautions are needed to remove it. Follow the steps below if a gown is grossly soiled.

- If wearing gloves, remove them. Dispose of them in the appropriate container. See Technique 9–4. *The gloves are likely to be more soiled than the gown and are therefore removed first.*

- Avoid touching soiled parts on the outside of the gown, if possible. The top part of the gown may be soiled, for example, if you have been holding an infant with a respiratory infection.

- Roll up the gown with the soiled part inside, and discard it in the appropriate container.

- Remove and discard the mask, if one has been worn, in the appropriate container.

- Wash hands when leaving the room.

KEY ELEMENTS OF GOWNING FOR ISOLATION PRECAUTIONS

- Put on a face mask, if required, before donning a gown, and remove the mask after removing the gown.
- Overlap the gown at the back to cover the uniform, and secure it with waist ties.
- Don gloves, if required, after putting on the gown, and remove them before removing the gown.
- Avoid touching the outside of a grossly contaminated gown when removing it.
- Wash hands after removing the gown.

Disposable Gloves

Disposable clean gloves are worn to protect the hands when the nurse is likely to handle any body substances, e.g., blood, urine, feces, sputum, mucous membranes, and nonintact skin. They are also indicated when caring for clients requiring strict isolation precautions. Nurses who have open sores or cuts on the hands should wear gloves for protection. Sterile gloves are used when the hands will come in contact with an open wound or when the hands might introduce microorganisms into a body orifice.

Technique 9–4 shows how to don and remove disposable gloves.

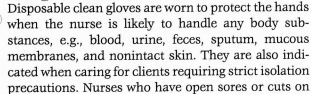

9-4   Donning and Removing Disposable Gloves

PURPOSES
- To prevent the transfer of microorganisms from the nurse's hands to the client
- To reduce the possibility of acquiring microorganisms on the hands that could be transmitted to others. While adequate hand washing usually prevents this transmission, gloves are also a practical means of prevention

▶ **Technique 9–4 Donning and Removing Disposable Gloves** *CONTINUED*

EQUIPMENT

☐ Pair of disposable gloves

INTERVENTION

1. Prepare to don gloves.

- Thoroughly wash and dry hands.

- Don a mask and a gown, if required.

2. Don gloves.

- No special technique is required to don disposable gloves.

- If you are wearing a gown, pull the gloves up to cover the cuffs of the gown. If you are not wearing a gown, pull the gloves up to cover the wrists.

3. Remove the gloves. No special technique is usually required to remove the gloves if the hands are to be washed afterward. If, however, there is a reason to prevent soilage of the hands (e.g., the nurse has a cut) follow the steps below.

- Remove the first glove by grasping it on its palmar surface just below the cuff, taking care to touch only glove to glove (Figure 9–8). *This keeps the soiled parts of the used gloves from touching the skin of the wrist or hand.*

- Pull the first glove completely off by inverting or rolling the glove inside out.

- Continue to hold the inverted removed glove by the fingers of the

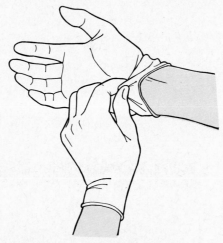

FIGURE 9–8 Plucking the palmar surface below the cuff of a contaminated glove.

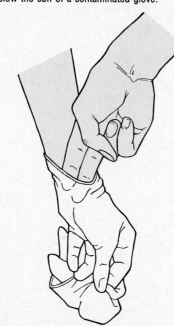

FIGURE 9–9 Inserting fingers to remove the second contaminated glove.

remaining gloved hand. Place the first two fingers of the bare hand inside the cuff of the second glove (Figure 9–9). *Touching the outside of the second soiled glove with the bare hand is avoided.*

- Pull the second glove off to the fingers by turning it inside out. This pulls the first glove inside the second glove. *The soiled part of the glove is folded to the inside to reduce the chance of transferring any microorganisms by direct contact.*

- Using the bare hand, continue to remove the gloves, which are now inside out, and dispose of them in the refuse container (Figure 9–10).

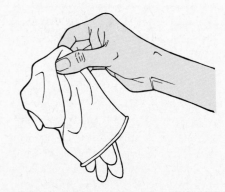

FIGURE 9–10 Holding contaminated gloves, which are inside out.

KEY ELEMENTS OF DONNING AND REMOVING DISPOSABLE GLOVES

- Pull glove cuffs well over the cuffs of a gown, if worn, or over the wrists if a gown is not worn.

- Invert or roll soiled gloves inside out when removing them, to prevent hand soiling.

Bagging

Most articles do not need to be bagged unless they are contaminated, or likely to be contaminated, with infective material such as pus, blood, body fluids, feces, or respiratory secretions. Soiled articles need to be enclosed in a sturdy impervious bag before they are removed from the room or cubicle of a client in isolation precautions. Some agencies use labels or bags of a particular color that designates them as infective wastes. Check agency policy.

The 1983 CDC guidelines recommend the following methods (Garner and Simmons 1983, p. 245):

- A single bag, if it is sturdy and impervious to microorganisms, and if the contaminated articles can be placed in the bag without soiling or contaminating its outside
- Double-bagging if the above conditions are not met

Technique 9–5 explains the steps in bagging articles.

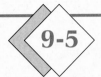

9-5   **Bagging Articles**

PURPOSE
- To prevent inadvertent exposure of health care workers to articles contaminated with infective material
- To prevent contamination of the environment

EQUIPMENT

- Bag(s) impervious to microorganisms and color-coded or with coded markers

---

INTERVENTION

1. Use the following CDC guidelines to handle and bag soiled items (Garner and Simmons 1984, pp. 109–10), or follow agency protocol.

- Place garbage and soiled *disposable* equipment, including dressings and tissues, in the plastic bag that lines the waste container. Some agencies separate dry and wet waste material and incinerate dry items, e.g., paper towels and disposable items. No special precautions are required for disposable equipment that is not contaminated.

- Place *nondisposable* or *reusable* equipment that is contaminated with infective material in a labeled bag before removing it from the client's room or cubicle, and send it to a central processing area for decontamination.

Some agencies may require that glass bottles or jars and metal items be placed in separate bags from rubber and plastic items. *Glass and metal can be sterilized in an autoclave, but rubber and plastic are damaged by this process and must be cleaned by other methods, e.g., gas sterilization.*

- Disassemble *special procedure trays* into component parts. *Some components can be discarded; others need to be sent to the laundry or central services for cleaning and decontaminating.*

- *Dishes* require no special precautions unless they are visibly contaminated with infective material (e.g., blood, drainage, or secretions). Bag any contaminated items before returning them to the food service depart-

ment. Soiled dishes can largely be prevented by encouraging clients to wash their hands before eating.

- Handle soiled *linen* as little as possible and with the least agitation possible before placing it in the client's laundry hamper. *This prevents gross microbial contamination of the air and/or persons handling the linen.*

- *Laboratory specimens*, if placed in a leak-proof container with a secure lid, need no special precautions. Use care when collecting specimens to avoid contaminating the outside of the container. Clean or disinfect specimen containers that are visibly contaminated on the outside before sending them to the laboratory.

▶

▶ **Technique 9–5 Bagging Articles** *CONTINUED*

- Bag *clothing* soiled with infective material before sending it home or to the agency laundry.

- Disinfect and destroy any *books, magazines, and toys* that are visibly contaminated. Do not allow children who have an infection that may be spread by contact transmission or by fomites to share toys with others.

- *Blood pressure equipment* needs no special precautions unless it becomes contaminated with infective material. If contaminated, follow agency protocol.

2. Use two bags for articles if the single bag is not sturdy or impervious to microorganisms or is soiled on the outside.

KEY ELEMENTS OF BAGGING ARTICLES

- Place refuse and all items soiled with infective material in bags that are sturdy and impervious to microorganisms (e.g., place linen in laundry hamper; place refuse, soiled *disposable* equipment, and soiled dressings in moisture-proof garbage container; place *nondisposable* equipment in plastic or paper containers).

- Disassemble special procedure trays before disposing of the equipment.

- Use two bags for articles if the single bag is soiled or not sturdy enough or not impervious to moisture.

- Ensure that all bags are appropriately labeled if not already color-coded or labeled.

Care of Severely Compromised Clients

Compromised clients are often infected by their own microorganisms, by microorganisms on the inadequately washed hands of health personnel, and by nonsterile items (food, water, air, and client care equipment). The 1983 CDC guidelines for severely compromised clients include (Garner and Simmons 1983, p. 254):

- Frequent and appropriate hand washing by all personnel before, during, and after client care

- Private rooms whenever possible

- Use of sterile gloves, sterile gowns, and masks by people caring for clients with major wounds or burns that cannot be enclosed by dressings

Surgical Hand Scrub

Nurses perform a surgical hand scrub to render the skin of the hands as free of microorganisms as possible. It is performed in operating rooms, delivery rooms, burn units, and in special diagnostic areas. The scrub lasts 5 to 10 minutes, depending on agency protocol. Research has indicated that the 5-minute initial scrub and the 3-minute consecutive scrubs with chlorhexidine gluconate (CHG) was an optimal regimen (Periera et al. 1990, p. 354). Brushes or sponges and antimicrobial agents are employed to remove bacteria on the hands.

The exact technique for a surgical hand scrub varies among agencies. The practices that follow should be carried out before beginning the scrub.

1. Keep nails short (to prevent glove punctures), clean, and free of nail polish. Do not wear artificial nails.

2. Ensure that hands and arms are free of cuts, abrasions, and other problems.

3. Ensure that the cap is in place and completely covers all the hair.

4. If a mask is needed, make sure it is in place before the scrub.

There are two types of surgical scrubs: the stroke-count scrub and the timed scrub. They both take about 5 minutes to complete. The stroke-count scrub involves a specific number of cleaning strokes for each aspect of the hands and arms. With the timed scrub, each area is scrubbed for a specific length of time. The fingers and hands are scrubbed, then the arms to 5 cm (2 in) above each elbow. Most agencies have specific recommended protocols regarding the surgical hand scrub.

Technique 9–6 describes how to perform a surgical hand scrub.

Performing a Surgical Hand Scrub

PURPOSE

- To render the hands and forearms as free as possible of microorganisms
- To apply an antimicrobial residue on the skin and reduce the growth of microorganisms for several hours

EQUIPMENT

- Antimicrobial solution
- Deep sink with foot, knee, or elbow controls
- Towels for drying the hands
- Nail-cleaning tool, such as a file or orange stick
- Two surgical scrub brushes
- Mask and cap

INTERVENTION

1. Prepare for the surgical hand scrub.

- Remove wristwatch and all rings, unless plain bands are allowed by agency protocol. Ensure that fingernails are trimmed. *A wristwatch and rings can harbor microorganisms and be damaged by water.*

- Make sure that sleeves are above the elbows.

- Ensure that the uniform is well-tucked in at the waist. *A loose-fitting uniform can contaminate the hands if it touches them.*

- Apply cap and face mask.

- Turn on the water, and adjust the temperature to lukewarm. *Warm water removes less protective oil from the skin than hot water. Soap irritates the skin more when hot water is used.*

2. Scrub the hands.

- Wet the hands and forearms under running water, holding the hands above the level of the elbows so that the water runs from the fingertips to the elbows (Figure 9–11). *The hands will become cleaner than the elbows. The water should run from the least contaminated to the most contaminated area.*

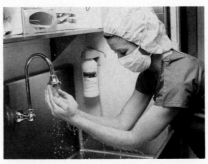

FIGURE 9–11 The hands are held higher than the elbows during a hand wash before sterile technique.

- Apply 2 to 4 ml (1 tsp) antimicrobial solution to the hands. Most agencies supply a liquid antimicrobial beside the sink. In some agencies, antimicrobial soap wafers are available.

- Use firm, rubbing, and circular movements to wash the palms and backs of the hands, the wrists, and the forearms. Interlace the fingers and thumbs, and move the hands back and forth. Continue washing for 20 to 25 seconds. *Circular strokes clean most effectively, and rubbing ensures a thorough and mechanical cleaning action. (Other areas of the hands still need to be cleaned, however.)*

- Hold the hands and arms under the running water to rinse thor-

oughly, keeping the hands higher than the elbows. *The nurse rinses from the cleanest to the least clean area.*

- Check the nails, and clean them with a file or orange stick if necessary. Rinse the nail tool after each nail is cleaned. *Sediment under the nails is removed more readily when the hands are moist. Rinsing the nail tool prevents the transmission of sediment from one nail to another.*

- Apply antimicrobial solution and lather the hands again. Using a scrub brush, scrub each hand for 45 seconds. Scrub each side of all fingers, including the skin between each of the fingers and the thumb, and the back and the palm of the hand. *Scrubbing loosens bacteria, including those in the creases of the hands.*

- Using the scrub brush, scrub from the wrists to 5 cm (2 in) above each elbow. Scrub all parts of the arms: lower forearm (15 seconds), upper forearm (15 seconds), and antecubital space to marginal area above elbows (15 seconds). Continue to hold the hands higher than the elbows. *Scrubbing thus proceeds from the*

▶

▶ **Technique 9–6 Performing a Surgical Hand Scrub** *CONTINUED*

cleanest area (hands) to the least clean area (upper arm).

• Discard the brush.

• Rinse hands and arms thoroughly so that the water flows from the hands to the elbows. *Rinsing removes resident and transient bacteria and sediment.*

• If a longer scrub is required, use a second brush and scrub each hand and arm with soap for the recommended time (e.g., each hand for 30 seconds, forearms for 45 seconds).

• Discard second brush, and rinse hands and arms thoroughly.

• Turn off the water with the foot or knee pedal.

3. Dry the hands and arms.

• Use a sterile towel to dry one hand thoroughly from the fingers to the elbow. Use a rotating motion. Use a second sterile towel to dry the second hand in the same manner. In some agencies towels are of a sufficient size that one half can be used to dry one hand and arm and the second

half for the second hand and arm. *Moist skin readily becomes chapped and subject to open sores. Thorough drying also makes it easier to don sterile gloves. The nurse dries the hands from the cleanest to the least clean area.*

• Discard the towels.

• Keep the hands in front and above the waist. *This position maintains the cleanliness of the hands and prevents accidental contamination.*

KEY ELEMENTS OF PERFORMING A SURGICAL HAND SCRUB

• Ensure that hands and arms are free of abrasions and jewelry and that nails are short, clean, and free of nail polish.

• Don mask and cap before the scrub.

• Always hold the hands higher than the elbows and above the waist.

• Use antimicrobial soap.

• Thoroughly scrub hands and then forearms for recommended times.

• Use firm, rubbing, circular movements and interlace fingers and thumbs; then use scrub brush.

• Clean nails with orange stick as required.

• Thoroughly rinse the hands and arms.

Sterile Field

A **sterile field** is a microorganism-free area. *Sterile* means free of microorganisms, including spores. Nurses often establish a sterile field by using the innermost side of a sterile wrapper or by using a sterile drape. When the field is established, sterile supplies and sterile solutions can be placed on it. Sterile forceps are used in many instances to handle and transfer the sterile supplies.

So that its sterility can be maintained, equipment is wrapped in a variety of materials. Commercially prepared items are frequently wrapped in plastic, paper, or glass. Commercially prepared sterile liquids for both internal and external use are often supplied in plastic or glass containers. Plastics are often pliable, usually transparent, impervious to dust, and relatively resistant to tearing. Liquids used in hospitals may be prepared commercially or in the hospital. In

the past, it was not unusual for sterile liquids, e.g., sterile water for irrigations, to be supplied in large glass containers and used many times. This practice is today considered undesirable because once a container has been opened, there can be no assurance that it is sterile. Liquids are preferably packaged in amounts adequate for one use only. Any leftover liquid is discarded. Hospital-packaged liquids are often sterilized in reusable containers; commercially packaged liquids are supplied in disposable containers. These containers normally have a seal over the cap, and often the word *sterile* is clearly marked on the top. If the cap has been tampered with or if the seal is broken, the liquid is considered unsterile. All containers should also be inspected for cracks.

Technique 9–7 describes how to establish and maintain a sterile field.

Establishing and Maintaining a Sterile Field

PURPOSE	• To maintain the sterility of supplies and equipment

EQUIPMENT

- ☐ Package containing a sterile drape
- ☐ Sterile equipment as needed, e.g., wrapped sterile gauze, wrapped sterile bowl, antiseptic solution, sterile forceps

INTERVENTION

1. Confirm the sterility of the package.

- Ensure that the package is clean and dry; if moist, it is considered contaminated and must be discarded.

- Check the sterilization expiration dates on the package, and look for any indications that it has been previously opened.

- Follow agency practice about the disposal of possibly contaminated packages.

2. Open the package.

To Open a Wrapped Package on a Surface:

- Place the package in the center of the work area so that the top flap of the wrapper opens away from you. *This position prevents you from subsequent reaching directly over the exposed sterile contents, which could contaminate them.*

- Reaching around the package (not over it), pinch the first flap on the outside of the wrapper between the thumb and index finger (Figure 9–12). With some folded packages, it may be necessary to grasp the uppermost flap at each corner. *Touching only the outside of the wrapper maintains the sterility of the inside of the wrapper.* Pull the flap open, laying it flat on the far surface.

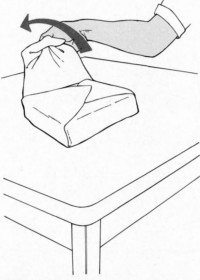

FIGURE 9–12 Opening the first flap of a sterile wrapped package.

- Repeat for the side flaps, opening the top one first. Use the right hand for the right flap, and the left hand for the left flap (Figure 9–13). *By using both hands, you avoid reaching over the sterile contents.*

- Pull the fourth flap toward you by grasping the corner that is turned down (Figure 9–14). Make sure that the flap does not touch your uniform. *If the inner surface touches any unsterile article, it is contaminated.*

To Open a Wrapped Package While Holding It:

- Hold the package in one hand with the top flap opening away from you.

- Using the other hand, open the

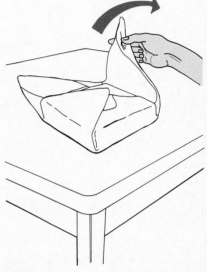

FIGURE 9–13 Opening the second flap to the side.

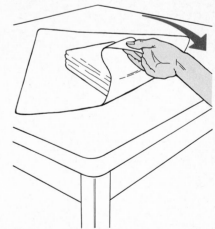

FIGURE 9–14 Pulling the last flap toward oneself by grasping the corner.

package as described above, pulling the corners of the flaps well back (Figure 9–15). *The hands are considered contaminated, and at no time should they touch the contents of the package.*

▶

▶ **Technique 9–7 Establishing and Maintaining a Sterile Field** CONTINUED

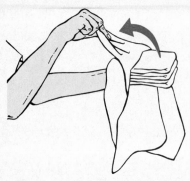

FIGURE 9–15 Opening a wrapped package while holding it.

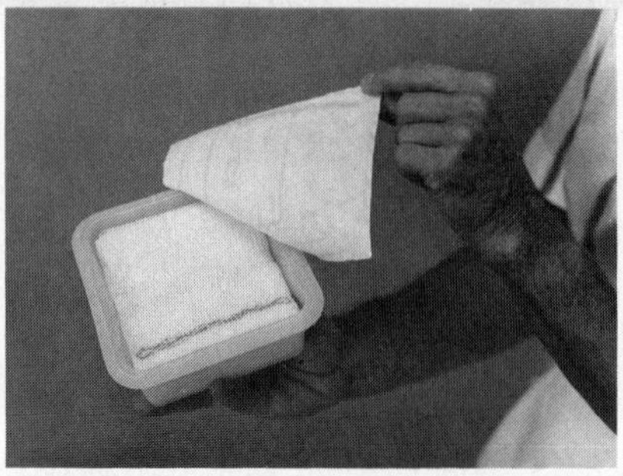

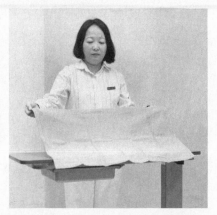

FIGURE 9–16 Opening a sterile package with an unsealed corner.

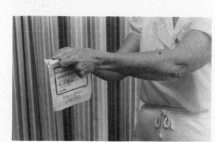

FIGURE 9–17 Opening a sterile package with a partially sealed edge.

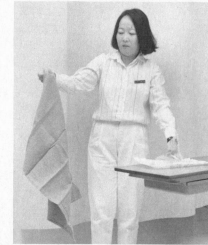

FIGURE 9–18 Allowing a drape to open freely without touching any articles.

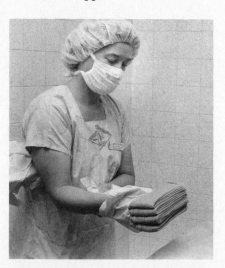

FIGURE 9–19 Placing a drape on a surface.

To Open Commercially Prepared Packages:

Commercially prepared sterile packages and containers usually have manufacturer's directions for opening.

- If the flap of the package has an unsealed corner, hold the container in one hand, and pull back on the flap with the other hand (Figure 9–16).

- If the package has a partially sealed edge, grasp both sides of the edge, one with each hand, and pull apart gently (Figure 9–17).

3. Rewrap the sterile package as required, e.g., for transport to the bedside.

- Rewrap in the *reverse* order to unwrapping. Close the proximal flap first to prevent reaching across the sterile field, the side flaps next, and the distal flap last.

4. Establish a sterile field by using a drape.

- Open the package containing the drape as described above.

- With one hand, pluck the corner of the drape that is folded back on the top.

- Lift the drape out of the cover, and allow it to open freely without touching any articles (Figure 9–18). *If the drape touches the outside of the package, the uniform, or any unsterile surface, it is considered contaminated.*

- Discard the cover.

- With the other hand, carefully pick up another corner of the drape, holding it well away from yourself.

- Lay the drape on a clean and dry surface, placing the bottom (i.e., the freely hanging side) farthest from you (Figure 9–19). *By placing the lowermost side farthest away, you avoid leaning over the sterile field and contaminating it.*

5. Add necessary sterile supplies.

To Add Wrapped Supplies to a Sterile Field:

- Open each wrapped package as described in the preceding steps.

- With the free hand, grasp the corners of the wrapper, and hold them against the wrist of the other hand (Figure 9–20). *The unsterile hand is now covered by the sterile wrapper.*

FIGURE 9–20 Adding wrapped sterile supplies to a sterile field.

▶ **Technique 9–7** *CONTINUED*

- Place the sterile bowl, drape, or other supply on the sterile field by approaching from an angle rather than holding the arm over the field.

- Discard the wrapper.

To Add Commercially Packaged Supplies to a Sterile Field:

- Open each package, e.g., gauze, as described above.

- Hold the package 15 cm (6 in) above the field, and allow the contents to drop on the field (Figure 9–21). Keep in mind that 2.5 cm (1 in) around the edge of the field is considered contaminated. *At a height of 15 cm (6 in), the outside of the package is not likely to touch and contaminate the sterile field.*

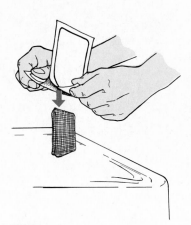

FIGURE 9–21 Adding a commercially packaged supply to a sterile field.

To Add Sterile Solution to a Sterile Bowl:

Sterile liquids (e.g., normal saline) frequently need to be poured into metal or nonabsorbent containers within a sterile field. Unwrapped bottles or flasks that contain sterile solution are considered sterile on the inside and contaminated on the outside, since the bottle may have been handled. Bottles used in an operating room may be sterilized on

the outside as well as the inside, however, and these are handled with sterile gloves.

- Before pouring any liquid, read the label three times to make sure you have the correct solution.

- Obtain the exact amount of solution, if possible. *Once a sterile container has been opened, its sterility cannot be ensured for future use unless it is used again immediately.*

- Read the label to confirm both the name of solution and its strength.

- Remove the lid or cap from the bottle, and invert the lid before placing it on a surface that is not sterile. *Inverting the lid maintains the sterility of the inside surface because it is not allowed to touch an unsterile surface.*

- Hold the bottle so that the label is uppermost. *Any solution that flows down the outside of the bottle during pouring will not damage or obliterate the label.*

- Hold the bottle of fluid at a height of 10 to 15 cm (4 to 6 in) over the bowl and to the side of the sterile field so that as little of the bottle as possible is over the field. *At this height, there is less likelihood of contaminating the sterile field by touching the field or by reaching an arm over it.*

- Pour the solution gently to avoid splashing the liquid. *If the sterile drape is on an unsterile surface, any moisture will contaminate the field by facilitating the movement of microorganisms through the sterile drape.*

- Replace the lid securely on the bottle if you plan to use it again, and provide the date and time of opening. Check agency protocol. *Replacing the lid immediately maintains the sterility of the inner*

aspect of the lid and the solution. In many agencies a sterile container of solution that is opened is used only once and then discarded.

6. Use sterile forceps to handle certain sterile supplies.

Forceps are commonly used for such techniques as changing a sterile dressing and shortening a drain. Transfer forceps are usually used to move a sterile article from one place to another, e.g., transferring sterile gauze from its package to a sterile dressing tray. Forceps are usually packaged and discarded or resterilized after use. Commonly used forceps include hemostats, or artery forceps (Figure 9–22), and tissue forceps (Figure 9–23).

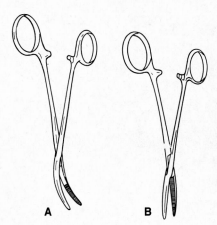

FIGURE 9–22 Hemostats: *A,* curved; *B,* straight.

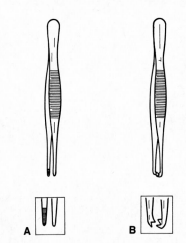

FIGURE 9–23 Tissue forceps: *A,* plain; *B,* toothed.

▶ **Technique 9–7 Establishing and Maintaining a Sterile Field** *CONTINUED*

- Keep the tips of wet forceps lower than the wrist at all times, unless you are wearing sterile gloves (Figure 9–24). *Gravity prevents liquids on the tips of the forceps from flowing to the handles*

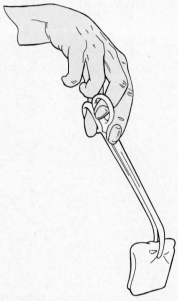

FIGURE 9–24 Holding forceps with an ungloved hand, keeping the tips lower than the handles.

and later back to the tips, thus making the forceps unsterile. The handles are unsterile once they are held by the bare hand.

- Hold sterile forceps above waist level. *There is less danger of contamination if the forceps are held near to eye level.*

- Hold sterile forceps within sight. *While out of sight, forceps may unknowingly become unsterile. Any such forceps should be considered unsterile.*

- When using forceps to lift sterile supplies out of a commercially prepared package, be sure that the forceps do not touch the edges or outside of the wrapper. *The edges and outside of the package are exposed to the air and handled and are thus unsterile.*

- When placing forceps whose handles were in contact with the bare hand, position the handles outside the sterile area. *The handles of these forceps harbor microorganisms from the bare hand.*

- Deposit a sterile item on a sterile field without permitting moist forceps to touch the sterile field when the surface under the absorbent sterile field is unsterile and a barrier drape is not used. A *barrier drape* is resistant to moisture (e.g., blood and antiseptics) and should be used whenever a procedure involves the use of liquids. *Made of chemically treated cotton or synthetic materials, barrier drapes prevent a sterile field from becoming unsterile when the drape becomes wet. It is known that a sterile cloth becomes unsterile when dampened (even with sterile water) if it is on an unsterile surface or has contact with any unsterile object. Microorganisms can move through a damp sterile cloth from an unsterile surface, contaminating the field. If the underlying surface is sterile (e.g., a plastic container), the field will not become unsterile when moist.*

KEY ELEMENTS OF ESTABLISHING AND MAINTAINING A STERILE FIELD

- Ensure the sterility of supplies before use.
- Use sterile waterproof barriers beneath sterile objects.
- Avoid reaching over exposed sterile contents unless the unsterile hand is covered with a sterile wrapper. Remember that a 2.5 cm (1 in) margin at each edge of an opened drape or wrap is considered unsterile.
- Keep all sterile objects within sight, above the waist, and away from the uniform.

- When adding sterile supplies to a sterile field, hold packages and liquids well above the sterile field 10 to 15 cm, or 4 to 6 in.
- Hold solution bottles with the label uppermost.
- Initially, place the lowermost side of a drape farthest from you.
- Handle sterile objects only with sterile forceps or sterile gloved hands.
- Always keep the tips of forceps lower than the wrists, unless wearing sterile gloves.

Sterile Gloves

Sterile gloves may be donned by the open method or the closed method. The open method is most frequently used outside the operating room, since the closed method requires that the nurse wear a sterile gown. Gloves are worn during many sterile procedures to maintain the sterility of equipment and protect a client's open wound.

Sterile gloves are packaged with a cuff often about 5 cm (2 in) and with the palms facing upward when the package is opened. The package usually indicates the size of the glove (e.g., size 6 or 7½). Gloves may or may not be used with sterile forceps. For example, when inserting a catheter, the nurse generally wears gloves and uses sterile forceps; when changing a dressing, the nurse uses sterile forceps but may not wear gloves.

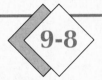

Latex and vinyl gloves are available to protect the nurse from contact with blood and body fluids. *Latex*

is more flexible than vinyl, molds to the wearer's hands, allows freedom of movement, and has the added feature of resealing tiny punctures automatically. Korniewicz et al. (1991, p. 39) recommend that nurses wear latex gloves when performing tasks (a) that demand flexibility; (b) that place stress on the material (e.g., turning stopcocks, handling sharp instruments or tape); and (c) that involve a high risk of exposure to pathogens (e.g., in intensive care units, the operating room, labor and delivery areas, infectious disease units, and emergency departments). *Vinyl* gloves should be chosen for tasks unlikely to stress the glove material, requiring minimal precision, and with minimal risk of exposure to pathogens (e.g., in ambulatory care settings, postoperative eye surgery units, and outpatient psychiatric units).

Technique 9–8 describes how to don and remove sterile gloves by the open method.

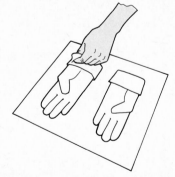

9-8 Donning and Removing Sterile Gloves (Open Method)

PURPOSES
- To enable the nurse to handle sterile objects freely
- To prevent clients at risk (e.g., those with open wounds) from becoming infected by microorganisms on the nurse's hands

---

EQUIPMENT
- Package of sterile gloves

INTERVENTION

1. Open the package of sterile gloves.

- Place the package of gloves on a clean dry surface. *Any moisture on the surface could contaminate the gloves.*

- Some gloves are packed in an inner as well as an outer package. Open the outer package without contaminating the gloves or the inner package. See Technique 9–7.

- Remove the inner package from the outer package.

- Open the inner package as above or according to the manufacturer's directions. Some manufacturers provide a numbered se-

quence for opening the flaps and folded tabs to grasp for opening the flaps. If no tabs are provided, pluck the flap so that the fingers do not touch the inner surfaces. *The inner surfaces, which are next to the sterile gloves, will remain sterile.*

2. Put the first glove on the dominant hand.

- If the gloves are packaged so that they lie side by side, grasp the glove for the dominant hand by its cuff (on the palmar side) with the thumb and first finger of the nondominant hand. Touch only the inside of the cuff (Figure 9–25). *The hands are not sterile. By touching only the inside of the*

FIGURE 9–25 Picking up the first sterile glove.

glove, the nurse avoids contaminating the outside.
or
If the gloves are packaged one on top of the other, grasp the cuff of the top glove as above, using the opposite hand.

▶

► **Technique 9–8 Donning and Removing Sterile Gloves (Open Method)** *CONTINUED*

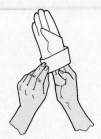

FIGURE 9–26 Putting on the first sterile glove.

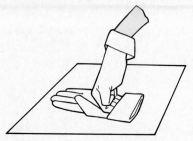

FIGURE 9–27 Picking up the second sterile glove.

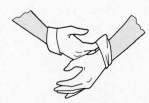

FIGURE 9–28 Putting on the second sterile glove.

- Insert the dominant hand into the glove and pull the glove on. Keep the thumb of the inserted hand against the palm of the hand during insertion (Figure 9–26). *If the thumb is kept against the palm, it is less likely to contaminate the outside of the glove.*

- Leave the cuff turned down.

3. Put the second glove on the nondominant hand.

- Pick up the other glove with the sterile gloved hand, inserting the gloved fingers under the cuff and holding the gloved thumb close to the gloved palm (Figure 9–27). *This helps prevent accidental contamination of the glove by the bare hand.*

- Pull on the second glove carefully. Hold the thumb of the gloved first hand as far as possible from the palm (Figure 9–28). *In this position, the thumb is less likely to touch the arm and become contaminated.*

- Adjust each glove so that it fits smoothly, and carefully pull the cuffs up by sliding the fingers under the cuffs.

4. Remove and dispose of used gloves.

- There is no special technique for removing sterile gloves. If they are soiled with secretions, remove them by turning them inside out. See Technique 9–4.

KEY ELEMENTS OF DONNING AND REMOVING STERILE GLOVES (OPEN METHOD)

- Ensure the sterility of the package.
- Place the sterile glove package on a clean, dry surface.
- Maintain the sterility of the gloves when opening the package.

- Touch only the inside of the cuff of the first glove to be donned.
- Pick up the second glove by inserting the gloved fingers under the cuff.

Sterile Gowns

Sterile gowning and closed gloving are chiefly carried out in operating or delivery rooms, where surgical asepsis is necessary. The closed method of gloving can be used only when a sterile gown is worn because the gloves are handled through the sleeves of the gown. In some agencies, gown and gloves are provided in a single sterile pack; in others, the gloves are provided in a separate package. Prior to these procedures, the nurse dons a hair cover and a mask, and performs a surgical hand wash.

Technique 9–9 describes the steps in donning a sterile gown and sterile gloves by the closed method.

9-9 Donning a Sterile Gown and Sterile Gloves (Closed Method)

PURPOSES

• To enable the nurse to work close to a sterile field and handle sterile objects freely
• To prevent clients at risk from becoming infected

EQUIPMENT

☐ A sterile pack containing a sterile gown and sterile gloves

INTERVENTION

Donning a Sterile Gown

1. Open the sterile pack.

• Remove the outer wrap from the sterile gloves, and drop the gloves in their inner sterile wrap on the sterile field established by the sterile outer wrapper. *If the inner wrapper is not touched, it will remain sterile.* See Technique 9–7, Step 2.

2. Carry out a surgical scrub for the length of time required by the agency.

• See Technique 9–6.

3. Put on the sterile gown.

• Grasp the sterile gown at the crease near the neck, hold it away from you, and permit it to unfold freely without touching anything, including the uniform. *The gown will be unsterile if its outer surface touches any unsterile articles.*

• Put the hands inside the shoulders of the gown, and work the arms partway into the sleeves without touching the outside of the gown (Figure 9–29).

• If donning sterile gloves by using the *closed* method (see below), work the hands down the sleeves only to the proximal edge of the cuffs.
or
If donning sterile gloves by using the *open* method, work the hands

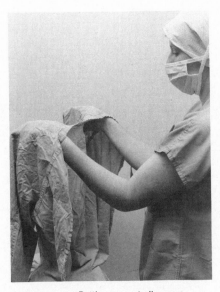

FIGURE 9–29 Putting on a sterile gown.

down the sleeves and through the cuffs.

• Have a coworker wearing a hair cover and mask grasp the neck ties without touching the outside of the gown and pull the gown upward to cover the neckline of your uniform in front and back. The coworker ties the neck ties. Gowning continues at Step 7.

Donning Sterile Gloves (Closed Method)

4. Open the sterile wrapper containing the sterile gloves.

• Open the sterile glove wrapper while the hands are still covered by the sleeves (Figure 9–30).

5. Put the glove on the nondominant hand.

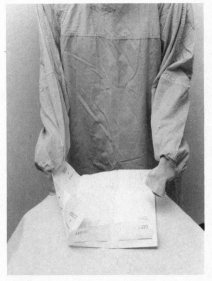

FIGURE 9–30 Opening the sterile glove wrapper.

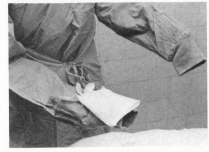

FIGURE 9–31 Positioning the first sterile glove, for the nondominant hand.

• With the *dominant* hand, pick up the *opposite* glove with the thumb and index finger, handling it through the sleeve.

• Lay the glove on the opposite gown cuff, thumb side down, with the glove opening pointed toward the fingers (Figure 9–31).

► Technique 9–9 Donning a Sterile Gown and Sterile Gloves CONTINUED

Position the nondominant hand palm upward inside the sleeve.

- Use the nondominant hand to grasp the cuff of the glove through the gown cuff, and firmly anchor it.

- With the dominant hand working through its sleeve, grasp the upper side of the glove's cuff, and stretch it over the cuff of the gown.

- Pull the sleeve up to draw the cuff over the wrist as you extend the fingers of the nondominant hand into the glove's fingers (Figure 9–32).

6. Put the glove on the dominant hand.

- Place the fingers of the gloved hand under the cuff of the remaining glove.

- Place the glove over the cuff of the second sleeve.

- Extend the fingers into the glove as you pull the glove up over the cuff (Figure 9–33).

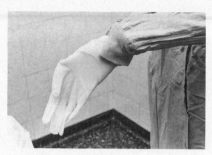

FIGURE 9–32 Pulling on the first sterile glove.

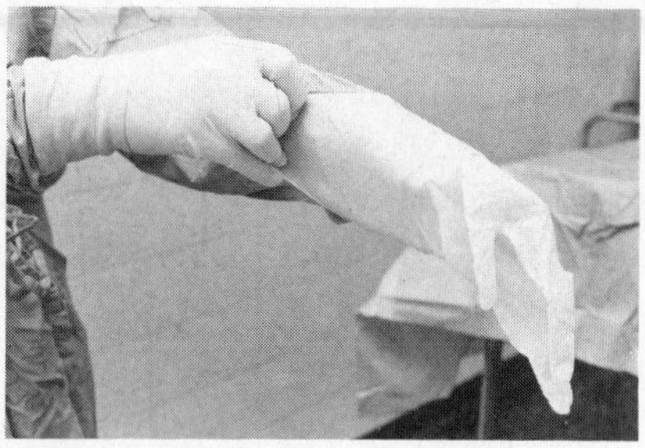

FIGURE 9–33 Extending the fingers into the second glove, for the dominant hand.

Completion of Gowning

7. Complete gowning as follows.

- Have a coworker who is masked and whose hair is covered hold the waist tie of your gown, using sterile gloves or a sterile forcep or drape. *This approach keeps the ties sterile.*

- Make a three-quarter turn, then take the tie, and secure it in front of the gown.

or

Have a coworker wearing sterile gloves take the two ties at each side of the gown and tie them at the back of the gown, making

sure that your uniform is completely covered. *Both methods ensure that the back of the gown remains sterile.*

- When worn, sterile gowns should be considered *sterile* in front from the chest to the level of the sterile field. The sleeves should be considered sterile from 2 inches above the elbow to the cuff, since the arms of a scrubbed person must move across a sterile field. Moisture collection and friction areas such as the neckline, shoulders, underarms, back, and sleeve cuff should be considered unsterile (AORN 1991, p. 482).

KEY ELEMENTS OF DONNING A STERILE GOWN AND STERILE GLOVES (CLOSED METHOD)

Gowning

- First put on a hair cover and mask and perform a surgical hand scrub.

- Keep the outer surface of the gown away from unsterile articles.

- Touch only the inside of the gown.

- If using the closed method of gloving, move the hands down the sleeves only to the proximal edge of the cuffs.

- Have a coworker fasten the neck ties, and then, using sterile gloves, forceps, or drape, secure the waist ties.

Gloving

- Use only the sterile gown cuff to manipulate the first sterile glove.

- Put on the nondominant glove first.

- Ensure the glove cuffs extend well over the gown cuffs.

CRITICAL THINKING CHALLENGE

An intravenous infusion has been ordered for Dennis Milton, a 33-year-old client who has AIDS. What specific precautions (gown, apron, mask, gloves, and so on) should you take to perform this procedure? After removing protective clothing, you note that you have blood on your arm. What should you do?

RELATED RESEARCH

Favero, M. S. June 1989. Preventing transmission of hepatitis B infection in health care facilities. *American Journal of Infection Control* 17(3): 168–71.

Maki, D. G.; Alvaredo, C.; and Hassemer, C. November 1986. Double-bagging of items from isolation rooms is unnecessary as an infection control measure: A comparative study of surface contamination with single- and double-bagging. *Infection Control* 7:535–37.

Newman, J. L., and Seitz, J. C. June 1990. Intermittent use of an antimicrobial hand gel for reducing soap-induced irritation of health care personnel. *American Journal of Infection Control* 18(3): 194–200.

Weinstein, S. A.; Gantz, N. M.; Pelletier, C.; and Hibert, D. October 1989. Bacterial surface contamination of patients' linen: Isolation precautions versus standard care. *American Journal of Infection Control* 17(5): 264–67.

REFERENCES

AORN. February 1991. Proposed recommended practices: Aseptic technique. *AORN Journal* 53(2): 480–87.

Beneson, A. S., editor. 1990. *Control of communicable diseases in man*. 15th ed. Washington, D.C.: American Public Health Association.

Garner, J. S., and Favero, M. S. 1985. *Guidelines for handwashing and hospital environmental control*. Washington, D.C.: U.S. Government Printing Office.

Garner, J. S., and Simmons, B. P. April 1984. CDC guidelines for the prevention and control of nosocomial infections: Guideline for isolation precautions in hospitals. *American Journal of Infection Control* 12:103–166.

Garner, J. S., and Simmons, B. P. July/August 1983. CDC guidelines for isolation precautions in hospitals. *Infection Control* 4:254–325.

Jackson, M. M., and Lynch, P. July 1991. An attempt to make an issue less murky: A comparison of four systems for infective precautions. *Infection Control and Hospital Epidemiology* 12:448–50.

Jackson, M. M., Lynch, P., McPherson, D.C., Cummings, M. J., and Greenawalt, N. C. September 1987. Why not treat all body substances as infectious? *American Journal of Nursing* 87:1137–39.

Konniewicz, D. M., Kirwin, M., and Larson, E. June 1991. Do your gloves fit the task? *American Journal of Nursing* 91:38–39, 40.

Larson, E. July 1989. Handwashing: It's essential—even when you use gloves. *American Journal of Nursing* 89:934–39.

Larson, E. L. 1989. Infection control. *Annual Review of Nursing Research*. :95–113.

Pereira, L. J., Lee, G. M., and Wade, K. J. December 1990. The effect of surgical handwashing routines on the microbial counts of operating room nurses. *American Journal of Infection Control* 18:354–70.

U.S. Department of Health and Human Services, Public Health Service. June 24, 1988, and June 23, 1989. Update: Universal precautions for prevention of transmission of human immunodeficiency virus, hepatitis B virus, and other blood-borne pathogens in health care settings. *Morbidity and Mortality Weekly Report* 37:377–82, 387–88; 38(S–6):9–18.

Williams, W. W. February 1984. CDC guidelines for the prevention and control of nosocomial infections: Guideline for infection control in hospital personnel. *American Journal of Infection Control* 12:34–57.

Vital Signs

OBJECTIVES

- Describe factors that affect the vital signs and accurate measurement of them

- Identify the normal ranges for each vital sign

- Identify the variations in normal body temperature, pulse, respirations, and blood pressure that occur from infancy to old age

- Identify factors affecting accuracy of measurement of each vital sign

- Identify common problems associated with each vital sign

- Describe advantages and disadvantages of using each body temperature site

- Identify indications and contraindications for using oral, rectal, and axillary body temperature sites

- Explain reasons for using specific pulse sites

- Describe five phases of Korotkoff's sounds

- Describe a method to determine appropriate blood pressure cuff size for clients

- Assess a client's vital signs accurately, using various sites and methods

- Record vital signs findings correctly

CONTENTS

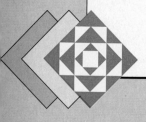

Vital Signs

The **vital**, or **cardinal**, **signs** are body temperature, pulse, respirations, and blood pressure. These signs, which should be looked at in total, enable health care workers to monitor the functions of the body. The signs reflect changes in function that otherwise might not be observed. Monitoring a client's vital signs should not be an automatic or routine procedure; it should be a thoughtful, scientific assessment. Vital signs, which should be evaluated with reference to the client's present and prior health status, are compared to accepted normal standards.

When and how often to assess a specific client's vital signs are chiefly nursing judgments, depending on the client's health status. Some agencies have policies about taking clients' vital signs, and physicians may specifically order assessment of a vital sign, e.g., "Blood pressure q2h." Ordered assessments, however, should be considered the minimum; nurses should measure clients' vital signs more often if their health status requires it. Examples of times to assess vital signs are listed in the box below.

Body Temperature

Body temperature is the balance between the heat produced by the body and the heat lost from the body. There are two kinds of body temperature: core temperature and surface temperature. **Core tempera-** ture is the temperature of the deep tissues of the body, e.g., cranium, thorax, abdominal cavity, and pelvic cavity. It remains relatively constant (37 C, 98.6 F). The **surface temperature** is the temperature of the skin, the subcutaneous tissue, and fat. It, by contrast, rises and falls in response to the environment.

The normal core body temperature is not an exact point on a scale but a range of temperatures. When measured orally, the average body temperature of an adult is between 36.7 C (98 F) and 37 C (98.6 F).

The body continually produces heat as a by-product of metabolism. The body uses carbohydrates, fats, and proteins to synthesize large quantities of adenosine triphosphate (ATP), which in turn is used as a source of energy by body cells. However, about 50% of the energy in food becomes heat rather than ATP, and the body produces further heat as it changes the food to ATP (Guyton 1986, p. 844). When the amount of heat produced by the body exactly equals the amount of heat lost, the person is in **heat balance** (Figure 10–1).

A number of factors affect the body's heat production. The most important are these five:

1. *Basal metabolic rate (BMR).* The **basal metabolic rate (BMR)** is the rate of energy utilization in the body required to maintain essential activities such as breathing.

Times to Assess Vital Signs

- On the client's admission to a health care agency, to obtain baseline data

- When a client has a change in health status or reports symptoms such as chest pain or feeling hot or faint

- According to a nursing or medical order

- Before and after surgery or an invasive diagnostic procedure

- Before and after the administration of a medication that could affect the respiratory or cardiovascular systems; e.g., before giving a digitalis preparation

- Before and after any nursing intervention that could affect the vital signs, e.g., ambulating a client who has been on bed rest

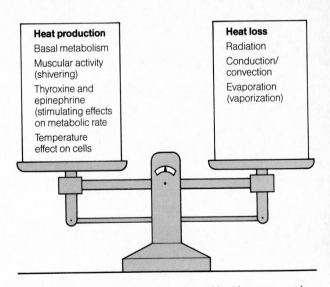

FIGURE 10–1 As long as heat production and heat loss are properly balanced, body temperature remains constant. Factors contributing to heat production (and temperature rise) are shown on the left side of the scale; those contributing to heat loss (and temperature fall) are shown on the right side of the scale. *Source:* Adapted from E. N. Marieb, *Human anatomy and physiology* (Redwood City, Calif.: Benjamin/Cummings, 1989). Adapted with permission.

2. *Muscle activity.* Muscle activity, including shivering, can greatly increase metabolic rate.

3. *Thyroxine output.* Increased thyroxine output increases the rate of cellular metabolism throughout the body. This effect is called **chemical thermogenesis**, the stimulation of heat production in the body through increased cellular metabolism.

4. *Epinephrine, norepinephrine, and sympathetic stimulation.* These immediately increase the rate of cellular metabolism in many body tissues.

5. *Increased temperature of body cells (fever).* Fever increases the cellular metabolic rate. For every 1 C (0.9 F) rise in temperature, about 12% more chemical reactions take place.

Heat is lost from the body through radiation, conduction, convection, and vaporization. Sweating, panting, lowering the environmental temperature, and wearing light clothing all promote heat loss. **Radiation** is the transfer of heat from the surface of one object to the surface of another without contact between the two objects. **Conduction** is the transfer of heat from one molecule in direct contact to another. The heat transfers to a molecule of lower temperature. The amount of heat transferred depends on the difference in temperature and the amount and duration of contact.

Convection is the dispersion of heat by air currents. There is usually a small amount of warm air adjacent to the body. This warm air rises and is replaced by cooler air, so people always lose a small amount of heat through convection. **Vaporization** is continuous evaporation of moisture from the respiratory tract and from the mucosa of the mouth and from the skin. (**Evaporation** is the conversion of a liquid into vapor.)

Regulation of Body Temperature

The system that regulates body temperature has three main parts: sensors in the shell and in the core, an integrator in the hypothalamus, and an effector system that adjusts the production and loss of heat. Most *sensors*, or *sensory receptors*, are in the skin, which is a major part of the shell. There are fewer receptors in the tongue, respiratory tract, and viscera. The skin has receptors of both cold and warmth; however, far more receptors detect cold than warmth (Guyton 1986, p. 854). Therefore, skin sensors detect cold more efficiently than warmth.

When the skin becomes chilled over the entire body, three physiologic processes to increase the body temperature take place:

1. Shivering increases heat production.

2. Sweating is inhibited to decrease heat loss.

3. Vasoconstriction decreases heat loss.

The receptors in the body's core, i.e., in the abdominal viscera, in the spinal cord, and in or around the large veins, respond only to the body's core temperature, not to the body's surface temperature. They also detect mainly cold rather than warmth. Thermoreceptors in the hypothalamus are likewise sensitive to the core temperature.

The **hypothalamic integrator**, the center that controls the core temperature, is located in the preoptic area of the hypothalamus. Some sensors are sensitive to heat, and some are sensitive to cold. Neurons transmit signals in response to signals from the sensors in the body shell. When the sensors in the hypothalamus detect heat, they send out signals to reduce the temperature, i.e., decrease heat production and increase heat loss. When the cold sensors are stimulated, the hypothalamus sends out signals to increase heat production and decrease heat loss.

The signals from the cold-sensitive receptors of the hypothalamus initiate *effectors* such as vasoconstriction, shivering, and the release of epinephrine, which increases cellular metabolism and hence heat production. Stimuli also suppress the release of thyroxine by the thyroid gland. When the warmth-sensitive receptors in the hypothalamus are stimulated, the effector system sends out signals that initiate sweating and peripheral vasodilation. Another part of the effector system is the somatic nervous system. When this system is stimulated, the person consciously makes appropriate adjustments, such as putting on additional clothing in response to cold or turning on a fan in response to heat.

Factors Affecting Body Temperature

Nurses should be aware of the factors that can affect a client's body temperature so that they can recognize normal temperature variations and understand the significance of body temperature measurements that deviate from normal. See Table 10–1 for a summary of the normal values of the vital signs at various ages. Among the factors that affect body temperature are the following:

- *Age.* The infant is greatly influenced by the temperature of the environment and must be protected from extreme changes. Children's temperatures continue to be more labile than those of adults until puberty. Studies by Kolanowski and Gunter indicate that many elderly people, particularly those over 75 years, are at risk of hypothermia (temperatures below 36 C, or 96.8 F) for a variety of reasons, such as lack of central heating, inadequate diet, loss of subcutaneous fat, lack of activity, and reduced thermoregulatory

TABLE 10–1   VARIATIONS IN VITAL SIGNS BY AGE

| Age | Average Temperature | Pulse Rate at Rest/Min | | Respiratory Rate/Min | Mean Blood Pressure |
		Average	Range		
Newborn	36.1–37.7 C 97.0–100.0 F (axilla)	125	70–190	30–80	78 systolic 42 diastolic by flush technique: 30–60
1 year	37.7 C 99.7 F	120	80–160	20–40	96 systolic 65 diastolic
2 years	37.2 C 98.9 F	110	80–130	20–30	100 systolic 63 diastolic
4 years		100	80–120	20–30	97 systolic 64 diastolic
6 years	37.0 C 98.6 F (oral)	100	75–115	20–25	98 systolic 65 diastolic
8 years		90	70–110		106 systolic 70 diastolic
10 years		90	70–110	17–22	110 systolic 72 diastolic
12 years		Male: 85 Female: 90	65–105 70–110	17–22	116 systolic 74 diastolic
14 years		Male: 80 Female: 85	60–100 65–105		120 systolic 76 diastolic
16 years		Male: 75 Female: 80	55–95 60–100	15–20	123 systolic 76 diastolic
18 years		Male: 70 Female: 75	50–90 55–95	15–20	126 systolic 79 diastolic
Adult		Same as 18 years		15–20	120 systolic 80 diastolic
Elderly (over 70 years)	36.0 C 96.8 F	Same as 18 years		15–20	Diastolic pressure may increase

Sources: Pulse rates: R. E. Behrman and V. C. Vaughan, III, editors, *Nelson textbook of pediatrics*, 12th ed. (Philadelphia: W. B. Saunders, 1983), p. 1100. G. H. Lowrey, *Growth and development of children*, 7th ed. (Chicago: Year Book, 1978), p. 450. For newborn and 1 year ages: National Heart, Lung, and Blood Institute, Task Force on Blood Pressure Control in Children: Report of the Task Force on Blood Pressure Control in Children, *Pediatrics* (May) 1987 (Suppl): 1–25.

efficiency. Elderly people are also particularly sensitive to extremes in the environmental temperature due to decreased thermoregulatory controls (Kolanowski and Gunter 1981, p. 362).

- *Diurnal variations.* Body temperatures normally change throughout the day, varying as much as 1.0 C (1.8 F) between the early morning and the late afternoon. The point of highest body temperature is usually reached between 2000 and 2400 hours (8:00 P.M. and midnight), and the lowest point is reached during sleep between 0400 and 0600 hours (4:00 and 6:00 A.M.).

- *Exercise.* Hard work or strenuous exercise can increase body temperature to as high as 38.3 to 40 C (101 to 104 F) measured rectally.

- *Hormones.* In women, progesterone secretion at the time of ovulation raises body temperature by about 0.35 C (0.5 F) above basal temperature (Olds, London, and Ladewig 1992, p. 176). Thyroxine, norepinephrine, and epinephrine also affect body temperature.

- *Stress.* Stimulation of the sympathetic nervous system can increase the production of epinephrine and norepinephrine, thereby increasing metabolic activity and heat production. Nurses may anticipate that a highly stressed or anxious client could have an elevated body temperature for that reason.

- *Environment.* Extremes in environmental temperatures can affect a person's temperature reg-

Clinical Signs of Fever

Onset (cold or chill stage)

- Increased heart rate
- Increased respiratory rate and depth
- Shivering due to increased skeletal muscle tension and contractions
- Pallid, cold skin due to vasoconstriction
- Cyanotic nail beds due to vasoconstriction
- Complaints of feeling cold
- "Gooseflesh" appearance of the skin due to contraction of the arrector pili muscles
- Cessation of sweating
- Rise in body temperature

Course

- Absence of chills
- Skin that feels warm
- Feelings of being neither hot nor cold
- Increased pulse and respiratory rates
- Increased thirst
- Mild to severe dehydration
- Simple drowsiness, restlessness, or delirium and convulsions due to irritation of the nerve cells
- Herpetic lesions of the mouth
- Loss of appetite with prolonged fever
- Malaise, weakness, and aching muscles due to protein catabolism

Defervescence (fever abatement)

- Skin that appears flushed and feels warm
- Sweating
- Decreased shivering
- Possible dehydration

Clinical Signs of Hypothermia

- Decreased body temperature
- Severe shivering (initially)
- Feelings of cold and chills
- Pale, cool, waxy skin
- Hypotension
- Decreased urinary output
- Lack of muscle coordination
- Disorientation
- Drowsiness progressing to coma

Hypothermia

Hypothermia is a core body temperature below the lower limit of normal. The ability of the hypothalamus to regulate temperature is greatly impaired when the body temperature falls below 34.5 C (94 F), and death usually occurs when the temperature falls below 34 C (93.2 F). With severe hypothermia, the rate of heat production in each cell declines substantially. Sleepiness and even coma are likely to develop, which depress the activity of heat control mechanisms further and prevent shivering. Clinical signs of hypothermia are shown in the box above.

Body Temperature Assessment Sites

There are a number of body sites for measuring body temperature. The three most common are oral, rectal, and axillary. Each of the sites has advantages and disadvantages. See Table 10–2. In recent years, the tympanic membrane site is also being used.

The body temperature is usually measured **orally** (by mouth). Traditionally, the oral method was not used for clients receiving oxygen, because the accuracy of the measurement was considered questionable. Evidence, however, suggests that oral readings are accurate in clients receiving oxygen by nasal cannula, aerosol mask, Venturi mask, and nasal prongs (Graas 1974, p. 1863; Hasler and Cohen 1982, p. 265).

Rectal temperature readings are considered to be the most accurate. In some agencies, taking temperatures rectally is contraindicated for clients with myocardial infarction. It is believed that inserting a rectal thermometer can produce vagal stimulation, which in turn can cause myocardial damage. Research, however, indicates that the rectal method has no deleterious effects on the heart (Creative Care Unit 1977, p. 997).

Measurements of temperature in the **axilla** (armpit) are about 0.65 C (1 F) less than the rectal tem-

ulatory systems. The limits of extreme heat that a person can tolerate vary according to humidity.

Alterations in Body Temperature

Pyrexia

A body temperature above the usual range is called **pyrexia, hyperthermia**, or (in lay terms) **fever**. A very high fever, e.g., 41 C (105.8 F) is called **hyperpyrexia**. Clinical signs of fever are shown in the box above.

TABLE 10–2 ADVANTAGES AND DISADVANTAGES OF THREE SITES FOR BODY TEMPERATURE MEASUREMENT

Site	Advantages	Disadvantages
Oral	Most accessible and convenient	Mercury-in-glass thermometers can be broken if bitten, thereby injuring the client. Therefore, it is contraindicted for infants, children under 6 years, and clients who are confused or who have convulsive disorders. Inaccurate if client has just eaten very hot or cold food or fluid or smoked.
		Inaccurate if client breathes through the mouth, therefore contraindicated for clients who have nasal surgery.
		Could injure the mouth following oral surgery.
Rectal	Most reliable measurement	Inconvenient and more unpleasant for clients; difficult for client who cannot turn to the side.
		Could injure the rectum following rectal surgery.
		Placement of the thermometer at different sites within the rectum yields different temperatures, yet placement at the same site each time is difficult.
		A rectal thermometer does not respond to changes in arterial temperatures as quickly as an oral thermometer, a fact that may be potentially dangerous for febrile clients, since misleading information may be acquired.
		Presence of stool may interfere with thermometer placement. If the stool is soft, the thermometer may be embedded in stool rather than against the wall of the rectum. If the stool is impacted, the depth of thermometer insertion may be insufficient.
		In newborns and infants, insertion of the rectal thermometer has resulted in ulcerations and rectal perforations. *Many agencies advise against using rectal thermometers on neonates.*
Axillary	Safest and most noninvasive	The thermometer must be left in place a long time to obtain an accurate measurement.

perature. Although the **axillary** temperature was considered less accurate than the rectal or oral method, studies now indicate that there is no clinically important difference in accuracy between axillary and rectal temperatures (Axillary temps safer 1978, p. 1081; Eoff and Joyce 1981, p. 1011; Schiffman 1982, p. 274; Martyn 1988, p. 32). The axilla is therefore the preferred site for temperature measurements in children, not only because it is easily accessible but also because there is less likelihood of rectal perforation and subsequent peritonitis (Axillary temps safer 1978, p. 1081; Eoff and Joyce 1981, p. 1010). Clients for whom the axillary method of temperature assessment is appropriate include newborns and infants, toddlers and preschoolers, clients with oral inflammation or wired jaws, clients recovering from oral surgery, clients who are breathing through their mouths (e.g., following nasal surgery), irrational clients, and clients for whom oral and rectal temperatures are contraindicated. However, axillary temperatures may be deceptively high in the cold-stressed neonate because of the metabolism of brown fat.

The **tympanic membrane**, or nearby tissue in the ear canal, is another core body temperature site. Tympanic membrane temperature readings average 1.1 to 1.5 F higher than oral temperature readings (Erikson and Yount 1991, p. 92). Like the sublingual oral site, the tympanic membrane has an abundant arterial blood supply, primarily from branches of the external carotid artery. Because temperature sensors applied directly to the tympanic membrane can be uncomfortable and involve risk of membrane injury or perforation, noninvasive *infrared thermometers* are now used.

Types of Thermometers
A common type of **thermometer** is a glass tube with a column of mercury inside it. Heat expands the mercury, thus expanding the column along the tube, where it can be measured against marked calibrations. Traditionally, body temperatures have been measured using *mercury-in-glass thermometers*. Oral thermometers may have long slender tips, short rounded tips, or pear-shaped tips (Figure 10–2). The

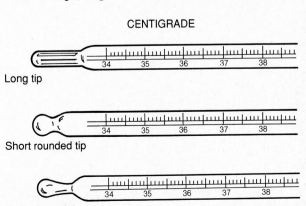

CENTIGRADE

Long tip

Short rounded tip

Pear-shaped tip

FIGURE 10–2 Three types of thermometer tips (Centigrade scale).

rounded thermometer can be used at the rectal as well as other sites. In some agencies, thermometers may be color coded; for example, blue-colored thermometers may be used for rectal temperatures and silver-colored ones for oral and axillary temperatures. *Disposable thermometers* are also manufactured; these are used only once.

Electronic thermometers offer another method of assessing body temperatures. They can provide a reading in only 2 to 60 seconds, depending on the model. The equipment consists of a battery-operated portable electronic unit, a probe that the nurse attaches to the unit, and a probe cover, which is usually disposable (Figure 10–3). Some models have a different circuit for each method of measurement, and the nurse needs to make sure that the correct circuit is switched on before taking the temperature.

Chemical disposable thermometers come in individual cases and are discarded after use. One type has small chemical dots at one end that respond to body heat by changing color, thereby providing a reading of the body temperature. The thermometer comes in a plastic case. To activate the chemicals, nurses hold the thermometer with the handle toward themselves, move the handle up and down, and then pull the plastic straight off the thermometer. The nurse then inserts the thermometer under the client's tongue, in the same way as a glass thermometer, and leaves it in place for the time recommended by the manufacturer (e.g., 45 seconds). After removing it, the nurse observes the dots for a change in color, noting the highest reading among the dots that have changed color (Figure 10–4). The chemical thermometer is discarded after use.

Temperature-sensitive tape may also be used to obtain a general indication of body surface temperature. When applied to the skin, usually of the forehead or abdomen, the tape responds by changing color. The skin area should be dry. After the length of time specified by the manufacturer (e.g., 15 seconds), a color appears on the tape. The nurse compares the color and then removes and discards the tape. This method is particularly useful at home and for infants whose temperatures are to be monitored for any reason. Skin strips may, however, register falsely elevated readings, so high readings should be validated with another temperature measurement device (Martyn 1988, p. 31).

Infrared thermometers sense body heat in the form of infrared energy given off by a heat source, which in the ear canal is primarily the tympanic membrane (Erikson and Yount 1991, p. 91). Because the infrared thermometer makes no contact with the tympanic membrane or moist mucous membrane, the risk of spreading infection is reduced. The ear canal has no mucous membrane and is dry.

To insert an infrared thermometer, the nurse places the probe tip into the outer portion of the ear canal just at the ear's opening. The probe tip seals the ear opening, and the nurse presses a button; in one or two seconds the temperature reading is digitized by computer onto a screen. Infrared thermometer probes are covered with comfortable disposable speculums that safely fit adults and infants. Covers can be applied and ejected without being touched.

Temperature Scales

The body temperature is measured in degrees on two scales: Celsius and Fahrenheit. The **Celsius**, or **centigrade**, scale normally extends from 34.0 to 42.0 C. The **Fahrenheit** scale usually extends from 94 to 108 F (Figure 10–5). Body temperatures rarely extend beyond these scales.

Technique 10–1 explains how to measure body temperature.

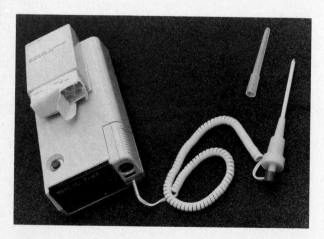

FIGURE 10–3 An electronic thermometer. Note the probe and the probe cover beside it.

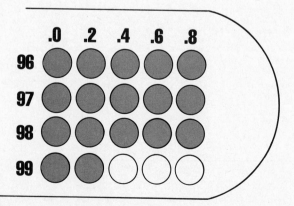

FIGURE 10–4 A chemical thermometer showing a reading of 99.2 F.

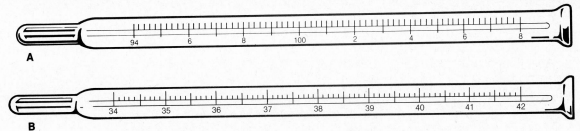

FIGURE 10–5   Thermometers. The upper one shows the Fahrenheit scale; the lower one, the Celsius (centigrade) scale.

Assessing Body Temperature Using a Mercury Thermometer

PURPOSES
- To establish baseline data for subsequent evaluation
- To identify whether the core temperature is within normal range
- To determine changes in the core temperature in response to specific therapies (e.g., antipyretic administration, immunosuppressive therapy, invasive procedure)
- To monitor clients at risk for alterations in temperature (e.g., clients at risk for infection or diagnosis of infection; those who have been exposed to temperature extremes; those with leukocyte count below 5000 or above 12,000)

ASSESSMENT FOCUS

Clinical signs of fever (see page 162); clinical signs of hypothermia (see page 162); site most appropriate for measurement (see pages 162–163); factors that may alter core body temperature (see pages 160–161).

EQUIPMENT
- Oral, rectal, or axillary thermometer
- Towel if the axillary site is being used
- Lubricant if the rectal site is being used
- Disposable gloves

INTERVENTION

1. Prepare the client.
- Ascertain which method of taking the temperature is appropriate for the client.

For an Oral Temperature
- Determine the time the client last took hot or cold food or fluids or smoked. *To obtain an accurate oral temperature reading, allow at least 5 minutes or amount of time according to agency protocol to elapse between a client's intake or smoking and the measurement.*

For a Rectal Temperature
- Assist the client to assume a lateral position. Place newborn in a lateral or prone position (Axillary temps safer in infants 1978, p. 1081). Place a young child in a lateral position with knees flexed, or prone across the lap.

- Provide privacy before folding the bedclothes back to expose the buttocks. *Privacy is essential, since exposure of the buttocks embarrasses most people.*

For an Axillary Temperature
- Expose the client's axilla. If the axilla is moist, dry it with the towel, using a patting motion. *Friction created by rubbing can raise the temperature of the axilla.*

2. Prepare the equipment.
- Remove the thermometer from its package, and check the temperature reading on the thermometer.
- Shake down the mercury (if necessary) by holding the thermometer between the thumb and

▶ **Technique 10–1 Assessing Body Temperature** CONTINUED

forefinger at the end farthest from the bulb. Snap the wrist downward.

- Repeat until the mercury is below 35 C (95 F).

3. Take the temperature.

For an Oral Temperature

- Place the thermometer or probe at the base of the tongue to the right or left of the frenulum, the posterior sublingual pocket (see Figure 10–6). *The thermometer needs to reflect the core temperature of the blood in the larger blood vessels of the posterior pocket.*

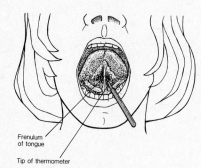

Frenulum of tongue

Tip of thermometer

FIGURE 10–6 The tip of an oral thermometer is placed beside the frenulum.

- Ask the client to close the lips, not the teeth, around the thermometer. *A client who bites the thermometer can break it and injure the mouth.*

- Leave the thermometer in place a sufficient time for the temperature to register or for the length of time recommended by the agency. The recommended time is 2 minutes (Baker et al. 1984, p. 111) or 3 minutes (Graves and Markarian 1980, p. 323). If an electronic oral thermometer is used, the client holds the thermometer under the tongue 10 to 20 seconds or until it completes registering.

For a Rectal Temperature

- Place some lubricant on a piece of tissue. Then apply lubricant to

the thermometer about 2.5 cm (1 in) above the bulb. *The lubricant facilitates insertion of the thermometer without irritating the mucous membrane.*

- Don a disposable glove on the dominant hand. With the nondominant hand, raise the client's upper buttock to expose the anus.

- Ask the client to take a deep breath, and insert the thermometer into the anus anywhere from 1.5 to 4 cm (0.5 to 1.5 in), depending on the age and size of the client (for example, 1.5 cm [0.5 in] for an infant, 2.5 cm [0.9 in] for a child, and 3.7 cm [1.5 in] for an adult). *Taking a deep breath often relaxes the external sphincter muscle, thus easing insertion.*

- Do not *force* insertion of the thermometer. *Inability to insert the thermometer into a newborn could indicate the rectum is not patent.*

- Hold the thermometer in place for 2 minutes (Nichols 1972, p. 1093) or for the length of time recommended by the agency. For neonates hold the thermometer in place for 5 minutes (Schiffman 1982, p. 276). Hold the young child firmly while the probe is in the rectum. *The thermometer may become displaced inside or outside of the anus if not held in place.*

For an Axillary Temperature

- Place the thermometer in the client's axilla (Figure 10–7).

- Assist the client to place the arm tightly across the chest to keep the thermometer in place.

- Leave the thermometer in place for 9 minutes (Nichols et al. 1966, p. 310). For infants and children, leave the thermometer

in place 5 minutes (Eoff and Joyce 1981, p. 1011).

- Remain with the client, and hold the thermometer in place if the client is irrational or very young.

4. Remove the thermometer.

- Remove the plastic sheath, or wipe the thermometer with a tissue. Wipe in a rotating manner toward the bulb. *The thermometer is wiped from the area of least contamination to that of greatest contamination.*

- Discard the tissue in a receptacle used for contaminated items.

5. Read the temperature.

- Hold the thermometer at eye level, and rotate it until the mercury column is clearly visible. The upper end of the mercury column registers the client's body temperature. On the Fahrenheit thermometer, each long line reflects 1 degree and each short line 0.2 degree. On the centigrade thermometer, each long line reflects 0.5 degree and each short line 0.1 degree.

6. Clean and shake down the thermometer.

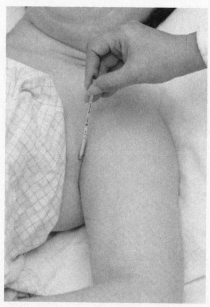

FIGURE 10–7 The bulb of the thermometer is placed in the center of the axilla.

► **Technique 10–1** *CONTINUED*

- Wash the thermometer in tepid, soapy water. Organic material such as mucus must be removed before the thermometer can be stored. *Organic materials on the thermometer can harbor micro-organisms.*

- Rinse the thermometer in *cold* water, dry it, and store it dry. *Hot water expands the mercury and may break the thermometer.*

- Shake down the thermometer, and return it to its container or discard it. Some agencies also have special equipment for spinning down the mercury levels.

- If the thermometer is to be disinfected before storage, use isopropyl alcohol 70%.

- Return an electronic thermometer to the battery base for recharging.

7. Document the temperature.

- Record the temperature to the nearest indicated tenth (for example, 98.4 F, 37.1 C) on a flowsheet or in a notebook. *Recording the temperature immediately ensures it is not forgotten.*

VARIATION: **Using an Electronic Thermometer**

- Remove the electronic unit from the battery charging area.

- Remove the temperature probe from the unit. If the probe is not attached, attach it to the appropriate circuit (oral, rectal, or axillary) in models that have separate circuits for each.

- Place a disposable cover securely on the probe.

- Warm up the machine by switching it on if removal of the probe does not automatically prepare the machine for functioning.

- Take the temperature as indicated above in Step 3.

- Listen for a sound indicating that the maximum measurement has been reached, and read the temperature on the dial or readout.

- Remove the thermometer.

- Remove and discard the probe cover.

EVALUATION FOCUS

The temperature measurement in relation to baseline data or normal range for age of client; time of day and any other influencing factors; relationship to other vital signs.

SAMPLE RECORDING

Date	Time	Notes
6/12/93	1600	Complains of feeling "hot." Skin warm and flushed. T 39.2 C orally, P 104, R 16. Tepid sponge bath given. ————————— Thomas W. Wilson, RN
	1630	T 38.8 C Skin remains warm but less flushed. Fluids encouraged. ————— Thomas W. Wilson, RN

KEY ELEMENTS OF ASSESSING BODY TEMPERATURE

For *oral* temperature measurement:

- Avoid taking oral temperatures of clients who are under age 6, irrational, unconscious, or who have oral pathology or surgery.

- Allow at least 5 minutes to elapse after a client's intake of hot or cold fluids or smoking.

- Place the tip of the thermometer at the base of the tongue to the right or left of the frenulum.

- Ask the client to hold a glass thermometer with the lips rather than the teeth.

For *rectal* temperature measurement:

- Avoid taking rectal temperatures on clients who have rectal pathology or convulsive disorders or who have had rectal surgery.

- Lubricate the thermometer or probe prior to insertion.

- Hold the child or infant firmly while the thermometer is in the rectum.

For *axillary* temperature measurement:

- Remain with the client, and hold the thermometer in place if the client is irrational or very young.

For *all* measurements:

- Wear gloves if in contact with body substances or secretions.

- Ensure the level of mercury in a glass thermometer is below 35 C or 95 F before insertion.

- Leave the thermometer in place for a time sufficient for the temperature to register.

- Assess the client for other signs of hyperthermia or hypothermia.

Pulse

The **pulse** is a wave of blood created by contraction of the left ventricle of the heart. The heart is a pulsatile pump, and the blood enters the arteries with each heartbeat, causing pressure pulses or pulse waves (Guyton 1986, p. 225). Generally, the pulse wave represents the stroke volume output and the compliance of the arteries. **Stroke volume output** is the amount of blood that enters the arteries with each ventricular contraction. **Compliance** of the arteries is the distensibility of the arteries, i.e., their ability to contract and expand. When a person's arteries lose their distensibility, as can happen in old age, greater pressure is required to pump the blood into the arteries.

In a healthy person, the pulse reflects the heartbeat, i.e., the **pulse rate** is the same as the rate of the ventricular contractions of the heart. However, in some types of cardiovascular disease, the heartbeat and pulse rates can differ. For example, a client's heart may produce very weak or small pulse waves that are not detectable in a peripheral pulse. In these instances, the nurse should assess the heartbeat *and* the peripheral pulse. See the section on assessing the apical pulse, later in this chapter. A **peripheral pulse** is a pulse located in the periphery of the body, e.g., in the foot, hand, or neck. The **apical pulse**, in contrast, is a central pulse; i.e., it is located at the apex of the heart.

The pulse rate is regulated by the autonomic nervous system (ANS). Impulses pass through the parasympathetic branch to the sinoatrial node (SA node), which is the pacemaker of the heart. These impulses decrease the heart rate. When body demands indicate a need for an increased heart rate, the impulses of the parasympathetic system are inhibited and the impulses of the sympathetic system increase.

Pulse Sites

The pulse is commonly taken in nine sites (Figure 10–8):

1. *Temporal*, where the temporal artery passes over the temporal bone of the head. The site is superior (above) and lateral to (away from the midline of) the eye.

2. *Carotid*, at the side of the neck below the lobe of the ear, where the carotid artery runs between the trachea and the sternocleidomastoid muscle.

3. *Apical*, at the apex of the heart. In an adult this is located on the left side of the chest, no more than 8 cm (3 in) to the left of the sternum (breastbone) and under the fourth, fifth, or sixth intercostal space (area between the ribs). For a child 7 to 9 years of

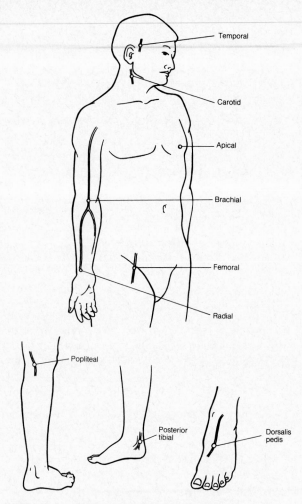

FIGURE 10–8 Nine sites commonly used for assessing a pulse.

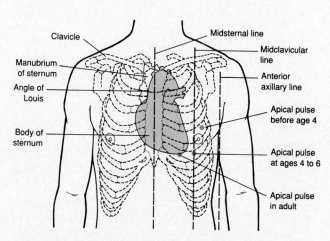

FIGURE 10–9 Location of the apical pulse for a child under 4 years, a child 4 to 6 years, and an adult.

age, the apical pulse is located between the fourth and fifth intercostal spaces. Before 4 years of age it is left of the midclavicular line (MCL); between 4 and 6 years it is at the MCL (Figure 10–9).

4. *Brachial*, at the inner aspect of the biceps muscle of the arm (especially in infants) or medially in the antecubital space (elbow crease).

5. *Radial*, where the radial artery runs along the radial bone, on the thumb side of the inner aspect of the wrist.

6. *Femoral*, where the femoral artery passes alongside the inguinal ligament.

7. *Popliteal*, where the popliteal artery passes behind the knee. This point is difficult to find, but it can be palpated if the client flexes the knee slightly (Figure 10–25, later in this chapter).

8. *Posterior tibial*, on the medial surface of the ankle where the posterior tibial artery passes behind the medial malleolus.

9. *Pedal (dorsalis pedis)*, where the dorsalis pedis artery passes over the bones of the foot. This artery can be palpated by feeling the dorsum (upper surface) of the foot on an imaginary line drawn from the middle of the ankles to the space between the big and second toes.

Some reasons for use of each site are given in Table 10–3. The radial site is most commonly used. It is easily found in most people and readily accessible.

Factors Affecting Pulse Rate

The rate of the pulse is expressed in beats per minute (BPM). A pulse rate varies according to a number of factors. The nurse should consider each of the following factors when assessing a client's pulse:

- *Age*. As age increases, the pulse rate gradually decreases. See Table 10–1 for specific variations in pulse rates from birth to adulthood.

- *Sex*. After puberty, the average male's pulse rate is slightly lower than the female's.

- *Exercise*. The pulse rate normally increases with activity. The rate of increase in the professional athlete is often less than in the average person because of greater cardiac size, strength, and efficiency.

- *Fever*. The pulse rate increases (a) in response to the lowered blood pressure that results from peripheral vasodilation associated with elevated body temperature and also (b) because of the increased metabolic rate.

- *Medications*. Some medications decrease the pulse rate, and others increase it. For example, cardiotonics (e.g., digitalis preparations) will decrease the heart rate, whereas epinephrine will increase it.

- *Hemorrhage*. Loss of blood from the vascular system (**hemorrhage**) normally increases pulse rate. An adult has about 5 liters of blood in the

TABLE 10–3 REASONS FOR USING SPECIFIC PULSE SITES

Pulse Site	Reasons for Use
Radial	Readily accessible and routinely used
Temporal	Used when radial pulse is not accessible
Carotid	Used for infants
	Used in cases of cardiac arrest
	Used to determine circulation to the brain
Apical	Routinely used for infants and children up to 3 years of age
	Used to determine discrepancies with radial pulse
	Used in conjunction with some medications
Brachial	Used to measure blood pressure
	Used during cardiac arrest for infants
Femoral	Used in cases of cardiac arrest
	Used for infants and children
	Used to determine circulation to a leg
Popliteal	Used to determine circulation to the lower leg
	Used to determine leg blood pressure
Posterial tibial	Used to determine circulation to the foot
Pedal	Used to determine circulation to the foot

system and can usually lose up to 10% without adverse effects.

- *Stress*. In response to stress, sympathetic nervous stimulation increases the overall activity of the heart. Stress increases the rate as well as the force of the heartbeat. Emotions such as fear and anxiety as well as the perception of severe pain stimulate the sympathetic system.

- *Position changes*. When a person assumes a sitting or standing position, blood usually pools in dependent vessels of the venous system. Pooling results in a transient decrease in the venous blood return to the heart and a subsequent reduction in blood pressure. These changes are primarily mediated through the sympathetic nervous system, increasing cardiac rate, force of the ventricular contractions, and tone of the veins and arteries.

Peripheral Pulse Assessment

When assessing the pulse, the nurse collects the following data: the rate, rhythm, volume, arterial wall elasticity, and presence or absence of bilateral equality. The *normal pulse rates* are shown in Table 10–1. An excessively fast heart rate, e.g., over 100 beats per minute in an adult, is referred to as **tachycardia**. A heart rate in an adult of 60 beats per minute or less is called **bradycardia**. If a client has either tachycardia or bradycardia, the nurse should assess the apical pulse.

The **pulse rhythm** is the pattern of the beats and the intervals between the beats. Equal time elapses between beats of a normal pulse. A pulse with an irregular rhythm is referred to as a **dysrhythmia** or **arrhythmia**. It may consist of random, irregular beats or a predictable pattern of irregular beats. When a dysrhythmia is detected, the nurse should assess the apical pulse. An electrocardiogram (ECG or EKG) is necessary to define the dysrhythmia further. Sinus arrhythmia is a common and often nonpathologic finding in many children (Whaley and Wong 1991, p. 273).

Pulse volume, also called the pulse strength or amplitude, refers to the force of blood exerted with each beat. Usually, pulse volume is the same with each beat. It can range from absent to bounding. A normal pulse can be felt with moderate pressure of the fingers and can be obliterated with greater pressure. A forceful or full blood volume that is obliterated only with difficulty is called a *full* or *bounding* pulse. A pulse that is readily obliterated with pressure from the fingers is referred to as *weak, feeble,* or *thready* (Figure 10–10). A pulse volume is usually measured on a scale of 0 to 3. See Table 10–4.

The *elasticity of the arterial wall* reflects its expansibility or its deformities. A healthy, normal artery feels straight, smooth, soft, and pliable. Elderly people often have inelastic arteries that feel twisted (tortuous) and irregular upon palpation. The elasticity of the arteries may not affect the pulse rate, rhythm, or volume, but it does reflect the status of the client's vascular system.

When assessing a peripheral pulse to determine the adequacy of blood flow to a particular area of the

TABLE 10–4   SCALE FOR MEASURING PULSE VOLUME

Scale	Description of Pulse
0	Absent, not discernible
1	Thready or weak, difficult to feel
2	Normal, detected readily, obliterated by strong pressure
3	Bounding, difficult to obliterate

body, the nurse should also assess the corresponding pulse on the other side of the body. The second assessment gives the nurse data with which to compare the pulses. For example, when assessing the blood flow to the right foot, the nurse assesses the right dorsalis pedis pulse and then the left dorsalis pedis pulse. If the client's right and left pulses are the same, the client's dorsalis pedis pulses are *bilaterally equal.*

A pulse is commonly assessed by palpation (feeling) or auscultation (hearing). The middle three fingertips are used for palpating all pulse sites except the apex of the heart. A stethoscope is used for assessing apical pulses and fetal heart tones. Increasingly, a Doppler ultrasound stethoscope (DUS; Figure 10–11) is used for pulses that are difficult to assess. The DUS headset has earpieces similar to standard stethoscope earpieces, but it has a long cord attached to a volume-controlled audio unit and an ultrasound transducer. The DUS detects movement of red blood cells through a blood vessel. In contrast to the conventional stethoscope, it excludes environmental sounds. It cannot detect blood flow in deep vessels or in those underlying bone, such as the vessels in the abdomen, thorax, or skull. The DUS is battery operated, and batteries must be replaced about every 6 months.

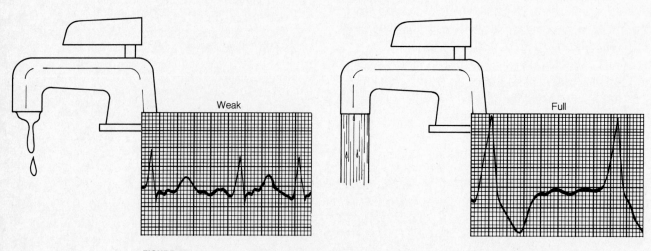

FIGURE 10–10 Two comparative electrocardiographs, one illustrating a weak pulse volume and one a full pulse volume.

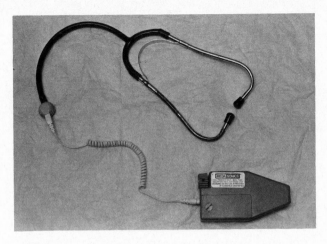

FIGURE 10–11 An ultrasound (Doppler) stethoscope.

A pulse is normally palpated by applying moderate pressure with the three middle fingers of the hand. The pads on the most distal aspects of the finger are the most sensitive areas for detecting a pulse. With excessive pressure, one can obliterate a pulse, whereas with too little pressure, one may not be able to detect it. Before the nurse assesses the *resting* pulse, the client should assume a comfortable position. The nurse should also be aware of the following:

- Any medication that could affect the heart rate.

- Whether the client has been physically active. If so, the nurse should wait 10 to 15 minutes until the client has rested and the pulse has slowed to its usual rate.

- Any baseline data about the normal heart rate for the client. For example, a physically fit athlete may have a heart rate below 60 BPM.

- Whether the client should assume a particular position, e.g., sitting. In some clients, the rate changes with the position because of changes in blood flow volume and autonomic nervous system activity.

A peripheral pulse, usually the radial pulse, is assessed by palpation for all individuals *except*:

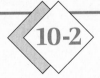

- Newborns and children up to 2 or 3 years. Apical pulses are assessed in these clients.

- Very obese or elderly clients, whose radial pulse may be difficult to palpate. Doppler equipment may be used for these clients, or the apical pulse is assessed.

- Individuals with heart disease, who require apical pulse assessment.

- Individuals in whom the circulation to a specific body part must be assessed; e.g., in clients who have undergone leg surgery, the pedal (dorsalis pedis) pulse is assessed.

Technique 10–2 provides guidelines for assessing peripheral pulses.

◀10-2▶ Assessing a Peripheral Pulse

PURPOSES

- To establish baseline data for subsequent evaluation
- To identify whether the pulse rate is within normal range
- To determine whether the pulse rhythm is regular and the pulse volume is appropriate
- To compare the equality of corresponding peripheral pulses on each side of the body
- To monitor and assess changes in the client's health status
- To monitor clients at risk for pulse alterations (e.g., those with a history of heart disease or experiencing cardiac arrhythmias, hemorrhage, acute pain, infusion of large volumes of fluids, fever)

ASSESSMENT FOCUS

Clinical signs of cardiovascular alterations, other than pulse rate, rhythm, or volume (e.g., dyspnea [difficult respirations], fatigue, pallor, cyanosis [bluish discoloration of skin and mucous membranes], palpations, syncope [fainting], impaired peripheral tissue perfusion as evidenced by skin discoloration and cool temperature); factors that may alter pulse rate (e.g., emotional status and activity level); site most appropriate for assessment.

► **Technique 10–2 Assessing a Peripheral Pulse** CONTINUED

EQUIPMENT

□ Watch with a second hand or indicator

□ If using Doppler ultrasound stethoscope, the transducer in the DUS probe, a stethoscope headset, and transmission gel

INTERVENTION

1. **Prepare the client.**

• Select the pulse point. Normally, the radial pulse is taken, unless it cannot be exposed or circulation to another body area is to be assessed.

• Assist the client to a comfortable resting position. When the radial pulse is assessed, the client's arm can rest alongside the body, the palm facing downward. Or, the forearm can rest at a 90° angle across the chest with the palm downward. For the client who can sit, the forearm can rest across the thigh, with the palm of the hand facing downward or inward. Positioning a child comfortably in the parent's arms or having the parent remain close by may decrease anxiety and yield more accurate results.

2. **Palpate and count the pulse.**

• Place two or three middle fingertips lightly and squarely over the pulse point (Figure 10–12). *Using the thumb is contraindicated because the thumb has a pulse that the nurse could mistake for the client's pulse.*

• If the pulse is regular, count for 30 seconds and multiply by 2. If it is irregular, count for 1 minute. If taking a client's pulse for the first time or when obtaining baseline data, count the pulse for a full minute. *An irregular pulse requires a full minute's count for a correct assessment.*

3. **Assess the pulse rhythm and volume.**

• Assess the pulse rhythm by noting the pattern of intervals between the beats. A normal pulse

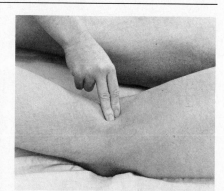
A

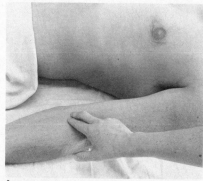
B

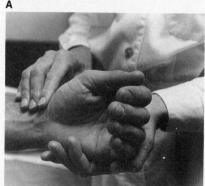
C

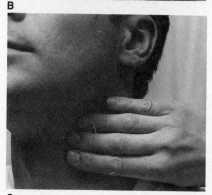
D

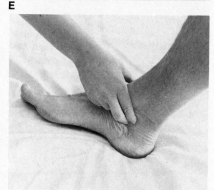
E

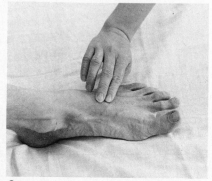
F

G

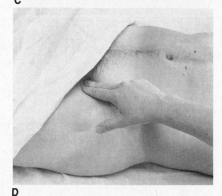

FIGURE 10–12 Assessing the pulses: *A*, brachial; *B*, radial; *C*, carotid; *D*, femoral; *E*, popliteal; *F*, posterior tibial; and *G*, pedal.

► **Technique 10–2** *CONTINUED*

has equal time periods between beats. If this is an initial assessment, assess for 1 minute.

- Assess the pulse volume. A normal pulse can be felt with moderate pressure, and the pressure is equal with each beat. A forceful pulse volume is full; an easily obliterated pulse is weak.

4. Assess the arterial wall.

- Compress the artery firmly, and run a finger distal to the heart along the artery (Figure 10–13). A normal arterial wall is smooth and straight.

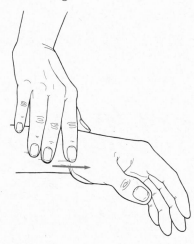

FIGURE 10–13 Assessing the status of the arterial wall.

5. Document and report pertinent assessment data.

- Record the pulse rate, rhythm, and volume, and the condition of the arterial wall. See sample recording below.

- Report to the nurse in charge pertinent data such as (a) pale skin color and cool skin temperature, (b) a pulse rate faster or slower than normal for the client, (c) a full, bounding, or weak pulse volume, (d) an irregular pulse rhythm, and (e) a tortuous arterial wall.

VARIATION: **Using a DUS**

- Plug the stethoscope headset into one of the two output jacks located next to the volume control. DUS units have jacks for two headpieces and accessory loudspeakers so that another person can listen to the signals.

- Apply transmission gel either to the probe (a device resembling a small transistor radio), at the narrow end of the plastic case housing the transducer, or to the client's skin. *Ultrasound beams do not travel well through air. The gel makes an airtight seal, which*

then promotes optimal ultrasound wave transmission.

- Press the "on" button.

- Hold the probe at a 45° angle against the skin over the pulse site. Use a light pressure, and keep the probe in contact with the skin. *Too much pressure can stop the blood flow and obliterate the signal.*

- Distinguish artery sounds from vein sounds. The artery sound (signal) is distinctively pulsating and has a pumping quality. The venous sound is like the wind, is intermittent, and varies with respirations. *Both artery and vein sounds are heard simultaneously through the DUS, since major arteries and veins are situated close together throughout the body.*

- If you have difficulty hearing arterial sounds, then reposition the probe.

- After assessing the pulse, remove all the gel from the probe to prevent damage to its surface. Clean the transducer with aqueous solutions. *Alcohol or other disinfectants may damage the face of the transducer.* Remove all gel from the client (Hudson 1983, p. 56).

EVALUATION FOCUS

The pulse rate in relation to baseline data or normal range for age of client; relationship of pulse rate and volume to other vital signs; pulse rhythm and volume in relationship to baseline data and health status; equality, rate, and volume in corresponding extremities if assessing peripheral pulses.

SAMPLE RECORDING

Date	Time	Notes
5/8/93	0900	Pale and listless. Pulse 116, weak and thready. Arterial wall feels soft and pliable. Reported above to Ms N. McNamara. ——— Sally M. Sahara, NS

KEY ELEMENTS OF ASSESSING A PERIPHERAL PULSE

- Ensure that the client is calm and quiet 10 to 15 minutes before pulse rate assessment to obtain accurate readings.
- Use the middle three fingertips to palpate the pulse rate, rhythm, volume, and arterial wall tension.
- Count an irregular pulse for 60 seconds.
- Report notable variations in the pulse promptly.

Apical Pulse Assessment

Assessment of the apical pulse is indicated for clients whose peripheral pulse is irregular as well as for clients with known cardiovascular, pulmonary, and renal diseases. Nurses commonly assess the apical pulse prior to administering medications that affect heart rate. The apical site is also used to assess the pulse for newborns, infants, and children up to 2 to 3 years old. Technique 10–3 presents guidelines for assessing the apical pulse.

10-3 Assessing an Apical Pulse

PURPOSES

- To obtain the heart rate of newborns, infants, and children 2 to 3 years old or of an adult with an irregular peripheral pulse
- To establish baseline data for subsequent evaluation
- To determine whether the cardiac rate is within normal range and the rhythm is regular
- To monitor clients with cardiac disease and those receiving medications to improve heart action

ASSESSMENT FOCUS

Clinical signs of cardiovascular alterations, other than pulse rate, rhythm, or volume (e.g., dyspnea, fatigue, pallor, cyanosis, syncope); factors that may alter pulse rate (e.g., emotional status, activity level).

EQUIPMENT

- Watch with a second hand or indicator
- Stethoscope with a bell-shaped or flat-disc diaphragm
- Antiseptic wipes
- If using ultrasound, a DUS, probe (transducer), and transmission gel

INTERVENTION

1. Position the client appropriately.

- Assist an adult or young child to a comfortable supine position with the head of the bed elevated, or to a sitting position on a chair, the edge of the bed, or the examination table.

- Place a baby in a supine position, and offer a pacifier if the baby is crying or restless. *Crying and physical activity will increase the pulse rate.* For this reason, take the apical pulse rate of infants and small children before assessing body temperature.

- Demonstrate the procedure to the child using a stuffed animal or doll, and allow the child to handle the stethoscope before beginning the procedure. *This will decrease anxiety and promote cooperation.*

- Expose the area of the chest over the apex of the heart.

2. Locate the apical impulse.

- This is the point over the apex of the heart where the apical pulse can be most clearly heard. It is also referred to as the point of maximal impulse (PMI). In 50% of the adult population, the apical impulse can be palpated (Malasanos et al. 1990, p. 337).

- Palpate the angle of Louis (the angle between the manubrium, the top of the sternum, and the body of the sternum). It is pal-

pated just below the suprasternal notch and is felt as a prominence (Figure 10–9, earlier).

- Place your index finger just to the left of the client's sternum, and palpate the second intercostal space.

- Place your middle or next finger in the third intercostal space, and continue palpating downward until you locate the apical impulse, usually about the fifth intercostal space, if the client is an adult or a child 7 years or older. If the client is a young child, palpate downward to the fourth intercostal space. *The apex of the heart is normally located in the fifth intercostal space in individ-*

▶ **Technique 10–3** *CONTINUED*

uals who are 7 years of age and over; it is in the fourth intercostal space in young children, and one or two spaces above the adult apex during infancy (Malasanos et al. 1990, p. 627).

- Palpate the apical impulse. For an adult, move your index finger laterally along the fifth intercostal space to the MCL. Normally, the apical impulse is palpable at or just medial to the MCL. For a young child, move your finger along the fourth intercostal space to a position between the MCL and the anterior axillary line (Figure 10–9, earlier).

3. Auscultate and count the heartbeats.

- Use antiseptic wipes to clean the earpieces and diaphragm of the stethoscope (Figure 10–14) if their cleanliness is in doubt. *The diaphragm needs to be cleaned and disinfected if soiled with body substances.*

- Warm the diaphragm of the stethoscope by holding it in the palm of the hand for a moment. *The metal of the diaphragm is usually cold and can startle the client when placed immediately on the chest.*

- Insert the earpieces of the stethoscope into your ears. The earpieces may be straight or bent. If they are bent, place them in the direction of the ear canals,

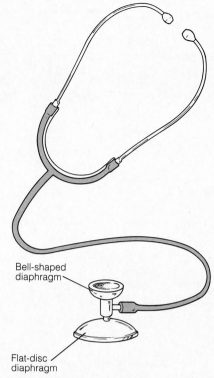

Bell-shaped diaphragm

Flat-disc diaphragm

FIGURE 10–14 A stethoscope with both bell-shaped and flat-disc diaphragms.

or slightly forward, to facilitate hearing.

- Place the diaphragm of the stethoscope over the apical impulse and listen for the normal S_1 and S_2 heart sounds, which are heard as "lub dub." Each lub dub is counted as one heartbeat. *The heartbeat is normally loudest over the apex of the heart. The two heart sounds are produced by closure of the valves of the heart.* The S_1 heart sound (lub) occurs when the atrioventricular valves close after the ventricles have been

sufficiently filled. The S_2 heart sound (dub) occurs when the semilunar valves close after the ventricles empty.

- Count the heartbeats for 30 seconds and multiply by 2 if the rhythm is regular; count the beats for 60 seconds if the rhythm is irregular or if the apical impulse is being taken on an infant or child. *A 60-second count provides a more accurate assessment of an irregular pulse than a 30-second count.*

4. Assess the rhythm and the strength of the heartbeat.

- Assess the rhythm of the heartbeat by noting the pattern of intervals between the beats. A normal pulse has equal time periods between beats.

- Assess the strength (volume) of the heartbeat. Normally, the heartbeats are equal in strength and can be described as strong or weak.

5. Document and report pertinent assessment data.

- Record the pulse site and rate, rhythm, and volume. See sample recording below.

- Report to the nurse in charge any pertinent data such as pallor, cyanosis, dyspnea, tachycardia, bradycardia, irregular rhythm, and reduced strength of the heartbeat.

EVALUATION FOCUS

The apical rate in relation to baseline data or normal range for the age of the client; relationship to other vital signs; apical pulse rhythm and volume in relationship to baseline data and health status.

SAMPLE RECORDING

Date	Time	Notes
1/26/93	0900	Apical pulse 56. Beats strong and equal. Digitoxin withheld. Notified Ms S. Santos, RN ———————————————— Tamara A. Jones, NS

▶ **Technique 10–3 Assessing an Apical Pulse** *CONTINUED*

KEY ELEMENTS OF ASSESSING AN APICAL PULSE

- Offer a pacifier if necessary to quiet a newborn or infant.
- Take the apical pulse of an infant or small child before assessing body temperature.

- Count the heartbeats for 60 seconds if the rhythm is irregular.
- Assess the rhythm and the strength of the heartbeat.

Apical-Radial Pulse Assessment

An apical-radial pulse may need to be assessed for clients with certain cardiovascular disorders. Normally, the apical and radial rates are identical. An apical pulse rate greater than a radial pulse rate can indicate that the thrust of the blood from the heart is too feeble for the wave to be felt at the peripheral pulse site, or it can indicate that vascular disease is preventing impulses from being transmitted. Any discrepancy between the two pulse rates needs to be reported promptly. The difference between the count of the apical pulse and the count of the radial pulse is known as the **pulse deficit**. In no instance is the radial pulse greater than the apical pulse.

An apical-radial pulse can be taken by two nurses or one nurse, although the two-nurse technique may be more accurate. Technique 10–4 describes how to assess an apical-radial pulse.

For infants, the *radial* and *femoral* pulses should be compared at least once during the first year of life to detect the presence of coarctation of the aorta or other cardiovascular problems (Stevens 1991, p. 205).

10-4   Assessing an Apical–Radial Pulse

PURPOSE	• To determine adequacy of peripheral circulation or presence of pulse deficit
ASSESSMENT FOCUS	Clinical signs of hypovolemic shock (hypotension, pallor, cyanosis, and cold, clammy, skin).

EQUIPMENT

- ▢ Watch with a second hand
- ▢ Stethoscope
- ▢ Antiseptic wipes

INTERVENTION

1. Position the client appropriately.

- Assist the client to assume the position described for taking the apical pulse. See Technique 10–3, Step 1.
- If previous measurements were taken, determine what position the client assumed, and use the same position. *This ensures an accurate comparative measurement.*

2. Locate the apical and radial pulse sites.

- In the two-nurse technique, one nurse locates the apical impulse by palpation or with the stethoscope while the other nurse palpates the radial pulse site. See Techniques 10–2 and 10–3.

3. Count the apical and radial pulse rates.

Two-Nurse Technique

- Place the watch where both nurses can see it. The nurse who is taking the radial pulse may hold the watch.
- Decide on a time to begin counting. A time when the second

► **Technique 10–4 Assessing an Apical–Radial Pulse** *CONTINUED*

hand is on 12, 3, 6, or 9 is usually selected. The nurse taking the radial pulse says "Start" at the designated time. *This ensures that simultaneous counts are taken.*

- Each nurse counts the pulse rate for 60 seconds. Both nurses end the count when the nurse taking the radial pulse says "Stop." *A full minute's count is necessary for accurate assessment of any discrepancies between the two pulse sites.*

- The nurse who assesses the apical rate also assesses the apical pulse rhythm and volume, i.e., whether the heartbeat is strong or weak. If the pulse is irregular, note whether the irregular beats come at random or at predictable times and create a regular irregularity.

- The nurse assessing the radial pulse rate also assesses the radial pulse rhythm and volume.

One-Nurse Technique

- Assess the apical pulse for 60 seconds.

- Assess the radial pulse for 60 seconds.

4. Document and report pertinent assessment data.

- Promptly report to the nurse in charge any notable changes from previous measurements or any discrepancy between the two pulses.

- Document the apical and radial (AR) pulse rates, rhythm, volume, and any pulse deficit.

- Record any other pertinent observations, such as pallor, cyanosis, or dyspnea.

- Check the physician's orders for any directions related to a discrepancy in the AR pulse rates.

EVALUATION FOCUS	Equality of apical and radial pulse rates; relationship to other vital signs, in particular respiratory rate and blood pressure; skin color and temperature.

SAMPLE RECORDING

Date	Time	Notes
12/2/93	1700	Skin pale, cold, and clammy. R 19 and shallow. BP 90/60. AR pulse 118/90. Radial pulse irregular, weak, and thready. Apical pulse regular. Dr. Wilson notified. ——————————————————— Inez N. Ortega, RN ——————————————————— Roy L. Steele, RN

KEY ELEMENTS OF ASSESSING AN APICAL–RADIAL PULSE

- Place the diaphragm of the stethoscope over the apical impulse.

- If two-nurse technique is being used, begin counting the pulse rates at the same time.

- Count both pulses for 60 seconds (simultaneously, if two nurses are present).

- Assess the rhythm and strength of each pulse.

Fetal Heart Assessment

The fetal heart rate (FHR) is audible as early as the tenth week of pregnancy, using the Doppler stethoscope with ultrasound. At about 18 to 20 weeks, the FHR can be heard by fetoscope or other stethoscope.

The FHR is usually about 140 beats per minute (BPM) with a normal range of 110 to 160 BPM. It can be detected during the early months of pregnancy at the midline of the abdomen over the mother's symphysis pubis (above the pubic hairline); later in the pregnancy, the location varies with the position of the fetus (Figure 10–15, on page 178).

FHRs are taken under these circumstances:

- If there is any concern about the health of the fetus

- On the client's admission

- Every hour during the onset of regular contractions of the uterus

- Every 30 minutes during cervical dilation

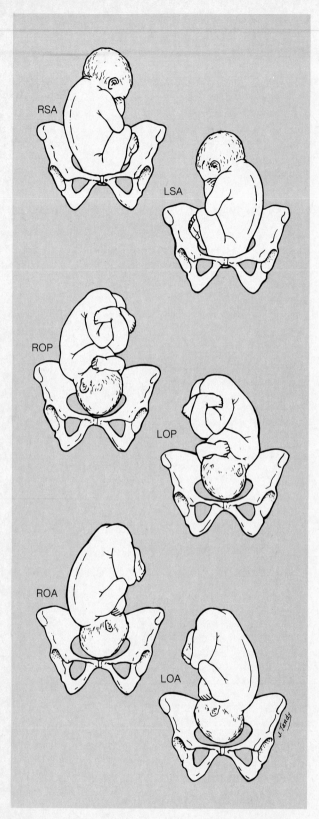

FIGURE 10–15 Six positions of the fetus: right sacrum anterior (RSA), right occiput posterior (ROP), right occiput anterior (ROA), left sacrum anterior (LSA), left occiput posterior (LOP), and left occiput anterior (LOA).

- Every 5 minutes or continually during the second stage of labor

- Immediately after the rupture of the uterine membranes

Because fetal heartbeats are most clearly transmitted through the back of the fetus, locations of maximum FHR intensity vary according to the position of the fetus (Figure 10–16).

The following kinds of stethoscopes are used in assessing FHRs:

- A fetal heart stethoscope (fetoscope) with a large weighted bell designed specifically for fetal heart auscultation (Figure 10–17). The weighted bell negates the need to hold the stethoscope in place, thus avoiding the noise of finger movement, which can interfere with auscultation. Some fetal heart stethoscopes can be adapted to monitor the mother's heart rate and blood pressure by substituting a smaller bell.

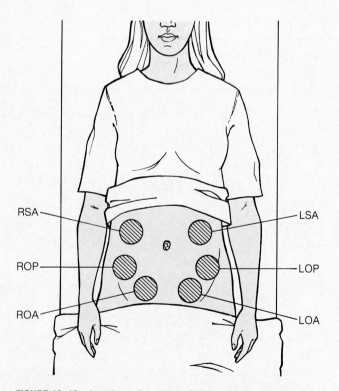

FIGURE 10–16 Locations of maximum FHR intensity according to the position of the fetus.

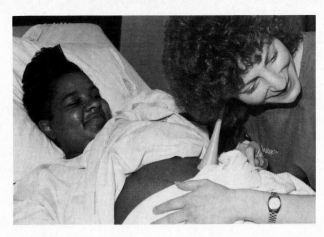

FIGURE 10–17 A fetoscope.

ducer is applied to the woman's abdomen in lieu of the bell of other fetoscopes.

Fetal position can be determined by palpating the woman's abdomen when the woman is at least 20 weeks pregnant. **Leopold's maneuvers** (Figure 10–18) are a systematic way of palpating the maternal abdomen. These maneuvers require frequent practice and skill and may be difficult to obtain on an obese person or on a person who has excessive amniotic fluid. Before performing the maneuvers, the nurse should have the woman empty her bladder and then position the woman supine with knees bent. There are four Leopold maneuvers:

- *First maneuver.* Determine the part of the fetus in the fundus by facing the woman and palpating the upper abdomen with both hands. Note the shape, consistency, and mobility of the palpated part. A fetal head feels firm, hard, and round and moves independently of the trunk. The buttocks feel irregular, softer, and are more difficult to move because they move with the trunk.

- *Second maneuver.* Locate the back, arms, and legs by moving the hands down toward the pelvis. The fetal back feels smooth and offers resistance as the nurse palpates; the arms, legs, and feet feel knobby and lumpy.

- A head stethoscope, which augments the fetal heart sounds; sounds are transmitted not only to the nurse's eardrums but also by bone conduction through the headpiece the nurse wears.

- A regular bell stethoscope held by rubber bands.

- A Doppler ultrasound stethoscope with probe (transducer) and transmission gel (Figure 10–11, earlier). The DUS is a more sensitive and reliable instrument than other fetoscopes. The trans-

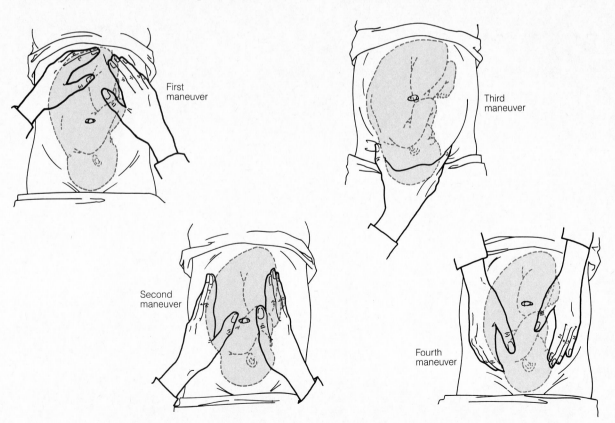

FIGURE 10–18 Leopold's maneuvers for determining fetal position and presentation.

- *Third maneuver.* Determine the part of the fetus presenting into the pelvis by placing one hand just above the symphysis pubis. Note whether the part palpated feels like the head or the buttocks. This maneuver is done to confirm the fetal position determined in the first maneuver.

- *Fourth maneuver.* Determine the degree of cephalic flexion and engagement in late stages of pregnancy by facing the woman's feet and palpating the lower abdomen with both hands. Move the fingers of both hands down the side of the uterus toward the pubis. Note the cephalic prominence, or brow.

Technique 10–5 describes how to assess the fetal heart.

10-5 Assessing a Fetal Heart

PURPOSES
- To establish baseline data in the initial assessment of the client
- To determine whether the rate is within normal range, the rhythm regular, and the beat strong
- To determine any change from previous measurements

ASSESSMENT FOCUS

Varies with gestation period.

EQUIPMENT

- Fetoscope, head stethoscope, regular bell stethoscope held by rubber bands, or a Doppler ultrasound stethoscope
- Soft tissues and aqueous solution, if Doppler equipment is used
- Watch with second hand

INTERVENTION

1. Position the client appropriately.

- Assist the woman to a supine position, and expose the abdomen.

2. Locate the maximum FHR intensity.

- Determine whether the area of maximum intensity is recorded on the client's chart or marked on the client's abdomen.
  or
  Perform Leopold's maneuvers to determine fetal position and locate its back (Figure 10–18, earlier).

3. Auscultate and count the FHR.

- Warm the hands and the head of the fetoscope before touching the client's abdomen.

- Place the bell of the fetoscope, the head stethoscope, or the regular stethoscope held by elastic bands firmly on the maternal abdomen over the area of maximum intensity of the FHR in accordance with the identified fetal position: right sacrum anterior (RSA), right occiput posterior (ROP), right occiput anterior (ROA), left sacrum anterior (LSA), left occiput posterior (LOP), and left occiput anterior (LOA) (Figure 10–16). *The FHR is best heard when sounds are transmitted through the fetus's back.*

- Listen to and identify the fetal heart tone.

- Differentiate the fetal heart tone from the uterine souffle by simultaneously taking the maternal radial pulse. The *uterine souffle* is the soft blowing sound made when the maternal heart propels the blood through the large blood vessels of the uterus. It synchronizes with the maternal heart rate and can be heard distinctly upon auscultation of the lower portion of the uterus.

- Differentiate the fetal heart tone from the *funic* (umbilical cord) *souffle,* a sharp hissing sound caused by blood rushing through the umbilical cord. It is equivalent to the fetal heart rate, that is, about 140 beats per minute.

- Count the FHR for at least 15 seconds whenever it is monitored during the gestation period before labor.

- During labor, count the FHR for 60 seconds during the relaxation period between contractions to determine the baseline FHR. Then count the FHR for 60 sec-

► **Technique 10–5** *CONTINUED*

onds during a contraction and for 30 seconds immediately following a contraction. *Signs of fetal distress may occur during a contraction but most often occur immediately after it. More than 160 or fewer than 120 beats per minute may indicate fetal distress.*

4. Assess the rhythm and the strength of the heartbeat.

- Assess the rhythm of the heartbeat by noting the pattern of intervals between the beats. A normal FHR has equal time periods between beats.

- Assess the strength (volume) of the heartbeat. Normally, the heartbeats are equal in strength and can be described as strong or weak.

- Assist the woman to listen to the FHR if she wishes.

5. Document and report pertinent assessment data.

- Record the FHR, including the rhythm and strength, on the appropriate record.

- If the fetal heart rate or strength is abnormal, report this immediately to the nurse in charge or physician, and initiate electronic fetal monitoring if appropriate.

VARIATION: Using a Doppler Stethoscope

- Follow the manufacturer's instructions about attaching the headset to the audio unit and transducer.

- Apply transmission gel to the woman's abdomen over the area on which the transducer is to be placed. *Gel creates an airtight seal between the skin and the transducer and promotes optimal ultrasound wave transmission.*

- In the early months of pregnancy, ask the client to drink plenty of fluids before the procedure to fill the bladder and improve ultrasound transmission. Later in the pregnancy, this may cause discomfort to the client.

- Place the earpieces of the headset in your ears, adjust the volume of the audio unit, hold that unit in one hand, and place the transducer on the mother's abdomen.

- After determining the FHR, remove the excess gel from the mother's abdomen and from the transducer with soft tissues.

- Clean the transducer with aqueous solutions. *Alcohol or other disinfectants may damage the face of the transducer.*

EVALUATION FOCUS | FHR in relation to baseline data and normal range; heartbeat rhythm and volume in relation to baseline data and health status.

SAMPLE RECORDING

Date	Time	Notes
9/14/93	1300	FHR 136 over right lower quadrant. Beats regular and strong. ————— ———————————————————————— Eva L. Mendez, SN

KEY ELEMENTS OF ASSESSING A FETAL HEART

- Locate area of maximum intensity.
- Use an appropriate stethoscope.
- Count the FHR (a) at least 15 seconds during the gestation period before labor, (b) for 60 seconds between and during contractions, and (c) for 30 seconds immediately following a contraction.
- Assess the rhythm and strength of the fetal heartbeat.
- Promptly report notable variations in the fetal heart rate, rhythm, or volume.

Respirations

Respiration is the act of breathing; it includes the intake of oxygen and the output of carbon dioxide. **External respiration** refers to the interchange of oxygen and carbon dioxide between the alveoli of the lungs and the pulmonary blood. **Internal respiration**, by contrast, takes place throughout the body; it is the interchange of these same gases between the circulating blood and the cells of the body tissues.

The term **inhalation** or **inspiration** refers to the intake of air into the lungs. **Exhalation** or **expiration** refers to breathing out or the movement of gases from the lungs to the atmosphere. **Ventilation** is another word that is used to refer to the movement of air in and out of the lungs. **Hyperventilation** refers to very deep, rapid respirations; **hypoventilation** refers to very shallow respirations.

There are basically two types of breathing that nurses observe: **costal breathing** (thoracic breathing) and **diaphragmatic breathing** (abdominal breathing). Costal breathing involves chiefly the external intercostal muscles and other accessory muscles, such as the sternocleidomastoid muscles. It can be observed by the movement of the chest upward and outward. By contrast, diaphragmatic breathing chiefly involves the contraction and relaxation of the diaphragm and is observed by the movement of the abdomen, which occurs as a result of the diaphragm's contraction and downward movement. Children under 7 years of age are primarily diaphragmatic breathers (Whaley and Wong 1991, p. 266).

Mechanics and Control of Breathing

During *inhalation* the following processes normally occur (Figure 10–19): The diaphragm contracts (flattens), the ribs move upward and outward, and the sternum moves outward, thus enlarging the thorax and permitting the lungs to expand. During *exhalation* (Figure 10–20), the diaphragm relaxes (its cur-

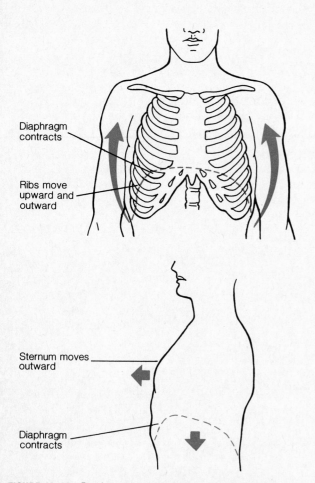

Diaphragm contracts

Ribs move upward and outward

Sternum moves outward

Diaphragm contracts

FIGURE 10–19 Respiratory inhalation: anterior and lateral views.

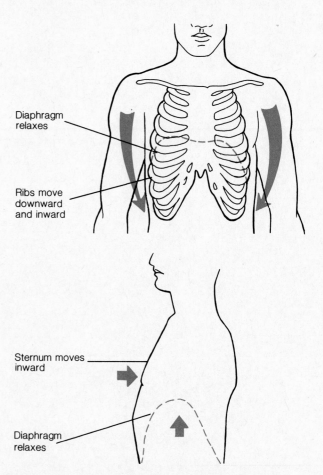

Diaphragm relaxes

Ribs move downward and inward

Sternum moves inward

Diaphragm relaxes

FIGURE 10–20 Respiratory exhalation: anterior and lateral views.

vature increases), the ribs move downward and inward, and the sternum moves inward, thus decreasing the size of the thorax as the lungs are compressed. Breathing is normally carried out automatically and effortlessly. Normal breathing is called **eupnea**. An inspiration normally lasts 1 to 1.5 seconds, and an expiration last 2 to 3 seconds. Difficult and labored breathing is known as **dyspnea**.

Respiration is controlled by (a) respiratory centers in the medulla oblongata and the pons of the brain and (b) by chemoreceptors located centrally in the medulla and peripherally in the carotid and aortic bodies. These centers and receptors respond to changes in the concentrations of oxygen (O_2), carbon dioxide (CO_2), and hydrogen (H^+) in the arterial blood.

Respiratory Assessment

Resting respirations should be assessed when the client is at rest because exercise affects respirations, increasing their rate and depth. Anxiety is likely to affect respiratory rate and depth as well. Respirations may also need to be assessed after exercise to identify the client's tolerance to activity. Before assessing a client's respirations, a nurse should be aware of

- The client's normal breathing pattern
- The influence of the client's health problems on respirations
- Any medications or therapies that might affect respirations
- The relationship of the client's respirations to cardiovascular function

The rate, depth, rhythm, and special characteristics of respirations should be assessed.

The *respiratory rate* is normally described in breaths per minute. A healthy adult normally takes between 15 and 20 breaths per minute. For the respiratory rates for different age groups, see Table 10–1. Several factors influence respiratory rate; some are listed in Table 10–5.

The *depth* of a person's respirations can be established by watching the movement of the chest. Respiratory depth is generally described as normal, deep, or shallow. *Deep respirations* are those in which a large

TABLE 10–5 MAJOR FACTORS INFLUENCING RESPIRATORY RATE

Factor	Influence
Exercise: increases metabolism	Increase
Stress: readies the body for "fight or flight"	Increase
Environment: increased temperature	Increase
Increased altitude: lower oxygen concentration	Increase
Certain medications, e.g., narcotic, analgesic	Decrease

volume of air is inhaled and exhaled, inflating most of the lungs. *Shallow respirations* involve the exchange of a small volume of air and often the minimal use of lung tissue. During a normal inspiration and expiration, an adult takes in about 500 ml of air.

Respiratory rhythm or **pattern** refers to the regularity of the expirations and the inspirations. Normally, respirations are evenly spaced. Respiratory rhythm can be described as *regular* or *irregular*. An infant's respiratory rhythm may be less regular than an adult's. Some disease conditions affect a person's respiratory rhythm.

Respiratory quality or **character** refers to those aspects of breathing that are different from normal, effortless breathing. Two of these are the amount of effort a client must exert to breathe and the sound of breathing. Usually, breathing does not require noticeable effort; some clients, however, breathe only with decided effort.

The sound of breathing is also significant. Normal breathing is silent, but a number of abnormal sounds such as a wheeze are obvious to the nurse's ear. Many sounds occur as a result of the presence of fluid in the lungs and are most clearly heard with a stethoscope. See Chapter 11, pages 244–250, for auscultation and percussion methods used to assess lung sounds. For details about altered breathing patterns and terms used to describe normal and abnormal patterns and sounds, see the box on page 184. Technique 10–6, on page 185, provides guidelines for assessing respirations.

Breathing Patterns and Sounds

Breathing Patterns

Rate

- *Eupnea*—normal respiration that is quiet, rhythmic, and effortless
- *Tachypnea*—Rapid respiration marked by quick, shallow breaths
- *Bradypnea*—abnormally slow breathing
- *Apnea*—cessation of breathing

Volume

- *Hyperventilation*—an increase in the amount of air in the lungs, characterized by prolonged and deep breaths; may be associated with anxiety
- *Hypoventilation*—a reduction in the amount of air in the lungs; characterized by shallow respirations

Rhythm

- *Cheyne-Stokes breathing*—rhythmic waxing and waning of respirations, from very deep to very shallow breathing and temporary apnea; often associated with cardiac failure, increased intracranial pressure, or brain damage

Ease or effort

- *Dyspnea*—difficult and labored breathing during which the individual has a persistent, unsatisfied need for air and feels distressed
- *Orthopnea*—ability to breath only in upright sitting or standing positions

Breath Sounds

Audible without amplification

- *Stridor*—a shrill, harsh sound heard during inspiration with laryngeal obstruction
- *Stertor*—snoring or sonorous respiration, usually due to a partial obstruction of the upper airway
- *Wheeze*—continuous, high-pitched musical squeak or whistling sound occurring on expiration and sometimes on inspiration when air moves through a narrowed or partially obstructed airway
- *Bubbling*—gurgling sounds heard as air passes through moist secretions in the respiratory tract

Audible by stethoscope

- *Crackles* (formerly called *rales*)—dry or wet crackling sounds simulated by rolling a lock of hair near the ear. Generally heard on inspiration as air moves through accumulated moist secretions. *Fine-to-medium* crackles occur when air passes through moisture in small air passages and alveoli. *Medium-to-coarse* crackles occur when air passes through moisture in brochioles, bronchi, and the trachea.
- *Gurgles* (formerly called *rhonchi*)—coarse, dry, wheezy, or whistling sound more audible during expiration as the air moves through tenacious mucus or narrowed bronchi
- *Pleural friction rub*—coarse, leathery, or grating sound produced by the rubbing together of inflamed pleura

Chest Movements

- *Intercostal retraction*—indrawing between the ribs
- *Substernal retraction*—indrawing beneath the breastbone
- *Suprasternal retraction*—indrawing above the breastbone
- *Supraclavicular retraction*—indrawing above the clavicles
- *Tracheal tug*—indrawing and downward pull of the trachea during inspiration
- *Flail chest*—the ballooning out of the chest wall through injured rib spaces; results in *paradoxical breathing*, during which the chest wall balloons on expiration but is depressed or sucked inward on inspiration

Secretions and Coughing

- *Hemoptysis*—the presence of blood in the sputum
- *Productive cough*—a cough accompanied by expectorated secretions
- *Nonproductive cough*—a dry, harsh cough without secretions

10-6 Assessing Respirations

PURPOSES

- To acquire baseline data against which future measurements can be compared
- To monitor abnormal respirations and identify changes
- To assess respirations before the administration of a medication such as morphine (an abnormally slow respiratory rate may warrant withholding the medication)
- To monitor respirations following the administration of a general anesthetic or any medication that influences respirations
- To monitor clients at risk for respiratory alterations (e.g., those with fever, pain, acute anxiety, chronic obstructive pulmonary disease, respiratory infection, pulmonary edema or emboli, chest trauma or constriction, brain stem injury)

ASSESSMENT FOCUS

Skin and mucous membrane color (e.g., cyanosis or pallor); position assumed for breathing (e.g., use of the orthopneic position); signs of cerebral anoxia (e.g., irritability, restlessness, drowsiness, or loss of consciousness); chest movements (e.g., retractions between the ribs or above or below the sternum); activity tolerance; chest pain; dyspnea; medications affecting respiratory rate.

EQUIPMENT

- ☐ Watch with a second hand or indicator

INTERVENTION

1. Determine the client's activity schedule.

- Choose a suitable time to monitor the respirations. *A client who has been exercising will need to rest for a few minutes to permit the accelerated respiratory rate to return to normal. An infant or child who is crying will have an abnormal respiratory rate and will need quieting before the accurate assessment of the respirations can be made.*

2. Observe or palpate and count the respiratory rate.

- Place a hand against the client's chest to feel the client's chest movements, or place the client's arm across the chest and observe the chest movements, while supposedly taking the radial pulse. Because young children are diaphragmatic breathers, observe the rise and fall of

the abdomen. *Awareness of respiratory rate assessment could cause the client voluntarily to alter the respiratory pattern.*

- Count the respiratory rate for 30 seconds if the respirations are regular. Count for 60 seconds if they are irregular. An inhalation and an exhalation count as one respiration.

3. Observe the depth, rhythm, and character of respirations.

- Observe the respirations for depth by watching the movement of the chest. During deep respirations a large volume of air is exchanged; during shallow respirations a small volume is exchanged.

- Observe the respirations for regular or irregular rhythm. Normally, respirations are evenly spaced.

- Observe the character of respirations—the sound they produce and the effort they require. Normally, respirations are silent and effortless.

4. Document and report pertinent assessment data.

- Document the respiratory rate, depth, rhythm, and character on the appropriate record. See sample below.
- Report to the nurse in charge:
  a. Respiratory rate significantly above or below the normal range
  b. An irregular respiratory rhythm
  c. Inadequate respiratory depth
  d. Abnormal character of breathing—orthopnea, wheezing, stridor, rales, or rhonchi
  e. Any complaints of dyspnea

►

▶ **Technique 10–6 Assessing Respirations** *CONTINUED*

EVALUATION FOCUS	The respiratory rate in relation to baseline data or normal range for age; relationship to other vital signs; respiratory depth, rhythm, and character in relation to baseline data and health status.

SAMPLE RECORDING

Date	Time	Notes
6/20/93	0900	R 38 and shallow. Dyspneic when talking. P 122. BP 94/60. Dr. Woo notified. ———————————————————————————— John P. Brown, NS

KEY ELEMENTS OF ASSESSING RESPIRATIONS

- Ensure that the client is resting and quiet and is unaware that the respiratory rate is being counted.

Blood Pressure

Arterial blood pressure is a measure of the pressure exerted by the blood as it pulsates through the arteries. Because the blood moves in waves, there are two blood pressure measures: the **systolic pressure**, which is the pressure of the blood as a result of contraction of the ventricles, i.e., the pressure of the height of the blood wave; and the **diastolic pressure**, which is the pressure when the ventricles are at rest. Diastolic pressure, then, is the lower pressure, present at all times within the arteries. The difference between the diastolic and systolic pressures is called the **pulse pressure**.

The average blood pressure of a healthy adult is 120/80 mm Hg. The blood pressure of infants and children varies with age and growth. "Normal" blood pressure must be evaluated on the basis of the child's sex and age and the size. A number of conditions are reflected by changes in blood pressure. The most common is **hypertension**, an abnormally high blood pressure over 140 mm Hg systolic and/or 90 mm Hg diastolic in the adult, when these are confirmed during a minimum of two consecutive visits by a client. **Hypotension**, or an abnormally low blood pressure, is a systolic pressure below 100 mm Hg in an adult.

Physiology of Arterial Blood Pressure

The arterial blood pressure is the result of the cardiac output times the resistance the blood encounters while it flows, i.e., the peripheral vascular resistance. **Cardiac output** is the amount of blood ejected by the heart with each ventricular contraction. A person's blood pressure is directly affected by the *volume* of blood in the systemic circulation. Blood flows in the vascular system along a *pressure gradient*. The pressure of the blood in the aorta, for example, is higher than the pressure in the arterioles, and in the arterioles it is higher than in the capillaries.

Peripheral resistance can increase blood pressure. The diastolic pressure especially is affected. The *size* of the arterioles and the capillaries determines in great part the peripheral resistance to the blood in the body. A **lumen** is a channel within a tube: the smaller the lumen of a vessel, the greater the resistance. Normally, the arterioles are in a state of partial constriction. Increased vasoconstriction raises the blood pressure, whereas decreased vasoconstriction lowers the blood pressure.

The arteries contain smooth muscles that permit them to contract, thus decreasing their **compliance** (distensibility). Arteries normally relax during systole and retract during diastole. The arteries account for most of the peripheral resistance. The major factor reducing arterial compliance is pathologic change affecting the arterial walls. The elastic and muscular tissues of the arteries are replaced with fibrous tissue; thus, the arteries lose much of their compliance. The condition, most common in middle-aged and elderly adults, is known as **arteriosclerosis**.

Viscosity is a physical property that results from friction of molecules in a fluid. In a viscous (or "thick") fluid, there is a great deal of friction among the molecules as they slide by each other. The blood pressure is higher when the blood is highly viscous, i.e., when the proportion of red blood cells to the blood plasma is high. This ratio is referred to as the **hematocrit**. The viscosity increases markedly when the hematocrit is more than 60 to 65%.

Factors Affecting Blood Pressure

- *Age.* Newborns have a mean systolic pressure of 78 mm Hg. The pressure rises with age, reaching a peak at the onset of puberty, and then tends to decline somewhat. One quick way to determine the normal systolic blood pressure of a child is to use the following formula (Evans 1983, p. 61):

Normal systolic BP = 80 + (2 × child's age in years)

In elderly people, elasticity of the arteries is decreased—the arteries are more rigid and less yielding to the pressure of the blood. This produces an elevated systolic pressure. Because the walls no longer retract as flexibly with decreased pressure, the diastolic pressure is also higher. Several baseline blood pressure readings should be taken in the elderly person who has an elevated blood pressure.

- *Exercise.* Physical activity increases both the cardiac output and hence the blood pressure; thus, a rest of 20 to 30 minutes following exercise is indicated before the blood pressure can be reliably assessed, unless the blood pressure during or after exercise is being assessed.

- *Stress.* Stimulation of the sympathetic nervous system increases cardiac output and vasoconstriction of the arterioles, thus increasing the blood pressure reading; however, severe pain can decrease blood pressure greatly and cause shock by inhibiting the vasomotor center and producing vasodilation.

- *Race.* Black males over 35 years have higher blood pressures than white males of the same age.

- *Obesity.* Pressure is consistently higher in some overweight and obese people than in people of normal weight (Overfield 1985, p. 46).

- *Sex.* After puberty, females usually have lower blood pressures than males of the same age; this difference is thought to be due to hormonal variations. After menopause, women generally have higher blood pressures than before.

- *Medications.* Many medications may increase or decrease the blood pressure; nurses should be aware of the specific medications a client is receiving and consider their possible impact when interpreting blood pressure readings.

TABLE 10–6   SELECTED CONDITIONS AFFECTING BLOOD PRESSURE

Condition	Effect	Cause
Fever	Increase	Increases metabolic rate
Stress	Increase	Increases cardiac output
Arteriosclerosis	Increase	Decreases artery compliance
Obesity	Increase	Increases peripheral resistance
Hemorrhage	Decrease	Decreases blood volume
Low hematocrit	Decrease	Decreases blood viscosity
External heat	Decrease	Increases vasodilation and thus decreases peripheral vascular resistance
Exposure to cold	Increase	Causes vasoconstriction and thus increases peripheral vascular resistance

- *Diurnal variations.* Pressure is usually lowest early in the morning, when the metabolic rate is lowest, then rises throughout the day and peaks in the late afternoon or early evening.

- *Disease process.* Any condition affecting the cardiac output, blood viscosity, and/or compliance of the arteries has a direct effect on the blood pressure. See Table 10–6 for selected conditions affecting blood pressure.

Blood Pressure Assessment

Equipment

Blood pressure is measured with a *blood pressure cuff*, a *sphygmomanometer*, and a *stethoscope*. The blood pressure cuff consists of a rubber bag that can be inflated with air, called the *bladder* (Figure 10–21). It is usually covered with cloth and has two tubes attached to it. One tube connects to a rubber bulb that inflates the bladder. When turned counterclockwise, a small valve on the side of this bulb releases the air in the bladder. When the valve is tightened (turned clockwise), air pumped into the bladder remains there. The other tube is attached to a sphygmomanometer.

The sphygmomanometer indicates the pressure of the air within the bladder. There are two types of sphygmomanometers: *aneroid* and *mercury* (Figure 10–22). The aneroid sphygmomanometer is a calibrated dial with a needle that points to the calibrations. The mercury sphygmomanometer is a calibrated cylinder filled with mercury. The pressure is indicated at the point to which the **meniscus** of the mercury (the crescent-shaped top surface of the column) rises. It is important to view the meniscus at eye level to avoid distortions in the reading.

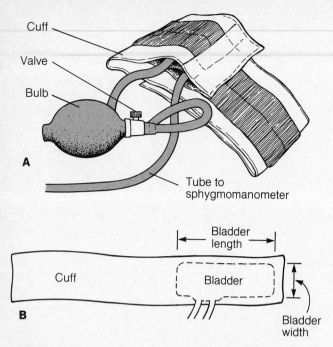

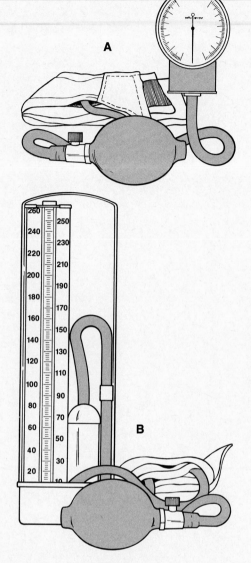

FIGURE 10–21 *A*, a blood pressure cuff and bulb; *B*, the bladder inside the cuff.

Some agencies use electronic sphygmomanometers, which eliminate the need to listen to the sounds of the client's systolic and diastolic blood pressures through a stethoscope. With some electronic sphygmomanometers, as the pressure in the cuff is lowered, a light flashes to indicate the systolic and diastolic pressures.

Ultrasound (Doppler) stethoscopes are also used to assess blood pressure (Figure 10–11, earlier). These are of particular value when blood pressure sounds are difficult to hear, e.g., in infants, obese clients, and clients in shock. The nurse applies transmission gel to a transducer probe, places the probe over the pulse point, and measures the blood pressure. A systolic blood pressure assessed with a DUS is recorded with a large D, e.g., 85D. Systolic pressure may be the only blood pressure obtainable with some ultrasound models.

Blood pressure cuffs come in various sizes, since the bladder must be the correct width and length for the client's arm. If the bladder is too narrow, the blood pressure reading will be erroneously elevated; if it is too wide, the reading will be erroneously low. The width should be 40% of the circumference, or 20% wider than the diameter of the midpoint of the limb on which it is used (American Heart Association 1987, p. 4). The bladder dimensions by arm circumference are shown in Table 10–7, the arm circumference, not the age of the client, should always determine bladder size. The nurse can also determine whether the width of a blood pressure cuff is appropriate: Lay the cuff lengthwise at the midpoint of the upper arm, and hold the outermost side of the

FIGURE 10–22 Blood pressure equipment: *A*, an aneroid manometer and cuff; *B*, a mercury manometer and cuff.

TABLE 10–7 RECOMMENDED BLOOD PRESSURE CUFF BLADDER DIMENSIONS BY ARM CIRCUMFERENCE

Adult Size	Arm Circumference (cm)	Cuff Size (cm)
Child (small)	<22	9 × 18
Adult (regular)	22–33	12 × 23
Adult (large)	33–41	15 × 33
Adult (thigh)	>41	18 × 36

Source: American Heart Association, *Recommendations for human blood pressure determination by sphygmomanometers,* Pub no. 701005 (American Heart Association, 1987), p. 10.

bladder edge laterally on the arm. With the other hand, wrap the width of the cuff around the arm, and ensure that the width is 40% of the arm circumference (Figure 10–23).

The length of the bladder also affects the accuracy of measurement. The bladder should be sufficiently long almost to encircle the limb and to cover at least two-thirds of its circumference.

Blood pressure cuffs are made of nondistensible material so that an even pressure is exerted around the limb. Most cuffs are held in place by hooks, snaps, or Velcro. Others have a cloth bandage that is long enough to encircle the limb several times; this type is closed by tucking the end of the bandage into one of the bandage folds.

Sites

The blood pressure is usually assessed in the client's arm using the brachial artery and a standard stethoscope. If the arm is very large or grossly misshapen and the conventional cuff cannot be properly applied,

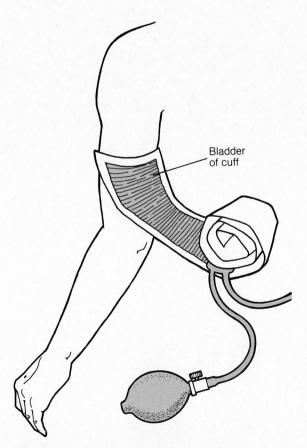

FIGURE 10–23 Determining that the bladder of a blood pressure cuff is 40% of the arm circumference, or 20% wider than the diameter of the midpoint of the limb.

leg or forearm measurements can be taken. To obtain a *leg blood pressure*, apply a standard-sized cuff over the lower leg, with the distal border of the cuff at the malleoli. Auscultate blood pressure sounds over the posterior tibial or dorsalis pedis arteries. To obtain a *thigh blood pressure*, apply an appropriate-sized cuff to the thigh, and auscultate the pulsations of the blood over the popliteal artery. To obtain a *forearm blood pressure*, apply an appropriate-sized cuff to the forearm 13 cm (5 in) from the elbow. Blood pressure sounds then can be heard over the radial artery.

Assessing the blood pressure on a client's thigh is usually indicated in these situations:

- The blood pressure cannot be measured on either arm, e.g., because of burns or other trauma.

- The blood pressure in one thigh is to be compared with the blood pressure in the other thigh.

- The blood pressure cuff is too large for the upper extremities.

- A child's thigh blood pressure should be compared with the arm blood pressure to detect coarctation of the aorta or other cardiovascular anomaly.

Blood pressure is *not* measured on a client's arm or thigh in the following situations:

- The shoulder, arm, or hand (or the hip, knee, or ankle) is injured or diseased.

- There is a cast or bulky bandage on any part of the limb.

- The client has had breast or axilla (or hip) surgery on that side.

- The client has an intravenous infusion or a blood transfusion running.

- The client has an arteriovenous fistula (e.g., for renal dialysis).

Methods

There are three *noninvasive indirect methods* of measuring blood pressure: the auscultatory, palpatory, and flush methods. The *auscultatory method* is most commonly used in hospitals, clinics, and homes. Required equipment is a sphygmomanometer, cuff, and a stethoscope. External pressure is applied to a superficial artery, and the nurse reads the pressure from the sphygmomanometer when the blood flow is first heard through a stethoscope. When carried out correctly, the auscultatory method is relatively accurate.

When taking a blood pressure using a stethoscope, the nurse identifies five phases in the series of sounds called **Korotkoff's sounds**. First, the nurse pumps the cuff up to about 30 mm Hg above the point where the last sound is heard; that is the point when the blood flow in the artery is stopped. Then the pressure is released slowly (2 to 3 mm Hg per sound), while the nurse observes the pressure readings on the manometer and relates them to the sounds heard through the stethoscope. Five phases occur (American Heart Association 1987, p. 4):

Phase 1. The period initiated by the first faint, clear tapping sounds. These sounds gradually become more intense. To ensure that they are not extraneous sounds, the nurse should identify at least two consecutive tapping sounds.
Phase 2. The period during which the sounds have a swishing quality.
Phase 3. The period during which the sounds are crisper and more intense.
Phase 4. The period during which the sounds become muffled and have a soft, blowing quality.
Phase 5. The point where the sounds disappear.

The American Heart Association (AHA 1987, p. 4) recommends that the systolic pressure be considered the point where the first tapping sound is heard (phase 1). In adults, the diastolic pressure is the point where the sounds become inaudible (phase 5). In children, however, the AHA recommends that diastolic pressure be considered to be the onset of phase 4, where the sounds become muffled. For complete accuracy, the phase 4 and 5 readings should be recorded. In agencies where phase 4 is considered the diastolic pressure of *adults*, three measures are recommended (systolic pressure, diastolic pressure, and phase 5). These may be referred to as systolic, first diastolic, and second diastolic pressures. The phase 5 (second diastolic pressure) reading may be zero; that is, the muffled sounds are heard even when there is no air pressure in the blood pressure cuff. In some instances, muffled sounds are never heard, in which case a dash is inserted where the reading would normally be recorded.

The *palpatory method* is sometimes used when Korotkoff's sounds cannot be heard and electronic equipment to amplify the sounds is not available, or when an auscultatory gap occurs. An **auscultatory gap**, which occurs particularly in hypertensive clients, is the temporary disappearance of sounds normally heard over the brachial artery when the cuff pressure is high and the reappearance of the sounds at a lower level. This temporary disappearance of sounds occurs in the latter part of phase 1 and phase 2 and may cover a range of 40 mm Hg. Instead of listening for the blood flow sounds, the nurse palpates the pulsations of the artery as the pressure in the cuff is released. The systolic pressure is read from the sphygmomanometer when the first pulsation is felt. A single whiplike vibration, felt in addition to the pulsations, identifies the point at which the pressure in the cuff nears the diastolic pressure. This vibration is no longer felt when the cuff pressure is below the diastolic pressure. To palpate the diastolic pressure, the nurse applies light to moderate pressure over the pulse point.

The *flush method* for determining blood pressure is another method used when Korotkoff's sounds cannot be heard by auscultation and electronic equipment is not available. The measurement is determined by a change in skin color when blood flow to an extremity resumes, i.e., when the extremity is no longer extremely pale but becomes reddened (vascular flush). This method is less reliable in clients with peripheral vascular disease or a circulatory problem of varied origin. The cuff is applied to the client's arm and the limb is wrapped in a bandage distally to proximally to force venous blood out of and restrict arterial flow into the extremity. The cuff is then inflated and the bandage is removed. The cuff pressure is released, and the nurse reads the pressure from the sphygmomanometer when the extremity flushes. This reading is the **mean blood pressure**, the midway point between the systolic and diastolic pressures.

Technique 10–7 gives guidelines for assessing blood pressure. Technique 10–8 describes how to assess an infant's blood pressure.

Assessing Blood Pressure (Arm)

PURPOSES

- To obtain a baseline measure of arterial blood pressure for subsequent evaluation
- To determine the client's hemodynamic status (e.g., stroke volume of the heart and blood vessel resistance)
- To identify and monitor changes in blood pressure resulting from a disease process and medical therapy (e.g., presence or history of cardiovascular disease, renal disease, circulatory shock, or acute pain; rapid infusion of fluids or blood products)

ASSESSMENT FOCUS

Signs and symptoms of hypertension (e.g., headache, ringing in the ears, flushing of face, nosebleeds, fatigue); signs and symptoms of hypotension (e.g., tachycardia, dizziness, mental confusion, restlessness, cool and clammy skin, pale or cyanotic skin); factors affecting blood pressure (e.g., activity, emotional stress, pain, and time the client last smoked or ingested caffeine).

EQUIPMENT

- Stethoscope or DUS Blood pressure cuff of the appropriate size (newborn, infant, child, small adult, adult, large adult, thigh)
- Sphygmomanometer

INTERVENTION

1. Prepare and position the client appropriately.

- Make sure that the client has not smoked or ingested caffeine within 30 minutes prior to measurement (U.S. Department of Health 1988, p. 5).

- Make sure that the bladder of the cuff encircles at least two-thirds of the arm and that the width of the cuff is appropriate

- Position the client in a sitting position unless otherwise specified. The arm should be slightly flexed with the palm of the hand facing up and the forearm supported at heart level. Readings in any other position should be specified. *The blood pressure is normally similar in sitting, standing, and lying positions, but it can vary significantly by position in certain persons and may need to be measured in all three positions. The*

blood pressure increases when the arm is below heart level and decreases when the arm above heart level.

- Expose the upper arm.

2. Wrap the deflated cuff evenly around the upper arm.

- Apply the center of the bladder directly over the medial aspect of the arm. *The bladder inside the cuff must be directly over the artery to be compressed if the reading is to be accurate.*

- For an adult, place the lower border of the cuff about 2.5 cm (1 in) above the antecubital space. The lower edge can be nearer the antecubital space of an infant.

3. If this is the client's initial examination, perform a preliminary palpatory determination of systolic pressure. The initial estimate tells the nurse the maximal

pressure to which the manometer needs to be elevated in subsequent determinations. It also prevents underestimation of the systolic pressure or overestimation of the diastolic pressure should an auscultatory gap occur.

- Palpate the brachial artery with the fingertips. The brachial artery is normally found medially in the antecubital space (Figure 10–24).

- Close the valve on the pump by turning the knob clockwise.

- Pump up the cuff until you no longer feel the brachial pulse. *At that pressure the blood cannot flow through the artery.*

- Note the pressure on the sphygmomanometer at which the pulse is no longer felt. *This gives an estimate of the maximum pressure required to measure the systolic pressure.*

▶ **Technique 10-7 Assessing Blood Pressure** CONTINUED

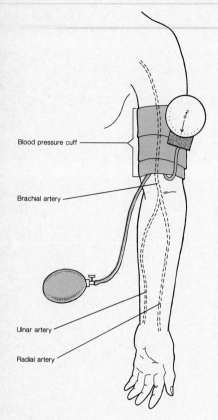

FIGURE 10-24 Location of the brachial artery.

• Release the pressure completely in the cuff, and wait 1 to 2 minutes before making further measurements. *A waiting period gives the blood trapped in the veins time to be released.*

4. Position the stethoscope appropriately.

• Insert the ear attachments of the stethoscope in your ears so that they tilt slightly forward. *Sounds are heard more clearly when the ear attachments follow the direction of the ear canal.*

• Ensure that the stethoscope hangs freely from the ears to the diaphragm. *Rubbing the stetho-*

scope against an object can obliterate the sounds of the blood within an artery.

• Place the diaphragm of the stethoscope over the brachial pulse. Use the bell-shaped diaphragm (Figure 10-14, earlier). *Since the blood pressure is a low-frequency sound, it is best heard with the bell-shaped diaphragm.* Hold the diaphragm with the thumb and index finger.

5. Auscultate the client's blood pressure.

• Pump up the cuff until the sphygmomanometer registers about 30 mm Hg above the point where the brachial pulse disappeared.

• Release the valve on the cuff carefully so that the pressure decreases at the rate of 2 to 3 mm Hg per second. *If the rate is faster or slower, an error in measurement may occur.*

• As the pressure falls, identify the manometer reading at each of the five phases.

• Deflate the cuff rapidly and completely.

• Wait 1 to 2 minutes before making further determinations. *This permits blood trapped in the veins to be released.*

• Repeat the above steps once or twice as necessary to confirm the accuracy of the reading.

6. Remove the cuff from the client's arm.

7. If this is the client's initial examination, repeat the procedure on the client's other arm.

• There should be a difference of no more than 10 mm Hg between the arms.

• The arm found to have the higher pressure should be used for subsequent examinations.

8. Document and report pertinent assessment data.

• Document the blood pressure according to agency policy. See sample that follows. Record two pressures in the form "130/80" where "130" is the systolic (phase 1) and "80" is the diastolic (phase 5) pressure. Record three pressures in the form "130/110/90," where "130" is the systolic, "110" is the first diastolic (phase

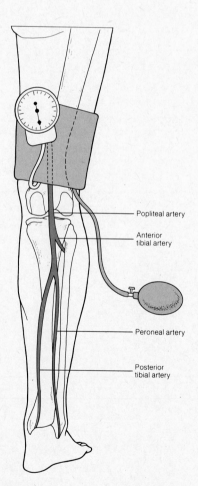

FIGURE 10-25 Location of the popliteal artery.

▶ **Technique 10–7** *CONTINUED*

4), and "90" is the second diastolic (phase 5) pressure. Use the abbreviations *RA* for right arm and *LA* for left arm. Record a difference of greater than 10 mm Hg in the arms.

- Report any significant change in the client's blood pressure to the nurse in charge. Also report these findings:

  a. Systolic blood pressure (of an adult) above 140 mm Hg

  b. Diastolic blood pressure (of an adult) above 90 mm Hg

  c. Systolic blood pressure (of an adult) below 100 mm Hg

VARIATION: Taking a Thigh Blood Pressure

- Help the client to assume a prone position. If the client cannot assume this position, measure the blood pressure while the client is in a supine position with the knee slightly flexed. *Slight flexing of the knee will facilitate placing the stethoscope on the popliteal space.*

- Expose the thigh, taking care not to expose the client unduly.

- Wrap the cuff evenly around the midthigh with the compression bladder over the posterior aspect

of the thigh. *The bladder must be directly over the artery if the reading is to be accurate.*

- If this is the client's initial examination, perform a preliminary palpatory determination of systolic pressure by palpating the popliteal artery (Figure 10–25). The systolic pressure in the popliteal artery is usually 10 to 40 mm Hg higher than that in the brachial artery because of use of a larger bladder; the diastolic pressure is usually the same.

- Auscultate the pressure as above.

EVALUATION FOCUS

The blood pressure in relation to baseline data, normal range for age, and health status; relationship to pulse and respirations.

SAMPLE RECORDING

Date	Time	Notes
8/14/93	1300	BP 130/90 in RA in bed-sitting position. P 115. R-20. Color pale. ———— Ruth P. O'Shea, SN

KEY ELEMENTS OF ASSESSING BLOOD PRESSURE

- Avoid taking the client's blood pressure measurement within 30 minutes after the client has eaten, smoked, or exercised.
- Wrap the cuff evenly and smoothly.
- Use a cuff of the appropriate size for the client.
- Avoid taking the measurement in a limb that is injured or diseased, is on the same side as breast or axillary (or hip) surgery, has an intravenous infusion running, has a bulky bandage or cast, or has an arteriovenous shunt.
- For an arm measurement, support the client's arm at heart level.

- For an initial examination, perform a preliminary palpatory determination of systolic blood pressure.
- After pumping up the cuff 30 mm Hg above the point where the brachial or popliteal pulse disappears, release the cuff pressure at the rate of 2 to 3 mm Hg per second.
- Wait 1 to 2 minutes before taking further measurements.
- Promptly report blood pressures indicative of hypotension (i.e., adult systolic pressure below 100 mm Hg) and hypertension (i.e., adult systolic pressure above 140 mm Hg and diastolic pressure above 90 mm Hg).

An Infant's Blood Pressure

The blood pressure of an infant can be measured by auscultation, palpation, ultrasound (Doppler technique), or flush technique. Auscultation is often difficult on infants under age 3, because Korotkoff's sounds are relatively inaudible, but it is the method of choice for children over 3 years of age. When the blood pressure cannot be auscultated, it can be palpated or measured by the flush technique. See page 190. Both of these methods reveal only a mean pressure between the systolic and diastolic pressures when the blood returns to the limb. The flush technique is largely being replaced by use of an ultrasound device. Some ultrasound models measure only systolic pressures; others measure both systolic and diastolic pressures.

When measuring an infant's blood pressure, the systolic pressure (phase 1) is noted when the first clear tapping sound is heard. Both phase 4 (muffling of sounds) and phase 5 (disappearance of sounds)

are recorded for the diastolic pressure. They are recorded in the form "118/78/68." If only phases 1 and 4 can be identified, they are recorded "118/78/0." This indicates that sounds were heard to the 0 point on the manometer.

When a cuff of the appropriate size is not available for an infant or child, it is preferable (a) to use an oversized cuff rather than an undersized one (wide cuffs apparently do not cause the low readings noted in adults [Whaley and Wong 1989, p. 138]) or (b) to use a different site that will accomodate the cuff size. For example, a radial pressure may be taken if the cuff is too small, or a thigh blood pressure may be taken if only a large cuff is available. Systolic blood pressure in the radial artery is usually 10 mm Hg lower than in the brachial artery; it is usually 10 mm Hg higher in the popliteal artery than in the brachial artery in children over age 1 year. Arm and thigh pressures are equal in children under age 1.

10-8 Assessing an Infant's Blood Pressure

PURPOSES

- To establish a baseline in the initial assessment of the infant
- To determine any change from previous measurements
- To determine the adequacy of the arterial blood pressure

ASSESSMENT FOCUS

Signs and symptoms of hypertension and hypotension; factors affecting blood pressure (see Technique 10-7)

EQUIPMENT

- Blood pressure cuff of a suitable size
- Sphygmomanometer (auscultatory method)
- Stethoscope (auscultatory method) or DUS
- Elastic bandage of suitable width to cover the limb distal to the cuff (flush method)

INTERVENTION

1. Prepare the infant/child appropriately.

- Explain each step of the procedure to children of preschool age and above, e.g., tell them how the cuff will feel (tight or like an arm hug) and to "watch the silver rise in the tube." When possible, demonstrate the procedure on a toy or your own arm.

- Be sure that the environment in

which the blood pressure measurement is to take place is quiet and reassuring to the infant. *Frightening sounds or sights can contribute to error in measurement, since anxiety and restlessness increase the blood pressure.*

- Allow time for the infant to recover from any activity or apprehension.

- Assist the child to a comfortable position. Infants and small chil-

dren may be more quiet if placed in a sitting position on the parent's lap.

- Expose the arm fully, if used, and then support it comfortably at the child's heart level.

2. Use the auscultation method for a child over 3 years of age.

- Follow the steps in Technique 10-7. The auscultatory method is essentially the same for children as for adults.

Technique 10–8 CONTINUED

- Identify the manometer reading at phases 1, 4, and 5 of Korotkoff's sounds. Phase 1 is the systolic pressure and phases 4 and 5 the diastolic pressures.

3. Use the palpation method, the flush technique, or a Doppler stethoscope when the blood pressure cannot be auscultated.

Palpation Method

- Place the cuff around the limb so that the lower edge is about 1 cm (0.4 in) above the antecubital space (Figure 10–26).
- Palpate the brachial pulse.
- Inflate the cuff to about 30 mm Hg beyond the point where the brachial pulse disappears.
- Release the cuff at the rate of 2 to 3 mm Hg per second, and identify the manometer reading at the point where the pulse returns in the brachial artery. This pressure is a mean pressure between the systolic and diastolic pressures.

Flush Technique

This procedure requires two people and a well-lighted room, so that the pressure at which the flush appears

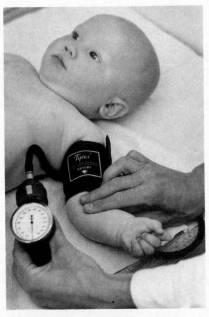

FIGURE 10–26 Taking an infant's blood pressure by palpation.

can be accurately determined.

- Place the cuff on the infant's wrist or ankle.
- Elevate the limb. *This promotes venous blood flow to the heart.*
- Wrap the limb distal to the cuff with an elastic bandage. Wrap firmly, starting at the fingers or toes and working up to the blood pressure cuff. *The bandage will*

force venous blood into the upper part of the limb and restrict arterial blood flow into the lower part of the limb.

- Lower the extremity to the heart level.
- Inflate the bladder of the cuff rapidly to about 200 mm Hg. *This stops arterial blood flow to the limb.*
- Remove the bandage. The limb should appear pale because of the absence of blood.
- Gradually release the pressure at no more than 5 mm Hg per second.
- Record the pressure at the appearance of a flush as the blood returns in the extremity distal to the cuff. This pressure is a mean blood pressure between the systolic and diastolic pressures.

Doppler Stethoscope

- See Technique 10–2, page 173, for information about using the DUS.
- Proceed to auscultate the blood pressure as described in Technique 10–7.

EVALUATION FOCUS

The blood pressure in relation to baseline data, normal range for age, and heart status; relationship to pulse and respiration.

KEY ELEMENTS OF ASSESSING AN INFANT'S BLOOD PRESSURE

- Use an appropriate cuff and site.
- Ensure that the infant/child is quiet and, if able, knows what to expect.
- For an arm measurement, place the arm at the heart level.
- When using the auscultatory method, record both phases 4 and 5 as the diastolic pressure.
- When performing the palpation technique, pump the cuff to about 30 mm Hg beyond the point where the brachial pulse disappears, and

release the cuff slowly (2 to 3 mm Hg per second until the pulse returns).

When performing the flush technique:

- Use a well-lighted room.
- Elevate the limb before wrapping it.
- Lower the limb to heart level.
- Inflate the bladder cuff rapidly to stop arterial blood flow.
- Gradually release the pressure, noting the point at which a flush appears.

CRITICAL THINKING CHALLENGE

In each of the following situations, the vital signs have been taken 4 hours apart. Based on your assessment of the vital signs, what nursing actions would you take?

a. 74-year-old male who is 3 days postoperative prostatectomy: 7:00 A.M.: T 99.6 (oral), P 84, R 16, BP 136/86. 11:00 A.M.: T 100.4 (oral), P 104, R 26, BP 134/82.

b. An infant whose umbilical hernia will be repaired the following day: 11:00 A.M.: T 98 (axillary), HR 104, R 28, BP NA. 3:00 P.M.: T 99 (axillary), H 106, R 28, BP NA.

c. A 32-year-old female who is immediate postoperative hysterectomy: 1:00 P.M. on return to floor from recovery: T 100.2 (tympanic membrane), P 84, R 16, BP 124/76. 5:00 P.M.: T 99 (oral), P 104, R 22, BP 90/60.

RELATED RESEARCH

Erickson, R. S., and Yount, S. T. March/April 1991. Comparison of tympanic and oral temperatures in surgical patients. *Nursing Research* 40:90–93.

Guiffre, M.; Heidenreich, T.; Carney-Gersten, P.; Dorsch, J. A.; and Heidenreich, E. May 1990. The relationship between axillary and core body temperature measurements. *Applied Nursing Research* 3:52–55.

Henneman, E. A., and Henneman, P. L. May 1989. Intricacies of blood pressure measurement: Reexamining the rituals. *Heart and Lung* 18:263–73.

Rebenson-Piano, M.; Holm, K.; Foreman, M. D.; and Kirchhoff, K. T. January/February 1989. An evaluation of two indirect methods of blood pressure measurement in ill patients. *Nursing Research* 38:42–45.

White, H. E.; Thurston, N. E.; Blackmore, K. A.; et al. October 1987. Body temperature in elderly surgical patients. *Research in Nursing and Health* 10:317–21.

REFERENCES

American Heart Association. 1980. *Recommendations for human blood pressure determination by sphygmomanometers.* Pub. no. 70–019–B, 80–100M, 9–81–100M. American Heart Association. National Center, 7320 Greenville Avenue, Dallas, Texas 75231.

Axillary temps safer in infants. June 1978. (Medical Highlights) *American Journal of Nursing* 78:1081.

Baker, N. C.; Cerone, S. B.; Gaze, N.; and Knapp, T. R. March/April 1984. The effect of type of thermometer and length of time inserted on oral temperature measurements of afebrile subjects. *Nursing Research* 33:109–11.

Behrman, R. E., and Vaughan, V. C. III, editors. 1983. *Nelson textbook of pediatrics.* 12th ed. Philadelphia: W. B. Saunders Co.

Creative Care unit. June 1977. Turnabout: Rectal temperatures for postcoronary patients. *American Journal of Nursing* 77:997.

Eoff, M. J., and Joyce, B. May 1981. Temperature measurement in children. *American Journal of Nursing* 81:1010–11.

Erickson, R. May/June 1980. Oral temperature differences in relation to thermometer and technique. *Nursing Research* 29:157–64.

Erickson, R. S., and Yount, S. T. March/April 1991. Comparison of tympanic and oral temperatures in surgical patients. *Nursing Research* 40:90–93.

Evans, M. J. March 1983. Tips for taking a child's blood pressure quickly. *Nursing 83:* 13:61.

Graas, S. October 1974. Thermometer sites and oxygen. *American Journal of Nursing* 74:1862–63.

Graves, R. D., and Markarian, M. F. September/October 1980. Three-minute intervals when using an oral mercury-in-glass thermometer without J-temperature sheaths. *Nursing Research* 29:323–24.

Guyton, A. C. 1986. *Textbook of medical physiology.* 7th ed. Philadelphia: W. B. Saunders Co.

Hasler, M. E., and Cohen, J. A. September/October 1982. The effect of oxygen administration on temperature assessment. *Nursing Research* 31:265–68.

Hudson, B. May 1983. Sharpen your vascular skills with the Doppler ultrasound stethoscope. *Nursing 83* 13:55–57.

Kolanowski, A., and Gunter, L. September/October 1981. Hypothermia in the elderly. *Geriatric Nursing* 2:362–65.

Lowrey, G. H. 1978. *Growth and development of children.* 7th ed. Chicago: Year Book.

Malasanos, L.; Barkauskas, V.; Moss, M.; and Stoltenberg-Allen, K. 1990. *Health assessment.* 4th ed. St. Louis: C. V. Mosby Co.

Marieb, E. N. 1989. *Human anatomy and physiology.* Redwood City, Calif.: Benjamin/Cummings.

Martyn, K. K., et al. 1988. Comparison of axillary, rectal, and skin-based temperature assessment in preschoolers. *Nurse Practitioner* 13(4): 31–33.

Merenstein, G. B.; Gardner, S. L.; and Blake, W. W. 1989. Heat balance. In Merenstein, G. B., and Gardner, S. L., editors. *Handbook of neonatal intensive care.* St. Louis: C. V. Mosby Co.

National Heart, Lung and Blood Institute, Task Force on Blood Pressure Control in Children. May 1987. Report of the second task force on blood pressure control in children. *Pediatrics* 39(Suppl): 1–25.

Nichols, G. A.; Ruskin, M. M.; Glor, B. A. K.; and Kelly, W. H. Fall 1966. Oral, axillary, and rectal determinations and relationships. *Nursing Research* 15:307–16.

Nichols, G. A. June 1972. Taking adult temperatures: Rectal measurement. *American Journal of Nursing* 72:1092–93.

Nursing Photobook Series. 1982. *Attending ob/gyn patients.* Springhouse, Pa.: Intermed Communications.

Olds, S. B.; London, M. L.; and Ladewig, P. A. 1992. *Maternal-newborn nursing: A family-centered approach.* 4th ed. Redwood City, Calif.: Addison-Wesley Publishing Co.

Overfield, T. 1985. *Biologic variation in health and illness.* Menlo Park, Calif.: Addison-Wesley Publishing Co.

Schiffman, R. F. September/October 1982. Temperature monitoring in the neonate: A comparison of axillary and rectal temperatures. *Nursing Research* 31:274–77.

Stevens, N. V. 1991. Measuring pulses. In Smith, D. P., editor. *Comprehensive child and family nursing skills.* St. Louis: C. V. Mosby Co.

U. S. Department of Health and Human Services, Public Health Service National Institutes of Health. May 1988. *The 1988 Report of the Joint National Committee on Detection, Evaluation, and Treatment of High Blood Pressure.* NIH Pub. no. 88–1088.

Whaley, L. F., and Wong, D. L. 1989. *Essentials of pediatric nursing,* 3rd ed. St. Louis: C. V. Mosby Co.

Whaley, L. F., and Wong, D. L. 1991. *Nursing care of infants and children.* 4th ed. St. Louis: C. V. Mosby Co.

11

Assessing Adult Health

OBJECTIVES

- Define terms associated with health assessment

- Describe ten components of a nursing health history

- Identify purposes of physical health examination

- Explain the four methods of examining

- Explain the significance of selected physical findings

- Identify expected outcomes of health assessment

- Identify the various steps in selected assessment procedures

- Describe suggested sequencing to conduct a physical health assessment in an orderly fashion

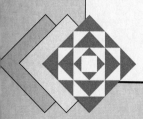

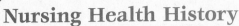

Nursing Health History

The nursing health history interview is the first part of the assessment of the client's health status and is usually carried out before the physical examination. This is a structured interview designed to collect specific health data and to obtain a detailed health record of the client. Its purposes are

• To elicit information about all the variables that may affect the client's health status

• To obtain data that help the nurse understand and appreciate the client's life experiences

• To initiate a nonjudgmental, trusting interpersonal relationship with the client

The nurse uses the data obtained in collaboration with the client to develop nursing diagnoses and subsequent plans for individualized care. Many health history forms are designed as checklists that the client fills out independently. The nurse then reviews the information with the client and clarifies or amplifies the data as needed. Components of the nursing history include (a) biographic data, (b) chief complaint or reason for visit, (c) history of present illness (current health status), (d) past history, (e) family history of illness, (f) review of systems, (g) life-style, (h) social data, (i) psychologic data, and (j) patterns of health care. Table 11–1 gives the common beliefs and practices of many different cultural groups.

TABLE 11–1   CULTURAL BEHAVIORS RELEVANT TO HEALTH ASSESSMENT

Cultural Group	Cultural Variations (Common Belief/Practice)	Nursing Implications
African Americans	Dialect and slang terms require careful communication to prevent error (i.e., "bad" may mean "good").	Question the client's meaning or intent.
Mexican Americans	Eye behavior is important. An individual who looks at and admires a child without touching the child has given the child the "evil eye."	Always touch the child you are examining or admiring.
Native Americans	Eye contact is considered a sign of disrespect and is thus avoided.	Recognize that the client may be attentive and interested even though eye contact is avoided.
Appalachians	Eye contact is considered impolite or a sign of hostility. Verbal patter may be confusing.	Avoid excessive eye contact. Clarify statements.
American Eskimos	Body language is very important. The individual seldom disagrees publicly with others. Client may nod yes to be polite, even if not in agreement.	Monitor own body language closely as well as client's to detect meaning.
Jewish Americans	Orthodox Jews consider excess touching, particularly from members of the opposite sex, offensive.	Establish whether client is an orthodox Jew and avoid excessive touch.
Chinese Americans	Individual may nod head to indicate yes or shake head to indicate no. Excessive eye contact indicates rudeness. Excessive touch is offensive.	Ask questions carefully, and clarify responses. Avoid excessive eye contact and touch.
Filipino Americans	Offending people is to be avoided at all cost. Nonverbal behavior is very important.	Monitor nonverbal behaviors of self and client, being sensitive to physical and emotional discomfort or concerns of the client.
Haitian Americans	Touch is used in conversation Direct eye contact is used to gain attention and respect during communication.	Use direct eye contact when communicating.
East Indian Hindu Americans	Women avoid eye contact as a sign of respect.	Be aware that men may view eye contact by women as offensive. Avoid eye contact.
Vietnamese Americans	Avoidance of eye contact is a sign of respect. The head is considered sacred; it is not polite to pat the head. An upturned palm is offensive in communication.	Limit eye contact. Touch the head only when mandated, and explain clearly before proceeding to do so. Avoid hand gesturing.

Source: Adapted from J. N. Gigen and R. E. Davidhizar, *Transcultural Nursing* (St. Louis: C. V. Mosby Co., 1991).

Physical Health Examination

A complete health assessment is generally conducted from the head to the toes; however, the procedure can vary in many ways according to the age of the individual, the severity of the illness, the preferences of the nurse, and the agency's priorities and procedures. Regardless of what procedure is used, the client's energy and time need to be considered. The health assessment is therefore conducted in a systematic and efficient manner that requires the fewest position changes for the client.

Frequently, nurses assess a specific body area instead of the entire body. These specific assessments are made in relation to client complaints, the nurse's own observation of problems, the client's presenting problem, nursing interventions provided, and medical therapies.

Preparing the Client

Most people need an explanation of the physical health examination. The nurse should explain when and where the examination will take place, why it is necessary, who will conduct it, and what will happen during the examination. The nurse should also inform the client of any special circumstances—for instance, the need to go to a different room or assume a special position—and tell the adult client that appropriate draping will be provided so that the body will not be unnecessarily exposed.

Most clients should empty their bladders before the examination. Doing so helps them feel more relaxed and facilitates palpation of the abdomen and pubic area. Since an empty rectum facilitates rectal examination, the client should be encouraged to defecate before a complete physical examination. If a urinalysis is required, the urine should be collected in a container for that purpose. Clients must often assume special positions during the health examination. See Table 11–2.

Dorsal and Horizontal Recumbent and Supine Positions

The appropriate drapes for a client in these positions usually include (a) a hospital gown or bath towel for the chest and (b) a bath blanket or sheet to cover the remainder of the body from the waist to the toes. The

TABLE 11–2 CLIENT POSITIONS AND BODY AREAS EXAMINED

Position	Description	Areas Examined	Cautions
Dorsal recumbent	Back-lying position with knees flexed and hips externally rotated; small pillow under the head	Head and neck, axillae, anterior thorax, lungs, breasts, heart, abdomen, extremities, peripheral pulses, vital signs, and vagina	May be difficult for clients who have cardiopulmonary problems to assume
Horizontal recumbent	Back-lying position with legs extended; small pillow under the head	Head, neck, axillae, anterior thorax, lungs, breasts, heart, extremities, peripheral pulses	Not used for abdominal assessment because of the increased tension of abdominal muscles
Dorsal (supine)	Back-lying position without a pillow	As for horizontal recumbent	Tolerated poorly by clients with cardiovascular and respiratory problems
Sitting	A seated position, back unsupported and legs hanging freely	Head, neck, posterior and anterior thorax, lungs, breasts, axillae, heart, vital signs, upper and lower extremities, reflexes	Elderly and weak clients may require support
Lithotomy	Back-lying position with feet supported in stirrups; the hips should be in line with the edge of the table	Female genitals, rectum, and female genital reproductive tract	May be difficult and tiring for elderly people
Genupectoral	Kneeling position with torso at a 90° angle to hips	Rectum	Uncomfortable position, tolerated poorly by clients who have respiratory problems
Sims'	Side-lying position with lowermost arm behind the body and uppermost leg flexed (see Chapter 20)	Rectum, vagina	Difficult for the elderly and people with limited joint movement
Prone	Face-lying position, with or without a small pillow	Posterior thorax, hip movement	Often not tolerated by the elderly and people with cardiovascular and respiratory problems

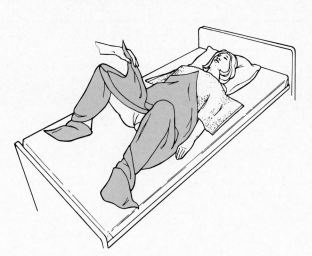

FIGURE 11-1 A client draped in a dorsal recumbent position.

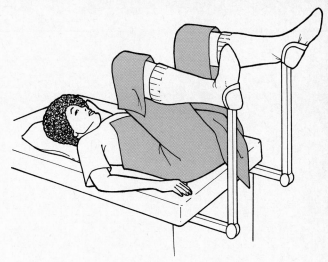

FIGURE 11-2 A client draped in the lithotomy position.

nurse places the bath towel across the chest, and the bath blanket or sheet diagonally over the person (Figure 11-1). If the client's perineal area is to be examined, opposite corners of the sheet are wrapped around the feet to cover the legs. The corner between the client's legs can be raised to expose the perineum at the appropriate time.

Sitting Position

This position is frequently assumed during examinations of the chest, neck, and head. The client requires a gown.

Lithotomy Position

The **lithotomy position** is frequently used for examinations of the vagina and sometimes for urinary catheterizations in woman.

The drapes usually used are (a) a gown for the upper body (optional), (b) a rectangular sheet or a **fenestrated drape** (a drape with an opening in its center), and (c) socks for the clients' feet (optional). The socks are put on the client before the feet are placed in the stirrups. The sheet is placed diagonally on the client so that the top part covers the client's chest and abdomen. The side corners are wrapped around the client's legs and feet (Figure 11-2). If the client is wearing socks, the drape need not cover the feet. The corner between the client's legs is lifted to expose the perineal area. A fenestrated drape is placed the same way as a rectangular sheet but with the opening directly over the area to be examined.

Genupectoral (Knee-Chest) Position

The **genupectoral position** is a kneeling position in which the head is turned to one side and the arms are held above the head. Special tables, provided in many agencies, support clients in this position.

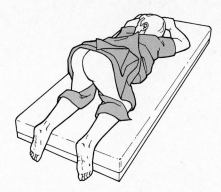

FIGURE 11-3 A fenestrated drape exposes only the anal area of a client in the genupectoral position.

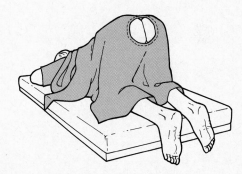

FIGURE 11-4 A client draped in the genupectoral position (rectangular drape).

The drapes required are (a) a hospital gown to cover the upper body, (b) socks to cover the feet and lower legs (optional), and (c) a fenestrated drape to cover the client's back, buttocks, and thighs. The hole in the drape exposes only the area to be examined (Figure 11-3). A rectangular drape can be used instead. The two lateral corners are tucked around the client's thighs. The corner between the thighs can then be lifted up to expose the area to be examined, e.g., the anus (Figure 11-4).

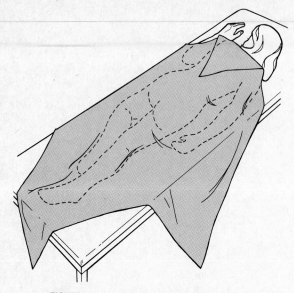

FIGURE 11–5 A client draped in Sims' position.

Sims' Position

In **Sims' position**, the lower arm is behind the client, and the upper arm is flexed at both the shoulder and the elbow. Both legs are also flexed, the upper one more so at the hip and the knee than the lower one.

The drape is usually one rectangular sheet, placed diagonally on the client (Figure 11–5). At the time of examination, the corner is folded back to expose the area. Because this position can be difficult for some clients to assume, particularly the elderly and the obese, it is normally not assumed until immediately before the examination.

Prone Position

A client in the **prone position** lies on the abdomen and usually turns the head to the side. See Figure 20–7 on page 490. A sheet to cover the client is required.

Methods of Examining

Four primary techniques are used in the physical examination: inspection, palpation, percussion, and auscultation. These are discussed throughout this chapter as they apply to each body system.

Inspection

Inspection is the visual examination, i.e., assessing by using the sense of sight. The nurse inspects with the naked eye and with a lighted instrument such as an **otoscope** (used to view the ear). Some authors consider the use of the senses of hearing and smell as part of the inspection (Malasanos, Barkauskas, and Stoltenberg-Allen 1990, p. 138). Nurses frequently use this technique to assess color, rashes, scars, body shape, facial expressions that may reflect emotions, and body structures, e.g., the inner eye. Inspection is an active process, not a passive one. The nurse must know what to look for and where. Inspection should be systematic, so that nothing is missed. Lighting must be sufficient; either natural or artificial light can be used.

Palpation

Palpation is the examination of the body using the sense of touch. The pads of the fingers are used because their concentration of nerve endings makes them highly sensitive to tactile discrimination. Palpation is used to determine (a) texture, e.g., of the hair; (b) temperature, e.g., of a skin area; (c) vibration, e.g., of a joint; (d) position, size, consistency, and mobility of organs or masses; (e) distention, e.g., of the urinary bladder; (f) presence and rate of peripheral pulses; and (g) tenderness or pain.

There are two types of palpation: light and deep. *Light* (superficial) palpation should always precede *deep* palpation, because heavy pressure on the fingertips can dull the sense of touch. For *light palpation*, the nurse extends dominant hand fingers parallel to the skin surface and presses gently downward while moving the hand in a circular fashion. If it is necessary to determine the details of a mass, the nurse presses lightly several times rather than holding the pressure.

Deep palpation is done with two hands (bimanually) or one hand. In deep bimanual palpation, the nurse extends the dominant hand as for light palpation, the places the fingerpads of the nondominant hand on the dorsal surfaces of the distal interphalangeal joint of the middle three fingers of the dominant hand (See Figure 11–6). The top hand applies pressure while the lower hand remains relaxed to perceive the tactile sensations. For deep palpation using one hand, the fingerpads of the dominant hand press over the area to be palpated. Often the other hand is used to support a mass or organ from below (Figure 11–7). Deep palpation is a technique used more commonly by nurse practitioners and clinical specialists than by nurses in general practice.

The effectiveness of palpation depends largely on the client's relaxation. Nurses can assist a client to relax by (a) gowning and/or draping the client appropriately; (b) positioning the client comfortably; (c) ensuring that their own hands are warm before beginning, e.g., running them under warm water if they are cold; and (d) commencing palpation with areas that are not painful. During palpation, the nurse should be sensitive to the client's verbal and facial expressions indicating discomfort.

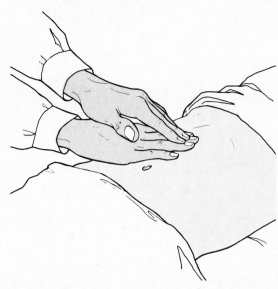

FIGURE 11–6 The position of the hands for deep bimanual palpation.

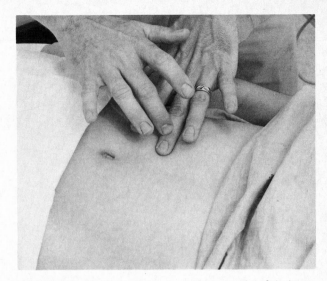

FIGURE 11–8 The position of the fingers for percussion. Only the middle finger of the nondominant hand is firmly in contact with the client's skin.

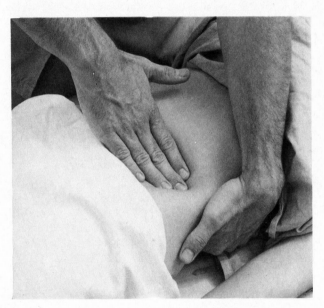

FIGURE 11–7 Deep palpation using the lower hand to support the body while the upper hand palpates the organ.

Percussion

Percussion is an assessment method in which the body surface is struck to elicit sounds that can be heard or vibrations that can be felt. There are two types of percussion: direct, or immediate, percussion and indirect, or mediate, percussion. In *direct percussion*, the nurse strikes the area to be percussed directly with the pads of two, three, or four fingers or with the pad of the middle finger. The strikes are rapid, and the movement is from the wrist. This technique is not generally used to percuss the thorax but is useful in percussing an adult's sinuses. The second

type, *indirect percussion*, is the striking of an object (e.g., a finger) held against the body area to be examined. In this technique, the middle finger of the non-dominant hand, referred to as the **pleximeter**, is placed firmly on the client's skin. Only the distal phalanx and joint of this finger should be in contact with the skin. Using the tip of the flexed middle finger of the other hand, called the **plexor**, the nurse strikes the pleximeter, usually at the distal interphalangeal joint (Figure 11–8). Some nurses may find a point between the distal and proximal joints to be a more comfortable pleximeter point. The striking motion should come from the wrist; the forearm remains stationary. The angle between the plexor and the pleximeter should be 90 degrees, and the blows must be firm, rapid, and short to obtain a clear sound.

Percussion is used to determine the size and shape of internal organs by establishing their borders. It indicates whether tissue is fluid-filled, air-filled, or solid. Percussion elicits five types of sound: flatness, dullness, resonance, hyperresonance, and tympany. **Flatness** is an extremely dull sound produced by very dense tissue, such as muscle or bone. **Dullness** is a thudlike sound produced by dense tissue, such as the liver, spleen, or heart. **Resonance** is a hollow sound such as that produced by lungs filled with air. **Hyperresonance** is not produced in the normal body. It is described as booming and can be heard over an emphysematous lung. **Tympany** is a musical or drumlike sound produced from an air-filled stomach. On a continuum, flatness reflects the most dense tissue (the least amount of air) and tympany the least dense tissue (the most amount of air). A percussion sound is described according to its intensity, pitch, duration, and quality. See Table 11–3 on page 204.

TABLE 11–3 PERCUSSION SOUNDS AND TONES

Sound	Intensity	Pitch	Duration	Quality	Example of Location
Flatness	Soft	High	Short	Extremely dull	Muscle, bone
Dullness	Medium	Medium	Moderate	Thudlike	Liver, heart
Resonance	Loud	Low	Long	Hollow	Lung
Hyperresonance	Very loud	Very low	Very long	Booming	Emphysematous lung
Tympany	Loud	High (distinguished mainly by musical timbre)	Moderate	Musical	Stomach filled with gas (air)

Auscultation

Auscultation is the process of listening to sounds produced within the body. Auscultation may be direct or indirect. *Direct auscultation* is the use of the unaided ear, e.g., to listen to a respiration wheeze or the grating of a moving joint. *Indirect auscultation* is the use of a stethoscope, which amplifies the sounds and conveys them to the nurse's ears. A stethoscope is used primarily to listen to sounds from within the body, e.g., bowel sounds or valve sounds of the heart.

The stethoscope should be 30 to 25 cm (12 to 14 in) long, with an internal diameter of about 0.3 cm (⅛ in). It should have both a flat-disc and a bell-shaped diaphragm. See Figure 10–14 on page 175. The flat-disc diaphragm best transmits high-pitched sounds, e.g., bronchial sounds, and the bell-shaped diaphragm best transmits low-pitched sounds, such as some heart sounds. The earpieces of the stethoscope should fit comfortably into the nurse's ears. The diaphragm of the stethoscope is placed firmly but lightly against the client's skin. If a client is very hairy, it may be necessary to dampen the hairs with a moist cloth so that they will lie flat against the skin and not cause scratching sounds.

Auscultated sounds are described according to their pitch, intensity, duration, and quality. The **pitch** is the frequency of the vibrations (the number of vibrations per second). Low-pitched sounds, e.g., some heart sounds, have fewer vibrations per second than high-pitched sounds, such as bronchial sounds. The **intensity** (amplitude) refers to the loudness or softness of a sound. Some body sounds are loud, e.g., bronchial sounds heard over the trachea, whereas others are soft, e.g., normal breath sounds heard in

the lungs. The **duration** of a sound is its length (long or short). The **quality** of sound is a subjective description of a sound, e.g., whistling, gurgling, or snapping.

Instrumentation

Illustrations of various equipment are shown throughout the chapter. Equipment is frequently set up on trays ready for use (Figure 11–9). All equipment required for the health examination should be clean, in good working order, and readily accessible. See Table 11–4.

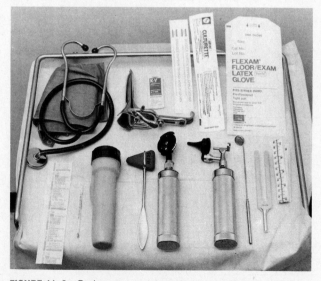

FIGURE 11–9 Equipment on a tray ready for a health examination.

TABLE 11–4 EQUIPMENT AND SUPPLIES USED FOR A HEALTH EXAMINATION

Instruments and Supplies	Purpose
Flashlight or penlight	To assist viewing of the pharynx and cervix or to determine the reactions of the pupils of the eye
Head mirror	To direct light to a specific body area, e.g., the pharynx
Laryngeal or dental mirror	To observe the pharynx and oral cavity
Nasal speculum	To permit visualization of the lower and middle turbinates; usually a penlight is used for illumination
Neurologic hammer	To test reflexes; often has a soft brush and needle in the handle that come out when it is unscrewed
Ophthalmoscope	A lighted instrument to visualize the interior of the eye
Otoscope	A lighted instrument to visualize the eardrum and external auditory canal (a nasal speculum may be attached to the otoscope to inspect the nasal cavities)
Percussion (reflex) hammer	An instrument with a rubber head to test reflexes
Smells (1 or 2 vials)	To test the sense of smell
Sphygmomanometer and cuff	To measure the blood pressure
Stethoscope	To auscultate body sounds, e.g., blood pressure, chest, bowel sounds
Thermometer	To measure body temperature
Tuning fork	A two-pronged metal instrument used to test hearing acuity and vibratory sense
Vaginal speculum (various sizes)	To assess the cervix and the vagina
Ayre spatula	To obtain a cervical scrape
Assorted containers and slides	For specimens
Cotton applicators	To obtain specimens
Disposable pads	To absorb liquid
Drapes	To cover the client
Gauze dressings	To cover wounds
Gloves (sterile and unsterile)	To protect the nurse
Lubricant	To ease insertion of instruments, e.g., vaginal speculum
Sterile safety pins	To test sensory function
Tongue blades (depressors)	To depress the tongue during assessment of the mouth and pharynx

General Survey

The nurse assesses many components of the general survey while taking the health history. Other data obtained as part of the survey include appearance and mental status, vital signs, and height and weight.

Mental status and the *level of consciousness* or state of awareness are often determined at the beginning of the physical examination. Ask the client to state name, the day or date, present location, and the reason for hospitalization or for seeking assistance. Record the client's ability to provide this information. For clients who are unable to speak, describe their specific responses to verbal and physical stimuli. See Neurologic Assessment, later in this chapter.

Appearance and Mental Status

The general appearance and behavior of an individual must be assessed in terms of culture, educational level, socioeconomic status, and current circumstances. For example, an individual who has recently experienced a personal loss may appropriately appear depressed. Also, the client's age, sex, and race are useful factors in interpreting findings that suggest increased risk for known conditions.

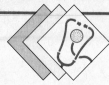

Assessing General Appearance and Mental Status

NURSING HISTORY FOCUS
Chronologic age, race, cultural background, and general health status; achievement of developmental tasks; body image concerns; self-esteem; educational level, thought processes; general health history; stressors (past and present); changes in personality, behavior, or memory; lifelong problems, e.g., poor job history, alcoholism, drug abuse, disciplinary problems.

ASSESSMENT	NORMAL FINDINGS	DEVIATIONS FROM NORMAL
General Appearance		
Observe body build, height, and weight in relation to the client's age, life-style, and health.	Varies with life-style	Excessively thin or obese
Observe the client's posture and gait, standing, sitting, and walking. See Chapter 21, page 498.	Relaxed, erect posture; coordinated movement	Tense, slouched, bent posture; uncoordinated movement; tremors
Observe the client's overall hygiene and grooming. Relate these to the person's activities prior to the assessment.	Clean, neat	Dirty, unkempt
Note body and breath odor in relation to activity level.	No body odor or minor body odor relative to work or exercise; no breath odor	Foul body odor; ammonia odor; acetone breath odor; foul breath
Observe for signs of distress in posture (e.g., bending over because of abdominal pain) or **facial expression** (e.g., wincing or labored breathing).		
Note obvious signs of health or illness (e.g., in skin color or breathing).	Healthy appearance	Pallor; weakness; obvious illness
Mental Status		
Assess the client's attitude.	Cooperative	Negative, hostile, withdrawn
Note the client's affect/mood; assess the appropriateness of the client's responses.	Appropriate to situation	Inappropriate to situation
Listen for quantity of speech (amount and pace), **quality** (loudness, clarity, inflection), **and organization** (coherence of thought, overgeneralization, vagueness).	Understandable, moderate pace Exhibits thought association	Rapid or slow pace Uses generalizations; lacks association; exhibits confabulation
Listen for relevance and organization of thoughts.	Logical sequence Makes sense; has sense of reality	Illogical sequence Flight of ideas; confusion

Vital Signs

Vital signs are measured (a) to establish baseline data against which to compare future measurements and (b) to detect actual and future health problems. See Chapter 10 for measurements of temperature, pulse, respirations, and blood pressure.

Height and Weight

In adults, the ratio of weight to height provides a general measure of health. By asking clients about their height and weight before actually measuring them, the nurse obtains some idea of the person's self-image. Excessive discrepancies between the client's responses and the measurements may provide clues to actual or potential problems in self-concept. It is also important that the nurse and client be aware of any weight gains or losses over a specific time period.

The nurse measures height with a measuring stick attached to weight scales or to a wall. The client removes the shoes and stands erect, with heels together, buttocks and head against the measuring stick, and eyes looking straight ahead. The nurse raises the L-shaped sliding arm on the weight scale until it rests on top of the client's head, or places a small flat object, such as a ruler or book, on the client's head. The edge of the ruler should abut the measuring guide. More accurate results can be obtained with a right-angled instrument.

Weight is usually measured when a client is admitted to a health agency and often regularly, e.g., each morning before breakfast. When accuracy is essential, the nurse should use the same scale each time (since every scale weighs differently), take the measurements at the same time each day, and make sure the client wears the same kind of clothing and no shoes. The client stands on a platform, and the weight is read from a digital display panel or a balancing arm. Clients who cannot stand are weighed on bed and chair scales (Figures 11–10 and 11–11). The bed scales have canvas straps or a stretcherlike apparatus. A machine lifts the client above the bed, and the weight is reflected either on a digital display panel or on a balance arm like that of a standing scale.

Standardized charts reflect average heights and weights of children and adults. See Table 11–5. It is important to remember that standardized charts reflect average heights and weights and provide only general guidelines for assessing growth, development, and nutritional status.

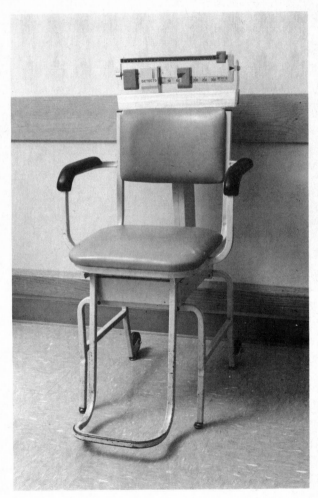

FIGURE 11–11   A chair scale.

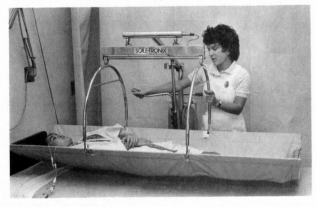

FIGURE 11–10   A bed scale.

TABLE 11-5 1983 METROPOLITAN HEIGHT AND WEIGHT TABLES, MEN AND WOMEN, AGES 25 TO 59

Men				Women			
	Weight (lb)*				Weight (lb)*		
Height	Small Frame	Medium Frame	Large Frame	Height	Small Frame	Medium Frame	Large Frame
5′ 2″	128–134	131–141	138–150	4′10″	102–111	109–121	118–131
5′ 3″	130–136	133–143	140–153	4′11″	103–113	111–123	120–134
5′ 4″	132–138	135–145	142–156	5′ 0″	104–115	113–126	122–137
5′ 5″	134–140	137–148	144–160	5′ 1″	106–118	115–129	125–140
5′ 6″	136–142	139–151	146–164	5′ 2″	108–121	118–132	128–143
5′ 7″	138–145	142–154	149–168	5′ 3″	111–124	121–135	131–147
5′ 8″	140–148	145–157	152–172	5′ 4″	114–127	124–138	134–151
5′ 9″	142–151	148–160	155–176	5′ 5″	117–130	127–141	137–155
5′10″	144–154	151–163	158–180	5′ 6″	120–133	130–144	140–159
5′11″	146–157	154–166	161–184	5′ 7″	123–136	133–147	143–163
6′ 0″	149–160	157–170	164–188	5′ 8″	126–139	136–150	146–167
6′ 1″	152–164	160–174	168–192	5′ 9″	129–142	139–153	149–170
6′ 2″	155–168	164–178	172–197	5′10″	132–145	142–156	152–173
6′ 3″	158–172	167–182	176–202	5′11″	135–148	145–159	155–176
6′ 4″	162–176	171–187	181–207	6′ 0″	138–151	148–162	158–179

*Weights at ages 25–59 based on lowest mortality. Weight in indoor clothing weighing 5 lb for men, 3 lb for women; height in shoes with 1″ heels

Source of basic data: 1979 build study, Society of Actuaries and Association of Life Insurance Medical Directors of America, 1980. Courtesy Metropolitan Life Insurance Company.

The Integument

The integument includes the skin, hair, and nails. The examination begins with a generalized inspection using a good source of lighting, preferably indirect natural daylight.

Skin

Assessment of the skin involves inspection and palpation. In some instances, the nurse may also need to use the olfactory sense to detect unusual skin odors; these are usually most evident in the skinfolds or in the axillae. Pungent body odor is frequently related to poor hygiene, **hyperhidrosis** (excessive perspiration), or **bromhidrosis** (foul-smelling perspiration). The entire skin surface may be assessed at one time or as each aspect of the body is assessed.

Pallor may be difficult to determine in clients with dark skin. It is usually characterized by the absence of underlying red tones in the skin and may be most readily seen in the buccal mucosa. In brown-skinned clients, pallor may appear as a yellowish brown tinge; in black-skinned clients, the skin may appear ashen gray. Pallor in people with light skins may also be evident in the face, the conjuctiva of the eyes, and the nails. **Cyanosis** (a bluish tinge) is most evident in the nail beds, lips, and buccal mucosa. In dark-skinned clients, close inspection of the palpebral conjunctiva and palms and soles may also show evidence of cyanosis. **Jaundice** (a yellowish tinge) may first be evident in the sclera of the eyes and then in the mucous membranes and the skin. Nurses should take care not to confuse jaundice with the normal yellow pigmentation in the sclera of a dark-skinned or black client. In these clients, the best place to inspect is the part of the sclera that is observable when the eye is open. If jaundice is suspected, the posterior part of the hard palate should also be inspected for a yellowish color tone. **Erythema** is a redness associated with a variety of rashes.

Dark-skinned clients have areas of lighter pigmentation, such as the palms, lips, and nail beds. Localized areas of hyperpigmentation (increased pigmentation) and hypopigmentation (decreased pigmentation) may also occur as a result of changes in the distribution of **melanin** (the dark pigment) or in

Selected Skin Lesions

Nurses are responsible for describing skin lesions accurately, as shown below. Medical diagnoses are given in parentheses.

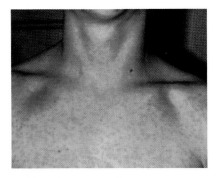

Diffuse discreet erythematous macules (rubella)

Diffuse varying-sized, confluent maculo-papular lesions (rubeola)

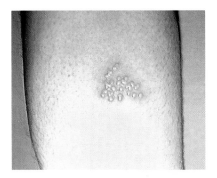

Clustered vesicles on an erythematous base (herpes simplex)

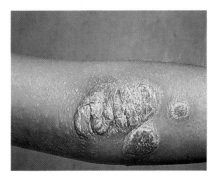

Grouped thick, silvery, scaly plaques (psoriasis)

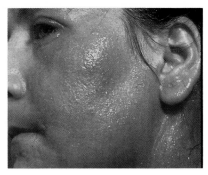

Diffuse edematous, bright erythema (contact dermatitis)

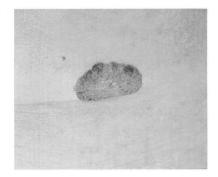

Circumscribed, oval, mottled, brown, slightly elevated lesion (sebborheic keratosis)

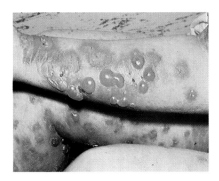

Grouped giant blisters on non-erythematous base (bullous pemphigoid)

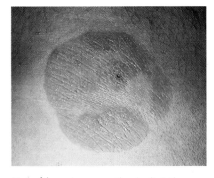

Coin-like, circumscribed, slightly elevated erythematous lesion (mycosis fungoides)

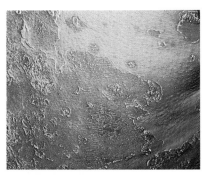

Irregular, varying-sized, pale erythematous patches with superficial fine scaling (pemphigus foliaceus)

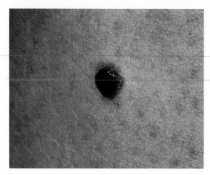

Solitary, deep brown, one-half inch nodule exhibiting a pale halo (malignant melanoma)

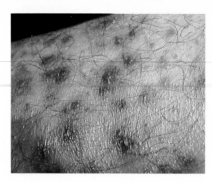

Purple discoloration with petechiae and ecchymoses (Henoch-Schönlein purpura)

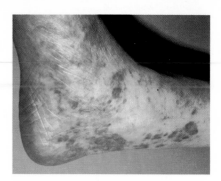

Extensive erythematous patches with small hemorrhagic nodules (Kaposi's sarcoma)

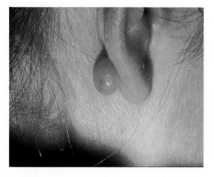

Solitary circumscribed, smooth, lentil-like papilloma (keloid)

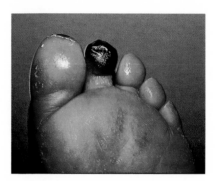

Distal half of toe exhibiting gangrene

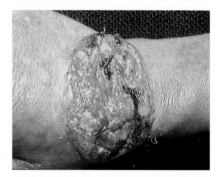

Fungating, ulcerating tumor exhibiting suppuration and necrosis (squamous cell carcinoma)

Decubitus Ulcers

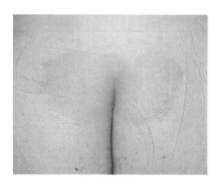

Stage I Non-blanchable erythema signalling potential ulceration

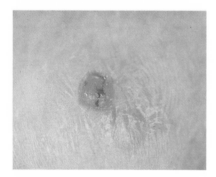

Stage II Abrasion, blister, or shallow crater involving the epidermis and possibly the dermis

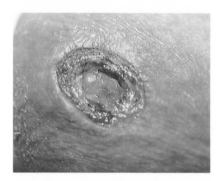

Stage III Deep ulcer exhibiting necrotic tissue and extending through the subcutaneous layer

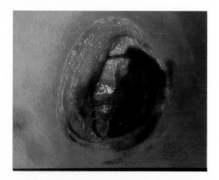

Stage IV Tissue necrosis and damage involving muscle, bone, or supporting structures

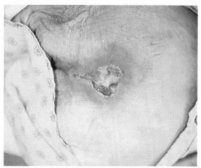

Kennedy terminal ulcer A large, pear-shaped coccygeal or sacral ulcer of sudden onset. Exhibits red, yellow, and black colors and indicates imminent death (Kennedy 1989, First National Pressure Ulcer Advisory Panel, Washington, D.C.)

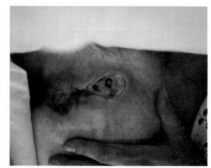

208b

TABLE 11–6 SKIN LESIONS

Type of Lesion	Description	Examples
PRIMARY		
Macule	A flat, circumscribed area of color with no elevation of its surface; 1 mm to 1 cm	Freckles, flat nevi (moles)
Patch	Same as macula, but larger than 1 cm	Port wine birthmark
Papule	A circumscribed, solid elevation of skin; less than 1 cm	Warts, acne, pimples
Plaque	Same as papule, but larger than 1 cm	Eczema
Nodule	A solid mass that extends deeper into the dermis than does a papule	Pigmented nevi
Tumor	A solid mass larger than a nodule	Epitheliomas
Vesicle	A circumscribed elevation containing serous fluid or blood; less than 1 cm	Blister, chickenpox
Bulla	A larger fluid-filled vesicle	Blister, second-degree burns
Pustule	A vesicle or bulla filled with pus	Acne vulgaris, impetigo
Wheal	A relatively reddened, elevated, localized collection of edema fluid; irregular in shape	Mosquito bites, hives
Telangiectasia	Dilated capillary; fine red lines	Seen chiefly in pregnancy and cirrhosis of the liver
Petechiae	Pinpoint red spots	May indicate a problem in blood-clotting mechanisms
SECONDARY		
Scale	Thickened epidermal cells that flake off	Dandruff, psoriasis
Crust	Dried serum or pus on the skin surface	Impetigo, scab on abrasion
Fissure	A linear crack	Athlete's foot
Erosion	Loss of all or part of the epidermis	Chickenpox and smallpox following rupture
Excoriation	Linear or hollowed out crusted area exposing dermis	Scratch, abrasion
Atrophy	A decrease in the volume of epidermis	Striae, aged skin
Scar	A formation of connective tissue	Healed wound
Ulcer	An excavation extending into the dermis or below	Stasis ulcer

the function of the melanocytes in the epidermis. An example of hyperpigmentation in a defined area is a birthmark; an example of hypopigmentation is vitiligo. *Vitiligo*, seen as patches of hypopigmented skin, is caused by the destruction of melanocytes in the area. *Albinism* is the complete or partial lack of melanin in the skin, hair, and eyes. Other localized color changes may indicate a problem such as edema or a localized infection. *Edema* is the presence of excess interstitial fluid. An area of edema appears swollen, shiny, and taut and tends to blanch skin color. Edema is most often an indication of impaired venous circulation and in some cases reflects cardiac dysfunction or vein abnormalities.

A skin lesion is a traumatic or pathologic interruption of the skin. There are many kinds of lesions. Nurses must observe the location (e.g., face), distribution (i.e., body region or location), configuration (the arrangement or position of several lesions) as well as color, shape, size, firmness, texture, and characteristics of individual lesions. See Table 11–6 for the different types of skin lesions.

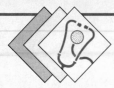

Assessing the Skin

NURSING HISTORY FOCUS

Pain or itching; presence and spread of any lesions, bruises, abrasions, pigmented spots; previous experience with skin problems; associated clinical signs; family history; presence of problems in other family members; related systemic conditions; use of medications, lotions, home remedies; excessively dry or moist feel to the skin; tendency to bruise easily; any association of the problem to season of year, stress, occupation, medications, recent travel, housing, personal contact, and so on; any recent contact with allergens, e.g., metal paint.

ASSESSMENT	NORMAL FINDINGS	DEVIATIONS FROM NORMAL
Inspect skin color (best assessed under natural light and on areas not exposed to the sun).	Varies from light to deep brown; from ruddy pink to light pink; from yellow overtones to olive	Pallor, cyanosis, jaundice, erythema
Inspect uniformity of skin color.	Generally uniform except in areas exposed to the sun; areas of lighter pigmentation (palms, lips, nail beds) in dark-skinned people	Areas of either hyperpigmentation or hypopigmentation (e.g., vitiligo, albinism, edema)
Assess edema, if present (i.e., location, color, temperature, shape, and the degree to which the skin remains indented or pitted when pressed by a finger). See the accompanying box.		
Inspect, palpate, and describe skin lesions (see Table 11–6 earlier). Palpate lesions to determine shape and texture. Describe lesions according to type or structure, color, distribution, and configuration. See the box below.	Freckles, some birthmarks, some flat and raised nevi; no abrasions or other lesions	Various interruptions in skin integrity

Scale for Describing Edema

- 1+ Barely detectable
- 2+ Indentation of less than 5 mm
- 3+ Indentation of 5 to 10 mm
- 4+ Indentation of more than 10 mm

Describing Skin Lesions

- *Type or structure.* Skin lesions are classified as *primary* (those that appear initially in response to some change in the external or internal environment of the skin) and *secondary* (those that do not appear initially but result from modifications such as chronicity, trauma, or infection of the primary lesion). For example, a vesicle (primary lesion) may rupture and cause an erosion (secondary lesion).
- *Color.* There may be no discoloration, one discrete color (e.g., red, brown, or black), or several colors, as with *ecchymosis* (a bruise), in which an initial dark red or blue color fades to a yellow color. When color changes are limited to the edges of a lesion, they are described as *circumscribed;* when spread over a large area, they are described as *diffuse*.
- *Distribution.* Distribution is described according to the location of the lesions on the body and symmetry or asymmetry of findings in comparable body areas.
- *Configuration.* Configuration refers to the arrangement of lesions in relation to each other. Configurations of lesions may be annular (arranged in a circle); clustered together or grouped; linear (arranged in a line); arc- or bow-shaped; merged together, or indiscrete; follow the course of cutaneous nerves; or meshed in the form of a network.

▶ **Assessing the Skin** *CONTINUED*

ASSESSMENT	NORMAL FINDINGS	DEVIATIONS FROM NORMAL
Observe and palpate skin moisture.	Moisture in skinfolds and the axillae (varies with environmental temperature and humidity, body temperature, and activity)	Excessive moisture (e.g., in hyperthermia); excessive dryness (e.g., in dehydration)
Palpate skin temperature. Compare the two feet and the two hands, using the backs of your fingers.	Uniform; within normal range	Generalized hyperthermia (e.g., in fever); generalized hypothermia (e.g., in shock); localized hyperthermia (e.g., in infection); localized hypothermia (e.g., in arteriosclerosis)
Note skin turgor (fullness or elasticity) by lifting and pinching the skin on an extremity.	When pinched, skin springs back to previous state	Skins stays pinched or tented or moves back slowly (e.g., in dehydration)

THE ELDERLY: PHYSICAL CHANGES OF THE SKIN

- Aging changes of the skin result from many factors: enzymatic changes in connective and epithelial tissues, heredity, inadequate nutrition from vascular changes, and endocrine changes. Aging changes in white skin occur at an earlier age than in black skin.
- The skin loses its elasticity and wrinkles. Wrinkles first appear on the skin of the face and neck, which are abundant in collagen and elastic fibers.
- The skin appears yellow-white (like parchment), thin, and translucent because of loss of dermis and subcutaneous fat. Atrophy of the epidermal structures results from degeneration of collagen and elastin.
- The skin is dry and flaky because sebaceous and sweat glands are less active. Dry skin is more prominent over the extremities, where circulation is not as efficient.
- The skin takes longer to return to its natural shape after being pinched between the thumb and finger. Because there is loss of skin turgor over the extremities, the skin of the forehead is recommended for the pinch-fold test for dehydration.
- Flat tan to brown-colored macules, referred to as *senile lentigines* or *melanotic freckles,* are normally apparent on the back of the hand and other skin areas that are exposed to the sun. These macules may be as large as 1 to 2 centimeters. They occur because cells lose their ability to spread out melanin.
- Warty lesions (*seborrheic keratosis*) with irregularly shaped borders and a scaly surface often occur on the face, shoulders, and trunk. These benign lesions begin as yellowish to tan and progress to a dark brown or black.
- *Vitiligo* tends to increase with age and is thought to result from an autoimmune response.
- Cutaneous tags (*acrochordons*) are most commonly seen in the neck and axillary regions. These skin lesions vary in size and are soft, often flesh colored, and pedicled.
- Visible, bright red, fine dilated blood vessels (*telangiectasias*) commonly occur as a result of the thinning of the dermis and the loss of support for the blood vessel walls.
- Pink to slightly red lesions with indistinct borders (*actinic keratoses*) may appear at about age 50, often on the face, ears, backs of the hands, and arms. They often become malignant.

Hair

Assessment of an individual's hair includes inspection of the hair, consideration of developmental changes, and determination of the individual's hair care practices and the factors influencing them. Much of the information about hair can be obtained by questioning the client.

Normal hair is resilient and evenly distributed. In people with several protein deficiency (kwashiorkor), the hair color is faded and appears reddish or bleached, and the texture is coarse and dry. Some therapies for cancer cause **alopecia** (hair loss), and some disease conditions affect the coarseness of hair.

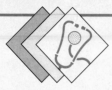

Assessing the Hair

NURSING HISTORY FOCUS
Recent use of hair dyes, rinses, or curling or straightening preparations; recent chemotherapy (if alopecia is present); presence of disease, such as hypothyroidism, which can be associated with dry, brittle hair.

ASSESSMENT	NORMAL FINDINGS	DEVIATIONS FROM NORMAL
Inspect the evenness of growth over the scalp.	Evenly distributed hair	Patches of hair loss (i.e., alopecia)
Inspect hair thickness or thinness.	Thick hair	Very thin hair (e.g., in hypothyroidism)
Inspect hair texture and oiliness.	Silky, resilient hair	Brittle hair (e.g., in hypothyroidism); excessively oily or dry hair
Note presence of infections or infestations by parting the hair in several areas.	No infection or infestation	Flaking, sores, lice, nits (louse eggs), and ringworm
Inspect amount of body hair.	Variable	Hirsutism in woman and children

THE ELDERLY: PHYSICAL CHANGES OF THE HAIR

- The age at which the scalp hair grays is influenced largely by genetic factors.
- There is loss of scalp, pubic, and axillary hair.

- In women, the hair of the eyebrows and some facial hair become coarse.
- Hairs of the eyebrows, ears, and nostrils become bristlelike and coarse.

Nails

Parts of the nail are shown in Figure 11–12. Nails are inspected for nail plate shape, angle between the nail and the nail bed, nail texture, nail bed color, and the intactness of the tissues around the nails.

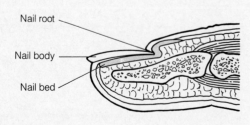
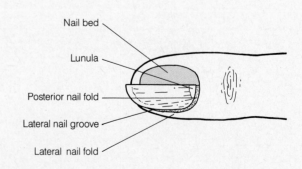

FIGURE 11–12 The parts of a nail.

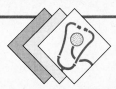

Assessing the Nails

NURSING HISTORY FOCUS
Presence of diabetes mellitus, peripheral circulatory disease, previous injury, or severe illness.

ASSESSMENT	NORMAL FINDINGS	DEVIATIONS FROM NORMAL
Inspect nail plate shape to determine its curvature and angle.	Convex curvature; angle between nail and nail bed of about 160° (Figure 11–13).	**Spoon** nail (Figure 11–14); **clubbing** (180° or greater) (Figure 11–15).

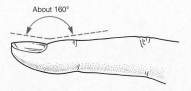

FIGURE 11–13   A normal nail, showing the convex shape and the nail plate angle of about 160°.

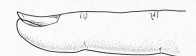

FIGURE 11–14   A spoon-shaped nail, which may be seen in clients with iron deficiency anemia.

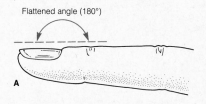

FIGURE 11–15   *A,* early clubbing; *B,* late clubbing. May be caused by long-term oxygen lack.

Inspect nail texture.	Smooth texture	Excessive thickness (e.g., result of poor circulation, iron deficiency anemia); excessive thinness or presence of grooves or furrows (e.g., in iron deficiency anemia); **Beau's lines** (transverse white lines or grooves; Figure 11–16).

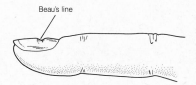

FIGURE 11–16   Beau's line on nail may result from severe injury or illness.

Inspect nail bed color.	Highly vascular and pink in light-skinned clients; dark-skinned clients may have brown or black pigmentation in longitudinal streaks	Bluish or purplish tint (may reflect cyanosis); pallor (may reflect poor arterial circulation)

▶

▶ **Assessing the Nails** *CONTINUED*

ASSESSMENT	NORMAL FINDINGS	DEVIATIONS FROM NORMAL
Inspect tissues surrounding nails.	Intact epidermis	**Hangnails; paronychia** (inflammation)
Perform blanch test to test capillary refill. Press two or more nails between your thumb and index finger; look for blanching and return of pink color to nail bed.	Prompt return of pink or usual color	Delayed return of pink or usual color (may indicate circulatory impairment)

THE ELDERLY: PHYSICAL CHANGES OF THE NAILS

- The nails grow more slowly and thicken.
- Longitudinal bands commonly develop, and the nails tend to split.

- Bands across the nails may indicate protein deficiency; white spots, zinc deficiency; and spoon shaped nails, iron deficiency.

Head

During an examination of the head, the nurse often inspects and palpates simultaneously, as well as auscultating. The nurse examines the skull, face, eyes, ears, nose, sinuses, mouth, and pharynx.

The Skull and Face

There is a large range of normal shapes of skulls. A normal head size is referred to as **normocephalic**. Names of areas of the head are derived from names of the underlying bones: frontal, parietal, occipital, mastoid process, mandible, maxilla, and zygomatic (Figure 11–17).

In adults, a large head may result from osteitis deformans or from acromegaly. **Osteitis deformans (Paget's disease)** is a disorder in which bony thickness increases. The skull, spine, pelvis, and femur are the usual sites of involvement. When the skull is involved, it appears enlarged, with prominent superficial veins, and often the hearing is impaired. **Acromegaly** is a disorder caused by excessive growth hormone secretion. The skull becomes thickened and enlarged, mandible length increases, the nose and forehead become more prominent, and the facial features look coarsened.

Many disorders cause a change in facial shape or condition. Kidney or cardiac disease can cause edema of the eyelids. Thyroid overactivity (hyperthyroidism) can cause **exophthalmus**, a protrusion of the eyeballs with elevation of the upper eyelids, resulting

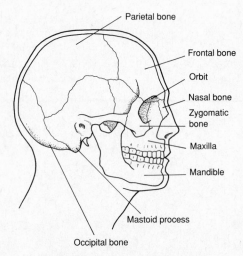

FIGURE 11–17   The bones of the head.

in a startled or staring expression. Thyroid underactivity (hypothyroidism, or **myxedema**) can cause a dry, puffy face with dry skin and coarse features, referred to as **myxedema facies**, and thinning of scalp hair and eyebrows. **Cushing's syndrome**, a disorder in which there is increased adrenal hormone production, can cause a round face with reddened cheeks, referred to as *moon face*, and excessive hair growth on the upper lips, chin, and sideburn areas. Intake of synthetic adrenal hormones also produces these changes. Prolonged illness, starvation, and dehydration can result in sunken eyes, cheeks, and temples.

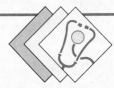

Assessing the Skull and Face

NURSING HISTORY FOCUS
Any past problems with lumps or bumps, itching, scaling, or dandruff; any history of loss of consciousness, dizziness, seizures, headache, facial pain, or injury; when and how any lumps occurred; length of time any other problem existed; any known cause of problem; associated symptoms, treatment, and recurrences.

ASSESSMENT	NORMAL FINDINGS	DEVIATIONS FROM NORMAL
Inspect the skull for size, shape, and symmetry. If skull is of abnormal size, measure its circumference just above the eyebrows.	Rounded (normocephalic and symmetrical, with frontal, parietal, and occipital prominences); smooth skull contour	Lack of symmetry; increased skull size with more prominent nose and forehead; longer mandible (may indicate excessive growth hormone or increased bone thickness)
Palpate the skull for nodules or masses and depressions. Use a gentle rotating motion with the fingertips. Begin at the front and palpate down the midline, then palpate each side of the head.	Smooth, uniform consistency; absence of nodules or masses	Sebaceous cysts; local deformities from trauma
Inspect the facial features (e.g., symmetry of structures and of the distribution of hair).	Symmetric or slightly asymmetric facial features; palpebral fissures equal in size; symmetric nasolabial folds	Increased facial hair; thinning of eyebrows; asymmetric features; exophthalmus; myxedema facies; moon face
Inspect the eyes for edema and hollowness.		Periorbital edema; sunken eyes
Note symmetry of facial movements. Ask the client to elevate the eyebrows, frown, or lower the eyebrows, close the eyes tightly, puff the cheeks, and smile and show the teeth. See Table 11–14 on page 274.	Symmetric facial movements	Asymmetric facial movements (e.g., eye on affected side cannot close completely); drooping of lower eyelid and mouth; involuntary facial movements (i.e., tics or tremors)

The Eyes and Vision

Many people consider vision the most important sense because it allows them to interact freely with their environment and enjoy the beauty of life around them. To maintain optimum vision, people need to have their eyes examined throughout life. It is recommended that people under age 40 have their eyes tested every 3 to 5 years, or more frequently if there is a family history of diabetes, hypertension, blood dyscrasia, or eye disease (e.g., glaucoma). After age 40, an eye examination is recommended every 2 years to rule out the possibility of glaucoma.

An eye assessment should be carried out as part of the client's initial physical examination; periodic reassesments need to be made for long-term care clients. Examination of the eyes commonly includes assessment of **visual acuity** (the degree of detail the eye can discern in an image), ocular movement, **visual fields** (the area an individual can see when looking straight ahead), and external structures. Most eye assessment procedures involve inspection. Consideration is also given to developmental changes and to individual hygienic practices, if the client wears contact lenses or an artificial eye. For the anatomic structures of the eye, see Figures 11–18 and 11–19.

Many people wear eyeglasses or contact lenses to correct common refractive errors of the lens of the eye. These errors include **myopia** (nearsightedness), **hyperopia** (farsightedness), and **presbyopia** (loss of elasticity of the lens and thus loss of ability to see close objects). Presbyopia begins at about 45 years of age. People notice that they have difficulty reading newsprint. Often two corrective lenses (bifocals) are

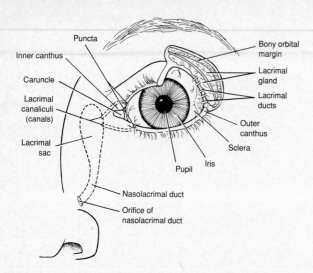

FIGURE 11–18 The external structures and lacrimal apparatus of the left eye.

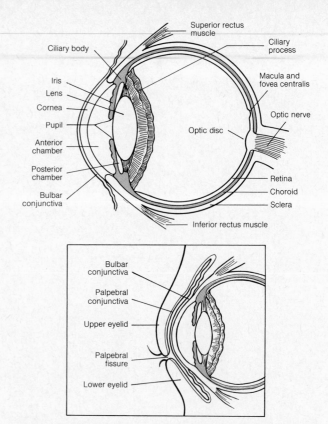

FIGURE 11–19 Anatomic structures of the right eye, lateral view.

required—one for near vision or reading, the other for far vision. **Astigmatism**, an uneven curvature of the cornea that prevents horizontal and vertical rays from focusing on the retina, is a common problem that may occur in conjunction with myopia and hyperopia.

Three types of eye charts are available to test visual acuity (Figure 11–20). The child acquires normal 20/20 vision by 6 years of age. Persons with denominators of 40 or more on the Snellen chart with or without corrective lenses need to be referred to an ophthalmologist.

Common inflammatory visual problems that nurses may encounter in clients include conjunctivitis, dacryocystitis, hordeolum, iritis, and contusions or hematomas of the eyelids and surrounding structures. **Conjunctivitis** (inflammation of the bulbar and palpebral conjunctiva) may result from foreign bodies, chemicals, allergenic agents, bacteria, or viruses. Redness, itching, tearing, and mucopurulent discharge occur. During sleep, the eyelids may become encrusted and matted together. **Dacryocystitis** (inflammation of the lacrimal sac) is manifested by tearing and a discharge from the nasolacrimal duct. **Hordeolum** (sty) is a redness, swelling, and tenderness of the hair follicle and glands that empty at the edge of the eyelids. **Iritis** (inflammation of the iris) may be caused by local or systemic infections and results in pain, tearing, and **photophobia** (sensitivity to light). **Contusions** or **hematomas** are "black eyes" resulting from injury.

Cataracts tend to occur in those over 65 years old. This opacity of the lens or its capsule, which blocks light rays, in frequently corrected by surgery. Cataracts may also occur in infants due to a malformation of the lens if the mother contracted rubella

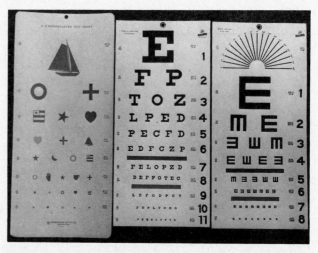

FIGURE 11–20 Three types of eye charts: the preschool children's chart (left), Snellen standard chart (center), and the Snellen E chart for clients unable to read (right).

in the first trimester of pregnancy. **Glaucoma** (a disturbance in the circulation of aqueous fluid, which causes an increase in intraocular pressure) is the most frequent cause of blindness in people over 40. It can be controlled if diagnosed early. Danger signs of glaucoma include blurred or foggy vision, loss of peripheral vision, difficulty focusing on close objects, difficulty adjusting to dark rooms, and seeing rainbow-colored rings around lights.

Eyelids that lie at or below the pupil margin are referred to as **ptosis** and are usually associated with aging, edema from drug allergy or systemic disease (e.g., kidney disease), congenital lid muscle dysfunction, neuromuscular disease (e.g., myasthenia gravis), and third cranial nerve impairment. Eversion, an outturning of the eyelid, is called **ectropion**; inversion, an inturning of the lid, is called **entropion**. These abnormalities are often associated with scarring injuries or the aging process.

Pupils are normally black, are equal in size (about 3 to 7 mm in diameter), and have round, smooth borders. Cloudy pupils are often indicative of cataracts. Enlarged pupils (**mydriasis**) may indicate injury or glaucoma, or result from certain drugs (e.g., atropine). Constricted pupils (**miosis**) may indicate an inflammation of the iris or result from such drugs as morphine or pilocarpine. Unequal pupils (**anisocoria**) may result from a central nervous system disorder; however, slight variations may be normal. The iris is normally flat and round. A bulging toward the cornea can indicate increased intraocular pressure.

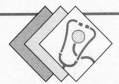

Assessing Eye Structures and Visual Acuity

NURSING HISTORY FOCUS
Family history of diabetes, hypertension, blood dyscrasia, or eye disease, injury, or surgery; client's last visit to an ophthalmologist; current use of eye medications; use of contact lenses or eyeglasses; hygienic practices for corrective lenses; current symptoms of eye problems (e.g., changes in visual acuity, blurring of vision, tearing, spots, photophobia, itching, or pain).

ASSESSMENT	NORMAL FINDINGS	DEVIATIONS FROM NORMAL
External Eye Structures		
Inspect the eyebrows for hair distribution and alignment and skin quality and movement (ask client to raise and lower the eyebrows).	Hair evenly distributed; skin intact Eyebrows symmetrically aligned; equal movement	Loss of hair; scaling and flakiness of skin Unequal alignment and movement of eyebrows
Inspect the eyelashes for evenness of distribution and direction of curl.	Equally distributed; curled slightly outward	Turned inward (see inversion of eyelid, below)
Inspect the eyelids for surface characteristics (e.g., skin quality and texture), **position in relation to the cornea, ability to blink, and frequency of blinking.** For proper visual examination of the upper eyelids, elevate the eyebrows with your thumb and index fingers, and have the client close the eyes (Figure 11–21). Inspect the lower eyelids while the client's eyes are closed.	Skin intact; no discharge; no discoloration Lids close symmetrically Approximately 15 to 20 involuntary blinks per minute; bilateral blinking When lids open, no visible sclera above corneas, and upper and lower borders of cornea are slightly covered	Redness, swelling, flaking, crusting, plaques, discharge, nodules, lesions Lids close asymmetrically, incompletely, or painfully Rapid, monocular, absent, or infrequent blinking Ptosis, ectropion, or entropion; rim of sclera visible between lid and iris (possible hyperthyroidism)

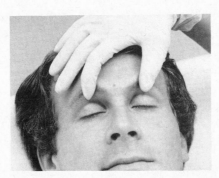

FIGURE 11–21 Inspecting the upper eyelids.

▶ Assessing Eye Structures and Visual Acuity *CONTINUED*

ASSESSMENT	NORMAL FINDINGS	DEVIATIONS FROM NORMAL
Inspect the bulbar conjunctiva (that lying over the sclera) **for color, texture, and the presence of lesions**. Retract the eyelids with your thumb and index finger, exerting pressure over the upper and lower bony orbits, and ask the client to look up, down, and from side to side.	Transparent; capillaries sometimes evident; sclera appears white (yellowish in dark-skinned clients)	Jaundiced sclera (e.g., in liver disease); excessively pale sclera (e.g., in anemia); reddened sclera; lesions or nodules (may indicate damage by mechanical, chemical, allergenic, or bacterial agents)
Inspect the palpebral conjunctiva (that lining the eyelids) by everting the lids. **Note color, texture, and the presence of lesions.** Evert both lower lids, and ask the client to look up. Then gently retract the lower lids with the index fingers.	Shiny, smooth, and pink or red	Extremely pale (possible anemia); extremely red (inflammation); nodules or other lesions
Evert the upper lids if a problem is suspected (see the box below).		

Everting the Upper Eyelid

- Ask the client to look down while keeping the eyes slightly open. *Closing the eyelids contracts the orbicular muscle, which prevents lid eversion.*

- Gently grasp the client's eyelashes with the thumb and index finger. Pull the lashes gently downward. *Upward or outward pulling on the eyelashes causes muscle contraction.*

- Place a cotton-tipped applicator stick about 1 cm above the lid margin, and push it gently downward while holding the eyelashes (Figure 11–22). These actions evert the lid, i.e., flip the lower part of the lid over on top of itself.

- Hold the margin of the everted lid or the eyelashes against the ridge of the upper bony orbit with the applicator stick or the thumb (Figure 11–23).

- Inspect the conjunctiva for color, texture, lesions, and foreign bodies.

- To return the lid to its normal position, gently pull the lashes forward, and ask the client to look up and blink.

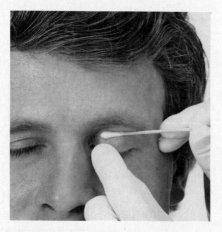

FIGURE 11–22 Everting the upper eyelid.

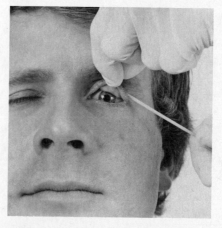

FIGURE 11–23 Holding the margin of the everted upper eyelid.

▶ **Assessing Eye Structures and Visual Acuity** *CONTINUED*

ASSESSMENT	NORMAL FINDINGS	DEVIATIONS FROM NORMAL
Inspect and palpate the lacrimal gland. See the box below.	No edema or tenderness over lacrimal gland	Swelling or tenderness over lacrimal gland
Inspect and palpate the lacrimal sac and nasolacrimal duct. See the box below.	No edema or tearing	Evidence of increased tearing; regurgitation of fluid on palpation of lacrimal sac

Palpating the Lacrimal Gland, Lacrimal Sac, and Nasolacrimal Duct

- Using the tip of your index finger, palpate the lacrimal gland (Figure 11–24).
- Observe for edema between the lower lid and the nose.

- Observe for evidence of increased tearing.
- Using the tip of your index finger, palpate inside the lower orbital rim near the inner canthus (Figure 11–25).

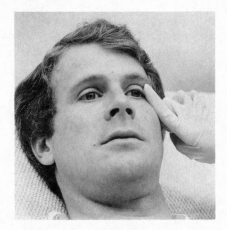

FIGURE 11–24   Palpating the lacrimal gland.

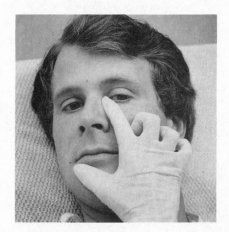

FIGURE 11–25   Palpating the lacrimal sac and nasolacrimal duct.

Inspect the cornea for clarity and texture. Ask the client to look straight ahead. Hold a penlight at an obligue angle to the eye, and move the light slowly across the corneal surface.	Transparent, shiny and smooth; details of the iris are visible In older people, a thin, grayish white ring around the margin, called arcus senilis, may be evident	Opaque; surface not smooth (may be the result of trauma or abrasion) Arcus senilis in clients under age 40 is abnormal
Perform the corneal sensitivity (reflex) test to determine the function of the fifth (trigeminal) cranial nerve. Ask the client to keep both eyes open and look straight ahead. With a wisp of cotton, approach from behind and beside the client, and lightly touch the cornea with the cotton wisp.	Client blinks when the cornea is touched, indicating that the trigeminal nerve is intact	One or both eyelids fail to respond

► **Assessing Eye Structures and Visual Acuity** *CONTINUED*

ASSESSMENT	NORMAL FINDINGS	DEVIATIONS FROM NORMAL
Inspect the anterior chamber for transparency and depth. Use the same oblique lighting as used to test the cornea.	Transparent No shadows of light on iris Depth of about 3 mm	Cloudy Crescent-shaped shadows on far side of iris Shallow chamber (possible glaucoma)
Inspect the pupils for color, shape, and symmetry of size. Pupil charts are available in some agencies. See Figure 11–26 for variations in pupil diameters.	Black in color; equal in size; normally 3 to 7 mm in diameter; round, smooth border, iris flat and round	Cloudiness, mydriasis, miosis, anisocoria; bulging of iris toward cornea

1 2 3   4   5   6   7   8   9   10

FIGURE 11–26 Variations in pupil diameters in millimeters.

Assess each pupil's direct and consensual reaction to light to determine the function of the third (oculomotor) and fourth (trochlear) cranial nerves. See the box below.	Illuminated pupil constricts (direct response) Nonilluminated pupil constricts (consensual response)	Neither pupil constricts Unequal responses Absent responses

---

Assessing Pupil Reactions

Direct and Consensual Reaction to Light

- Partially darken the room.
- Ask the client to look straight ahead.
- Using a penlight or flashlight and approaching from the side, shine a light on the pupil.
- Observe the response of the illuminated pupil. It should constrict (direct response).
- Again shine the light on the pupil, and observe the response of the other pupil. It should also constrict (consensual response).

Reaction to Accommodation

- Hold an object (a penlight or pencil) about 10 cm (4

in) from the bridge of the client's nose.
- Ask the client to look first at the top of the object and then at a distant object (e.g., the far wall) behind the penlight. Alternate the gaze from the near to the far object.
- Observe the pupil response. The pupils should constrict when looking at the near object and dilate when looking at the far object.
- Next, move the penlight or pencil toward the client's nose. The pupils should converge.

To record normal assessment of the pupils, use the abbreviation PERRLA (pupils equally round and react to light and accommodation).

Assess each pupil's reaction to accommodation. See the box above.	Pupils constrict when looking at near object; pupils dilate when looking at far object; pupils converge when near object is moved toward nose	One or both pupils fail to constrict, dilate, or converge
Visual Fields		
Assess peripheral visual fields to determine function of the retina and neuronal visual pathways to the brain and second (optic) cranial nerve. See the box on page 221.	When looking straight ahead, client can see objects in the periphery	Visual field smaller than normal (possible glaucoma); one-half vision in one or both eyes (indicates nerve damage)
Extraocular Muscle Tests		
Assess six ocular movements to determine eye alignment and coordination. These can be performed on clients over 6 months of age. See the box on page 221.	Both eyes coordinated, move in unison, with parallel alignment End-point **nystagmus** (rapid involuntary movement of the eyeball on the extreme lateral gaze)	Eye movements not coordinated or parallel; one or both eyes fail to follow a penlight in specific directions, (e.g., **strabismus** (cross-eye or squint) Nystagmus other than end-point (may indicate neurologic impairment)

▶ **Assessing Eye Structures and Visual Acuity** *CONTINUED*

Assessing Peripheral Visual Fields

- Have the client sit directly facing you at a distance of 60 to 90 cm (2 to 3 ft).

- Ask the client to cover the right eye with a card and look directly at your nose.

- Cover or close your eye directly opposite the client's covered eye (i.e., your left eye), and look directly at the client's nose.

- Hold an object (e.g., a penlight or pencil) in your fingers, extend your arm, and move the object into the visual field from various points in the periphery (Figure 11–27). The object should be at an equal distance from the client and yourself. Ask the client to tell you when the moving object is first spotted.

  a. To test the *temporal field* of the left eye, extend and move your right arm in from the client's right periphery. Temporally, peripheral objects can be seen at right angles (90°) to the central point of vision.

  b. To test the *upward field* of the left eye, extend and move the right arm down from the upward periphery. The upward field of vision is normally 50° because the orbital ridge is in the way.

  c. To test the *downward field* of the left eye, extend and move the right arm up from the lower periphery. The downward field of vision is normally 70° because the cheekbone is in the way.

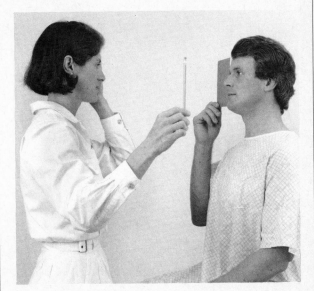

FIGURE 11–27 Assessing the client's left peripheral visual field.

  d. To test the *nasal field* of the left eye, extend and move your left arm in from the periphery. The nasal field of vision is normally 50° away from the central point of vision because the nose is in the way.

- Repeat the above steps for the right eye, reversing the process.

Assessing the Six Ocular Movements

- Stand directly in front of the client, and hold the penlight at a comfortable distance, e.g., 30 cm (1 ft) in front of the client's eyes.

- Ask the client to hold the head in a fixed position facing you and to follow the movements of the penlight with the *eyes only*.

- Move the penlight in a slow, orderly manner through the six cardinal fields of gaze, i.e., from the center of the eye along the lines of the arrows in Figure 11–28 and back to the center.

- Stop the movement of the penlight periodically so that nystagmus can be detected.

These six positions are used because six muscles guide the movements of each eye. Four *rectus* muscles (superior, inferior, lateral, and medial) move the eye in the direction indicated Two *oblique* muscles (superior and inferior) rotate the eyeball on its axis. Cranial nerves III (oculomotor), IV (trochlear), and VI (abducens) innervate these muscles. Moving the object through the six positions can identify a nonfunctioning muscle or associated cranial nerve.

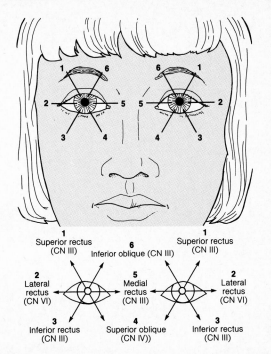

FIGURE 11–28 The six muscles that govern eye movement.

► **Assessing Eye Structures and Visual Acuity** *CONTINUED*

ASSESSMENT	NORMAL FINDINGS	DEVIATIONS FROM NORMAL
Perform the cover-uncover patch test to determine eye alignment. See the box below.	Uncovered eye does not move from fixed point when other eye is covered Newly uncovered eye, if well aligned, does not move when index card is removed	Uncovered eye moves to focus on fixed point, indicating it was *not* well aligned before other eye was covered; it is shifting from a lateral to central gaze Newly uncovered eye moves to focus on fixed point, indicating it was *not* well aligned when covered; muscle weakness is apparent when eye turns outward while covered; as eye is uncovered, it quickly moves inward to bring itself back in alignment
Perform the corneal light reflex test to determine eye alignment. See the box below.	Light reflection appears at symmetric spots in both eyes	Light reflection appears at different spots in each eye (asymmetric)

Testing Eye Alignment

Cover-Uncover Patch Test

- Ask the client to stare straight ahead at a fixed point, e.g., at a penlight held 15 cm (6 in) in front of the eyes.
- Cover one of the client's eyes with an eye cover or index card while observing the uncovered eye.
- Remove the eye cover, and observe the newly uncovered eye for movement.

- Repeat the above steps for the other eye.
- Test each eye several times to confirm your findings.

Corneal Light Reflex Text
- Darken the room.
- Ask the client to stare straight ahead.
- Shine a penlight on the bridge of the nose.
- Observe the light reflection in both corneas.

Visual Acuity

Assess near vision by providing adequate lighting and asking the client to read from a magazine or newspaper held at a distance of 36 cm (14 in). If the client normally wears corrective lenses, the glasses or lenses should be worn during the test.	Able to read newsprint	Difficulty reading newsprint unless due to aging process
Assess distance vision by asking the client to wear corrective lenses, unless they are used for reading only, i.e., for distances of only 36 cm (12 to 14 in). See the box below.	20/20 vision on Snellen chart from age 6 onward	Denominator of 40 or more on Snellen chart with corrective lenses

---

Assessing Distance Vision

- Ask the client to stand or sit 6 m (20 ft) from a Snellen chart, cover the eye not being tested, and identify the letters on the Snellen chart.
- Take three readings: right eye, left eye, both eyes.
- Record the readings of each eye and both eyes, i.e., the smallest line from which the person is able to read one-half or more of the letters.

At the end of each line of the Snellen chart are standardized numbers (fractions). The top line is 20/200. The numerator (top number) is always 20, the distance the person stands from the chart. The denominator (bottom number) is the distance from which the normal eye can read the chart. Therefore, a person who has 20/40 vision, can see at 20 feet from the chart what a normal-sighted person can see at 40 feet from the chart. Visual acuity is recorded as "s̄c" (without correction), or "c̄c" (with correction). You can also indicate how many letters were misread in the line, e.g., "visual acuity 20/40—2c̄c" indicates that two letters were misread in the 20/40 line by a client wearing corrective lenses.

▶ **Assessing Eye Structures and Visual Acuity** *CONTINUED*

ASSESSMENT	NORMAL FINDINGS	DEVIATIONS FROM NORMAL
Perform functional vision tests if the client is unable to see the top line (20/200) of the Snellen chart. See the box below.		Functional vision only (e.g., light perception, hand movements, counting fingers at 1 ft)

Performing Functional Vision Tests

Light Perception

Shine a penlight into the client's eye from a lateral position, and then turn the light off. Ask the client to tell you when the light is on or off. If the client knows when the light is on or off, the client has light perception, and the vision is recorded as "LP."

Hand Movements (H/M)

Hold your hand 30 cm (1 ft) from the client's face, and move it slowly back and forth, stopping it periodically.

Ask the client to tell you when your hand stops moving. If the client knows when your hand stops moving, record the vision as "H/M 1 ft."

Counting Fingers (C/F)

Hold up some of your fingers 30 cm (1 ft) from the client's face, and ask the client to count your fingers. If the client can do so, note on the vision record "C/F 1 ft."

THE ELDERLY: PHYSICAL CHANGES OF THE EYES AND VISION

Visual Acuity

- Visual acuity decreases as the lens of the eye ages and becomes more opaque and loses elasticity.
- The ability of the iris to accommodate to darkness and dim light diminishes.
- Peripheral vision diminishes.
- The adaptation to light (glare) and dark decreases.
- Accommodation to far objects often improves, but accommodation to near objects decreases.
- Color vision declines; older people are less able to perceive purple colors and to discriminate pastel colors.
- Many older people wear corrective lenses; they are most likely to have hyperopia. Visual changes are due to loss of elasticity (presbyopia) and transparency of the lens.
- The number of vitreous floaters increases with age.

External Eye Structures

- The skin around the orbit of the eye may darken.
- The eyeball may appear sunken because of the decrease in orbital fat.
- Skinfolds of the upper lids may seem more prominent, and the lower lids may sag.

- The eyes may appear dry and lusterless because of the decrease in tear production from the lacrimal glands.
- A thin, grayish white arc or ring (*arcus senilis*) appears around part or all of the cornea. It results from an accumulation of a lipid substance on the cornea. The cornea tends to cloud with age.
- The iris may appear pale with brown discolorations as a result of pigment degeneration.
- The conjunctiva of the eye may appear paler than that of younger adults and may take on a slightly yellow appearance because of the deposition of fat.
- Pupil reaction to light and accommodation is normally symmetrically equal but may be less brisk.
- The pupils can appear smaller in size, unequal, and irregular in shape because of sclerotic changes in the iris.

Internal Eye Structures

- The fundus may be yellower in appearance and lack luster.
- The blood vessels narrow slightly.
- The macula and fovea are less bright.

The Ears and Hearing

Assessment of the ear includes direct inspection and palpation of the external ear, inspection of the remaining parts of the ear by an **otoscope**, and determination of auditory acuity. The ear is usually assessed during an initial physical examination; periodic reassessments may be necessary for long-term clients or those with hearing problems.

The ear is divided into three parts: external ear, middle ear, and inner ear. The external ear includes the **auricle**, or **pinna**, the external auditory canal, and the **tympanic membrane**, or eardrum (Figure 11–29. Landmarks of the auricle include the **lobule** (earlobe), **helix** (the posterior curve of the auricle's upper aspect), **anthelix** (the anterior curve of the auricle's upper aspect), **tragus** (the cartilaginous protrusion at the entrance to the ear canal), **triangular fossa** (a depression of the antihelix), and **external auditory meatus** (the entrance to the ear canal). Although not part of the ear, the **mastoid**, a bony prominence behind the ear, is another important landmark (Figure 11–30). The external ear canal is curved, is about 2.5 cm (1 in) long in the adult, and ends at the tympanic membrane. It is covered with skin that has many fine hairs, glands, and nerve endings. The glands secrete **cerumen** (earwax), which lubricates and protects the canal.

The middle ear is an air-filled cavity that starts at the tympanic membrane and contains three **ossicles** (bones of sound transmission): the **malleus** (hammer), which is the most easily seen, the **incus** (anvil), and the **stapes** (stirrups) (Figure 11–29). The **eustachian tube**, another part of the middle ear, connects the middle ear to the nasopharynx. The tube stabilizes the air pressure between the external atmosphere and the middle ear, thus preventing rupture of the tympanic membrane and discomfort produced by marked pressure differences.

The inner ear contains the **cochlea**, a seashell-shaped structure essential for sound transmission and hearing, and the **vestibule** and **semicircular canals**, which contain the organs of equilibrium (Figure 11–29).

Sound transmission and hearing are complex processes. In brief, sound can be transmitted by air conduction or bone conduction. Air-conducted transmission occurs by this process:

1. A sound stimulus enters the external canal and reaches the tympanic membrane.

2. The sound waves cross the tympanic membrane and reach the ossicles.

3. The sound waves travel from the ossicles to the opening in the inner ear (oval window).

4. The cochlea receives the sound vibrations.

5. The stimulus travels to the auditory nerve (the eighth cranial nerve) and the cerebral cortex.

Bone-conducted sound transmission occurs when skull bones transport the sound directly to the auditory nerve.

The curvature of the external ear canal differs with age. In the infant and toddler, the canal has an upward curvature. By age 3, the ear canal assumes the more downward curvature of adulthood.

Audiometric evaluations, which measure hearing at various decibels, are recommended for the elderly. A common hearing deficit with age is loss of ability to hear high-frequency sounds, such as *f, s, sh,* and

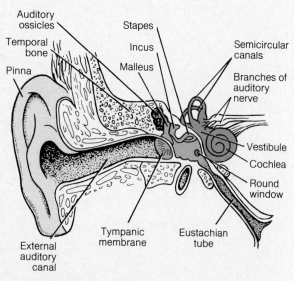

FIGURE 11–29 Anatomic structures of the external, middle, and inner ear.

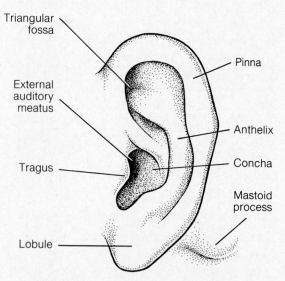

FIGURE 11–30 Landmarks of the external ear.

ph. This neurosensory hearing deficit does not respond well to use of a hearing aid.

To inspect the external ear canal and tympanic membrane, the nurse inserts an **otoscope** (Figure 11–31) into the external auditory canal.

In some practice settings, the nurse does not perform otoscopic examinations. In others, the nurse's examination is limited to inspection of the external ear canal and the color of the tympanic membrane.

Advanced practitioners use tuning fork tests to assess whether the client's hearing loss is a conduction, sensorineural, or mixed problem. *Conduction hearing loss* is the result of interrupted transmission of sound waves through the outer and middle ear structures. Possible causes are a tear in the tympanic membrane or an obstruction, due to swelling or other causes, in the auditory canal. *Sensorineural hearing loss* is the result of damage to the inner ear, the auditory nerve, or the hearing center in the brain. *Mixed hearing loss* is a combination of conduction and sensorineural loss.

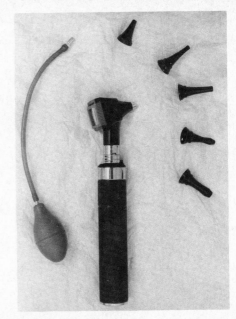

FIGURE 11–31 An otoscope with ear specula and an air insufflator.

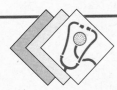

Assessing the Ears and Hearing

NURSING HISTORY FOCUS

Family history of hearing problems or loss; presence of any ear problems; medication history, especially if there are complaints of ringing in ears; any hearing difficulty: its onset, factors contributing to it, and how it interferes with activities of daily living; use of a corrective hearing device: when and from whom it was obtained.

ASSESSMENT	NORMAL FINDINGS	DEVIATIONS FROM NORMAL
Auricles **Inspect the auricles for color, symmetry of size, and position.** To inspect position, note the level at which the superior aspect of the auricle attaches to the head in relation to the eye.	Color same as facial skin	Bluish color of earlobes (e.g., cyanosis); pallor (e.g., frostbite); excessive redness (inflammation or fever)
	Symmetric position. Line drawn from lateral angle of eye to point where top part of auricle joins head is horizontal; imaginary line drawn from the top to the bottom of the ear varies no more than 10° from the vertical (Figure 11–32)	Low-set ears (associated with a congenital abnormality, such as Down syndrome)

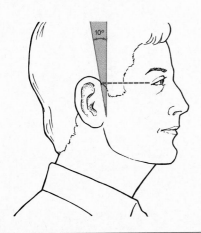

FIGURE 11–32 Normal ear alignment and ear angle.

▶ **Assessing the Ears and Hearing** *CONTINUED*

ASSESSMENT	NORMAL FINDINGS	DEVIATIONS FROM NORMAL
Palpate the auricles for texture, elasticity, and areas of tenderness.	Mobile, firm, and not tender; pinna recoils after it is folded	Lesions (e.g., cysts); flaky, scaly skin (e.g., seborrhea); tenderness when moved or pressed (may indicate inflammation or infection of external ear)
• Pull the auricle upward, downward, and backward.		
• Fold the pinna forward (it should recoil).		
• Push in on the tragus.		
• Apply pressure to the mastoid process.		
External Ear Canal and Tympanic Membrane		
Using an otoscope, inspect the external ear canal for cerumen, skin lesions, pus, and blood and the tympanic membrane for color.	Distal third contains hair follicles and glands Dry cerumen, grayish-tan color; or sticky, wet cerumen in various shades of brown	Redness and discharge Scaling Excessive cerumen obstructing canal
• Attach a speculum to the otoscope.		
• Use the largest diameter that will fit the ear canal without causing discomfort. *This achieves maximum vision of the entire ear canal and tympanic membrane.*		
• Tip the client's head away from you, and straighten the ear canal. For an adult, straighten the ear canal by pulling the pinna up and back (Figure 11–33). *Straightening the ear canal facilitates vision of the ear canal and the tympanic membrane.*		

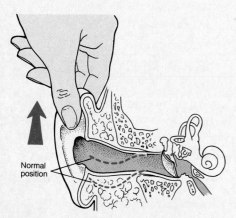

Normal position

FIGURE 11–33 Straightening the ear canal of an adult by pulling the pinna up and back.

▶ **Assessing the Ears and Hearing** *CONTINUED*

ASSESSMENT	NORMAL FINDINGS	DEVIATIONS FROM NORMAL

• Hold the otoscope either (a) right side up, with your fingers between the otoscope handle and the client's head or (b) upside down, with your fingers and the ulnar surface of your hand against the client's head (Figure 11–34). *This stabilizes the head and protects the eardrum and canal from injury if a quick head movement occurs.*

• Gently insert the tip of the otoscope into the ear canal, avoiding pressure by the speculum against either side of the ear canal. *The inner two-thirds of the ear canal is bony; if the speculum is pressed against either side, the client will experience discomfort.*

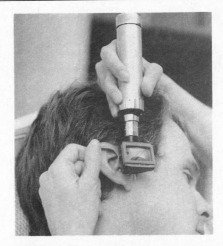

FIGURE 11–34   Inserting an otoscope.

Inspect the tympanic membrane.

• Inspect the membrane for color and gloss.	Pearly gray color, semitransparent	Pink to red, some opacity Yellow-amber White Blue or deep red Dull surface

Gross Hearing Acuity Tests

Assess client's response to normal voice tones. If client has difficulty hearing the normal voice, proceed with the following tests.	Normal voice tones audible	Normal voice tones not audible (e.g., requests nurse to repeat words or statements, leans toward the speaker, turns the head, cups the ears, or speaks in loud tone of voice)

Assess client's response to whispered voice. This test is used for screening purposes only, because maintaining consistency in the whispered voice is difficult.

• Stand 30 to 60 cm (1 to 2 ft) from the client in a position where the client cannot read your lips. Ask the client to occlude one ear by putting a finger in it.

• Whisper some nonconsecutive numbers and have the client tell you what was heard. Increase the loudness of the whisper until the client can identify at least 50% of the numbers. Repeat the process with the other ear. *Nonconsecutive numbers are used so that the client cannot anticipate what number will follow.*	Able to repeat nonconsecutive numbers	Unable to repeat 50% of numbers whispered

▶

► **Assessing the Ears and Hearing** *CONTINUED*

ASSESSMENT	NORMAL FINDINGS	DEVIATIONS FROM NORMAL
Perform the watch tick test. The ticking of a watch has a higher pitch than the human voice.	Able to hear ticking in both ears	Unable to hear ticking in one or both ears
• Have the client occlude one ear. Out of the client's sight, place a ticking watch 2 to 3 cm (1 to 2 in) from the unoccluded ear.		
• Ask whether the client can hear it. Repeat with the other ear.		
Tuning Fork Tests		
Perform Weber's test to assess bone conduction. See the box below. Note findings as Weber positive and indicate whether right or left ear.	Sound is heard in both ears or is localized at the center of the head (Weber negative)	Sound is heard better in impaired ear, indicating a bone-conductive hearing loss (e.g., due to obstruction of ossicles), *or* sound is heard better in ear without a problem, indicating a sensorineural disturbance (nerve or inner ear damage)

Performing Tuning Fork Tests

Weber's Test

This test assesses bone conduction by testing the lateralization (sideward transmission of sounds)

• Hold the tuning fork at its base. Activate it by tapping the fork gently against the back of your hand near the knuckles or by stroking the fork between your thumb and index fingers. It should be made to ring softly.

• Place the base of the vibrating fork on top of the client's head (Figure 11–35) and ask where the client hears the noise.

Rinne Test

This test compares air conduction to bone conduction.

• Ask the client to block the hearing in one ear intermittently by moving a fingertip in and out of the ear canal.

• Hold the handle of the activated tuning fork on the mastoid process of one ear (Figure 11–36) until the client states that the vibration can no longer be heard.

• Immediately hold the still vibrating fork prongs in front of the client's ear canal (Figure 11–37). Push aside the client's hair if necessary. Ask whether the client now hears the sound. Sound conducted by air is heard more readily than sound conducted by bone. The tuning fork vibrations conducted by air are normally heard longer.

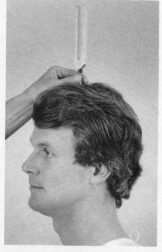

FIGURE 11–35 Placing the base of the tuning fork on the client's skull (Weber's test).

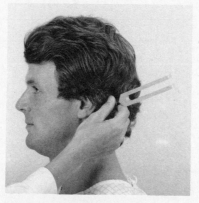

FIGURE 11–36 Placing the base of the tuning fork on the mastoid process (Rinne test).

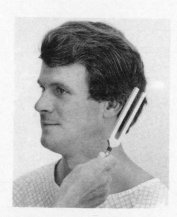

FIGURE 11–37 Placing the tuning fork prongs in front of the client's ear canal (Rinne test).

▶ **Assessing the Ears and Hearing** *CONTINUED*

ASSESSMENT	NORMAL FINDINGS	DEVIATIONS FROM NORMAL
Conduct the Rinne test to compare air conduction to bone conduction. See the box on page 228.	Air-conducted hearing is greater than bone-conducted hearing, i.e., AC > BC (positive Rinne)	Bone conduction time is equal to or longer than the air conduction time, i.e., BC > AC or BC = AC (negative Rinne; indicates a conductive hearing loss)

THE ELDERLY: PHYSICAL CHANGES OF THE EARS AND HEARING

- The skin of the ear may appear dry and be less resilient because of the loss of connective tissue.
- Increased coarse and wirelike hair growth occurs along the helix, anthelix, and tragus.
- The pinna increases in both width and length, and the earlobe elongates.
- Earwax is drier.
- The tympanic membrane is more translucent and less flexible. The intensity of the light reflex may diminish slightly.
- Sensorineural hearing loss occurs.
- Generalized hearing loss (presbycusis) occurs in all frequencies, although the first symptom is the loss of high-frequency sounds: the *f, s, sh,* and *ph* sounds. To such persons, conversation can be distorted and result in what appears to be inappropriate or confused behavior.

The Nose and Sinuses

A nurse can inspect the nasal passages very simply with a flashlight. However, a nasal *speculum,* which is a lighted instrument, facilitates examination of the nasal chambers.

Assessment of the nose includes inspection and palpation of the external nose (the upper third of the nose is bone; the remainder is cartilage); patency of the nasal cavities; and inspection of the nasal cavities.

Major structures of the nose are shown in Figure 11–38. The nasal turbinates increase the surface of the mucous membrane in the nares. The clefts between the turbinates are called meati. Each meatus is named for the adjacent turbinate, e.g., the inferior meatus is near the inferior turbinate. The nurse also inspects and palpates the facial sinuses (Figure 11–39 on page 231). Advanced practitioners may perform transillumination of the sinuses.

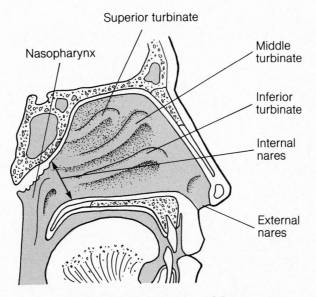

FIGURE 11–38 Major structures of the nose.

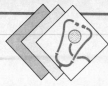

Assessing the Nose and Sinuses

History of allergies, difficulty breathing through the nose, sinus infections, injuries to nose or face, nosebleeds; any medications taken; any changes in sense of smell.

ASSESSMENT	NORMAL FINDINGS	DEVIATIONS FROM NORMAL
Nose		
Inspect the external nose for any deviations in shape, size, or color and flaring or discharge from the nares.	Symmetric and straight No discharge or flaring Uniform color	Asymmetric Discharge from nares Localized areas of redness or presence of skin lesions
Lightly palpate the external nose to determine any areas of tenderness, masses, and displacements of bone and cartilage.	Not tender; no lesions	Tenderness on palpation; presence of lesions
Determine patency of both nasal cavities. Ask the client to close the mouth, exert pressure on one naris, and breathe through the opposite naris. Repeat the procedure to assess patency of the opposite naris.	Air moves freely as the client breathes through the nares	Air movement is restricted in one or both nares
Inspect the nasal cavities using a flashlight or a nasal speculum as follows:		
• Tip the client's head back.		
• If using a speculum, hold it in your nondominant hand, and place your index finger on the side of the nose to stabilize its position. Use your dominant hand to position the head and hold the light.		
• Inspect the lining of the nares (mucosa) and the coarse hairs that filter the air. Observe for the presence of redness, swelling, growths, and discharge.	Mucosa pink Clear, watery discharge No lesions	Mucosa red, edematous Abnormal discharge (e.g., purulent) Presence of lesions (e.g., polyps)
• Inspect the position of the nasal septum between the nasal chambers, noting in particular any deviation to right or left.	Nasal septum intact and in midline	Septum deviated
Facial Sinuses		
Palpate the maxillary and frontal sinuses for tenderness.	Not tender	Tenderness in one or more sinuses
Transilluminate the frontal sinuses by placing a penlight against the inner aspect of the supraorbital ridge of the frontal bone (see Figure 11–39). This is best done in a darkened room.	Sinuses are well outlined, contain air, and light up equally	Fluid in sinuses appears darker on transillumination

► **Assessing the Nose and Sinuses** *CONTINUED*

ASSESSMENT	NORMAL FINDINGS	DEVIATIONS FROM NORMAL
Transilluminate the maxillary sinuses by placing a penlight in the mouth and shining it to the left and to the right.	As above	As above

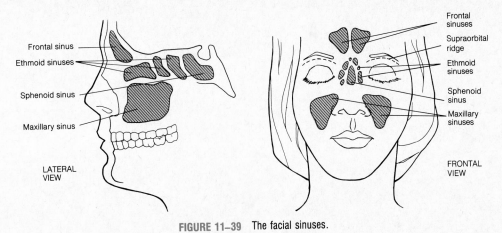

FIGURE 11–39   The facial sinuses.

THE ELDERLY: PHYSICAL CHANGES OF THE NOSE AND SENSE OF SMELL

- The sense of smell markedly diminishes because of a decrease in the number of olfactory nerve fibers and atrophy of the remaining fibers. Older persons are less able to identify and discriminate odors.

- Nosebleeds may result from hypertensive disease or other arterial vessel changes.

The Mouth and Oropharynx

The mouth and pharynx are composed of a number of structures: lips, inner and buccal mucosa, the tongue and floor of the mouth, teeth and gums, hard and soft palate, uvula, salivary glands, tonsillar pillars, and tonsils. Anatomic structures of the mouth are shown in Figure 11–40.

By age 25, most people have all their permanent teeth (Figure 11–41). For information about structures of the teeth, see Chapter 16, page 402.

Normally, three pairs of salivary glands empty into the oral cavity: the parotid, submandibular, and sublingual glands (Figure 11–40). The *parotid gland* is the largest and empties through the Stensen's duct opposite the second molar. The *submandibular gland* empties through Wharton's duct, which is situated at the side of the frenulum on the floor of the mouth. The *sublingual salivary gland* lies in the floor of the mouth and has numerous openings.

Dental **caries** (cavities) and **periodontal disease (pyorrhea)** are two problems that most fre-

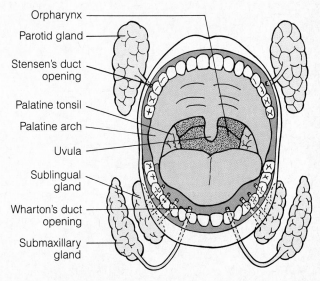

FIGURE 11–40   Anatomic structures of the mouth.

quently affect the teeth. Both problems are commonly associated with plaque and tartar deposits. **Plaque** is an *invisible* soft film that adheres to the enamel surface of teeth; it consists of bacteria, molecules of saliva, and remnants of epithelial cells and leukocytes. When plaque is unchecked, tartar (dental calculus) forms. **Tartar** is a visible, hard deposit of plaque and dead bacteria that forms at the gum lines. Tartar buildup can alter the fibers that attach the teeth to the gum and eventually disrupt bone tissue. Periodontal disease is characterized by **gingivitis** (red, swollen *gingiva*, i.e., gum) bleeding, receding gum lines, and the formation of pockets between the teeth and gums. In advanced periodontal disease, the teeth are loose, and pus is evident when the gums are pressed.

Other problems nurses may see are **glossitis** inflammation of the tongue), **stomatitis** (inflammation of the oral mucosa), and **parotitis** (inflammation of the parotid salivary gland). The accumulation of foul matter (food, microorganisms and epithelial elements) on the teeth and gums is referred to as **sordes**.

Physical examination of the mouth includes inspection and palpation techniques. The CDC recommends that the nurse wear gloves when in contact with the buccal mucosa. Equipment needed for assessment of the mouth and pharynx includes tongue blade, gauze squares (2 × 2), a penlight or flashlight, and disposable gloves.

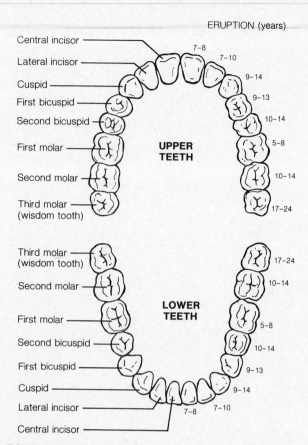

FIGURE 11–41 Permanent teeth and their times of eruption (stated in years).

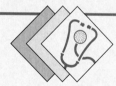

Assessing the Mouth and Oropharynx

NURSING HISTORY FOCUS
Routine pattern of dental care, last visit to dentist; length of time ulcers or other lesions have been present; any denture discomfort; any medications client is receiving.

ASSESSMENT	NORMAL FINDINGS	DEVIATIONS FROM NORMAL
Lips and Buccal Mucosa		
Inspect the outer lips for symmetry of contour, color, and texture. Ask the client to purse the lips as if to whistle.	Uniform pink color (darker, e.g., bluish hue, in Mediterranean groups and dark-skinned clients) Soft, moist, smooth texture Symmetry of contour Ability to purse lips	Pallor; cyanosis Blisters; generalized or localized swelling; fissures, crusts, or scales (may result from excessive moisture, nutritional deficiency, or fluid deficit) Inability to purse lips (indicative of facial nerve damage)
Inspect and palpate the inner lips and buccal mucosa for color, moisture, texture, and the presence of lesions. See the box on page 233.	Uniform pink color (freckled brown pigmentation in dark-skinned clients) Moist, smooth, soft, glistening, and elastic texture (drier oral mucosa in elderly due to decreased salivation)	Pallor; white patches (leukoplakia) Excessive dryness Mucosal cysts; irritations from dentures; abrasions, ulcerations; nodules

▶ **Assessing the Mouth and Oropharynx** *CONTINUED*

Inspecting and Palpating the Inner Lip, Buccal Mucosa, Teeth, and Gums

Inner Lip and Front Teeth

- Ask the client to relax the mouth, and, for better visualization, pull the lip outward away from the teeth.
- Grasp the lip on each side between the thumb and index finger (Figure 11–42).
- Palpate any lesions for size, tenderness, and consistency.
- Inspect the front teeth and gums.

Buccal Mucosa and Back Teeth

- Ask the client to open the mouth. Using a tongue blade, retract the cheek (Figure 11–43). View the surface buccal mucosa from top to bottom and back to front. A flashlight or penlight will help illuminate the surface. Repeat the procedure for the other side.
- Ask the client to open the mouth again. Using a fingercot (or gloves) and a penlight, move a finger along the inside cheek. Another finger may be moved outside the cheek.

- Examine the back teeth. For proper vision of the molars, use the index fingers of both hands to retract the cheek (Figure 11–44). Ask the client to relax the lips and first close, then open, the jaw. Closing the jaw assists in observation of tooth alignment and loss of teeth; opening the jaw assists in observation of dental fillings and caries. Observe the number of teeth, tooth color, the state of fillings, dental caries, and tartar along the base of the teeth. Note the presence and fit of partial or complete dentures.

Gums

- Inspect the gums around the molars. Observe for bleeding, color, retraction (pulling away from the teeth), edema, and lesions.
- Assess the texture of the gums by gently pressing the gum tissue with a tongue blade.

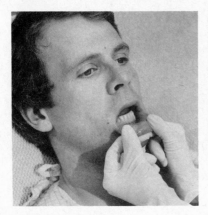
FIGURE 11–42 Inspecting the mucosa of the lower inner lip.

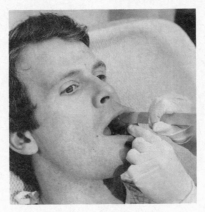
FIGURE 11–43 Inspecting the buccal mucosa using a tongue blade.

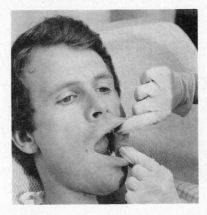
FIGURE 11–44 Inspecting the back teeth.

Teeth and Gums

Inspect the teeth and gums while examining the inner lips and buccal mucosa. See the box above.

32 adult teeth	Missing teeth Ill-fitting dentures
Smooth, white, shiny tooth enamel	Brown or black discoloration of the enamel (may indicate staining or the presence of caries)
Pink gums (bluish or dark patches in dark-skinned clients)	Excessively red gums
Moist, firm texture to gums	Spongy texture; bleeding; tenderness (may indicate periodontal disease)
No retraction of gums (pulling away from the teeth)	Receding, atrophied gums; swelling that partially covers the teeth
Smooth, intact dentures	Ill-fitting dentures; irritated and excoriated area under dentures

Inspect the dentures. Ask the client to remove complete or partial dentures. Inspect their condition, noting in particular broken or worn areas.

▶

▶ **Assessing the Mouth and Oropharynx** *CONTINUED*

ASSESSMENT	NORMAL FINDINGS	DEVIATIONS FROM NORMAL
Tongue/Floor of the Mouth		
Inspect the surface of the tongue for position, color, and texture. Ask the client to protrude the tongue.	Central position	Deviated from center (may indicate damage to hypoglossal [twelfth cranial] nerve)
	Pink color (some brown pigmentation on tongue borders in dark-skinned clients); moist; slightly rough; thin whitish coating	Smooth red tongue (may indicate iron, vitamin B_{12}, or vitamin B_3 deficiency) Dry, furry tongue (associated with fluid deficit)
	Smooth, lateral margins; no lesions	Nodes, ulcerations, discolorations (white or red areas); areas of tenderness
Inspect tongue movement. Ask the client to roll the tongue upward and move it from side to side.	Moves freely; no tenderness	Restricted mobility
Inspect the base of the tongue, the mouth floor, and the frenulum. Ask the client to place the tip of the tongue against the roof of the mouth.	Smooth tongue base with prominent veins Varicosities (tiny bluish-black or purple swollen areas) in elderly people	Swelling, ulceration
Palpate the tongue and floor of the mouth for any nodules, lumps, or excoriated areas. To palpate the tongue, use a piece of gauze to grasp its tip (stabilizes it), and with the index finger of your other hand, palpate the back of the tongue, its borders, and its base (Figure 11–45).	Smooth with no palpable nodules	Swelling, nodules

To assess function of the glossopharyngeal and hypoglossal nerves, see the Neurologic Assessment, later in this chapter.

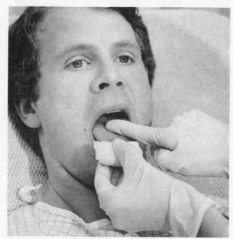

FIGURE 11–45   Palpating the tongue.

Salivary Glands		
Inspect salivary duct openings for any swelling or redness. See the discussion of salivary glands, page 231.	Same as color of buccal mucosa and floor of mouth	Inflammation (redness and swelling)
Palates and Uvula		
Inspect the hard and soft palate for color, shape, texture, and the presence of bony prominences. Ask the client to open the mouth wide and tilt the head backward. Then, depress tongue with a tongue blade as necessary, and use a penlight for appropriate visualization.	Light pink, smooth, soft palate Lighter pink hard palate, more irregular texture	Discoloration (e.g., jaundice or pallor) Palates the same color Irritations Bony growths (exostoses) growing from the hard palate

► **Assessing the Mouth and Oropharynx** *CONTINUED*

ASSESSMENT	NORMAL FINDINGS	DEVIATIONS FROM NORMAL
Inspect the uvula for position and mobility while examining the palates. To observe the uvula, ask the client to say "ah" so that the soft palate rises.	Positioned in midline of soft palate	Deviation to one side from tumor or trauma; immobility (may indicate damage to trigeminal (fifth cranial) nerve or vagus (tenth cranial) nerve
Oropharynx and Tonsils		
Inspect the oropharynx for color and texture. Inspect one side at a time to avoid eliciting the gag reflex. To expose one side of the oropharynx, press a tongue blade against the tongue on the same side about halfway back while the client tilts the head back and opens the mouth wide. Use a penlight for illumination, if needed.	Pink and smooth posterior wall	Reddened or edematous; presence of lesions, plaques, or exudate
Inspect the tonsils (behind the fauces) **for color, discharge, and size.**	Pink and smooth No discharge Of normal size (see the box below for a grading system to describe the size of tonsils)	Inflamed Presence of discharge Swollen
Elicit the gag reflex by pressing the posterior tongue with a tongue depressor.	Present	Absent (may indicate problems with glossopharyngeal or vagus nerves)

Grading System to Describe Size of Tonsils

- Grade 1 (normal): The tonsils are behind the tonsillar pillars, i.e., the soft structures supporting the soft palate.
- Grade 2: The tonsils are between the pillars and the uvula.

- Grade 3: The tonsils touch the uvula.
- Grade 4: One or both tonsils extend to the midline of the oropharynx.

THE ELDERLY: PHYSICAL CHANGES OF THE MOUTH AND SENSE OF TASTE

- The oral mucosa may be drier than that of younger persons because of decreased salivary gland activity. Decreased salivation occurs only in elderly people taking prescribed medications such as antidepressants, antihistamines, decongestants, diuretics, antihypertensives, tranquilizers, antispasmodics, and antineoplastics. Extreme dryness is associated with dehydration.
- Some receding of the gums occurs, giving an appearance of increased toothiness.
- There may be a brownish pigmentation to the gums, especially in black persons.
- Taste sensations diminish. Sweet and salty tastes are lost first. Elderly persons may add more salt and sugar

to food than they did when they were younger. Diminished taste sensation is due to atrophy of the taste buds and a decreased sense of smell. It indicates diminished function of the fifth and seventh cranial nerves.

- Tiny purple or bluish black swollen areas (varicosities) under the tongue, known as *caviar spots*, are not uncommon.
- The teeth may show signs of staining, erosion, chipping, and abrasions due to loss of dentin. Tooth loss occurs as a result of dental disease.
- The gag reflex may be slightly sluggish.

The Neck

Examination of the neck includes the muscles, lymph nodes, trachea, thyroid gland, carotid arteries, and jugular veins. Areas of the neck are defined by the sternocleidomastoid muscles, which divide each side of the neck into two triangles: the anterior and posterior (Figure 11–46). The trachea, thyroid gland, anterior cervical nodes, and carotid artery lie within the anterior triangle (the carotid artery runs parallel and anterior to the sternocleidomastoid muscle); Figure 11–47). The posterior lymph nodes lie within the posterior triangle (Figure 11–48).

Each sternocleidomastoid muscle extends from the upper sternum and the medial third of the clavicle to the mastoid process of the temporal bond behind the ear (Figure 11–46). These muscles turn and laterally flex the head. Each trapezius muscle extends from the occipital bone of the skull to the lateral third of the clavicle. These muscles draw the head to the side and back, elevate the chin, and elevate the shoulders to shrug them.

Lymph nodes in the neck that collect lymph from the head and neck structures are grouped serially and referred to as *chains*. See Figure 11–48 and Table 11–7. The deep cervical chain is not shown in Figure 11–48 because it lies beneath the sternocleidomastoid muscle.

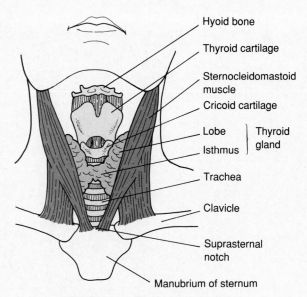

FIGURE 11-47 Structures of the neck.

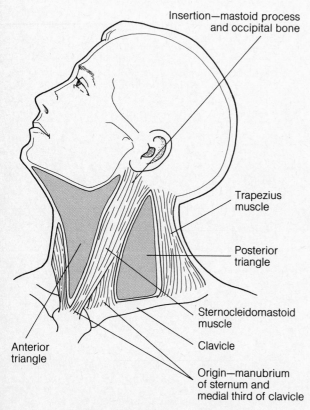

FIGURE 11-46 Major muscles of the neck.

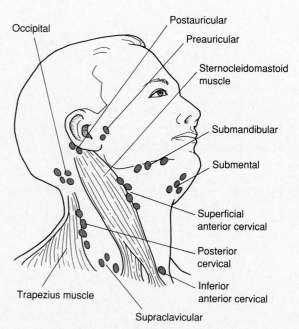

FIGURE 11-48 Lymph nodes of the neck.

TABLE 11–7   LYMPH NODES OF THE HEAD AND NECK

Node Center	Location	Area Drained
HEAD		
Occipital	At the posterior base of the skull	The occipital region of the scalp and the deep structures of the back of the neck
Postauricular (mastoid)	Behind the auricle of the ear over or in front of the mastoid process	The parietal region of the head and part of the ear
Preauricular	In front of the tragus of the ear	The forehead and upper face
FLOOR OF MOUTH		
Submandibular (submaxillary)	Along the medial border of the lower jaw, halfway between the angle of the jaw and the chin	The chin, upper lip, cheek, nose, teeth, eyelids, part of the tongue and of the floor of the mouth
Submental	Behind the tip of the mandible, in the midline, under the chin	The anterior third of the tongue, gums, and floor of the mouth
NECK		
Superficial (anterior) cervical chain	Along and anterior to the sternocleidomastoid muscle	The skin and neck
Posterior cervical chain	Along the anterior aspect of the trapezius muscle	The posterior and lateral regions of the neck, occiput, and mastoid
Deep cervical chain	Under the sternocleidomastoid muscle	The larynx, thyroid gland, trachea, and upper part of the esophagus
Supraclavicular	Above the clavicle, in the angle between the clavicle and the sternocleidomastoid muscle	The lateral regions of the neck and lungs

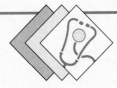

Assessing the Neck

NURSING HISTORY FOCUS
Any problems with neck lumps; neck pain or stiffness; when and how any lumps occurred; any previous diagnoses of thyroid problems: over- or underfunction of the thyroid; tests taken, test results, medications ordered, former and current dosages, and any other treatments provided (e.g., surgery, radiation).

ASSESSMENT	NORMAL FINDINGS	DEVIATIONS FROM NORMAL
Neck Muscles		
Inspect the neck muscles (sternocleidomastoid and trapezius) for abnormal swellings or masses. Ask the client to hold the head erect.	Muscles equal in size; head centered	Unilateral neck swelling; head tilted to one side (indicates presence of masses, injury, muscle weakness, shortening of sternocleidomastoid muscle, scars)
Observe head movement. Ask client to	Coordinated, smooth movements with no discomfort	Muscle tremor, spasm, or stiffness
• Move the chin to the chest (determines function of the sternocleidomastoid muscle).	Head flexes 45°	Limited range of motion; painful movements; involuntary movements (e.g., up-and-down nodding movements associated with Parkinson's disease)
• Move the head back so that the chin points upward (determines function of the trapezius muscle).	Head hyperextends 60°	Head hyperextends less than 60°

▶ Assessing the Neck CONTINUED

ASSESSMENT	NORMAL FINDINGS	DEVIATIONS FROM NORMAL
• Move the head so that the ear is moved toward the shoulder on each side (determines function of the sternocleidomastoid muscle).	Head laterally flexes 40°	Head laterally flexes less than 40°
• Turn the head to the right and to the left (determines function of the sternocleidomastoid muscle).	Head laterally rotates 70°	Head laterally rotates less than 70°
Assess muscle strength.		
• Ask the client to turn the head to one side against the resistance of your hand. Repeat with the other side (determines the strength of the sternocleidomastoid muscle).	Equal strength	Unequal strength
• Shrug the shoulders against the resistance of your hands (determines the strength of the trapezius muscles).	As above	As above
Lymph Nodes		
Palpate the entire neck for enlarged lymph nodes, using the guidelines shown in the box below.	Not palpable	Enlarged, palpable, possibly tender (associated with infection and tumors)

Palpating Neck Lymph Nodes

- Face the client, and bend the client's head forward slightly or toward the side being examined to relax the soft tissue and muscles.

- Palpate the nodes using the pads of the fingers. Move the fingertips in a gentle rotating motion.

- When examining the submental and submandibular nodes, place the fingertips under the mandible on the side nearest the palpating hand, and pull the skin and subcutaneous tissue laterally over the mandibular surface so that the tissue rolls over the nodes.

- When palpating the supraclavicular nodes, have the client bend the head forward to relax the tissues of the anterior neck and to relax the shoulders so that the clavicles drop. Use your hand nearest the side to be examined when facing the client, i.e., your left hand for the client's right nodes. Use your free hand to flex the client's head forward if necessary. Hook your index and third fingers over the clavicle lateral to the sternocleidomastoid muscle (Figure 11–49).

- When palpating the anterior cervical nodes and posterior cervical nodes, move your fingertips slowly in a forward circular motion against the sternocleidomastoid and trapezius muscles, respectively.

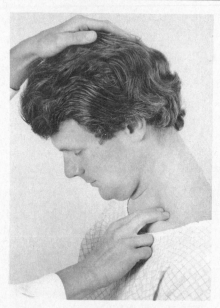

FIGURE 11–49 Palpating the supraclavicular lymph nodes.

- To palpate the deep cervical nodes, bend or hook your fingers around the sternocleidomastoid muscle.

▶ Assessing the Neck *CONTINUED*

ASSESSMENT	NORMAL FINDINGS	DEVIATIONS FROM NORMAL
Trachea		
Palpate the trachea for lateral deviation. Place your fingertip or thumb on the trachea in the suprasternal notch (see Figure 11–47, earlier), and then move your finger laterally to the left and the right in spaces bordered by the clavicle, the anterior aspect of the sternocleidomastoid muscle, and the trachea (Figure 11–50).	Central placement in midline of neck; spaces are equal on both sides	Deviation to one side, indicating possible neck tumor; thyroid enlargement; enlarged lymph nodes

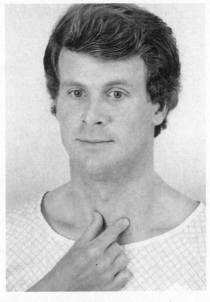

FIGURE 11–50   Palpating the trachea for lateral deviation.

ASSESSMENT	NORMAL FINDINGS	DEVIATIONS FROM NORMAL
Thyroid Gland		
Inspect the thyroid gland.		
• Stand in front of the client.		
• Observe the lower half of the neck overlying the thyroid gland for symmetry and visible masses.	Not visible on inspection	Visible diffuseness or local enlargement
• Ask the client to hyperextend the head and swallow. If necessary, offer a glass of water to make it easier for the client to swallow. This action determines how the thyroid and cricoid cartilages move and whether swallowing causes a bulging of the gland.	Gland ascends during swallowing but is not visible	Gland is not fully movable with swallowing
Palpate the thyroid gland for smoothness. Note any areas of enlargement, masses, or nodules. See the box on page 240 for palpation methods.	Lobes may not be palpated If palpated, lobes are small, smooth, centrally located, painless, and rise freely with swallowing	Solitary nodules
If enlargement of the gland is suspected, auscultate over the thyroid area for a bruit (a soft rushing sound created by turbulent blood flow). Use the bell-shaped diaphragm of the stethoscope.	Absence of bruit	Presence of bruit (see page 255 for further discussion of bruits)

▶

▶ **Assessing the Neck** *CONTINUED*

Palpating the Thyroid Gland

Stand in front of or behind the client, and ask the client to lower the chin slightly. *Lowering the chin relaxes the neck muscles, facilitating palpation.*

Posterior Approach

- Place your hands around the client's neck, with your fingertips on the lower half of the neck over the trachea (Figure 11–51).

- Ask the client to swallow (taking a sip of water, if necessary), and feel for any enlargement of the *thyroid isthmus* as it rises. The isthmus lies across the trachea, below the cricoid cartilege. See Figure 11–47, earlier.

- To examine the right thyroid lobe, have the client lower the chin slightly and turn the head slightly to the right (the side being examined). With your left fingers, displace the trachea slightly to the right. With your right

fingers, palpate the right thyroid lobe (Figure 11–52). Have the client swallow while you are palpating.

- Repeat the last step, in reverse, to examine the left thyroid lobe.

Anterior Approach

- Place the tips of your index and middle fingers over the trachea, and palpate the thyroid isthmus as the client swallows.

- To examine the right thyroid lobe, have the client lower the chin slightly and turn the head slightly to the right. With your right fingers, displace the trachea slightly to the client's right (your left). With your left fingers, palpate the right thyroid lobe (Figure 11–53).

- To examine the left thyroid lobe, repeat the above step in reverse.

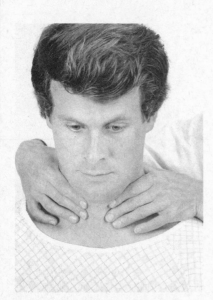

FIGURE 11–51 Placement of fingertips over the trachea to begin palpation of the thyroid gland (posterior approach).

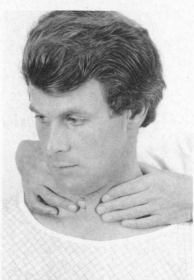

FIGURE 11–52 Palpating the right thyroid lobe (posterior approach).

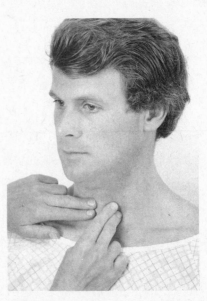

FIGURE 11–53 Palpating the right thyroid lobe (anterior approach).

Physical Assessment

Integument
- Skin
- Hair
- Nails

Neurologic System
- Level of consciousness
- Mental status
- Cranial nerves
- Reflexes
- Motor function
- Sensory function

Cardiovascular System
- Heart
- Peripheral vascular system

Musculoskeletal System
- Muscles
- Bones
- Joints

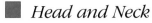

Head and Neck
- Skull
- Face
- Eyes and vision
- Ears and hearing
- Nose and sinuses
- Mouth and oropharynx
- Neck muscles
- Lymph nodes
- Trachea
- Thyroid gland

Thorax and Lungs

Breasts and Axillae

Abdomen
- Intestines
- Liver
- Spleen
- Kidneys
- Bladder

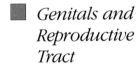

Genitals and Reproductive Tract

Female
- Inguinal lymph nodes
- External genitals
- Internal genitals

Male
- Penis
- Scrotum
- Inguinal area

Rectum and Anus

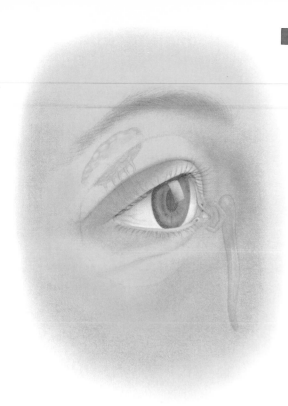

■ Eyes and Vision

- Inspect the external eye structures.
  - Eyebrows for hair distribution and alignment, skin quality, and movement
  - Eyelashes for evenness of distribution and direction of curl
  - Eyelids for surface characteristics, position, and movement
  - Palpebral and bulbar conjunctiva for color, texture, and lesions
  - Lacrimal apparatus for edema or tenderness
  - Cornea for clarity and texture
  - Anterior chamber for transparency and depth
  - Pupils for color, size, and equality

- Test visual acuity.
- Test peripheral visual fields.
- Test extraocular movements.
- Using an opthalmoscope, inspect the internal eye structures.
  - Red reflex through the pupil
  - Optic disc and cup for color, size, and shape
  - Retinal blood vessels for size, color, pattern, and arteriovenous crossings
  - Retinal background for color and surface characteristics
  - Macula and fovea centralis for color and surface characteristics

■ Ears and Hearing

- Inspect the auricles for color, texture, symmetry of size, position, and angle.
- Palpate the auricles for texture, elasticity, and areas of tenderness.
- Using an otoscope, inspect the external ear canals for cerumen, inflammation, scaling, foreign bodies, or other lesions.
- Using an otoscope, inspect each internal ear.
  - Tympanic membrane for color and gloss
  - Appearance of the annulus, pars flaccida, pars tensa, malleus, umbo, and light reflex
- Test hearing acuity.
  - Gross hearing acuity by response to voice tones
  - Tuning fork tests (Weber, Rinne, Schwabach tests)

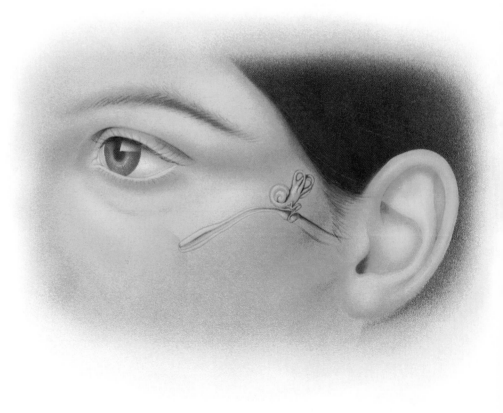

Nose and Sinuses

- Inspect the mucosa for redness, swelling, growths, discharge, and nasal polyps.
- Inspect the nasal septum for deviation.
- Palpate the external nose for tenderness.
- Palpate the maxillary and frontal sinuses for tenderness.
- Transilluminate the maxillary and frontal sinuses for the presence of air or fluid.

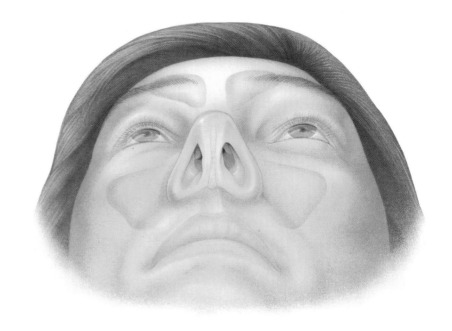

Neck

- Inspect the neck muscles for swellings or masses.
- Assess neck movement and strength of muscles.
- Palpate for enlarged lymph nodes.
- Palpate trachea for position.
- Inspect and palpate thyroid gland for symmetry and masses.

Mouth and Oropharynx

Mouth

- Inspect the lips for symmetry of contour, color, and texture.
- Using gloves, inspect the inner mucosa and the buccal mucosa for color, moisture, texture, and lesions; palpate the mucosa.
- Inspect the teeth for color, presence of fillings, dental caries, partial or complete dentures, and tartar.
- Inspect the gums for bleeding, color, retraction, edema, and lesions; palpate the gums to determine firmness and texture.
- Inspect the tongue for color, size, texture, position, mobility, and coating.
- Palpate the tongue and floor of the mouth for tenderness, nodules, lumps, or excoriated areas.
- Examine the hard and soft palates for color, shape, texture, and the presence of bony prominences.
- Observe the uvula for position and mobility.
- Inspect the salivary gland openings for swelling or redness.

Oropharynx

- Inspect the palatine arches for redness, lesions, and plaques.
- Inspect the tonsils for color, discharge, and size.
- Inspect the oropharynx for edema, inflammation, lesions, or exudate.
- Assess the gag reflex.

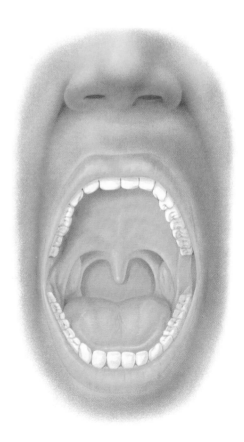

Peripheral Vascular System

- Measure the blood pressure.
- Assess all pulses for rate, rhythm, and volume.
- Palpate the following pulses:
  - Temporal
  - Carotids
  - Radial
  - Femoral
  - Popliteal
  - Posterior tibial
  - Pedal
- Palpate all pulses, except carotids, bilaterally and simultaneously.
- Inspect and auscultate the carotid pulses.

- Inspect the jugular veins for pulsations and distention.
- Inspect the peripheral veins for the presence and/or appearance of superficial veins when limbs are dependent and when limbs are elevated.
- Assess peripheral leg veins for signs of redness, tenderness, or edema.
- Assess peripheral perfusion, noting the color, temperature, and appearance of the skin of the hands and feet.
- Test capillary refill.

Heart

- Determine the location of the atria (base) and ventricles (apex) of the heart.
- Inspect and palpate the aortic, pulmonic, tricuspid, and apical areas for the presence of abnormal pulsations or lifts or heaves.
- Inspect and palpate the epigastric area for abdominal aortic pulsations.
- Standing at the client's right, use both the diaphragm and the bell to auscultate for heart sounds at the aortic, pulmonic, tricuspid, and apical areas.
- At each area of auscultation, distinguish both the S1 and S2 sounds.

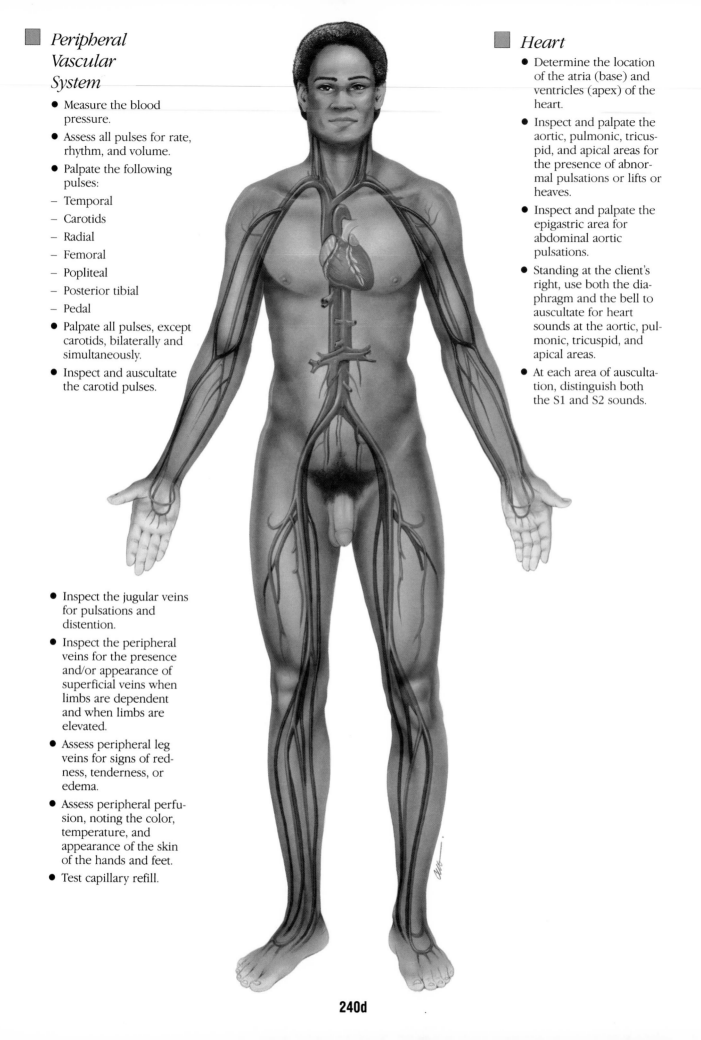

240d

Musculoskeletal System

- Observe body posture standing and sitting.
- Observe muscles and tendons for contractures.
- Inspect the muscles for size bilaterally.
- Palpate muscles at rest to determine tonicity.
- Test muscle strength.
- Observe muscles for fasciculations and tremors.
- Inspect each joint for swelling.
- Palpate each joint for tenderness, smoothness of movement, swelling, crepitation, and the presence of nodules.
- Determine the range of motion of the body joints bilaterally.

Neurologic System

- Assess level of consciousness.
- Assess mental status.
  - Assess for aphasias and related language deficits
  - Determine orientation to time, place, and person
  - Assess attitude and affect
  - Evaluate attention span and calculation
  - Listen for lapses in memory
  - Test judgment
  - Assess abstract reasoning
- Assess cranial nerve function.
- Test deep tendon reflexes.
  - Biceps
  - Triceps
  - Brachioradialis
  - Patellar
  - Achilles
  - Plantar (Babinski)
- Test motor function.
  - Conduct gross motor and balance tests
  - Conduct fine motor tests for the upper and lower extremities
- Assess sensory function.
  - Assess light touch sensation and tactile location
  - Assess pain sensation
  - Test temperature sensation
  - Test vibratory sense
  - Test for kinesthetic sensation
  - Test tactile discrimination

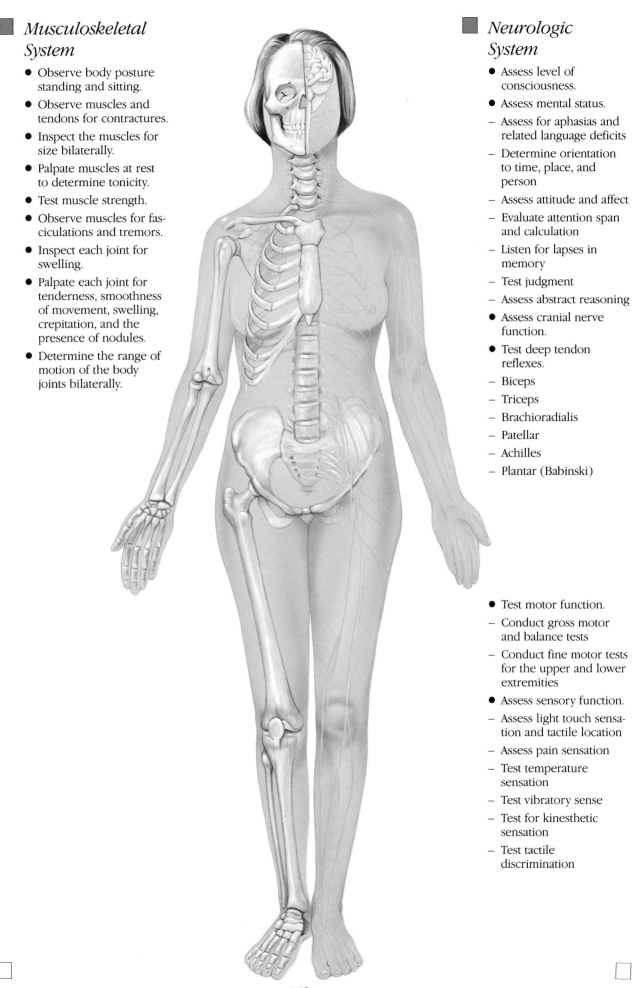

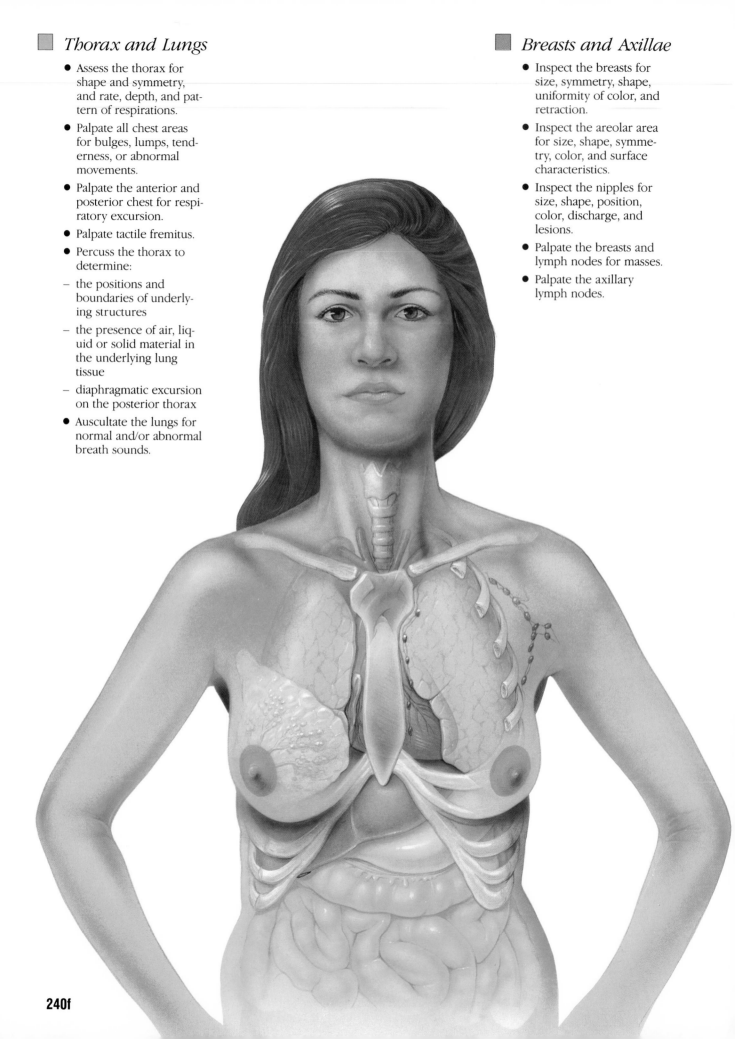

Thorax and Lungs

- Assess the thorax for shape and symmetry, and rate, depth, and pattern of respirations.
- Palpate all chest areas for bulges, lumps, tenderness, or abnormal movements.
- Palpate the anterior and posterior chest for respiratory excursion.
- Palpate tactile fremitus.
- Percuss the thorax to determine:
  - the positions and boundaries of underlying structures
  - the presence of air, liquid or solid material in the underlying lung tissue
  - diaphragmatic excursion on the posterior thorax
- Auscultate the lungs for normal and/or abnormal breath sounds.

Breasts and Axillae

- Inspect the breasts for size, symmetry, shape, uniformity of color, and retraction.
- Inspect the areolar area for size, shape, symmetry, color, and surface characteristics.
- Inspect the nipples for size, shape, position, color, discharge, and lesions.
- Palpate the breasts and lymph nodes for masses.
- Palpate the axillary lymph nodes.

◼ Female Genitals and Reproductive Tract

- Inspect the amount, distribution, and characteristics of pubic hair.
- Inspect the pubic skin for parasites, inflammation, swelling, and lesions.
- Palpate the inguinal lymph nodes for enlargement and tenderness.
- Using gloves, inspect the clitoris, urethral orifice, and vaginal orifice for lesions, discharge, and inflammation.
  - Palpate Bartholin's glands
  - Assess the integrity of the pelvic musculature
- Insert a vaginal speculum and examine the internal genitals.
  - Inspect the cervix for shape of the os, color, size, and position
  - Obtain a specimen for a Papanicolaou smear
  - Inspect the vaginal walls for color, texture, and secretions

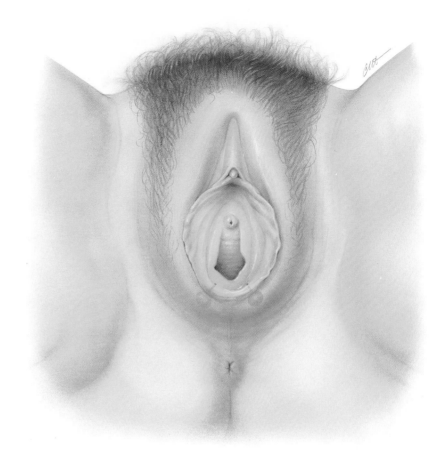

◼ Male Genitals and Reproductive Tract

- Observe the amount, distribution, and characteristics of pubic hair.
- Using gloves, inspect the penile shaft, glans, and urethral meatus for lesions, nodules, swelling, inflammation, and discharge.
- Observe the color and position of the urethral meatus.
- Inspect the scrotum for appearance, general size, and symmetry.
- Palpate the scrotum, testicles, epididymis, and spermatic cord for swelling, irregularities, and tenderness.
- Inspect the inguinal areas for hernias.
- Palpate for inguinal and femoral hernias.

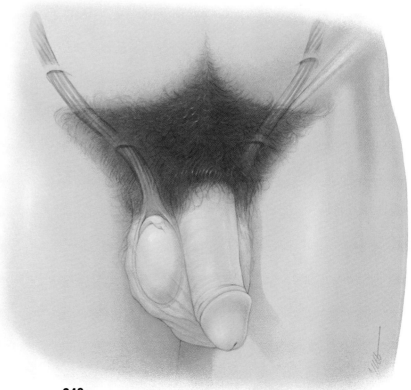

240g

Abdomen

- Inspect the abdomen for skin integrity, contour, and symmetry.
- Observe any movements associated with respiration, peristalsis, or aortic pulsations.
- Auscultate the abdomen for bowel sounds, vascular sounds, and any peritoneal friction rubs.
- Percuss the abdomen for tympany and dullness.
- Percuss the abdomen to determine liver and spleen size.
- Percuss the abdomen to detect areas of tenderness over the liver and kidney.
- Percuss the abdomen to define the outline of a distended bladder.
- Palpate the liver, spleen and kidneys to determine position and size.
- Palpate the abdomen to detect tenderness, presence of masses, and distention.

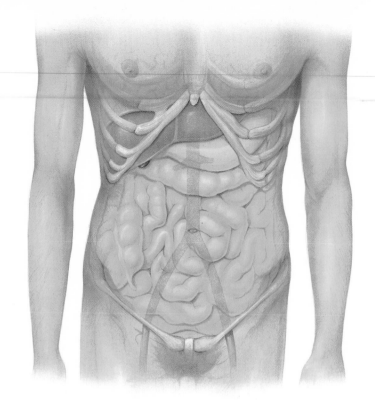

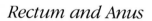

Rectum and Anus

- Using gloves, spread the buttocks with both hands and inspect the anus and surrounding tissue for skin lesions, fissures, ulcers, protruding hemorrhoids, fistula openings, and rectal prolapse.
- Ask the client to bear down and note any bulges, rectal prolapse, polyps, internal hemorrhoids, or rectal fissures.
- Using a gloved, lubricated index finger, palpate for nodules, masses, and tenderness.
- Ask the client to tighten the anal sphincter and note the tone.
- In the male, palpate the prostate gland.
- In the female, palpate the cervix of the uterus.

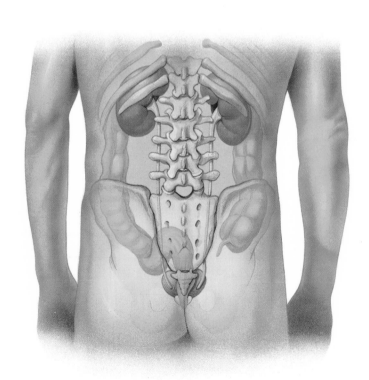

The Thorax and Lungs

Assessing the thorax and lungs is frequently critical to assessing the client's aeration status. Changes in the respiratory system can come about slowly or quickly. In clients with chronic obstructive pulmonary disease (COPD), such as chronic bronchitis, emphysema, and asthma, changes are frequently gradual; however, in clients who are acutely ill, e.g., those who have a **pneumothorax** (accumulation of gas or fluid in the pleural cavity), changes occur quickly, and death can result if immediate action is not taken. For information about the mechanics of breathing, see Chapter 10, page 182.

The client's posture is important to note. Some people with chronic respiratory problems tend to bend forward or even prop their arms on a support to elevate their clavicles. This posture is an attempt to expand the chest fully and thus breathe with less effort.

Chest Wall Landmarks

Before beginning the assessment, the nurse must be familiar with a series of imaginary lines on the chest wall and be able to locate the position of each rib and some spinous processes. These landmarks help the nurse to identify the position of underlying organs, e.g., lobes of the lung, and to record abnormal assessment findings. Figure 11–54 shows the anterior, lateral, and posterior series of lines. The *midsternal line* is a vertical line running through the center of the sternum. The *midclavicular lines* (right and left) are vertical lines from the midpoints of the clavicles. The *anterior axillary lines* (right and left) are vertical lines from the anterior axillary folds (Figure 11–54, A). Figure 11–54, B shows the three imaginary lines of the lateral chest. The *posterior axillary line* is a vertical line from the posterior axillary fold. The *midaxillary line* is a vertical line from the apex of the axilla. The anterior axillary line is described above. Figure 11–54, C shows the posterior chest landmarks. The *vertebral line* is a vertical line along the spinous processes. The *scapular lines* (right and left) are vertical lines from the inferior angles of the scapulae.

Locating the position of each rib and certain spinous processes is essential for identifying underlying lobes of the lung. Figures 11–55, 11–56, and 11–57 show an anterior view, right and left lateral views, and a posterior view of the chest and underlying lungs. Each lung is first divided into the upper and lower lobes by an oblique fissure that runs from the level of the spinous process of the third thoracic vertebra (T-3) to the level of the sixth rib at the midclavicular line (Figure 11–55). The right upper lobe is abbreviated RUL; the right lower lobe, RLL. Similarly, the left upper lobe is abbreviated LUL; the left lower lobe,

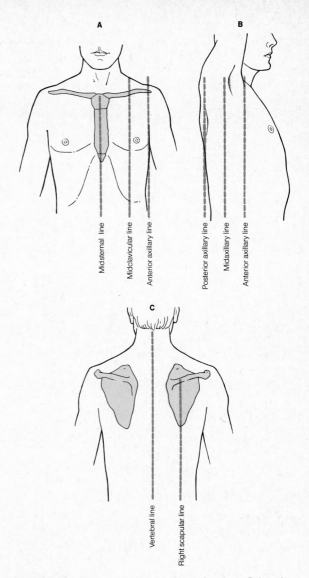

FIGURE 11–54 Chest wall landmarks: *A*, anterior chest; *B*, lateral chest; *C*, posterior chest.

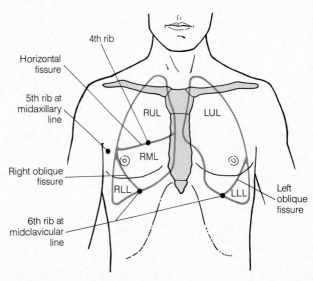

FIGURE 11–55 Anterior chest landmarks and underlying lungs.

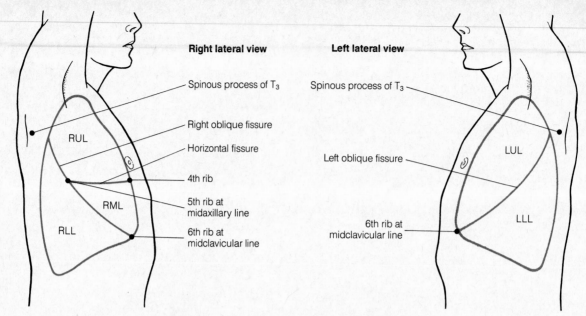

FIGURE 11–56 Lateral chest landmarks and underlying lungs.

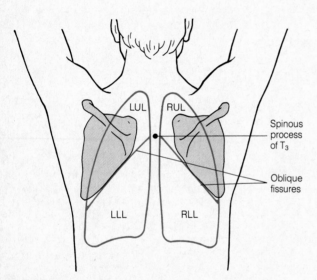

FIGURE 11–57 Posterior chest landmarks and underlying lungs.

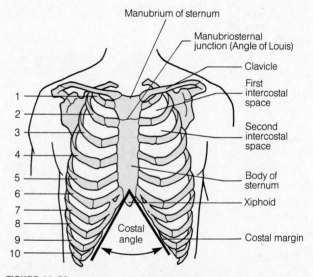

FIGURE 11–58 Location of the anterior ribs in relation to the angle of Louis and the sternum.

LLL. The right lung is further divided by a minor fissure into the right upper lobe and right middle lobe (RML). This fissure runs anteriorly from the right midaxillary line at the level of the fifth rib to the level of the fourth rib.

These specific landmarks, i.e., T-3 and the fourth, fifth, and sixth ribs, are located as follows. The starting point for locating the ribs anteriorly is the **angle of Louis**, the junction between the body of the **sternum** (breastbone) and the **manubrium** (the handlelike superior part of the sternum that joins with the clavicles). The superior border of the second rib attaches to the sternum at this manubriosternal junction (Figure 11–58). The nurse can identify the manu-

brium by first palpating the clavicle and following its course to its attachment at the manubrium. The nurse then palpates and counts distal ribs and intercostal spaces (ICS) from the second rib. It is important to note that an ICS is numbered according to the number of the rib immediately *above* the space. When palpating for rib identification, the nurse should palpate along the midclavicular line rather than the sternal border, because the rib cartilages are very close at the sternum. Only the first seven ribs attach directly to the sternum.

The counting of ribs is more difficult on the posterior than on the anterior thorax. For identifying underlying lung lobes, the pertinent landmark is

T-3. The starting point for locating T-3 is the spinous process of the seventh cervical vertebra (C-7), also referred to as the *vertebra prominens* (Figure 11–59). When the client flexes the neck anteriorly, a prominent process can be observed and palpated. This is the spinous process of the seventh cervical vertebra. If two spinous processes are observed, the superior one is C-7, and the inferior one is the spinous process of the first thoracic vertebra (T-1). The nurse then palpates and counts the spinous processes from C-7 to T-3. Each spinous process up to T-4 is adjacent to the corresponding rib number; e.g., T-3 is adjacent to the third rib. After T-4, however, the spinous processes project obliquely, causing the spinous process of the vertebra to lie, not over its correspondingly numbered rib, but over the rib below. Thus, the spinous process of T-5 lies over the body of T-6 and is adjacent to the sixth rib.

Chest Shape and Size

In the infant, the thorax is rounded; i.e., the diameter from the front to the back (anteroposterior) is equal to the transverse diameter. It is also cylindrical, having a nearly equal diameter at the top and the base. When a child reaches 6 years, the anteroposterior diameter has decreased in proportion to the transverse one. In adults, the thorax is oval. Its anteroposterior diameter is two times smaller than its transverse diameter (Figure 11–60). The overall shape of the thorax is elliptical; i.e., its diameter is smaller at the top than at the base. In the elderly, kyphosis and osteoporosis alter the size of the chest cavity as the ribs move downward and forward.

There are several deformities of the chest (Figure 11–61 on page 244). **Pigeon chest (pectus cari-**

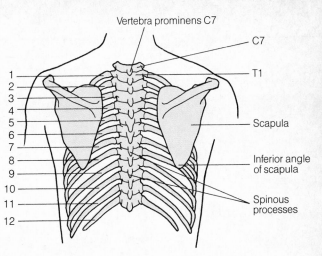

FIGURE 11–59 Location of the posterior ribs in relation to the spinous processes of the vertebrae.

natum), a permanent deformity, may be caused by rickets. Pigeon chest is characterized by a narrow transverse diameter, an increased anteroposterior diameter, and a protruding sternum. A **funnel chest (pectus excavatum)**, a congenital defect, is the opposite of pigeon chest in that the sternum is depressed, narrowing the anteroposterior diameter. Because the sternum points posteriorly in clients with a funnel chest, abnormal pressure on the heart may result in altered function. A **barrel chest,** in which the ratio of the anteroposterior to lateral diameter is 1 to 1, is seen in clients with thoracic **kyphosis** (excessive convex curvature of the thoracic spine) and **emphysema** (chronic pulmonary condition in which the air sacs, or alveoli, are dilated and distended). **Scoliosis** is a lateral deviation of the spine.

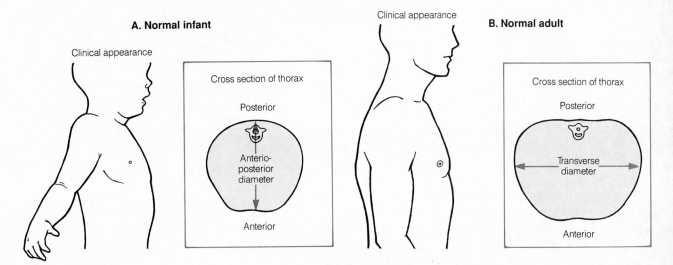

FIGURE 11–60 Configurations of the thorax showing anteroposterior diameter and transverse diameter: *A*, infant; *B*, adult.

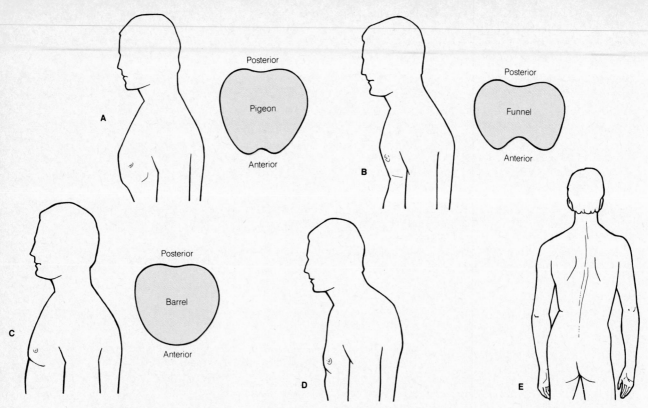

FIGURE 11–61 Chest deformities: *A*, pigeon chest; *B*, funnel chest; *C*, barrel chest; *D*, kyphosis; *E*, scoliosis.

Breath Sounds

Abnormal or adventitious breath sounds occur when air passes through narrowed airways or airways filled with fluid or mucus, or when pleural linings are inflamed. See Table 11–8 for normal breath sounds. Adventitious sounds are often superimposed over normal sounds. The three types of adventitious sounds—crackles (previously referred to as rales or **crepitations**), gurgles, and pleural friction rub—are described in the box on page 184 and Table 11–9. Absence of breath sounds over some lung areas is also a significant finding that is associated with collapsed and surgically removed lobes.

Assessment of the lungs and thorax includes all methods of examination: inspection, palpation, percussion, and auscultation. The following are needed for the examination: (a) stethoscope, (b) a marking pencil, and (c) a centimeter ruler. For efficiency, the nurse usually examines the posterior chest first, then the anterior chest. For posterior and lateral chest examinations, the client is uncovered to the waist and in a sitting positon. A sitting or lying position may be used for anterior chest examination. The sitting position is preferred because it maximizes chest expansion. Good lighting is essential, especially for chest inspection.

TABLE 11–8 NORMAL BREATH SOUNDS

Type	Description	Location	Characteristics
Vesicular	Soft-intensity, low-pitched, "gentle sighing" sounds created by air moving through smaller airways (bronchioles and alveoli)	Over peripheral lung; best heard at base of lungs	Best heard on inspiration, which is about 2.5 times longer than the expiratory phase (5:2 ratio)
Bronchovesicular	Moderate-intensity and moderate-pitched "blowing" sounds created by air moving through larger airways (bronchi)	Between the scapulae and lateral to the sternum at the first and second intercostal spaces	Equal inspiratory and expiratory phases (1:1 ratio)
Bronchial (tubular)	High-pitched, loud, "harsh" sounds created by air moving through the trachea	Anteriorly over the trachea; not normally heard over lung tissue	Louder than vesicular sounds; have a short inspiratory phase and long expiratory phase (1:2 ratio)

TABLE 11-9   ADVENTITIOUS BREATH SOUNDS

Name	Description	Cause	Location
Crackles (rales)	Fine, short, interrupted crackling sounds; alveolar rales are high-pitched; bronchial rales are lower-pitched. Sound can be simulated by rolling a lock of hair near the ear. Best heard on inspiration but can be heard on both inspiration and expiration. May not be cleared by coughing.	Air passing through fluid or mucus in any air passage.	Most commonly heard in the bases of the lower lung lobes.
Gurgles (rhonchi)	Continuous, low-pitched, coarse, gurgling, harsh, louder sounds with a moaning or snoring quality. Best heard on expiration but can be heard on both inspiration and expiration. May be altered by coughing.	Air passing through narrowed air passages as a result of secretions, swelling, tumors.	Loud sounds can be heard over most lung areas but predominate over the trachea and bronchi.
Friction rub	Superficial grating or creaking sounds heard during inspiration and expiration. Not relieved by coughing.	Rubbing together of inflamed pleural surfaces.	Heard most often in areas of greatest thoracic expansion (e.g., lower anterior and lateral chest).
Wheeze	Continuous, high-pitched, squeaky musical sounds. Best heard on expiration. Not usually altered by coughing.	Air passing through a constricted bronchi as a result of secretions, swelling, tumors.	Heard over all lung fields.

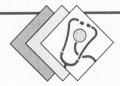

Assessing the Thorax and Lungs

NURSING HISTORY FOCUS
Family history of illness, including cancer, allergies, tuberculosis; life-style, including smoking and occupational hazards (e.g., inhaling fumes); any medications being taken; current problems, (e.g., swellings, coughs, wheezing, pain).

ASSESSMENT	NORMAL FINDINGS	DEVIATIONS FROM NORMAL
Posterior Thorax		
Inspect the shape and symmetry of the thorax from posterior and lateral views. Compare the anteroposterior diameter to the lateral diameter.	Anteroposterior to lateral diameter in ratio of 1:2 Chest symmetric	Barrel chest; increased anteroposterior to lateral diameter Chest asymmetric
Inspect the spinal alignment for deformities. Have the client stand. From a lateral position, observe the three normal curvatures: (cervical, thoracic, and lumbar). From the posterior, drop a plumb line from the occiput of the skull to the gluteal cleft.	Spine vertically aligned	Exaggerated spinal curvatures (kyphosis, lordosis); lateral deviation of spine (scoliosis)
Palpate the posterior thorax.		
• For clients who have no respiratory complaints, rapidly assess the temperature and integrity of all chest skin.	Skin intact; uniform temperature	Skin lesions; areas of hyperthermia

▶

▶ **Assessing the Thorax and Lungs** *CONTINUED*

ASSESSMENT	NORMAL FINDINGS	DEVIATIONS FROM NORMAL
• For clients who do have respiratory complaints, palpate all chest areas for bulges, tenderness, or abnormal movements. Avoid deep palpation for painful areas, especially if a fractured rib is suspected. *In such a case, deep palpation could lead to displacement of the bone fragment against the lungs.*	Chest wall intact; no tenderness; no masses	Lumps, bulges; depressions; areas of tenderness; movable structures (e.g., rib)
Palpate the posterior chest for respiratory excursion (thoracic expansion). Place the palms of both your hands over the lower thorax with your thumbs adjacent to the spine and your fingers stretched laterally (Figure 11–62). Ask the client to take a deep breath while you observe the movement of your hands and any lag in movement.	Full and symmetric chest expansion (i.e., when the client takes a deep breath, your thumbs should move apart an equal distance and at the same time; normally the thumbs separate 3 to 5 cm [1 1/2 to 2 in] during deep inspiration)	Asymmetric and/or decreased chest expansion

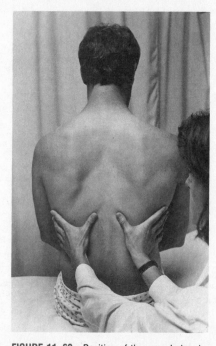

FIGURE 11–62 Position of the nurse's hands when assessing respiratory excursion on the posterior thorax.

Palpate the chest for vocal (tactile) fremitus, the faintly perceptible vibration felt through the chest wall when the client speaks. • Place the palmar surfaces of your fingertips or the ulnar aspect of your hand or closed fist on the posterior chest, starting near the apex of the lungs (Figure 11–63, position A).	Bilateral symmetry of vocal fremitus Fremitus is heard most clearly at the apex of the lungs Low-pitched voices of males are more readily palpated than higher pitched voices of females	Decreased or absent fremitus (associated with pneumothorax) Increased fremitus (associated with consolidated lung tissue, as in pneumonia)

▶ **Assessing the Thorax and Lungs** *CONTINUED*

ASSESSMENT	NORMAL FINDINGS	DEVIATIONS FROM NORMAL
• Ask the client to repeat such words as "blue moon" or "one, two, three." • Repeat the two steps, moving your hands sequentially to the base of the lungs, through positions B–E in Figure 11–63. • Compare the fremitus on both lungs and between the apex and the base of each lung, using either one hand and moving it from one side of the client to the corresponding area on the other side *or* using two hands that are placed simultaneously on the corresponding areas of each side of the chest.	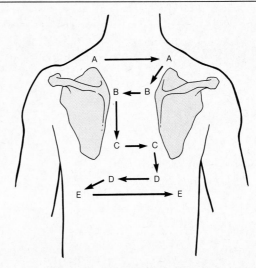 **FIGURE 11–63** Areas and sequence for palpating tactile fremitus on the posterior chest.	
Percuss the thorax. See the box on page 248.	Percussion notes resonate, except over scapula Lowest point of resonance is at the diaphragm (i.e., at the level of the eighth to tenth rib posteriorly) *Note:* percussion on a rib normally elicits dullness	Asymmetry in percussion Areas of dullness or flatness over lung tissue (associated with consolidation of lung tissue or a mass)
Percuss for diaphragmatic excursion (movement of the diaphragm during maximal inspiration and expiration). See the box on page 248.	Excursion is 3 to 5 cm (1 to 2 in) bilaterally in females and 5 to 6 cm (2 to 3 in) in males Diaphragm is usually slightly higher on the right side	Restricted excursion (associated with lung disorder)
Auscultate the chest using the flat-disc diaphragm of the stethoscope (best for transmitting the high-pitched breath sounds). • Use the systematic zigzag procedure used in percussion (Figure 11–64). • Ask the client to take slow, deep breaths through the mouth. Listen at each point to the breath sounds during a complete inspiration and expiration. • Compare findings at each point with the corresponding point on the opposite side of the chest.	Vesicular and bronchovesicular breath sounds (see Table 11–8)	**Adventitious breath sounds** (e.g., crackles, rhonchi, wheeze, friction rub; see Table 11–9) Absence of breath sounds (associated with collapsed and surgically removed lung lobes)

▶

► **Assessing the Thorax and Lungs** *CONTINUED*

ASSESSMENT	NORMAL FINDINGS	DEVIATIONS FROM NORMAL

Percussing the Thorax

Percussing for Normal Thorax Sounds

Percussion of the thorax is performed to determine whether underlying lung tissue is filled with air, liquid, or solid material and to determine the positions and boundaries of certain organs. Because percussion penetrates to a depth of 5 to 7 cm (2 to 3 in), it detects superficial rather than deep lesions. Percussion sounds and tones are described in Table 11–3, earlier.

- Ask the client to bend the head and fold the arms forward across the chest. *This separates the scapula and exposes more lung tissue to percussion.*

- Percuss in the intercostal spaces at about 5 cm (2 in) intervals in a systematic sequence (Figure 11–64). Figure 11–65 shows normal percussion sounds in the posterior chest.

- Compare one side of the lung with the other.

- Percuss the lateral thorax every few inches, starting at the axilla and working down to the eighth rib.

Percussing for Diaphragmatic Excursion

- Ask the client to take a deep breath and hold it while you percuss downward along the scapular line until dullness is produced at the level of the diaphragm. Mark this point with a marking pencil, and repeat the procedure on the other side of the chest.

- Ask the client to take a few normal breaths and then expel the last breath completely and hold it while you percuss upward from the marked point to assess and mark the diaphragmatic excursion during deep expiration on each side.

- Measure the distance between the two marks.

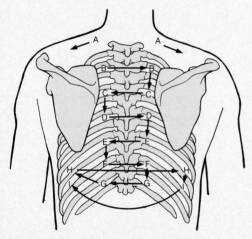

FIGURE 11–64 Sequence for posterior chest percussion.

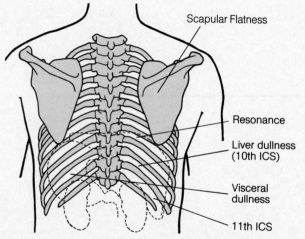

FIGURE 11–65 Normal percussion sounds on the posterior chest.

Anterior Thorax

Inspect breathing patterns (e.g., respiratory rate and rhythm).

See Chapter 10, page 183

See Chapter 30, page 739, for abnormal breathing patterns and sounds

Inspect the costal angle (angle formed by the intersection of the costal margins) **and the angle at which the ribs enter the spine.**
Palpate the anterior chest (see posterior chest palpation).

Costal angle is less than 90°, and the ribs insert into the spine at approximately a 45° angle (see Figure 11–58, earlier)

Costal angle is widened (associated with chronic obstructive pulmonary disease)

► **Assessing the Thorax and Lungs** *CONTINUED*

ASSESSMENT	NORMAL FINDINGS	DEVIATIONS FROM NORMAL
Palpate the anterior chest for respiratory excursion. • Place the palms of both your hands on the lower thorax, with your fingers laterally along the lower rib cage and your thumbs along the costal margins (Figure 11–66). • Ask the client to take a deep breath while you observe the movement of your hands.	Full symmetric excursion; thumbs normally separate 3 to 5 cm (1 1/2 to 2 in)	Asymmetric and/or decreased respiratory excursion

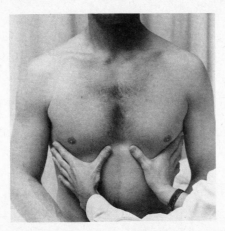

FIGURE 11–66 Position of nurse's hands when assessing respiratory excursion on the anterior thorax.

ASSESSMENT	NORMAL FINDINGS	DEVIATIONS FROM NORMAL
Palpate tactile fremitus in the same manner as for the posterior chest and using the sequence shown in Figure 11–67. If the breasts are large and cannot be retracted adequately for palpation, this part of the examination is usually omitted.	Same as posterior vocal fremitus Fremitus is normally decreased over heart and breast tissue	Same as posterior fremitus

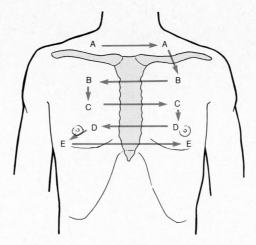

FIGURE 11–67 Areas and sequence for palpating tactile fremitus on the anterior chest.

ASSESSMENT	NORMAL FINDINGS	DEVIATIONS FROM NORMAL
Percuss the anterior chest systematically. • Begin above the clavicles in the supraclavicular space, and proceed downward to the diaphragm (Figure 11–68).	Percussion notes resonate down to the sixth rib at the level of the diaphragm but are flat over areas of heavy muscle and bone, dull on areas over the heart and the liver, and tympanic over the underlying stomach (Figure 11–69)	Asymmetry in percussion notes Areas of dullness or flatness over lung tissue

►

▶ **Assessing the Thorax and Lungs** *CONTINUED*

ASSESSMENT	NORMAL FINDINGS	DEVIATIONS FROM NORMAL

- Compare one side of the lung to the other.
- Displace female breasts for proper examination.

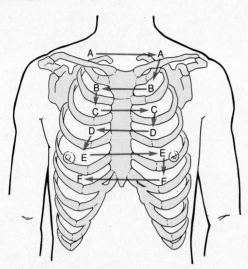

FIGURE 11–68 Sequence for anterior chest percussion.

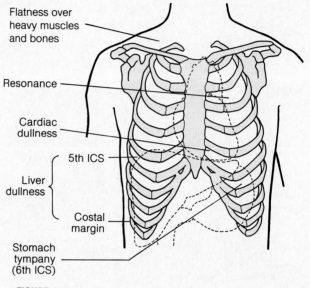

FIGURE 11–69 Normal percussion sounds on the anterior chest.

Auscultate the trachea (Figure 11–70).	Bronchial and tubular breath sounds (see Table 11–8 on page 244)	Adventitious breath sounds (see Table 11–9 on page 245)

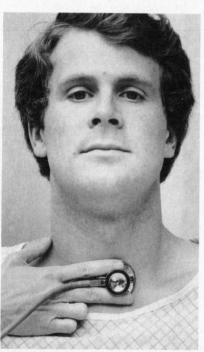

FIGURE 11–70 Auscultating the trachea.

Auscultate the anterior chest. Use the sequence used in percussion (see Figure 11–68), beginning over the bronchi between the sternum and the clavicles.	Bronchovesicular and vesicular breath sounds (see Table 11–8)	Adventitious breath sounds (see Table 11–9)

THE ELDERLY: PHYSICAL CHANGES OF THE THORAX AND BREATHING PATTERNS

- The thoracic curvature may be accentuated (kyphosis) because of osteoporosis and changes in cartilage, resulting in collapse of the vertebrae.
- The anteroposterior diameter of the chest widens, giving the person a barrel-chested appearance. This is due to loss of skeletal muscle strength in the thorax and diaphragm and constant lung inflation from excessive expiratory pressure on the alveoli.
- Breathing rate and rhythm are unchanged at rest; the rate normally increases with exercise but may take longer to return to the preexercise rate.
- Inspiratory muscles become less powerful, and the inspiration reserve volume decreases. A decrease in depth of respiration is therefore apparent.
- Expiration may require the use of accessory muscles. The expiratory reserve volume significantly increases

because of the increased amount of air remaining in the lungs at the end of a normal breath.
- Deflation of the lung is incomplete.
- Small airways lose their cartilaginous support and elastic recoil; as a result, they tend to close, particularly in basal or dependent portions of the lung.
- Elastic tissue of the alveoli loses its stretchability and changes to fibrous tissue. This thicker alveolar membrane decreases the pulmonary diffusion capacity. As a result, arterial oxyhemoglobin saturation and PaO_2 are slightly lower than those of young adults. Exertional capacity also decreases.
- Cilia in the airways decrease in number and are less effective in removing mucus; elderly clients are therefore at greater risk for pulmonary infections.

The Cardiovascular and Peripheral Vascular Systems

Heart

Heart function can be assessed to a large degree by findings in the history, by symptoms such as shortness of breath, by the client's general appearance (e.g., cyanosis and edema of the legs suggest impaired function), and by pulse rate, rhythm, and quality. Direct examination of the heart, however, offers more specific information, including the heart sounds, the heart size, and such findings as lifts, heaves, or **murmurs** (more prolonged sounds during systole and diastole). Nurses assess heart functions through observations (inspection), palpation, and auscultation, in that sequence. Auscultation is more meaningful when other data are obtained first. The heart is usually assessed during an initial physical assessment; periodic reassessments may be necessary for long-term or at-risk clients or those with cardiac problems. Heart examinations are usually performed while the client is in a semireclined position. The practitioner stands at the client's right side, where palpation of the cardiac area is facilitated and optimal inspection allowed.

To assess the client's heart, the nurse must first determine its exact location. In the average adult, most of the heart lies behind and to the left of the sternum. A small portion (the right atrium) extends

to the right of the sternum. The upper portion of the heart (both atria), referred to as its **base**, lies toward the back. The lower portion (the ventricles), referred to as its **apex**, points forward. The apex of the left ventricle actually touches the anterior chest wall at or medial to the left midclavicular line (MCL) and at or near the fifth left intercostal space (LICS), which is slightly below the left nipple. See Figure 10–9 on page 168. This point where the apex touches the anterior chest wall is known as the **point of maximal impulse (PMI)**.

The **precordium**, the area of the chest overlying the heart, is inspected and palpated simultaneously for the presence of abnormal pulsations or lifts or heaves. The terms **lift** and **heave**, often used interchangeably, refer to a rising along the sternal border with each heartbeat. A lift occurs when cardiac action is very forceful (overactive). It should be confirmed by palpation with the palm of the hand. Enlargement or overactivity of the left ventricle produces a heave lateral to the apex, whereas enlargement of the right ventricle produces a heave at or near the sternum.

Several heart sounds can be heard by auscultation. Only the first and second heart sounds (S_1 and S_2) will be emphasized in this book. The normal first two heart sounds are produced by closure of the valves of the heart. The first heart sound, S_1, occurs when the atrioventricular (A-V) valves close. These valves close when the ventricles have been sufficiently filled. Although the right and left A-V valves do not close simultaneously, the closures occur closely enough to be heard as one sound (S_1), a dull, low-pitched sound described as "lub." After the ventricles empty their blood into the aorta and pulmonary arteries, the semilunar valves close, producing the second heart sound, **S_2**, described as "dub." S_2 has a higher pitch than S_1 and is also shorter. These two sounds, S_1 and S_2 ("lub-dub"), occur within 1 second or less, depending on the heart rate.

The two heart sounds are audible anywhere on the precordial area, but they are best heard over the aortic, pulmonic, tricuspid, and apical areas (Figure 11–71). Each area is associated with the closure of heart valves: the aortic area with the aortic valve (inside the aorta as it arises from the left ventricle); the pulmonic area with the pulmonic valve (inside the pulmonary artery as it arises from the right ventricle); the tricuspid area with the tricuspid valve (between the right atrium and ventricle); and the apical (mitral) area with the mitral valve (between the left atrium and ventricle).

Associated with these sounds are systole and diastole. **Systole** is the period in which the ventricles contract. It begins with the first heart sound and ends at the second heart sound. Systole is normally shorter than diastole. **Diastole** is the period in which the ventricles relax. It starts with the second sound and ends at the subsequent first sound. Normally no sounds are audible during these periods (Figure 11–72). The experienced nurse, however, may perceive extra heart sounds (S_3 and S_4) during diastole. Both sounds are low in pitch and heard best at the apical site, with the bell of the stethoscope, and with the client lying on the left side. S_3 occurs early in diastole right after S_2 and sounds like "lub-dub-*ee*" (S_1, S_2, S_3) or "Kentuc-*ky*." It often disappears when the client sits up. S_3 is normal in children and young

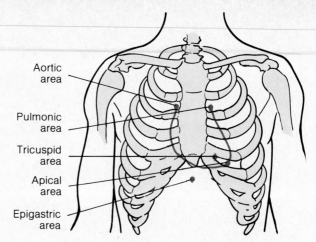

FIGURE 11–71 Anatomic sites of the precordium.

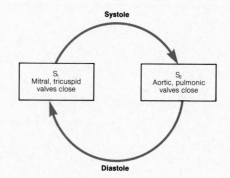

FIGURE 11–72 Relationship of heart sounds to systole and diastole.

adults. In older adults it may indicate heart failure. S_4 is rarely heard in healthy clients. It occurs near the very end of diastole just before S_1 and creates the sound of "*dee*-lub-dub" (S_4, S_1, S_2) or "*Ten*-nessee." S_4 may be heard in many elderly clients and can be a sign of hypertension.

Normal heart sounds are summarized in Table 11–10.

TABLE 11–10 NORMAL HEART SOUNDS

Sound or Phase	Description	Area			
		Aortic	**Pulmonic**	**Tricuspid**	**Apical**
S_1	Dull, low-pitched, and longer than S_2; sounds like "lub"	Less intensity than S_2	Less intensity than S_2	Louder than or equal to S_2	Louder than or equal to S_2
S_2	High-pitched, snappy, and shorter than S_1; creates sound of "dub"	Louder than S_1	Louder than S_1; abnormal if louder than the aortic S_2 in adults over 40	Less intensity than or equal to S_1	Less intensity than or equal to S_1
Systole	Normally silent interval between S_1 and S_2				
Diastole	Normally silent interval between S_2 and next S_1				

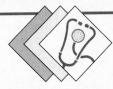

Assessing the Cardiovascular System

NURSING HISTORY FOCUS

Family history of incidence and age of heart disease, high cholesterol levels, high blood pressure, stroke, obesity, congenital heart disease, and rheumatic fever; client's past history of rheumatic fever, heart murmur, heart attack, or heart failure; present symptoms indicative of heart disease, e.g., fatigue, dyspnea, orthopnea, edema, cough, chest pain, palpitations, syncope, hypertension, wheezing, hemoptysis; presence of diseases that affect heart, e.g., obesity, diabetes, lung disease, endocrine disorders; life-style habits that are risk factors for cardiac disease, e.g., smoking, alcohol intake, eating and exercise patterns, areas and degree of stress perceived.

ASSESSMENT	NORMAL FINDINGS	DEVIATIONS FROM NORMAL
Simultaneously inspect and palpate the precordium for the presence of abnormal pulsations, lifts, or heaves. To locate the valve areas of the heart, see the box below.		
• Inspect and palpate the aortic and pulmonic areas, observing them at an angle and to the side, to note the presence or absence of pulsations. *Observing these areas at an angle increases the likelihood of seeing pulsations.*	No pulsations, although some people have aortic pulsations	Pulsations
• Inspect and palpate the tricuspid area for pulsations and heaves or lifts.	No pulsations No lift or heave	Pulsations Diffuse lift or heave, indicating enlarged or overactive right ventricle
• Inspect and palpate the apical area for pulsation, noting its specific location (it may be displaced laterally or lower) and diameter. If displaced laterally, record the distance between the apex and the MCL in centimeters.	Pulsations visible in 50 % of adults and palpable in most PMI in fifth LICS at or medial to MCL Diameter of 1 to 2 cm (1/3 to 1/2 in) No lift or heave	PMI displaced laterally or lower (indicates enlarged heart) Diameter over 2 cm (indicates enlarged heart or aneurysm) Diffuse lift or heave lateral to apex (indicates enlargement or overactivity of left ventricle)
• Inspect and palpate the epigastric area at the base of the sternum for abdominal aortic pulsations.	Aortic pulsations	Bounding abdominal pulsations (e.g., aortic aneurysm)

Locating the Aortic, Pulmonic, Tricuspid, and Apical Areas of the Precordium

- Locate the angle of Louis. It is felt as a prominence on the sternum.
- Move your fingertips down each side of the angle until you can feel the second intercostal spaces. The client's right second intercostal space is the *aortic area*, and the left second intercostal space is the *pulmonic area*.
- From the pulmonic area, move your fingertips down three left intercostal spaces along the side of the sternum. The left fifth intercostal space close to the sternum is the *tricuspid* or *right ventricular area*.
- From the tricuspid area, move your fingertips laterally 5 to 7 cm (2 to 3 in) to the left midclavicular line (LMCL). This is the *apical* or *mitral area, or PMI.* If you have difficulty locating the PMI, have the client roll onto the left side to move the apex closer to the chest wall.

▶ **Assessing the Cardiovascular System** *CONTINUED*

ASSESSMENT	NORMAL FINDINGS	DEVIATIONS FROM NORMAL
Auscultate the heart in all four anatomic sites: aortic, pulmonic, tricuspid, and apical (mitral). Auscultation need not be limited to these areas; however, the nurse may need to move the stethoscope to find the most audible sounds for each client. The box below describes the steps involved in auscultating the heart.	S_1: Usually heard at all sites Usually louder at apical area S_2: Usually heard at all sites Usually louder at base of heart **Systole:** Silent interval Slightly shorter duration than diastole at normal heart rate (60 to 90 beats/min) **Diastole:** silent interval Slightly longer duration than systole at normal heart rates S_3 in children and young adults S_4 in many older adults	Increased or decreased intensity Varying intensity with different beats Increased intensity at aortic area Increased intensity at pulmonic area Sharp-sounding ejection clicks S_3 in older adults S_4 may be a sign of hypertension

Auscultating the Heart

- Eliminate all sources of room noise. *Heart sounds are of low intensity, and other noise hinders the nurse's ability to hear them.*

- Keep the client in a supine position with head elevated 30° to 45°.

- Use both the flat-disc diaphragm and the bell-shaped diaphragm to listen to all areas.

- In every area of auscultation, distinguish both S_1 and S_2 sounds.

- When auscultating, concentrate on one particular sound at a time in each area: the first heart sound, followed by systole, then the second heart sound, then diastole. Systole and diastole are normally silent intervals.

- Later, reexamine the heart while the client is in the upright sitting position. *Certain sounds are more audible in certain positions.*

THE ELDERLY: PHYSICAL CHANGES OF THE HEART

- If no disease is present, heart size remains the same size throughout life.

- Cardiac output and strength of contraction decrease, thus lessening the older person's activity tolerance.

- The heart rate returns to its resting rate more slowly after exertion than it did when the individual was younger.

- S_4 heart sound is considered normal in older adults.

- Extra systoles commonly occur. Ten or more systoles per minute are considered abnormal.

- Sudden emotional and physical stresses may result in cardiac arrhythmias and heart failure.

Peripheral Vascular System

Assessment of the peripheral vascular system includes measurement of the blood pressure; palpation of peripheral pulses; inspection, palpation, and auscultation of the carotid pulse; inspection of the jugular and peripheral veins; and inspection of the skin and tissues to determine **perfusion** (passage of blood constituents through the vessels) to the extremities. Certain aspects of peripheral vascular assessment are often incorporated into other parts of the assessment procedure. For example, blood pressure is usually measured at the beginning of the physical

examination (see the section on assessing blood pressure in Chapter 10).

Pulse sites and pulse assessments are described in Chapter 10. Figures 10–8 and 10–12 illustrate the sites for palpating the peripheral pulses.

The *cartoid arteries* supply oxygenated blood to the head and neck (Figure 11–73). Since they are the only source of blood to the brain, prolonged occlusion of one of these arteries can result in serious brain damage. The carotid pulses correlate with central aortic pressure, thus reflecting cardiac function better than the peripheral pulses. When cardiac output is

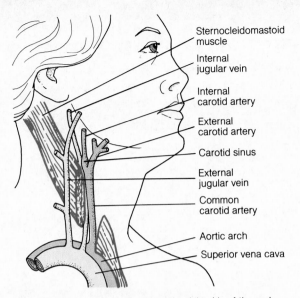

Sternocleidomastoid muscle
Internal jugular vein
Internal carotid artery
External carotid artery
Carotid sinus
External jugular vein
Common carotid artery
Aortic arch
Superior vena cava

FIGURE 11–73 Arteries and veins of the right side of the neck.

for a thrill. A **bruit** (a blowing or swishing sound) is created by turbulence of blood flow due either to a narrowed arterial lumen (a common development in older people) or to a condition, such as anemia or hyperthyroidism, that elevates cardiac output. A **thrill**, which frequently accompanies a bruit, is a vibrating sensation like the purring of a cat or water running through a hose. It, too, indicates turbulent blood flow due to arterial obstruction.

The *jugular veins* drain blood from the head and neck directly into the superior vena cava and right side of the heart (Figure 11–73). The external jugular veins are superficial and may be visible above the clavicle. The internal jugular veins lie deeper along the carotid artery and may transmit pulsations onto the skin of the neck. Normally, external neck veins are distended and visible when a person lies down; they are flat and not as visible when a person stands up, because gravity encourages venous drainage. By inspecting the jugular veins for pulsations and distention, the nurse can assess the adequacy of function of the right side of the heart and venous pressure. Bilateral jugular vein distention (JVD) may indicate right-sided heart failure.

diminished, the peripheral pulses may be difficult or impossible to feel, but the carotid pulse should be felt easily.

The carotid is also auscultated for a bruit, and if a bruit is found, the carotid artery is then palpated

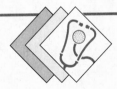

Assessing the Peripheral Vascular System

NURSING HISTORY FOCUS
Past history of heart disorders, varicosities, arterial disease, and hypertension; life-style, specifically exercise patterns, activity patterns and tolerance, smoking habits, and use of alcohol.

ASSESSMENT	NORMAL FINDINGS	DEVIATIONS FROM NORMAL
Peripheral Pulses		
Palpate the peripheral pulses (except the carotid pulse) **on both sides of the client's body simultaneously and systematically** to determine the symmetry of pulse volume. If you have difficulty palpating some of the peripheral pulses, use a Doppler ultrasound probe.	Symmetric pulse volumes Full pulsations	Asymmetric volumes (indicate impaired circulation) Absence of pulsation (indicates arterial spasm or occlusion) Decreased, weak, thready pulsations (indicate impaired cardiac output) Increased pulse volume (may indicate hypertension, high cardiac output, or circulatory overload)
Carotid Arteries		
Palpate the carotid artery, using extreme caution. See the accompanying box.	Symmetric pulse volumes Full pulsations, thrusting quality Quality remains same when client breathes, turns head, and changes from sitting to supine position Elastic arterial wall	Asymmetric volumes (possible stenosis or thrombosis) Decreased pulsations (may indicate impaired left cardiac output) Increased pulsations Thickening, hard, rigid, beaded, inelastic walls (indicate arteriosclerosis)

► **Assessing the Peripheral Vascular System** CONTINUED

ASSESSMENT	NORMAL FINDINGS	DEVIATIONS FROM NORMAL
Auscultate the carotid artery to determine the presence of a bruit. See the box below.	No sound heard on auscultation	Presence of bruit in one or both arteries (suggests occlusive artery disease)

Palpating and Auscultating the Carotid Artery

Palpation

- Palpate only one carotid artery at a time. *This ensures adequate cerebral blood flow through the other and thus prevents possible ischemia. Ischemia is a deficiency of blood in a body part due to constriction or obstruction of a blood vessel.*

- Avoid exerting too much pressure and massaging the area. *Pressure can occlude the artery and carotid sinus massage can precipitate bradycardia. The carotid sinus is a small dilation at the beginning of the internal carotid artery just above the bifurcation of the common carotid artery, in the upper third of the neck.*

- Ask the client to turn the head slightly toward the side being examined. *This makes the carotid artery more accessible.*

Auscultation

- Turn the client's head slightly away from the side being examined. *This facilitates the placement of the stethoscope.*

- Auscultate the carotid artery on one side and then the other.

- Listen for the presence of a bruit.

- If you hear a bruit, gently palpate the artery to determine the presence of a thrill.

Jugular Veins

Inspect the jugular veins for distention while the client is placed in a semi-Fowler's position (30° to 45° angle), with the head supported on a small pillow. **If jugular distention is present, assess the jugular venous pressure (JVP).**	Veins not visible (indicating right side of heart is functioning normally)	Veins visibly distended (indicating advanced cardiopulmonary disease) Bilateral measurements above 3 cm are considered elevated (may indicate right-sided heart failure) Unilateral distention (may be caused by local obstruction)

- Locate the highest visible point of distention of the internal jugular vein. Although either the internal or the external jugular vein can be used, the internal jugular vein is more reliable. *The external jugular vein is more easily affected by obstruction or kinking at the base of the neck.*

- Measure the vertical height of this point in centimeters from the sternal angle (the point at which the clavicles meet; Figure 11–74).

- Repeat the steps above on the other side.

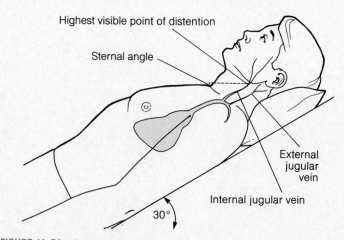

FIGURE 11–74 Assessing the highest point of distention of the internal jugular vein.

Peripheral Veins

Inspect the peripheral veins in the arms and legs for the presence and/or appearance of superficial veins when limbs are dependent and when limbs are elevated.	In dependent position, distention and nodular bulges at calves are present When limbs are elevated, veins collapse (veins may appear tortuous or distended in older people)	Distended veins in the anteromedial part of thigh and/or lower leg or on posterolateral part of calf from knee to ankle

Assessing the Peripheral Vascular System *CONTINUED*

ASSESSMENT	NORMAL FINDINGS	DEVIATIONS FROM NORMAL
Assess the peripheral leg veins for signs of phlebitis. See the box below.	Limbs not tender Symmetric in size	Tenderness on palpation Pain in calf muscles with forceful dorsiflexion of the foot (positive Homans') Warmth and redness over vein Swelling of one calf or leg

Assessing Peripheral Leg Veins for Signs of Phlebitis

- Inspect the calves for redness and swelling over vein sites.
- Palpate the calves for firmness or tension of the muscles, the presence of edema over the dorsum of the foot, and areas of localized warmth. *Palpation augments inspection findings, particularly in higher pigmented people in whom redness may not be visible.*
- Push the calves from side to side to test for tenderness.
- Firmly dorsiflex the client's foot while supporting the entire leg in extension (Homans' test), or have the person stand or walk.

Peripheral Perfusion

Inspect the skin of the hands and feet for color, temperature, edema, and skin changes.	Skin color pink	Cyanotic (venous insufficiency) Pallor that increases with limb elevation Dusky red color when limb is lowered (arterial insufficiency) Brown pigmentation around ankles (arterial or chronic venous insufficiency)
	Skin temperature not excessively warm or cold	Skin cool (arterial insufficiency)
	No edema	Marked edema (venous insufficiency) Mild edema (arterial insufficiency)
	Skin texture resilient and moist	Skin thin and shiny or thick, waxy, shiny, and fragile, with reduced hair and ulceration (venous or arterial insufficiency)
Assess the adequacy of arterial flow if arterial insuffiency is suspected. See the box below.	Buerger's test: Original color returns in 10 seconds; veins in feet or hands fill in about 15 seconds	Delayed color return or mottled appearance; delayed venous filling; marked redness of arms or legs (indicates arterial insufficiency)
	Capillary refill test: Immediate return of color	Delayed return of color (arterial insufficiency)

Assessing the Adequacy of Arterial Blood Flow

Buerger's Test (Arterial Adequacy Test)

- Assist the client to a supine position. Ask the client to raise one leg or one arm about 30 cm (1 ft) above heart level, move the foot or hand briskly up and down for about 1 minute, and then sit up and dangle the leg or arm.
- Observe the time elapsed until return of original color and vein filling. Original color normally returns in 10 seconds, and the veins fill in about 15 seconds.

Capillary Refill Test

- Squeeze the client's fingernail and toenail between your fingers sufficiently to cause blanching.
- Release the pressure, and observe how quickly normal color returns. Color normally returns immediately.

Other Assessments

- Inspect the fingernails for changes indicative of circulatory impairment. See the section on assessment of nails, earlier in this chapter.
- See also peripheral pulse assessment, earlier.

THE ELDERLY: PHYSICAL CHANGES IN THE PERIPHERAL VASCULAR SYSTEM

- The overall effectiveness of blood vessels decreases as smooth muscle cells are replaced by connective tissue. The lower extremities are more likely to show signs of arterial and venous impairment because of the more distal and dependent position.

- Proximal arteries become thinner and dilate.

- Peripheral arteries become thicker and dilate less effectively because of arteriosclerotic changes in the vessel walls.

- Blood vessels lengthen and become more tortuous and prominent. Varicosities occur more frequently.

- In some instances, arteries may be palpated more easily because of the loss of supportive surrounding tissues. Often, however, the most distal pulses of the lower extremities are more difficult to palpate because of decreased arterial perfusion.

- Systolic and diastolic blood pressures increase, but the increase in the systolic pressure is greater. As a result, the pulse pressure widens. Any client with a blood pressure reading above 140/90 should be referred for follow-up assessments.

- Peripheral edema is frequently observed and is most commonly the result of chronic venous insufficiency or low protein levels in the blood (hypoproteinemia).

- Carotid artery assessment is an essential aspect of peripheral vascular examination in the older adult.

The Breasts and Axillae

The breasts of men and women need to be inspected and palpated. Men have some glandular tissue beneath each nipple, a potential site for malignancy, whereas mature women have glandular tissue throughout the breast. During adolescence, asymmetric development is not unusual, because one breast may develop more rapidly than the other. Boys may have some breast development in early adolescence. Stages of breast development are shown in the box below. In females, the largest portion of glandular breast tissue is located in the upper outer quadrant of each breast. From this quadrant there is a projection of breast tissue into the axilla, called the **axillary tail of Spence** (Figure 11–75). The majority of breast tumors are located in this upper outer breast quadrant and in the tail of Spence. During assessment, the nurse can localize specific findings by using this division of the breast into quadrants and the axillary tail.

Five Stages of Breast Development*

- Stage 1 Elevation of the nipple
- Stage 2 Enlargement of the areola
- Stage 3 Enlargement of the breast
- Stage 4 Projection of the areola and nipple
- Stage 5 Recession of the areola by about age 14 or 15, leaving only the nipple projecting

*The 2-year transient breast growth that occurs in males reaches only the second stage.

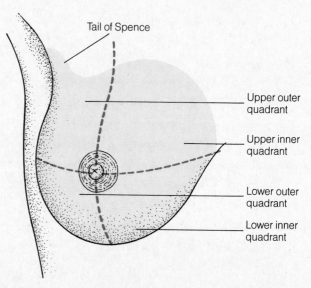

FIGURE 11–75 Four breast quadrants and the axillary tail of Spence.

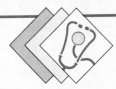

Assessing the Breasts and Axillae

NURSING HISTORY FOCUS

History of breast self-examination; technique used and when performed in relation to the menstrual cycle; history of breast masses and what was done about them; any pain or tenderness in the breasts and relation to menstrual cycle; any discharge from the nipple; medication history (some medications, e.g., oral contraceptives, steroids, digitalis, and diuretics, may cause nipple discharge; others, e.g., exogenous estrogens and phenothiazine, are associated with the development of cysts or cancer, respectively); risk factors for development of breast cancer (e.g., mother, sister, aunt, or grandmother with breast cancer; menarche before age 13; menopause after age 50; age 35 or more at first pregnancy).

ASSESSMENT	NORMAL FINDINGS	DEVIATIONS FROM NORMAL
Inspect the breasts for size, symmetry, and contour or shape while the client is in a sitting position.	Females: Rounded shape; slightly unequal in size; generally symmetric Males: Breasts even with the chest wall; if obese, may be similar in shape to female breasts	Recent change in breast size; swellings; marked asymmetry
Inspect the skin of the breast for localized discolorations or hyperpigmentation, retraction or dimpling, localized hypervascular areas, swelling or edema (Figure 11–76).	Skin uniform in color (same in appearance as skin of abdomen or back) Skin smooth and intact Diffuse symmetric horizontal or vertical vascular pattern in light-skinned people **Striae** (stretch marks); moles and nevi	Localized discolorations or hyperpigmentation Retraction or dimpling (result of scar tissue or an invasive tumor Unilateral, localized hypervascular areas (associated with increased blood flow) Swelling or edema appearing as pig skin or orange peel due to exaggeration of the pores

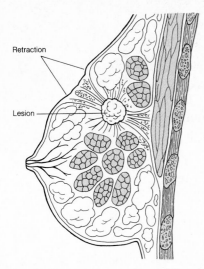

FIGURE 11–76 A lesion causing retraction of the skin.

Accentuate any retraction by having the client

- Raise the arms above the head.
- Push the hands together, with elbows flexed (Figure 11–77).
- Press the hands down on the hips (Figure 11–78).

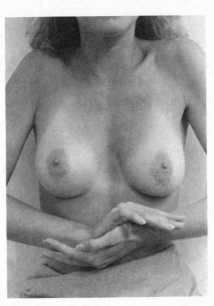

FIGURE 11–77 Pushing the hands together to accentuate retraction of breast tissues.

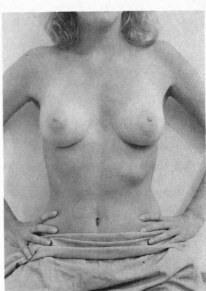

FIGURE 11–78 Pressing the hands down on the hips to accentuate retraction of breast tissue.

▶ **Assessing the Breasts and Axillae** *CONTINUED*

ASSESSMENT	NORMAL FINDINGS	DEVIATIONS FROM NORMAL
Inspect the areola area for size, shape, symmetry, color, surface characteristics, and any masses or lesions.	Round or oval and bilaterally the same Color varies widely, from light pink to dark brown Irregular placement of sebaceous glands on the surface of the areola (Montgomery's tubercles)	Any asymmetry, mass, or lesion
Inspect the nipples for size, shape, position, color, discharge, lesions.	Round, everted, and equal in size; similar in color; soft and smooth; both nipples point in same direction No discharge, except for colostrum in pregnant females Inversion of one or both nipples that is present from puberty	Asymmetrical size and color Presence of discharge, crusts, or cracks Recent inversion of one or both nipples
Palpate the axillary, subclavicular, and supraclavicular lymph nodes (Figure 11–79) while the client sits with the arms abducted and supported on the nurse's forearm. For palpation of clavicular lymph nodes, see page 278. Use the palmar surfaces of all fingertips to palpate the four areas of the axilla: • the edge of the greater pectoral muscle (musculus pectoralis major) along the anterior axillary line, • the thoracic wall in the midaxillary area, • the upper part of the humerus, and • the anterior edge of the latissimus dorsi muscle along the posterior axillary line.	No tenderness, masses, or nodules	Tenderness, masses, or nodules

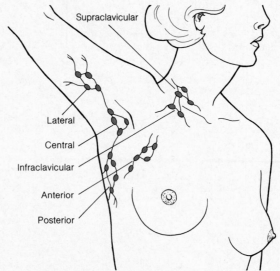

FIGURE 11–79 Lymph nodes that drain the breast tissues.

Palpate the breast for masses, tenderness, and any discharge from the nipples. See the box on page 261 for palpation methods.	No tenderness, masses, nodules, or nipple discharge	Tenderness, masses, nodules, or nipple discharge
Palpate the areola and the nipples for masses. Compress each nipple to determine the presence of any discharge. If discharge is present, milk the breast along its radii to identify the discharge-producing lobe. Assess any discharge for amount, color, consistency, and odor. Note also any tenderness on palpation.	No tenderness, masses, nodules, or nipple discharge	Tenderness, masses, nodules, or nipple discharge
Palpate the male breasts and the axillary lymph nodes when the client is supine.	As above for female client	As above for female client

▶ **Assessing the Breasts and Axillae** *CONTINUED*

Palpating the Breast

Palpation of the breast may be performed while the client is supine or sitting. For clients who have a past history of breast masses, who are at high risk for breast cancer, or who have pendulous breasts, examination in both positions is recommended (Malasanos, Barkauskas, and Stoltenberg-Allen 1990, p. 289).

Bimanual Palpation

A bimanual technique is often preferred, particularly if the breasts are large. The nondominant hand is placed under the breast, and the dominant hand palpates the breast. This bimanual technique can be most effective in detecting small deep masses. The client is in the *sitting* position. The bimanual technique is performed as follows:

• If the client reports a breast lump, start with the "normal" breast to obtain baseline data that will serve as a comparison to the reportedly involved breast.

• Press the palmar surface of the middle three fingertips (held together) on the skin surface, starting at the periphery of the breast (Figure 11–80).

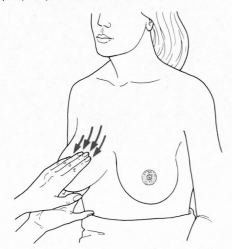

FIGURE 11–80 Bimanual breast palpation with the client in a sitting position.

• Use a smooth rotary motion or back-and-forth technique to press the breast tissue against the other hand.

• Palpate from the periphery to the areola.

• Move from the peripheral starting point around the breast systematically until all breast surfaces are thoroughly surveyed.

• Pay particular attention to the upper outer quadrant area and the tail of Spence, where about 50% of breast cancers develop.

One-Handed Palpation

• This technique is often performed after bimanual palpation, with the client in the *supine* position. *In the*

supine position, the breasts flatten evenly against the chest wall, facilitating palpation. It is performed as follows:

• To enhance flattening of the breast, instruct the client to abduct the arm and place her hand behind her head. Then place a small pillow or rolled towel under the client's shoulder.

• Use the fingertips of one hand, and visualize the breast as a clock (Figure 11–81).

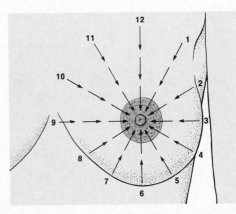

FIGURE 11–81 Pattern for palpating a breast, using the clock to describe the location of any masses.

• Palpate the breast tissue along the hands of the clock, moving from the periphery toward the areola.

• Choose any starting point for palpation, but start and end at a fixed point to ensure that all breast surfaces are assessed.

• If you detect a mass, record the following data:

a. *Location:* the exact location relative to the clock (as in Figure 11–81) and the distance from the nipple in centimeters.

b. *Client's position:* whether the arms were raised or lowered and whether the client was sitting or supine. The position can change the perceived location of the mass.

c. *Size:* the length, width, and thickness of the mass in centimeters. If you are unable to determine the discrete edges, record this fact.

d. *Mobility:* whether the mass is movable or fixed. If it is fixed, determine whether it is firmly or moderately fixed, if possible.

e. *Consistency:* whether the mass is hard or soft.

f. *Surface:* whether the surface is smooth or irregular.

g. *Tenderness:* whether palpation is painful.

h. *Shape:* whether the mass is round, discoid, regular, or irregular.

THE ELDERLY: PHYSICAL CHANGES OF THE BREASTS

- In the postmenopausal female, breasts change in shape and often appear pendulous or flaccid; they lack the firmness they had in younger years.

- The presence of breast lesions may be detected more readily because of the decrease in connective tissue.

- General breast size remains the same. Although glandular tissue atrophies, the amount of fat in breasts (predominantly in the lower quadrants) increases in most women.

The Abdomen

Description of abdominal findings is facilitated by two commonly used methods of subdivision: quadrants and nine regions. To divide the abdomen into quadrants, the nurse imagines two lines: a vertical line from the xiphoid process to the pubic symphysis, and a horizontal line across the umbilicus (Figure 11–82). These quadrants are labeled right upper quadrant (*1*), left upper quadrant (*2*), right lower quadrant (*3*), and left lower quadrant (*4*). Using the second method, division into nine regions, the nurse imagines two vertical lines that extend superiorly from the midpoints of the inguinal ligaments, and two horizontal lines, one at the level of the edge of the lower ribs and the other at the level of the iliac

crests (Figure 11–83). Specific organs or parts of organs lie in each abdominal region. See Tables 11–11 and 11–12.

In addition, practitioners often use certain landmarks to locate abdominal signs and symptoms. These are the xiphoid process of the sternum, the costal margins, the midline (a line drawn from the tip of the sternum through the umbilicus to the pubic symphysis), the anterosuperior iliac spine, the inguinal ligaments (Poupart's ligaments), and the superior margin of the pubic symphysis (Figure 11–84).

Assessment of the abdomen involves all four methods of examination (inspection, auscultation, palpation, and percussion). Of these, beginning practitioners usually perform only inspection and *auscultation*. In some agencies, the nurse also performs *palpation*. Check agency protocol.

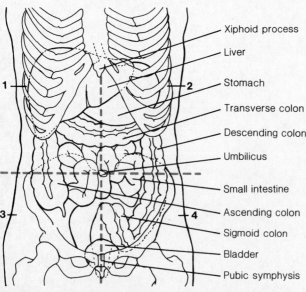

FIGURE 11–82 The four abdominal regions and the underlying organs: *1*, right upper quadrant; *2*, left upper quadrant; *3*, right lower quadrant; *4*, left lower quadrant.

Xiphoid process
Liver
Stomach
Transverse colon
Descending colon
Umbilicus
Small intestine
Ascending colon
Sigmoid colon
Bladder
Pubic symphysis

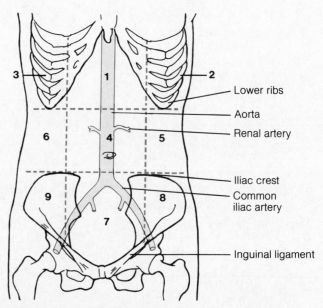

FIGURE 11–83 The nine abdominal regions: *1*, epigastric; *2*, *3*, left and right hypochondriac; *4*, umbilical; *5*, *6*, left and right lumbar; *7*, suprapubic and hypogastric; *8*, *9*, left and right inguinal or iliac.

Lower ribs
Aorta
Renal artery
Iliac crest
Common iliac artery
Inguinal ligament

TABLE 11–11 ORGANS IN THE FOUR ABDOMINAL QUADRANTS

RIGHT UPPER QUADRANT	**LEFT UPPER QUADRANT**
Liver	Left lobe of liver
Gallbladder	Stomach
Duodenum	Spleen
Head of pancreas	Upper lobe of left kidney
Right adrenal gland	Pancreas
Upper lobe of right kidney	Left adrenal gland
Hepatic flexure of colon	Splenic flexure of colon
Section of ascending colon	Section of transverse colon
Section of transverse colon	Section of descending colon
RIGHT LOWER QUADRANT	**LEFT LOWER QUANDRANT**
Lower lobe of right kidney	Lower lobe of left kidney
Cecum	Sigmoid colon
Appendix	Section of descending colon
Section of ascending colon	Left ovary
Right ovary	Left fallopian tube
Right fallopian tube	Left ureter
Right ureter	Left spermatic cord
Right spermatic cord	Part of uterus (if enlarged)
Part of uterus (if enlarged)	

TABLE 11–12 ORGANS IN THE NINE ABDOMINAL REGIONS

RIGHT HYPOCHONDRIAC	**EPIGASTRIC**	**LEFT HYPOCHONDRIAC**
Right lobe of liver	Aorta	Stomach
Gallbladder	Pyloric end of stomach	Spleen
Part of duodenum	Part of duodenum	Tail of pancreas
Hepatic flexure of colon	Pancreas	Splenic flexure of colon
Upper half of right kidney	Part of liver	Upper half of left kidney
Suprarenal gland		Suprarenal gland
RIGHT LUMBAR	**UMBILICAL**	**LEFT LUMBAR**
Ascending colon	Omentum	Descending colon
Lower half of right kidney	Mesentery	Lower half of left kidney
Part of duodenum and jejunum	Lower part of duodenum	Part of jejunum and ileum
	Part of jejunum and ileum	
RIGHT INGUINAL	**HYPOGASTRIC (PUBIC)**	**LEFT INGUINAL**
Cecum	Ileum	Sigmoid colon
Appendix	Bladder (if enlarged)	Left ureter
Lower end of ileum	Uterus (if enlarged)	Left spermatic cord
Right ureter		Left ovary
Right spermatic cord		
Right ovary		

When assessing the abdomen, the nurse performs inspection first, followed by auscultation, palpation, and/or percussion. **Auscultation is done before palpation and percussion** because palpation and percussion cause movement or stimulation of the bowel, which can increase bowel motility and thus heighten bowel sounds, creating false results.

To facilitate validity of observations and enhance client comfort, the nurse asks the client to urinate before beginning the assessment and assists the client to a supine position, with the arms placed comfortably at the sides. The nurse also places small pillows beneath the knees and the head. This position and an empty bladder prevent tension in the abdominal muscles. By contrast, the abdominal muscles tense when the client is sitting or supine with knees and arms extended and with hands clasped behind the head.

The nurse should ensure that the room is warm and expose only the client's abdomen from chest line to the pubic area to avoid chilling and shivering, which can tense the abdominal muscles. An examining light, a tape measure (metal or unstretchable cloth), a water-soluble skin-marking pencil, and a stethoscope are necessary for the examination.

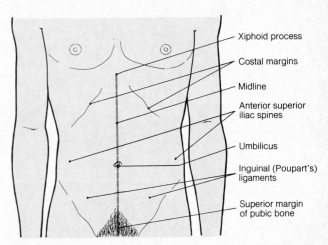

- Xiphoid process
- Costal margins
- Midline
- Anterior superior iliac spines
- Umbilicus
- Inguinal (Poupart's) ligaments
- Superior margin of pubic bone

FIGURE 11–84 Landmarks commonly used to identify abdominal areas.

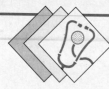

Assessing the Abdomen

NURSING HISTORY FOCUS

Incidence of abdominal pain: its location, onset, sequence, and chronology; its quality (description); its frequency; associated symptoms (e.g., nausea, vomiting, diarrhea); bowel habits; incidence of constipation or diarrhea (have client describe what client means by these terms); change in appetite, food intolerances, and foods ingested in last 24 hours; specific signs and symptoms (e.g., heartburn, flatulence and/or belching, difficulty swallowing, hematemesis, blood or mucus in stools, and aggravating and alleviating factors); previous problems and treatment (e.g., stomach ulcer, gallbladder surgery, history of jaundice).

ASSESSMENT	NORMAL FINDINGS	DEVIATIONS FROM NORMAL
Inspection of the Abdomen		
Inspect the abdomen for skin integrity (refer to the discussion about skin assessment, earlier in this chapter).	Unblemished skin Uniform color Silver-white striae or surgical scars	Presence of rash or other lesions Tense, glistening skin (may indicate ascites, edema) Purple striae (associated with Cushing's disease)
Inspect the abdomen for contour and symmetry.		
• Observe the abdominal contour (profile line from the rib margin to the pubic bone) while standing at the client's side when the client is supine.	Flat, rounded (convex), or scaphoid (concave)	Distended
• Ask the client to take a deep breath and to hold it (makes an enlarged liver or spleen more obvious).	No evidence of enlargement of liver or spleen	Evidence of enlargement of liver or spleen
• Assess the symmetry of contour while standing at the foot of the bed.	Symmetric contour	Asymmetric contour, e.g., localized protrusions around umbilicus, inguinal ligaments, or scars (possible hernia or tumor)
• If a hernia is suspected, ask the client to raise the head and shoulders from the pillow without using the arms for support (increases intra-abdominal pressure and may cause upward protrusion of the hernia).	No appearance of bulges or marked ridges	Bulges or masses appear
• If distention is present, measure the abdominal girth by placing a tape around the abdomen at the level of the umbilicus (Figure 11–85).		

FIGURE 11–85 Measuring the abdominal girth at the level of the umbilicus.

▶ Assessing the Abdomen *CONTINUED*

ASSESSMENT	NORMAL FINDINGS	DEVIATIONS FROM NORMAL
Observe abdominal movements associated with respiration, peristalsis, or aortic pulsations.	Symmetric movements caused by respiration Visible peristalsis in very lean people Aortic pulsations in thin persons at epigastric area	Limited movement due to pain or disease process Visible peristalsis in nonlean clients (with bowel obstruction) Marked aortic pulsations
Auscultate of the Abdomen **Auscultate the abdomen for bowel sounds, vascular sounds, and peritoneal friction rubs.** The auscultation procedure is shown in the box below.	Audible bowel sounds Absence of arterial bruits Absence of friction rub	Absent or hypoactive bowel sounds Hyperactive bowel sounds Loud bruit over aortic area (possible aneurysm) Bruit over renal or iliac arteries Friction rub

---

Auscultating the Abdomen

Warm the hands and the stethoscope diaphragms. *Cold hands and a cold stethoscope may cause the client to contract the abdominal muscles, and these contractions may be heard during auscultation.*

For Bowel Sounds

- Use the flat-disc diaphragm. *Intestinal sounds are relatively high-pitched and best accentuated by the flat-disc diaphragm. Only light pressure with the stethoscope is adequate to detect sounds.*

- Ask when the client last ate. *The frequency of sounds relates to the state of digestion or the presence of food in the gastrointestinal tract. Shortly after or long after eating, bowel sounds may normally increase. They are loudest when a meal is long overdue. Four to 7 hours after a meal, bowel sounds may be heard continuously over the ileocecal valve area while the digestive contents from the small intestine empty through the valve into the large intestine.*

- Place the flat-disc diaphragm of the stethoscope in each of the four quadrants of the abdomen over all the auscultatory sites shown in Figure 11–86. Many nurses begin in the lower right quadrant in the area of the cecum.

- Listen for active bowel sounds—irregular gurgling noises occurring about every 5 to 20 seconds. The duration of a single sound may range from less than a second to more than several seconds.

- Normal bowel sounds are described as *audible.* Alterations in sounds are described as *absent* or *hypoactive,* i.e., extremely soft and infrequent (e.g., one per minute), and *hyperactive* or *increased,* i.e., high-pitched, loud, rushing sounds that occur frequently (e.g., every 3 seconds) also known as *borborygmi.* Absence of sounds indicates a cessation of intestinal motility. Hypoactive sounds indicate decreased motility

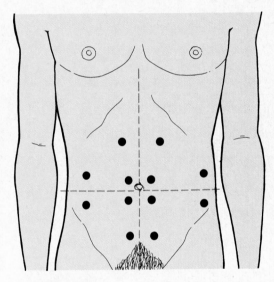

FIGURE 11–86 Auscultation sites of the abdomen.

and are usually associated with manipulation of the bowel during surgery, inflammation, paralytic ileus, or late bowel obstruction. Hyperactive sounds indicate increased intestinal motility and are usually associated with diarrhea, an early bowel obstruction, or the use of laxatives.

- If bowel sounds appear to be absent, listen for 3 to 5 minutes before concluding that they are absent. *Because bowel sounds are so irregular, a longer time and more sites are used to confirm absence of sounds.*

For Vascular Sounds

Use the bell of the stethoscope over the aorta, renal arteries, and iliac arteries as follows, and listen for bruits.

continued on page 266

▶ **Assessing the Abdomen** *CONTINUED*

Auscultating the Abdomen CONTINUED

- Auscultate the aorta superior to the umbilicus.

- Auscultate the renal arteries at or to the left and right of the upper abdominal midline or farther toward the flank.

- Auscultate the iliac arteries to the left and right of the abdominal midline below the umbilicus. See Figure 11–83, earlier, to locate these areas.

Peritoneal Friction Rubs

Peritoneal friction rubs sound like two pieces of leather rubbing together. Friction rubs may be caused by infectious or abnormal growth processes, including metas-

tases. Listen for peritoneal friction rubs at the various auscultating sites, especially above the liver and spleen. *The liver and spleen have large surface areas in contact with the peritoneum; thus they are most frequently the beginning sites for friction rubs.*

- To auscultate the splenic site, place the stethoscope over the left lower rib cage in the anterior axillary line, and ask the client to take a deep breath. *A deep breath may accentuate the sound of a friction rub area.*

- To auscultate the liver site, place the stethoscope over the lower right rib cage.

Palpating the Abdomen

Palpation is used to detect tenderness, the presence of masses or distention, and the outline and position of abdominal organs (e.g., the liver, spleen, and kidneys). Two types of palpation are used: light and deep. In some practice settings, palpation is limited to light abdominal palpation to assess tenderness and bladder palpation to assess for distention. Before palpation, (a) ensure that the client's position is appropriate for relaxation of the abdominal muscles, and (b) warm the hands. *Cold hands can elicit muscle tension and thus impedes palpatory evaluation.*

Light Palpation

- Hold the palm of your hand slightly above the client's abdomen, with your fingers parallel to the abdomen.

- Depress the abdominal wall lightly, about 1 cm or to the depth of the subcutaneous tissue, with the pads of your fingers (Figure 11–87).

- Move the finger pads in a slight circular motion.

- If the client is extremely ticklish, place the client's hand under or over your hand. *This may decrease the degree of ticklishness and resulting muscle tenseness.*

- Note areas of slight tenderness or superficial pain, large masses, and muscle guarding. To determine areas of tenderness, ask the client to tell you about them, watch for changes in the client's facial expressions, and note areas of muscle guarding. When the client complains of overall abdominal tenderness, use a cotton wisp for palpation to help the client identify specific pain areas.

Deep Palpation

- Palpate sensitive areas last.

- Press the distal half of the palmar surface of the fingers of one hand into the abdominal wall.
  or
  Use the bimanual method of palpation discussed earlier in this chapter, page 202.

- Depress the abdominal wall about 4 to 5 cm (1.5 to 2.0 in) or an appropriate distance beyond subcutaneous tissue (Figure 11–88).

- Note masses and the structure of underlying contents. If a mass is present, determine its size, location, mobility, contour, consistency, and tenderness. Normal abdominal structures that may be mistaken for masses include the lateral borders of the rectus abdominis muscles; the feces-filled ascending, descending, or sigmoid colon; the aorta; the uterus; the common iliac artery; and the sacral promontory.

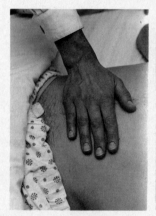
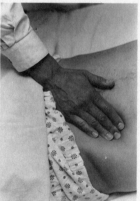

FIGURE 11–87 Light palpation of the abdomen.

FIGURE 11–88 Deep palpation of the abdomen.

▶ Assessing the Abdomen *CONTINUED*

ASSESSMENT	NORMAL FINDINGS	DEVIATIONS FROM NORMAL
Palpation of the Abdomen		
Perform light palpation first to detect areas of tenderness and/or muscle guarding. Systematically explore all four quadrants. See the box on page 266 for palpation technique.	No tenderness; relaxed abdomen with smooth, consistent tension	Tenderness and hypersensitivity Superficial masses Localized areas of increased tension
Perform deep palpation over all four quadrants. See the box on page 266.	Tenderness may be present near xiphoid process, over cecum, and over sigmoid colon	Generalized or localized areas of tenderness Mobile or fixed masses
Palpation of the Liver		
Palpate the liver to detect enlargement and tenderness. See palpation methods in the box below.	May not be palpable	Enlarged (abnormal finding, even if liver is smooth and not tender)
	Border feels smooth	Smooth but tender; nodular or hard

Palpating the Liver

Two bimanual approaches are used in palpation of the liver. In using the first method, place one hand along the anterior rib cage and the other hand on the posterior rib cage.

- Stand on the client's right side.

- Place your left hand on the posterior thorax at about the eleventh or twelfth rib. This hand is used to push upward and provide support of underlying structures for the subsequent anterior palpation.

- Place your right hand along the rib cage at about a 45° angle to the right of the rectus abdominis muscle or parallel to the rectus muscle with the fingers pointing toward the rib cage (Figure 11–89).

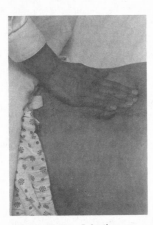

FIGURE 11–89 Palpating the liver.

- While the client exhales, exert a gradual and gentle downward and forward pressure beneath the costal margin until you reach a depth of 4 to 5 cm (1 1/2 to 2 in). *During expiration, the abdominal wall relaxes, facilitating deep palpation.*

- Maintain your hand position, and ask the client to inhale deeply. *This makes the liver border descend and moves the liver into a palpable position.*

- While the client inhales, feel the liver border move against your hand. It should feel firm and have a regular contour. If you do not palpate the liver initially, ask the client to take two or three more deep breaths while you maintain or apply slightly more palpation pressure. Livers are harder to palpate in obese, tense, or very physically fit people.

- If the liver is enlarged, i.e., palpable below the costal margin, measure the number of centimeters it extends below the costal region.

A *second* method is the bimanual palpation method discussed on page 202, in which one hand is superimposed on the other (Figure 11–6, earlier). The techniques and principles used above apply to that method as well.

► **Assessing the Abdomen** *CONTINUED*

ASSESSMENT	NORMAL FINDINGS	DEVIATIONS FROM NORMAL
Palpation of the Bladder **Palpate the area above the pubic symphysis** if the client's history indicates possible urinary retention (Figure 11–90).	Not palpable	Distended and palpable as smooth, round, tense mass (indicates urinary retention)

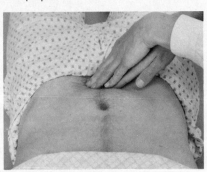

FIGURE 11–90 Palpating the bladder.

THE ELDERLY: PHYSICAL CHANGES IN THE GASTROINTESTINAL TRACT

- The rounded abdomens of many older persons are due to an increase in adipose tissue and a decrease in muscle tone.

- The abdominal wall is slacker and thinner, making palpation easier and more accurate than in younger clients. Muscle wasting and loss of fibroconnective tissue occur.

- The side-effects of drugs are often manifested in the gastrointestinal tract, e.g., nausea, vomiting, and diarrhea.

- The pain threshold in the elderly is often greater; major abdominal problems such as appendicitis or other acute emergencies may therefore go undetected.

- Gastrointestinal pain needs to be differentiated from cardiac pain. Gastrointestinal pain may be located in the chest or abdomen, whereas cardiac pain is usually located in the chest. Factors aggravating gastrointestinal pain are usually related to either ingestion or lack of food intake; gastrointestinal pain is usually relieved by antacids, food, or assuming an upright position. Common factors that can aggravate cardiac pain are activity or anxiety; cardiac pain is relieved by rest or nitroglycerin.

Esophagus

- Esophageal motility may decrease and, if it is severe, it can cause discomfort as food passes through the esophagus.

- Difficulty swallowing (dysphagia), a common complaint of older adults, must be differentiated from heartburn or regurgitation. Questions about food getting "stuck in the throat" or the ability to swallow liquid foods versus solid foods can clarify these symptoms.

- Many older individuals have increased esophageal spasms and less efficient action of the lower esophageal sphincter.

Stomach

- Gastric acid secretion decreases, and emptying time of the stomach is delayed, resulting in indigestion and intolerance to certain foods. Decreases in the production of pancreatic enzymes also contribute to complaints of indigestion and anorexia.

Intestines

- Stool passes through the intestines at a slower rate in elderly clients, and the perception of stimuli that produce the urge to defecate often diminishes.

- Fecal incontinence may occur in confused or neurologically impaired older adults.

- Many older persons erroneously believe that the absence of a daily bowel movement signifies constipation. When assessing for constipation, the nurse must consider the client's diet, activity, medications, characteristics and ease of passage of feces, as well as the frequency of bowel movements.

- The incidence of colon cancer is higher among older adults than younger adults. Symptoms include a change in bowel function, rectal bleeding, and weight loss. Changes in bowel function, however, are associated with many factors, such as diet, exercise, and medications.

- Decreased absorption of oral medications often occurs with aging.

Liver

- The liver changes minimally with age, as does the gallbladder. Liver function tests are unaltered.

- Impaired metabolism of some drugs may occur with aging.

The Musculoskeletal System

The musculoskeletal system encompasses the muscles, bones, and joints. The completeness of an assessment of this system depends largely on the needs and problems of the individual client. The nurse usually assesses the musculoskeletal system for muscle strength, tone, size and symmetry of muscle development, and fasciculations and tremors. A **fasciculation** is an abnormal contraction (shortening) of a bundle of muscle fibers. A **tremor** is an involuntary trembling of a limb or body part. Tremors may involve large groups of muscle fibers or small bundles of muscle fibers. An *intention tremor* becomes more apparent when an individual attempts a voluntary movement, e.g., holding a cup of coffee. A *resting tremor* is more apparent when the client is at rest and diminishes with activity.

Bones are assessed for normalcy of form. Joints are assessed for tenderness, swelling, thickening, **crepitation** (a crackling, grating sound), presence of nodules, range of motion. The amount of joint movement can be measured by a **goniometer**, a device that measures the angle of the joint in degrees. See (Figure 11–91). Body posture is assessed for normalcy in standing and sitting positions. For information about body posture see Chapter 21.

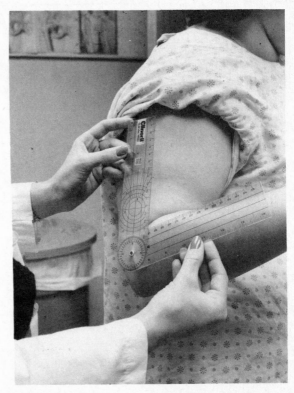

FIGURE 11–91 A goniometer used to measure joint range of motion.

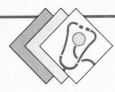

Assessing the Musculoskeletal System

NURSING HISTORY FOCUS

History or presence of muscle pain: onset, location, character, associated phenomena (e.g., redness and swelling of joints), and aggravating and alleviating factors; any limitations to movement or inability to perform activities of daily living; previous sports injuries; any loss of function without pain.

ASSESSMENT	NORMAL FINDINGS	DEVIATIONS FROM NORMAL
Muscles		
Inspect the muscles for size. Compare the muscles on one side of the body (e.g., of the arm, thigh, and calf) to the same muscle on the other side. For any discrepancies, measure the muscles with a tape.	Equal size on both sides of body	**Atrophy** (a decrease in size) or **hypertrophy** (an increase in size)
Inspect the muscles and tendons for contractures.	No contractures	Malposition of body part (e.g., a foot fixed in dorsiflexion)
Inspect the muscles for fasiculations and tremors. Inspect any tremors of the hands and arms by having the client hold the arms out in front of the body.	No fasiculations or tremors	Presence of fasiculation or tremor

▶

▶ **Assessing the Musculoskeletal System** *CONTINUED*

ASSESSMENT	NORMAL FINDINGS	DEVIATIONS FROM NORMAL
Palpate muscles at rest to determine muscle tonicity (the normal condition of tension, or tone, of a muscle at rest).	Normally firm	Atonic (lacking tone)
Palpate muscles while the client is active and passive for flaccidity, spasticity, and smoothness of movement.	Smooth coordinated movements	**Flaccidity** (weakness or laxness) or **spasticity** (sudden involuntary muscle contraction)
Test muscle strength. See tests in the box below. Compare the right side with left side.	Equal strength on each body side	25% or less of normal strength

---

Testing and Grading Muscle Strength

Muscle/Activity

Deltoid: Client holds arm up and resists while nurse tries to push it down.
Biceps: Client fully extends each arm and tries to flex it while nurse attempts to hold arm in extension.
Triceps: Client flexes each arm and then tries to extend it against the nurse's attempt to keep arm in flexion.
Wrist and finger muscles: Client spreads the fingers and resists as the nurse attempts to push the fingers together.
Grip strength: Client grasps the index and middle fingers of the examiner while the nurse tries to pull the fingers out.
Hip muscles: Client is supine, both legs extended; client raises one leg at a time while the nurse attempts to hold it down.
Hip abduction: Client is supine, both legs extended. Nurse's hands are on the lateral surface of each knee; client is asked to spread the legs apart against the nurse's resistance.
Hip adduction: Client is in same position as for hip abduction; the nurse's hands are now placed between the knees; client is asked to bring the legs together against the nurse's resistance.

Hamstrings: Client is supine, both knees bent. Client resists while the nurse attempts to straighten them.
Quadriceps: Client is supine, knee partially extended; client resists while the nurse attempts to flex the knee.
Muscles of the ankles and feet: Client resists while the nurse attempts to dorsiflex the foot and again resists while the nurse attempts to flex the foot.

Grading Muscle Strength

0: 0% of normal strength; complete paralysis.
1: 10% of normal strength; no movement, contraction of muscle is palpable or visible.
2: 25% of normal strength; full muscle movement against gravity, with support.
3: 50% of normal strength; normal movement against gravity.
4: 75% of normal strength; normal full movement against gravity and against minimal resistance.
5: 100% of normal strength; normal full movement against gravity and against full resistance.

Bones

Inspect the skeleton for normal structure and deformities.	No deformities	Bones misaligned
Palpate the bones to locate any areas of edema or tenderness.	No tenderness or swelling	Presence of tenderness or swelling (may indicate fractures, neoplasms, or osteoporosis)

Joints

Inspect the joints for swelling.	No swelling	One or more swollen joints
Palpate each joint for tenderness, smoothness of movement, swelling, crepitation, presence of nodules.	No tenderness, swelling, crepitation, or nodules. Joints move smoothly	Presence of tenderness, swelling, crepitation, or nodules

ASSESSMENT	NORMAL FINDINGS	DEVIATIONS FROM NORMAL
Assess joint range of motion. Table 21–2, page 501, lists the types of joint movements. • Ask the client to move selected body parts as shown in Table 21–2, page 501. Measure the amount of movement by a goniometer, as indicated.	Varies to some degree in accordance with person's genetic makeup and degree of physical activity	Limited range of motion in one or more joints

---

THE ELDERLY: PHYSICAL CHANGES IN THE MUSCULOSKELETAL SYSTEM

• Muscle mass decreases progressively with age, but there are wide variations among different individuals.

• The decrease in speed, strength, resistance to fatigue, reaction time, and coordination in the older person is due to a decrease in nerve conduction and muscle tone.

• The bones become more fragile, and osteoporosis leads to a loss of total bone mass. As a result, elderly people are predisposed to fractures and compressed vertebrae.

• In most elderly people, osteoarthritic changes in the joints can be observed.

The Neurologic System

The nervous system integrates all other body systems, but it also depends on the appropriate functioning of peripheral organs from which it receives internal and external environmental stimuli. A thorough neurologic examination may take 1 to 3 hours; however, routine screening tests are usually done first. If the results of these tests are questionable, more extensive evaluations are made. Three major considerations determine the extent of a neurologic exam: (a) the client's chief complaints, (b) the client's physical condition (i.e., level of consciousness and ability to ambulate), because many parts of the exam require movement and coordination of the extremities, and (c) the client's willingness to participate and cooperate.

Examination of the neurologic system includes assessment of (a) mental status, (b) level of consciousness, (c) the cranial nerves, (d) reflexes, (e) motor function, and (f) sensory function.

Parts of the neurologic assessment are performed throughout the health examination. For example, the nurse performs a large part of the mental status assessment during the taking of the history and when observing the client's general appearance. In addition, the nurse assesses the function of many cranial nerves. Cranial nerves II, III, IV, V (opthalmic branch), and XI are assessed with the eyes and vision tests and cranial nerve VIII (cochlear branch) is assessed with the ears and hearing.

Nursing History Focus

The client is assessed for presence of pain in the head, back, or extremities: onset and aggravating and alleviating factors; disorientation to time, place, or person: speech disorder; any history of loss of consciousness, fainting, convulsions, trauma, tingling or numbness, tremors or tics, limping, paralysis, uncontrolled muscle movements, loss of memory, mood swings, or problems with smell, vision, taste, touch, or hearing.

Mental Status

Assessment of mental status reveals the client's general cerebral function. These functions include intellectual (cognitive) as well as emotional (affective) functions. Affective behavior is discussed in the general survey at the beginning of this chapter.

If problems with use of language, memory, concentration, thought processes, or attention span and memory are noted during the nursing history, a more extensive examination is required during neurologic assessment. Major areas of mental status assessment include language, orientation, memory, and attention span and calculation.

Language

Any defects in or loss of the power to express oneself by speech, writing, or signs or to comprehend spoken or written language due to disease or injury of the cerebral cortex is called **aphasia**. Aphasias can be categorized as sensory or receptive aphasia and motor or expressive aphasia.

Sensory/receptive aphasia is the loss of the ability to comprehend written or spoken words. Two types of sensory aphasia are auditory or acoustic aphasia and visual aphasia. Clients with *auditory aphasia* have lost the ability to understand the symbolic content associated with sounds. Clients with *visual aphasia* have lost the ability to understand printed or written figures.

Motor/expressive aphasia involves loss of the power to express oneself by writing, making signs, or speaking. Clients may find that even though they can recall words, they have lost the ability to combine speech sounds into words.

To assess language deficits related to aphasia:

1. Point to common objects, and ask the client to name them.

2. Ask the client to read some words and to match the printed and written words with pictures.

3. Ask the client to respond to simple verbal and written commands, e.g., "point to your toes" or "raise your left arm."

It is also important to identify speech patterns. A pattern of repeating the same response as different questions are asked is called **perseveration. Paraphasia** is speech that is appropriately expressive but contains many incorrect words.

Orientation

Determine the client's orientation to *time, place* and *person* by tactful questioning. Orientation is easily assessed by asking the client the city and state or residence, time of day, date, day of the week, duration of illness, and names of family members. More direct questioning may be necessary for some people; e.g., "Where are you now?" "What day is it today?" Most people readily accept these questions if initially the nurse asks, "Do you get confused at times?"

Memory

Listen for lapses in memory. First, ask the client about difficulty with memory. If problems are apparent, three categories of memory are tested: immediate recall, recent memory, and remote memory.

To assess *immediate recall:*

- Ask the client to repeat a series of three digits, e.g., 7-4-3, spoken slowly.

- Gradually increase the number of digits, e.g., 7-4-3-5, 7-4-3-5-6, and 7-4-3-5-6-7-2, until the client fails to repeat the series correctly.

- Start again with a series of three digits, but this time ask the client to repeat them backward. The

average person can repeat a series of five to eight digits in sequence and four to six digits in reverse order.

To assess *recent memory:*

- Ask the client to recall the recent events of the day, such as how the client got to the clinic. This information must be validated, however.

- Ask the client to recall information given early in the interview, e.g., the name of a doctor.

- Provide the client with three facts to recall, e.g., a color, an object, an address, or a three-digit number, and ask the client to repeat all three. Later in the interview, ask the client to recall all three items.

To assess *remote memory,* ask the client to describe a previous illness or surgery, e.g., 5 years ago, or a birthday or anniversary.

Attention Span and Calculation

Test the ability to concentrate or attention span by asking the client to recite the alphabet or to count backward from 100. Test the ability to calculate by asking the client to subtract 7 or 3 progressively from 100; i.e., 100, 93, 86, 79, or 100, 97, 94, 91. This standard test is often referred to as the *serial sevens* or *serial threes test.* Normally, an adult can complete the serial sevens test in about 90 seconds with three or fewer errors. Because educational level and language or cultural differences affect calculating ability, this test may be inappropriate for some people.

Changes in mental function in elderly people are shown in the box on page 273.

Level of Consciousness

Level of consciousness (LOC) can lie anywhere along a continuum from a state of alertness to coma. A fully alert client responds to questions spontaneously; a comatose client may not respond to verbal stimuli. The Glasgow Coma Scale was originally developed to predict recovery from a head injury; however, it is used today to assess LOC. It tests in three major areas: eye response, motor response, and verbal response. An assessment totaling 15 points indicates the client is alert and completely oriented. A comatose client scores 7 or less. See Table 11–13.

Cranial Nerves

For the specific functions and assessment methods of each cranial nerve, see Table 11–14 on page 274. The nurse needs to be aware of these functions to detect abnormalities. (The names and order of the cranial nerves can be recalled by remembering this

THE ELDERLY: CHANGES IN MENTAL FUNCTION

- A decline in mental status is not a normal result of aging. Changes are more the result of physical or psychologic disorders (e.g., fever, fluid and electrolyte imbalances).
- Intelligence and learning ability are unaltered with age. Many factors, however, inhibit learning (e.g., anxiety, illness, pain, cultural barrier).
- Short-term memory is often less efficient. Long-term memory is usually unaltered.

- Because old age is often associated with loss of support persons, depression is a common disorder. It may be manifested by mood changes, weight loss, anorexia, constipation, and early morning awakening.
- The stress of being in unfamiliar situations can cause confusion in the elderly person.

sentence: "On old Olympus's treeless top, a Finn and German viewed a hop." The first letter of each word in the sentence is the same as the first letter of the names of the cranial nerves.)

Reflexes

A **reflex** is an automatic response of the body to a stimulus. It is not voluntarily learned or conscious. The deep tendon reflex (DTR) is activated when a tendon is stimulated (tapped) and its associated muscle contracts. The quality of a reflex response varies among individuals and by age. As a person ages reflex responses may become less intense.

Reflexes are tested using a percussion hammer. The response is described on a scale of 0 to +4. See the box below for a scale describing reflex responses. Experience is necessary to determine appropriate scoring for an individual. When assessing reflexes, it is important for the nurse to compare one side of the body with the other to evaluate the symmetry of response.

Several reflexes are normally tested during a physical examination. These are (a) the biceps reflex, (b) the triceps reflex, (c) the brachioradialis reflex, (d) the patellar reflex, (e) the Achilles reflex, and (f) the plantar (Babinski) reflex.

Biceps Reflex

The biceps reflex tests the spinal cord level C-5, C-6.

1. Partially flex the client's arm at the elbow, and rest the forearm over the thighs, placing the palm of the hand down.

2. Place the thumb of your nondominant hand horizontally over the biceps tendon.

3. With your other hand, hold the percussion hammer between thumb and index finger.

4. Deliver a blow (slight downward thrust) with the percussion hammer to your thumb.

TABLE 11–13 LEVELS OF CONSCIOUSNESS: GLASGOW COMA SCALE

Faculty Measured	Response	Score★
Eye opening	Spontaneous	4
	To verbal command	3
	To pain	2
	No response	1
Motor response	To verbal command	6
	To painful stimuli:	
	• Localizes pain	5
	• Flexes and withdraws	4
	• Assumes decorticate posture	3
	• Assumes decerebrate posture	2
	• No response	1
Verbal response (arouse client with painful stimuli, if necessary)	Oriented, converses	5
	Disoriented, converses	4
	Uses inappropriate words	3
	Makes incomprehensible sounds	2
	No response	1

*Coma is defined as a score of 7 or less. A score of 3 or 4 indicates an 85% chance of dying or remaining vegetative. A score of 11 or more suggests an 85% chance of moderate disability or good recovery.

Source: Adapted from G. Teasdale and B. Bennett, Assessment of coma and impaired consciousness: A practical scale, *Lancet* 1974; 2(7872):81.

Scale for Grading Reflex Responses

- 0 No reflex response
- +1 Minimal activity (hypoactive)
- +2 Normal response
- +3 More active than normal
- +4 Maximum activity (hyperactive)

TABLE 11–14 CRANIAL NERVE FUNCTIONS AND ASSESSMENT METHODS

Cranial Nerve	Name	Type	Function	Assessment Method
I	Olfactory	Sensory	Smell	Ask client to close eyes and identify different mild aromas, such as coffee, tobacco, vanilla, oil of cloves, peanut butter, orange, lemon, lime, chocolate.
II	Optic	Sensory	Vision and visual fields	Ask client to read Snellen chart; check visual fields by confrontation; and conduct an ophthalmoscopic examination.
III	Oculomotor	Motor	Extraocular eye movement (EOM); movement of sphincter of pupil; movement of ciliary muscles of lens	Assess six ocular movements and pupil reaction.
IV	Trochlear	Motor	EOM, specifically moves eyeball downward and laterally	Assess six ocular movements.
V	Trigeminal			
	Ophthalmic branch	Sensory	Sensation of cornea, skin of face, and nasal mucosa	While client looks upward, lightly touch lateral sclera of eye to elicit blink reflex; to test light sensation, have client close eyes, wipe a wisp of cotton over client's forehead and paranasal sinuses; to test deep sensation, use alternating blunt and sharp ends of a safety pin over same areas.
	Maxillary branch	Sensory	Sensation of skin of face and anterior oral cavity (tongue and teeth)	Assess skin sensation as for ophthalmic branch above.
	Mandibular branch	Motor and sensory	Muscles of mastication; sensation of skin of face	Ask client to clench teeth.
VI	Abducens	Motor	EOM; moves eyeball laterally	Assess directions of gaze.
VII	Facial	Motor and sensory	Facial expression; taste (anterior two thirds of tongue)	Ask client to smile, raise the eyebrows, frown, puff out cheeks, close eyes tightly; ask client to identify various tastes placed on tip and sides of tongue: sugar (sweet), salt, lemon juice (sour), and quinine (bitter); identify areas of taste.
VIII	Auditory			
	Vestibular branch	Sensory	Equilibrium	Assessment methods are discussed with cerebeller functions (in next section).
	Cochlear branch	Sensory	Hearing	Assess client's ability to hear spoken word and vibrations of tuning fork.
IX	Glossopharyngeal	Motor and sensory	Swallowing ability and gag reflex, tongue movement, taste (posterior tongue)	Use tongue blade on posterior tongue while client says "ah" to elicit gag reflex; apply tastes on posterior tongue for identification; ask client to move tongue from side to side and up and down.
X	Vagus	Motor and sensory	Sensation of pharynx and larynx; swallowing; vocal cord movement	Assessed with cranial nerve IX; assess client's speech for hoarseness.
XI	Accessory	Motor	Head movement; shrugging of shoulders	Ask client to shrug shoulders against resistance from your hands and turn head to side against resistance from your hand (repeat for other side).
XII	Hypoglossal	Motor	Protrusion of tongue	Ask client to protrude tongue at midline, then move it side to side.

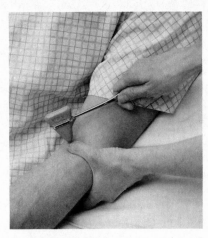

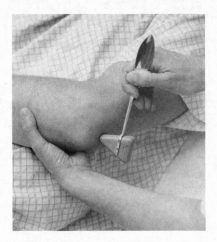

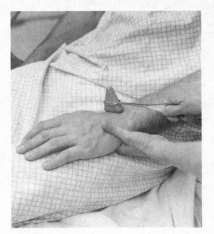

FIGURE 11–92 Assessing the biceps reflex.   FIGURE 11–93 Assessing the triceps reflex.   FIGURE 11–94 Assessing the brachioradialis reflex.

5. Observe the normal slight flexion of the elbow, and feel the bicep's contraction through your thumb (Figure 11–92).

Triceps Reflex
The triceps reflex tests the spinal cord level C-7, C-8.

1. Flex the client's arm at the elbow, and support it in the palm of your nondominant hand.

2. Palpate the triceps tendon about 2 to 5 cm (1 to 2 in) above the elbow.

3. Deliver a blow with the percussion hammer directly to the tendon (Figure 11–93).

4. Observe the normal slight extension of the elbow.

Brachioradialis Reflex
The brachioradialis reflex tests the spinal cord level C-3, C-6.

1. Rest the client's arm in a relaxed position on your forearm or on the client's own leg.

2. Deliver a blow with the percussion hammer directly on the radius 2 to 5 cm (1 to 2 in) above the wrist or the styloid process, the bony prominence on the thumb side of the wrist (Figure 11–94).

3. Observe the normal flexion and supination of the forearm. The fingers of the hand may also extend slightly.

Patellar Reflex
The patellar reflex tests the spinal cord level L-2, L-3, L-4.

1. Ask the client to sit on the edge of the examining table so that the legs hang freely.

2. Locate the patellar tendon directly below the patella (kneecap).

3. Deliver a blow with the percussion hammer directly to the tendon (Figure 11–95).

4. Observe the normal extension or kicking out of the leg as the quadriceps muscle contracts.

5. If no response occurs and you suspect the client is not relaxed, ask the client to interlock the fingers and pull. This action often enhances relaxation so that a more accurate response is obtained.

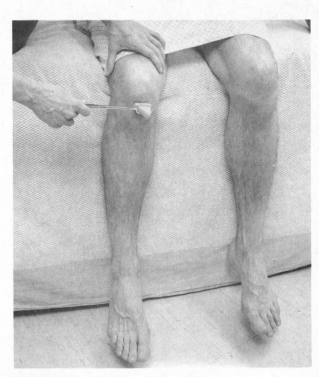

FIGURE 11–95 Assessing the patellar reflex.

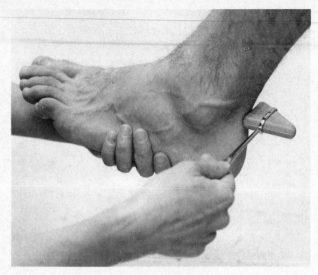

FIGURE 11–96 Assessing the Achilles reflex.

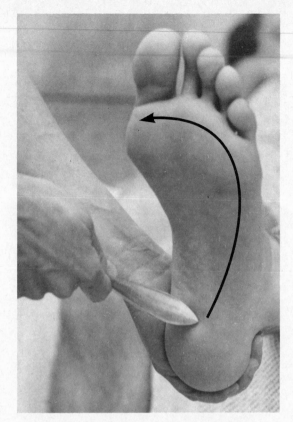

FIGURE 11–97 Assessing the plantar (Babinski) reflex.

Achilles Reflex

The Achilles reflex tests the spinal cord level S-1, S-2.

1. With the client in the same position as for the patellar reflex, slightly dorsiflex the client's ankle by supporting the foot lightly in the hand.

2. Deliver a blow with the percussion hammer directly to the Achilles tendon just above the heel (Figure 11–96).

3. Observe and feel the normal plantar flexion (downward jerk) of the foot.

Plantar (Babinski) Reflex

The plantar, or Babinski, reflex is superficial. It may be absent in adults without pathology or overridden by voluntary control.

1. Use a moderately sharp object, such as the handle of the percussion hammer, a key, or the dull end of a pin or applicator stick.

2. Stroke the lateral border of the sole of the client's foot, starting at the heel, continuing to the ball of the foot, and then proceeding across the ball of the foot toward the big toe (Figure 11–97).

3. Observe the response. Normally, all five toes bend downward; this reaction is negative Babinski. In an abnormal Babinski response the toes spread outward and the big toe moves upward. Positive Babinski is abnormal after the child ambulates.

Motor Function

Neurologic assessment of the motor system evaluates proprioception and cerebellar function. Structures involved in proprioception are the proprioceptors, the posterior columns of the spinal cord, the cerebellum, and the vestibular apparatus (which is innervated by cranial nerve VIII) in the labyrinth of the internal ear.

Proprioceptors are sensory nerve terminals, occurring chiefly in the muscles, tendons, joints, and the internal ear, that give information about movements and position of the body. Stimuli from the proprioceptors travel through the posterior columns of the spinal cord. Deficits of function of the posterior columns of the spinal cord result in impairment of muscle and position sense. Clients with such an impairment often must watch their own arm and leg movements to ascertain the position of the limbs.

The cerebellum (a) helps to control posture; (b) acts with the cerebral cortex to make body movements smooth and coordinated; and (c) controls skeletal muscles to maintain equilibrium.

Cerebellar disorders cause certain characteristics and common symptoms of **ataxia**: impairment of position sense, lack of muscle coordination, tremors, disturbance of equilibrium, disturbance in the timing of movements, and disturbance of gait. Tremors are especially pronounced toward the end of movements. Clients with cerebellar disease also have difficulty performing rapid skilled movements, alternating movements such as supinating and pronating the hands, and starting and stopping motions.

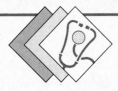

Assessing Motor Function

ASSESSMENT	NORMAL FINDINGS	DEVIATIONS FROM NORMAL
Gross Motor and Balance Tests There are several gross motor function and balance tests. Generally, the Romberg test and one other are used.		
WALKING GAIT Ask the client to **walk across the room and back**, and assess the client's gait.	Has upright posture and steady gait with opposing arm swing; walks unaided, maintaining balance	Has poor posture and unsteady, irregular, staggering gait with wide stance; bends legs only from hips; has rigid or no arm movements
ROMBERG TEST Ask the client to **stand with feet together and arms resting at the sides**, first with eyes open, then closed. Stand close during this test to prevent the client from falling.	Negative Romberg's: May sway slightly but is able to maintain upright posture and foot stance	Positive Romberg's: Cannot maintain foot stance; moves the feet apart to maintain stance If client cannot maintain balance with the eyes shut, client may have sensory ataxia If balance cannot be maintained whether the eyes are open or shut, client may have cerebellar ataxia
STANDING ON ONE FOOT WITH EYES CLOSED Ask the client to **close the eyes and stand on one foot and then the other**. Stand close to the client during this test.	Maintains stance for at least 5 seconds	Cannot maintain stance for 5 seconds
HEEL-TOE WALKING Ask the client to **walk a straight line, placing the heel of one foot directly in front of the toes of the other foot**.	Maintains heel-toe walking along a straight line	Assumes a wider foot gait to stay upright
TOE OR HEEL WALKING Ask the client to **walk several steps on the toes and then on the heels**.	Able to walk several steps on toes or heels	Cannot maintain balance on toes or heels
Fine Motor Tests for the Upper Extremities		
FINGER-TO-NOSE TEST Ask the client to **abduct and extend the arms at shoulder height and rapidly touch the nose alternately with one index finger and then the other**. The client repeats the test with the eyes closed if the test is performed easily.	Repeatedly and rhythmically touches the nose (Figure 11–98)	Misses the nose or gives lazy response

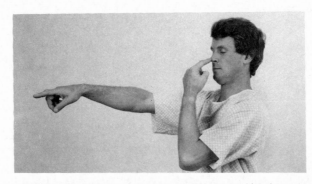

FIGURE 11–98 A test of fine motor coordination: touching the nose.

► Assessing Motor Function *CONTINUED*

ASSESSMENT	NORMAL FINDINGS	DEVIATIONS FROM NORMAL
ALTERNATING SUPINATION AND PRONATION OF HANDS ON KNEES Ask the client to **pat both knees with the palms of both hands and then with the backs of the hands alternately** at an ever-increasing rate.	Can alternately supinate and pronate hands at rapid pace	Performs with slow, clumsy movements and irregular timing; has difficulty alternating from supination to pronation
FINGER TO NOSE AND TO THE NURSE'S FINGER Ask the client to **touch the nose and then your index finger**, held at a distance at about 45 cm (18 in), **at a rapid and increasing rate**.	Performs with coordination and rapidity	Misses the finger and moves slowly
FINGERS TO FINGERS Ask the client to **spread the arms broadly at shoulder height and then bring the fingers together at the midline**, first with the eyes open and then closed, first slowly and then rapidly.	As above	Moves slowly and is unable to touch fingers consistently
FINGERS TO THUMB (SAME HAND) Ask the client to **touch each finger of one hand to the thumb of the same hand** as rapidly as possible (Figure 11–99).	Rapidly touches each finger to thumb with each hand	Cannot coordinate this fine discrete movement with either one or both hands

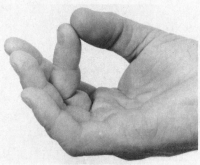

FIGURE 11–99   A test of fine motor coordination: touching the tip of each finger with the thumb.

Fine Motor Tests for the Lower Extremities

Ask the client to lie supine and to perform these tests.

► **Assessing Motor Function** *CONTINUED*

ASSESSMENT	NORMAL FINDINGS	DEVIATIONS FROM NORMAL
HEEL DOWN OPPOSITE SHIN Ask the client to **place the heel of one foot just below the opposite knee and run the heel down the shin to the foot**. Repeat with the other foot (Figure 11–100). The client may also use a sitting position for this test.	Demonstrates bilateral equal coordination	Has tremors or is awkward; heel moves off shin

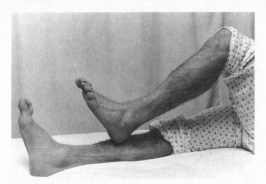

FIGURE 11–100   Running the heel down the shin to the foot.

ASSESSMENT	NORMAL FINDINGS	DEVIATIONS FROM NORMAL
TOE OR BALL OF FOOT TO THE NURSE'S FINGER Ask the client to **touch your finger with the large toe of each foot** (Figure 11–101).	Moves smoothly, with coordination	Misses your finger; cannot coordinate movement

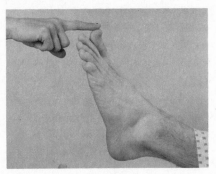

FIGURE 11–101   Touching the toes to the nurse's finger.

Sensory Function

Sensory functions include touch, pain, temperature, position, and tactile discrimination. The first three are routinely tested in a few locations. Generally, the face, arms, legs, hands, and feet are tested for touch and pain, although all parts of the body can be tested. If the client complains of numbness, peculiar sensations, or paralysis, the practitioner should check sensation more carefully over flexor and extensor surfaces of limbs, mapping out clearly any abnormality of touch or pain by examining responses in the area about every 2 cm (1 in). This is a lengthy procedure. Abnormal responses to touch stimuli include loss of sensation (**anesthesia**); more than normal sensation (**hyperesthesia**); less than normal sensation (**hypoesthesia**); or an abnormal sensation such as burning, pain, or the feel of an electric shock (**paresthesia**).

A more detailed neurologic examination includes position sense, temperature sense, and tactile discrimination. Three types of tactile discrimination are generally tested: **one- and two-point discrimination**, the ability to sense whether one or two areas of the skin are being stimulated by pressure; **stereognosis**, the act of recognizing objects by touching and manipulating them; and **extinction**, the failure to perceive touch on one side of the body when two symmetrical areas of the body are touched simultaneously.

To assess sensory function, the nurse needs the following equipment:

- Wisps of cotton to assess light touch sensation

- Sterile safety pin or sterile hypodermic needle to assess pain sensation

- Test tubes of hot and cold water for skin temperature assessment (optional)

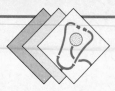

Assessing Sensory Functions

ASSESSMENT	NORMAL FINDINGS	DEVIATIONS FROM NORMAL

Light-Touch Sensation

Compare the light-touch sensation of symmetric areas of the body. *Sensitivity to touch varies among different skin areas.*

Light tickling or touch sensation

Anesthesia, hyperesthesia, hypoesthesia, and paresthesia

- Ask the client to close the eyes and to respond by saying "yes" or "now" whenever the client feels the cotton wisp touching the skin.

- With a wisp of cotton, lightly touch one specific spot and then the same spot on the other side of the body (Figure 11–102).

- Test areas on the forehead, cheek, hand, lower arm, abdomen, foot, and lower leg. Check a specific area of the limb first (i.e., the hand before the arm and the foot before the leg), because the sensory nerve may be assumed to be intact if sensation is felt at its most peripheral part.

- Ask the client to point to the spot where the touch was felt. *This demonstrates whether the client is able to determine tactile location (point localization),* i.e., can accurately perceive where the client was touched.

- If areas of sensory dysfunction are found, determine the boundaries of sensation by testing responses about every 2.5 cm (1 in) in the area. Make a sketch of the sensory loss area for recording purposes.

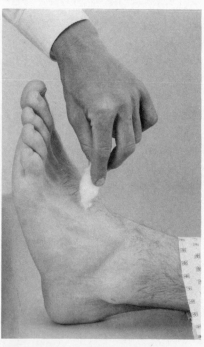

FIGURE 11–102 Assessing light-touch sensation.

Pain Sensation

Assess pain sensation as follows:

- Ask the client to close the eyes and to say "sharp," "dull," or "don't know" when the sharp or dull end of the safety pin or needle is felt.

- Alternately use the sharp and dull end of the sterile pin or needle to lightly prick designated anatomic areas at random, e.g., hand, forearm, foot, lower leg, abdomen. The face

Able to discriminate "sharp" and "dull" sensations

Areas of reduced, heightened, or absent sensation (map them out for recording purposes)

► **Assessing Sensory Functions** *CONTINUED*

ASSESSMENT	NORMAL FINDINGS	DEVIATIONS FROM NORMAL

is not tested in this manner (Figure 11–103). *Alternating the sharp and dull ends of the instrument more accurately evaluates the client's response. A sterile safety pin or needle is used to avoid the risk of infection.*

- Allow at least 2 seconds between each test to prevent summation effects of stimuli, i.e., several successive stimuli perceived as one stimulus.

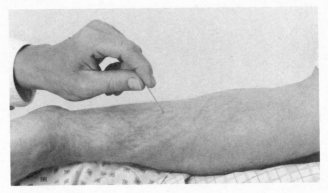

FIGURE 11–103 Assessing pain sensation with a pin.

Temperature Sensation

Temperature sensation is not routinely tested if pain sensation is found to be within normal limits. If pain sensation is not normal or is absent, testing sensitivity to temperature may prove more reliable.

- Touch skin areas with test tubes filled with hot or cold water.

- Have the client respond say saying "hot," "cold," or "don't know."

Able to discriminate between "hot" and "cold" sensations

Areas of dulled or lost sensation (when sensations of pain are dulled, temperature sense is usually also impaired because distribution of these nerves over the body is similar)

Position or Kinesthetic Sensation

Commonly, the middle fingers and the large toes are tested for the *kinesthetic sensation* (sense of position).

- To test the fingers, support the client's arm with one hand, and hold the client's palm in the other; to test the toes, place the client's heels on the examining table.

- Ask the client to close the eyes.

- Grasp a middle finger or a big toe firmly between your thumb and index finger, and exert the same pressure on both sides of the finger or toe while moving it.

- Move the finger or toe until it is up, down, or straight out, and ask the client to identify the position (Figure 11–104).

- Use a series of brisk up-and-down movements before bringing the finger or toe suddenly to rest in one of the three positions.

Can readily determine the position of fingers and toes

Unable to determine the position of one or more fingers or toes

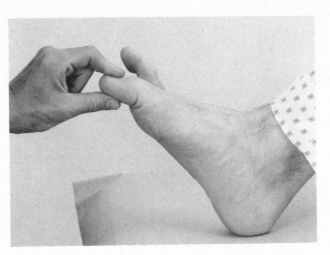

FIGURE 11–104 Testing position (kinesthetic sensation).

► **Assessing Sensory Functions** *CONTINUED*

ASSESSMENT	NORMAL FINDINGS	DEVIATIONS FROM NORMAL
Tactile Discrimination For all tests, the client's eyes need to be closed.		
ONE- AND TWO-POINT DISCRIMINATION Alternately stimulate the skin with two pins simultaneously and then with one pin. Ask whether the client feels one or two pinpricks.	Perception varies widely in adults over different parts of the body. Normally, a person can distinguish between a one- and two-point stimulus within the following minimum distances: Fingertips, 2.8 mm Palms of hands, 8–12 mm Chest, forearm, 40 mm Back, 50–70 mm Upper arm, thigh, 75 mm Toes, 3–8 mm	Unable to sense whether one or two areas of the skin are being stimulated by pressure
STEREOGNOSIS Place familiar objects, such as a key, paper clip, or coin, in the client's hand, and ask the client to identify them.	Able to recognize specific objects	Unable to recognize specific objects
If the client has a motor impairment of the hand and is unable to manipulate an object, write a number or letter on the client's palm, using a blunt instrument, and ask the client to identify it.	Able to identify numbers or letters written on palm	Unable to identify numbers or letters written on palm
EXTINCTION PHENOMENON Simultaneously stimulate two symmetric areas of the body, such as the thighs, the cheeks, or the hands.	Both points of stimulus are felt	Failure to perceive touch on one side of the body when two symmetric areas of the body are touched simultaneously (frequently noted in clients with lesions of the sensory cortex)

THE ELDERLY: CHANGES IN THE NEUROLOGIC SYSTEM

- Because older clients tire more easily than younger clients, a total neurologic assessment is often done at a different time than the other parts of the physical assessment.

- Although there is a progressive decrease in the number of functioning neurons in the central nervous system and in the sense organs, the older client usually functions well because of the abundant reserves in the number of brain cells.

- Impulse transmission and reaction to stimuli are slower in elderly clients.

- Many elderly clients generally have some impairment of hearing, vision, smell, temperature and pain sensation, memory, and mental endurance.

- Coordination changes in older clients, including a reduced speed of fine finger movements. Standing balance remains intact, and Romberg's test remains negative.

- Reflex responses may slightly increase or decrease in the older client. Many show loss of the Achilles reflex, and the plantar reflex may be difficult to elicit.

- When testing sensory function, the nurse needs to give the older client time to respond. Normally, older clients have unaltered perception of light touch and superficial pain, decreased perception of deep pain, and decreased perception of temperature stimuli. Many also reveal a decrease or absence of position sense in the large toes.

The Female Genitals and Inguinal Lymph Nodes

In adult females, the examination of the genitals and reproductive tract includes assessment of the inguinal lymph nodes and inspection and palpation of the external genitals.

Completeness of the assessment of the genitals and reproductive tract depends on the needs and problems of the individual client. *In many practice settings, nurses perform only inspection of the external genitals.*

Assessment of adolescent girls is limited to an inspection of the external genitals, unless the girl is sexually active. If so, an annual Papanicolaou test (Pap test) is advised for detecting cancer of the cervix and uterus. If the adolescent is sexually active and has an increased or abnormal vaginal discharge, specimens should be taken to check for sexually transmitted disease. Examination of the internal genitals by vaginal speculum, and collection of specimens, are discussed in Chapter 14. The accompanying box shows the five stages of pubic hair development during puberty.

Examination of the genitals usually creates uncertainty and apprehension in females, and the lithotomy position required can cause embarrassment. The nurse must explain each part of the examination in advance and perform the examination in an objective and efficient manner. Appropriate draping is essential to prevent undue exposure of the client, and good lighting is essential for the nurse to ensure accuracy of inspection. The nurse wears disposable gloves for this genital examination to prevent the transfer of microorganisms from the client to the nurse and from the nurse to other clients.

Five Stages of Pubic Hair Development in Females

- Stage 1 Preadolescence. No pubic hair except for fine body hair.
- Stage 2 Usually occurs at ages 11 and 12. Sparse, long, slightly pigmented curly hair develops along the labia.
- Stage 3 Usually occurs at ages 12 and 13. Hair becomes darker in color and curlier and develops over the pubic symphysis.
- Stage 4 Usually occurs between ages 13 and 14. Hair assumes the texture and curl of the adult but is not as thick and does not appear on the thighs.
- Stage 5 Sexual maturity. Hair assumes adult appearance and appears on the inner aspect of the upper thighs.

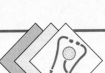

Assessing the Female Genitals and Inguinal Lymph Nodes

NURSING HISTORY FOCUS

Age of onset of menstruation, last menstrual period (LMP), regularity of cycle, duration, amount of daily flow, and whether menstruation is painful; incidence of pain during intercourse; vaginal discharge; number of pregnancies, number of live births, labor or delivery complications; urgency and frequency of urination at night, blood in urine, painful urination, incontinence; history of sexually transmitted disease, past and present.

ASSESSMENT	NORMAL FINDINGS	DEVIATIONS FROM NORMAL
Inspect the distribution, amount, and characteristics of pubic hair.	There are wide variations; generally kinky in the menstruating adult, thinner and straighter after menopause Distributed in the shape of an inverse triangle Hair growth should not extend over the abdomen	Scant pubic hair (may indicate hormonal problem)

▶

▶ **Assessing the Female Genitals** *CONTINUED*

ASSESSMENT	NORMAL FINDINGS	DEVIATIONS FROM NORMAL
Inspect the skin of the pubic area for parasites (e.g., lice), **inflammation, swelling, and lesions** (e.g., fissures, excoriations, scars from episiotomies, varicosities, leukoplakia). To assess pubic skin adequately, separate the labia majora and labia minora.	Pubic skin intact, no lesions Skin of vulva area slightly darker than the rest of the body Labia round, full, and relatively symmetric in adult females; labia atrophied and flatter in older females	Lice, lesions, scars, fissures, swelling, erythema, or leukoplakia
Inspect the clitoris, urethral orifice, and vaginal orifice when separating the labia minora.	Clitoris does not exeed 1 cm in width and 2 cm in length Urethral orifice appears as a small slit and is the same color as surrounding tissues No inflammation, swelling, or discharge	Presence of lesions (the clitoris is a common site for syphilitic chancres in younger females and cancerous lesions in older females) Presence of inflammation, swelling, or discharge
If there is inflammation or discharge at the urethral orifice, palpate the Skene's (paraurethral) glands on either side of the urethral orifice.	Not palpable No discharge	Pain; tenderness; urethral discharge

- Insert a gloved index finger, palm uppermost, into the entrance of the vagina about 2.5 cm (1 in).

- While pressing gently upward, palpate for Skene's glands, then draw the finger outward (Figure 11–105). This maneuver will milk the urethra of any discharge.

- Observe for any discharge.

- If discharge is present, take a specimen, and then change gloves before proceeding with further examination.

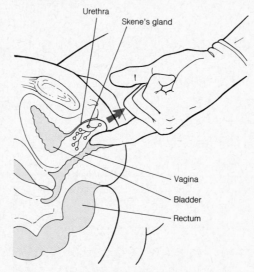

FIGURE 11–105 Palpating Skene's glands.

	Not tender or palpable	Tender and palpable

Palpate Bartholin's glands (located on the posterior aspect of the vaginal orifice).

- Insert a gloved finger into the entrance of the vagina.

- Move the finger to the lateral and posterior aspect of the vagina.

- Palpate against the thumb at the posterior aspect of the labia majora (Figure 11–106).

- Repeat for the other side.

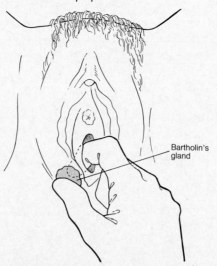

FIGURE 11–106 Palpating Bartholin's gland.

▶ **Assessing the Female Genitals** *CONTINUED*

ASSESSMENT	NORMAL FINDINGS	DEVIATIONS FROM NORMAL
Assess the pelvic musculature while your gloved finger is in the vaginal orifice. • Place two gloved fingers (index and middle finger) into the vagina. • Ask the client to constrict her vaginal orifice. • Ask the client to bear down while your fingers spread the vaginal wall laterally. Observe the vaginal wall for bulges.	Good tone; a **nulliparous** female (one who has never had a child) will probably have a high degree of muscle tone, whereas a **multiparous** female will have less tone Walls intact No bulges	**Cystocele** (bulging of the anterior vaginal wall as a result of a prolapse of the anterior wall and the bladder) **Rectocele** (bulging of the posterior vaginal wall as a result of a prolapse of the posterior wall and the rectum) **Enterocele** (bulging from the posterior fornix as a result of prolapse of the pouch of Douglas into the vagina)
Palpate the inguinal lymph nodes (Figure 11–107). Use the pads of the fingers in a rotary motion, noting any enlargement or tenderness.	No enlargement or tenderness	Enlargement and tenderness

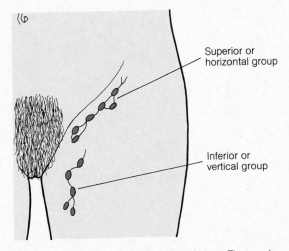

Superior or horizontal group

Inferior or vertical group

FIGURE 11–107 Lymph nodes of the groin area. The superior group drains the skin of the abdominal wall, the external genitals, anal canal, and lower vagina. The inferior group receives lymph from the medial aspect of the leg and foot.

THE ELDERLY: CHANGES IN THE FEMALE GENITOURINARY SYSTEM

• Loss of pubic hair and a flattening of the labia occur.

• The vulva atrophies as a result of a reduction in vascularity, elasticity, adipose tissue, and estrogen levels. Because the vulva is more fragile, it is more easily irritated.

• The vaginal wall becomes thinner and less vascular, and the vagina appears pink, dry, and smooth, with fewer rugae. Atrophic vaginal tissue may readily bleed from trauma of speculum insertion.

• The vaginal environment becomes drier and more alkaline, resulting in an alteration of the type of flora present and a predisposition to vaginitis. Dyspareunia (difficult or painful coitus) is also a common occurrence.

• The cervix and uterus decrease in size. The cervix may be narrow, and the examiner may be unable to palpate the uterus during the pelvic examination.

• The fallopian tubes and ovaries atrophy.

• Ovulation and estrogen production cease.

• Vaginal bleeding unrelated to estrogen therapy is abnormal in older women.

• Prolapse of the uterus frequently occurs in older females, especially those who have had multiple pregnancies.

• Older females may be arthritic and find the lithotomy position uncomfortable. A semilithotomy position may be necessary.

The Male Genitals

In adult males, complete examination should include assessment of the external genitals, the presence of any hernias, and the prostate gland. As with females, *nurses in some practice settings performing routine assessment of clients may assess only the external genitals.* The male reproductive and urinary systems (Figure 11–108) share the urethra, which is the passageway for both urine and semen. Therefore, in physical assessment of the male, these two systems are frequently assessed together.

Examination of the male genital organs by a female practitioner (physician or nurse) is becoming increasingly common. Formerly, most examinations of men were done by men. Most male clients accept examination by a female, especially if she is emotionally comfortable with herself about performing it and does so in a matter-of-fact and competent manner. If the female nurse does not feel comfortable about this part of the examination or if the client is reluctant to be examined by a female, the nurse should refer this part of the examination to a male practitioner.

The techniques of inspection and palpation are used to examine the male genitals. Equipment needed includes gloves and a penlight to transilluminate any mass. The client may be in a lying or sitting position.

Development of secondary sex characteristics is also assessed in relationship to the client's age. See Table 11–15 for the five stages of the development of pubic hair, the penis, and the testes/scrotum during puberty.

All clients should be screened for the presence of inguinal or femoral hernias. A **hernia** is a protrusion of the intestine through the inguinal wall or canal. The loop of bowel may even extend down to the scro-

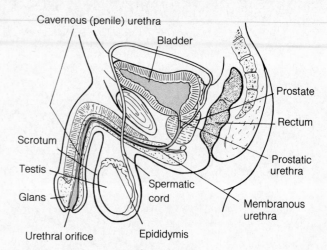

FIGURE 11–108 The male urogenital tract.

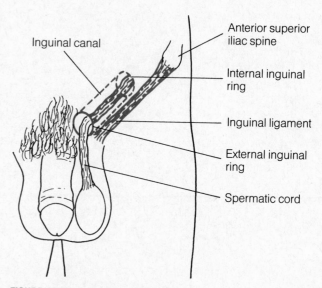

FIGURE 11–109 Structures of the inguinal area.

TABLE 11–15	FIVE STAGES OF DEVELOPMENT OF PUBIC HAIR, PENIS, AND TESTES/SCROTUM (12 TO 16 YEARS)		
Stage	**Pubic Hair**	**Penis**	**Testes/Scrotum**
1 (pre-adolescent)	None, except for body hair like that on the abdomen	Size is relative to body size, as in childhood	Size is relative to body size, as in childhood
2	Scant, long, slightly pigmented at base of penis	Slight enlargement occurs	Becomes reddened in color and enlarged
3	Darker, begins to curl and becomes more coarse; extends over pubic symphysis	Elongation occurs	Continuing enlargement
4	Continues to darken and thicken; extends on the sides, above and below	Increase in both breadth and length; glans develops	Continuing enlargement; color darkens
5	Adult distribution that extends to inner thighs, umbilicus, and anus	Adult appearance	Adult appearance

tum. Structures of the inguinal canal are shown in Figure 11–109. An *indirect inguinal hernia* is a loop of bowel that enters the internal inguinal ring. It may stay in the canal, exit through the external ring, or pass into the scrotum. A *direct inguinal hernia* enters the inguinal canal directly through a weakness in the abdominal wall just behind the external inguinal ring. It does not pass through the inguinal canal. A *femoral hernia* is more common in women. It is lower and more lateral than an inguinal hernia and may look like an enlarged lymph node.

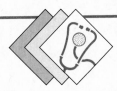

Assessing the Male Genitals and Inguinal Area

NURSING HISTORY FOCUS
Usual fluid intake and output, voiding patterns and any changes, bladder control, urinary incontinence, frequency, urgency, abdominal pain; any symptoms of sexually transmitted disease; any swellings that could indicate presence of hernia; family history of nephritis, malignancy of the prostate, or malignancy of the kidney.

ASSESSMENT	NORMAL FINDINGS	DEVIATIONS FROM NORMAL
Pubic Hair **Inspect the distribution, amount, and characteristics of pubic hair.**	Triangular distribution, often spreading up the abdomen	Scant amount or absence of hair
Penis **Inspect the penile shaft and glans penis for lesions, nodules, swellings and inflammation.**	Penile skin intact Appears slightly wrinkled and varies in color as widely as other body skin Foreskin easily retractable from the glans penis Small amount of thick white **segma** between the glans and foreskin	Presence of lesions, nodules, swellings, or inflammation
Inspect the urethral meatus for swelling, inflammation, and discharge. • Compress or ask the client to compress the glans slightly to open the urethral meatus to inspect it for discharge. • If the client has reported a discharge, instruct the client to strip the penis from the base to the urethra (i.e., grasp the base of the penis, with the thumb at the front and fingers behind, and while applying moderate pressure, move the thumb and fingers slowly down the shaft of the penis.	Pink and slitlike appearance Positioned at the tip of the penis	Inflammation; discharge Variation in meatal locations (e.g., **hypospadias**, on the underside of the penile shaft, and **epispadias**, on the upper side of the penile shaft)
Palpate the penis for tenderness, thickening, and nodules. Use your thumb and first two fingers.	Smooth and semifirm Is slightly movable over the underlying structures	Presence of tenderness, thickening, or nodules Immobility

► **Assessing the Male Genitals** *CONTINUED*

ASSESSMENT	NORMAL FINDINGS	DEVIATIONS FROM NORMAL
Scrotum		
Inspect the scrotum for appearance, general size, and symmetry.	Scrotal skin is darker in color than that of the rest of the body and is loose	Discolorations; any tightening of skin (may indicate edema or mass)
• To facilitate inspection of the scrotum during a physical examination, ask the client to hold the penis out of the way.	Size varies with temperature changes (the dartos muscles contract when the area is cold and relax when the area is warm)	Marked asymmetry in size
• Inspect all skin surfaces by spreading the rugated surface skin and lifting the scrotum as needed to observe posterior surfaces.	Scrotum appears asymmetric (left testis is usually lower than right testis)	
Palpate the scrotum to assess status of underlying testes, epididymis, and spermatic cord. Palpate both testes simultaneously for comparative purposes. The palpation procedure is outlined in the box below.	Testicles are rubbery, smooth, and free of nodules and masses	Testicles are enlarged, with uneven surface (possible tumor)
	Testis is about 2 × 4 cm (0.7 × 1.5 in)	Testis has swelling that transilluminates (possible hydrocele)
	Epididymis is resilient, normally tender, and softer than the spermatic cord	Epididymis is nonresilient and painful
	Spermatic cord is firm	

Palpating the Scrotum

• Using your first two fingers and thumb, palpate each testis for size, consistency, shape, smoothness, and presence of masses. During assessment of male adolescents, establish the descent of the testicles into the scrotum; note undescended testes.

• Palpate the epididymis between your thumb and index finger. It is located at the top of the testis and extends behind it.

• Palpate the spermatic cord between thumb and index finger. It is usually found at the top lateral portion of the scrotum and feels firm.

• If swelling, irregularities, or nodules are detected during the scrotal examination, attempt to transilluminate the lesion. This is done by darkening the room and shining a flashlight behind the scrotum through the mass. Serous fluid causes the light to show with a red glow; tissue or blood does not transilluminate.

• Describe all scrotal masses in terms of their size, shape, placement, consistency, tenderness, and presence of transillumination.

ASSESSMENT	NORMAL FINDINGS	DEVIATIONS FROM NORMAL
Inguinal Area		
Inspect both inguinal areas for bulges while the client is standing, if possible.	No swelling or bulges	Swelling or bulge (possible inguinal or femoral hernia)
• First, have the client remain at rest.		
• Next, have the client hold the breath and strain or bear down as though having a bowel movement. *Bearing down may make the hernia more visible.*		

▶ **Assessing the Male Genitals** *CONTINUED*

ASSESSMENT	NORMAL FINDINGS	DEVIATIONS FROM NORMAL
Palpate hernias as described in the box below.	No palpable bulge	Palpable bulge in the area

Palpating a Hernia

Direct Hernia

- Using your right hand for the client's right side or left hand for the client's left side, advance your index finger into the loose scrotal skin and over the external inguinal ring (Figure 11–110).
- Instruct the client to bear down.
- If a hernia is present, a palpable bulge will appear in the area.

Indirect Hernia

- Attempt to move the index or little finger into the path of the inguinal canal (Figure 11–109, earlier) while the client flexes the knee on the same side.
- When your finger has moved as far as possible, ask the client to bear down.
- If a hernia is present, it will be felt as a mass of tissue touching the finger and withdrawing from it.

Fermoral Hernia

- Palpate the inguinal area directly again, first while the client is at rest and then while the client bears down.
- If a hernia is present, a bulge will be felt most prominently when the client bears down.

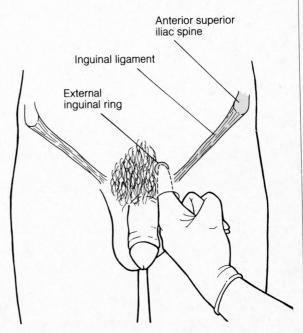

FIGURE 11–110   Palpating for the presence of an inguinal hernia.

THE ELDERLY: CHANGES IN THE MALE GENITOURINARY SYSTEM

Genitals

- The penis decreases in size with age; the size and firmness of the testes decrease.
- Testosterone is produced in smaller amounts.
- More time and direct physical stimulation are required for the older male to achieve an erection, but the elderly man can maintain the erection for longer periods before ejaculation than he could at a younger age.
- Seminal fluid is reduced in amount and viscosity.

Urinary Bladder

- In the elderly male client, urinary frequency, nocturia, dribbling, and problems with beginning and ending the stream are usually the result of prostatic enlargement.

The Rectum and Anus

Rectal examination, an essential part of every comprehensive physical examination, involves inspection and palpation (digital examination). The extent of the assessment of the rectum and anus depends on the rectal problems stated by the client in the nursing history. *In many practice settings, the nurse performs only inspection of the anus.* An interior view of the rectum and anal canal are shown in Figure 27–1 on page 658.

A left lateral or Sims' position with the upper leg acutely flexed is required for the examination. For females, a dorsal recumbent position with hips externally rotated and knees flexed or a lithotomy position may be used. For males, a standing position while the client bends over the examining table may also be used. This position is commonly used to examine the prostate gland. For all rectal examinations the nurse should wear gloves (Malasanos, Barkauskas, and Stoltenberg-Allen 1990, p. 389).

Because digital examination can cause apprehension and embarrassment in the client, it is important that the nurse (a) help the client relax by encouraging the client to take slow, deep breaths (tension can cause spasms of the anal spincters, making the examination uncomfortable), (b) inform the client about potential sensations such as feelings of defecation or passing gas, (c) assure the client that an accident is very unlikely, (d) proceed with the examination in a competent and gentle way, and (e) drape the client appropriately to prevent undue exposure of body parts.

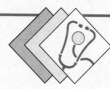

Assessing the Rectum and Anus

NURSING HISTORY FOCUS

History of bright blood in stools, tarry black stools, diarrhea, constipation, abdominal pain, excessive gas, hemorrhoids, or rectal pain; family history of colorectal cancer; when last stool specimen for occult blood was performed and the results; and, if not obtained during the genitourinary examination, any signs or symptoms of prostate enlargement (e.g., slow urinary stream, hesitance, frequency, dribbling, and nocturia).

ASSESSMENT	NORMAL FINDINGS	DEVIATIONS FROM NORMAL
Inspect the anus and surrounding tissue for color, integrity, and skin lesions. Then, ask the client to bear down as though defecating. *Bearing down creates slight pressure on the skin that may accentuate rectal fissures, rectal prolapse, polyps, or internal hemorrhoids.* Describe the location of all abnormal findings in terms of a clock, with the 12 o'clock position toward the pubic symphysis.	Intact perianal skin; usually slightly more pigmented than the skin of the buttocks Anal skin is normally more pigmented, coarser, and moister than perianal skin and is usually hairless	Presence of fissures (cracks), ulcers, excoriations, inflammations, abscesses, protruding **hemorrhoids** (dilated veins seen as reddened protrusions of the skin), lumps or tumors, fistula openings, or **rectal prolapse** (varying degrees of protrusion of the rectal mucous membrane through the anus)
Palpate the rectum for anal sphincter tonicity, nodules, masses, and tenderness. See the box on page 291 for palpation technique.	Anal sphincter has good tone	Hypertonicity of the anal sphincter (may occur in the presence of an anal fissure or other lesion that causes contraction) Hypotonicity of anal sphincter (may occur after rectal surgery or result from a neurologic deficiency)
	Rectal wall is smooth and not tender	Rectal wall is tender and nodular

► **Assessing the Rectum and Anus** *CONTINUED*

ASSESSMENT	NORMAL FINDINGS	DEVIATIONS FROM NORMAL

Palpating the Rectum

- Lubricate your index finger, and instruct the client to bear downward as though having a bowel movement. *This relaxes the anal sphincter.*
- Slowly insert your finger into the anus and into the rectum in the direction of the umbilicus. The anal canal (distance from the anal opening to the anorectal junction) is short (less than 3 cm [about 1 in]). The posterior wall of the rectum follows the curve of the coccyx and sacrum. The nurse's finger is usually able to palpate a distance of 6 to 10 cm (over 2 to 4 in).

- Never force digital insertion. If lesions are painful or bleeding occurs, discontinue the examination.
- Ask the client to tighten the anal sphincter around your finger, and note the tone of the anal sphincter.
- Rotate the pad of the index finger along the anal and the rectal walls, feeling for nodules, masses, and tenderness.
- Note the location of any abnormalities of the rectum (e.g., "anterior wall, 2 cm proximal to the internal anal sphincter").

ASSESSMENT	NORMAL FINDINGS	DEVIATIONS FROM NORMAL
On withdrawing the finger from the rectum and anus, observe it for feces.	Brown color	Presence of mucus, blood, or black tarry stool
Palpate the prostate gland (if the client is male) through the anterior wall of the rectum (Figure 11–111). You should be able to feel the median sulcus, which divides the gland into two lobes.	No tenderness Edges are discrete Gland is about 4 cm (1 1/2 in) in diameter, firm, rubbery, smooth, and mobile	Enlarged; not movable Nodular surface; tenderness

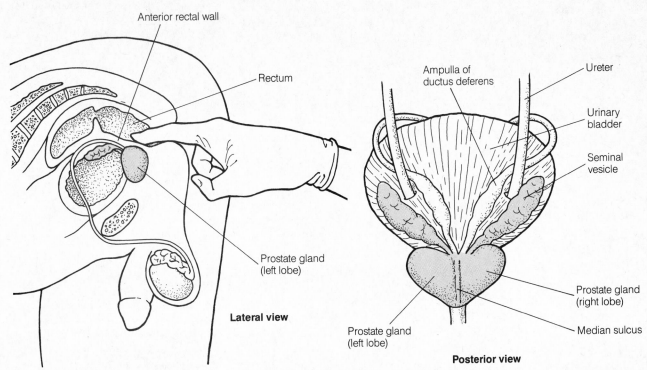

FIGURE 11–111 Palpating the prostate gland through the anterior wall of the rectum.

▶ **Assessing the Rectum and Anus** *CONTINUED*

ASSESSMENT	NORMAL FINDINGS	DEVIATIONS FROM NORMAL
Palpate the cervix (if the client is female) through the anterior rectal wall (Figure 11–112).	Smooth, round, firm, and movable; no tenderness Size is 2 to 3 cm (about 1 in)	Enlargement or tenderness of cervix; nodular surface

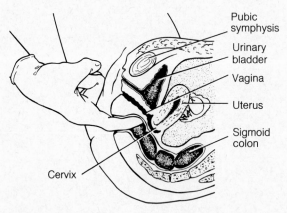

FIGURE 11–112 Palpating the cervix through the anterior rectal wall.

CRITICAL THINKING CHALLENGE

In the following situations, is a complete physical examination indicated, or might a partial exam be done? If only a partial exam is needed, which components of the exam should be included?

a. Mary Jost, a 39-year-old female, just admitted to the nursing unit for evaluation of a breast mass

b. Kevin Brantley, a 22-year-old college student, admitted to the health clinic with a possible broken left arm sustained during a basketball game

c. Charlotte Evans, a 66-year-old female who was hospitalized 3 days ago for congestive heart failure

REFERENCES

Bates, B. 1987. *A guide to physical examination.* 4th ed. Philadelphia: J. B. Lippincott Co.

Becker, K. L. March 1988. Get in touch and in tune with cardiac assessment, Part 1. *Nursing 88* 18:51–55.

Becker, K. L., and Stevens, S. A. June 1988. Performing in-depth abdominal assessment. *Nursing 88* 18:59–63.

Berliner, H. October 1986 and November 1986. Aging skin. (2 parts.) *American Journal of Nursing* 86:1138–41; 1259–61.

Block, G. J., and Nolan, J. W. 1986, *Health assessment for professional nursing: A developmental approach.* 2d ed. Norwalk, Conn.: Appleton-Century-Crofts.

Bowers, A. C., and Thompson, J. M. 1988 *Clinical manual of health assessment.* 3d ed. St. Louis. C. V. Mosby Co.

Burggraf, V., and Donlon, B. September 1985. Assessing the elderly, system by system. Part 1. *American Journal of Nursing* 85:974–84.

Ebersole, P., and Hess, P. 1989 *Toward healthy aging.* 3d ed. St. Louis: C. V. Mosby Co.

Hays, A. M., and Borger, F. October 1985. Assessing the elderly: A test in time. Part 2. *American Journal of Nursing* 85:1107–11.

Henderson, M. L. October 1985. Assessing the elderly: Altered presentations. Part 2. *American Journal of Nursing* 85:1103–6.

Malasanos, L.; Barkauskas, V.; and Stoltenberg-Allen, K. 1990. *Health assessment.* 4th ed. St. Louis: C. V. Mosby Co.

McConnell, E. A. August 1988. Getting the feel of lymph node assessment. *Nursing 88* 18:54–57.

Miracle, V. A. April 1988. Get in touch and in tune with cardiac assessment, Part 2. *Nursing 88* 18:41–47.

Nettles-Carlson, B. September/October 1989. Early detection of breast cancer . . . mammography, clinical breast examination (CBE) and breast self-examination. *Journal of Obstetric, Gynecologic, and Neonatal Nursing* 18:373–81.

Parrino, T. A. September 30, 1987. The art and science of percussion. *Hospital Practice* 22:25–28, 32, 34.

Rice, E. M. May/June 1989. Geriatric assessment. *Advances in Clinical Care* 4:8–15.

Santo-Novak, D. A. August 1988. Seven keys to assessing the elderly. *Nursing 88* 18:60–63.

Smith, C. E. February 1988. Assessing bowel sounds: More than just listening. *Nursing 88* 18:42–43.

Stark, J. L. July 1988. A quick guide to urinary tract assessment. *Nursing 88* 18:56–58.

Stevens, S. A., and Becker, K. L. January 1988. How to perform picture-perfect respiratory assessment. *Nursing 88* 18:57–63.

———. September 1988 and October 1988. A simple, step-by-step approach to neurologic assessment. (2 parts.) *Nursing 88* 18:53–61; 51–58.

Taylor, D. L. January 1985. Clinical applications: Assessing heart sounds. *Nursing 85* 15:51–53.

———. March 1985. Clinical applications: Assessing breath sounds *Nursing 85* 15:60–62.

Teasdale, G., and Bennett, B. 1974. Assessment of coma and impaired consciousness: A practical scale. *Lancet* 2(7872):81.

12

Assessing Infant and Child Health

OBJECTIVES

- Identify the purposes of a comprehensive child health assessment

- Explain the relevance of age and development-specific findings in determining the overall status of the pediatric client

- Describe the sequence of a developmentally appropriate physical examination of a pediatric client

CONTENTS

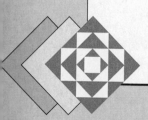

Nursing Health History

The nursing health history for the newborn or pediatric client has a different emphasis from the history of the adult client. In contrast to the adult client, the following areas will be highlighted: (a) birth history; (b) attainment of developmental milestones; (c) nutrition; (d) specific dates of immunization; (e) sleep patterns; (f) school readiness; and (g) elimination. Specific purposes for the health history of a newborn or pediatric client are

- To obtain data related to the child's interactions with family or guardians

- To initiate a nonjudgmental, trusting, interpersonal relationship with the client (and parents or guardians)

The nurse should consider the following age-specific elements of the health history.

Identifying Data
The nurse should include the child's name, address, telephone number, parents' names and home/work telephone numbers, child's date of birth (DOB), birthplace, sex, race, ethnic origin, names and ages of siblings, name of school attended, and current grade in school.

When assessing a newborn or young pediatric client, the nurse should recognize that the parent may be the primary source of data. (Note: Hereafter, the term *parent* is used to indicate all parental support persons or other family members or guardians). If the child is able to communicate, the nurse should always include the child's concerns. When determining the chief complaint or history of present illness, the nurse should also include the child's perceptions when possible.

Past History
Birth history: This should include information about prenatal status, e.g., complications, drug use, exposure to X rays, labor and delivery, postnatal status, e.g., hyperbilirubinemia. Childhood illnesses: Determine age, complications, and recent exposure. Specifically determine ear infections. Developmental milestones: Determine milestones such as cooing, babbling, crawling, and so on. Immunizations: The nurse should record all that are outstanding or in progress so that the required series of injections can be completed or further immunizations withheld if the child's immunosuppressive status so indicates. Data should include any adverse reactions that may contraindicate further immunizations. Allergies:

Allergic reactions common in childhood include eczema, allergic rhinitis, asthma, urticaria, and insect hypersensitivity.

Life-Style and Social Data
Providing private opportunities for the child or adolescent to respond to questions about family relationships and friendships allows possible disclosure of concerns the youth is uncomfortable or afraid to discuss while the parent is present, e.g., parental abuse or concerns related to an adoptive parent or stepparent. The youth may also be hesitant to discuss personal habits (e.g., smoking, use of illegal substances, intake of snacks and junk foods, sexual activity) in front of the parent. Sleep patterns should also be carefully assessed.

Cross-cultural Considerations
The nurse should recognize that older children, particularly adolescents, may not manifest the traditional values and habits of their parents. In addition, individual variations may exist among persons of the same culture.

Educational History
Specific data related to the child or adolescent's current educational institution, school performance, learning styles, and school readiness of the preschooler (e.g., ease of separation from parents, attention span) should be included.

Work History
The nurse should obtain information about the client's work-study experiences or after-school employment, including the risk of exposure to toxic substances.

Psychological Data
Knowledge about the child's usual temperament, e.g., easy, difficult, slow to warm up, helps the nurse determine whether unusual behaviors are reactions to the stress of a new situation or the result of illness.

Nutritional History
During infancy, breast versus bottle-feeding, or a combination of both methods, should be recorded. Frequency, duration, positioning, and the use of vitamin, mineral, and fluoride supplements should also be noted. The introduction of solid food, including the infant's age, food type and amount, and reaction to the food, should be included. For the older child, a 24-hour recall or 7-day diary is a helpful method of determining the child's appetite, food preferences,

desired amount of food, food jags, and food fads. Cultural practices should be considered when making recommendations regarding the child's diet.

Family History

A family history should include presence of cardiac disease, hypertension, cancer, diabetes, stroke, blood disorders, asthma, allergy, cystic fibrosis, alcoholism, obesity, mental illness, mental retardation, seizures, learning disabilities, birth defects, and sudden infant death syndrome (SIDS). A genogram or family tree may also be completed.

Review of Systems

The review of systems will be brief for most children unless the child has chronic or multiple conditions. Ask the parent or child certain key questions in the following areas:

General: Significant weight loss or gain, change in energy level, presence of fatigue, hyperactivity, or change in behavior.

Skin: Color change (pallor or cyanosis), rashes, lesions, birthmarks, change in moles, acne, or bruising.

Head: Head injury or headache and the use of bike helmet.

Eyes: Visual ability at school, strabismus, pain, discharge, and reading problems. Does child sit at least 10 ft away from television? Does child wear glasses? When was the last eye examination?

Ears: Hearing function and incidence of ear infections (number since birth and number within last six months).

Nose and Sinuses: Frequency of colds in one year (3–6 is considered within the normal range). Nasal stuffiness, snoring, discharge, nosebleeds, and allergies.

Mouth and Throat: Streptococcal infection, hoarseness, dental problems. When was the last dental examination and dental prophylaxis?

Breasts: For preadolescent girls, determine onset of pubertal change. For older adolescents, determine whether they have been taught American Cancer Society (ACS) approved methods of breast self-examination (BSE).

Respiratory: Croup, bronchiolitis, asthma, pneumonia, or chronic cough.

Cardiac: Activity tolerance compared with peers. Presence of a congenital heart defect or a murmur. Is the blood pressure within the normal range as described by the National Heart, Lung, and Blood Institute?

Gastrointestinal: Frequency of bowel movements, diarrhea, constipation, abdominal pain, stool color and consistency, and history of pinworms.

Genitourinary System: Urine color, stream, history of urinary tract infection, method of toilet training, day and night dryness, and enuresis. For the adolescent male, has testicular self-examination been discussed? For the preadolescent female, has menses occurred? Has sex education been provided by the parent and/or school? Are secondary sex characteristics present?

Musculoskeletal System: History of injuries, scoliosis screening.

Neurologic System: Were developmental milestones attained on time? Are cognitive or behavior issues a concern? Determine history of headache, head injury, or convulsions.

Hematologic System: Exposure to radiation or toxins in utero or postnatally, history of excessive bruising, epistaxis, or lymphadenopathy.

Physical Health Examination

The physical examination of a newborn or child (hereafter referred to as the pediatric client) will vary from that of an adult, depending on the age and size. Comprehensive child health assessment requires the appreciation and recognition of children as unique individuals. This chapter provides an overview of the additional considerations necessary for performing comprehensive health assessment of the newborn or pediatric client. In-depth descriptions of assessment techniques may be found in Chapter 11. The adolescent client's physical examination is similar to the adult's, unless physical or developmental growth delays indicate otherwise.

The health assessment of infants and children includes not only the assessment of physical status but also the administration of developmental tests to determine cognitive, psychosocial, language, and motor skills. The nurse's observational skills, and tools such as the Brazelton Neonatal Behavior Assessment Scale and the Denver Developmental Screening Test II (Denver II) assist in detecting developmental delay in infants and preschoolers. The student is referred to other texts for specialized information.

The physical exam of the pediatric client should begin with the least invasive or least uncomfortable procedures. This organization prevents disruption of the examination due to crying, agitation, or fear, which can alter results of vital signs, chest auscultation, abdominal assessment, or other findings. For example, the mouth and ears should be examined last. Inspection and auscultation are generally performed before palpation and percussion, because the latter may distress the infant or young child. If the client is quiet, the nurse may start with chest auscultation; if the child is active, the nurse may begin with the extremities. The nurse should assess vital signs when the pediatric client is as calm and as inactive as possible. See Chapter 10 for vital sign measurement techniques.

Parental presence will provide comfort and reduce fear and anxiety. Permit the 6- month- to 3-year-old child to remain on the parent's lap for as much of the examination as possible. Allowing the child to manipulate assessment equipment or to perform a simultaneous assessment of a stuffed animal or doll may allay the toddler's or preschooler's fears and may facilitate the examination process.

Special care must be taken when performing examination techniques with pediatric clients from certain ethnic backgrounds. For example, many Hispanic or Latino clients believe that inspecting and commenting on the features of a child without touching the child is placing an "evil eye" on the child. Before beginning the examination, determine cultural concerns that may relate to the client and, if in doubt, proceed in a manner that will elicit as little offense as possible.

Before beginning the examination and before each assessment step, explain the procedure to the child and parent and address any concerns or questions that arise. Explain the need for special positioning or draping, and inform the child and parent if their assistance will be required to facilitate the examination process. Explain that most examinations are not painful and that care will be taken to maintain comfort and to preserve the child's modesty. Use clear, simple terms, and demonstrate using a doll or stuffed animal to promote clear communication.

General Survey

Observations made during the general survey of a pediatric client must take into account age-specific developmental norms. For example, assessment of the mental status and state of awareness of a pediatric client might be impeded by the child's age and limited ability to communicate, as well as by the child's reluctance to cooperate and communicate with the unfamiliar nurse.

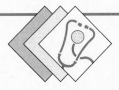

Assessing General Appearance and Mental Status

ASSESSMENT	NORMAL FINDINGS	DEVIATIONS FROM NORMAL
Note the client's size in relation to age. For children under 2 years of age, adjust chronologic age (CA) for prematurity by subtracting the number of weeks premature from the child's chronologic age: CA − (40 − number of weeks of gestation) = adjusted age.	Size appropriate for age	Small or large size for age
Note the child's race. Physical features alone may not indicate race. Consult history for designated race.	Distinct coloring or features indicating race	
Observe the client's body build in relation to age-specific norms and general health, as well as cultural differences.	Varies with age and developmental stage; the newborn infant and the young child may have more fatty tissue than the preadolescent, adolescent, or adult	Excessively thin or obese
Observe the client's posture and gait, lying, sitting, standing, and walking (if ambulatory).	Newborn or infant generally rests with knees and arms slightly flexed The toddler or young child may have a broad-based gait until 3 to 4 years of age	Hyperactivity or flaccidity Spastic gait; limp; knock-knees after 6 years or bowlegs after 18 months (see musculoskeletal assessment)

► **Assessing General Appearance and Mental Status** *CONTINUED*

ASSESSMENT	NORMAL FINDINGS	DEVIATIONS FROM NORMAL
Observe the client's general hygiene and grooming status. Consider recent activities. The young child's grooming often depends on adult support; adolescent grooming concerns are similar to those of an adult.	Clean and neat	Soiled, wrinkled clothing; dirty skin (may be a sign of neglect, knowledge deficit, or lack of finances)
Assess for excessive body and breath odor. Question recent food intake, and consider possible source of unusual breath odor.	No foul body odor or minimal skin odor, particularly if perspiration present; no breath odor	Ammonia, acetone, or foul breath odor
Observe for signs of distress with movement or stimulation.	Calm facial expression	Crying, withdrawal, or wincing, particularly in response to palpation of body part
Note signs of healthy skin, e.g., color, temperature, moisture.	Healthy appearance	Pallor, flushing, jaundice, or cyanosis
Note activity level and breathing pattern.		Weakness or inactivity; obvious distress or illness
Inspect the child's genitals.	Sex organs clearly male or female	Ambiguous genitals; unclear gender
Mental Status		
Observe the client's attitude in the parent's presence. Note the client's response to the situation and personnel.	Infants and young children may withdraw from strangers and unfamiliar procedures	Very withdrawn or hostile, or nonresponsive to parents
Monitor the child's interaction with parents or family.	May vary with personality of child and age; generally should respond warmly to parent (situation may alter)	Inappropriate for situation; different as reported from usual state
Note articulation, quantity, and organization of the child's speech.	Clarity and vocabulary appropriate for the child's age	Poor verbal skills (may indicate organic or developmental delay)
Note the child's thought processes and ability to express questions or needs. Nonverbal behaviors may be observed with infants.	Appropriate for developmental level	Autistic behavior; confusion; nonresponsiveness

Body Measurements

Height or Length and Weight

In infants and growing children, height and weight provide an index of normal or abnormal growth. In addition, height and weight measurements are essential in calculating body surface area to determine safe dosages of medications. Standardized growth charts provide baseline data and guidelines for assessment; however, variations from these norms may not always indicate illness. Average height and weight gains per year of life are shown in Table 12–1 on page 301. See also Figures 12–1 and 12–2.

Length The average length of a white newborn in the United States is about 50 cm (20 in). At birth, black infants tend to be shorter than white infants. This range is from 47.5 to 52.5 cm (19 to 21 in). Female babies are on the average smaller than male babies.

Two recumbent lengths are the crown-to-rump length (the sitting length) and the head-to-heel length (from the top of the head to the base of the heels; Figure 12–3 on page 301). Normally the crown-to-rump length is approximately the same as the head circumference. By 6 months, infants gain another 13.75 cm (5.5 in) of height. By 12 months, they add another 7.5 cm (3 in). Rate of increase in height is

BOYS FROM BIRTH TO 36 MONTHS

LENGTH FOR AGE

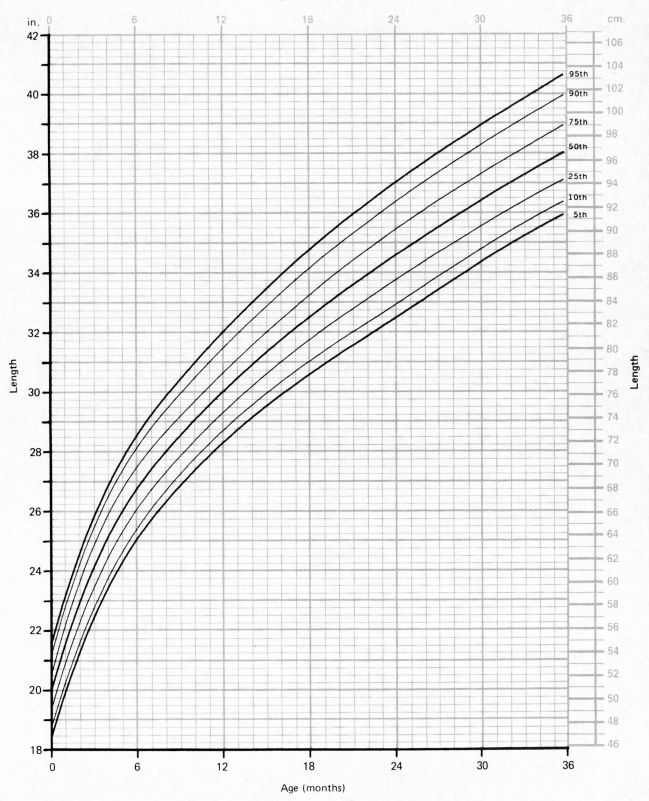

FIGURE 12–1 Growth chart for boys from birth to 36 months.
Source: S. R. Mott, S. R. James, and A. M. Sperhac, *Nursing care of children and families*, 2d ed. (Redwood City, Calif.: Addison-Wesley Nursing, 1990), p. 1911.

GIRLS FROM BIRTH TO 36 MONTHS

LENGTH FOR AGE

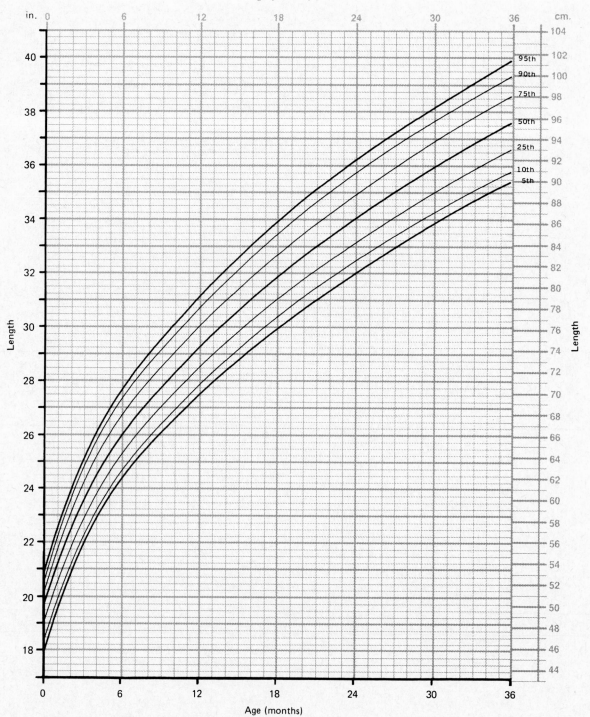

Source: National Center Health Statistics, Department of HEW

FIGURE 12–2 Growth chart for girls from birth to 36 months.
Source: S. R. Mott, S. R. James, and A. M. Sperhac, *Nursing care of children and families,* 2d ed. (Redwood City, Calif.: Addison-Wesley Nursing, 1990), p. 1908.

TABLE 12-1 AVERAGE HEIGHT AND WEIGHT GAIN PER YEAR OF LIFE

Age	Linear growth per year	Weight gain per year
0–12 months	10 in (25 cm)	13–18 lb (6–8 kg)
13–24 months	5 in (12.5 cm)	5–8 lb (2.5 kg)
25–36 months	4 in (10 cm)	4–6 lb (2 kg)
37–48 months	3 in (8 cm)	3–5 lb (1–2 kg)
4 years to puberty	2.0–2.5 in (5.0–6.5 cm)	4–6 lb (2–3 kg)

Source: S. R. Mott, S. R. James, and A. M. Sperhac, *Nursing care of children and families,* 2d ed. (Redwood City, Calif.: Addison-Wesley Nursing, 1990), p. 1505.

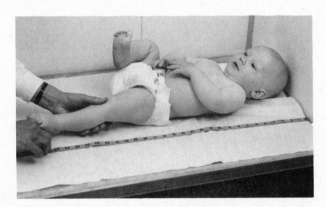

FIGURE 12–3 Measuring an infant, head to heel.

Measuring the Recumbent Length of an Infant

- Remove the infant's shoes. It is unnecessary to undress the infant, but remove any bulky outdoor clothing so that the infant can lie horizontally with the knees extended.

- Reassure the infant with a soothing voice and gentle, sure movements.

- Place a clean protector on the measuring surface. *This protects the infant from microorganisms present on the measuring board.*

- Place the infant supine on the measuring surface parallel to the measuring rule. Do not leave the infant, because the child may roll off. The measuring surface must be firm to make an accurate measurement.

- Have the infant face the ceiling, and press the top of the head against an upright structure that is at point zero on the measuring scale.

- Make sure the infant's knees are extended.

- Place the ruler or measuring square against the soles of the feet at a right angle to the measuring board.

- Determine the point on the measuring board to which the ruler or measuring square comes.

- Take the infant off the measuring surface.

- Put shoes and any clothes removed back on, and put the infant in a safe place.

largely influenced by the baby's size at birth and by nutrition.

Measuring the recumbent length of infants, especially newborns, is difficult because the legs are flexed and tensed. Guidelines are provided in the accompanying box. The following equipment is needed:

- Horizontal measuring board or a measure, usually calibrated in centimeters

- Brace for the feet (e.g., a box), if a measuring board is not available

- Ruler or measuring square

- Clean protector for the scale

Weight At birth, most babies weigh from 2.7 to 3.8 kg (6.0 to 8.5 lb); white infants tend to weigh more than infants of other races. A number of factors can affect the child's weight at birth. These include the mother's life-style (e.g., nutrition, substance abuse), age, heredity, and the weeks of gestation. Just after birth, most infants lost 5% to 10% of their birth weight because of fluid loss. This weight loss is normal, and infants usually regain that weight in about 1 week. After several days, babies usually gain weight at the rate of 5 to 7 ounces weekly for 6 months. By 5 months of age infants usually reach twice their birth weight

and three times their birth weight by age 12 months. Guidelines for measuring an infant's weight are provided in the box on page 302. A special scale with a tray is used to weigh infants (Figure 12–4). The tray is covered with a paper protector each time an infant is weighed to prevent both cross-contamination and heat loss from conduction.

Measuring the Weight of an Infant

- Remove the infant's clothing. In most instances, the infant's naked weight is taken. Often the infant's weight is measured in association with hygienic care. If for some reason an infant cannot be unclothed at the time, the clothes are later weighed separately, and that weight is deducted from the earlier weight to determine the infant's naked weight.

- Reassure the infant with a soothing voice and gentle, sure movements.

- Drape the scale tray with the paper protector. *The protector prevents the transfer of microorganisms from one infant to another using the same scale.*

- Check that the scale registers zero, and adjust it if necessary.

- Gently lift and place the infant on the tray.

- Hold one hand about an inch above but not touching the baby. Use the other hand to adjust the scale. Never leave an infant unattended. *The nurse holds one hand over the baby for safety reasons but avoids touching the baby because this would distort the weight measurement.*

- Determine the weight.

- Clothe and return the infant to the crib.

Head and Chest Circumferences

Assessment of head circumference is of particular importance in infants and children to determine the growth rate of the skull and the brain. An infant's head should be measured at every visit to the physician or nurse until the child is 2 years old. Head measurement of children 3 years or older usually does not need to be done routinely; however, this measurement should be taken during initial examinations of young children (Figure 12–5 and Figures 12–1 and 12–2, earlier).

Normal head circumferences (**normocephaly**) are often related to chest circumferences. At birth, the average infant's head circumference is 35 cm (14 in) and generally varies only 1 or 2 cm (0.5 in). The chest circumference of the newborn is usually less than the head circumference by about 2.5 cm (1 in). One exception occurs during the first 24 hours of life, when head molding and overriding sutures from delivery may create a slightly smaller head circumference than that of the chest. A molded head contour returns to normal within 48 to 72 hours. The head circumference increases 12 cm in the first 12 months of life.

As the infant grows, the chest circumference becomes larger than the head circumference. At about 9 or 10 months, the head and chest circum-

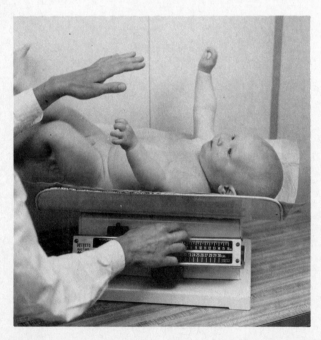

FIGURE 12–4 Weighing an infant. The scale is balanced before each weighing, with the protective pad in place. The caregiver's hand is poised above the infant as a safety measure.

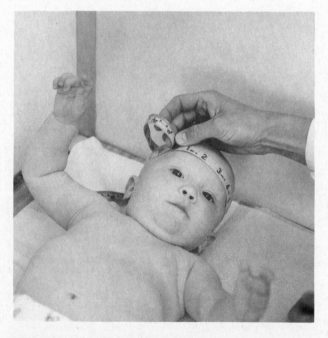

FIGURE 12–5 Measuring an infant's head circumference around the skull, above the eyebrows.

ferences are about the same, and after 1 year of age the chest circumference is larger.

Abnormalities in the circumference of a head are referred to as **macrocephaly** (a large head) or **microcephaly** (a small head). The former is often the result of excessive cerebrospinal fluid within the skull (**hydrocephalus**).

Guidelines for measuring head and chest circumferences are provided in the accompanying box.

The Integument

The Skin

Bluish pigmentation in the gums, nailbeds, and buccal mucosa are normal findings in dark-skinned clients. Areas of hyperpigmentation over the buttocks, known as Mongolian spots, are a normal finding. In contrast, cafe au lait spots should be carefully evaluated. While lower extremity bruising is expected with active children, extensive bruises may be an indication of abuse, problems with equilibrium resulting in falls, or coagulation abnormalities. Newborns may evidence bruising or localized edema in the presenting part because of the trauma of birth, which usually resolves during the newborn period.

Measuring Head and Chest Circumferences

- Reassure the infant with a soothing voice and gentle, sure movements.
- Place the infant in a recumbent position on a firm surface, e.g., a crib or examining table.

Head Circumference

- Place the tape under the infant's head.
- Apply the tape snugly around the greatest circumference of the head:

  a. Posteriorly at the level of the occipital protuberances.
  b. Anteriorly at the midforehead level just above the eyebrows.

- If the head has an abnormal shape, as in hydrocephalus, position the tape over whatever points on the forehead or occiput give the greatest circumference.

Chest Circumference

- Place the tape under the infant's back.
- Apply the tape snugly around the chest at the level of the xiphoid cartilage (at the nipple line) and at right angles to the spinal column. Make sure the tape is at the same level in the front and back.

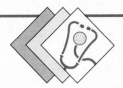

Assessing the Skin

ASSESSMENT	NORMAL FINDINGS	DEVIATIONS FROM NORMAL
Inspect for skin color, noting uniformity. Consider ethnicity. Inspect skin in natural or soft lighting.	Varies from light to dark pink or brown; yellow or olive undertones; pink nail beds	Bruise or port-wine stain Cyanosis; ashen gray lips in dark-skinned clients
	Mongolian spots, in Asian and black infants; jaundice from 24 hours after birth to 2 weeks	Cafe au lait spots; jaundice at birth or within 12 hours of birth
	Uniform, except for suntanned areas or palms and soles of dark-skinned clients	Hyperpigmentation or hypopigmentation, pallor, albinism
Inspect skin turgor. Pinch forehead skin, and extremities. Note edema—location, degree of pitting, and so on.	Elastic texture; skin springs back when pinched	Poor skin elasticity; skin remains tented when pinched or returns to original state slowly
	Newborns: Localized edema at presenting part	Generalized edema or severe periorbital edema

▶ **Assessing the Skin** *CONTINUED*

ASSESSMENT	NORMAL FINDINGS	DEVIATIONS FROM NORMAL
Assess skin lesions and texture. Palpate lesions to determine shape and texture. Note color and distribution. (See the box on skin lesions on p. 209 in Chapter 11.)	Newborns: May have fine hair, milia, cheesy vernix, or desquamation over the skin surface; capillary hemangiomas on face and neck Adolescent: May have acne	Raised hemangiomas on areas other than face or neck Lack of subcutaneous fat (indicates malnutrition) Subcutaneous nodules (may indicate juvenile arthritis)
Assess skin moisture. Observe and palpate the skin.	Moist skinfold areas under arms and perineum	Either excessive moisture or excessive dryness
Assess skin temperature. Palpate skin over body areas.	Warm, uniform skin temperature over body surfaces	Wide variation in skin temperature between upper extremities and lower extremities (may indicate cardiovascular anomaly); localized warmth (may indicate inflammation)

The Hair and Nails

The amount of hair varies from one newborn to another. The color and texture of a child's hair often changes 2 to 3 months after birth. Patches of hair loss may indicate trauma or be a sign of extended pressure to an area of the scalp. Hair loss (alopecia) may be noted in pediatric clients undergoing cancer treatment. The nurse should inspect a child's hair and scalp closely for insect or lice infestation, lesions, and signs of trauma. Nails are assessed for nail bed color, shape, and texture.

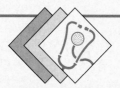

Assessing the Hair

ASSESSMENT	NORMAL FINDINGS	DEVIATIONS FROM NORMAL
The Hair		
Inspect the evenness of hair growth over the scalp. Note areas of hair loss.	Evenly distributed hair	Patchy losses of hair (alopecia)
Note thickness of hair.	Thick hair	Very thin hair
Inspect hair texture and oiliness (appropriate for ethnic group).	Silky, resilient hair or strong, springing curls in some ethnic groups	Dry, brittle hair
Note the presence of infection or infestations by examining the scalp in several areas.	No infection or infestation	Flaking, sores, lice, nits (louse eggs), or ringworm
Inspect hair growth over body surfaces.	Evenly distributed, faint hair over body surfaces; more hair in the pubic area, under the arms, and on eyebrows and lashes	Heavy hair growth over skin surface; tufts of hair over spine or sacrum; absence of pubic hair at adolescence

▶ **Assessing the Hair** *CONTINUED*

ASSESSMENT	NORMAL FINDINGS	DEVIATIONS FROM NORMAL
The Nails		
Inspect nail bed color.	Pink nail beds	Yellowing of the nail beds (meconium stained)
Inspect nail plate shape and texture.	Convex curvature; normal length; and smooth texture	Broad nail beds (may indicate chromosomal anomalies); short, jagged edges (may indicate nail biting); pitted nails (may indicate fungus or psoriasis); brittle, thin, or excessively thick nails (indicate poor circulation, iron deficiency, or poor hydration)

The Head

Assessment of the head includes inspection, palpation, and auscultation. The nurse must remember to ask parental permission before touching the child's head; in some cultures, this action is considered inappropriate.

Skull and Face

The heads of most newborn babies are misshapen because of the molding of the head that occurs during vaginal deliveries. Molding of the head is made pos-sible by **fontanelles** (unossified membranous gaps) in the bone structure of the skull and by overriding of the **sutures** (junction lines of the skull bones). Within a week, a newborn's head usually regains its symmetry, a fact that reassures parents.

The eight bones of the cranium are separated by sutures, which gradually ossify during childhood. These bones are the frontal bone, the occipital bone, two parietal and two temporal bones, and the sphenoid and ethmoid bones (Figure 12–6). Six fontanelles are present at birth, but the two most prominent ones are the frontal (anterior) and the occipital (posterior) ones. The posterior fontanelle

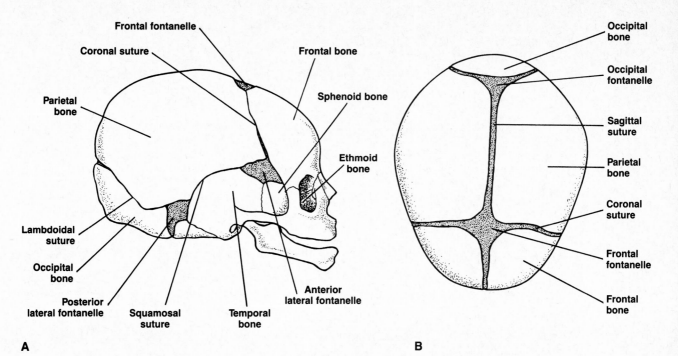

FIGURE 12–6 The bones of the skull showing the fontanelles and the suture lines: *A*, lateral view; *B*, superior view.

between the parietal bones and the occipital bone is the smaller of the two (1 to 2 cm in diameter) and is generally closed by 1 to 8 weeks after birth. The posterior fontanelle may not be palpated for a few hours after birth because of the overriding of the sutures during delivery. The larger anterior fontanelle (4 to 6 cm in diameter and diamond-shaped) can increase in size for several months after birth. After 6 months, the size gradually decreases until closure occurs between 9 and 18 months.

Ideally, the nurse examines the infant's head for symmetry of shape and for palpation of the fontanelles while the infant is sitting comfortably in the mother's lap. Normally, in a crying, coughing, or vom-iting infant, the anterior fontanelle has a certain tenseness, fullness, and bulging, indicating increased intracranial pressure. Continual bulging is abnormal and is associated with tumors or infections of the brain or hydrocephalus due to obstruction of the cerebrospinal fluid circulation in the ventricles. Depression of the anterior fontanelle generally indicates dehydration.

Forehead prominence may indicate a genetic condition. Skull assymetry may be the result of in utero position or extended periods of lying in one position, possibly due to poor health, lack of parental care, or neglect.

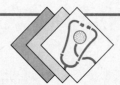

Assessing the Skull and Face

ASSESSMENT	NORMAL FINDINGS	DEVIATIONS FROM NORMAL
Inspect the skull for its shape and symmetry.	Symmetric	Asymmetric
Palpate the anterior and posterior fontanelles.	A fontanelle may bulge with crying, coughing, or vomiting	Continuous bulging, full, or tense fontanelles; sunken or depressed fontanelles (may be dehydration)
Assess head control.	Voluntary head control after 6 months of age	Poor head control; head tilt (may indicate hearing or vision deficit)
Assess facial features. Note symmetry of movement, eyebrows, and eyelashes.	Symmetric features and movement; or slight asymmetry	Asymmetric facial features; increased or sparse facial hair; myxedema of face; drooping eyes/lips
Assess frontal, ethmoid, and maxillary sinuses.	No tenderness	Tenderness (may indicate infection or inflammation)

The Eyes and Vision

Visual abilities are present at birth. The newborn can follow large moving objects, is attracted to black–white contrast, can fixate on certain stimuli for 4 to 10 seconds, and can react to changes in the intensity of light. The pupils of the newborn respond slowly, however, and the eyes cannot focus on objects further than 20 inches away. By 3 months of age, vision has developed so that the eyes coordinate both horizontally and vertically. By 4 months of age, the infant recognizes familiar objects and follows moving objects. At 6 years of age, visual acuity is comparable to that of an adult. Preschool children are generally farsighted until their eyes grow and become **emmetropic** (refracting normally and focusing objects on the retina).

The visual assessment may produce discomfort or agitation in the child and should be performed near the end of the physical examination. Visual assessment of an infant should be performed shortly after birth and at routine checkups and is limited to the ability to fixate and follow an object, and pupillary constriction or dilation in response to light. Children under 4 years of age can be tested for vision by asking them to match a specified object with an identical object or picture of the object. The examiner should approach the testing process as a game and praise the child throughout the process for cooperation and effort.

Special vision charts are available for children, as well as decorative pads for covering one eye while testing the other. When using the visual acuity charts, the nurse begins by asking the child to indicate the direction of the largest letter or object to determine whether the child understands the testing process. When using the Snellen E chart (see Figure 11–20, page 216), for example, the nurse asks the child to indicate the direction the letter is pointing and to compare the legs of the E to three fingers on the hand. The nurse asks the child to turn the fingers in the same direction as the letter. For preschoolers who may have difficulty identifying direction, use a large duplicate letter E and have them turn it to match the letter on the chart. For the other charts, the child identifies the object or letter on the specified line. Children should have their first professional vision evaluation before age 4 or 5 years and biannual exam-inations throughout the school years. Learning difficulties in school often indicate a visual deficit.

Normal vision for the newborn is estimated to range from 20/200 to 20/400; at 2 months to 6 months, it is approximately 20/200; and from 6 months to 1 year of age and older, acuity may range from 2/40–60 to 20/20. **Binocular vision** (ability to focus on images with both eyes) is present by 3 to 6 months of age. Children under 8 years of age may normally have **hyperopia** (farsightedness). **Strabismus** (crossed eyes) requires a referral to an ophthalmologist to determine whether an eye muscle disorder is present. Early identification and treatment of this condition is essential to prevent **amblyopia** (lazy eye) and permanent vision loss in the affected eye. Eye shapes vary according to race. In Asians an upward palpebral slant is often normal; however, alterations in the epicanthal folds and palpebral slant may also be characteristic of Down syndrome. Children with wide nasal bridges or epicanthal folds may appear to have strabismus. This mistaken condition is known as *pseudostrabismus*; however, further testing is needed to confirm the diagnosis.

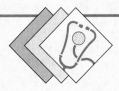

Assessing Eye Structures and Visual Acuity

ASSESSMENT	NORMAL FINDINGS	DEVIATIONS FROM NORMAL
External Eye Structures		
Assess eyebrows, eyelids, and eye-lashes for growth, symmetry, and movement. Use a "Can you do this?" approach: Demonstrate raising and lowering of eyebrows on request. With infants, you need to watch for spontaneous movement.	Symmetric structures with equal movement	Asymmetric structures or unequal movement
Examine eyelids and eyelashes for position, mobility, and lesions.	Eyelashes have upward and outward curve	Inversion of the lashes; **ptosis** (drooping eyelids) or incomplete closure Sty Excessive blinking
	"Setting sun" phenomenon (sclera visible above the iris) may be normal in newborn, particularly premature infants	Marked visibility of sclera above the iris (may indicate pathology)
	Hypertelorism (wide spacing between eyes) may be a normal variant, unless other facial anomalies are present	Hypertelorism with epicanthal folds and upward palpebral slant

▶ **Assessing the Eye Structures and Visual Acuity** *CONTINUED*

ASSESSMENT	NORMAL FINDINGS	DEVIATIONS FROM NORMAL
Assess the conjunctiva. Observe the upper conjunctiva by gently pushing the eyelid upward. Examine the lower conjunctiva by pulling the lower lid down while the child looks up.	Pink and glossy appearance	Pallor, redness, or discharge—with or without odor; jaundice
Inspect the cornea for clarity and texture.	Transparent, shiny, and smooth	Opaque, red, irregular surface (may indicate abrasion)
Assess pupillary reaction. Ask the child to focus on a distant light or object while another object or penlight is brought closer to the child's face; observe pupillary response—direct and consensual.	PERRLA Pupil constricts as object or light draws near	Sluggish or asymmetric reaction to light (may indicate increased intracranial pressure) Strabismus (after 6 months of age) **Nystagmus** (involuntary rapid movement of the eyeball)
Assess the lens for clarity.	Clear lens	Opaque lens
Visual Acuity		
Assess near vision. If the child is old enough and able to read, ask the child to read from material held at 36 cm (14 in) distance, with glasses worn, if applicable. Ask a young child to match letters or objects in a book with identical objects.	Able to read or match letters or objects	Difficulty matching letters or objects (may be related to age and immaturity)
Assess distant vision. Use the Snellen E or other age-appropriate chart. Perform test without corrective lenses first. For a young child, an assistant may be needed to occlude the eye for testing.	20/40–60 to 20/20	Difference of two or more lines between eyes (refer client to ophthalmologist)
• For a 3-year-old, begin with the 20/50 line, and if the child is successful, proceed to the 20/40 and so on. Ask the child to read alternate lines from right to left, then left to right to avoid memorization of letters.	20/40 to 20/20	20/50 or less (should be referred)
• For a 4-year-old, begin with the 20/40 line.	20/20 to 20/30	20/40 or less (should be referred)
Assess light perception. For infants, move a penlight across the field of vision, and observe for head movement. A colorful toy may be used. Assess older children by shining a penlight in the eyes and asking the child to indicate when the light is on or off.	Eyes and head follow light Nystagmus in extreme lateral position	No response to object or light Presence of nystagmus without light stimulation indicates greater pathology
Determine visual fields. Using a game approach, hold your hand or your "wiggling" fingers 30 cm (1 ft) from the child's face, and move the hand slowly back and forth, stopping periodically. Ask the child to identify when the hand or fingers stop or move.	Identifies movement or lack of movement Results for young children may be limited to level of understanding	Unable to identify movement

The Ears and Hearing

The ears of infants and young children should be assessed at the end of the physical examination, because invasive procedures are involved. Examination of the external ear canal is important to determine the presence of **otitis externa** (inflammation of the external auditory canal). Tenderness of the tragus may indicate otitis externa. During insertion of the otoscope, the examiner should use restraint if resistive activity is noted. Placing the child in the parent's lap or on a table with an assistant firmly holding the child's upper and lower extremities may ensure a safe, stable procedure. The ear canal of a child under 2 to 3 years of age curves upward, so the pinna must be pulled down and back to facilitate examination of the external canal and tympanic membrane (Figure 12–7). For children over 3 years of age, the pinna is pulled up and back to straighten the ear canal, because the ear canal normally curves down and forward. Crying neonates, infants, and young children may normally exhibit slight erythema of the tympanic membrane. Children with upper airway infections are at high risk for ear infections because the ear canal in children is shorter and the eustachian tube is straighter, which allows easier pas-

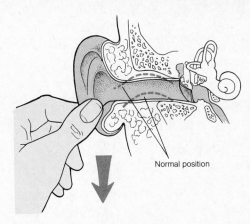

FIGURE 12–7 Straightening the ear canal of a child by pulling the pinna down and back.

sage of organisms from the pharynx into the ear canal. Native Americans, Eskimos, and children with Down syndrome have a higher incidence of otitis media than other pediatric groups.

An audiologist can conduct brain stem auditory-evoked response screening (BAERS) tests on all children from birth through adolescence. In addition, visual response audiometry can be used after 7 months.

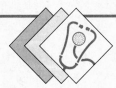

Assessing the Ears and Hearing

ASSESSMENT	NORMAL FINDINGS	DEVIATIONS FROM NORMAL
Examine the auricles for color, symmetry, and position.	Color same as facial skin Dark-skinned infants may exhibit darker coloring of the posterior auricle during the initial months Symmetric position	Cyanosis, pallor, excessive redness Protruding pinna; Low-set ears
Palpate the auricles for texture, elasticity, and areas of tenderness.	Mobile, firm and not tender; pinna recoils after it is folded	Lesions such as cysts; flaky, scaly, skin (e.g., seborrhea); tenderness when moved or pressed may indicate inflammation or infection of the external canal
Using an otoscope (see Figure 11–34) **inspect the external ear canal for skin lesions, pus, and blood and tympanic membrane for color.**	Clear ear passage; translucent, pearly gray tympanic membrane	Foreign bodies; dull gray or yellow tympanic membrane; purulent discharge
Assess hearing.		
• Test the infant by noting whether the infant turns in response to a noise or music.	Turns in response to noise	No response to noise

▶

▶ **Assessing the Ears and Hearing** *CONTINUED*

ASSESSMENT	NORMAL FINDINGS	DEVIATIONS FROM NORMAL
• Have older children respond to a whisper test, or a portable audiometer; use of game with silly words might be most effective. Explain that Rinne and Weber tests are games to detect when the "hummingbird" is nearby (see Chapter 11 and Figures 11–35, 11–36, and 11–37 for testing techniques). Accuracy in the Rinne and Weber tests require that the child be able to understand the test and communicate as questioned. These tests are rarely used before school age.	Child might giggle in response to whispered words Rinne: Air-conducted hearing is greater than bone-conducted hearing; record AC > BC Weber: Sound heard in both ears equally well	No response, or states unable to hear clearly Rinne: Bone-conducted hearing greater than air-conducted hearing Weber: Sound lateralizes to one ear

The Nose and Sinuses

Infants are obligatory nose breathers; a child who appears to breathe better through the mouth should therefore be assessed for closely **choanal atresia** (congenital occlusion of the openings between the nasal cavities and the nasopharynx), nasal polyps, septal deviation, or other obstruction. Children with chronic allergies often develop a crease across the bridge of the nose due to the constant pushing against the nose in response to itching. **Epistaxis** (nose bleeding) may be a result of nose picking, allergy, or blood dyscrasias.

Pain or tenderness on palpation of the sinuses is a sign of sinusitis. Maxillary and ethmoid sinuses are developed at birth. The frontal sinuses develop by age 7 or 8, and the sphenoid sinus develops after puberty.

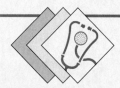

Assessing the Nose and Sinuses

ASSESSMENT	NORMAL FINDINGS	DEVIATIONS FROM NORMAL
Inspect the external nose for color, size, shape, discharge, and flaring. Tilt the head back, push the tip of the nose up, and illuminate the nares with a flashlight.	Symmetric nares, patent bilaterally	Flat nares
Examine sinuses with a flashlight. Transillumination may not be successful in children because of the small size of the sinuses.	No tenderness	Nasal flaring; osbtruction
Assess sense of smell. As a game, have the child identify familiar scents.	Correctly identifies scent	Unable to identify scent or states unable to smell

The Mouth and Oropharynx

Teeth begin to erupt at about 6 months of age. By 30 months of age, all 20 deciduous teeth have usually erupted (Figure 12–8) and between 5 and 6 years of age, they often begin to shed. Permanent teeth begin to erupt at approximately 6 years of age and continue until all 32 teeth are present. Delayed tooth eruption may indicate systemic disease. Variations in the timing of tooth eruption, however, may be normal and are often hereditary. A child may have a **malocclusion** (an overbite or underbite) due to thumb sucking or overcrowding of teeth. Flattened tooth surfaces may be due to **bruxism** (teeth grinding), which may occur as a result of anxiety.

Congenital malformation of the lip or soft palate (cleft lip or palate) is usually evident at birth or discovered shortly thereafter. An abnormally high palatal arch may be associated with a congenital disorder and may result in speech difficulty. The white nodules often found in the palate of the newborn (**Epstein's pearls**) are a normal finding. Tonsils are generally small in infancy, appear large in preschool years, and become smaller as the child ages toward puberty.

The mouth and oropharynx of an infant or child should be assessed at the latter part of the physical examination. The infant may need to be restrained; however, the nurse may elicit the child's cooperation through the use of games. The nurse may need a tongue blade to open the mouth of a reluctant child for examination of the oropharynx.

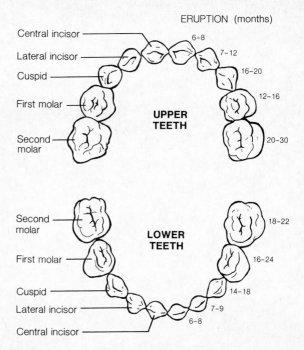

FIGURE 12–8 Temporary teeth and their times of eruption (stated in months).

Assessing the Mouth and Oropharynx

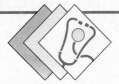

ASSESSMENT	NORMAL FINDINGS	DEVIATIONS FROM NORMAL
Examine the outer lip for symmetry, color, contour, and texture.	Symmetric, intact, smooth lip surface	Cleft lip; lip asymmetry
Observe and palpate the inner lip and oral mucosa.	Moist, smooth mucosa	**Koplik's spots** (red spots indicating prodromal stage of measles); white patches (indicate candida, or thrush)
Inspect the teeth and gum line.	Black line on gums of dark-skinned children may be normal	Delayed tooth eruption; malocclusion; bruxism; black line on gums of fair-skinned children (may indicate lead poisoning)
Inspect the tongue surface and base and the undersurface and floor of the mouth. Note mobility of the tongue; observe as the child cries or speaks.	Tongue in central position. Smooth tongue base with visible veins. Tongue extends to the gum line	Excessive protrusion (glossoptosis). Tongue-tied (tongue attached to the frenulum)

▶ **Assessing the Mouth and Oropharynx** *CONTINUED*

ASSESSMENT	NORMAL FINDINGS	DEVIATIONS FROM NORMAL
Inspect salivary duct openings. Note degree of salivation.	Same color as buccal mucosa Drooling (up to 2 years of age)	Redness and swelling of ducts Excessive drooling after 2 years of age
Inspect the hard and soft palate for color, shape, and texture.	Pink, smooth, moist; intact surface	Cleft palate (varying severity)
Note the position of the uvula.	Midline of the soft palate	Deviated to one side
Note the color and texture of the oropharynx.	Pink and smooth oral surface	Irregular oral surface; lesions, redness
Elicit the gag reflex.	Gag reflex present	Gag reflex absent
Note the size and color of the tonsils (for size description, see the box on p. 235 in Chapter 11). If child has a croupy cough, do not probe oropharynx. *This may cause complete airway obstruction.*	Tonsils the same color as mucosa; no discharge	Enlarged tonsils; redness; lesions; discharge

The Neck

The neck is short in infancy, lengthening at 2 to 3 years of age. Head control is related to control of neck muscles. **Tonic neck reflex** (Fencer's position) is normal until 6 months of age. It is a reflex in which, when the head is forcibly turned to one side, the arm and leg on that side are extended while the opposite limbs are flexed. An infant will not crawl until the tonic neck reflex disappears. The thyroid gland is generally not palpable until adolescence. To determine neck mobility, the nurse should use "Simon Says" or a similar game involving a demonstration–return demonstration approach.

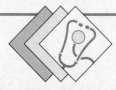

Assessing the Neck

ASSESSMENT	NORMAL FINDINGS	DEVIATIONS FROM NORMAL
Inspect neck muscles for masses or swelling.	No masses or swelling	Neck weakness; masses; swelling; short or webbed neck; distended veins
Note neck range of motion—forward, back, right, and left. Have child turn and shrug shoulders against your hand.	Full range of motion without resistance Tonic neck reflex	Resistant neck movement/stiffness Persistent tonic neck reflex beyond 6 months of age
Note jaw size.	Appropriate size	Abnormally large (**macrognathia**) or abnormally small jaw (**micrognathia**)
Palpate the lymph nodes (refer to the box on p. 238 in Chapter 11 and Figure 11–48). Press gently but firmly, noting the location, size, tenderness, mobility, and color. For cervical nodes, tilt the child's head upward.	Small (less than 1 cm), nontender, movable nodes; usually nonpalpable after puberty	Enlarged nodes (> 2 cm); fixed, red, or tender nodes

▶ **Assessing the Neck** *CONTINUED*

ASSESSMENT	NORMAL FINDINGS	DEVIATIONS FROM NORMAL
Assess the trachea. Gently place your thumb and finger on each side of the trachea, and slide them up and down.	At the midline or slightly right of the midline	May be deviated if child or infant has **atelectasis** (collapse of lung tissue)
Inspect and palpate the thyroid gland.	Nonpalpable in young children; not visible but smooth and may be palpable in older children	Palpable gland in children, enlarged gland in adolescent

The Thorax and Lungs

In the assessment of infants and children, marked disproportion of the chest is evident when chest circumference is compared to head circumference (see page 302). The lung assessment of an infant or child normally reveals **hyperresonance** (booming sound) due to the thinness of the chest wall. Breath sounds are usually harsher or louder in children for the same reason. Absent or diminished breath sounds should be considered abnormal and should be further investigated. The nurse may note retraction of the chest in the infant or young child with respiratory congestion or obstruction. In children under 6 or 7 years of age, respirations are abdominal. Older children are commonly thoracic breathers, although males tend to be abdominal breathers. Abdominal breathing may be a sign of pathology.

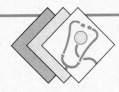

Assessing the Thorax and Lungs

ASSESSMENT	NORMAL FINDINGS	DEVIATIONS FROM NORMAL
Inspect and palpate the thorax.	Neonates: circular, barrel chest (anteroposterior: transverse diameter of 1:1); see Figure 11–60A on page 243 Older child: oval chest (ratio near 1:2)	Marked disproportion, asymmetry, pectus excavatum (funnel chest), pectus carinatum (pigeon breast), scoliosis, kyphosis; atrophy or hypertrophy of chest muscles
Observe the symmetry of chest movement in respiration.	Symmetric respirations—abdominal in children under 6 years, thoracic in older children	Asymmetric chest movements
Palpate for tactile fremitus. Assess infants when they are crying or spontaneously verbalizing. Use requested vocalizations for older children.	Moderate fremitus palpable; easily felt in infants	Reduced, absent, or increased fremitus
Auscultate the lung. Make deep breathing a game for the child, e.g., blowing out candles on a cake. Infants and young children might require the use of a small or bell-shaped stethoscope diaphragm because of the tight fit over the ribs.	Clear breath sounds	Adventitious breath sounds indicating lung or airway inflammation or obstruction
Inspect the spinal alignment for any deformities.	Spine aligned in a vertical line when client stands	Spinal curvatures: kyphosis, lordosis, or scoliosis

The Cardiovascular and Peripheral Vascular Systems

In children younger than 8 years of age, the heart lies more horizontally, with the apex left of the nipple line. The point of maximal impulse (PMI) may therefore be located higher than the fifth left intercostal space and more medially than the midclavicular line. In children, a pleural friction rub will stop if the breath is held, whereas a precordial friction rub will persist. An S_3 gallop rhythm is often normal in children because of vibrations during ventricular filling. An S_4 heart sound is rarely normal in a child and should be evaluated further. Figure 12–9 shows heart auscultation sites.

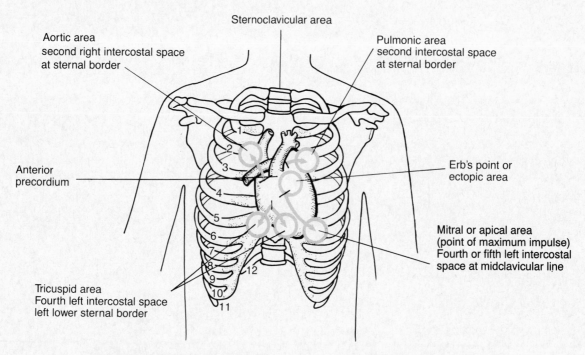

Sternoclavicular area

Aortic area
second right intercostal space
at sternal border

Pulmonic area
second intercostal space
at sternal border

Anterior
precordium

Erb's point or
ectopic area

Mitral or apical area
(point of maximum impulse)
Fourth or fifth left intercostal
space at midclavicular line

Tricuspid area
Fourth left intercostal space
left lower sternal border

FIGURE 12–9 Pediatric cardiac assessment.
Source: S. R. Mott, S. R. James, and A. M. Sperhac, *Nursing care of children and families*, 2d ed. (Redwood City, Calif.: Addison-Wesley Nursing, 1990), p. 378.

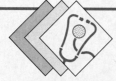

Assessing the Cardiovascular and Peripheral Vascular Systems

ASSESSMENT	NORMAL FINDINGS	DEVIATIONS FROM NORMAL
The Cardiovascular System		
Inspect and palpate the chest to locate the PMI.	PMI at fifth intercostal space at midclavicular line in children 8 years or older; may be higher and more medial in younger child	PMI in different location (may indicate hypertrophy)
Systematically examine the entire chest surface for pulsations, thrills, heaves, and lifts.	Absence of any heaves, lifts, or other pulsations	Other pulsations, thrills, lifts, or heaves

▶ **Assessing the Cardiovascular and Peripheral Vascular Systems** *CONTINUED*

ASSESSMENT	NORMAL FINDINGS	DEVIATIONS FROM NORMAL
Auscultate chest for heart sounds, murmurs, ejection clicks, or friction rubs.	Normal S_1 and S_2; S_3 may be noted	S_4 (should be further evaluated)
Peripheral Pulses		
Palpate the peripheral pulses (except the carotid), **and note skin temperature** on both sides of the body simultaneously.	Symmetric pulses bilaterally; symmetric skin temperature bilaterally	Asymmetric pulses or temperature
Palpate the carotid artery. Gently palpate one side of the neck at a time for pulsation. In the infant, pulsation may be difficult to determine because of the shortness of the neck.	Strong and regular pulse	Absent or weak pulse
Auscultate the carotid artery for bruit. Turn the client's head to the side opposite that being examined to promote access.	No sounds audible	Bruit present
Assess the femoral pulse. Palpate the groin area for pulsation.	Strong, regular pulse	Absent or diminished pulses (may indicate **coarctation of the aorta** (severe narrowing of the aorta) Bounding pulse (may indicate **patent ductus arteriosis**)
Veins		
Assess the jugular veins. With the child in a semi-Fowler's position, turn the head first to one side then the other. Note whether veins are visible.	Veins not visible (neck size and length may inhibit examination)	Veins visibly distended
Peripheral Perfusion		
Assess the capillary refill. Press nail or skin area until pale; release, and note the time it takes for color to return.	Capillary refill to normal within 3 to 5 seconds Absence of edema	Capillary refill delayed Edema (may indicate poor venous return or renal problems)

The Breasts and Axillae

Newborns may display breast enlargement with a white discharge from the nipples, often referred to as *witch's milk*, as a normal result of a maternal estrogenic effect. This effect should disappear within 1 to 2 weeks. In late childhood, usually during the pre-adolescent period, girls should be monitored for breast asymmetry as well as breast masses. **Gynecomastia** in male teens usually results from obesity or early changes of puberty but could also result from a hormonal imbalance or exposure to marijuana. Early or late development of secondary sex characteristics should be further assessed. Refer to the box on p. 258 in Chapter 11 for stages of breast development.

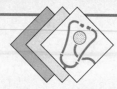

Assessing the Breasts and Axillae

ASSESSMENT	NORMAL FINDINGS	DEVIATIONS FROM NORMAL
Inspect the nipples, and note the size and symmetry of the breasts. For adolescent girls, delay breast assessment during premenstrual time. Assess for pregnancy if indicated.	"Witch's milk" in infant; gynecomastia in newborns or obese males Breast may be nodular during menses	Discharge in older children Masses, redness, discoloration, or tenderness not associated with menses
Note the color and texture of the skin of the breasts.	Smooth, uniform skin surface and color; areola and nipple are often darker and slightly irregular in texture because of sebaceous glands	Localized discolorations; swelling or edema
Examine and palpate the axillary and infraclavicular lymph nodes.	Absence of masses	Masses or nodules

The Abdomen

Children are often ticklish and may need to be distracted during the examination to prevent tensing of abdominal muscles. Flexing the child's knees will assist in relaxing the abdomen. The nurse should prevent or minimize crying, if possible, to prevent disruption of abdominal assessment. Children commonly point to the umbilical area if asked where the pain is; therefore, any other area the child might indicate is very significant. Because children under the age of 6 are usually abdominal breathers, suspect per-

itoneal discomfort if this pattern is *not* noted. Pulsations may be present in the abdominal area, particularly in thin children. Peristalsis is not usually visible and may be a sign of an intestinal obstruction. Normal infants and young children exhibit a "potbelly" contour that often disappears by age 3 to 5. Umbilical hernias less than 5 cm in size are common up to 1 to 2 years of life, particularly in black infants.

In infants, the liver may normally extend 1 to 2 cm below the right costal margin; the spleen may extend 1 to 2 cm below the left costal margin.

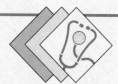

Assessing the Abdomen

ASSESSMENT	NORMAL FINDINGS	DEVIATIONS FROM NORMAL
Inspect and palpate the surface of the abdomen for contour, symmetry, movement, and skin integrity.	Smooth skin surface without bulges or palpable mobility; rounded contour in young children	Bulges, masses, rashes, asymmetry, pulsation, distention, fluid waves, or visible peristalsis
Palpate below the right costal margin to determine the liver border.	Infants: 1 to 3 cm below the right costal margin Older children: not palpable	Palpable enlargement or masses
Auscultate for bowel sounds, vascular sounds, or friction rubs.	Active bowel sounds	Absence of bowel sounds; presence of bruit or friction rub
Palpate the bladder if urinary retention is suspected. Gently palpate the lower abdominal/suprapubic area.	Not palpable	Distended bladder (smooth, round, tense mass palpated)

The Musculoskeletal System

Muscle hypertrophy in a young child can be an early sign of **Duchenne muscular dystrophy** (a genetically acquired disease that causes gradual progressive muscle wasting). The range of motion of the hips of infants and children must be assessed during the neonatal period and throughout childhood to prevent lifelong disability. Congenital dislocation, or *subluxation*, must be ruled out as early as possible. The legs should be assessed for **femoral torsion** (medial or lateral rotation often responsible for toeing in or toeing out). Abnormal femoral torsion may correct spontaneously prior to age 6 years if the child is discouraged from sitting in the preferred "TV squat" position. Encourage such children to use the tailor position; if this position is painful, encourage them to sit with the legs extended.

Young children often have **genu varum** (bowlegs) through toddlerhood (1 to 2 years of age) (Figure 12–10, *A*). **Genu valgum** (knock-knees) is normal from 2 to 7 years of age and is due to overcompensation for genu varum (Figure 12–10, *B*). A broad-based gait is normal until 3 years of age. Feet may be flat until the child has been walking for 1 to 2 years. Mild degrees of foot deformity tend to correct

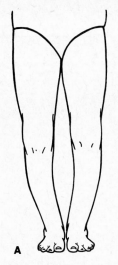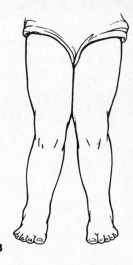

FIGURE 12–10 *A*, Genu varum (bowlegs); *B*, Genu valgum (knock-knees). *Source:* S. R. Mott, S. R. James, and A. M. Sperhac, *Nursing care of children and families*, 2d ed. (Redwood City, Calif.: Addison-Wesley Nursing, 1990), p. 387.

themselves passively. A spinal curve that is evident when the child stands upright but disappears when the child bends forward usually indicates poor posture, not congenital scoliotic curvature.

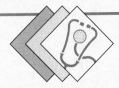

Assessing the Musculoskeletal System

ASSESSMENT	NORMAL FINDINGS	DEVIATIONS FROM NORMAL
Inspect and palpate the muscles for size, tonicity, and strength. Examine the tendons for contractures.	Uniform and strong; without contracture	Atrophy; hypertrophy; spastic or flaccid muscles; contractures
Tests for congenital dislocation of the hip.		
• Perform *Ortolani's test* (Figure 12–11) on a firm surface while the baby is relaxed. Flex the hips and knees to a 90° angle, one at a time. Grasp the thigh with your middle finger over the greater trochanter, and lift the thigh to bring the femoral head from its dislocated posterior position opposite the acetabulum. Simultaneously, gently abduct the thigh, reducing the femoral head into the acetabulum.	Negative test	Ortolani's click (audible "clunk" that indicates reduction)

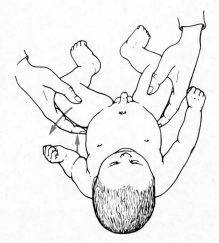

FIGURE 12–11 Ortolani's (reduction) test to assess congenital dislocation of the hip. *Source:* S. R. Mott, S. R. James, and A. M. Sperhac, *Nursing care of children and families*, 2d ed. (Redwood City, Calif.: Addison-Wesley Nursing; 1990), p. 386.

▶ Assessing the Musculoskeletal System *CONTINUED*

ASSESSMENT	NORMAL FINDINGS	DEVIATIONS FROM NORMAL
• Perform *Barlow's test* (Figure 12–12, *A*). If the femoral head is in the acetabulum, determine hip instability by grasping the thigh as in Ortolani's test and adducting with gentle downward pressure.	Negative test	Dislocation palpable as the femoral head slips out of the acetabulum

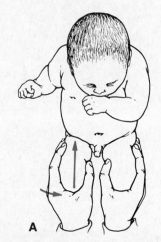

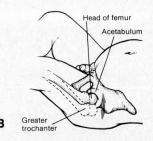

FIGURE 12–12   *A*, Barlow's (dislocation) test to assess congenital hip dislocation; *B*, Normal position of the femur in the acetabulum and position when femur dislocates (dotted lines). *Source:* S. R. Mott, S. R. James, and A. M. Sperhac, *Nursing care of children and families*, 2d ed. (Redwood City, Calif.: Addison-Wesley Nursing, 1990), p. 386.

ASSESSMENT	NORMAL FINDINGS	DEVIATIONS FROM NORMAL
Assess the legs for symmetry (Figure 12–10, *A & B*).	Genu varum or valgum before the age of 6 or 7	Genum varum or valgum after age 7
Monitor the feet. Check the arch by trying to slide one finger under the child's medial arch.	Flat feet in children under 18 months of age; one finger allowed under the medial arch	Finger not allowed under arch, or more than one finger fits under arch (high arch); clubfoot (**talipes**); **pes valgus/ varus** (toeing in/out)

The Neurologic System

A child's nervous system matures at different rates, and physical endurance and ability to cooperate varies from child to child. When assessing the neurologic integrity of the infant or young child, therefore, the examiner needs to modify most testing approaches and interpret findings cautiously to ensure the accuracy of the results. A standard neurologic examination is not likely to yield valid results before middle childhood. (Mott, James, and Sperhac 1990, p. 338). The examiner should approach all tests as games to encourage the child's full cooperation, giving careful consideration to the child's developmental stage and potential capabilities to avoid frustration.

As with the adult examination, many aspects of the neurologic examination are integrated with other systems. For example, several cranial nerves are assessed during the eye and ear examinations. Head abnormalities, irregularities of the spine, limited range of motion, asymmetry of spontaneous movements, and abnormal postures can all reflect a problem with the nervous system. A helpful tool for assessing neurodevelopmental status in an infant and young child is the Revised Denver Developmental Screening Test (Denver II). This test includes gross and fine motor skills, language skills, and social skills and compares the findings with other children the same age.

Areas assessed during the neurologic examination include the cranial nerves, reflexes, motor system, and sensory function. Cranial function tests to assess cranial nerve function in young children are shown in Table 12–2.

Reflexes

During the assessment of reflexes, children should be instructed to relax the side of the body being tested; the child might be distracted by a toy during the test. The basic reflexes tested in adults are also tested in children (see Chapter 11).

Neonates are tested to determine the maturation or normality of the nervous system. A hyperactive response might indicate hypertonicity, whereas a hypoactive response might indicate nerve damage or muscle weakness. Deep tendon reflexes should be assessed for symmetry. The presence of one abnormal reflex finding should elicit a more thorough examination of neonatal reflexes, because a group of abnormal reflexes often indicates the presence of neurologic damage—congenital anomaly or intraventricular hemorrhage (IVH) resulting in cerebral palsy. Some of the common neonatal reflexes tested are included in the following section.

TABLE 12–2 TESTING CRANIAL NERVE FUNCTION IN YOUNG CHILDREN

Cranial nerves	Procedures and observations
CN II	Use the Snellen E or Picture Chart to test vision. Test visual fields while immobilizing the head as needed.
CN III, IV, and VI	Move an object through the cardinal points of gaze and have the child follow it with the eyes.
CN V	Observe bilateral jaw strength while the child chews a cookie or cracker. Touch the child's forehead and cheeks with cotton and watch the child bat it away.
CN VII	Observe the child's face when smiling, frowning, and crying. Ask the child to show the teeth. Demonstrate puffed cheeks and ask the child to imitate.
CN VIII	Observe the child turn to sounds such as a bell or whisper. Whisper a commonly used word, such as "doggie," behind the child's back and have the child repeat the word.
CN IX and X	Elicit the gag reflex
CN XI and XII	Ask an older child to stick out the tongue and shrug the shoulders or raise the arms.

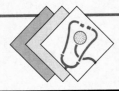

Assessing Neonatal Reflexes

ASSESSMENT	NORMAL FINDINGS	DEVIATIONS FROM NORMAL
Assess the blinking reflex. Shine a bright light or flash your finger quickly in front of the infant's eyes.	Blinks, closes eyes	No response
Assess the rooting reflex. Lightly touch the cheek, close to the mouth.	Turns head toward the side touched; reflex usually disappears after 4 months	No response
Assess the palmar grasp reflex. Press your finger or a small object against the palm of the hand from the ulnar side.	Fingers curl around the object	Weak or absent response
Assess the plantar/toe grasping reflex. Press your finger against the sole of the foot.	Plantar flexion in all toes; disappears after first year	Weak response or absence of response
Assess the tonic neck reflex. Place the infant on the back, and turn the head to one side.	Arm and leg on the side the infant faces extend; opposite extremities flex May be present at birth or by 2 months; disappears by 6 months	Weak response, absence of response, or persistence after 6 months

▶

▶ **Assessing Neonatal Reflexes** *CONTINUED*

ASSESSMENT	NORMAL FINDINGS	DEVIATIONS FROM NORMAL
Assess the startle reflex. Clap your hands loudly to startle the child.	Arms spread out, elbows flex, and hands remain flexed; disappears by 4 months	Absence indicates hearing loss
Assess the Moro reflex. While the child lies supine, raise the head slightly, and then release it suddenly; or hold infant up horizontally, and then lower infant suddenly. The head must be in the midline.	Sudden extension and abduction of extremities; fanning of fingers, with index finger and thumb forming a "C" shape, followed by flexion and adduction of extremities; legs may weakly flex; infant may cry Disappears after age 3-4 months; usually strongest during first 2 months	Persistence of Moro reflex past age 6 months (may indicate brain damage) Asymmetric Moro reflex (may suggest injury to brachial plexus, clavicle, or humerus)
Assess the Babinski reflex. Gently stroke the sole of the foot.	Fanning and extension of the toes (opposite in adults)	Incorrect or absent response

Motor Function

Infants gain control over the extremities in a cephalocaudal order—head and neck to legs and feet. Fine motor control is gained in a proximal to distal order—arms, then hands, then fingers. When assessing the cerebellar function of a child, the nurse must consider that fine motor coordination is not fully developed until 4 to 6 years of age. Younger children will not be able to perform sophisticated fine motor function tests; however, a pincer grasp should be present at 9 months and a child should be able to stack blocks at 12 months. For 2- to 8-year-old children, motor function is routinely tested by having them copy specific shapes. As with other testing, the use of a game such as "Can you do as I do?" with return demonstration might promote cooperation and accuracy in testing. See motor function in Chapter 11, page 276.

Sensory Function

In children who are too young to cooperate with sensory function testing, assessment is limited to pain perception. Familiar objects should be used to determine the child's ability to recognize the items; again, a game approach is the most appropriate. Usually children can identify some numbers and letters, as well as geometric shapes, by preschool age. Cortical motor integration, the ability to recognize objects through senses, can be tested in several ways. Children may be asked to copy a picture or attempt to draw the toy or piece of furniture shown. Refer to Chapter 11 for other testing techniques.

The Female Genitals and Inguinal Lymph Nodes

Internal pelvic examination is generally not performed in children unless sexual abuse is suspected. Ambiguous genitals with palpable masses, which may be testes, are monitored from early infancy by a urologist. Advanced or delayed development of secondary sexual characteristics should be referred for further evaluation. Refer to Chapter 11 for specific assessment techniques.

The Male Genitals

An enlarged penis in an infant or child may indicate congenital pathology. The prepuce may be tight in an uncircumcised infant and should not be forced over the penis during assessment. By 3 to 4 years of age, the foreskin should easily retract over the penis. A poor urinary stream may indicate urethral stenosis. A small scrotum with midline separation may indicate ambiguity of the genitals. Undescended testes should spontaneously descend in most children by 1 year of age. Refer to Chapter 11 for full assessment of male genital and inguinal areas.

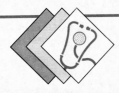

Assessing the Male Genitals

ASSESSMENT	NORMAL FINDINGS	DEVIATIONS FROM NORMAL
Palpate the scrotum to note the presence of the testes.	Undescended testes in infant younger than 1 year	Undescended testes in child over 1 year (cryptorchidism)
Assess the inguinal area for hernias and palpable inguinal lymph nodes.	Absence of bulges	Bulges in inguinal area that increase with crying or coughs
	Nonpalpable lymph nodes or nodes less than 1 cm, soft and mobile	Lymph nodes greater than 1 cm, firm to hard, and immobile

The Rectum and Anus

Neonates may be born with a number of anorectal malformations. Blind rectal pouches may appear normal and are often not detected until symptoms, such as failure to pass stool, are noted. Performance of a rectal temperature could lead to discovery of such conditions; however, radiographic examination is the usual method of diagnostic evaluation. Digital examination could lead to the discovery of an anal stenosis (constricted anal opening). Refer to Chapter 11 for a description of the rectal examination.

REFERENCES

Bates, B. 1987. *A guide to physical examination*. 5th ed. Philadelphia: J. B. Lippincott Co.

Behrman R. E., and Vaughan, V. C. III. 1983. *Nelson Textbook of Pediatrics*. 12th ed. Philadelphia: W. B. Saunders Co.

Giger, J. N., and Davidhizar, R. E. 1991. *Transcultural nursing*. St. Louis: Mosby Year Book.

James, S. R., and Mott, S. R. 1988. *Child health nursing: Essential care of children and families*. Menlo Park, Calif.: Addison-Wesley Publishing Co.

Malasanos, L.; Barkauskas, V.; and Stoltenberg-Allen, K. 1990. *Health assessment*. 4th ed. St. Louis: C. V. Mosby Co.

Mott, S. R.; James, S. R.; and Sperhac, A. M. 1990. *Nursing care of children and families*. 2d ed. Redwood City, Calif.: Addison-Wesley Nursing.

Olds, S. B.; London, M. L.; and Ladewig, P. W. 1992. *Maternal-newborn nursing: A family centered approach*. 4th ed. Menlo Park, Calif.: Addison-Wesley Nursing.

Smith, D. P., editor. 1991. *Comprehensive child and family nursing skills*. St. Louis: Mosby Year Book.

Whaley, L. and Wong, D. 1990. *Clinical manual of pediatric nursing*. 3d ed. St. Louis: C. V. Mosby Co.

Whaley, L., and Wong, D. 1991. *Nursing care of infants and children*. 4th ed. St. Louis: Mosby Year Book.

13

Assessing Maternal Health During the Perinatal Period

OBJECTIVES

- Define terms associated with assessment of the woman during the childbearing period

- Identify the purposes of maternal physical assessment

- Identify the components of maternal physical assessment during the antepartal, intrapartal, and postpartal periods

- Explain the significance of selected findings

- Identify expected outcomes of the maternal assessment during each phase of childbearing

- Describe the suggested sequence of a systematic maternal assessment

CONTENTS

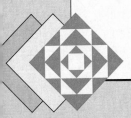

Introduction

Assessing maternal and fetal status is imperative to detecting and managing any complications that arise during each stage of pregnancy. The overall goals are to assist the mother to a full-term delivery and to promote optimal health of the mother and infant. A variety of techniques, equipment, and nursing assessments are used to evaluate the status of the pregnancy.

Many physiologic changes take place throughout **gestation** (pregnancy), labor, delivery, and the postpartal recovery period. The uterus, the organ of childbearing, undergoes the most profound changes. Changes also take place in other body systems and help shape the course of the pregnancy. Moreover, the entire process of childbearing affects the psychologic well-being of both the woman and the family.

To fully understand normal variations in pregnancy, as well as deviations from the norm, the nurse should first be familiar with normal findings in the nonpregnant female. (Components of normal adult physical assessment are described in Chapter 11.) The process of maternal physical assessment is ongoing and begins with the woman's initial contact with the health care system. The assessment consists of the interview, general observation of psychophysiologic status, the physical examination, and the evaluation of laboratory data.

Nursing Health History

All of the components of the health history discussed in Chapter 11 (Assessing Adult Health) apply to the maternity client, in addition to obstetric information. See the box on the next page for obstetrical data.

The estimated date of delivery (EDD) is calculated by *Nagele's rule*. The woman determines the first day of her last menstrual period, subtracts 3 months from that date, then adds 7 days. The following is an example:

Formula	Calculation
First day of last period	October 23
Minus 3 months	July 23
Plus 7 days	July 30th (EDD)

Physical Health Examination

The physical health examination is discussed in this chapter only as it relates to adaptations during the **perinatal period** (from the 28th week of gestation through 28 days after delivery); so the student should refer to Chapter 11 for techniques of adult physical examination not discussed here.

Nurses should be particularly careful to conduct in-depth assessments on high-risk maternity clients, e.g., women who are grossly overweight, who are over 35 or under 17 years old, who smoke or are substance abusers, or who have a preexisting medical condition.

Although health care workers need to intrude upon what many women view as the very essence of physical privacy during the maternity experience, providing privacy cannot be overemphasized. The nurse should make a concerted effort to ascertain that the client does not feel she has been violated and treated without dignity.

The woman should empty her bladder before the examination in the intrapartal and postpartal periods and as required during labor.

The client must assume a number of positions during the assessment (see Chapter 11). During the perinatal period, most assessments take place in the lithotomy position.

The nurse should be alert to problems that may arise during the physical examination, such as **vaso-vagal syncope** and **supine hypotensive syndrome**. As the uterus enlarges, it compresses venous return in the inferior vena cava, resulting in a decrease in arterial blood pressure (Figure 13–1). This phenomenon, referred to as supine hypotensive syndrome (vena caval syndrome) can be corrected by repositioning the client to her left side to relieve pressure on the vessel. The nurse must know beforehand how to manage the client experiencing these problems, because time will not allow the caregiver to consult references.

A variety of specimens are obtained for laboratory evaluation during the perinatal period. Contact with body fluids and secretions occurs frequently in the overall physical examination of the obstetric client. The nurse should adhere closely to universal precautions when examining the client.

In addition to the instruments used in the adult physical examination, some specialized instruments such as a fetoscope, internal and external electronic fetal monitoring devices, and Doppler ultrasound stethoscope are used.

The nurse should determine agency protocol regarding pelvic examinations that require the use of the vaginal speculum. Most speculum examinations are performed by the physician with the nurse functioning as an assistant, warming and lubricating the speculum before use and ensuring that slides and culture plates are available for specimens.

Nursing Health History: Obstetrical Data

Personal Data

- Acceptance of pregnancy
- Personal preferences about the birth
- Plans for child care following birth

Current Medical History

- Blood type and Rh factor, if known
- Record of immunizations (especially rubella)

Family Medical History

- Occurrence of multiple births
- Occurrence of cesarean births

Partner's History

- Presence of genetic conditions or diseases
- Age
- Significant health problems
- Attitude toward the pregnancy

Occupational History

- Occupation
- Exposure to harmful substances
- Opportunity for regular lunch, breaks
- Provision for maternity leave

Gynecologic History

- Previous infections: vaginal, cervical, tubal, sexually transmitted
- Previous surgery
- Age of menarche
- Regularity, frequency, and duration of menstrual flow
- History of dysmenorrhea
- Sexual history

- Contraceptive history (If birth control pills were used, did pregnancy immediately follow cessation of pills? If not, how long after?)
- Date of last Pap smear; any history of abnormal Pap smear

Current Pregnancy

- First day of last normal menstrual period (LMP)
- Presence of cramping, bleeding, or spotting since LMP
- Client's opinion about when conception occurred and when infant is due
- Client's attitude toward pregnancy (Is it planned, wanted?)
- Results of pregnancy test, if completed
- Any discomforts since LMP, e.g., nausea, vomiting, urinary frequency

Past Pregnancies

- Number of pregnancies
- Number of abortions, spontaneous or induced
- Number of living children
- History of preceding pregnancies: length of pregnancy, length of labor and birth, type of birth (vaginal, forceps or silastic cup, cesarean, and so on), client's perception of the experience, complications (antepartal, intrapartal, postpartal)
- Perinatal status of previous children: Apgar scores, birth weights, general development, complications, feeding patterns (breast/bottle)
- Blood type and Rh factor (if negative, medication after birth to prevent sensitization)
- Prenatal education classes, resources

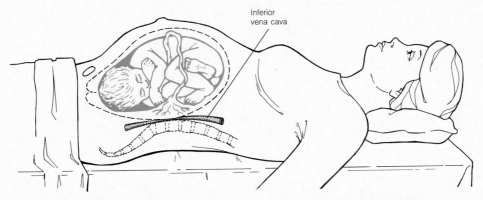

FIGURE 13–1 Supine hypotensive syndrome. The expanding uterus compresses the vena cava and critically reduces blood return to the heart.
Source: S.B. Olds, M.L. London, P.W. Ladewig, *Maternal-newborn nursing: A family-centered approach*, 4th ed. (Redwood City, Calif.: Addison-Wesley Nursing, 1992), p. 293.

The Antepartal Period

The antepartal (prenatal) period lasts about 40 weeks and is subdivided into three trimesters. The nursing history data pertinent to each trimester follows.

First Trimester

Complete health history; the status of various discomforts frequently occurring during the first trimester (e.g., nausea and vomiting, general malaise, urinary frequency, breast discomfort and changes, and emotional changes, i.e., mood swings); nutritional patterns; understanding of importance and schedule of prenatal visits; general knowledge level about health promotion, life-style habits that may affect pregnancy outcome, normal and abnormal manifestations of pregnancy, and problems to be immediately reported; and the support of family or significant others.

Second Trimester

Status of progress since the client's last visit; the status of problems or discomforts frequently experienced during the second trimester (e.g., headaches, heartburn, flatulence, constipation, various skin changes, backache, varicosities, interruption of normal sleeping patterns); the status of fetal movement (**quickening**); and abdominal discomforts and vaginal discharge.

Third Trimester

Status of progress since the last visit; the nature of contractions and vaginal discharge; clinical signs indicating impending labor; and the status of problems or discomforts frequently experienced during the third trimester (e.g., urinary frequency and urgency, shortness of breath, lower extremity edema and varicosity, leg cramping, restlessness, increased anxiety and fear, body image concerns, and general fatigue).

Physiologic and Psychologic Changes During Pregnancy

Vital Signs

Accelerated cardiovascular and metabolic function causes a variety of changes that affect vital signs. Circulating volume increases by 50%. Vasodilation of peripheral vasculature and variations in hormone levels result in a slight decrease in blood pressure. The nurse should assess vital signs on each visit and evaluate them in relation to each other. Abnormal values may reflect complications of pregnancy, such as pregnancy-induced hypertension, as well as client anxiety.

Height and Weight

Water retention, protein, carbohydrate, fat metabolism, and dietary habits may result in weight gain and the development of complications. The nurse should obtain the client's weight on every visit. Many of the strict limits on weight gain that were imposed in previous decades have been lifted, because more is now known about weight gain in relation to body build and metabolic rate. The ranges presented in this chapter represent general recommendations.

The Thorax and Lungs

As pregnancy progresses, the uterus pushes the diaphragm upward in the thorax, infringing on diaphragmatic expansion. In the assessment, the nurse may note a slight increase in respiratory effort as the body attempts to adapt to this change.

The Cardiovascular System

Circulating volume progressively increases, resulting in an increased workload on the heart. The heart is displaced upward and slightly left as the uterus enlarges and places pressure on the diaphragm. Variations in heart sounds auscultated during pregnancy usually disappear following delivery. A previous history of cardiovascular problems warrants a more in-depth assessment and follow-up of the client.

The Peripheral Vascular System

As return flow to the heart increases, varicosities and dependent edema of the lower extremities are likely to develop. Therefore, it is important that the nurse assess the lower extremities carefully. The nurse should consider the client's peripheral vascular status in combination with the vital signs and cardiopulmonary findings.

The Breasts and Axillae

The breasts should be inspected and palpated on prenatal visits. Most of the changes in the breast occur as preliminary steps to milk production. The breasts may become larger, sensitive to light touch, and tender because of changes in the mammary duct system. Because of the incidence of breast cancer, the nurse should encourage the woman to continue practicing breast self-examination (BSE) during pregnancy. Although the physiologic changes of the breast may make breast examination somewhat difficult, the woman is more likely to be the first to note significant variations as they occur in her own body.

The Abdomen

As the abdominal wall stretches to accommodate the enlarging uterus, the appearance of the abdominal skin changes significantly.

During most of the first trimester, the nurse can assess the abdomen using the usual techniques for abdominal assessment. As the pregnancy progresses, the uterus essentially becomes an abdominal organ. At this point, abdominal assessment extends to include a focus on the status of the **fundus** (the upper part of the uterus located between the fallopian tubes) and fetus.

Assessment of the uterus will reveal changes in the organ's size, location, and structure. Hormonal stimulus stretches the muscle fibers of the organ as fetus matures, causing the uterus to enlarge and hypertrophy. The uterus is displaced into the abdominal cavity during the second trimester and rises progressively until the last few weeks of gestation. In the last 3 to 4 weeks of gestation, the uterus begins to descend as the fetus drops into the pelvic cavity in preparation for delivery. The wall of the uterus becomes thinner and softer. The nurse inspects, measures, and palpates the fundus.

The position, movement, and heart rate of the fetus are also detected as the fundus is assessed.

The Genitourinary and Reproductive Systems

As the uterus continues to rise, it displaces the bladder upward and laterally, often causing discomfort, especially in the last trimester.

The cervix, vagina, and genitals are examined as part of the pelvic examination. During pregnancy, the cervix develops a **mucous plug** that obstructs the **cervical os** (cervical opening) to protect the fetus from infection. The mucous plug is expelled early in labor.

The vascularity and secretions of the vagina increase. The vaginal walls also thicken in preparation for their function as the birth canal. Assessing the integrity of the vagina is crucial to ensuring safe delivery of the child.

The Rectum and Anus

The enlargement of the uterus places considerable pressure on the rectum; however, defecation usually does not significantly change.

Psychoemotional Status

The woman may express a variety of responses when she learns she is pregnant; therefore, the nurse must consider a number of factors surrounding the client's history when assessing her psychoemotional status. An initial negative response to pregnancy may be normal, one phase in the process of integrating the new status.

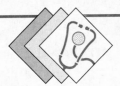

Assessing During the Antepartal Period

ASSESSMENT	NORMAL FINDINGS	DEVIATIONS FROM NORMAL
General Appearance **Determine age and race.**		
Observe body build in relation to muscle mass, skeletal frame, and height and weight.	Varies with age and general medical condition	Excessive thinness or obesity
Assess body language, posture, and gait.	Relaxed, erect posture; coordinated movement; lordosis in last few weeks of pregnancy from pressure of the uterus	Uncoordinated movement; facial grimacing
Note obvious signs of discomfort.	Varies according to the individual's pain threshold	Unrelieved or extreme discomfort

► **Assessing During the Anteparтal Period** *CONTINUED*

ASSESSMENT	NORMAL FINDINGS	DEVIATIONS FROM NORMAL
Vital Signs		
Obtain blood pressure. Note position of client when obtaining blood pressure. Use caution when taking blood pressure during the second and third trimesters. During these trimesters, do not place the client in the supine position. See supine hypotensive syndrome on page 324.	Readings consistent with prepregnancy state, or minor variations as follows: **Systolic:** Decrease of 5 to 10 mm/Hg during the first and second trimesters **Diastolic:** Decrease of 5 to 10 mm/Hg during the first and second trimesters Blood pressure increases slightly during third trimester	**Systolic:** Increase of 30 mm/Hg *or* **Diastolic:** Increase of 15 mm/Hg or more (Increases frequently associated with pregnancy-induced hypertension; Decreases with supine hypotensive syndrome)
Determine body temperature.	Normal prepregnancy values	Elevation (may be related to vaginal or urinary tract infection)
Obtain the radial pulse.	Increase of 15 to 20 beats per minute of usual resting rate, beginning at about 3½ months of pregnancy Slight irregularities on occasion (related to sympathetic system variations)	Decrease (may be associated with supine hypotensive syndrome if combined with decrease in blood pressure) Frequent or persistent pulse irregularity (may indicate cardiac problem)
Determine respiratory rate.	Consistent with prepregnancy state; minimal increases of about 2 breaths per minute	Increased rate; hyperventilation
Height and Weight		
Weigh the client.	Appropriate for height and age	Inappropriate for height and age
Assess progression of the client's weight during each trimester.	Average: 22 to 28 pounds First trimester: Small weight gain (2 to 4 pounds) Second trimester: Rapid increase in rate and amount of gain (12 to 14 pounds) Third trimester: Slight decline in rate of weight gain (8 to 10 pounds)	Gain of 6.0 pounds or more per month (associated with pregnancy-induced hypertension and fluid retention) Gain of less than 22 pounds (indicates insufficient utilization of nutrients, which can jeopardize fetal health)
Thorax and Lungs		
Inspect, palpate, and percuss the chest, noting diaphragmatic expansion and character of respirations.	Symmetric expansion Thoracic breathing as pregnancy progresses Respiratory depth slightly deeper, with increased ventilatory effort Slight shortness of breath in third trimester occurs in 60% to 70% of women	Asymmetric expansion; barrel chest or funnel chest (e.g., respiratory pathology, chronic obstructive pulmonary disease)
Auscultate breath sounds.	Lungs clear in all fields	Adventitious sounds (rales, wheezes, rhonchi); absent breath sounds
Heart		
Auscultate heart sounds.	Systolic murmur common in 75% to 90% of women; split S_1 heart sound; S_3 often heard	Gallop rhythm with S_4 gallop

► Assessing During the Antepartal Period *CONTINUED*

ASSESSMENT	NORMAL FINDINGS	DEVIATIONS FROM NORMAL
Peripheral Vascular System		
Assess for varicosities and edema in client's extremities and face, especially around the eyes. Observe degree and location of edema.	Mild varicose veins in latter pregnancy Edema in hands and ankles in late second and third trimester	Marked edema Lower extremities reddened, hot, painful (may indicate thrombophlebitis)
Breasts and Axillae		
Inspect and palpate the breasts, noting size, color, status of breast discharge, and vascularity.	Increase in breast size; darkened areolar area; nipple erection; secretion of colostrum near end of first trimester; general lumpiness throughout breasts (nodular); formation of **striae** (stretch marks)	Palpable axillary nodes; hard breast nodes Painful, edematous, reddened, or cracked nipples (may indicate infection)
Abdomen		
Inspect and palpate the abdomen, determining the size and contour and the appearance of the skin.	Nonpalpable and nontender on initial visit Purple striae on **primigravida**, silver striae on **multigravida** No masses or nodules **Linea nigra** (black line in center of abdomen)	Acute tenderness with guarding of abdomen Palpable masses or nodules (may indicate cancer or **ectopic pregnancy**)
Auscultate abdominal sounds. Note normal bowel sounds.	Normal bowel sounds	Absence of bowel sounds
Assess fundal height by measuring in centimeters from the top of the symphysis pubis to the top of the fundus (Figure 13–2).	Expected fundal height based on gestational week (Figure 13–3) 12 weeks: Fundus at symphysis pubis 20 weeks: Fundus at level of umbilicus After 20 weeks: Fundus approximates weeks of gestation (Example: Fundal height of 28 cm indicates 28 weeks of gestation)	Increased fundal height (associated with multiple pregnancy, polyhydramnios, hydatidiform moles) Decreased fundal height (associated with fetal growth retardation, fetal demise, fetal abnormalities) Variations also associated with errors in calculation of gestational week

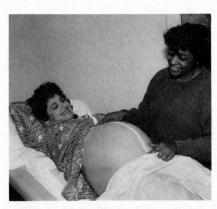

FIGURE 13–2 Measuring fundal height.
Source: S.B. Olds, M.L. London, P.W. Ladewig, *Maternal-newborn nursing: A family-centered approach*, 4th ed. (Redwood City, Calif.: Addison-Wesley Nursing, 1992), p. 332.

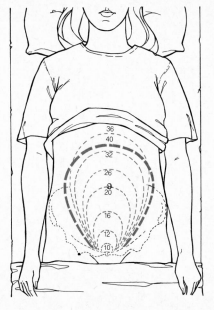

FIGURE 13–3 Fundal height approximations during specific gestational weeks.
Source: S.B. Olds, M.L. London, P.W. Ladewig, *Maternal-newborn nursing: A family-centered approach*, 4th ed. (Redwood City, Calif.: Addison-Wesley Nursing, 1992), p. 300.

►

▶ **Assessing During the Antepartal Period** *CONTINUED*

ASSESSMENT	NORMAL FINDINGS	DEVIATIONS FROM NORMAL
Note the status of contractions (intermittent tightening and shortening of uterine muscle fibers) by palpating with the fingertips. (See the section on assessment of contractions during the intrapartal period for additional information).	**Braxton Hicks contractions**: Painless and irregular during the first trimester; stronger, more regular during last few weeks but may be present throughout pregnancy	**Preterm labor** contractions prior to expected delivery date (every 10 minutes or less)
Determine the fetal position (relationship of the presenting part of the fetus to the mother's pelvis) by palpating the abdomen using the technique for Leopold's maneuvers (refer to Chapter 10, page 179).	**Cephalic presentation**: Left occipitoanterior or right occipitoanterior presentation of the **vertex** (top of the head)	**Breech presentation** (buttocks or feet) or **transverse lie** (shoulder)
Assess the fetal tones, noting the rate and the quadrant in which they are heard. The sounds are muffled because they must be auscultated through the mother's thick abdominal wall. A quiet environment facilitates differentiating fetal heart tones from other abdominal sounds (refer to Chapter 10, page 180).	120 to 160 beats per minute; sounds muffled	Greater than 160 or less than 120 (may indicate fetal distress); absence of fetal tones is often associated with fetal death

Genitourinary System

BLADDER

Palpate the lower abdomen for bladder distention. Note: Have the client empty the bladder before palpation.	Nonpalpable	Palpable Client needs to void (indicates urinary retention)

VAGINA

Observe the status of vaginal discharge and appearance of vagina.	Slight increase in white discharge; no change in color of white discharge No redness or inflammation of vagina	Changes in color, amount, and consistency of discharge: More than usual amount of discharge; bloody, pink, mucous, or watery discharge (may be signs of preterm labor) Yellowish white discharge (may indicate infection) Brownish spotting 48 hours after vaginal examination; bloody discharge (may indicate **abruptio placentae**, i.e., placental separation) Redness or irritation of vagina (may indicate infection, inflammation)

CERVIX

Inspect the cervix using a sterile speculum. Note color, shape of os, and position in relation to the uterus and vagina.	4 to 6 weeks: **Goodell's sign** (softening of cervix) 8 to 11 weeks: Chadwick's sign (bluish discoloration)	Absence of Goodell's sign (may indicate cancer, previous cryotherapy)

PERINEUM

Spread the buttocks apart, and inspect the perineum, noting any redness, irritation, or lesions.	No redness or irritation; normal color Absence of lesions or varicosities	Redness and irritation Presence of lesions or varicosities

▶ **Assessing During the Antepartal Period** *CONTINUED*

ASSESSMENT	NORMAL FINDINGS	DEVIATIONS FROM NORMAL
Rectum and Anus **Inspect and palpate the anal opening.** • Assist the client to a lateral position. • Lift the buttocks to inspect carefully for hemorrhoids.	No tears, masses, or tenderness	Masses or nodules (may indicate cancer); hemorrhoids; rectal prolapse
Psychoemotional Status **Assess the client's psychoemotional state.** Note general affect and mood, as well as verbal and nonverbal cues.	Positive response; actions consistent with acceptance of pregnancy; mild anxiety	Prolonged negative response; apathy; anger; denial; depression
Laboratory Evaluation **Obtain specimen for urinalysis.** • Ask the client to void and obtain a clean-catch midstream urine specimen (refer to Chapter 28, p. 688). • Test the urine with a dipstick for ketones, protein, albumin, and glucose. Otherwise, forward to laboratory. **Obtain blood for laboratory analysis as indicated:** • Chemistry profiles • Hematology profiles • Rubella titer • VDRL • HIV and HBV status • Blood type • Rh status	Negative for albumin and protein and glucose Straw-colored or yellow; no sediment, hematuria, or foul odor	Positive for albumin or protein (suggests **preeclampsia**) Positive for glucose (suggests gestational diabetes) Concentrated urine (suggests inadequate fluid intake) Presence of sediment, foul odor, and blood (suggests urinary tract infection)

The Intrapartal Period

The **intrapartal** period is marked by the onset of labor and terminates with the beginning stages of physiologic restabilization of the client. It is divided into four stages of labor.

First Stage of Labor

The first is marked by the onset of true labor contractions and ends with full **cervical dilation** (opening) of 10 centimeters.

This stage of labor is subdivided into three phases based on the progress of cervical dilation and **effacement** (cervical muscle thinning). The three phases are:

• latent—0 to 3 centimeters cervical dilation
• active—4 to 7 centimeters cervical dilation
• transition—8 to 10 centimeters cervical dilation

As indicated by the term *transition*, the end of this phase of cervical dilation marks the change from the first stage of labor to the second. Table 13–1 highlights various parameters for determining labor status. Table 13–2 compares the contractions of a woman in labor with those of a woman not in labor.

Second Stage

The second stage of labor extends from full cervical dilation to the delivery of the infant. The nurse places special emphasis on assessing fetal status as the fetus moves through the birth canal.

TABLE 13–1 ASSESSING THE STATUS OF CONTRACTIONS AND CERVICAL DILATION

	Latent Phase	Active Phase	Transitional Phase
Frequency	5–30 min	3–5 min	2–3 min
Duration	10–30 sec	30–45 sec	45–60 sec
Contraction intensity	Mild (slightly tight; moderately pliable)	Moderate (firm but not rigid)	Strong (maximum contractility; hard and rigid)
Cervical dilation	0–3 cm	4–7 cm	8–10 cm

TABLE 13–2 COMPARISON OF CONTRACTION PATTERNS OF THE WOMAN IN LABOR AND THE WOMAN NOT IN LABOR*

Woman in Labor	Woman Not in Labor
Contractions occur at regular intervals: 3 to 5 minutes apart.	Contractions occur at irregular intervals.
Intervals between contractions shorten.	Intervals between contractions lengthen or remain unchanged; no distinct pattern.
Intensity heightens gradually.	Intensity diminishes or remains unchanged.
Progressive dilation and effacement of the cervix.	No change in status of dilation and effacement.
Bloody show frequently present.	Absence of bloody show.
Membranes may be ruptured.	Membranes are not ruptured.
Pain occurs primarily in the back.	Pain occurs primarily in area of groin and lower abdomen.
Pain unrelieved by mild sedation and rest.	Pain relieved or reduced by mild sedation and rest.

*These comparisons are to be used as guidelines only, because individual labor patterns vary greatly. The only *true* measure of labor efficacy is the cervical examination.

Third Stage

The third stage of labor extends from the birth of the infant to placental delivery. During this stage, the placenta separates from the endometrial lining and is expelled. Following this, maternal circulating blood volume increases as pooled blood returns to the central circulation. The sudden increase in blood volume increases the risk of embolism. Hemodynamic indicators must be monitored closely in this stage as the cardiovascular system attempts to restabilize immediately after the birth of the infant.

Fourth Stage

Stage four of labor is the beginning of the **puerperium**, or **postpartal** period, in which the woman's body begins the healing process of reestablishing its normal prepregnant status. It extends 1 to 4 hours after birth. Because stage four addresses the postpartal condition of the woman, it is discussed in combination with the postpartum period, later in this chapter.

Complications may quickly present themselves during any of the stages of labor. Their rapid course of development necessitates close and accurate assessment by the nurse.

Nursing History Focus

The nursing history focus during the intrapartal period primarily addresses the status of labor and contractions, maternal adjustment during labor, and the condition of the fetus. The status of the woman in relation to previous pregnancies may affect the length of the intrapartal period. Multigravidas tend to move through the intrapartal period faster than primigravidas.

History information obtained at varying stages centers around the following indicators:

- Vital signs

- Characteristics of contractions

- The nature of fetal movement and fetal heart rate

- Status of **rupture of membranes** (spontaneous breaking of the amniotic sac)
- Characteristics of vaginal discharge
- Status of discomfort or comfort
- Maternal emotional response to labor and contractions as they progress
- Physiologic complications during pregnancy
- Adequacy of maternal pelvis and history of orthopedic problems
- Psychoemotional response of significant others

The accompanying box highlights some of the most important questions for the nurse to ask during a phone call assessment of possible precipitate labor.

Quick Phone Assessment of Precipitate Delivery Presentation

- Date due?
- Doctor or midwife?
- Gravida/Para status?
- Bag of water broken? (Any water or blood from vagina?)
- Frequency of contractions?
- Duration of contractions?
- Any chronic medical problems?
- Distance away from hospital?
- Who is with you?

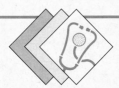

Assessing During the Intrapartal Period

ASSESSMENT	NORMAL FINDINGS	DEVIATIONS FROM NORMAL
First Stage of Labor		
VITAL SIGNS		
Assess blood pressure, pulse, respirations, and fetal heart tones every 15 minutes.	Blood pressure and pulse consistent with prepregnant state Fetal heart tones from 120 to 160 beats/minute Increased respiratory rate; hyperventilation as labor progresses	Increased blood pressure Fetal heart rate < 120 or > 160 beats/minute Decreased blood pressure and increased pulse (associated with hemorrhage or supine hypotensive syndrome)
Assess temperature every 2 hours following the rupture of membranes.	Consistent with prepregnant status.	Elevated temperature after membrane rupture (suggests infection)
Assess the status of pain, discomfort, and anxiety.	Varies with individual	Unrelieved or excessive; nausea and vomiting, rectal pressure, and hyperventilation
CONTRACTIONS **Assess the state of contractions throughout labor**, noting frequency, duration, and intensity.		
• Time the frequency or regularity of the contractions, i.e., the number of minutes from the beginning of one contraction to the beginning of the next contraction.	Latent phase: Every 5 to 30 minutes Active phase: Every 3 to 5 minutes Transition phase: Every 2 to 3 minutes	Irregular, long intervals between contractions (indicative of false labor, Braxton Hicks contractions)

▶ **Assessing During the Intrapartal Period** *CONTINUED*

ASSESSMENT	NORMAL FINDINGS	DEVIATIONS FROM NORMAL
• Time the length or duration of each contraction in seconds from the on-set of the contraction to the end of that contraction. The end of the con-traction is marked by relaxation of the uterus and abdomen.	Latent phase: 10 to 30 seconds Active phase: 30 to 45 seconds Transition phase: 45 to 60 seconds	Contractions greater than 90 seconds (indicates uterine tetany)
• Determine the quality of the strength of each contraction. Document the contractions as mild, moderate, or strong in intensity, based on the fol-lowing criteria:		
Mild—fundus slightly tight as it stretches; still some pliability noted.	Mild in latent phase of labor	
Moderate—fundus firm but not rigid, examiner unable to make indentation.	Moderate in active phase of labor	
Strong—maximum intensity; fundus hard.	Strong in transition phase of labor	
(See Table 13–2 on page 332 for a com-parison of patterns of contractions for the woman in labor and the woman not in labor.)		
Assist the client to empty the bladder to minimize discomfort and maximize confirmation of fetal position as the re-mainder of the examination continues.		
Apply sterile gloves, and perform a vaginal examination (if agency proto-col permits) to assess the status of membranes (intact or ruptured), vaginal secretions, bloody show, cervical dila-tion, and effacement.		
VAGINAL SECRETIONS **Assess vaginal secretions.**	Increased as labor progresses; be-comes bloody show	Copious bleeding in early stages
MEMBRANE RUPTURE **Assess the status of the membrane rupture.**	May rupture any time during the labor period	
Note the color, amount, consistency, and odor of the amniotic fluid, and the time that the water breaks.	Consistency: Watery Color: Clear or pale-straw colored	Consistency: Viscous (indicates infec-tion) Color: Greenish brown (indicates that hypoxic episode has occurred; meco-nium passage follows hypoxic episode) Yellowish color (indicates occurrence of hypoxia 36 hours before membrane rupture or fetal hemolytic disease) Port-wine color (suggests abruptio placentae)

► **Assessing During the Intrapartal Period** *CONTINUED*

ASSESSMENT	NORMAL FINDINGS	DEVIATIONS FROM NORMAL
	Amount: 500 to 1200 ml	More than 1200 ml (indicative of **poly-hydramnios**) Less than 500 ml (indicative of **oligo-hydramnios**)
	Odor: No odor	Odor (associated with infection)
Perform the nitrazine tape test to verify the acidity (pH) of the fluid from the ruptured membrane. • Don sterile gloves. • Obtain a small amount of vaginal secretions with a long cotton-tipped applicator from an area of pooled secretions. • Place a sample of the secretions on the nitrazine paper. • Note any changes in color on the test paper.	Ruptured membranes: Varying shades of blue, such as blue-green, dark blue, or bluish gray (indicates alkaline amniotic fluid if membranes have ruptured)	Membranes intact: Varying shades of yellow (indicates acidic fluid, e.g., vaginal secretions or urine)
BLOODY SHOW **Assess for the presence of bloody show.** It begins as a small discharge of light pink mucus secretions and progresses to copious amounts as labor progresses to full cervical dilation.	Scant to copious amount as labor progresses	Marked bleeding in large amounts during early phase of labor
PERINEUM **Assess the perineum** in relation to the general appearance.	Slight bulging	

CERVICAL DILATION
Assess cervical dilation in centimeters relative to the amount of time spent in each phase of dilation.

• Insert the index and middle fingers up to the cervix, and palpate the cervical os. Estimate the amount of dilation (opening of cervical os, circumference) in centimeters (Figure 13–4) by comparing to a centimeter scale. (A measurement scale is usually posted on the clinical unit for immediate access.)

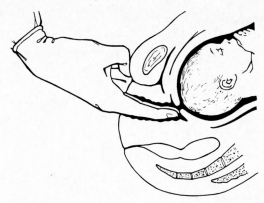

FIGURE 13–4 Determining cervical dilation. *Source:* S.B. Olds, M.L. London, P.W. Ladewig, *Maternal-newborn nursing: A family-centered approach*, 4th ed. (Redwood City, Calif.: Addison-Wesley Nursing, 1992), p. 615.

• Note the amount of time spent in each phase of cervical dilation:

ASSESSMENT	NORMAL FINDINGS	DEVIATIONS FROM NORMAL
Latent phase	0 to 3 cm dilation 6 to 10 hours' duration	Inadequate dilation for the amount of time spent in each phase (suggests ineffective uterine contractility, inadequate fetal position).
Active phase	4 to 7 cm dilation 3 hours	Rapid labor, i.e., less than 3 to 3½ hours (increases the risk of severe vaginal and
Transition phase	8 to 10 cm dilation 1 to 2 hours	perineal tears and precipitate delivery

► **Assessing During the Intrapartal Period** *CONTINUED*

ASSESSMENT	NORMAL FINDINGS	DEVIATIONS FROM NORMAL
CERVICAL EFFACEMENT **Assess the status of cervical efface-ment** (Figure 13–5). • Palpate the shortness and thinness of cervical canal tissue. • Determine how close the cervix is to becoming 100% effaced.	Precedes dilation in the primigravida; precedes or occurs in conjunction with dilation in the multigravida Progressive effacement	Lack of cervical pliability (rigidity) de-laying or interfering with cervical thinning

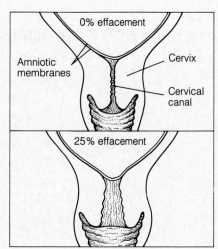

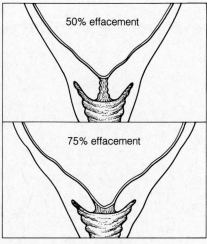

A. Cervix near the end of pregnancy but before labor. Top, primigravida; bottom, multipara.

B. Beginning effacement of cervix. Note dilation of internal os and funnel-shaped cervical canal. Top, primigravida; bottom, multipara.

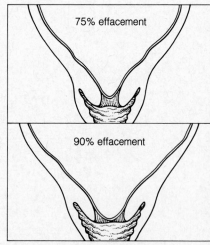

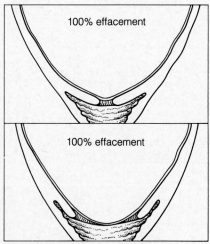

C. Further effacement of cervix. Top, primigravida; bottom, multipara.

D. Cervical canal obliterated, i.e., the cervix is completely effaced. Top, primigravida; bottom, multipara.

FIGURE 13–5 Cervical effacement. *Source:* S.B. Olds, M.L. London, P.W. Ladewig, *Maternal-newborn nursing: A family-centered approach*, 4th ed. (Redwood City, Calif.: Addison-Wesley Nursing, 1992), p. 615.

► **Assessing During the Intrapartal Period** *CONTINUED*

ASSESSMENT	NORMAL FINDINGS	DEVIATIONS FROM NORMAL
FETAL PARAMETERS **Determine the fetal parameters**, noting the presenting part, station, and fetal heart rate.		
PRESENTING PART **Assess for the presenting part**, using the techniques of Leopold's maneuvers (see Chapter 10, page 179) along with vaginal palpation.		
Palpate the dilated cervix to outline the fetal structure presenting at the cervical opening (Figure 10–15, page 178, shows examples of various fetal presentations).	Cephalic presentation	Malpresentations: transverse lie; breech
STATION **Determine the fetal station**, the relationship of the presenting part to the ischial spines of the mother's pelvis. See the box below.		

Determining Fetal Station

- Identify the ischial spines.
- Palpate to determine whether the presenting part is above or below the ischial spines.
- Using the ischial spines as a zero point, estimate the number of centimeters above or below the ischial spines the presenting part lies. Use a scale of −1 to −5 to indicate the position above the ischial spines and +1 to +5 for the position below the ischial spines (Figure 13–6).

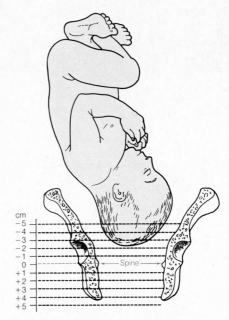

FIGURE 13–6 Measuring the station of the fetal head. In this view, the station is −2/−3. *Source:* S.B. Olds, M.L. London, P.W. Ladewig, *Maternal-newborn nursing: A family-centered approach*, 4th ed. (Redwood City, Calif.: Addison-Wesley Nursing, 1992), p. 581.

►

▶ **Assessing During the Intrapartal Period** *CONTINUED*

ASSESSMENT	NORMAL FINDINGS	DEVIATIONS FROM NORMAL
Second Stage of Labor		
FETAL HEART RATE AND VITAL SIGNS **Assess fetal heart, blood pressure, and pulse every 5 minutes.** Obtain the data between contractions. The heart location changes as the fetus descends down the birth canal (Figure 13–7).	Fetal rate 120 to 160 beats/minute	Bradycardia (indicates cord compression or prolapse); tachycardia (indicates hypoxic fetus)

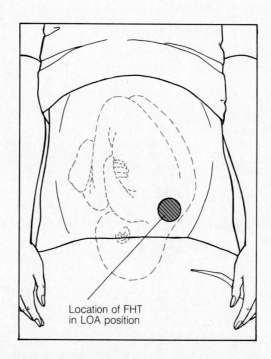

FIGURE 13–7 Location of fetal heart in relation to fetal position.
Source: S.B. Olds, M.L. London, P.W. Ladewig, *Maternal-newborn nursing: A family-centered approach*, 4th ed. (Redwood City, Calif.: Addison-Wesley Nursing, 1992), p. 626.

ASSESSMENT	NORMAL FINDINGS	DEVIATIONS FROM NORMAL
CROWNING **Assess for crowning**, the appearance of the fetal head at the vaginal opening.		
DURATION OF STAGE TWO **Note the duration of the second stage of labor** by documenting the time that the second stage begins and ends.	Primigravida: 25 minutes to 2 hours Multigravida: Few minutes to 1 hour	Prolonged duration in stage two
Third Stage of Labor		
VITAL SIGNS **Assess vital signs.**	Prepregnant values; normal pulse rate or slight bradycardia	Elevated blood pressure (hypertension); decreased blood pressure (indicates hemorrhage)
STATUS OF BLEEDING **Assess amount of blood loss** and relation to vital signs.	No excessive blood loss	Excessive blood loss

The Postpartal Period

The postpartal period, or puerperium, begins after the delivery of the placenta (after stage three of labor) and continues for approximately 6 weeks. The hallmark of this period is the process of uterine **involution**, the process of the uterus returning to its normal state. As this process evolves, other physiologic changes take place to bring the woman to a complete physical recovery. **Postpartal hemorrhage** (blood loss of 500 ml or more after vaginal delivery, or more than 1000 ml after cesarean) is most likely to occur within the first 1 to 2 hours after delivery. The nurse must be skillful in assessing the client during this crucial time. The nurse should also monitor the client's urinalysis, hemoglobin, and hematocrit. The Rh status, and the need for Rh_o (D) immune globulin (RhoGAM) should be determined. If the mother is negative and the father is positive, RhoGAM should be administered as an antibody titer within 72 hours after delivery. (Note: Many women are not sure of or willing to acknowledge who the father is. RhoGAM is also given at 28 weeks' gestation prophylactically to Rh-negative women to avoid sensitization if hemorrhage during pregnancy occurs.)

Women who undergo cesarean sections should undergo a postoperative surgical assessment in addition to the postpartal assessment. Gastrointestinal, genitourinary, cardiovascular, and respiratory assessments should be expanded to include other components of these system assessments.

The nurse must also take the woman's psychologic status into consideration during this stage. As she recovers from the impact of pregnancy and delivery, she must also adapt to life-style changes that the addition of a new family member demands.

Vital Signs

Several factors influence fluctuations in the status of circulating volume, which in turn influence the client's vital signs:

- Blood returned to the maternal circulation immediately following placental delivery
- Amount of **lochia** (vaginal discharge)
- General status of hydration
- Fluid loss from postpartum diuresis

As these changes occur, the vital signs should remain normal as the body adapts. The nurse must correlate abnormal vital signs with these physiologic changes, however.

The temperature may be slightly elevated (i.e., 37.8 to 38°C) within the first 24 postpartal hours because of fluid loss and lack of oral intake during labor. After 24 hours, the temperature should stabilize to the client's normal range. A temperature of 38°C or higher on any 2 of the next 9 days strongly suggests postpartal infection.

Bowel Sounds

Abdominal stretching during pregnancy results in loss of muscle tone. Bowel sounds diminish within the first few hours because of decreased abdominal muscle tone, the use of analgesics during labor, and the hormonal influence of progesterone. Bowel elimination may be affected by many factors, including diminished abdominal muscle tone, fluid status, recent food and fluid intake, and perineal pain and discomfort. Women who have had cesarean sections may have an additional risk for decreased abdominal muscle tone and peristaltic activity.

The Uterus

As the process of uterine involution occurs, the nurse assesses changes in the uterine muscle in terms of fundal height, position, and tone. Figure 13–8 illustrates the expected pattern of uterine involution as it returns to its normal position in the pelvic cavity.

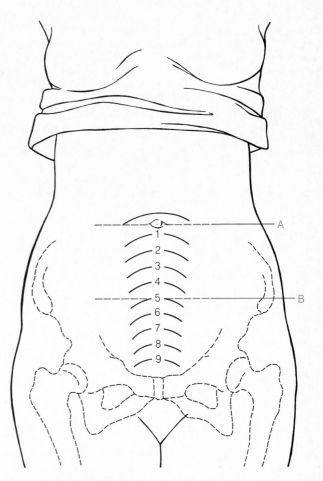

FIGURE 13–8 Involution of the uterus. *Source:* S.B. Olds, M.L. London, P.W. Ladewig, *Maternal-newborn nursing: A family-centered approach*, 4th ed. (Redwood City, Calif.: Addison-Wesley Nursing, 1992), p. 1068.

The Bladder

Two to 3 days following delivery, postpartum diuresis begins as the body rids itself of about 3 liters of accumulated fluid volume. This excess in fluid is a result of extracellular accumulation during pregnancy. Urine output increases significantly during this time.

The bladder is assessed along with the fundus. Bladder retention may interfere with the process of proper involution and predispose the woman to postpartal hemorrhage. Trauma to urinary tract tissue associated with the birth process results in urethral bruising and swelling and an increase in bladder capacity. This in turn results in urinary retention, and subsequent catheterization may be necessary. Urinary retention is a risk factor for the development of urinary tract infection.

Vaginal Discharge (Lochia)

The vagina is assessed in relation to its appearance and the discharge of lochia. Trauma to the birth canal as the fetus passes causes bruising, lacerations, and general tissue irritation.

As the endometrial lining heals, lochia is discharged through the vaginal canal. The lochia consists mainly of epithelial tissue, red blood cells, white blood cells, and traces of **decidua** (lining from the endometrium). Lochia discharge should follow an expected pattern of variation in appearance and usually ceases in about 3 to 4 weeks. Lochia is assessed when the fundus is assessed.

The Perineum

Tissue trauma to the perineum during birth may result in perineal bruising and/or the need for an episiotomy.

The Breasts

The breasts undergo change as the process of **lactation** (milk production) begins. Hormonal variations in estrogen, progesterone, and prolactin stimulate the process of lactation. Estrogen and progesterone levels drop, and prolactin levels increase. **Colostrum** is secreted from the breasts for the first day or two, and then breast milk is secreted. As the mammary ducts fill with milk, the breasts may become engorged and tender.

The Peripheral Vascular System

Residual effects of the prolonged pooling of fluid in the lower extremities during pregnancy and the intrapartal period may reduce venous return. In addition, limited activity during labor and the early puerperium may result in venous stasis.

Level of Comfort

Generalized soreness from the trauma of childbirth may last for several days. Uterine contractions occur at intervals, contributing to **afterpains** of a cramplike nature. Afterpains are more common in the multigravida because of structural changes in the uterus with previous births. If the mother is breast-feeding, afterpains may worsen when oxytocin is released as the infant sucks the breast. Women who have had cesarean deliveries may experience additional discomfort because of disrupted tissue integrity from surgical incision. The nurse should provide general comfort measures and give analgesics as necessary to minimize discomfort.

Psychoemotional Status

The woman experiences a wide range of thoughts and emotions as she attempts to cope successfully with her childbirth experience and the changes in life-style that the addition of a new family member may require. The latter part of pregnancy, along with the physical and psychologic strain of labor and delivery, is emotionally draining. Initially, the woman's physiologic needs must be met through sleep and food and fluid intake.

After these needs have been met, the client's attention shifts to the infant and significant others. Mother-infant bonding and family support systems are important in the transition to motherhood. The nurse assesses the client's patterns of interaction with the new infant, the spouse, and other family members and her knowledge regarding care of the new infant, so that teaching and learning needs can be addressed.

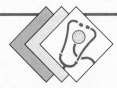

Assessing During the Postpartal Period

ASSESSMENT	NORMAL FINDINGS	DEVIATIONS FROM NORMAL
Vital Signs		
Assess the client's blood pressure, pulse, and respirations. Assess parameters frequently or as indicated by client condition and agency protocol for the first 24 hours: usually at least every 15 minutes during the fourth stage of labor followed by 30-minute and hourly checks for the next 3 to 4 hours, then progressively every 4, 6, and 8 hours.	Normal range of prepregnancy values Bradycardia may persist for 2 to 3 days	Increased blood pressure Decreased blood pressure (related to hemorrhage) Increased pulse (suggests hemorrhage, pain, and/or anxiety)
Assess the client's temperature.	Normal range for the client	Elevated finding (indicates dehydration, excessive fatigue from stress of labor and delivery, infection)
Abdomen		
Assess bowel sounds.	Active, slightly hypoactive; bowel movement 2 to 3 days postpartum	Absent
Note the status of the abdominal dressing and the appearance of the abdominal incision if the client had a cesarean section.	No redness, heat, swelling, drainage, or discoloration of incision	Redness, heat, discoloration, drainage, or odor
Uterus		
Assess the tone, height, and position of the fundus. Position and height are determined in relation to the umbilicus. See the box on page 342.	Firm In the midline, at or slightly below the umbilicus 1 to 2 hours postdelivery, followed by progressive decline of approximately 1 cm per day	**Boggy** (soft and spongy) (potential hemorrhage) Failure to involute to normal state in appropriate time (may indicate infection, bladder displacement, or bleeding) Displaced from midline (bladder distended)
If the fundus is soft and boggy, apply massage. See the box on page 342.		
Bladder		
Assess the status of the bladder at the same time the fundus is being assessed. • Palpate the fundus as described in the box. • Palpate for bladder distension in the lower abdomen. • Have the client void if the fundus is displaced from the midline or the bladder is palpable. • Catheterize, if necessary.	Voiding adequate quantity of urine (postpartum diuresis approximately 3000 ml 2 to 3 days after birth); bladder nonpalpable	Bladder palpable (feels like balloon)

▶

▶ Assessing During the Postpartal Period *CONTINUED*

ASSESSMENT	NORMAL FINDINGS	DEVIATIONS FROM NORMAL

Assessing and Massaging the Postpartal Fundus

- Place the client on back with knees flexed. Cup your dominant hand, and apply pressure to the abdomen right below the umbilicus.

- Place your nondominant hand around the area of the symphysis pubis, and press into the lower abdomen.

- Note the position, tone, and height of the uterus in relation to the umbilicus.

- Estimate fundal height by determining the number of fingerbreaths above or below the umbilicus.

- If the fundus is displaced, have the client void, and reassess the fundus.

- If the fundus is soft and boggy, massage as follows (Figure 13–9):

a. Place client on back with knees flexed (lithotomy position).

b. While cupping the lower part of the fundus under the umbilicus, place the palmar surface of your other hand over the top of the fundus.

c. With gentle pressure, rotate the upper hand over the fundus, aiming the strokes toward the vagina.

d. Continue to rotate your hand over the fundus until it becomes firm (feels like a grapefruit) and contracted at midline and clots have been expressed. Do not overmassage.

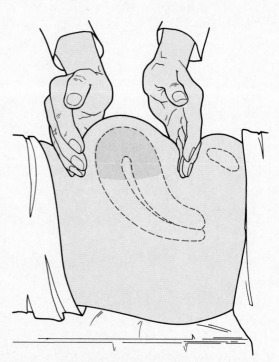

FIGURE 13–9 Palpating the fundus of the uterus.
Source: S.B. Olds, M.L. London, P.W. Ladewig, *Maternal-newborn nursing: A family-centered approach*, 4th ed. (Redwood City, Calif.: Addison-Wesley Nursing, 1992), p. 684.

Vaginal Discharge (Lochia)

Assess lochia in terms of color, amount, consistency, and odor at the same time the fundus is being assessed.

- Lower the perineal pad.

- Inspect the lochia discharge while palpating the fundus.

- Have the client roll to the side, or lift the buttocks and check for blood under the client.

- Note the number of perineal pads used, and quantify the amount of bleeding (Figure 13–10).

Day 1 to 3: Lochia rubra (dark red discharge with clots and debris); moderate amount; fleshy odor
Day 4 to 7: Lochia serosa (thin; light; moderate amount; rusty brown color)
Day 7 to 10: Lochia alba (thin, whitish bone to light yellow); fleshy, stale odor; scant to moderate amount

Bright red discharge of blood with or without clotting (hemorrhage)
Excessive amount (more than 1 pad fully saturated per hour)
Blood released in spurts or coming out in jet-stream fashion (suggests cervical tear)
Foul odor (suggests infection)

► **Assessing During the Postpartal Period** *CONTINUED*

ASSESSMENT	NORMAL FINDINGS	DEVIATIONS FROM NORMAL

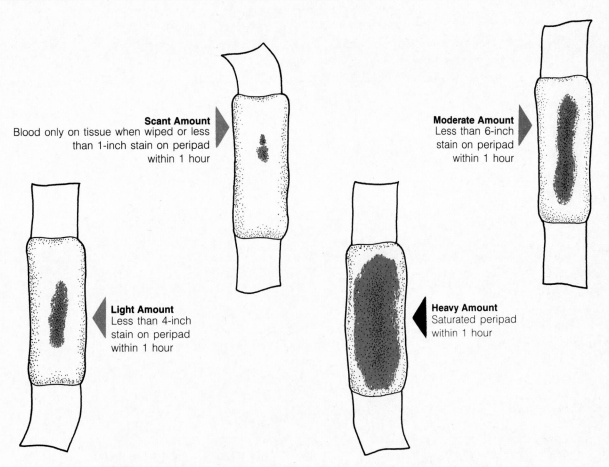

Scant Amount
Blood only on tissue when wiped or less than 1-inch stain on peripad within 1 hour

Moderate Amount
Less than 6-inch stain on peripad within 1 hour

Light Amount
Less than 4-inch stain on peripad within 1 hour

Heavy Amount
Saturated peripad within 1 hour

FIGURE 13–10 Suggested guidelines for assessing lochia volume. *Source:* H. Jacobson, A standard for assessing lochia volume, *American Journal of Maternal Child Nursing*, May/June 1985, 10:175. American Journal of Nursing Company. Used with permission. All rights reserved.

Perineum

Assess the perineum.

- Remove excess lochia with a clean washcloth.

- Have the client roll to the side and flex the top leg.

- Inspect the perineum for abnormalities.

- Note intactness of the episiotomy. Note the general appearance of episiotomy.

Minimal to no edema; absence of discoloration; sutures intact; no tears noted No redness, excessive swelling, foul odor, or discoloration of episiotomy

Edema; erythema or hematoma; tears noted; incisions/sutures not intact

Breasts

Assess the breasts each shift or as indicated by the client's condition.

Day 1: Soft with colostrum secretion
Day 2: Firm, taut, painful, distended, slightly lumpy; may begin milk secretion
Day 3 to 4: Milk secretion
Nipples intact; no redness or cracking

Failure to follow normal progression of milk production from colostrum secretion to milk secretion

Nipples cracked, painful

►

▶ **Assessing During the Postpartal Period** *CONTINUED*

ASSESSMENT	NORMAL FINDINGS	DEVIATIONS FROM NORMAL
Peripheral Vascular System		
Assess for Homans' sign of the legs by dorsiflexing the feet one at a time. (See Chapter 11, page 257, for other assessment procedures related to peripheral vascular assessment.)	Negative: Absence of pain in calf when dorsiflexed	Positive: Calf/leg pain on dorsiflexion
Level of Comfort		
Assess the client's general state of comfort or discomfort.	General soreness, with mild abdominal, breast, and perineal discomfort to varying degrees	Severe pain unrelieved with adequate analgesics
Psychoemotional Status		
Note the general affect and mood of the client.	Initially concerned with basic physical requirements of sleep and food Mood swings first few days after birth Postpartum blues (postpartum depression) third or fourth day	Prolonged periods of either anxiety or depression
Note response of mother to newborn.	Interacting with infant through cuddling and talking	Does not hold infant
Assess the family support system.	Positive interactions with spouse and/ or family	Absence of interaction with others
Assess the learning needs of the client in relation to care for self and infant after discharge.	Vary with individual	
• Note verbal and nonverbal clues while giving care to the client.		
• Note mother's ability and interest in performing specific tasks of infant care.		

REFERENCES

Bobak, I. M.; Jensen, M. D.; and Zalar, M. K. 1989. *Maternity and gynecologic care: The nurse and the family.* 4th ed. St. Louis: C. V. Mosby Co.

Engstrom, J. L. May/June 1988. Measurement of fundal height. *Journal of Obstetric, Gynecologic, and Neonatal Nursing* 17:172–173.

May, K., and Mahlmeister, L. 1990. *Comprehensive maternity nursing: Nursing process and the childbearing family.* 2d ed. Philadelphia: J. B. Lippincott Co.

McKay, S., and Roberts, J. 1985. Second stage labor: What is normal? *Journal of Obstetric, Gynecologic, and Neonatal Nursing* 14: 101–6.

Olds, S. B.; London, M. L.; and Ladewig, P. W. 1992. *Maternal-newborn nursing.* 4th ed. Redwood City, Calif.: Addison-Wesley Nursing.

Suddarth, D. S. 1991. *The Lippincott manual of nursing practice.* 5th ed. Philadelphia: J. B. Lippincott Co.

Special Studies

OBJECTIVES

- Define terms related to selected special procedures used in diagnosing and treating clients

- Describe the purposes and sequencing of selected procedures

- Identify assessment data required for specific procedures

- Identify education needs of clients undergoing certain tests and treatments

- Outline measures to prepare the client physically for specific procedures

- Identify the nursing responsibilities during selected procedures

- Describe guidelines for evaluating and recording the client's responses after special procedures

CONTENTS

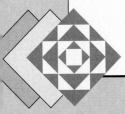

NURSING PROCESS GUIDE
SPECIAL STUDIES

ASSESSMENT

Determine

- Vital signs before, during, and after the procedure

- Client's knowledge of the procedure and ability to maintain the required position or hold breath if needed

- Relevant laboratory tests

- Pertinent health factors, e.g., the presence of dyspnea, that could present a problem during the study

- Any drug allergies, particularly allergies to drugs contained in local anesthetics and skin antiseptics

See also assessment data required for specific procedures throughout this chapter.

PLANNING

Client Goals

The client will

- Experience optimum comfort.

- Experience no injury.

- Be prepared physically and psychologically for the study.

Outcome Criteria

The client

- Reports minimal discomfort during the study.

Nursing Responsibilities For All Special Procedures

Tests and treatments are frightening to many people. They may fear pain, the results of tests, or their reactions to either the pain or the findings. Fear of the unknown increases these misgivings. It is important that the nurse be aware of the needs of clients and support persons and be prepared to help them meet these needs. For special studies, the nurse's chief concern is the client.

The nurse's function during special studies can be divided into three areas: preparing the client and/or the support persons, monitoring and assisting the client during the procedure, and caring for the client after the procedure. The nurse's responsibilities include:

- Determining if a consent form has been signed. Some agencies require a signed consent from the client for special procedures.

- Coordinating the services of personnel from other departments who are involved in the procedure, assisting in scheduling, and helping the client meet schedules.

- Ensuring that the client understands the procedure and the preparation involved. A well-prepared client is likely to experience the least possible discomfort during the tests.

 • Donning gloves if there is a risk of contacting body fluids.

- Assessing the client before, during, and after the procedure.

- Ensuring that certain pretest interventions are administered or completed. This helps assure success of the study performed.

- Supporting and enhancing the client's safety throughout the procedure.

- Labeling any specimens and arranging for them to be sent immediately to the laboratory. Incorrect identification of specimens can lead to subsequent error of diagnosis or therapy for the client.

- Providing required nursing intervention after the procedure.

Removal of Body Fluids and Tissues

A number of fluids and tissues may be removed for diagnostic purposes. Table 14–1 lists common procedures. Normally, a physician performs the procedure at the bedside, in an examining room, or sometimes in the emergency department of a hospital. All the procedures described here involve inserting an instrument, often a needle, through the skin and withdrawing some fluid or tissue. The fluid or

TABLE 14–1   COMMON STUDIES INVOLVING REMOVAL OF BODY FLUID OR TISSUES

Name	Type of Specimen	Source	Common Tests
Lumbar puncture	Spinal fluid	Subarachnoid space of the spinal canal	Pressure, appearance, sugar, protein, cell count, bacteria, Queckenstedt-Stookey test
Abdominal paracentesis	Ascitic fluid	Peritoneal cavity	Cell count, cells, specific gravity, protein
Thoracentesis	Pleural fluid	Pleural cavity	Cell count, protein
Bone marrow biopsy	Bone marrow	Iliac crest, posterior superior iliac spine, or sternum	Cells, iron
Liver biopsy	Liver tissue (needle biopsy specimen)	Liver	Carcinoma, cells
Amniocentesis	Amniotic fluid	Amniotic sac	Fetal maturity, genetic abnormalities
Vaginal examination	Cells	Cervical os or vaginal floor	Papanicolaou test for carcinoma

tissue is usually placed in a special container and sent to the hospital laboratory for examination. Although the techniques for taking specimens are considered safe, complications can occur with each of them.

Techniques 14–1 through 14–7 describe how to assist with a lumbar puncture, abdominal paracentesis, thoracentesis, bone marrow biopsy, liver biopsy, amniocentesis, and vaginal examination.

Lumbar Puncture

In a **lumbar puncture** (LP, or spinal tap), cerebrospinal fluid (CSF) is withdrawn through a needle inserted into the **subarachnoid space** of the spinal canal between the third and fourth lumbar vertebrae or between the fourth and fifth lumbar vertebrae. At this level the needle avoids damaging the spinal cord and major nerve roots (Figure 14–1). During a lumbar puncture, the physician frequently takes CSF pressure readings using a **manometer**, a glass or plastic tube calibrated in millimeters. A Queckenstedt-Stookey

test may also be done while the manometer is in place. When the veins in the neck are compressed on one or both sides, there is a rapid rise in the pressure of the cerebrospinal fluid of healthy persons, and this

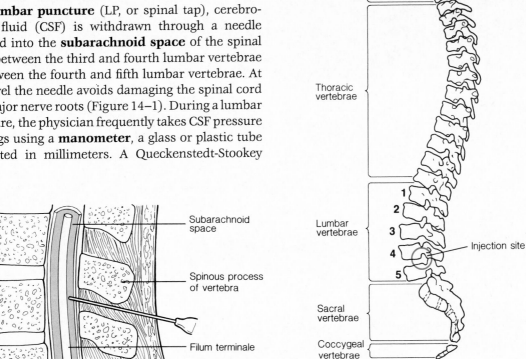

FIGURE 14–1 A diagram of the vertebral column, indicating a site for insertion of the lumbar puncture needle into the subarachnoid space of the spinal canal.

rise quickly disappears when pressure is taken off the neck. But when there is a block in the vertebral canal the pressure of the cerebrospinal fluid is minimally or not affected by this maneuver. If the nurse is not

supporting the client in position, the nurse may be asked to exert digital (finger) pressure on one or both of the internal jugular veins for this test (Figure 14–2).

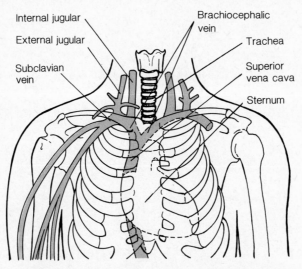

FIGURE 14–2   Location of the internal jugular vein for the Queckenstedt-Stookey test.

 14-1   **Assisting with a Lumbar Puncture**

PURPOSES
- To obtain a CSF specimen
- To take CSF pressure readings

ASSESSMENT FOCUS
Baseline vital signs; neurologic status; presence of headache; allergies to skin antiseptics or anesthetic agents.

EQUIPMENT

□ Sterile lumbar puncture set containing
  Sterile sponges or gauze squares
  Skin antiseptic
  Drapes (one may be fenestrated)
  Syringe and needle to administer the local anesthetic (A 2-ml syringe and #24 and #22 needles are often provided)

Spinal needle 5 to 12.5 cm (2 to 5 in) long, with stylet. The shorter needles are used for infants.
Manometer
Three-way stopcock (a valve between the spinal needle and the manometer that regulates the flow of CSF by shutting off the CSF drainage, allowing the CSF to flow either into the manometer or out into a receptacle)

Specimen containers and labels
Local anesthetic, e.g., 1% procaine (if not included in preassembled set, a vial or ampule of it must be obtained)
Small dressing
□ Face masks (optional)
□ Sterile gloves
□ Examining light, if needed

► **Technique 14–1** *CONTINUED*

INTERVENTION

Preprocedure

1. Explain the procedure to the client and support persons.

- Tell the client

  a. That the physican will be taking a small sample of spinal fluid from the lower spine.

  b. That a local anesthetic will be given so that the client will feel little pain.

  c. When and where the procedure will occur, e.g., at the bedside or in the treatment room.

  d. Who will be present, i.e., the physician and the nurse.

  e. How much time is involved, e.g., about 15 minutes.

- In addition, tell the client what to expect during the procedure. The client may feel slight discomfort (like a pinprick) when the local anesthetic is injected and a sensation of pressure when the spinal needle (Figure 14–3) is being inserted. Remind the client that it is important to remain still and in one position throughout the procedure. A restless client or a child will need to be held to prevent movement.

2. Prepare the client.

- Have the client empty the bladder and bowels prior to the pro-

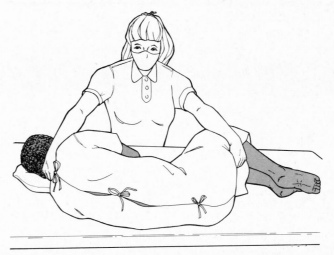

FIGURE 14–4   Supporting the client for a lumbar puncture.

cedure. *This prevents unnecessary discomfort.*

- Position the client laterally with the head bent toward the chest, the knees flexed onto the abdomen, and the back at the edge of the bed or examining table (Figure 14–4). Place a very small pillow under the client's head to maintain the horizontal align-

ment of the spine. *In this position the back is arched, increasing the spaces between the vertebrae so that the spinal needle can be inserted readily.*

- Drape the client to expose only the lumbar spine.

- Open the lumbar puncture set (Figure 14–5) if requested to do so by the physician.

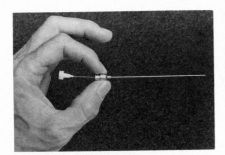

FIGURE 14–3   A spinal needle with the stylet protruding from the hub.

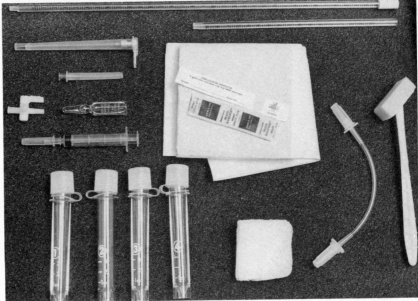

FIGURE 14–5   A preassembled lumbar puncture set. Note the manometer at the top of the set.

► **Technique 14–1 Assisting with a Lumbar Puncture** CONTINUED

During the Procedure

3. Support and monitor the client throughout.

- Stand in front of the client, and support the back of the neck and knees if the client needs help remaining still (Figure 14–4).

- Reassure the client throughout the procedure by explaining what is happening. Encourage the client to breathe normally and to relax as much as possible. *Excessive muscle tension, coughing, or changes in breathing can increase CSF pressure, giving a false reading.*

- Observe the client's color, respirations, and pulse during the lumbar procedure.

4. Handle specimen tubes appropriately.

- Don gloves before handling test tubes. *The outside may have been in contact with the CSF.*

- Label the specimen tubes in sequence if they are not already la-beled. While handling the tubes, take care to prevent contamination of the physician's sterile gloves, the sterile field, and yourself. *The CSF may contain virulent microorganisms, e.g., organisms that cause meningitis.*

5. Place a small sterile dressing over the puncture site. *This helps prevent infection after the needle is removed.*

Postprocedure

6. Ensure the client's comfort and safety.

- Assist the client to a dorsal recumbent position with only one head pillow. The client remains lying down for 8 to 24 hours, until the spinal fluid is replaced. Determine the recommended time this position should be maintained. *Some clients experience a headache following a lumbar puncture, and the dorsal recumbent position tends to prevent or alleviate it.*

- Determine whether analgesics are ordered and can be given for headaches.

7. Monitor the client.

- Observe for swelling or bleeding at the puncture site.

- Determine whether the client feels faint.

- Monitor changes in neurologic status.

- Determine whether the client is experiencing any numbness, tingling, or pain radiating down the legs. *This may be due to nerve irritation.*

8. Transport the specimens to the laboratory.

9. Document the procedure on the client's chart. Include the date and time it was performed; the name of the physician; the color, character, and amount of CSF obtained; the pressure readings; the number of specimens obtained; and the nurse's assessments and interventions.

EVALUATION FOCUS	Vital signs; neurologic status; status of puncture site; complaints of discomfort or feelings of numbness or tingling in the lower extremities.

SAMPLE RECORDING

Date	Time	Notes
5/24/93	1500	Lumbar puncture performed by Dr Guido. Four 2 ml specimens of cloudy serous CSF sent to lab. Initial pressure 130 mm. Closing pressure 100 mm. No apparent discomfort. Resting. ——————— Sarah D. Nicols, NS

KEY ELEMENTS OF ASSISTING WITH A LUMBAR PUNCTURE

- Determine allergies of the client.
- Assess the client's neurologic status and vital signs before the procedure.
- Position the client laterally with the neck, spine, and knees flexed.
- Assist the client to remain still throughout the procedure. Hold a restless client or child to prevent movement.

- Encourage the client to avoid coughing and to breathe normally when CSF pressure readings are taken.
- Maintain asepsis.
- Monitor vital signs and neurologic status following the procedure.
- Promptly report adverse changes in vital signs and neurologic status.

Abdominal Paracentesis

Normally the peritoneum creates just enough peritoneal fluid for lubrication. The fluid is continuously formed and absorbed into the lymphatic system. However, in some disease processes, a large amount of fluid accumulates in the cavity; this condition is called **ascites**. Normal ascitic fluid is serous, clear, and light yellow in color. An **abdominal paracentesis** is carried out to obtain a fluid specimen for laboratory study and to relieve pressure on the abdominal organs due to the presence of excess fluid. See Table 14–1, earlier.

The procedure is carried out by a physician with the assistance of a nurse. Strict sterile technique is followed. A common site for abdominal paracentesis is midway between the umbilicus and the symphysis pubis on the midline (Figure 14–6). The physician makes a small incision with a scalpel, inserts the **trocar** (a sharp, pointed instrument) and **cannula** (tube), and then withdraws the trocar, which is inside the cannula (Figure 14–7). Tubing is attached to the cannula and the fluid flows through the tubing into a receptacle. If the purpose of the paracentesis is to obtain a specimen, the physician may use a long aspirating needle attached to a syringe rather than making an incision and using a trocar and cannula. Normally about 1500 ml is the maximum amount of fluid drained at one time, to avoid hypovolemic shock. The fluid is drained very slowly for the same reason. Some fluid is placed in the specimen container before the cannula is withdrawn. The small incision may or may not be sutured; in either case, it is covered with a small sterile bandage.

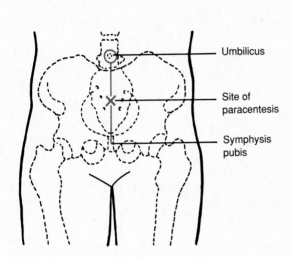

FIGURE 14–6 A common site for an abdominal paracentesis.

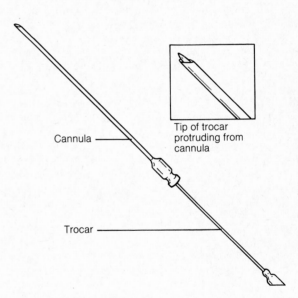

FIGURE 14–7 A trocar and cannula may be used for an abdominal paracentesis.

14-2 Assisting with an Abdominal Paracentesis

PURPOSES
- To obtain a fluid specimen
- To relieve abdominal pressure due to excess fluid

ASSESSMENT FOCUS

Baseline vital signs; degree of ascites in the abdomen (weigh the client and measure the abdominal girth at the level of the umbilicus); general appearance and health status; allergies to skin antiseptic or anesthetic agents.

▶ **Technique 14–2 Assisting with an Abdominal Paracentesis** *CONTINUED*

EQUIPMENT

☐ Sterile set containing
    Sterile sponges or gauze squares with an antiseptic solution
    Drape or drapes (one may be fenestrated)

2-ml syringe and #24 and #22 needles
Small scalpel, needle holder, and sutures
Receptacle for the fluid
Aspirating set or aspirating needle

Local anesthetic
☐ Specimen containers and labels
☐ Masks (optional)
☐ Sterile gloves
☐ Nonsterile disposable gloves for the nurse

INTERVENTION

Preprocedure

1. Prepare the client.

- Explain the procedure to the client. Normally, an abdominal paracentesis is not painful, and, when a client has considerable ascites, the procedure can relieve discomfort caused by the fluid. The procedure to remove ascitic fluid usually takes 30 to 60 minutes. Obtaining a specimen usually takes about 15 minutes. Emphasize the importance of remaining still during the procedure. Include in your explanation when and where the procedure will occur and who will be present.

- Have the client void just before the paracentesis. *This lessens the possibility of puncturing the urinary bladder.* Notify the physician if the client cannot void.

- Help the client assume a sitting position in bed or in a chair. *This allows the fluid to accumulate in the lower abdominal cavity, and the force of gravity and the pressure of the abdominal organs will help the flow of the fluid from the cavity.* Some clients may be able to sit on the edge of the bed with pillows to support the back.

- Cover the client to expose only the necessary area. If using a fenestrated drape, place the opening at the site where the fluid will be removed.

During the Procedure

2. Assist and monitor the client.

- Support the client verbally, and describe the steps of the procedure as needed.

- Observe the client closely for signs of distress, e.g., abnormal pulse rate, skin color, and blood pressure. Observe for signs of hypovolemic shock induced by the loss of fluid: pallor, dyspnea, diaphoresis (profuse perspiration), and a drop in blood pressure.

- Place a small sterile dressing over the site of the incision after the cannula or aspirating needle is withdrawn. *This prevents bleeding or leakage of fluid.*

Postprocedure

3. Monitor the client closely.

- Observe for hypovolemic shock (see step 2).

- Observe the puncture site regularly for leakage.

- Observe the client for any scrotal edema.

- Monitor vital signs, urine output, and drainage from the puncture site every 15 minutes for at least 2 hours and every hour for four hours thereafter, or as the client's condition indicates.

- Measure the abdominal girth with a tape measure in the same place it was measured preprocedure.

4. Document all relevant information.

- Record the procedure on the client's chart, including the date and time; the name of the physician; the girth of the client's abdomen before and after the procedure; the color, clarity, and amount of drained fluid; and any nursing assessments and interventions.

5. Transport the correctly labeled specimens to the laboratory.

► **Technique 14–2** *CONTINUED*

<table>
<tr>
<td>**EVALUATION FOCUS**</td>
<td>Abdominal girth; weight; vital signs; urine output; drainage from puncture area; signs of infection (elevated body temperature); signs of internal hemorrhage (lowered blood pressure, accelerated pulse, hard, boardlike abdomen).</td>
</tr>
</table>

SAMPLE RECORDING

Date	Time	Notes
7/18/93	1400	Paracentesis performed by Dr Johnson, 300 ml clear serosanguinous fluid obtained. Abdominal girth at umbilical level 114 cm before, 109 cm after. Specimen sent to laboratory. P 72, BP 120/85. Slight pallor. Resting comfortably. ——————————————— Roxanne J. Tuttle, NS

KEY ELEMENTS OF ASSISTING WITH AN ABDOMINAL PARACENTESIS

- Determine allergies.
- Assess the client's vital signs before the procedure, and monitor the pulse, respiratory rate, and blood pressure during and following the procedure.
- Weigh the client before and after the procedure.
- Measure the client's abdominal girth before and after the procedure.

- Have the client void before the procedure.
- Ensure that the client is positioned appropriately and remains still throughout the procedure.
- Maintain asepsis.
- Promptly report signs of shock and elevated body temperature.

Thoracentesis

Normally, only sufficient fluid to lubricate the pleura is present in the pleural cavity. However excessive fluid can accumulate as a result of injury, infection, or other pathology. In such a case or in a case of pneumothorax, a physician may perform a **thoracentesis** to remove the excess fluid or air to ease breathing. Thoracentesis is also performed to introduce chemotherapeutic drugs intrapleurally.

The physician and the assisting nurse follow strict sterile technique. The physician attaches a syringe and/or stopcock to the aspirating needle. The stopcock must be in the closed position so that no air will enter the pleural space. The physician inserts the needle through the intercostal space to the pleural cavity. In some instances, the physician threads a small plastic tube through the needle and then withdraws the needle. (The tubing is less likely to puncture the pleura.)

If a syringe is used to receive the fluid, the plunger is pulled out to draw out the pleural fluid as the stopcock is opened. If a large container is used to receive the fluid, the tubing is attached from the stopcock to the adapter on the receiving bottle. When the adapter and stopcock are opened, negative pressure in the container created by a pump or suction machine will draw the fluid from the pleural cavity. After the fluid has been withdrawn, the physician removes the needle or plastic tubing.

14-3 Assisting with a Thoracentesis

Before the thoracentesis, note any orders for medication. A cough suppressant is sometimes ordered to be given 30 minutes before the procedure. An analgesic may also be ordered.

PURPOSES

- To remove excess fluid or air from the pleural cavity
- To introduce chemotherapeutic drugs intrapleurally

ASSESSMENT FOCUS

Baseline vital signs; respirations for bilateral depth and chest movement during inspiration; any differences in chest expansion between the sides; dyspnea, abnormal breath sounds, coughing, or chest pain; character and amount of sputum if cough is productive; allergies to skin antiseptics or anesthetic agents.

EQUIPMENT

- Sterile set containing
  Sterile sponges or gauze squares
  Skin antiseptic
  Drape or drapes (one may be fenestrated)
  2-ml syringe and #24 and #22 needles
  Receptacle for the fluid (50-ml

  syringe and #16 needle or an airtight container)
  Three-way stopcock
  Two-way stopcock with connecting tubing
  Thoracentesis needle, usually a #15 needle about 5 to 7.5 cm (2 to 3 in) long

  Specimen container and label
  Local anesthetic
  Specimen containers and labels
- Sterile gloves
- Disposable gloves for the nurse
- Masks (optional)

INTERVENTION

Preprocedure

1. Prepare the client.

- Explain the procedure to the client. Normally, a thoracentesis is not painful, although the client may experience a feeling of pressure when the needle is inserted. The procedure may bring considerable relief if breathing has been difficult. The procedure takes only a few minutes, depending primarily on the time it takes for the fluid to drain from the pleural cavity. To avoid puncturing the lungs, it is important for the client not to cough while the needle is inserted. Include in your explanation when and where the procedure will occur and who will be present.

- Help the client assume a comfortable position. This is usually a sitting position with the arms

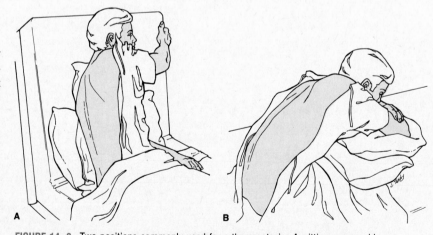

FIGURE 14–8 Two positions commonly used for a thoracentesis: *A*, sitting on one side with the arm held to the front and up; *B*, sitting and leaning forward over a pillow.

above the head, which spreads the ribs and enlarges the intercostal space. Two positions commonly used are one in which the arm is elevated and stretched forward (Figure 14–8, *A*) and one in which the client leans for-

ward over a pillow (Figure 14–8, *B*). To make sure that the needle is inserted below the fluid level when fluid is to be removed (or above any fluid if air is to be removed), the physician will palpate the chest and select the ex-

▶ **Technique 14–3** *CONTINUED*

act site for insertion of the needle. A site on the lower posterior chest is often used to remove fluid, and a site on the upper anterior chest is used to remove air.

- Cover the client as needed with a bath blanket. If using a fenestrated drape, place the opening at the site of the thoracentesis.

During the Procedure

2. Support and monitor the client throughout.

- Support the client verbally, and describe the steps of the procedure as needed.
- Observe the client for signs of distress, such as dyspnea, pallor, and coughing. If the client becomes distressed or has to cough, the procedure is halted briefly.

3. Place a small sterile dressing over the site of the puncture.

Postprocedure

4. Monitor the client.

- Assess pulse rate and respiratory rate and skin color. *A shift in the mediastinum (e.g., heart and large blood vessels) can occur with removal of large amounts of fluid.* Signs of mediastinal shift include pallor, accelerated pulse rate, dyspnea, accelerated respiration rate, and dizziness.
- Observe changes in the client's cough, sputum, respiratory depth, breath sounds, and note complaints of chest pain.

5. Position the client appropriately.

- Some agency protocols recommend that the client lie on the unaffected side with the head of the bed elevated 30° for at least 30 minutes. *This position facilitates expansion of the affected lung and eases respirations.*

6. Document all relevant information.

- Record the thoracentesis on the client's chart, including the date and time; the name of the physician; the amount, color, and clarity of fluid drained; and nursing assessments and interventions provided.

7. Transport the specimens to the laboratory.

EVALUATION FOCUS

Respiratory rate, depth, and bilateral chest movement; bilateral breath sounds; vital signs; evidence of cyanosis or dyspnea; complaints of chest pain.

SAMPLE RECORDING

Date	Time	Notes
4/18/93	1500	Thoracentesis performed by Dr Sargent. 275 ml of cloudy serosanguineous fluid removed. Specimen sent to laboratory. R 32, shallow and wet. P 76. Skin pale. Coughing occasionally. Small amount of thick white sputum. Resting more comfortably. ———————————— Ron L. Landry, NS

KEY ELEMENTS OF ASSISTING WITH A THORACENTESIS

- Determine allergies.
- Assess the client's vital signs before the procedure.
- Administer cough suppressant if ordered before the procedure.
- Ensure that the client is positioned appropriately.

- Ensure that the client avoids coughing during needle insertion.
- Monitor the client's pulse rate, respiratory rate, chest movements, and breath sounds following the procedure.
- Promptly report signs of mediastinal shift, absence of breath sounds, and sudden chest pain.

Bone Marrow Biopsy

A bone marrow biopsy is the removal of a specimen of bone marrow for laboratory study. The biopsy is used to detect specific diseases of the blood, e.g., pernicious anemia and leukemia. The bones of the body commonly used for a bone marrow biopsy are the sternum and the iliac crests (Figure 14–9).

The physician introduces a bone marrow needle with stylet through the skin and bone into the red marrow of the spongy bone (Figure 14–10). Once the needle is in the marrow space, the stylet is removed and a 10-ml syringe is attached to the needle. The plunger is withdrawn until 1 to 2 ml of marrow has been obtained. The physician replaces the stylet in the needle, withdraws the needle, and places the specimen in test tubes and/or on glass slides.

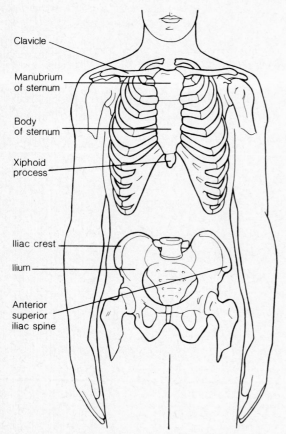

FIGURE 14–9   The sternum and the iliac crests are common sites for a bone marrow biopsy.

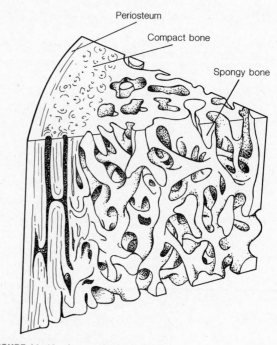

FIGURE 14–10   A cross section of a bone.

 14-4   # Assisting with a Bone Marrow Biopsy

PURPOSE	• To obtain a bone marrow sample to check for abnormal blood cell development
ASSESSMENT FOCUS	Baseline vital signs; allergies to skin antiseptics or anesthetic agents.

EQUIPMENT

- A sterile set containing
  Drape or drapes (one is often
    fenestrated)
  Antiseptic
  Local anesthetic

2-ml syringe and #25 needle
10-ml syringe
Bone marrow needle with stylet
Sterile gauze squares
Test tubes and/or glass slides

- Masks (optional)
- Sterile gloves
- Disposable, nonsterile gloves
  for the nurse
- Specimen containers and labels

Technique 14–4 *CONTINUED*

INTERVENTION

Preprocedure

1. Prepare the client.

- Explain the procedure. The client may experience pain when the marrow is aspirated. There may be a crunching sound when the needle is pushed through the cortex of the bone. The entire procedure usually takes 15 to 30 minutes. Include in your explanation when and where the procedure will occur and who will be present.

- Help the client assume a supine position (with one pillow if desired) for a biopsy of the sternum (sternal puncture) or a prone position for a biopsy of either iliac crest. Fold the bedclothes back or drape the client to expose the area.

During the Procedure

2. Monitor and support the client throughout.

- Describe the steps of the procedure as needed, and provide verbal support.

- Observe the client for pallor, diaphoresis, and faintness due to bleeding or pain.

3. Place a small dressing over the site of the puncture after the needle is withdrawn.

- Some agency protocols recommend direct pressure over the site for 5 to 10 minutes to prevent bleeding.

Postprocedure

4. Monitor the client.

- Assess for discomfort and bleeding from the site. The client may experience some tenderness in the area. Bleeding and hematoma formation need to be assessed for several days. Report any bleeding or pain to the nurse in charge.

- Provide an analgesic as needed and ordered.

5. Document all relevant information.

- Record the procedure, including the date and time of the procedure, the name of the physician, and any nursing assessments and interventions.

6. Transport the specimens to the laboratory.

EVALUATION FOCUS

Vital signs and puncture site for bleeding.

SAMPLE RECORDING

Date	Time	Notes
8/19/93	0900	Bone marrow biopsy from right iliac crest performed by Dr Rosenthal. Site dry, no apparent bleeding. No complaints of discomfort. Specimen sent to the laboratory. ——————————— Donna S. Lambert, NS

KEY ELEMENTS OF ASSISTING WITH A BONE MARROW BIOPSY

- Determine any allergies.
- Assess the client's vital signs before and after the procedure.
- Position the client appropriately.
- Maintain asepsis.
- Assess the client for bleeding and hematoma formation following the procedure.
- Promptly report excessive bleeding and hematoma formation at the puncture site.

Liver Biopsy

A liver biopsy is a short procedure, generally performed at the client's bedside, in which a sample of liver tissue is aspirated. A physician inserts a needle in the intercostal space between two of the right lower ribs and into the liver (Figure 14–11) or through the abdomen below the right rib cage (subcostally). The client exhales and stops breathing while the physician inserts the biopsy needle, injects a small amount of sterile normal saline to clear the needle of blood or particles of tissue picked up during insertion, and aspirates liver tissue by drawing back on the plunger of the syringe. After the needle is withdrawn, the nurse applies pressure to the site to prevent bleeding, often by positioning the client on the biopsy site.

Because many clients with liver disease have blood clotting defects and are prone to bleeding, prothrombin time and platelet count are normally taken well in advance of the test. If the test results are abnormal, the biopsy may be contraindicated.

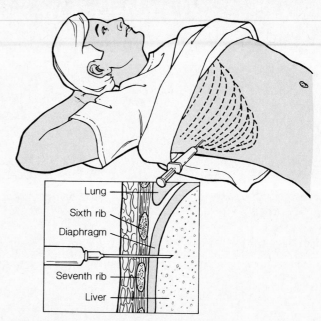

FIGURE 14–11   A common site for a liver biopsy.

14-5   Assisting with a Liver Biopsy

PURPOSES

- To obtain data about the nature of liver disease
- To facilitate diagnosis
- To gain information about specific changes in liver tissue

ASSESSMENT FOCUS

Client's ability to hold the breath for up to 10 seconds and remain still while the biopsy needle is inserted; prothrombin time and platelet count; allergies to skin antiseptics and anesthetic agents.

EQUIPMENT

- Sterile liver biopsy set containing
  Sterile sponges or gauze squares with an antiseptic solution
  2-ml syringe and a #22 and #25 needle (6 in)

- Large biopsy syringe and needle
  Drapes
  Local anesthetic
  Sterile normal saline
  Specimen container with formalin

- Face masks (optional)
- Sterile gloves
- Disposable gloves for the nurse
- Specimen containers and labels

INTERVENTION

Preprocedure

1. Prepare the client.

- Give preprocedural medications as ordered. *Vitamin K may be given for several days before the biopsy to reduce the risk of hemorrhage. Vitamin K may be lacking in some clients with liver disease. It is essential for the production of prothrombin, which is a requisite for blood clotting.*

- Explain the procedure. Tell the client

  a. What the physician will do, i.e., take a small sample of liver tissue by putting a needle into the client's side or abdomen.

  b. That a sedative and local anesthetic will be given, so the client will feel no pain.

▶ **Technique 14–5** *CONTINUED*

c. When and where the procedure will occur.

d. Who will be present.

e. The time required.

f. What to expect as the procedure is being performed; e.g., the client may experience mild discomfort when the local anesthetic is injected and slight pressure when the biopsy needle is inserted.

• Ensure that the client fasts for at least 2 hours before the procedure.

• Administer the appropriate sedative about 30 minutes beforehand or at the specified time.

• Help the client assume a supine position, with the upper right quadrant of the abdomen exposed. Cover the client with the bedclothes so that only the abdominal area is exposed.

During the Procedure

2. Monitor and support the client throughout.

• Support the client in a supine position.

• Instruct the client to take a few deep inhalations and exhalations and to hold the breath after the final exhalation for up to 10 seconds as the needle is inserted, the biopsy obtained, and the needle withdrawn. *Holding the breath after exhalation immobilizes the chest wall and liver and keeps the diaphragm in its highest position, avoiding injury to the diaphragm and laceration of the liver.*

• Instruct the client to resume breathing when the needle is withdrawn.

• Apply pressure to the site of the puncture. *Pressure will help stop any bleeding.*

3. Apply a small dressing to the site of the puncture.

Postprocedure

4. Position the client appropriately.

• Assist the client to a right side-lying position with a small pillow or folded towel under the biopsy site (Figure 14–12). Instruct the client to remain in this position for several hours. *The right lateral position compresses the biopsy site of the liver against the chest wall and minimizes the escape of blood or bile through the puncture site by applying pressure to the area.*

5. Monitor the client.

• Assess the client's vital signs— i.e., pulse, respirations, blood pressure—every 15 minutes for the first hour following the test or until the signs are stable. Then monitor vital signs every hour for 24 hours or as needed. *Complications of a liver biopsy are rare, but hemorrhage from a perforated blood vessel can occur.*

• Determine whether the client is experiencing abdominal pain. *Severe abdominal pain may indicate bile peritonitis (an inflammation of the peritoneal lining of the abdomen caused by bile leaking from a perforated bile duct).*

• Check the biopsy site for localized bleeding. Pressure dressings may be required if bleeding does occur.

6. Document all relevant information.

• Record the procedure, including the date and time it was performed, the name of the physician, and all nursing assessments and interventions.

7. Transport the specimens to the laboratory.

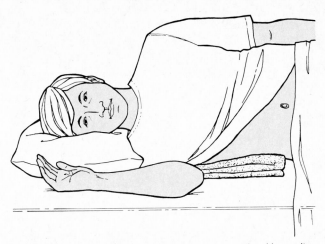

FIGURE 14–12   The position to provide pressure on a liver biopsy site.

EVALUATION FOCUS   Vital signs; bleeding from puncture site; complaints of abdominal pain.

▶ **Technique 14–5 Assisting with a Liver Biopsy** *CONTINUED*

SAMPLE RECORDING

Date	Time	Notes
2/13/93	1000	Liver biopsy performed by Dr Martinez. Specimen sent to laboratory. P 86, R 16 and regular, BP 110/76/70. Small amount bleeding at site (0.3 cm diameter). Resting comfortably in right lateral position. ————— Theresa A. Milligan, NS

KEY ELEMENTS OF ASSISTING WITH A LIVER BIOPSY

- Determine any allergies.
- Assess the client's vital signs before the procedure.
- Before the procedure, determine the client's ability to hold the breath for up to 10 seconds.
- Ensure that the client's prothrombin time and platelet count are normal before the procedure.
- Ensure that preprocedural medications (e.g., vitamin K) are given as ordered.
- Maintain asepsis.

- Instruct the client to exhale and stop breathing during needle insertion and the biopsy.
- Apply pressure to the puncture site after the procedure.
- Position the client appropriately following the procedure.
- Monitor vital signs and signs of hemorrhage after the procedure.
- Promptly report excessive bleeding at the biopsy site, signs of shock, or severe abdominal pain.

Amniocentesis

An amniocentesis is the removal of a specimen of amniotic fluid from the amniotic sac in the uterus. The procedure, possible after the fourteenth week of pregnancy, requires sterile technique. The physician inserts a needle through the abdominal wall and withdraws amniotic fluid (Figure 14–13). After the needle is withdrawn, a small dressing is placed over the puncture site. Immediately before amniocentesis is performed, the abdomen is scanned by ultrasound to locate the placenta, fetus, and an adequate pocket of fluid. Identification of an appropriate needle insertion site is essential to avoid puncturing the fetus, placenta, umbilical cord, and uterine arteries. Transabdominal or suprapubic sites may be used. After a suprapubic tap, the fluid obtained should be checked for protein content with a dipstick because there is a possibility that urine was obtained. Amniotic fluid has a high protein content, an abnormal finding in urine. A blood sample is also taken before amniocentesis to compare the results with a postprocedure blood sample to assess potential fetomaternal hemorrhage.

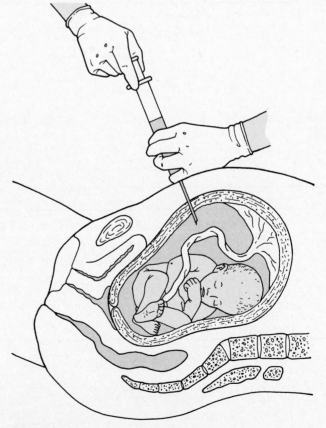

FIGURE 14–13 The site for an amniocentesis.

14-6 Assisting with an Amniocentesis

PURPOSES	• To obtain a specimen of amniotic fluid to determine fetal health and maturity • To induce abortion
ASSESSMENT FOCUS	Fetal heart sounds; maternal vital signs; allergies to skin antiseptics or anesthetic agents.

EQUIPMENT

- Sterile amniocentesis tray containing
  Sterile sponges or gauze squares with antiseptic
  10-ml and 20-ml syringes and #22 gauge spinal needle with stylet

- Drapes
  Betadine or other cleaning agent
  A local anesthetic
  Three specimen containers (amber-colored or covered with tape)

- Face masks
- Sterile gloves
- Disposable gloves for the nurse
- Fetal monitor

INTERVENTION

Preprocedure

1. Gather data.

- Ensure that the results of the ultrasound showing the position of the placenta are available.

2. Prepare the client.

- Assist the woman to a supine position.

- If the women is pregnant more than 20 weeks, ask her to empty her bladder. *This makes it less likely that the needle will puncture the bladder.* If the woman is pregnant less than 20 weeks, emptying the bladder is not necessary. *A full bladder helps brace the uterus.*

- Explain the procedure to the client. Tell the client that

  a. The procedure takes only 10 minutes.

  b. It is usually painless.

- Drape the abdomen so that the upper portion of the abdomen is exposed.

- Assess the woman's vital signs and the fetal heart rate (FHR).

- Give any ordered preprocedure medications.

During the Procedure

3. Monitor and support the woman and fetus.

- Monitor the woman's vital signs, and observe for signs of labor.

- Monitor the FHR.

- Wash the antiseptic off the abdomen after the needle is withdrawn.

4. Apply a small dressing to the puncture site.

Postprocedure

5. Monitor the woman and fetus.

- Take the woman's vital signs (BP, pulse, respirations) regularly. *Fetomaternal hemorrhage can be a complication.*

- Monitor the FHR, and observe for signs of hemorrhage. Continue monitoring until normal, usually for 1 hour.

- Observe the puncture site for bleeding.

- Instruct the woman to notify the physician at the first sign of labor, bleeding, or infection.

- Position the client on her left side. *This increases venous return and cardiac output, thus permitting the restoration of normal circulation before the client arises.*

6. Document all relevant information.

- Include the date and time the procedure was performed, name of the physician, and all nursing assessments and interventions.

EVALUATION FOCUS	Woman's vital signs; FHR; signs of premature labor or infection.

▶ **Technique 14–6 Assisting with an Amniocentesis** *CONTINUED*

SAMPLE RECORDING

Date	Time	Notes
6/6/93	0800	Amniocentesis performed by Dr K. Champion. Full explanation given to woman. Fetal position determined by sonogram. 30 ml clear fluid withdrawn and sent to laboratory. BP 130/86, P 84, R 18, F H R 122. FHR monitored continuously by fetal monitor for 1 hour. No evidence of vaginal bleeding or leakage from puncture site. Remained in left lateral position for 20 min. before rising. ——————————— Roberta S. Snakee, RN
	0815	Turned without discomfort. FHR 130, BP 126/80, P. 76, R. 16. No signs of labor or bleeding. ——————————— Roberta S. Snakee, RN

KEY ELEMENTS OF ASSISTING WITH AN AMNIOCENTESIS

- Determine any allergies.
- Assess the woman's vital signs and the FHR before the procedure.
- Ensure that the results of the ultrasound showing placenta position are available.
- Maintain asepsis.

- Apply a bandage to the puncture site after the needle is withdrawn.
- Monitor vital signs and FHR following the procedure.
- Promptly report any signs of bleeding, labor, or hemorrhage.

Vaginal Examination

A vaginal examination is the examination of the internal female genitals: the cervix and the vagina. After the woman is draped in lithotomy position, the physician inserts the vaginal speculum. (Figure 14–14). After visualizing the cervix, the physician takes smear specimens from the sites (Figure 14–15) and then withdraws the speculum while observing the vagina. In some instances, the physician then inserts gloved fingers into the vagina to palpate the uterus and ovaries for any abnormalities.

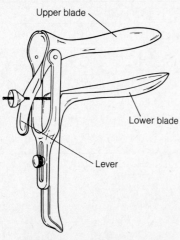

FIGURE 14–14 A vaginal speculum.

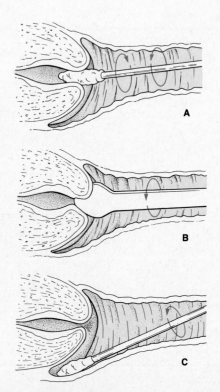

FIGURE 14–15 Methods of obtaining Pap smears: *A,* Endocervical. A cotton swab is inserted into the cervical os and rotated clockwise and counterclockwise in the os. *B,* Cervical scrape. An Ayre spatula with the longer end inserted into the cervical os is rotated to scrape cells from the outer surface. *C,* Vaginal smear or pool. A cotton-tipped applicator or elongated spatula is inserted along the vaginal floor.

14-7 Assisting with a Vaginal Examination

PURPOSES
- To inspect the internal female genitals
- To obtain a specimen for cytology studies

ASSESSMENT FOCUS
> Evidence of any bleeding or discomfort; discharge from the vagina.

EQUIPMENT
- Good lighting (a flashlight may be necessary to view the cervix)
- Drapes
- Disposable gloves
- Vaginal speculum of the correct size (a virgin or a sexually inactive older woman will probably require a small speculum; otherwise the size of the speculum required depends on the individual's sexual and obstetric history.
- Warm water
- Lubricant
- Supplies for cytology studies Cotton applicators

Normal saline solution
Ayre spatula (for a cervical scrape)
Slides
Fixative spray or solution for the specimen

INTERVENTION

Preprocedure

1. Prepare the client.

- Advise the client not to douche prior to the procedure.
- Explain the procedure. It should take only 5 minutes and is normally not painful.
- Assist the client to a lithotomy position as needed, and drape her appropriately.

During the Procedure

2. Support the client.

- Explain the procedure as needed.
- Encourage the client to take deep breaths. *These will help the pelvic muscles relax.*

Postprocedure

3. Monitor and assist the client.

- Assist the client from the lithotomy position.

- Assist client with perineal care as needed. See Technique 15–2, page 385.
- Observe any discharge from the vagina.

4. Document the procedure.

- Include the date and time it was performed, the name of the physician, and any nursing assessments and interventions.

EVALUATION FOCUS
> Discomfort; vaginal discharge.

SAMPLE RECORDING

Date	Time	Notes
2/18/93	1315	Vaginal examination by Dr R. Groves. Three specimens taken for Pap. smear examination. No vaginal bleeding or discomfort. ——— Ginny Black, RN

KEY ELEMENTS OF ASSISTING WITH A VAGINAL EXAMINATION
- Advise the client not to douche before the procedure.
- Position and drape clients in lithotomy position.
- Observe any vaginal discharge.

Studies Involving Visual Inspection

Visual inspection or direct visualization techniques involve the use of special instruments called **endoscopes**, through which interior parts of the body can be seen. Originally, endoscopes were straight, rigid, metal tubes. Today, most endoscopes are fiberoptic; i.e., they are flexible, easily maneuvered, brightly lighted tubes. These fiberoptic endoscopes, or fiberscopes, make examination easier to perform and more comfortable for the client. Some endoscopes are equipped with a camera that takes color photographs, which can be studied following the examination; others allow the attachment of a second eyepiece (Figure 14–16) so that another diagnostician or student can observe the procedure simultaneously.

Endoscopes and the examinations performed with them assume their names from the body part to be examined. For example, a *bronchoscope* is used to visualize the bronchi of the lungs, and the examination is called a *bronchoscopy*. Endoscopic examinations are usually performed in surgery or special treatment rooms. They generally take about 30 to 60 minutes to complete. See Table 14–2 for nursing responsibilities before, during, and after each type of endoscopic examination.

Laryngoscopy and **bronchoscopy** are sterile procedures using a laryngoscope and bronchoscope, respectively. A general or local anesthetic may be given before the examination. If a general anesthetic is given, routine preoperative care is given. A local anesthetic, if given, is sprayed on the client's pharynx to prevent gagging; alternatively, the client gargles with an anesthetic to anesthetize the throat. The bronchoscope is then inserted to visualize the larynx or bronchi. In some cases, a section of tissue is taken for biopsy. For this procedure, the client usually lies supine on the examining table. See Table 14–2 for nursing interventions before, during, and after the examination.

Esophagoscopy (visual examination of the esophagus), **gastroscopy** (visual examination of the stomach), and **duodenoscopy** (visual examination of the duodenum) are performed with a gastroscope. This is a clean rather than a sterile procedure. The preparation and care of the client are the same as for laryngoscopy and bronchoscopy. During these procedures, a tissue sample may be taken for biopsy, and samples of secretions may be taken for study of digestive enzymes. See Table 14–2 for nursing interventions.

Cystoscopy is the visualization of the interior of the urinary bladder; this examination requires insertion of a cystoscope into the bladder via the urethra. It is a sterile procedure. A general or local anesthetic is given, and the preparation is similar to that for

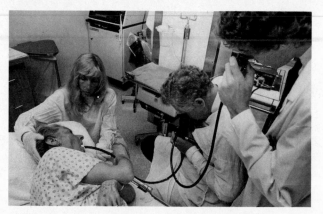

FIGURE 14–16 An endoscopic procedure in progress.

bronchoscopy. During cystoscopy, catheters may be inserted up the ureters into each kidney. Contrast medium is then injected into the kidneys, and X-ray photographs are taken. This procedure is known as **retrograde pyelography**. The X-ray film shows the kidney calyces, the kidney pelvis, the ureters, and the urinary bladder. When a pyelogram is to be taken, the client is given laxatives and enemas to free the intestines of feces and gas. **Intravenous pyelography (IVP)** or **urography (IVU)** is roentgenography of the kidneys after the injection of dye into the arterial system. An intravenous pyelogram shows the same structures as a retrograde pyelogram. This examination does not require an anesthetic and normally lasts about 1 hour. See Table 14–2 for nursing interventions.

Anoscopy, **proctoscopy**, **sigmoidoscopy**, and **colonoscopy** are endoscopic procedures of the mucosa of the anus, rectum, sigmoid colon, and colon, respectively. A proctoscope or sigmoidoscope is used to examine the anus, rectum, and sigmoid colon. A colonoscope is used to examine the large bowel.

Preparation generally includes the administration of laxatives or enemas begun the evening before to clear the bowel of feces. General anesthesia is not usually necessary, although the client may experience some discomfort. The client assumes a knee-chest position on a special examining table during the examination.

Studies Involving the Measuring of Electric Impulses

A number of machines measure and record electric impulses. The **electrocardiograph** receives impulses from the heart, the **electroencephalograph** from the brain, and the **electromyograph** from the muscles. All these machines have electrodes that attach

TABLE 14–2   NURSING INTERVENTIONS FOR ENDOSCOPIC EXAMINATIONS

Examination	Preprocedure	During Procedure	Postprocedure
Laryngoscopy or bronchoscopy	Explain the procedure, and clarify concerns of the client. Explain that a local spray or gargle will be given or that some medications will be injected through a needle in the vein, that the client will rest the teeth against a small plastic mouthpiece, that the procedure is painless but some pressure may be felt. Explain that the test will take about 30 to 60 minutes. Assess vital signs, sputum, and character of respirations for baseline data. Remove dentures, necklaces, earrings, hairpins, and combs. Ensure good oral hygiene. Ensure nothing by mouth 6 to 8 hours beforehand. Confirm that the client is not allergic to any medications that will be given. Administer analgesic, sedative, antianxiety agent, and medication to dry secretions, if ordered.	Assist the physician as required, e.g., to hold the head piece or to move the client's head. Monitor the client's pulse and respirations. Support the client using touch and verbal communication.	1. Monitor vital signs every 30 minutes or as needed during the recovery period, and compare results to baseline data. 2. Withhold fluids until the gag reflex is restored and the client is conscious. 3. Position the client as ordered or indicated. Place the unconscious client in the lateral position so that secretions are not aspirated. 4. Inspect the client's sputum for blood caused by tissue damage. 5. Observe the client for signs of dyspnea, stridor, and shortness of breath, which may result from laryngeal edema or laryngospasm. 6. Provide ice chips and warm saline gargles or throat lozenges, and administer ordered analgesics as required for throat discomfort. 7. Advise the client to contact the physician if there is difficulty with breathing, blood in sputum, fever, or pain.
Esophagoscopy, gastroscopy, and duodenoscopy	As above for bronchoscopy, with the exception of assessing sputum. Explain that the client may feel pressure in the stomach as the tube is moved about and fullness or bloating, like that after eating a large meal.	As above for bronchoscopy. Administer oral simethicone (Mylicon) before test if ordered; it decreases air bubbles in the stomach. If atropine is given intravenously to reduce gastrointestinal spasm, carefully monitor the client's pulse rate. Atropine increases the heart rate.	1. Follow steps 1 to 3 and 6, as for bronchoscopy. 2. Inspect emesis for blood and test it for occult blood if agency practice indicates. 3. Advise the client to contact the physician if client has persistent difficulty swallowing, pain, fever, blood in vomitus, or black stools.
Cystoscopy	Assess vital signs, frequency of urination, dysuria, amount and consistency of urine for baseline data. Administer enema if ordered. A clear bowel is necessary if X-ray films are planned. Ensure nothing by mouth for 6 to 8 hours or only IV fluids if general anesthetic is being given. Ensure appropriate fluid intake, if ordered, for the client having a local anesthetic to ensure an adequate flow of urine for the collection of specimens. Administer sedative and medication to dry secretions, if ordered.	Support the client emotionally. Monitor vital signs. Label specimens, if taken, appropriately. Assist the physician as requested.	1. Monitor vital signs, urination, and urine, and compare with baseline data. 2. Position the unconscious client appropriately (as above for bronchoscopy). 3. Inspect the client's urine for blood and report bright red bleeding. 4. Report inability to urinate by 8 hours. 5. Encourage increased fluid intake to decrease irritation of urinary tissue. 6. If dyes were used in the procedure, warn the client that the urine may be an unusual color.

TABLE 14–2 Endoscopic Examinations *CONTINUED*

Examination	Preprocedure	During Procedure	Postprocedure
			7. Administer analgesics, as ordered, for pain.
			8. If the client is discharged, advise the client to report persistent difficulty passing urine, bright blood in urine, pain, or fever.
Anoscopy, proctoscopy, sigmoidoscopy, and colonoscopy	Assess vital signs and consistency of feces for baseline data.	Support the client physically in the knee-chest position, as needed.	1. Monitor vital signs and compare with baseline data.
	Ensure appropriate preexamination diet and fluid intake. Some agencies provide a light evening meal the day before and only fluid the day of the examination	Monitor pulse and respiratory rates.	2. Inspect the next few stools for blood.
	Administer laxative, if ordered, the evening before.	Label specimens, if taken, appropriately.	3. Allow the client to rest. This procedure may be physically and emotionally tiring.
	Administer enemas until returns are clear or suppository as ordered the morning of the examination.	Support the client emotionally. Acknowledge feelings the client experiences, e.g., cramps, and assure the client that they are not unusual.	4. Provide fluids and food.
	Ensure that the client voids before the examination. The pressure during the procedure may injure a full bladder.		
	Administer sedative beforehand, if ordered.		
	Just before the endoscope is inserted explain (a) that the client will experience the sensation of having to move the bowels due to the pressure of the instrument, and (b) that the client may experience some abdominal cramping when air is introduced to distend the bowel.		

to the body parts. The electrodes are sensitive to electric activity, which is recorded graphically. The graphic reading can also be shown on an oscilloscope screen.

Electrocardiography

An **electrocardiogram** (ECG or EKG) is a graph of electric impulses from the heart. The heart muscle is said to be *polarized*, or charged, when it is at rest. When the muscle cells of the ventricles and the atria contract, they *depolarize*, or lose their charge. During a resting stage, they regain their electric charge, or *repolarize*. Cardiac depolarization and repolarization are recorded on an electrocardiogram.

The heartbeat is normally initiated at the *sinoatrial (SA) node*, which is located in the upper aspect of the right atrium. The SA node is often referred to as the pacemaker of the heart. The impulse it initiates radiates over the atria, causing them to contract. It is then picked up by the *atrioventricular (AV) node*, situated at the base of the atrial septum. The impulse travels from the AV node down two bundle branches throughout the ventricles of the heart. The SA and AV nodes and the bundle branches have dense networks of *Purkinje's fibers*, modified cardiac tissue that helps conduct the impulse. As the impulse travels throughout this system, the ventricles contract or depolarize. Figure 14–17 shows a normal electrocardiogram and indicates the intervals of depolarization and repolarization. The P wave arises when the impulse from the SA node causes the atria to contract or depolarize. The QRS wave occurs with contraction and depolarization of the ventricles. The T wave rep-

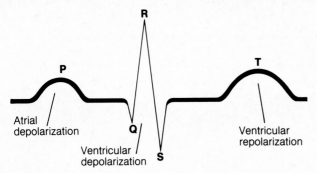

FIGURE 14-17 Schematic of a normal electrocardiogram.

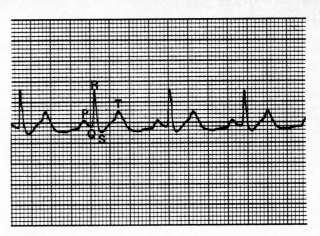

FIGURE 14-18 A normal electrocardiogram.

resents the resting or repolarization of the ventricles. Repolarization of the atria occurs during the QRS segment of the graph; it is normally not seen on an ECG. The ECG is produced on finely lined paper. The horizontal lines represent the voltage of the electric impulse, and the vertical lines represent time (Figure 14–18). The graph waves can be abnormal in size, position, and form when cardiac pathology exists.

Clients who require ECGs may go to a special department of a hospital or laboratory. If the client is very ill, a portable ECG machine can be brought to the bedside in a home or hospital. If the client is critically ill, the heart may be monitored continually. For such clients, a *cardiac monitor* is used. This machine shows cardiac waves on an oscilloscope.

An electrocardiogram is usually taken by a nurse-technician or physician. Electrodes are attached by leads to the electrocardiograph. The electrodes are attached to the client's body by paste, suction cups, or tape. One electrode is attached to the lower part of each limb, and a fifth electrode is moved to six different positions on the chest. The first position is on the right sternal border; subsequent positions follow the general outline of the heart around to the left sternal border and laterally as far as the midaxillary line (Figure 14–19). The heart's electric impulses register on a graph that the machine produces during the procedure. A physician interprets the graph after the test.

Electroencephalography

Electroencephalograms (EEGs) are recordings of electric activity in the brain. Electroencephalographs have leads to electrodes that attach to the client's scalp with paste or small needles. The person lies in a dorsal recumbent position in a darkened room and may be asked to hyperventilate. Readings may also be taken while the client sleeps. If performed on a sleeping client, the test may take 2 hours; otherwise it lasts no more than 1 hour. The test is normally

painless, although the client may feel occasional pin-pricks if needle electrodes are used in the scalp.

Preparation for an EEG varies. Some agency protocols require that the client not take stimulants, such as coffee, or depressants, such as alcohol, on the day of the test. Usually the client takes no medications prior to the test, and the hair is shampooed to remove traces of hair spray, hair creams, and the like.

Electromyography

An **electromyogram (EMG)** is a record of the electric potential created by the contraction of a muscle. Two electrodes are attached with paste or small needles to the skin over the muscle. This test is used to

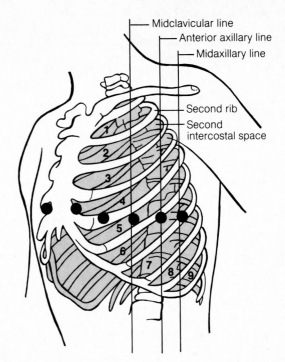

FIGURE 14-19 The placement of electrodes on the chest of an adult for electrocardiography.

discern muscle abnormalities such as **fasciculation** (abnormal contraction involving the whole motor unit). No special preparation is necessary for this procedure. The client may experience some discomfort when the needle electrodes are inserted and some residual discomfort if many muscles are tested.

Often a **nerve conduction study** is done in conjunction with the EMG. This procedure determines the excitability and conduction velocities of motor and sensory nerves and the presence of disease of the peripheral nerves. A stimulating electrode and a recording electrode are placed over specific sites to test a specific nerve. The distance between the electrodes and the time required for a nerve impulse to pass from the point of stimulation to the point of recording are precisely measured. Conduction velocity is then calculated. The client will experience the discomfort of mild electric shock during this procedure, but there should be no residual discomfort.

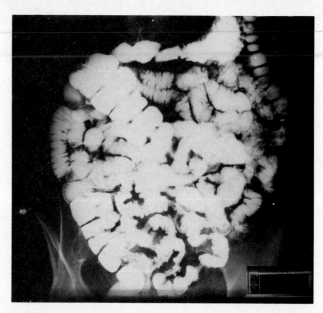

FIGURE 14–20 An X-ray film of the small and large intestines filled with a contrast medium.

Studies Involving Roentgenography

Roentgen rays (X rays) are part of the spectrum of electromagnetic radiation. They travel at the speed of light and have considerably shorter wavelengths than light or radio waves. This distinctive property enables radiation to penetrate organs and tissues according to their thickness and density.

It is the differential absorption of X rays by the various tissues that makes roentgenography diagnostically useful. *Contrast agents* can be introduced to make certain body parts, e.g., the digestive tract and blood vessels, visible on the film. Contrast materials (solids, liquids, or gaseous substances) must absorb either more or fewer X rays than the surrounding tissues. Commonly used contrast agents are compounds of iodine, barium, air, and carbon dioxide. Iodine and barium absorb more X rays than soft tissues; air and carbon dioxide absorb fewer. Contrast materials are introduced into the body in four ways to view specific organs:

1. Orally or rectally for the digestive tract (esophagus, stomach, intestines) and gallbladder (Figure 14–20)

2. Intravenously for the blood vessels, bile ducts, and kidneys

3. Into the subarachnoid space for the spine and the ventricles of the brain

4. Through a nasotracheal tube or bronchoscope for the bronchial tree (This method has been used infrequently since the advent of fiberoptic bronchoscopy, which has increased the area available to direct visual examination.)

Radiography of the gastrointestinal tract often involves fluroscopy as well as a radiographic examination. **Fluoroscopy** is an examination during which X rays are used to visualize body structures on a screen. A fluroscope is a machine for examining internal structures by viewing the shadows they cast on the fluorescent screen after X rays travel through the structures. The following radiographic studies are frequently carried out:

- Gastrointestinal tract: pharynx and esophagus, upper gastrointestinal tract (**barium swallow**), and lower gastrointestinal tract (**barium enema**). See Table 14–3.

- Gallbladder (**cholecystography**) and bile ducts (**cholangiography**). See Table 14–4 on page 370.

- Urinary tract (**intravenous pyelography [IVP]**; or **intravenous urography [IVU]**). See Table 14–5 on page 371.

- Central nervous system (**myelography**). See Table 14–5.

- Vascular system (**angiography**). See Table 14–5.

TABLE 14–3 STUDIES OF THE GASTROINTESTINAL TRACT

Name	Description	Nursing Interventions	
		Preprocedure Teaching	**Postprocedure**
Barium swallow (usually part of an upper GI series)	The client swallows barium, and the pharynx and esophagus are outlined.	Procedure lasts 30 minutes. Client will be given a chalky substance (liquid barium) to drink.	Encourage fluids and activity to prevent constipation. Observe stool for whitish color, indicating client has passed barium in stool. Notify physician if barium not passed in 2 to 3 days (a laxative may be required).
Upper gastrointestinal (GI) series	The client swallows barium, and X-ray films are taken of its course through the esophagus, stomach, and duodenum.	Client must fast 4 to 6 hours before the examination. The client will be given a chalky substance (liquid barium) to drink. Procedure lasts from 30 minutes to 1 hour. Client may experience a feeling of fullness. Client may need to assume several positions on the X-ray table.	Encourage fluids and activity to prevent constipation. Observe stool for whitish color, indicating client has passed barium in stool. Client may require a laxative or enema if client is constipated or does not pass barium in 2 to 3 days.
Lower gastrointestinal series (barium enema)	A barium enema is given, and X-ray films are taken of the large intestine.	A laxative may be given the night before the test. Liquids are restricted after midnight before the test. Enemas or suppositories are given on the morning of the test to clean the bowel. The barium enema creates a feeling of fullness, and the client will feel the urge to defecate. Test usually lasts 30 to 45 minutes. There may be some cramping. Special tubes with balloons are often used to help the client retain the barium. The client will be asked to assume various positions, e.g., lying on the left side, then moving to the right side. Client will probably pass the barium at the X-ray department.	Provide a rest period afterward because procedure is fatiguing. Encourage fluids to prevent constipation. Observe stool for passage of barium, and assess regularity of movements. Notify physician if barium not passed in 2 to 3 days. An enema may be required if client does not pass all the barium.

TABLE 14-4 STUDIES OF THE GALLBLADDER AND BILE DUCTS

Name	Description	Nursing Interventions	
		Preprocedure	**Postprocedure**
Cholecystography (oral cholecystography)	X-ray films are taken of the gallbladder after a contrast dye has been given orally.	A fat-free supper is given the evening before. Check for allergy to the contrast dye, which contains iodine. A laxative may be given the evening before, or an enema the morning of the test. Six or more contrast pills (e.g., Telepaque) are given at 5-minute intervals the evening before the test, each with 4 to 6 oz water. The client fasts from midnight the evening before but may drink water. Explain that: • A fatty drink may be given during the test. • No discomfort is usually felt. • The procedure lasts about 30 to 45 minutes.	Provide a rest period. The client resumes a regular diet. A snack can be provided if the client is hungry. Assess allergy to the contrast dye.
Intravenous cholangiography	X-ray films are taken of the bile ducts after dye has been administered intravenously.	The client fasts from midnight the evening before the test but may drink water. The bowel is cleaned with a laxative the evening before or with an enema the morning of the test. Check for allergy to iodine contained in the dye. Explain that: • Iodine dye is given intravenously in the X-ray department. A test for allergy is given in the arm before the test. Study lasts 3 to 4 hours.	Assess for allergy to the dye. Observe IV site for bleeding, tenderness.
Percutaneous transhepatic cholangiography	A needle is inserted through the abdominal wall into the biliary radicle, and a contrast agent is injected. Test distinguishes between obstructive and nonobstructive jaundice.	As above for intravenous cholangiography. Explain that procedure lasts about 30 minutes.	Monitor vital signs q15 minutes for 1 hour, q30 minutes for 4 hours, and then q4 hours until client is stable. Encourage bed rest. Position client on right side to place pressure on the puncture site to prevent bleeding. Monitor puncture site for bleeding.
Postoperative cholangiography	Dye is injected through the T-tube, and X-ray films are taken and fluoroscopy is done to determine if common bile duct is unobstructed.	As above for intravenous cholangiography.	If T-tube is in place, clamp or attach to drainage as ordered. If T-tube is removed, apply sterile dressing.

TABLE 14–5   RADIOGRAPHIC STUDIES: INTRAVENOUS PYELOGRAPHY, ANGIOGRAPHY, MYELOGRAPHY

Name	Description	Nursing Interventions	
		Preprocedure	Postprocedure
Intravenous pyleography or urography (IVP, IVU)	An intravenous injection of radiopaque material is given to examine the kidneys and ureters.	A strong laxative (e.g., castor oil) is given the afternoon before the test to clear the bowel of fecal material, which can obstruct the view of the urinary structures. The client fasts from midnight prior to the test. Check for allergy to iodine. Explain that: • An intravenous injection will be administered in the X-ray department. • The procedure lasts about 1 hour.	Encourage fluid intake. The client resumes a regular diet. Provide for rest, since the laxative and fasting can cause weakness. Observe for reactions to the radiopaque dye.
Angiography, e.g., cerebral angiography (vascular system of the brain), coronary arteriography (coronary arteries of the heart), renal angiography (vascular system of the kidneys), pulmonary angiography (vascular system of the lungs).	A radiopaque material is injected into an artery or vein to examine portions of the vascular system.	For some of these procedures, a catheter may be inserted into an artery or vein prior to the injection of radiopaque material. Before some procedures, the client is given a sedative. The client fasts from midnight prior to the test. A strong laxative may be given the evening before certain tests (e.g., renal arteriography). Client will be tested for allergy to iodine. The time needed for these procedures varies. Some may take up to 3 hours.	Bed rest is generally maintained for up to 12 hours. Monitor the client's radial pulse, respirations, and blood pressure every 15 to 30 minutes until they stabilize. Monitor peripheral pulses distal to the injection site. Observe the injection site for bleeding and swelling. Cold pack may prevent swelling. Determine any discomfort experienced by the client.
Myelography	A contrast material is injected into the subarachnoid space, and X-ray films are taken of the spinal cord, nerve roots, and vertebrae.	Fasting may be required from midnight prior to the test. The client may be given a sedative prior to the procedure. Explain that: • A radiopaque oil dye is injected via a lumbar puncture in the X-ray department. • The client will assume various positions, e.g., on the side for a lumbar puncture, then prone, and then tilted on X-ray table equipped with shoulder and foot supports. • Some pain may be felt when the oil is removed, due to irritation of the nerve roots. The procedure may last about 2 hours.	The client is generally positioned flat in bed for 24 hours to minimize headache and/or nausea, but may be positioned with the head elevated above the level of the spine if the dye has not been completely removed. This prevents the dye from moving to the head and causing an inflammation of the meninges (meningitis). Monitor vital signs and neurologic status, e.g., complaints of numbness, pain, or tingling in the extremities; muscle weakness. Monitor urinary output.

Mammography is radiologic examination of breast tissue (Figure 14–21). It may be done with or without injection of a contrast agent and is performed as a screening test or to study suspicious areas before a mass is distinguishable.

Xerography or **xeromammography** is mammography using a xerographic plate instead of film. The advantages of xerography are that smaller doses of radiation are used and that the images of blood vessel patterns and tissue densities are more distinct. **Thermography** is a noninvasive screening procedure usually done before mammography. It measures and records the temperature distribution, especially areas of heat, of breast tissue.

The nurse's role in assisting with an X-ray procedure is largely to prepare the client for the examination and to provide follow-up care. Nursing responsibilities include:

* Refer to the physician's order sheet to determine the specific study ordered and the specific preparatory measures.

* Determine where the examination is to be carried out. Most X-ray examinations are performed in a radiology department. However, some scanning procedures that use radioactive materials are carried out in the nuclear medicine department of a hospital or at a community clinic.

* Determine whether medications are to be given or are canceled prior to the test. For example, a diabetic client whose diet is altered for a barium enema may have an insulin dosage canceled the morning of the test. For a diabetic client, the roentgenography may be scheduled early in the day to prevent undue disruption of routine insulin administration and diet.

* Determine the client's allergies to iodine. The oral contrast agents (e.g., Telepaque tablets) used for gallbladder X-ray films are iodine compounds. Most of the intravenous contrast agents used for angiograms and intravenous urography also contain iodine compounds.

* Provide the follow-up care required for each procedure, e.g., a laxative as ordered following an upper gastrointestinal series, or instruct the client about follow-up care. See Tables 14–3 to 14–6.

* Monitor hospitalized clients closely for discomfort and potential complications related to the procedure, e.g., allergic reactions to contrast dye.

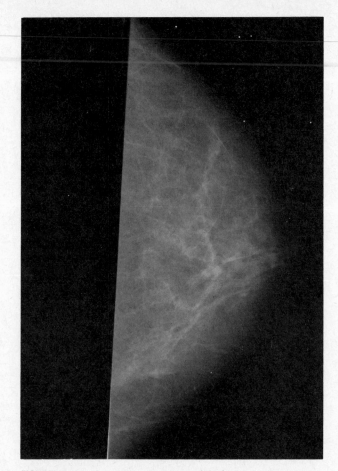

FIGURE 14–21 A normal mammogram of the breast.

* Provide or advise adequate rest periods following the procedure. Many diagnostic procedures are tiring, and in some instances several procedures are carried out on consecutive days. For example, a sigmoidoscopy may be done one day, a barium enema the next day, and a barium swallow the third day.

"High Tech" Studies

Nuclear Medicine (Radioisotopes)

The instruments and **radioisotopes** (radioactive tracers) used in nuclear medicine are constantly changing, but the fundamental principles remain the same. A basic principle is that body constituents are dynamic, not static. Isotopes enter into the same chemical reactions and metabolic processes as stable elements.

In nuclear medicine techniques, radioactive substances that have an affinity for specific body tissues

TABLE 14–6 RADIOISOTOPE STUDIES: ORGAN SCANS

Description	Preparation	Follow-Up Care
A scanning examination of a body organ following oral or intravenous administration of a radioactive substance. The specific organ to be examined gives the scan its name, e.g., brain scan, liver scan, lung scan.	Restless clients, e.g., children, may be given a sedative prior to the procedure. Assure the client there is no need to fear exposure to radiation; it is less than that acquired from the usual X-ray procedure. A radioactive substance is given orally or intravenously. Depending on the substance used, a blocking agent may also be given to prevent uptake of the radioactive substance by organs other than the one being studied, and to ensure that the substance goes into the organ being studied, e.g.: • Lugol's solution (iodine) is given to block uptake by the thyroid (given orally with juice, since its taste is unpleasant), or a potassium compound may be given to clients allergic to iodine. • Mercaptomerin sodium is given (intramuscularly) to block uptake by the kidneys. Check for allergies to the blocking agents used. Explain that: • The scan is performed in the nuclear medicine department. • There will be a brief waiting period while the radioactive substance is distributed. • There is no discomfort with the procedure. • The client will be asked to assume various positions and must remain still while the scans are taken.	Additional scans may be performed at subsequent intervals, e.g., 2 hours, 24 hours, 48 hours, and 72 hours. Assess allergic reaction to the blocking agent. It may range from mild to severe, depending on the agent used.

are introduced orally or intravenously. The scanning device may be a **scintillation counter** or a **scintillation camera**. The scintillation scanner has a probe that is passed back and forth over the body area being studied; the scintillation camera produces many images in rapid sequence, showing the transit of the isotope through blood vessels.

Radioisotopes are administered in extremely small doses, e.g., one billionth of a gram. For this reason, the body absorbs minimal amounts of radi-ation, and normal body cells are not damaged. The procedure is painless and has three steps:

1. Oral or intravenous intake of the radioisotope

2. A waiting period from 1 to 48 hours, during which the isotope is assimilated by the organ being studied

3. The scanning procedure, during which the client must remain still
See Table 14–6.

Computerized Axial Tomography (CAT or CT Scan)

Computerized axial tomography is a painless, non-invasive X-ray procedure with the unique capability of distinguishing minor differences in the radiodensity of soft tissues (Figure 14–22). For example, CAT scans can be used to distinguish liver tissue from tumor or brain tissue from hematoma. Dense substances appear white; low-density substances appear dark. The organ to be studied gives the scan its name, e.g., brain scan, liver scan, lung scan.

In this technique, a planar slice of the body is subjected to sequential sweeps, or **scans**, of a narrow X-ray beam. The unabsorbed beam emerging through the tissues is measured by a radiation detector. Data obtained are stored in a computer, which produces an image, called a **tomogram**, on a viewing apparatus or printout machine. Photographs of the image can be reproduced.

The CAT scan provides a three-dimensional view of the area under study. The scanner rotates 1° at a time through a 180° arc in about 5 minutes. At least five consecutive scans, or "cuts," of sequential parts of the organ are usually taken. Following this initial scan, the client is usually given an intravenous injection of an iodine-containing contrast material, and the entire scan is repeated. This second scan is referred to as a "contrast enhancement" scan. The entire scanning procedure takes about 1 hour. The client must remain still throughout the scan to prevent false computer results. See Table 14–6 for preparation and follow-up care.

Ultrasonography (Ultrasound)

Ultrasonography (**ultrasound**), another noninvasive technique, uses high-frequency sound waves well above the upper limit of human hearing. During this procedure, which has no known harmful effects, acoustic densities of tissues are measured. In contrast to usual radiography, ultrasound reveals the depth of a structure below the skin and the anteroposterior dimension of masses. Sound waves travel at different speeds, depending on the density of the structures through which they pass. Because sound is poorly conducted by gases and is well reflected by bone, structures containing air (such as the lung) or surrounded by bone (such as the pelvis) are difficult to examine with ultrasound.

In this technique, a transducer or probe is used as both an emitter and a receiver. The probe is moved over the structure being examined, and an ultrasound beam is directed into the body. Echoes (sounds reflected back to the probe) are translated into a dis-

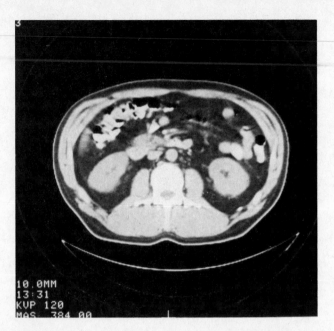

FIGURE 14–22 A CAT scan showing a midabdomen cross section. The spine is at the base; the kidneys are to the right and left of the spine.

play unit for observation and photographic recording. The test usually takes 20 to 45 minutes.

Before many ultrasound examinations, the client requires no physical preparation. Food and fluids are withheld 8 to 10 hours before examination of the abdominal organs, and some physicians may order an enema or other agent to decrease the amount of intestinal gas, which impedes the sound reflection. For examinations of the pelvic organs, the client must have some urine in the bladder to facilitate better visualization. Inform the client to void 4 hours before the procedure and then not to void until after the procedure. If this is difficult for the client, 2 hours without voiding may be acceptable if the client drinks several glasses of fluid before the examination. The client also needs to know the following:

- Mineral oil or water-soluable jelly will be spread over the skin. The oil prevents air from becoming trapped between the probe and the skin and facilitates acoustic contact.

- The procedure is painless. The client will merely feel the probe moving over the skin.

- The client will be asked to change positions on the table to allow visualization of the organ from different angles.

- During a scan of upper abdominal organs, the client may be asked periodically to inhale deeply and hold the breath for a few seconds. Inspiration displaces upper abdominal organs downward.

CRITICAL THINKING CHALLENGE

Following thoracentesis, Murray Thompson complains of shortness of breath and expectorates blood-tinged sputum. He wears an expression of fear. What action should the nurse take?

RELATED RESEARCH

Hartfield, M. T.; Cason, C. L.; and Cason, G. J. July/ August 1982. Effects of information about a threatening procedure on patients' expectations and emotional distress. *Nursing Research* 31:202–5.

REFERENCES

Bryne, C. J.; Saxton, D. F.; Pelikan, P. K.; and Nugent, P. M. 1986. *Laboratory tests: Implications for nursing care.* 2d ed. Menlo Park, Calif.: Addison-Wesley Publishing Co.

Davenport, D. O'G. June 1987. Computerized monitoring systems. *Nursing Clinics of North America* 22:495–501.

Kozier, B.; Erb, G.; and Olivieri, R. 1991. *Fundamentals of nursing: Concepts, process and practice.* Redwood City, Calif.: Addison-Wesley Publishing Co.

The Nurses' Reference Library. 1986. *Diagnostics.* 2d ed. Springhouse, Pa.: Intermed Communications.

Questions and answers about the CT scan exam: Patient education aid. April 15, 1985. *Patient Care* 19:185.

Rudolphi, D. M. April 1990. Duplex scanning. *American Journal of Nursing* 90:123–24.

Thrasher, S. B. September 1989. "What I didn't know really hurt me." . . . Preparing patients for diagnostic tests. *RN* 52:49–50.

15

OBJECTIVES

- Identify the major structures and functions of the skin

- Describe variations that occur in the skin according to age

- Identify relevant assessment data for the skin

- Identify common problems of the skin

- Perform techniques included in this chapter

- Explain reasons underlying selected steps of the techniques

- Document relevant information about the client, including all nursing assessments and interventions

Skin Hygiene

CONTENTS

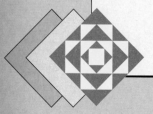

NURSING PROCESS GUIDE
SKIN HYGIENE

ASSESSMENT

Determine

- Presence of pain, itching, tingling, or numbness
- Previous experience with skin problems and associated clinical signs
- Presence of problems in other family members
- Related systemic conditions
- Use of medications, lotions, home remedies
- History of easy bruising
- Possible relation of a problem to season of year, stress, occupation, medications, recent travel, housing, personal contact, and so on
- Any recent contact with allergens, e.g., metal paint
- History of surgeries or other skin trauma
- Skin color, uniformity of color, texture, **turgor** (fullness and elasticity), temperature, presence of lesions, skin breakdown (see Chapter 11, page 210)
- Skin care practices (e.g., usual showering or bathing times, hygienic products routinely used (or *not* used because of skin problems)
- Self-care abilities (e.g., any problems managing hygienic practices)
- Allergic tendencies

Identify clients at risk:

- *Clients with alterations in nutritional status*, such as emaciation and insufficient protein intake. In emaciated individuals, subcutaneous fat is sufficient to provide padding or support over bony prominences to withstand normal stress or pressure. Individuals with inadequate protein intake are also prone to skin breakdown, since protein is essential for the building, maintenance, and repair of all body tissues.

- *Immobilized clients*. When a person cannot change position, e.g., if the person is paralyzed or unconscious, or does not change position for prolonged periods (1 or 2 hours), blood circulation, which carries essential nutrients to the skin, is reduced. Without essential nutrients, tissues of the skin are ultimately destroyed.

- *Clients with altered hydration*. In dehydrated individuals, the skin becomes excessively dry, and skin turgor is diminished. Both conditions make the skin less resistant to injury.

- *Clients with altered sensation*. Loss of sensation in a body area may be the result of paralysis or other neurologic disease. Loss of sensation reduces a person's ability to discern injurious heat and cold and to feel the tingling (pins and needles) that signals loss of circulation. This loss makes the person prone to skin damage.

- *Presence of secretions or excretions on the skin*. An accumulation of secretions, such as perspiration and sebum, or excretions, such as urine or feces, is irritating to the skin, harbors microorganisms, and makes an individual prone to skin breakdown and infection.

- *Presence of mechanical devices*. The presence of restraints, casts, or braces that create pressure or a shearing force can alter skin integrity considerably.

- *Clients with altered venous circulation*. Stasis of venous blood in the lower extremities, which is associated with varicose veins, can cause **stasis dermatitis** (inflammation of the skin) on the feet and around the ankles. This dermatitis is characterized by redness, dryness, itching, and swelling. Ultimately, skin tissues become **ischemic** (deficient of blood) and **necrotic** (dying), and ulcerations form.

RELATED DIAGNOSTIC CATEGORIES

- Self-care deficit: Bathing/hygiene
- Self-care deficit: Dressing/grooming
- Impaired skin integrity
- High risk for Impaired skin integrity
- Impaired tissue integrity
- Knowledge deficit

PLANNING

Client Goals
The client will

- Improve or maintain skin cleanliness.
- Restore or maintain skin integrity.
- Maintain circulation to the skin.
- Improve or maintain a sense of well-being.

Outcome Criteria
The Client

- Has intact, pink, smooth, soft, and hydrated skin.
- Has good tissue turgor.
- Has warm skin.
- Verbalizes less discomfort.
- Describes factors, when known, that contribute to skin alterations.
- Demonstrates hygienic and other interventions to maintain skin integrity.
- Describes interventions to prevent specific skin problems.
- Expresses positive statements about sense of well-being.
- Completes bathing/hygiene and dressing/grooming self-care activities independently.

Hygienic Care

Hygiene is the science of health and its maintenance. Personal hygiene is one aspect of self-care by which people maintain health. Hygiene is a highly personal matter determined by individual values and practices. It is also influenced by cultural, social, familial, and individual factors, as well as by the person's knowledge of health and hygiene and perceptions of personal comfort and needs.

Hygiene involves care of the skin, hair, nails, teeth, oral and nasal cavities, eyes, ears, and perineal and genital areas.

People who are very ill often are unable or lack the energy to bathe or brush their teeth, for example. They require assistance to carry out many hygienic activities. Nurses commonly use the following terms to describe kinds of hygienic care.

Early morning care is provided to clients as they awaken in the morning. Usually, it consists of providing a urinal or bedpan to the client confined to bed, washing the face and hands, and giving oral care. *Morning care* is provided after clients have breakfast. It usually includes the provision of a urinal or bedpan (to clients who are not ambulatory), a bath or shower, perineal care, back massage, and oral, nail, and hair care. Making the client's bed is part of morning care. *Afternoon care* may be provided, for example, when clients return from physiotherapy or diagnostic tests. Providing a bedpan or urinal, washing the hands and face, and assisting with oral care refresh clients. *Hour of sleep (HS) care* is provided to clients before they retire for the night. It usually involves providing for elimination needs, washing face and hands, giving oral care, and giving a back massage.

Skin

The skin is the largest organ of the body. It serves five major functions:

1. It protects underlying tissues from injury by preventing the passage of microorganisms. The skin and mucous membrane are considered the body's first line of defense.

2. It regulates the body temperature. Cooling of the body occurs through the heat loss process of evaporation of perspiration and by radiation and conduction of heat from the body when the blood vessels of the skin are vasodilated.

3. It secretes **sebum**, an oily substance that (a) softens and lubricates the hair and skin, (b) prevents the hair from becoming brittle, (c) decreases water loss from the skin when the external humidity is low, (d) lessens the amount of heat lost from the skin, and (e) has a **bactericidal** (bacteria-killing) action.

4. It transmits sensations through nerve receptors, which are sensitive to pain, temperature, touch, and pressure.

5. It produces and absorbs vitamin D in conjunction with ultraviolet rays from the sun, which activate a vitamin D precursor present in the skin.

The normal skin of a healthy person has transient microorganisms that are not usually harmful. Adults usually have some resident micrococci, bacteria of the genera *Corynebacterium* and *Propionibacterium*, and a genus of fungi, *Pityrosporon*. Children also have gram-positive, spore-forming rods and *Neisseria* bacteria. Transient microorganisms vary considerably from one person to another.

Sudoriferous (sweat) glands are on all body surfaces except the lips and parts of the genitals. The body has from two to five million sweat glands, and all are present at birth. They are most numerous on the palms of the hands and the soles of the feet. The secretion of these glands is odorless, but when decomposed or acted upon by bacteria on the skin, it takes on a musky, unpleasant odor.

Developmental Changes

In early embryonic life, the skin is a single layer of cells. Other layers develop quickly. The skin of an infant is thinner than that of an adult and usually mottled. In light-skinned infants the skin varies from pink to red and becomes ruddy when the baby cries. Babies who are genetically dark skinned are lightly pigmented at birth. Dark bluish areas due to the presence of pigmented cells in the deeper skin layers are often apparent on the lower back or buttocks of dark-skinned babies. These are referred to as **mongolian spots** (no relation to mongolism) and usually disappear spontaneously during the first year. Skin pigmentation gradually increases until about 6 to 8 weeks of age. Sweat glands begin to function at about 1 month of age.

In adolescence, the sebaceous glands increase in activity as a result of higher hormone levels. The hair follicle openings enlarge to accomodate the greater amount of sebum. The apocrine glands begin to secrete at puberty and respond to emotional stimulation. They become more active before and after monthly menses and to secrete less after menopause.

Older people also experience skin changes. The skin tends to become thinner and drier, with fine wrinkling and some inelasticity. This process occurs at various ages, from 40 on. The elderly person's skin typically shows wrinkles, sagging, pigmentations, and **keratotic spots** (horny growths, such as warts or calluses, that usually appear on areas exposed to the sun). The skin is also less resilient—that is, when it is pinched, it returns to place more slowly than the skin of a younger person.

Common Problems

Nurses frequently observe skin problems in clients. Some need to be brought to a physician's attention; others require minimal care; and still others eventually disappear spontaneously.

Erythema (redness) is associated with a variety of rashes and infections. **Petechiae** (pinpoint red areas) are caused by intradermal hemorrhages, whereas **ecchymoses** (bruises) are collections of blood beneath the skin. Initially, ecchymoses are bluish purple, firm, and tender; as the blood is reabsorbed, they become yellowish and soften.

Acne is an inflammatory condition of the **sebaceous glands** (the glands that secrete sebum). It commonly occurs in adolescence. A hair follicle becomes obstructed, causing sebum to accumulate in the follicle, and a **comedo** (blackhead) forms. The sebaceous gland is eventually destroyed, releasing fatty acids into the surrounding tissues. This causes an inflammation and the acne nodule.

In the newborn, **milia**, small white nodules (whiteheads) due to clogged sebaceous glands, are commonly present on the nose and sometimes the cheeks for several weeks. **Miliaria rubra**, a prickly heat rash, appears most often on the face, neck, and trunk, and in the diaper area of infants. It is due to excessive heat and will disappear if the baby is kept cooler, often with fewer clothes. Mongolian spots (discussed earlier under Developmental Changes) generally disappear without treatment as the baby gets older.

Hemangiomas are vascular lesions present at birth. There are several types. The nurse notes and records the size, shape, exact color (such as pink or port-wine color), and elevation (whether flat or raised from the skin) of any hemangiomas observed.

Diaper rash, also referred to as **ammonia dermatitis**, is caused by skin bacteria reacting with urea, a product related to ammonia and excreted in the urine. The reaction is irritating to the baby's **perineum** and buttocks, causing them to become red and sore. Most diaper rashes can be prevented by keeping the buttocks clean and dry. Protective ointments containing zinc oxide may also be preventive.

General Guidelines for Skin Care

1. *An intact, healthy skin is the body's first line of defense.* Nurses need to ensure that all skin care measures prevent injury and irritation. Scratching the skin with jewelry or long, sharp fingernails is avoided. Harsh rubbing or use of rough towels and washcloths can cause tissue damage, particularly when the skin is irritated or when circulation or sensation is diminished. Bottom bedsheets are kept taut and free from wrinkles to reduce friction and abrasion to the skin. Top bed linens are arranged to prevent undue pressure on the toes. When necessary, bed cradles or footboards are used to keep bedclothes off the feet.

2. *The degree to which the skin protects the underlying tissues from injury depends on the general health of the cells, the amount of subcutaneous tissue, and the dryness of the skin.* Skin that is poorly nourished and dry has less ability to protect and is more vulnerable to injury. When the skin is dry, lotions or creams with lanolin are applied, and bathing is limited to once or twice a week. For back rubs, lotion is used rather than alcohol. The greater the amount of subcutaneous tissue, the more padding there is, particularly over bony prominences. Nurses also assess the client's nutritional and fluid intake. When either one is deficient, nurses should take measures if possible to improve it.

3. *Moisture in contact with the skin for a period of time can result in increased bacterial growth and irritation.* After a bath, the nurse dries the client's skin carefully, paying particular attention to areas such as the axillae, the groin, beneath the breasts, and between the toes, where the potential for irritation is greatest. A nonirritating dusting powder, such as cornstarch, tends to reduce moisture and can be applied to these areas after they are dried. Clients who are incontinent of urine or feces or perspire excessively, should receive immediate cleaning to prevent skin irritation.

4. *Body odors are caused by resident skin bacteria acting on body secretions.* Cleanliness is the best deodorant. Commercial deodorants and antiperspirants can be applied only after the skin is cleaned. Deodorants diminish odors, whereas antiperspirants reduce the amount of perspiration. Neither is applied immediately after shaving, because of the possibility of skin irritation. Nor are they used on skin that is already irritated.

5. *Skin sensitivity to irritation and injury varies among individuals and in accordance with their health.* Generally, skin sensitivity is greater in infants, very young children, and the elderly. A person's nutritional status also affects sensitivity. Emaciated or obese per-

sons tend to experience more skin irritation and injury. The same tendency is seen in individuals with inadequate dietary habits and insufficient fluid intake. Even in healthy persons, skin sensitivity is highly variable. Some people's skin is sensitive to chemicals in skin care agents and cosmetics. Hypoallergenic cosmetics and soaps or soap substitutes are now available for these people. The nurse needs to ascertain whether the client has any sensitivities and what agents are appropriate to use.

Bathing and Skin Care

Bathing removes accumulated oil, perspiration, dead skin cells, and some bacteria. The nurse can appreciate the quantity of oil and dead skin cells produced when observing the skin of a person after the removal of a cast that has been on for 6 weeks. The skin is crusty, flaky, and dry underneath the cast. Applications of oil over several days are usually necessary to remove the debris.

Excessive bathing, however, can interfere with the intended lubricating effect of the sebum, causing dryness of the skin. This is an important consideration of people, e.g., the elderly, who produce limited sebum.

In addition to cleaning the skin, bathing also stimulates circulation. A warm or hot bath dilates superficial arterioles, bringing more blood and nourishment to the skin. Vigorous rubbing has the same effect. Rubbing with long smooth strokes from the distal to proximal parts of extremities (from the point farthest from the body to the point closest) is particularly effective in facilitating venous blood flow.

Bathing also produces a sense of well-being. It is refreshing and relaxing and frequently improves morale, appearance, and self-respect. Some people take a morning shower for its refreshing, stimulating effect. Others prefer an evening bath because it is relaxing. These effects are more evident when a person is ill. For example, it is not uncommon for clients who have had a restless or sleepless night to feel relaxed, comfortable, and sleepy after a morning bath.

Bathing offers an excellent opportunity for the nurse to assess ill clients. The nurse can observe the condition of the client's skin and physical conditions such as sacral edema or rashes. While assisting a client with a bath, the nurse can also assess the client's psychosocial needs, e.g., orientation to time and ability to cope with the illness. Learning needs, such as a diabetic client's need to learn foot care, can also be assessed.

There are generally two categories of baths given to clients: cleaning and therapeutic. *Cleaning baths*

are given chiefly for hygienic purposes and include these types:

- *Complete bed bath.* The nurse washes the entire body of a dependent client in bed.

- *Self-help bed bath.* Clients confined to bed are able to bathe themselves with help from the nurse for washing the back and perhaps the feet.

- *Partial bath (abbreviated bath).* Only parts of the client's body that might cause discomfort or odor, if neglected, are washed: the face, hands, axillae, perineal area, and back. Omitted are the arms, chest, abdomen, legs, and feet. The nurse provides this care for dependent clients and assists self-sufficient clients confined to bed by washing their backs. Some ambulatory clients prefer to take a partial bath at the sink. The nurse can assist them by washing their backs.

- *Tub bath.* Tub baths are preferred to bed baths, because washing and rinsing are easier in a tub. Tubs are also used for therapeutic baths. The amount of assistance the nurse offers depends on the abilities of the client. Many agencies have specially designed tubs for dependent clients. These tubs greatly reduce the work of the nurse in lifting clients in and out of the tub and have greater benefits than a sponge bath in bed.

- *Shower.* Many ambulatory clients are able to use shower facilities and require only minimal assistance from the nurse.

The water should feel comfortably warm to the client. People vary in their sensitivity to heat; generally, the temperature should be 43 to 46 C (110 to 115 F). Most clients will verify a suitable temperature. The water for a bed bath should be changed at least once.

Therapeutic baths are given for physical effects, such as to soothe irritated skin or to treat an area (e.g., the perineum). Medications may be placed in the water. A therapeutic bath is generally taken in a tub one-third or one-half full, about 114 liters (30 gal). The client remains in the bath for a designated time, often 20 to 30 minutes. If the client's back, chest, and arms are to be treated, these areas need to be immersed in the solution. The bath temperature is generally included in the order; 37.7 to 46 C (100 to 115 F) may be ordered for adults and 40.5 C (105 F) is usually ordered for infants. Commonly used types of therapeutic baths include saline, oatmeal, and sodium bicarbonate.

Because of the increasing acuity of hospitalized clients, many clients receive intravenous therapy. The nurse needs to pay special attention when changing the client's gown after the bath (or whenever the gown becomes soiled). General guidelines (see the box below) for changing the gown may be modified to suit the equipment in use.

Technique 15–1 provides guidelines for bathing adult and pediatric clients.

Changing a Hospital Gown for a Client with an Intravenous Infusion

- Slip the gown completely off the arm without the infusion and onto the tubing connected to the arm with the infusion.
- Holding the container above the client's arm, slide the sleeve up over the container to remove the used gown.
- Place the clean gown sleeve for the arm with the infusion over the container as if it were an extension of the client's arm, from the inside of the gown to the sleeve cuff.

- Rehang the container. Slide the gown carefully over the tubing toward the client's hand.
- Guide the client's arm and tubing into the sleeve, taking care not to pull on the tubing.
- Assist the client to put the other arm into the second sleeve of the gown, and fasten as usual.
- Count the rate of flow of the infusion to make sure it is correct before leaving the bedside.

 15-1 # Bathing an Adult or Pediatric Client

Before commencing to bathe a client, determine: (a) the type of bath the client needs, and what assistance the clients requires, and (b) other care the client is receiving, such as roentgenography or physiotherapy, so that the bath can be coordinated with those activities to prevent undue fatigue, and (c) the bed linen required by the client.

 When bathing a client who is HIV positive, the caregiver should wear gloves when in the presence of body fluids or open lesions.

PURPOSES
- To clean and deodorize the skin
- To stimulate circulation to the skin
- To produce a sense of well-being
- To promote relaxation and comfort
- To prevent or eliminate unpleasant body odors

ASSESSMENT FOCUS

Condition of the skin (color, texture and turgor, presence of pigmented spots, temperature, lesions, excoriations, and abrasions); fatigue; presence of pain and need for adjunctive measures, e.g., an analgesic before the bath; range of motion of the joints and any other aspects of health that affect the bathing process.

EQUIPMENT

- Bedpan or urinal
- Changing table
- Bath blanket
- Gloves (if giving perineal care)
- Washcloth

- Soap
- Basin
- Water between 43 and 46 C (110 and 115 F) for adults, 38 and 40 C (100 and 105 F) for children
- Two bath towels

- Additional bed linen and towels, if required
- Hygienic supplies such as lotion, powder, and deodorant
- Clean gown or pajamas as needed

▶ **Technique 15–1 Bathing an Adult or Pediatric Client** CONTINUED

INTERVENTION

1. Prepare the client and the environment.

▶ • Invite a parent or family member to participate if desired.

• Close the windows and doors to make sure that the room is free from drafts. *Air currents increase loss of heat from the body by convection.*

• Provide privacy by drawing the curtains or closing the door. *Hygiene is a personal matter.* Some agencies provide signs indicating the need for privacy.

• Offer the client a bedpan or urinal or ask whether the client wishes to use the toilet or commode. *The client will be more comfortable after voiding, and voiding before cleaning the perineum is advisable.*

• During the bath, assess each area of the skin carefully.

For a Bed Bath

2. Prepare the bed, and position the client appropriately.

▶ • Place the bed in the high position. Place an infant or small child on a changing table or elevated crib. *This avoids undue strain on the nurse's back.*

• Remove the top bed linen, and replace it with the bath blanket. If the bed linen is to be reused, place it over the bedside chair. If it is to be changed, place it in the linen hamper.

• Assist the client to move near you. *This facilitates access without undue reaching and straining.*

• Remove the gown.

3. Make a bath mitt with the washcloth (Figure 15–1). *A bath mitt retains water and heat better than a cloth loosely held.*

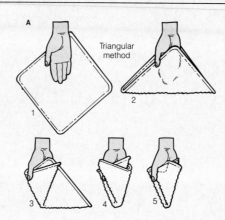

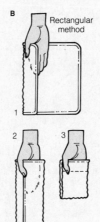

FIGURE 15–1 Making a bath mitt: *A,* triangular method; *B,* rectangular method.

• Triangular method: (1) Lay your hand on the washcloth; (2) fold the top corner over your hand; (3,4) fold the side corners over your hand; (5) tuck the second corner under the cloth on the palmar side to secure the mitt.

• Rectangular method: (1) Lay your hand on the washcloth, and fold one side over your hand; (2) fold the second side over your hand; (3) fold the top of the cloth down, and tuck it under the folded side against your palm to secure the mitt.

4. Wash the face.

• Place one towel across the client's chest.

• Wash the client's eyes with water only, and dry them well. Use a separate corner of the washcloth for each eye. *Using separate corners prevents transmitting microorganisms from one eye to the other.* Wipe from the inner to the outer canthus. *Cleaning from the inner to the outer canthus prevents secretions from entering the nasolacrimal ducts.*

• Ask whether the client wants soap used on the face. *Soap has a drying effect, and the face, which is exposed to the air more than other body parts, tends to be drier.*

• Wash, rinse, and dry the client's face, neck, and ears.

5. Wash the arms and hands.

• Place the bath towel lengthwise under the arm. *It protects the bed from becoming wet.*

• Wash, rinse, and dry the arm, using long, firm strokes from distal to proximal areas (from the point farthest from the body to the point closest. *Firm strokes from distal to proximal areas increase venous blood return.*

• Wash the axilla well. Repeat for the other arm. (Omit the arms for a partial bath.) Exercise caution if an intravenous infusion is present, and check its flow after moving the arm.

• Place a towel directly on the bed, and put the basin on it. Place the client's hands in the basin. *Many clients enjoy immersing their hands in the basin and washing themselves.* Assist the client as needed to wash, rinse, and dry the hands, paying particular attention to the spaces between the fingers.

6. Wash the chest and abdomen.

• Fold the bath blanket down to the client's pubic area, and place

▶ **Technique 15–1** *CONTINUED*

the towel alongside the chest and abdomen.

- Wash, rinse, and dry the chest and abdomen, giving special attention to the skinfold under the breasts. Keep the chest and abdomen covered with the towel between the wash and the rinse.

- Replace the bath blanket when the areas have been dried. (Omit the chest and abdomen for a partial bath. However, the creases under a woman's breasts may require bathing if they are irritated.) Avoid undue exposure when washing the chest and abdomen. For some clients, it may be preferable to wash the chest and the abdomen separately. In that case, place the bath towel horizontally across the abdomen first and then across the chest.

7. Wash the legs and feet.

- Wrap one of the client's legs and feet with the bath blanket, ensuring that the pubic area is well covered (Figure 15–2).

- Place the bath towel lengthwise under the other leg, and wash that leg. Use long, smooth, firm strokes, washing from the ankle to the knee to the thigh. *Washing from distal to proximal areas stimulates venous blood flow.*

- Rinse and dry that leg, reverse the coverings, and repeat for the

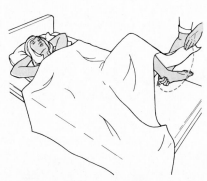

FIGURE 15-2 Draping one leg of the client.

other leg. (Omit legs and feet for a partial bath.)

- Wash the feet by placing them in the basin of water.

- Dry each foot. Pay particular attention to the spaces between the toes. If you prefer, wash one foot after that leg, before washing the other leg.

- Obtain fresh, warm bath water now or when necessary. *The temperature of the water in the basin cools relatively rapidly, and the water becomes soapy.*

8. Wash the back and perineum.

- Assist the client to turn to a prone position or side-lying position facing away from you, and place the bath towel lengthwise alongside the back and buttocks.

- Wash and dry the back, buttocks, and upper thighs, paying particular attention to the gluteal folds. Give a back rub (see Technique 15–3). Avoid undue exposure of the client, as for the abdomen and chest. See above.

- Assist the client to the supine position, and determine whether the client can wash the genital-perineal area independently. If the client cannot do so, drape the client as shown in Figure 15–3 on page 386, and wash the area. See Technique 15–2.

9. Assist the client with grooming aids such as powder, lotion, or deodorant.

- Use powder sparingly. Release as little as possible into the atmosphere. *This will avoid irritation of the respiratory tract by powder inhalation.*

- Help the client to put on a clean gown or pajamas.

- Assist the client to care for hair, mouth, and nails. Some people

prefer or need mouth care prior to the bath.

10. Document pertinent data.

- Record assessments, such as excoriation in the folds beneath the breasts or reddened areas over bony prominences and progress in relief of previous problems.

- Record the type of bath given (i.e., complete, partial, or self-help). This is usually recorded on a flow sheet.

For a Tub Bath or Shower

11. Prepare the client and the tub.

- Fill the tub about one-third to one-half full of water at 43 to 46 C (110 to 115 F). *Sufficient water is needed to cover the perineal area.*

- Cover all intravenous catheters or wound dressings with plastic coverings, and instruct client to prevent wetting area as much as possible.

- Secure assistance with holding a pediatric client as indicated. *Holding may be necessary to minimize contamination of open skin areas.*

- Apply a rubber bath mat or towel to the floor of the tub, if safety strips are not on tub floor. *These prevent slippage of the client during the bath or shower.*

- Use a small basin or large sink for a small child. *Smaller containers decrease the danger of slippage of an active child and possible drowning.*

12. Assist the client into the shower or tub.

- Assist the client taking a standing shower with the initial adjustment of the water temperature and water flow pressure, as needed.

▶

► **Technique 15–1 Bathing an Adult or Pediatric Client** CONTINUED

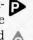

- If the client requires considerable assistance with a tub bath, a second nurse may be needed to help the client into and out of the tub or to hold the client in a sitting position throughout the bath. Instruct the client to hold the handbar while you support the upper trunk under the axillae. To provide support as the client sits down in the tub, fold a towel lengthwise, and place it around the chest under both axillae; then hold the ends securely at the back as the client sits. It may be helpful to seat the client on the edge of the tub or on a chair beside the tub before transferring the client into the tub.

- Explain how the client can signal for help, and leave the client for 2 to 5 minutes.

- Never leave an infant or small pediatric client unattended in a tub. *Slippage and drowning can occur in a matter of seconds and in very little water.*

13. Assist the client with washing and getting out of the tub.

- Wash the client's back, lower legs, and feet, if necessary.

- Assist the client out of the tub. If the client is unsteady, drain the tub of water before the client attempts to get out of it, and place a bath towel over the client's shoulders. *Draining the water first lessens the likelihood of a fall. The towel prevents chilling.*

14. Dry the client, and assist with follow-up care.

- Follow step 9.

- Assist the client back to the room, and provide a back rub if the client is spending long periods in bed. See Technique 15–3.

- Clean the tub or shower in accordance with agency practice, discard used linen in the laundry hamper, and place the "unoccupied" sign on the door.

15. Document pertinent data.

- Follow step 10.

EVALUATION FOCUS

Client tolerance of procedure (note respiratory rate and effort, and pulse rate); status of skin (dryness, turgor, lesions, and so on); client strength and percentage of bath done without assistance.

SAMPLE RECORDING

Date	Time	Notes
6/6/93	0800	Full bath, P 56, R 20 unchanged. Skin moist, decreased turgor. Sacral skin reddened; no broken areas. Lotion applied to sacrum. No complaints of pain during or after bathing. Range of motion exercises carried out on lower extremities. ———————————— Rozelle Ho, SN

KEY ELEMENTS OF BATHING AN ADULT OR PEDIATRIC CLIENT

For Bed Bath

- Determine allergies to soap; detergents; bath oils; skin creams, powders, and lotions; and deodorants or antiperspirants.

- Prevent undue exposure of the client.

- Clean eyes with water only, proceeding from the inner to the outer canthus. Use separate corners of the washcloth for each eye.

- Use firm strokes on the extremities from distal to proximal areas to stimulate venous blood flow.

- Thoroughly rinse and dry areas with creases and skinfolds, e.g., beneath the breasts, gluteal folds, between toes and fingers, and perineum.

For a Tub Bath or Shower

- Instruct the client how to call for assistance.

- Use safety precautions when assisting clients into and out of a tub.

Perineal–Genital Care

Perineal–genital care is also referred to as *perineal care* or *peri-care*. Perineal care is a part of the bed bath that may be an embarrassing procedure for many clients. Nurses also may find it embarrassing initially, particularly with clients of the opposite sex. Most clients who require a bed bath from the nurse are able to clean their own genital areas with minimal assistance. The nurse may need to hand a moistened washcloth and soap to the client, rinse the washcloth, and provide a towel.

Because some clients are unfamiliar with terminology for the genitals and perineum, it may be difficult for nurses to explain what is expected. Most clients, however, understand what is meant if the nurse simply says, "I'll give you a washcloth to finish your bath." Older clients may be familiar with the term *private parts*. Whatever expression the nurse uses, it needs to be one that the client understands and one that is comfortable for the nurse to use.

The nurse needs to provide perineal care efficiently and matter-of-factly. Some nurses wear gloves while providing this care for the comfort of the client and to protect themselves from infection. Technique 15–2 explains how to provide perineal–genital care.

15-2 Providing Perineal–Genital Care

PURPOSES
- To remove normal perineal secretions and odors
- To prevent infection, e.g., when an indwelling catheter is present
- To promote client comfort

ASSESSMENT FOCUS

Presence of irritation, excoriation, inflammation, swelling; excessive discharge; odor; pain or discomfort; presence of urinary or fecal incontinence; recent rectal or perineal surgery; presence of indwelling catheter; perineal–genital hygiene practices; self-care abilities.

EQUIPMENT

Perineal–genital care provided in conjunction with the bed bath
- Bath towel
- Bath blanket
- Disposable gloves
- Bath basin two-thirds filled with water at 43 to 46 C (110 to 115 F)
- Soap

- Washcloth
- Protective ointment as required

Special perineal–genital care
- Bath towel
- Bath blanket
- Disposable gloves
- Cotton balls or swabs

- Solution bottle, pitcher, or container filled with warm water or a prescribed solution
- Bedpan to receive rinse water
- Moisture-resistant bag or receptacle for used cotton swabs
- Perineal pad

INTERVENTION

1. Prepare the client.

- Offer the client an appropriate explanation, being particularly sensitive to any embarrassment felt by the client.

- Determine whether the client is experiencing any discomfort in the genital-perineal area.

- Fold the top bed linen to the foot of the bed, and fold the gown up to expose the genital area.

- Place a bath towel under the client's hips so that the lower end can be used to dry the anterior perineum, while the upper end can dry the rectal area. *The bath towel also prevents the bed from becoming soiled.*

2. Position and drape the client, and clean the upper inner thighs.

For females

- Position the female in a back-lying position, with the knees

▶

▶ **Technique 15–2 Providing Perineal–Genital Care** *CONTINUED*

flexed and spread well apart (abducted).

- Cover her body and legs with the bath blanket. Drape the legs by tucking the bottom corners of the bath blanket under the inner sides of the legs (Figure 15–3). *Minimum exposure lessens embarrassment and helps to provide warmth.* Bring the middle portion of the base of the blanket up over the pubic area.

- Don gloves, and wash and dry the upper inner thighs.

For males

- Position the male client in a supine position with knees slightly flexed and hips slightly externally rotated.

- Don gloves, and wash and dry the upper inner thighs.

3. **Inspect the perineal area**.

- Note particular areas of inflammation, excoriation, or swelling, especially between the labia in females and the scrotal folds in males.

- Also note excessive discharge or secretions from the perineal-genital orifices and the presence of odors.

4. **Wash and dry the perineal–genital area**.

For females

- Clean the labia majora. Then spread the labia to wash the folds between the labia majora and the labia minora (Figure 15–4). *Secretions that tend to collect around the labia minora facilitate bacterial growth.*

- Use separate quarters of the washcloth for each stroke, and wipe from the pubis to the rectum. For menstruating women and clients with indwelling catheters, use cotton balls or gauze. Take a clean ball for each stroke. *Using separate quarters of the*

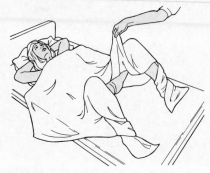

FIGURE 15–3 Draping the client for perineal-genital care.

washcloth or new cotton balls or gauzes prevents the transmission of microorganisms from one area to the other. Wiping is done from the area of least contamination (the pubis) to the area of greatest contamination (the rectum).

- Rinse the area well. You may place the client on a bedpan and pour a pitcher of warm water over the area. Dry the perineum thoroughly, paying particular attention to the folds between the labia. *Moisture supports the growth of many microorganisms.*

For males

- Wash and dry the penis, using firm strokes. *Handling the penis firmly may prevent an erection.*

- If the client is uncircumcised, retract the prepuce (foreskin) to expose the glans penis (the tip of the penis) for cleaning. Replace the foreskin after cleaning the glans penis (Figure 15–5.). *Retracting the foreskin is necessary*

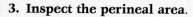

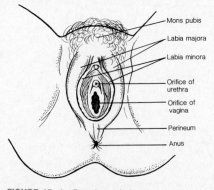

FIGURE 15–4 Female genitals.

to remove the smegma that collects under the foreskin and facilitates bacterial growth.

- Wash and dry the scrotum. The posterior folds of the scrotum may need to be cleaned with the buttocks. *The scrotum tends to be more soiled than the penis because of its proximity to the rectum; thus it is usually cleaned after the penis is cleaned.*

5. **Inspect perineal orifices for intactness**.

- Inspect particularly around the urethra in clients with indwelling catheters. *A catheter may cause excoriation around the urethra.*

- Apply protective ointment, if necessary.

6. **Clean between the buttocks.**

- Assist the client to turn on the side facing away from you.

- Pay particular attention to the anal area and posterior folds of the scrotum in males. Clean the anus with toilet tissue before washing it, if necessary.

- Dry the area well.

- Apply protective ointments, such as petroleum jelly, if necessary.

- For postdelivery females, apply a perineal pad as needed from front to back. *This prevents contamination of the vagina and urethra from the anal area.*

7. **Document any assessments such as redness, swelling, or discharge.**

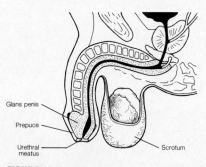

FIGURE 15–5 Male genitals.

▶ **Technique 15–2** *CONTINUED*

EVALUATION FOCUS	Perineal–genital skin integrity; presence of inflammation, excoriation, swelling, discharge; localized areas of tenderness.

SAMPLE RECORDING

Date	Time	Notes
7/10/93	0900	Perineal care given. Circular reddened area about 2.5 cm diameter to left of urethral orifice. No discharge no odor. ———— Patricia L. Snow, SN

KEY ELEMENTS OF PROVIDING PERINEAL–GENITAL CARE

- Carefully inspect the perineal and urethral areas for irritation or signs of excoriation and the presence of any discharge.
- Don gloves.

- Thoroughly rinse and dry the perineal area, paying particular attention to skinfold areas.
- Apply ointment to protect excoriated areas.

Back Rubs

Back rubs, or massage of the back, have two chief objectives: to relax and relieve tension (sedative effect), and to stimulate blood circulation to the tissues and the muscles. Friction from the rubbing produces heat at the skin surface. Heat dilates the peripheral blood vessels in the area, thus increasing the blood supply to the area. Because tissues are under pressure when a client is in bed and muscles are usually relaxed, stimulation of the circulation is essential so that the tissues obtain nutrients and oxygen.

Emollient creams and lotions are frequently used to lubricate the skin during back rubs. Unless another agent is specifically ordered, lotion is preferred because of its lubricating action on the skin. Powder is sometimes used. Alcohol preparations are cooling, but they are used infrequently today. Although they are refreshing and toughen skin by hardening the skin protein, they tend to dry the skin, and very dry skin is likely to crack. Breaks in the skin can predispose to **decubitus ulcers**. Alcohol preparations are particularly undesirable for use on elderly clients, whose skin is usually dry. Dehydrated and poorly nourished clients may also not benefit from an alcohol back rub.

The position of choice for a back rub is the prone position (lying on the stomach). The second preferred position is the side-lying position; its disadvantage is the difficulty of massaging the lateral aspect of the hip on which the client is lying, and the client must be turned to the other side.

Other pressure points on the body that generally benefit from massage and the application of lotions are the elbows, knees, and heels. Sometimes massage of the anterior aspects of both iliac crests of very thin clients is also indicated. Nurses are advised not to rub tender, reddened areas on the lower legs of clients, particularly the calves. Redness, tenderness, and heat, particularly along the course of a vein, may indicate a thrombus (blood clot) in the area. Massage might dislodge the clot, which could travel to the heart or the lung, causing a myocardial or pulmonary embolus. This can present a very serious problem. Technique 15–3 provides guidelines for giving a back rub.

15-3 Giving a Back Rub

Before commencing a back rub, determine (a) previous assessments of the skin, (b) special lotions to be used, and (c) positions contraindicated for the client.

PURPOSES
- To promote relaxation and comfort
- To stimulate blood circulation to the tissues in the area, thereby preventing decubitus ulcers
- To relieve muscle tension and/or pain

ASSESSMENT FOCUS
> Areas of potential impaired skin integrity; behavior indicating or complaints of muscle tension.

EQUIPMENT
- Lotion, alcohol, or powder
- Towel

INTERVENTION

1. Prepare the client.

- Assist the client to move to the near side of the bed within your reach.

- Establish which position the client prefers. The prone position is recommended for a back rub. A client who cannot assume this position assumes a side-lying position but will need to turn to the other side for you to complete the massage.

- Expose the back from the shoulders to the inferior sacral area.

2. Massage the back.

- Pour a small amount of lotion onto the palms of your hands, and hold it for a minute, or place the container in a bath basin filled with warm water. *Back rub preparations tend to feel uncomfortably cold to people. Holding warms the solution, so that it will be more comfortable.*

- Rub in a circular motion over the sacral area.

- Move your hands up the center of the back and then over both scapulae.

- Massage in a circular motion over the scapulae.

- Move your hands down the sides of the back.

- Massage the areas over the right and left iliac crests (Figure 15–6).

- Repeat above for 3 to 5 minutes, obtaining more lotion as necessary.

- While massaging the skin, inspect for (a) whitish or reddened skin areas that do not disappear after rubbing and (b) broken or raw skin areas, especially on the elbows or heels.

- Massage directly over pressure areas gently and only if there is no evidence of underlying tissue damage. If there is evidence of pressure, massage around the area, not directly on it. *Vigorous massage over bony prominences*

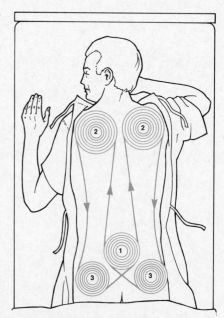

FIGURE 15–6 One suggested pattern for a back massage.

can increase damage in nutrient-deprived tissues.

- Pat dry any excess solution with a towel.

3. Document assessments.

EVALUATION FOCUS
> Areas of redness; broken skin areas; skin dryness.

► **Technique 15–3** *CONTINUED*

Date	Time	Notes
7/7/93	1600	Back rubs with lotion provided q 3h. Whitened area 1.5 cm diameter over right ilium. Positioned on left side. No broken areas. No discomfort verbalized. — ————————————————— Natalie McLean, SN

KEY ELEMENTS OF GIVING A BACK RUB

- Massage pressure areas gently and only if there is no evidence of underlying tissue damage.
- Inspect skin areas of pressure points for whitened or reddened areas that do not disappear after rubbing.
- Measure the size of broken and raw skin areas.

Infant Hygiene Care

Practices in the hygienic care of infants vary considerably. For example, in some agencies the nurse bathes the newborn when it is first admitted to the nursery; in others, the nurse simply removes any birth debris from the infant's face, for aesthetic reasons, and then diapers and wraps the baby warmly in a blanket. Some agencies require that the nurse remove the **vernix caseosa** (the whitish, cheesy, greasy protective material found on the skin at birth), whereas others do not. When the newborn's status is stabilized, daily hygienic care often includes a sponge bath until the umbilical cord stump falls off. Cord care and, for some male infants, circumcision care are also required. The cord stump usually falls off spontaneously in 5 to 8 days, but it may remain up to 2 weeks. Technique 15–4 explains how to give an infant sponge bath.

After the cord stump has separated and the umbilicus is healed, the infant's body can be immersed in a tub of water. New parents need information from the nurse about this basic hygienic care. Many agencies provide bath demonstrations and opportunities for new parents to ask questions before they leave the hospital. Technique 15–5 describes how to give an infant tub bath. Technique 15–6 describes how to change a diaper.

 Giving an Infant Sponge Bath

 Before commencing the infant's sponge bath, determine (a) if the infant is HIV positive and is stooling or has open skin lesions, (b) whether the infant's eyes, face, and scalp are to be washed before or after the infant is undressed (agency protocols vary), (c) whether the infant requires a complete or partial bath, (d) whether the baby's weight is to be taken in conjunction with the bath; and (e) whether the infant's temperature is to be taken after the bath.

PURPOSES
- To remove the vernix caseosa that covers the skin of the fetus, particularly from creases and folds, such as under the foreskin of the glans penis in male babies and between the labia in female babies, if required
- To clean the skin, including the scalp, genitals, and buttocks
- To provide care for the umbilical cord stump
- To assess the skin, healing of the cord stump and circumcision incision, and general physical growth and functioning

►

▶ **Technique 15–4 Giving an Infant Sponge Bath** *CONTINUED*

ASSESSMENT FOCUS	Dry, cracked, or peeling skin areas; cradle cap on the scalp; signs of redness at the cord stump or a foul-smelling discharge around the umbilicus; diaper rash, healing of circumcision, overall color of skin.

EQUIPMENT

- Basin with bath water at 38 to 40 C (100 to 105 F)
- Gloves (optional)
- Towel to place under the baby during the bath
- Disposable cups
- Soft washcloth or absorbent pad
- Cotton balls
- Moisture-resistant bag
- Mild, nonperfumed soap in a container
- Soft-bristled brush or baby comb
- Isopropyl alcohol
- Bath blanket or towel to cover the infant
- Mild lotion or baby oil if needed for dry skin
- Shirt and/or nightgown
- Diaper

INTERVENTION

1. Prepare the environment.

- Wash hands before handling a newborn, because infants have few defenses against unfamiliar microorganisms.

- Ensure that the room is warm and free of drafts. *This is particularly important when caring for newborns, because their temperature-regulating mechanisms are not completely developed.*

- Measure the temperature of the water with a bath thermometer, or test it against the inside of your wrist or elbow.

- Don gloves, if necessary.

2. Prepare the infant.

- Remove the infant's diaper, and wipe away any feces on the baby's perineum with tissues.

- Reassure the infant before and during the bath by talking in soothing tones, and hold the infant firmly but gently.

- Undress the infant, and bundle it in a supine position in a towel.

- Place small articles such as safety pins out of the infant's reach.

- Ascertain the infant's weight and vital signs. They are often measured in conjunction with a bath.

3. Wash the infant's head.

- Clean the baby's eyes with water only, using a washcloth or cotton balls. Use a separate corner of the washcloth or a separate ball for each eye. Wipe from the inner to the outer canthus. Some nurses prefer to wash the infant's eyes, face, and scalp *before* the infant is undressed. Dispose of cotton balls in moisture-resistant bag. *Using a separate corner or ball prevents the transmission of microorganisms from one eye to the other. Wiping away from the inner canthus avoids wiping debris into the nasolacrimal duct.*

- Wash and dry the baby's face using water only. Soap may be used to clean the ears. *Soap can be very irritating to the eyes.*

- Pick the baby up using the football hold; that is, hold the baby against your side, supporting the body with your forearm and the head with the palm of your hand (Figure 15–7). Position the baby's head over the washbasin, and lather the scalp with a mild soap. Massage the lather over the scalp using the soft-bristled brush, the baby comb, or your fingertips. *This loosens any dry scales from the scalp and helps to*

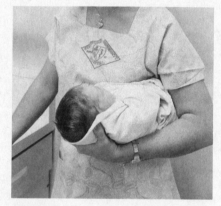

FIGURE 15–7 Using a football hold to carry an infant.

prevent cradle cap. If cradle cap is present, it may be treated with baby oil, a dandruff shampoo, or ointment prescribed by the physician.

- Rinse and dry the scalp well. Place the baby supine again.

4. Wash the infant's body.

- Wash, rinse, and dry each arm and hand, paying particular attention to the axilla. Avoid excessive rubbing. Dry thoroughly. *Rubbing can cause skin irritation, and moisture can cause excoriation of the skin.*

▶ **Technique 15–4** CONTINUED

- Wash, rinse, and dry the baby's chest and abdomen.

- Keep the baby covered with the bath blanket or towel between washing and rinsing. *Covering the infant prevents chilling.*

- Clean the base of the umbilical cord with a cotton ball dipped in 70% isopropyl alcohol. Other antiseptics, such as povidone-iodine (Betadine) are also used. *Using alcohol promotes drying and prevents infection.*

- Wash, rinse, and dry the baby's legs and feet. Expose only one leg and foot at a time. Give special attention to the areas between the toes. *Keeping exposure to a minimum maintains the baby's warmth.*

- Turn the baby on the stomach or side. Wash, rinse, and dry the back.

5. Clean the genitals and anterior perineum.

- Place the baby on the back. Clean and dry the genitals and anterior perineal area from front to back. *The rectal area is cleaned last because it is the most contaminated.*

- Clean the folds of the groin.

- For females, separate the labia, and clean between them. Clean the genital area from front to back, using moistened cotton balls. Use a clean swab for each stroke. *The smegma that collects between the folds of the labia (and under the foreskin in males) facilitates bacterial growth and should be removed. Lotions, powders,* *and so on, can also accumulate between the labia and need to be removed. Clean swabs are used to avoid spreading microorganisms from the rectal area to the urethra.*

- If a male infant is uncircumcised, retract the foreskin if possible, and clean the glans penis, using a moistened cotton ball. If the foreskin is tight, do not forcibly retract it. Gentle pressure on a tight foreskin over a period of days or weeks may accomplish eventual retraction. **Phimosis** (narrowness of the opening of the foreskin) may require correction by circumcision. After swabbing, replace the foreskin to prevent edema (swelling) of the glans penis. Clean the shaft of the penis and the scrotum. In some agencies, the foreskin is not retracted.

- If a male infant has been recently circumcised, clean the glans penis by gently squeezing a cotton ball moistened with clear water over the site. Note any signs of bleeding or infection. In some agencies, petroleum jelly or a bactericidal ointment is applied to the circumcision site. Avoid applying excessive quantities of ointment. *Excess ointment may obstruct the urinary meatus.*

- Apply A and D Ointment (lanolin and petrolatum) to the perineum according to agency protocol. *This helps prevent diaper rash.*

6. Clean the posterior perineum and buttocks.

- Grasp both of the baby's ankles, raise the feet, and elevate the buttocks.

- Wash and rinse the area with the washcloth.

- Dry the area, and apply ointment, according to agency policy. Do not apply powder. *The baby may inhale particles of powder, which can irritate the respiratory tract.*

7. Check for dry, cracked, or peeling skin, and apply a mild baby oil or lotion as required.

8. Dress and position the infant.

- Clothe the baby in a shirt (if the temperature of the environment warrants it) and/or nightgown and a diaper. Place the diaper below the cord site. *Exposing the cord site to the air will promote healing.*

- Until the umbilicus and circumcision are healed, position the baby on its side in the crib with a rolled towel or diaper behind the back for support. *This position allows more air to circulate around the cord site, facilitates drainage of mucus from the mouth, and is more comfortable for circumcised babies.*

- After the umbilicus and circumcision are healed, place the baby in a safe position.

- Cover and bundle the baby with a blanket, if the environmental temperature permits. *This gives the baby a sense of security as well as providing warmth.*

9. Record any significant assessments.

EVALUATION FOCUS

Reddened areas or skin rashes; color and consistency of stool; state of cord stump; state of circumcision incision.

▶ **Technique 15–4 Giving an Infant Sponge Bath** *CONTINUED*

SAMPLE RECORDING

Date	Time	Notes
3/3/93	0900	Bathed infant. Skin moist, slightly jaundiced. Umbilicus healing well, no discharge. Responsive to tactile stimulation ——————— Laurie Law, SN

KEY ELEMENTS OF GIVING AN INFANT SPONGE BATH

- Provide a room that is warm and free of drafts.
- Keep small articles out of the infant's reach.
- Use cotton balls or washcloth and water only to clean the eyes and face.
- Clean the eyes from the inner canthus to the outer canthus, using a separate corner of the washcloth or cotton ball for each eye.
- Use the football hold to support the infant when washing the scalp over the wash basin.
- Thoroughly rinse and dry areas with creases and skinfolds, e.g., gluteal folds and between the fingers and toes.

- Prevent undue exposure of the baby between washing and rinsing body parts.
- Clean the base of the umbilical cord and circumcision site according to agency practice.
- Remove smegma from between the labia and under the foreskin.
- Clean the rectal area last.
- Apply ointment as required to the perineal area and buttocks.

15-5 Giving an Infant Tub Bath

 Before commencing an infant tub bath, determine (a) if the infant is HIV positive, (b) whether the baby's weight and temperature are to be measured in conjunction with the bath, and (c) any skin problems and other progress assessments that need to be made.

PURPOSES
- To clean and deodorize the skin
- To stimulate circulation to the skin
- To provide a sense of well-being
- To assess the skin, reflexes, and so on

ASSESSMENT FOCUS

Skin color, texture, turgor, and temperature; presence of lesions or skin breakdown (see Chapter 11, page 210).

EQUIPMENT
- Tub with bath water at 38 to 40 C (100 to 105 F)
- Towel to place under the baby before and after the bath and to dry the infant
- Soft washcloth or absorbent pad
- Cotton balls

- Bag in which to dispose of used cotton balls
- Mild, nonperfumed soap in a container
- Soft-bristled brush
- Bath blanket or towel to cover the infant before and after the bath

- Mild lotion or baby oil if needed for dry skin
- Shirt and/or nightgown
- Diaper

▶ **Technique 15–5 Giving an Infant Tub Bath** *CONTINUED*

INTERVENTION

1. Prepare the bath area.

- Prepare a flat, padded surface in the bath area on which to dress and undress the infant. It should be high enough so that you or the parent can avoid stooping, which can produce back strain. Usually parents use a counter or table top in the bathroom or kitchen, unless a bathinette is available. Cover the surface with a towel.

- Assemble all supplies needed so that they are within easy reach. *A baby left unattended or out of sight for even a few seconds can move or fall from the bath area. Keep supplies out of reach of the infant, however. Small articles, such as safety pins, can be hazardous to an active and curious infant.*

- For small infants, use a wash basin.

- Place the tub or basin near the dressing surface to prevent exposure and chilling when transferring the baby in and out of the tub. Be sure the room is warm and free from drafts.

- Measure the temperature of the water with a bath thermometer, or test it against the inside of your wrist or elbow.

2. Clean the infant's eyes and face before placing the infant in the tub.

- Follow Technique 15–4, step 3.

3. Pick up and place the infant in the tub.

- Pick up and hold the baby securely, with the head and shoulders supported on one forearm and the hips and buttocks supported on the other hand (Figure 15–8). *Young infants have not developed sufficiently to hold their heads up alone.*

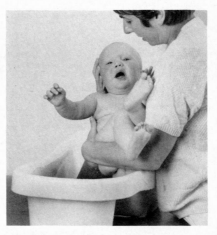

FIGURE 15–8   Holding an infant while placing him in a tub.

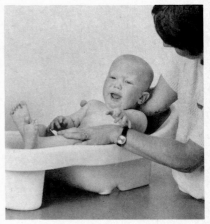

FIGURE 15–9   Keeping the infant's head and back supported during a tub bath.

- Gradually immerse the baby into the tub. *This gives the infant time to adjust to the water.*

4. Wash the infant.

- Keeping the baby's head and back supported on your forearm (Figure 15–9), lather the scalp with a mild soap. Massage the lather over the scalp, using the soft-bristled brush or your fingertips. Rinse the scalp well. *This loosens any dry scales from the scalp and helps prevent cradle cap.* If cradle cap is present, it may be treated with mineral oil, a dandruff shampoo, or ointment prescribed by the physician.

- Soap and rinse the baby's trunk, extremities, genitals, and perineal area with your free hand. Hold the baby as shown in Figure 15–9 throughout. If the baby enjoys the bath, this can be done in a leisurely manner.

5. Remove the infant from the tub, and dry the infant well.

- Remove the baby from the tub by the hold shown in Figure 15–8, and quickly bundle the

baby in a towel. *It is important to avoid chilling the infant.*

- Gently pat the baby dry, giving special attention to the body creases and folds. *Rubbing can cause skin irritation.*

- Apply baby oil or lotion to dry, cracked, or peeling areas.

6. Ensure the infant's comfort and safety.

- Clothe the baby in a shirt (if the temperature of the environment warrants it) and/or a nightgown and a diaper.

- Place the baby in a side-lying position in the crib. *This position facilitates the drainage of mucus from the mouth.*

- Cover and bundle the baby with a blanket, if the environmental temperature permits. *This gives the baby a sense of security as well as providing warmth.*

7. Document all pertinent information.

- Record any significant observations, such as reddened areas or skin rashes, and the color and consistency of the stool.

▶

► **Technique 15–5 Giving an Infant Tub Bath** CONTINUED

EVALUATION FOCUS

See Assessment Focus.

SAMPLE RECORDING

Date	Time	Notes
3/5/93	1010	Tub bath given. Skin clear, moist, warm. No reddened areas. ———— Laurie Law, SN

KEY ELEMENTS OF GIVING AN INFANT TUB BATH

- Clean the baby's eyes and face before placing the infant in the tub.
- Hold the baby appropriately and securely when lifting the infant into and out of the tub and while bathing the infant.
- Immerse the baby gradually into the tub, and allow time for adjustment to the water temperature.

- Thoroughly rinse and dry body areas with creases and skinfolds.
- Apply baby oil or lotion to dry, cracked, or peeling areas.
- Clothe the baby appropriately according to the environmental temperature.

15-6 Changing a Diaper

When a diaper becomes soiled with either urine or feces, it should be changed promptly so that the baby's skin does not become irritated by the waste products. The infant's perineal–genital area is washed and thoroughly dried before a clean diaper is applied.

 Before commencing to change the diaper, determine (a) whether the infant is HIV positive, (b) type of diaper required, and (c) any special precautions, e.g., not elevating buttocks by lifting legs, need for a stool specimen.

PURPOSES

- To maintain the infant's comfort and cleanliness
- To maintain the integrity of the skin by preventing irritation from urine and/or feces

ASSESSMENT FOCUS

Condition of the skin around the perineum and buttocks; amount, color, and odor of the urine and feces; state and progress of circumcision.

EQUIPMENT

- Clean disposable or cloth diaper
- Receptacle for the soiled diaper
- Commercially prepared wipes
- or a basin with warm water, 38 to 40 C (100 to 105 F)
- Soap
- Washcloth
- Towel
- Mild lotion or protective ointment, e.g., zinc oxide
- Gloves in accordance with agency protocol

▶ **Technique 15–6 Changing a Diaper** *CONTINUED*

INTERVENTION

1. Fold a clean diaper, if using a cloth diaper.

• Three methods can be used to fold diapers: rectangular, triangular, or kite (Figures 15–10 to 15–12). When using the rectangular method, provide an extra thickness of material either at

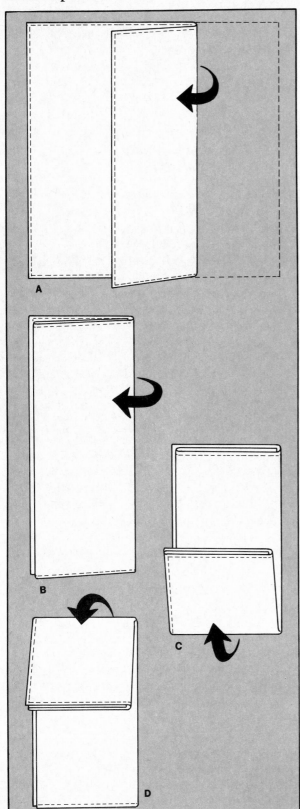

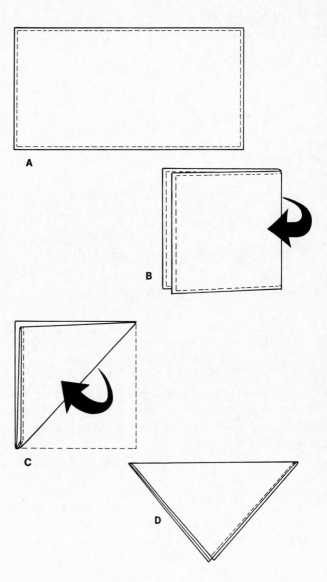

FIGURE 15–11 The triangular method of folding a diaper: *A*, Fold a square cloth to a rectangular shape; *B*, fold the cloth again to form a square; *C*, bring opposite corners together to form a triangle; *D*, apply the triangle with the fold at the waist.

FIGURE 15–10 The rectangular method of folding a diaper: *A*, *B*, Fold the diaper into a rectangle by bringing the sides over; *C*, fold the bottom edge up to provide the thickness in front; or *D*, fold the top edge down to provide the thickness at the back.

► **Technique 15–6 Changing a Diaper** CONTINUED

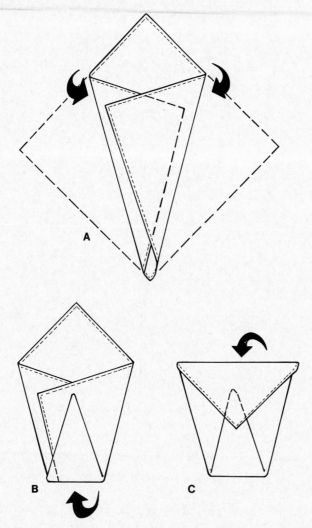

FIGURE 15–12 The kite method of folding a diaper: *A,* Make a triangle by folding the side corners to the center; *B,* bring the bottom corner up to the center; *C,* fold down the top corner.

the front (for boys) or the back (for girls) for additional absorbency. It may also be placed at the front for girls who are positioned on their stomachs for sleep (so that the urine runs to the front).

2. Position and handle the infant appropriately.

- Place the infant in a supine position on a clean, flat surface near the assembled supplies.

- Handle the infant slowly and securely, and speak in soothing tones. *Slow movements and soothing voice tones will help calm any of the infant's fears.*

3. Remove the soiled diaper.

- Place your fingers between the baby's skin and the diaper, and unpin the diaper on each side. Close the pins, and place them out of reach of the infant. *The fingers protect the baby from being pricked as the pins are removed. Babies may grab the pins and place them in their mouths if the pins are within reach.*

- Pull the front of the diaper down between the infant's legs.

- Grasp the infant's ankles with one hand, and lift the buttocks (Figure 15–13).

- Use the clean portion of the diaper to wipe any excess urine or feces from the buttocks. Wipe from anterior to posterior. *Wiping toward the posterior of the infant wipes away the urethral orifice and decreases the possibility of transferring microorganisms to the urinary tract.*

- Remove the diaper. Lower the baby's buttocks. Dispose of the diaper. Do not let the infant out of your sight or reach. *The infant could roll over and off the changing surface.*

4. Clean the buttocks and anal-genital area.

- Use warm water and soap or commercial cleansing tissues.

- Clean toward the posterior as in step 3, above. *Cleaning removes remaining urine and feces, which can irritate the skin.*

- Rinse and dry the area well with the towel. *Drying well prevents irritation of the skin by moisture.*

- Apply a protective ointment or lotion to the perineum and buttocks, especially to the skin creases.

5. Apply the clean diaper, and fasten it securely.

- Lay the diaper flat on a clean surface with the folded edges up, and place the baby on the center of the diaper width so that the

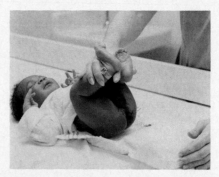

FIGURE 15–13 Lifting the infant's buttocks to remove a soiled diaper.

▶ **Technique 15–6** CONTINUED

back edge of the diaper is at waist level.

or

Grasp the baby's ankles with one hand and raise the baby's legs and buttocks. Place the diaper under the baby so that the back edge is at waist level.

- Draw the diaper up between the baby's legs to the waist in front.

- Fold the diaper below the umbilicus until the infant's cord stump has healed. *This promotes drying and healing of the stump site and minimizes possible infection from wet diapers.*

- Fasten the diaper at the waist

with tape provided so that it fits snugly. If using safety pins for cloth diapers, hold your fingers between the baby and the diaper while pinning. *The fingers protect the baby from being pricked with the pins.*

- Position the pins either vertically or horizontally. *The horizontal position is suggested when the child is old enough to sit. The pins are then less likely to poke the body. The vertical position is suggested for diapers pinned at the sides rather than at the front, if the infant does not yet sit up.*

- Insert the diaper pins so that they face upward or outward. *If*

a pin opens inadvertently, it will not puncture the baby's thigh or abdomen.

6. Ensure infant comfort and safety.

- Dress the infant with additional clothes as required.

- Return the infant to the crib.

7. Document all pertinent information.

- Record stool and/or urine observations on the record sheet and/or the infant's chart.

- Record other pertinent observations, such as skin redness, on the patient's record.

EVALUATION FOCUS | See Assessment Focus.

KEY ELEMENTS OF CHANGING A DIAPER

- Change soiled diapers promptly to prevent skin irritation.
- Fold the clean diaper appropriately to accommodate the infant's size, or use a clean commercial disposable diaper.
- Handle the infant slowly and securely, and never let the infant out of your sight or reach.
- When unpinning a diaper, place your fingers between the baby's skin and the diaper.
- Keep pins out of reach of the infant.
- Clean excess urine or feces from the buttocks and perineum using a clean portion of the soiled diaper and wiping from anterior to posterior.

- Clean the buttocks and anal-genital area using warm water and soap or commercial cleaning tissues.
- Thoroughly rinse and dry the area well.
- Apply protective skin ointments or lotions as needed.
- Apply and securely fasten the diaper.
- If using safety pins, hold your fingers between the baby and the diaper while pinning. Place the pins either horizontally or vertically at the infant's sides and facing upward or outward.

CRITICAL THINKING CHALLENGE

John Lee is a 44-year-old male who was admitted to the nursing unit following a myocardial infarction. His physician has ordered complete bed rest. Mr. Lee refuses to allow the nurse to bathe him and asks to take a shower in the bathroom. What would be your response and why?

REFERENCES

Freinkel, R. K. July 1988. Caring for your skin. *Diabetes Forecast* 41:76–78, 81.

Gooch, J. October 1989. Skin hygiene. *Professional Nurse* 5:13, 16, 18.

Hill, M. J. February 1990. The skin: Anatomy and physiology. *Dermatology Nursing* 2:13–17.

Joachim, G. April 1983. Step-by-step massage techniques. *Canadian Nurse* 79:32–33.

Kozier, B., Erb, G.; and Olivieri, R. 1991. *Fundamentals of nursing: Concepts, process and practice.* 4th ed. Redwood City, Calif.: Addison-Wesley Publishing Co.

Miller, C. A. May/June 1991. Ins and outs of skin care. *Geriatric Nursing* 12:111–12, 156.

Wagnild, G., and Manning, R. W. December 1985. Convey respect during bathing procedures. *Journal of Gerontological Nursing* 11:6–10.

16

Mouth, Eye, and Ear Care

OBJECTIVES

- Identify variations in the mouth, eyes, and ears from infancy to old age

- Describe common problems of the mouth, eyes, and ears

- Identify essential information required to assess mouth, eyes, and ears

- Identify reasons underlying selected steps of each technique

- Safely perform the techniques outlined in this chapter

- Appropriately communicate and document relevant information about the client

CONTENTS

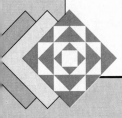

NURSING PROCESS GUIDE
MOUTH, EYE, AND EAR CARE

MOUTH CARE: ASSESSMENT

Determine

- History or presence of sore, swollen, or bleeding gums; toothaches, or difficulty swallowing

- Whether dentures are worn and type (upper, lower, or partial)

- Date of last dental examination and frequency of dental appointments

Assess

- Color and texture of outer lips, inner lips, buccal mucosa, gingiva, tongue, palates, and orophanynx (see Chapter 11, page 232)

- Presence of lesions, such as sordes, leukoplakia, or ulcerations

- Teeth for number, presence of cavities, status of fillings, presence of tartar, integrity of dentures

- Gag reflex by pressing the posterior tongue with a tongue blade

- Mouth care practices (e.g., usual products used, frequency of brushing and flossing teeth)

- Self-care abilities (e.g., any problems managing mouth care)

Identify clients at risk of developing oral problems:

- Confused, comatose, and depressed clients, who may lack the knowledge or ability to maintain oral hygiene

- Clients receiving oxygen or those with nasogastric tubes, who are likely to develop dry oral mucous membranes

- Those who have had oral or jaw surgery, who are prone to developing infections and require meticulous oral hygiene

- Individuals whose nutritional intake is inadequate, whose intake of refined sugars is excessive, and who have a family history of periodontal disease

- Persons who have dry mucous membranes aggravated by poor fluid intake, alcohol use, high salt intake, anxiety, and many medications (e.g., diuretics, laxatives, major tranquilizers, certain antidepressants, antihypertensives, antispasmodics, antihista

mines, and chemotherapeutic agents used to treat cancer)

RELATED DIAGNOSTIC CATEGORIES

- Self-care deficit: Oral hygiene

- Impaired tissue integrity

- High risk for Infection

- Knowledge deficit (correct oral hygiene practices)

PLANNING

Client Goals

The client will

- Maintain or improve oral hygienic practices.

- Maintain or restore mucous membrane hydration.

- Improve or maintain a sense of well-being.

Outcome Criteria

The client

- Has an intact, smooth, well-hydrated oral mucosa of uniform color.

- Has no inflammation of the oral mucosa.

- Has firm, well-hydrated, nonbleeding gums of uniform color.

- Has a well-hydrated tongue without inflammation.

- Has smooth and well-hydrated lips.

- Verbalizes no oral discomfort.

- Has teeth free of food particles and plaque.

- Demonstrates appropriate brushing and flossing techniques.

- Describes interventions that prevent tooth decay and dental plaque.

- Expresses positive feelings about sense of well-being and appearance.

EYE CARE: ASSESSMENT

Determine

- History or presence of eye infection, eye pain, excessive tearing, difficulty seeing, double vision, blurring, sensitivity to light, cataracts, itching, spots in front of eyes, injury, or surgery

- Whether eyeglasses are worn for near or far vision and when prescribed

Continued on page 401

Nursing Process Guide CONTINUED

- Whether contact lenses are worn, type of lens worn (soft, hard, gas permeable), and when prescribed
- Presence of eye prostheses
- Date of last eye examination and frequency of eye examinations
- Name, dosage, and frequency of any eye medications

Assess

- All external eye structures for signs of inflammation, excessive drainage, encrustations, or other obvious abnormalities (see Chapter 11, page 217)
- Hygienic practices for contact lenses (e.g., how often worn in a given day, insertion and removal procedures, cleaning and storage procedures)
- Artificial eye care practices
- Self-care abilities (e.g., any problems managing contact lenses or artificial eye)

RELATED DIAGNOSTIC CATEGORIES

- High risk for Infection
- High risk for Injury
- Self-care deficit (contact lenses or artificial eye insertion, removal, and cleaning)
- Knowledge deficit (contact lens or artificial eye insertion, removal, and cleaning)

PLANNING

Client Goals
The client will

- Maintain the integrity of the cornea, conjunctiva, and/or prosthesis.
- Prevent eye injury and infection.

Outcome Criteria
The client

- Has clear conjunctiva and white sclera without inflammation.
- Has reduced secretions on eyelids.
- Reports no tearing.
- Verbalizes no eye discomfort.
- Demonstrates appropriate methods of caring for contact lenses.
- Describes interventions to prevent eye injury and infection.

EAR CARE: ASSESSMENT

Determine

- History or presence of any infection, loss of hearing, pain, discharge, or ringing in the ears
- Medication history, especially if client is experiencing ringing in the ears
- Whether a hearing aid is worn and any problems experienced
- Date of last ear/hearing examination and frequency of examinations
- How ears are protected if there is exposure to high noise levels in the work environment

Assess

- External ear structures for signs of inflammation, excessive drainage, discomfort, or other obvious abnormalities (see Chapter 11, page 225)
- Hearing aid care practices (e.g., cleaning and storage procedures)
- Self-care abilities (e.g., any problems managing hearing aid)

RELATED DIAGNOSTIC CATEGORIES

- High risk for Injury
- High risk for Infection
- Self-care deficit (hearing aid removal, cleaning, and insertion)

PLANNING

Client Goals
The client will

- Prevent ear injury and infection.
- Maintain optimal hearing acuity.

Outcome Criteria
The client

- Describes measures to prevent ear injury and infection.
- Demonstrates appropriate methods of caring for a hearing aid.
- Verbalizes no ear discomfort.
- Wears a hearing aid throughout the day.
- Expresses positive feelings about wearing a hearing aid.

The Mouth

Mucous membrane, which is continuous with the skin, lines the digestive, urinary, reproductive, and respiratory tracts and the conjunctiva of the eye. It is an epithelial tissue and forms mucus, concentrates bile, and secretes or excretes enzymes, for example, in the digestive tract. It serves four general functions: (1) protection, (2) support for associated structures, (3) absorption of nutrients into the body (in the digestive tract), and (4) secretion of mucus, enzymes, and salts.

The mouth (oral cavity) is bordered by the lips anteriorly, the cheeks laterally, and the pharynx posteriorly. The cheeks contain several accessory muscles of **mastication** (chewing), which keep food from escaping the masticating motions of the teeth. The tongue, containing numerous taste buds, extends from the floor of the mouth and is attached to it by a fold of mucous membrane called the **frenulum**. The tongue helps to mix saliva, keeps food pressed between the teeth for chewing, and pushes food into the pharynx for swallowing. The **palate** (roof of the mouth) has two parts: the anterior portion (hard palate) and the posterior portion (soft palate), which ends in a free projection called the **uvula** that marks the opening of the mouth into the pharynx.

The mouth contains two sets of **dentures** (teeth). Teeth are necessary to masticate food, so that it can be swallowed and digested in the stomach. Each tooth has a number of parts: the crown, the root, and the pulp cavity. The **crown** is the exposed part of the tooth, which is outside the gum. It is covered with a hard substance called **enamel**. The internal part of the crown below the enamel is ivory colored and is referred to as **dentin** (Figure 16–1). The **root** of a tooth is embedded in the jaw, and is covered by a bony tissue called **cementum**. The **pulp cavity** in the center of the tooth contains the blood vessels and nerves.

Assessment of the mouth is covered in Chapters 11 and 12.

Developmental Changes

Teeth usually appear 5 to 8 months after birth. By the time children are 2 years old, they usually have all 20 of their temporary teeth. See Figure 12–8 on page 311. At about age 6 or 7, children start losing their deciduous teeth, which are gradually replaced by the 32 permanent teeth. See Figure 11–41 on page 232. By age 25, most people have all their permanent teeth.

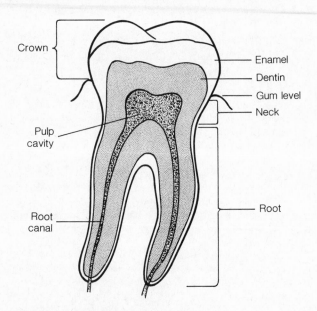

FIGURE 16–1 The anatomic parts of a tooth.

The incidence of periodontal disease increases during pregnancy, because an increase in female hormones affects gingival tissue and increases its reaction to bacterial plaque. Many pregnant women manifest increased redness and swelling of the **gingiva** (the gum) and increased bleeding from the gingival **sulcus** (the groove between the surface of the tooth and the gum) during brushing.

Elderly people may have few permanent teeth left, and many have dentures. Some people lose all their own teeth by age 70, mainly because of periodontal disease rather than dental caries; however, caries are also common in the middle-aged adult. Preventive dental care is important.

Some receding of the gums and a brownish pigmentation of the gums occur with age. Because saliva production decreases with age, dryness of the oral mucosa is a common finding in older people.

Common Problems

Dental caries and periodontal disease are problems frequently encountered in adult clients. For further information about these problems, as well as plaque, tartar, and inflammatory problems of the mouth, see Chapter 11, page 231.

Oral Hygiene

Good oral hygiene includes daily stimulation of the gums, mechanical scrubbing of the teeth, flushing of the mouth, and regular checkups by a dentist. The nurse is often in a position to help people to maintain oral hygiene by helping or teaching them to clean the teeth and oral cavity, by inspecting whether clients (especially children) have done so, or by actually providing mouth care to clients who are ill or incapacitated. The nurse can also be instrumental in identifying and referring problems that require the intervention of a dentist or oral surgeon. Specific measures to teach clients to prevent tooth decay and periodontal disease are shown in the accompanying box.

Thorough brushing of the teeth is important in preventing tooth decay. The mechanical action of brushing removes food particles that can harbor and incubate bacteria. It also stimulates circulation in the gums, thus maintaining their healthy firmness. The brushing of teeth needs to be demonstrated to children by age 2, when their teeth appear. Until the child can manipulate the toothbrush effectively, however, parents need to help the child to do this. The technique most recently recommended for brushing teeth is called the **sulcular technique**, which removes plaque and cleans under the gingival margins. An effective **dentifrice** (paste or powder used to clean or polish the teeth) can be made by combining two parts of table salt to one part of baking soda, and many toothpastes are marketed, any of which can be used. See Technique 16–1 for brushing and flossing teeth.

CLIENT TEACHING

Measures to Prevent Tooth Decay

- Brush your teeth thoroughly after meals and at bedtime. Assist children or inspect their mouths to be sure the teeth are clean. If you cannot brush your teeth after eating, vigorously rinse your mouth with water.
- Floss your teeth daily.
- Ensure an adequate intake of nutrients, particularly calcium, phosphorus, vitamins A, C, and D, and fluoride.
- Avoid sweet foods and drinks between meals. Take them in moderation at meals.
- Eat coarse, fibrous foods (cleansing foods), such as fresh fruits and raw vegetables.
- Take a fluoride supplement daily until age 14 or 16, unless the drinking water is fluoridated.
- Have topical fluoride applications as prescribed by the dentist.
- Have a checkup by a dentist every 6 months.
- Have your child visit the dentist for the first time at about age 2½ or 3, so that the child learns not to fear such visits.

16-1 Brushing and Flossing the Teeth

PURPOSES
- To remove food particles from around and between the teeth
- To remove dental plaque
- To enhance the client's feelings of well-being
- To prevent sordes and infection of the oral tissues

ASSESSMENT FOCUS
Self-care abilities; presence of tooth caries; gum inflammation; halitosis; status of oral mucosa and lips; usual mouth care practices.

EQUIPMENT

- Towel
- Gloves
- Curved basin
- Toothbrush
- Cup of tepid water
- Dentifrice
- Mouthwash
- Dental floss, at least two pieces 20 cm (8 in) in length
- Floss holder (optional)

▶ **Technique 16–1 Brushing and Flossing the Teeth** CONTINUED

INTERVENTION

1. Prepare the client.

- Explain the procedure.

- Assist the client to a sitting position in bed, if health permits. If not, assist the client to a side-lying position with the head on a pillow so that the client can spit out the rinse water.

2. Prepare the equipment.

- Place the towel under the client's chin.

- Don gloves. *Wearing gloves while providing mouth care prevents the nurse from acquiring infections, such as AIDS, particularly if oral bleeding is present. They also prevent transmission of microorganisms to the client.*

- Moisten the bristles of the toothbrush with tepid water, and apply the dentifrice to the toothbrush.

- Use small toothbrushes for children. A soft toothbrush is recommended. Most people have a flavor preference and have their own dentifrice. For the person who does not have dentifrice, use a mixture of salt and baking soda.

- For the client who must remain in bed, place or hold the curved basin under the client's chin, fitting the small curve around the chin or neck.

- Inspect the mouth and teeth.

3. Brush the teeth.

- Hand the toothbrush to the client, or brush the client's teeth as follows.

  a. Hold the brush against the teeth with the bristles at a 45° angle (Figure 16–2). The tips of the outer bristles should rest against and penetrate under the gingival sulcus (Figure 16–3). The

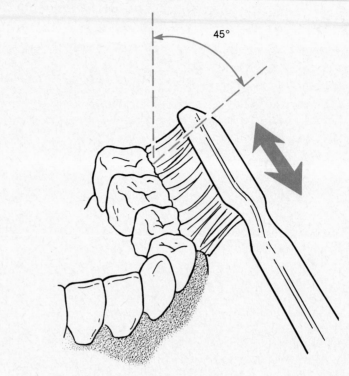

FIGURE 16–2 The sucular technique: placing the bristles at a 45° angle against the teeth.

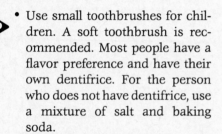

FIGURE 16–3 Directing the tips of the outer bristles under the gingival margins.

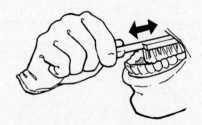

FIGURE 16–4 Brushing the biting surfaces of the teeth.

brush will clean under the sulcus of two or three teeth at one time. *This sulcular technique removes plaque and cleans under the gingival margins.*

  b. Move the bristles back and forth using a vibrating or jiggling motion, from the sulcus to the crowns of the teeth.

  c. Repeat until all outer and inner surfaces of the teeth and sulci of the gums are cleaned.

  d. Clean the biting surfaces by moving the brush back and forth over them in short strokes (Figure 16–4).

  e. If the tongue is coated, brush it gently with the toothbrush. *Brushing removes accumulated materials and coatings. A coated*

▶ **Technique 16–1** *CONTINUED*

tongue may be caused by poor oral hygiene and low fluid intake. Brushing gently and carefully helps prevent gagging or vomiting.

- Hand the client the water cup or mouthwash to rinse the mouth vigorously. Then ask the client to spit the water and excess dentifrice into the basin. Some hospitals supply a standard mouthwash. Alternatively, a mouth rinse of normal saline or diluted hydrogen peroxide can be an effective cleaner and moisturizer. *Vigorous rinsing loosens food particles and washes out already loosened particles.*

- Repeat the steps above until the mouth is free of dentifrice and food particles.

- Remove the curved basin, and help the client wipe the mouth.

4. Floss the teeth.

- Assist the client to floss independently, or floss the teeth as follows. Waxed floss is less likely to fray than unwaxed floss; particles between the teeth attach more readily to unwaxed floss than to waxed floss. Some believe that waxed floss leaves a residue on the teeth and that plaque then adheres to the wax.

  a. Wrap one end of the floss around the third finger of each hand. (Figure 16–5).

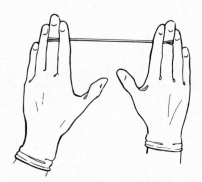

FIGURE 16–5 Stretching the floss between the third finger of each hand.

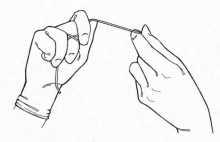

FIGURE 16–7 Flossing the lower teeth by using the index fingers to stretch the floss.

  b. To floss the upper teeth, use your thumb and index finger to stretch the floss (Figure 16–6). Move the floss up and down between the teeth from the tops of the crowns to the gum and along the gum lines as far as possible. Make a "C" with the floss around the tooth edge being flossed. Start at the back on the right side and work around to the back of the left side, or work from the

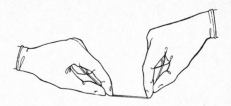

FIGURE 16–6 Flossing the upper teeth by using the thumbs and index fingers to stretch the floss.

center teeth to the back of the jaw on either side.

  c. To floss the lower teeth, use your index fingers to stretch the floss (Figure 16–7).

- Give the client tepid water or mouthwash to rinse the mouth and a curved basin in which to spit the water.

- Assist the client in wiping the mouth.

5. Remove and dispose of equipment appropriately.

- Remove and clean the curved basin.

- Remove and discard the gloves.

6. Document assessment of the teeth, tongue, gums, and oral mucosa. Include any problems such as sordes or inflammation and swelling of the gums. Brushing and flossing teeth are not usually recorded.

EVALUATION FOCUS	Health status of teeth, gums, tongue, oral mucosa, tongue, and lips.

KEY ELEMENTS OF BRUSHING AND FLOSSING THE TEETH

- Wear gloves when performing oral assessment or administering oral care.

- Assess the status of all oral structures.
- Use correct technique when brushing teeth.

Artificial Dentures

Some people have artificial teeth in the form of a plate—a complete set of teeth for one jaw. A person may have a lower plate and/or an upper plate. When only a few artificial teeth are needed, the individual may have a bridge rather than a plate. A bridge may be fixed or removable. Artificial teeth are fitted to the individual and usually will not fit another person. People who wear dentures or other oral prostheses should be encouraged to use them. Those who do not wear their prostheses are prone to shrinkage of the gums, which results in further tooth loss.

Most people prefer privacy when they take their artificial teeth out to clean them. Many do not like to be seen without their teeth; one of the first requests of many postoperative clients is "May I have my teeth in, please?"

Like natural teeth, artificial dentures collect microorganisms and food. They need to be cleaned regularly, at least once a day. They can be removed from the mouth, scrubbed with a toothbrush, rinsed, and reinserted. Some people use a dentifrice, while others use commercial cleaning compounds for plates. Technique 16–2 describes how to clean artificial dentures.

16-2 · Cleaning Artificial Dentures

Before commencing to clean artificial dentures, determine (a) areas in the mouth that require ongoing assessment, and (b) whether the client has upper and lower dentures.

PURPOSES
- To remove food particles and microorganisms from artificial teeth
- To prevent infection of the oral tissues
- To enhance the client's feeling of well-being

ASSESSMENT FOCUS

Health status of gums, oral mucosa, and tongue; condition of dentures.

EQUIPMENT

- Gloves
- Tissue or piece of gauze
- Denture container
- Clean washcloth
- Toothbrush or stiff-bristled brush
- Dentifrice or denture cleaner
- Tepid water
- Container of mouthwash
- Curved basin
- Towel

INTERVENTION

1. Prepare the client.

- Assist the client to a sitting or side-lying position.

2. Remove the dentures.

- Don gloves. *Wearing gloves protects the nurse from infection.*

- If the client cannot remove the dentures, take the tissue or gauze, and grasp the upper plate at the front teeth with your thumb and second finger, and move the denture up and down slightly (Figure 16–8). *The slight*

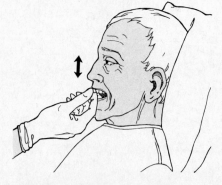

FIGURE 16–8 Removing the top dentures by first breaking the suction.

movement breaks the suction that holds the plate on the roof of the mouth.

- Lower the upper plate, move it out of the mouth, and place it in the denture container.

- Lift the lower plate, turning it so that the left side, for example, is slightly lower than the right, to remove the plate from the mouth without stretching the lips. Place the lower plate in the denture container.

▶ **Technique 16–2** *CONTINUED*

- Remove a partial denture by exerting equal pressure on the border of each side of the denture, not on the clasps, which can bend or break.

3. Clean the dentures.

- Take the denture container to a sink. Take care not to drop the dentures. *They may break.* Place a washcloth in the bowl of the sink. *A washcloth prevents damage if the dentures are dropped.*

- Using a toothbrush or special stiff-bristled brush, scrub the dentures with the cleaning agent and tepid water. *Hot water is not used because heat will change the shape of some dentures.*

- Rinse the dentures with tepid running water. *Rinsing removes the cleaning agent and food particles.*

- If the dentures are stained, soak them in a commercial cleaner. Be sure to follow the manufacturer's directions. To prevent corrosion, dentures with metal parts should not be soaked overnight. Home substitutes for commercial cleaner are the following mixtures:

  a. 5 to 10 ml (1 to 2 tsp) white vinegar and 240 ml (1 cup) warm water.
  or

  b. 5 ml (1 tsp) chlorine bleach, 10 ml (2 tsp) water softener, and 240 ml (1 cup) warm water. It is essential to mix water softener with the bleach to prevent denture corrosion and to rinse well before replacing in the mouth.

4. Inspect the dentures and the mouth.

- Observe the dentures for any rough, sharp, or worn areas that could irritate the tongue or mucous membranes of the mouth, lips, and gums.

- Inspect the mouth for any redness, irritated areas, or indications of infection.

- Assess the fit of the dentures. People who have them should see a dentist at least once a year to check the fit, occlusion, and the presence of any irritation to the soft tissues of the mouth. Clients who need repairs to their dentures or new dentures may need a referral for financial assistance to correct problems.

5. Return the dentures to the mouth.

- Offer some mouthwash and a curved basin to rinse the mouth. If the client cannot insert the dentures independently, insert

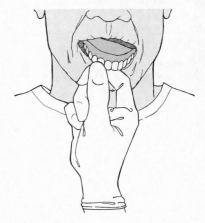

FIGURE 16–9 Inserting the dentures at a slight angle.

the plates one at a time. Hold each plate at a slight angle while inserting it, to avoid injuring the lips (Figure 16–9).

6. Assist the client as needed.

- Wipe the client's hands and mouth with the towel.

- If the client does not want to or cannot wear the dentures, store them in a denture container with water. Label the cup with the client's name and identification number.

7. Remove and discard gloves.

8. Document all relevant information.

- Document all assessments, and include any problems, such as an irritated area on the mucous membrane.

EVALUATION FOCUS	Condition of the oral mucosa, gums, tongue, and lips; condition of the dentures.

KEY ELEMENTS OF CLEANING ARTIFICIAL DENTURES

- Wear gloves.
- Place a washcloth in the bowl of the sink before cleaning dentures.
- Use tepid (not hot) water to clean dentures.
- Avoid soaking dentures with metal parts in commercial cleaners for lengthy periods.

- Inspect dentures for rough or sharp areas.
- Assess the oral mucosa and gums for reddened or irritated areas.
- Provide an appropriately labeled container to store dentures.

Special Oral Care

For the client who is unconscious or has excessive dryness, sores, or irritations of the mouth, it may be necessary to clean the oral mucosa and tongue, in addition to cleaning the teeth. Agency practices differ in regard to special mouth care and the frequency with which it is provided. Depending on the health of the client's mouth, special care may be needed every 2 to 8 hours.

Mouth care for unconscious people is very important, because their mouths tend to become dry and consequently predisposed to infections. Dryness occurs because the client cannot take fluids by mouth, is often breathing through the mouth, or may be receiving oxygen, which tends to dry the mucous membranes.

The nurse can use commercially prepared applicators of lemon juice and oil to clean the mucous membranes. If these are unavailable, a gauze square rolled around the index finger and dipped into lemon juice and oil or into mouthwash solution usually suffices. Long-term use can lead to further dryness of the mucosa and changes in tooth enamel, however. Applicator swabs or tongue blades covered with gauze may also be used. Mineral oil is generally contraindicated, because aspiration of it can initiate an infection (lipid pneumonia). Hydrogen peroxide can be used prior to the lemon juice and oil, if necessary. This agent, which should be diluted 1:1 with water, is effective in removing encrustations that coat the tongue.

Technique 16–3 focuses on oral care for the unconscious person but may be adapted for conscious persons who are seriously ill or have mouth problems.

16-3 Providing Special Oral Care

PURPOSES
- To maintain the continuity of the lips, tongue, and mucous membranes of the mouth
- To prevent oral infections
- To clean and moisten the membranes of the mouth and lips

ASSESSMENT FOCUS

Status of the oral mucosa, lips, tongue, and teeth; presence of halitosis.

EQUIPMENT

- Towel
- Curved basin
- Gloves
- Bite-block to hold the mouth open and teeth apart (optional)
- Toothbrush

- Cup of tepid water
- Dentifrice or denture cleaner
- Tissue or piece of gauze to remove dentures (optional)
- Denture container as needed
- Mouthwash

- Rubber-tipped bulb syringe
- Applicators and cleaning solution for cleaning the mucous membranes
- Petroleum jelly (Vaseline) or cold cream

INTERVENTION

1. Prepare the client.

- Position the unconscious client in a side-lying position, with the head of the bed lowered. *In this position, the saliva automatically runs out by gravity rather than being aspirated into the lungs.* This position is the one of choice for the unconscious client receiving mouth care. If the client's head cannot be lowered, turn it to one side. *The fluid will readily run out of the mouth or pool in the side of the mouth, where it can be suctioned.*

- Place the towel under the client's chin.

- Place the curved basin against the client's chin and lower cheek to receive the fluid from the mouth (Figure 16–10).

- Don gloves.

2. Clean the teeth, and rinse the mouth.

- If the person has natural teeth, brush the teeth as described earlier. Brush gently and carefully to avoid injuring the gums. If the client has artificial teeth, clean them as described earlier.

► **Technique 16–3** *CONTINUED*

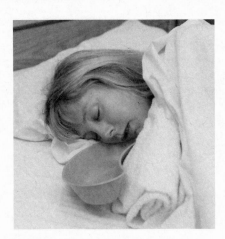

FIGURE 16–10 Position of client and placement of curved basin when providing special mouth care.

- Rinse the client's mouth by drawing about 10 ml of water or mouthwash into the syringe and injecting it gently into each side of the mouth. *If the solution is injected with force, some of it may flow down the client's throat and be aspirated into the lungs.*

- Watch carefully to make sure that all the rinsing solution has run out of the mouth into the basin. If not, suction the fluid from the mouth. See the section on or-opharyngeal suctioning in Chapter 31, p. 766. *Fluid remaining in the mouth may be aspirated into the lungs.*

- Repeat rinsing until the mouth is free of dentifrice, if used.

3. Inspect and clean the oral tissues.

- If the tissues appear dry or un-clean, clean them with the applicators or gauze and cleaning solution. If hydrogen peroxide is used, rinse the mouth thorough-ly before applying oil and lemon juice. *The gums and mucosa can become spongy from prolonged action of hydrogen peroxide.* Oil and lemon juice are recommend-ed for short-term use only.

- Picking up one oil applicator, wipe the mucous membrane of one cheek. If no commercially prepared applicators are avail-able, wrap a small gauze square around your index finger, and moisten it with oil and lemon so-lution. Discard the applicator or gauze in a waste container, and with a fresh one clean the next area. *Using separate applicators for each area of the mouth pre-vents the transfer of microorgan-isms from one area to another.*

- Clean all the mouth tissues in an orderly progression, using sep-arate applicators: the cheeks, roof of the mouth, base of the mouth, and tongue.

- Observe the tissues closely for inflammation and dryness.

- Rinse the client's mouth as de-scribed above.

- Remove and discard gloves.

4. Ensure client comfort.

- Remove the basin, and dry around the client's mouth with the towel. Replace artificial den-tures, if indicated.

- Lubricate the client's lips with petroleum jelly or cold cream. *Lubrication prevents cracking and subsequent infection.*

5. Document pertinent data.

- Record special oral hygiene and pertinent observations.

- Report problems to the nurse in charge.

EVALUATION FOCUS	Status of oral tissues, lips, and tongue; any irritation, dryness, or lesions.

SAMPLE RECORDING

Date	Time	Notes
4/7/93	1500	Special mouth care using oil and lemon juice q2h. Outer aspect of lower right gum remains reddened and swollen. No discharge. —— Sally R. Nolan, SN

KEY ELEMENTS OF PROVIDING SPECIAL ORAL CARE

- Wear gloves.
- Position the unconscious client appropriately to prevent aspiration of fluid.
- Avoid using mineral oil.
- Dilute hydrogen peroxide, if used, with an equal amount of water.

- Administer rinsing solution carefully to prevent aspiration, and ensure that all solution is drained or removed.
- Use separate applicators for each part of the mouth.
- Assess all mouth tissues.

The Eyes

The eyes are extremely important organs. The **lacrimal glands**, situated in a depression in the frontal bone at the upper outer angle of the eye orbit, produce lacrimal fluid, which continually washes the eyes. See Figure 11–18 on page 216. This fluid drains through the **lacrimal ducts** onto the **conjunctiva** at the upper outer corner of the eye and then through **lacrimal canaliculi** (canals) to the **lacrimal sac**, which is situated in the inner **canthus**, the angular junction of the eyelids at the corner of the eye. From the lacrimal sac the fluid drains through the **nasolacrimal duct** to the inferior meatus of the nose. The fluid keeps the eyeball moist and helps wash away foreign particles. Excessive lacrimal fluid forms tears.

Developmental Changes

Visual abilities are present at birth; the newborn can follow large moving objects, is attracted to black-white contrast, can fixate on certain stimuli for 4 to 10 seconds, and can react to changes in the intensity of light. The pupils of the newborn respond slowly, however, and the eyes cannot focus on close objects. By 3 months of age, vision has developed so that the eyes are coordinated both horizontally and vertically. By 4 months, the infant recognizes familiar objects and follows moving objects. At 6 years of age, visual acuity is comparable to that of an adult. Preschool children are generally farsighted until their eyes grow in length and become **emmetropic** (refracting normally and focusing objects on the retina).

Loss of visual acuity occurs in elderly people as the lens of the eye ages, becomes more opaque, and loses elasticity. Other changes include loss of ability of the iris to accommodate in darkness and dim light, loss of peripheral vision, and difficulty in distinguishing similar colors.

Common Problems

In children, **strabismus** is the most common congenital problem. The muscles of the two eyes are not coordinated, and, when the child has one eye directed straight ahead, the other eye may be directed inward, outward, or upward. The eyes appear crossed. Eyeglasses or eye exercises may be used to correct strabismus; in some cases, surgery is performed on the eye muscles.

Eye Care

Dried secretions that have accumulated on the lashes need to be softened and wiped away. Hospital nurses soften dried secretions by placing a sterile cotton ball moistened with sterile water or normal saline over

---

Eye Care for the Comatose Client

When a comatose client's corneal reflex is impaired, eye care is essential to keep moist the areas of the cornea that are exposed to air.

- Administer moist compresses to cover the eyes as ordered, e.g., every 2 to 4 hours.
- Clean eyes with saline solution and cotton balls. Wipe from the inner to outer canthus. This prevents debris from being washed into the nasolacrimal duct.
- Use a new cotton ball for each wipe. This prevents extending infection in one eye or to the other eye.
- Instill ophthalmic ointment into the lower lids. This keeps the eyes moist.
- Close the client's eyelids, and then put a small amount of mineral oil on the outer eyelids to lubricate and protect the skin.
- If the client's corneal reflex is absent, keep the eyes closed by placing an eye pad soaked in the saline solution over each eye and securing these with non-allergenic tape. These pads should *not* be so tight as to provide pressure on the eyes.

---

the lid margins. The nurse then wipes the loosened secretions from the inner canthus of the eye to the outer canthus to prevent the particles and fluid from draining into the lacrimal sac and nasolacrimal duct.

For the client who is unconscious and lacks a blink reflex or cannot close the eyelids completely, the nurse must prevent drying and irritation of the cornea. Lubricating eye drops may be administered if ordered by the physician. An eye patch may also be placed over the affected eye or eyes. See the box above for providing eye care for the comatose client.

Eyeglass Care

It is essential that the nurse exercise caution when cleaning eyeglasses to prevent breaking or scratching the lenses. Glass lenses can be cleaned with warm water and dried with a soft tissue that will not scratch the lenses. Plastic lenses are easily scratched and require special cleaning solutions and drying tissues. When not being worn, all glasses should be placed in a case labeled appropriately, and stored in the client's bedside table drawer.

Contact Lens Care

Contact lenses, thin curved discs of hard or soft plastic, fit on the cornea of the eye directly over the pupil.

They float on the tear layer of the eye. For some people, there are several advantages of contact lenses over eyeglasses: (a) they cannot be seen and thus have cosmetic value; (b) they are highly effective in correcting some astigmatisms; (c) they are safer than glasses for some physical activities; (d) they do not fog, as eyeglasses do; and (e) they provide better vision in many cases.

Contact lenses may be either hard or soft or a compromise between the two types—gas-permeable lenses. *Hard contact lenses* are made of a rigid, unwettable, airtight plastic that does not absorb water or saline solutions. They usually cannot be worn for more than 12 to 14 hours and are rarely recommended for first-time wearers.

Soft contact lenses cover the entire cornea. Being more pliable and soft, they mold to the eye for a firmer fit. The duration of extended-wear varies by brand from 1 to 30 days or more. Eye specialists recommend that long-wear brands be removed and cleaned at least once a week. These lenses require scrupulous care and handling.

Gas-permeable lenses are rigid enough to provide clear vision but are more flexible than the traditional hard lens. They permit oxygen to reach the cornea, thus providing greater comfort, and will not cause serious damage to the eye if left in place for several days.

Most clients normally care for their own contact lenses. In general, each lens manufacturer provides detailed cleaning instructions. Depending on the type of lens and cleaning method used, warm tap water, normal saline, or special rinsing or soaking solutions may be used.

Seriously ill people who have had their contact lenses removed will not need them reinserted until they become more active in their care and require their lenses to see properly.

Most users have a special container for their lenses. Some contain a solution so that the lenses are stored wet; in others, the lenses are dry. Each lens container has a slot with a label indicating whether it is for the right or left lens. It is essential that the correct lens be stored in the appropriate slot so that it can be worn in the correct eye.

Techniques 16–4 and 16–5 describe how to insert and remove contact lenses.

16-4 Inserting Contact Lenses (Hard and Soft)

Before inserting contact lenses, determine (a) the client's own practices regarding cleaning and inserting the lenses, and (b) any reasons for not inserting the lenses.

PURPOSE

• To enhance the client's visual acuity

ASSESSMENT FOCUS

> Presence of eye inflammation, infection, discomfort, or excessive tearing; when lenses were last worn and cleaned; cleanliness of the lenses; any scratches on the lenses.

EQUIPMENT

☐ Client's lens storage case
☐ Gloves (optional)
☐ Wetting agent

INTERVENTION

1. Take the client's lens storage case, and select the correct lens for the eye. *Each lens is ground to fit the individual eye and correct its visual defect.*

• Start with the right eye. *Always starting with the right eye establishes a habit so that incorrect placement of each lens is avoided.*

• Don gloves, if desired.

To Insert Hard Lenses

2. Lubricate the lens.

• Put a few drops of sterile wetting solution on the right lens. Solutions of saline, methyl cellulose,

▶ Technique 16–4 Inserting Contact Lenses CONTINUED

or polyvinyl alcohol are frequently used. *Wetting solution helps the lens to glide over the cornea, thus reducing the risk of injury.*

- Spread the wetting solution on both surfaces of the lens by using your thumb and index finger or an absorbent applicator, or place the lens in the palm of your hand and spread the solution with your index finger.

3. Insert the lens.

- Ask the client to tilt the head backward.

- Place the lens convex side down on the tip of your dominant index finger (the right, if you are righthanded; Figure 16–11).

- Separate the upper and lower eyelids of the right eye with the thumb and index finger of your nondominant hand (Figure 16–11). When separating the eyelids, ⓢ exert gentle pressure with your fingers over the supraorbital and infraorbital bony prominences. *This prevents direct pressure, discomfort, and injury to the eyeball.*

- Place the lens as gently as possible on the cornea, directly over the iris and the pupil.

- Repeat the above steps for the other lens.

4. If the lens is off center, center the lens.

- Separate the eyelids, using the index or middle finger of the left hand to lift the upper lid and the index or middle finger of the right hand to depress the lower lid.

- Locate the lens, and ask the client to gaze in the opposite direction (Figure 16–12).

- Gently push the lens in the direction of the cornea, using a finger or the eyelid margins.

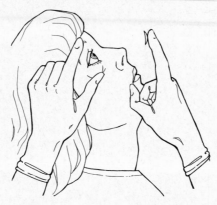

FIGURE 16–11   Inserting a hard contact lens.

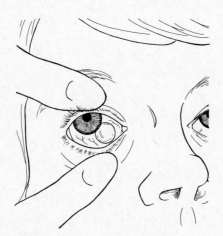

FIGURE 16–12   Locating a lens that is off center by separating the eyelids and asking the client to gaze in the opposite direction.

- Ask the client to look slowly toward the lens. The lens will slide easily onto the cornea as the client looks toward it.

To Insert Soft Lenses

5. Keep the dominant finger dry for insertion.

- Remove the lens from its saline-filled storage case with your nondominant hand. *Because "water-loving" soft contact lenses have a natural attraction to wet surfaces, the lens will adhere more readily to the moist eye if the finger is dry.*

6. Position the lens correctly for insertion.

For A Regular Soft Lens

- Hold the lens at the edge be-

tween your thumb and your index finger.

- Flex the lens slightly. The lens is in the correct position if the edges point inward. If the edges point outward, it is in the wrong position (i.e., inside out) and must be reversed (Figure 16–13). *A lens placed on the eye inside out is less comfortable (an edge sensation may be felt), tends to fold on the eye, can drop to a lower position on the eye, and may move excessively on blinking.*

For an Ultrathin Soft Lens

- Do not flex an ultrathin lens. Instead, put the lens on your placement finger and allow it to dry slightly for a few seconds.

Correct

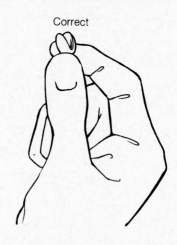

Inside out

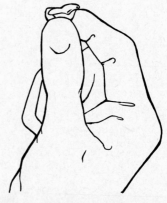

FIGURE 16–13   Checking the position of a soft contact lens before insertion.

▶ **Technique 16–4** *CONTINUED*

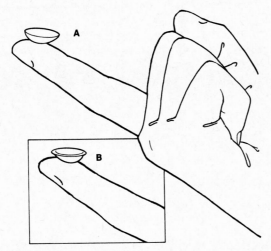

FIGURE 16-14 Checking the position of an ultrathin contact lens before insertion: *A*, position is correct, i.e., edges are turned upward; *B*, lens is inside out and must be reversed.

- Closely inspect the lens to see whether the edges turn upward (Figure 16–14, *A*). If they turn downward (Figure 16–14, *B*), the lens is inside out and must be reversed. *Flexing an ultrathin lens may cause the lens to fold and stick together.*

7. Wet the lens with saline solution using your nondominant fingers.

- See step 2 for hard lenses.

8. Insert the lens.

- Ensure that your placement finger is dry. This is particularly important for ultrathin soft lenses.

- Place the lens convex side down on the tip of your dominant index finger.
- Insert the lens in the same manner as a hard contact lens.

9. Store lens equipment appropriately.

- Replace the lens container, lens cleaner, and wetting solution in the drawer of the bedside table.

10. Document pertinent information.

- Record insertion of the contact lenses if a nurse is required to remove them; otherwise, this is not normally recorded (consult agency protocol).
- Record all assessments, and report to the nurse in charge any problems observed in the eyes or the lenses.
- Record on the nursing care plan the time for the lenses to be removed.

EVALUATION FOCUS	Discharge from eyes; color and clarity of conjunctiva; discomfort; tearing; client's perception of sight.

SAMPLE RECORDING

Date	Time	Notes
10/10/93	2100	Contact lenses inserted in both eyes. Slight white discharge from inner canthus R eye. Upper eyelid R eye reddened. No discomfort. States can read now. ———————————————— Marilyn S. McLean, SN

KEY ELEMENTS OF INSERTING CONTACT LENSES

- Before insertion, assess the eyes for irritation.
- Make sure the correct lens is selected for the eye, i.e., right lens for right eye.
- Ensure that the lenses are cleaned and moistened with wetting solution before insertion.
- Before insertion, allow ultrathin lenses to air dry a few seconds, and do not flex them.
- Make sure your placement finger is dry before handling soft lenses.

- Retract the eyelids by using the pads of your fingertips, and exert pressure only on the bony orbits above and below the eye, not on the eye.
- Place the concave side of the lens against the cornea.
- Make sure the lens is centered over the pupil and iris.
- Use aseptic technique.

16-5 Removing Contact Lenses (Hard and Soft)

PURPOSES
- To prevent eye damage from prolonged lens wearing
- To prevent loss of the lenses

ASSESSMENT FOCUS
> Any eye irritation; length of time lens has been in place.

EQUIPMENT
- ☐ Gloves (optional)
- ☐ Flashlight (optional)
- ☐ Cotton applicator dipped in saline (optional)
- ☐ Lens storage case; or, if not available, two small medicine cups or specimen containers partially filled with normal saline solution and marked "L lens" and "R lens."

INTERVENTION

1. Locate the position of the lens. *The lens must be positioned directly over the cornea for proper removal.*

- Don gloves, if needed.

- Ask the client to tilt the head backward.

- Retract the upper eyelid with your index finger, and ask the client to look up, down, and from side to side.

- Retract the lower eyelid with your index finger, and ask the client to look up and down and from side to side.

- Use a flashlight if necessary to find a colorless soft lens.

2. Reposition a displaced lens.

- Ask the client to look straight ahead.

- Using your index fingers, gently exert pressure on the inner margins of the upper and lower lids, and move the lens back onto the cornea.
  or
  Using a cotton-tipped applicator dipped in saline, gently move the lens into place.

To Remove Hard Lenses

3. Separate the upper and lower eyelids.

- Use both thumbs or index fingers to separate the upper and lower eyelids of one eye until they are beyond the edges of the lens (Figure 16–15). Exert pressure toward the bony orbit above and below the eye. *Retraction of the eyelids against the bony orbit prevents direct pressure, discomfort, and injury to the eyeball.*
  or
  Use the middle finger to retract the upper eyelid and the thumb of the same hand to retract the lower lid. *Using one hand for retraction keeps the other hand free to receive the lens.*

4. Remove the lens.

- Gently move the margins of both the lower eyelid and the upper eyelid toward the lens. *The margins of the lids trap the edges of the lens.*

- Hold the top eyelid stationary at the edge of the lens, and lift the bottom edge of the contact lens by pressing the lower lid at its margin firmly under the lens (Figure 16–16). *Pressure exerted under the edge of the lens interrupts the suction of the lens on the cornea.*

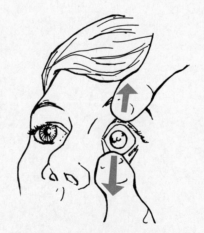

FIGURE 16–15 Separating the eyelids until they are beyond the edges of a hard lens.

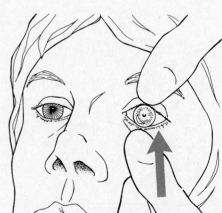

FIGURE 16–16 Holding the top lid stationary at the edge of a hard lens and lifting the bottom edge of the lens by pressing the lower lid at its margin.

▶ **Technique 16–5** *CONTINUED*

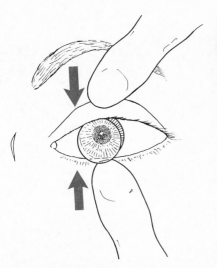

FIGURE 16–17 Sliding a hard lens out of the eye by moving both eyelids toward each other.

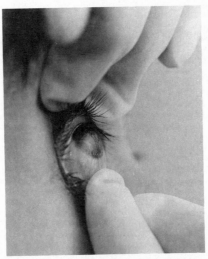

FIGURE 16–18 Moving a soft lens down to the inferior part of the sclera.

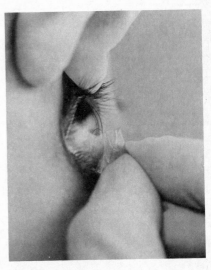

FIGURE 16–19 Removing a soft lens by pinching it between the pads of the thumb and index finger.

- After the lens is slightly tipped, slide the lens off and out of the eye by moving both eyelids toward each other (Figure 16–17).

- Grasp the lens with your index finger and thumb, and place it in the palm of your hand.

- To avoid lens mixups, place the first lens in its designated cup in the storage case before removing the second lens.

- Repeat the above steps for the other lens.

To Remove Soft Lenses

5. Separate the eyelids.

- Ask the client to look upward at the ceiling and keep the eye opened wide.

- Retract the lower or upper lid with one or two fingers of your *nondominant* hand.

- Using the index finger of your dominant hand, move the lens down to the inferior part of the sclera (Figure 16–18). *Moving the lens onto the sclera reduces the risk of damage to the cornea.*

6. Remove the lens.

- Gently pinch the lens between the pads of the thumb and index finger of your dominant hand (Figure 16–19). *Pinching causes the lens to double up, so that air enters underneath the lens, breaking the suction and allowing removal. The pads of the fingers are used to prevent scratching the eye or the lens with the fingernails.*

- Place the lens in the palm of your hand.

- For *ultrathin* lenses, open the lens with the thumb and index finger *immediately* on removal. *This keeps the edges from sticking together.*

- Repeat the above steps for the other lens.

7. Clean and store the lenses appropriately.

- Clean the lenses according to manufacturer's instructions.

- Place the lens in the correct slot in its storage case. The slots are labeled for right and left lenses.

- Be sure each lens is centered in the storage case. *If the lens is not centered, it may crack, chip, or tear.* Tighten or close the cover.

- Place the contact lens container in the drawer of the bedside table. *The lenses and the case should never be exposed to direct sunlight or extreme heat, because these can dry or warp them.*

8. Document all relevant information.

- Document the removal of the lenses prior to surgery or when this is a nursing responsibility.

- Document all assessments and problems, such as redness of the conjunctiva, and report problems to the nurse in charge.

▶ **Technique 16–5 Removing Contact Lenses** *CONTINUED*

EVALUATION FOCUS	Absence of eye inflammation; adequacy of visual acuity with lenses inserted; integrity of lenses; eye comfort.

SAMPLE RECORDING

Date	Time	Notes
3/22/93	2100	Contact lenses removed. No redness of eyelids or conjunctiva noted. Both lenses intact. ———————————————— Anita R. Rodriguez, SN

KEY ELEMENTS OF REMOVING CONTACT LENSES

- Ensure that lens storage cases are appropriately labeled and that the correct lens is stored in the appropriate slot.
- Keep lenses and storage cases away from extreme heat and sunlight.

- Exert pressure only on the bony orbits above and below the eye, not on the eye.
- Always use the pads of the fingers when handling eye structures and lenses.
- Use aseptic technique.

Artificial Eyes

Artificial eyes are usually made of glass or plastic. Some are permanently implanted; others are removed regularly for cleaning. Most clients who wear a removable artificial eye follow their own care regimen. Even for an unconscious client, daily removal and cleaning are not necessary. If the nurse notices problems, e.g., redness of the surrounding tissues, drainage from the eye socket, or crusting on the eyelashes, or if the client is scheduled for surgery, the nurse must remove the eye from the socket; clean the eye, the socket, and the surrounding tissues; and then reinsert the eye unless otherwise directed. Clients whose mobility is impaired by injury or paralysis may also require assistance. Sterile supplies are usually used in a hospital when removing and inserting an artificial eye, but this is not usually a sterile procedure. Technique 16–6 explains how to remove, clean, and insert an artificial eye.

16-6 **Removing, Cleaning, and Inserting an Artificial Eye**

Before removing, cleaning, and inserting an artificial eye, determine the client's routine eye care practices.

PURPOSES	• To maintain the integrity of the eye socket and eyelids • To prevent infection of the eye socket and surrounding tissues • To assess the tissues and sockets for irritation or infection • To maintain the client's self-esteem
ASSESSMENT FOCUS	Client's care regimen; inflammation of surrounding tissues; drainage from the eye socket; crusting of the eyelashes.

▶ **Technique 16–6** *CONTINUED*

EQUIPMENT

- ☐ Small labeled storage container, such as a denture or specimen container
- ☐ Gloves (optional)
- ☐ Small rubber bulb, a syringe bulb, or a medicine dropper bulb (optional)
- ☐ Soft gauze or cotton wipe
- ☐ Bowl of warm normal saline

INTERVENTION

1. Remove the eye.

- Make sure that the container in which the prosthesis will be stored has been lined to cushion the eye and prevent scratches. Also, be sure to use sterile supplies. (This is not a sterile procedure, however.)

- Assist the client to a sitting or supine position, if the client's health permits.

- Identify the eye to be removed, and don gloves, if indicated.

- If the client has an effective method for removing the eye, follow that method. *Most people can remove their own eyes under normal circumstances, and they may have a convenient method.*

- Otherwise:

  a. Pull the lower eyelid down over the infraorbital bone with your dominant thumb, and exert slight pressure below the eyelid (Figure 16–20).
  or

  b. Compress a small rubber bulb, and apply the tip directly on the eye. Gradually decrease the finger pressure on the bulb, and draw the eye out of the socket. *Compression squeezes the air out of the bulb, causing a negative pressure inside the bulb. When the finger pressure is released, the suction of the bulb counteracts the suction holding the eye in the socket.*

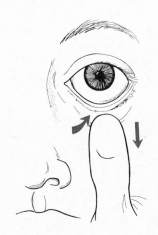

FIGURE 16–20 Removing an artificial eye by retracting the lower eyelid and exerting slight pressure below the eyelid.

- Receive the eye with the other hand, and place it carefully in the container. Do not scratch or drop the eye.

2. Clean the eye and the socket.

- Expose the socket by raising the upper lid with the index finger and pulling the lower lid down with the thumb.

- Clean the socket with soft gauze or cotton wipes and normal saline. Pat dry.

- Wash the tissue around the eye, stroking from the inner to the outer canthus using a fresh gauze for each wipe. *This direction of stroking avoids washing any debris down the lacrimal canaliculi, if they are still intact.* Be sure to wash crusts off the upper and lower lids and eyelashes.

- Dry the tissues gently, in the direction described in the step above, using dry wipes.

- Wash the artificial eye gently with the warm normal saline, and dry it with dry wipes.

- If the eye is not to be inserted, place it in the lined container filled with water or saline solution, close the lid, label the container with the client's name and room number, and place it in the drawer of the bedside table.

3. Reinsert the eye.

- Ensure that the eye is moistened with water or saline. *Moisture facilitates insertion by reducing friction.*

- Using the thumb and index finger of one hand, retract the eyelids, exerting pressure on the supraorbital and infraorbital bones (Figure 16–21).

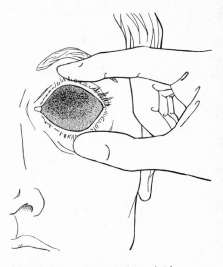

FIGURE 16–21 Exposing the socket by retracting the upper and lower eyelids.

▶ **Technique 16–6 Artificial Eyes** *CONTINUED*

- With the thumb and index finger of the other hand, hold the eye so that the front of it is toward the palm of your hand (Figure 16–22). Slip the eye gently into the socket, and release the lids. The eye should fit securely under the lids.

4. Document pertinent information.

- Record the removal, cleaning, and/or insertion of an artificial eye prior to surgery or for a helpless person. Otherwise, these procedures are not usually recorded.

- Document any assessments and problems, and report them to the nurse in charge.

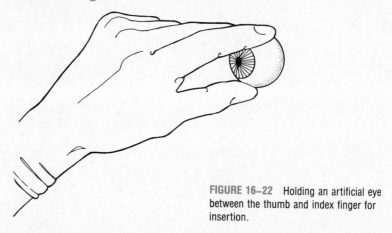

FIGURE 16–22 Holding an artificial eye between the thumb and index finger for insertion.

EVALUATION FOCUS	Clean appearance and uniform pale pink color of tissues in the eye socket; absence of encrustations on the eyelids; scratches or rough areas on eye.

KEY ELEMENTS OF REMOVING, CLEANING, AND INSERTING AN ARTIFICIAL EYE

- Handle the eye prosthesis carefully to prevent damage to it.
- Use aseptic technique.

- Safely store in an appropriately labeled container a prosthesis that is not reinserted in the socket.

The Ears

The ear is divided into three parts: external ear, middle ear, and inner ear. For details about the ears and hearing, see Chapter 11, page 224.

Developmental Changes

The curvature of the external ear canal differs with age. In the infant and toddler, the canal has an upward curvature. By age 3, the ear canal assumes the more downward curvature of adulthood. See Figures 12–7 on page 309 and 11–33 on page 226.

Common Problems

Mechanical blockages of the external ear canal most commonly arise from a buildup of cerumen or from foreign bodies lodged in the canal. Children are notorious for inserting small objects in their ears. Signs of blockage are pain and some loss of hearing.

The most common traumatic stress to the eardrum involves exposure to loud noises. Frequent close exposure to loud music or machines is associated with a high potential for hearing loss.

Cleaning the Ears

The auricles of the ear are cleaned during the bed bath. The nurse or client must remove excessive cerumen that is visible or that causes discomfort or hearing difficulty. Visible cerumen may be loosened and removed by retracting the auricle downward. If this measure is ineffective, irrigation is necessary (see the section on otic irrigation in Chapter 35, page 842). Clients need to be advised never to use bobby pins, toothpicks, or cotton-tipped applicators to remove cerumen. Bobby pins and toothpicks can injure the ear canal and rupture the tympanic membrane; cotton-tipped applicators can cause wax to become impacted within the canal.

Care of Hearing Aids

A hearing aid is a battery-powered, sound amplifying device used by hearing-impaired persons. It consists of a microphone that picks up sound and converts it to electric energy, an amplifier that magnifies the electric energy electronically, a receiver that converts the amplified energy back to sound energy, and an earmold that directs the sound into the ear.

For correct functioning, hearing aids require appropriate handling during insertion and removal, regular cleaning of the earmold, and replacement of dead batteries. With proper care, hearing aids generally last 5 to 10 years. Earmolds generally need readjustment every 2 to 3 years.

16-7   Removing, Cleaning, and Inserting a Hearing Aid

PURPOSE	• To maintain proper hearing aid function
ASSESSMENT FOCUS	Any problems with the hearing aid; hearing aid care practices; presence of inflammation, excessive wax or drainage, or discomfort in external ear canal.

EQUIPMENT

- Client's hearing aid
- Soap, water, and towels or a damp cloth
- Pipe cleaner or toothpick (optional)
- New battery (if needed)

INTERVENTION

1. Remove the hearing aid.

- Turn the hearing aid off, and lower the volume. The on/off switch may be labeled "O" (off), "M" microphone, "T" (telephone), or "TM" (telephone/microphone). *The batteries continue to be used if the aid is not turned off.*

- Remove the earmold by rotating it slightly forward and pulling it outward.

- If the aid is not to be used for several days, remove the battery. *Removal prevents corrosion of the aid from battery leakage.*

- Store the hearing aid in a safe place. Avoid exposure to heat and moisture. *Proper storage prevents loss or damage.*

2. Clean the earmold.

- Detach the earmold *if possible.* Disconnect the earmold from the receiver of a body hearing aid or from the hearing aid case of behind-the-ear and eyeglasses aids where the tubing meets the hook of the case. Do not remove the earmold if it is glued or secured by a small metal ring. *Removal facilitates cleaning and prevents inadvertent damage to the other parts.*

- If the earmold is *detachable,* soak it in a mild soapy solution. Rinse and dry it well. Do not use isopropyl alcohol because it can cause damage to the hearing aid.

- If the earmold is *not detachable*

or is for an in-the-ear aid, wipe the earmold with a damp cloth.

- Check that the earmold opening is patent. Blow any excess moisture through the opening or remove debris (e.g., earwax) with a pipe cleaner or toothpick.

- Reattach the earmold if it was detached from the rest of the hearing aid.

3. Insert the hearing aid.

- Determine from the client if the earmold is for the left or the right ear.

- Check that the battery is inserted in the hearing aid. Turn off the hearing aid, and make sure the volume is turned all the way

▶ **Technique 16–7 Hearing Aids** *CONTINUED*

down. *A volume that is too loud is distressing.*

- Inspect the earmold to identify the ear canal portion. Some earmolds are fitted for only the ear canal and concha; others are fitted for all the contours of the ear. The canal portion, common to all, can be used as a guide for correct insertion.

- Line up the parts of the earmold with the corresponding parts of the client's ear.

- Rotate the earmold slightly forward, and insert the ear canal portion.

- Gently press the earmold into the ear while rotating it backward.

- Check that the earmold fits snugly by asking the client if it feels secure and comfortable.

- Adjust the other components of a behind-the-ear or body hearing aid.

- Turn the hearing aid on, and adjust the volume according to the client's needs.

4. Correct problems associated with improper functioning.

- If the sound is weak or there is no sound:

  a. Ensure that the volume is turned high enough.

  b. Ensure that the earmold opening is not clogged.

  c. Check the battery by turning the aid on, turning up the volume, cupping your hand over the earmold, and listening. A constant whistling sound indicates the battery is functioning. If necessary, replace the bat-

tery. Be sure that the negative (−) and positive (+) signs on the battery match those on the aid.

  d. Ensure that the ear canal is not blocked with wax, which can obstruct sound waves.

- If the client reports a whistling sound or squeal after insertion:

  a. Turn the volume down.

  b. Ensure that the earmold is properly attached to the receiver.

  c. Reinsert the earmold.

5. Document pertinent data.

- The removal and the insertion of a hearing aid are not normally recorded.

- Report and record any problems the client has with the hearing aid.

EVALUATION FOCUS

Absence of inflammation; wax buildup or discomfort in external ear canal; adequacy of hearing acuity with aid inserted; comfort of aid when inserted.

KEY ELEMENTS OF REMOVING, CLEANING, AND INSERTING A HEARING AID

- Store the aid in a dry, safe place. Turn the aid off when not in use, and remove the battery if it is not to be used for lengthy periods, e.g., several days.

- Avoid exposure of the aid to heat, moisture, sprays, and aerosols.

- Avoid using isopropyl alcohol for cleaning.

- Before inserting an aid, make sure the volume is turned all the way down.

CRITICAL THINKING CHALLENGE

Sally Nelson is an 86-year-old female who has been admitted to the extended care facility following hospital treatment for a right-sided cerebral vascular accident (CVA). She has impaired movement of the left arm and leg. She also has difficulty speaking and eating and has periods of confusion. After giving her mouth care, you note that there is still an offensive odor coming from her mouth. What do you think is causing the odor? What would you say to Mrs. Nelson? What actions would you take?

RELATED RESEARCH

Harrell, J. S., and Damon, J. F. December 1989. Prediction of patient's need for mouth care. *Western Journal of Nursing Research* 11(6): 748–56.

Ismail, A. I., and Szpunar, S. M. December 1990. The prevalence of total tooth loss, dental cavities, and periodontal disease among Mexican Americans, Cuban Americans, and Puerto Ricans: Findings from HHANES 1982–1984. *American Journal of Public Health* 80 (Suppl): 66–70.

Kenny, S. A. December 1990. Effects of two oral care protocols on the incidence of stomatitis in hemotology patients. *Cancer Nursing* 13(6): 345–53.

Poland, J. M. April 1987. Comparing moi-stir to lemon glycerin swabs. *American Journal of Nursing* 87:422, 424.

REFERENCES

Bhaskar, S. N.; Lilly, G. E.; and Pratt, L. W. January 3, 1990. A practical high-yield mouth exam. *Patient Care* 24(2): 53–57, 60, 62.

Blaney, G. M. September/October 1986. Mouth care—basic and essential, *Geriatric Nursing* 7:242–43.

Bocking, H.; Sercombe, A. K.; Kenny, M.; Butlin, T.; and Back, A. May 2–8, 1990. Making sense of . . . artificial eyes. *Nursing Times* 86(18): 40–41.

Carden, R. G. February 1985. The ins and outs of contact lenses. *RN* 48:48–50.

Harrison, K. W. May/June 1989. Gas permeable lenses: A growing trend. *Journal of Ophthalmic Nursing and Technology.* 8(3): 108–10.

Hauk, L. September/October 1986. Enabling clients to manage dentures. *Geriatric Nursing* 7:254–55.

Kamenir, S., and Fothergill, R. December 1982. Hands-on skills for dealing with hearing aids. *Canadian Nurse* 78:44–45.

Longman, A. L., and Dewalt, E. M. September/October 1986. A guide for oral assessment: Nursing assistants working in long-term care facilities. *Geriatric Nursing* 7:252–53.

Marieb, E. N. 1989. *Human anatomy and physiology.* Redwood City, Calif.; Benjamin/Cummings.

Ofstehage, J. C., and Magilvy, K. September/October 1986. Oral health and aging. *Geriatric Nursing* 7:238–41.

Ophthalmic issues. April 1988. Facts and myths: Misconceptions about eye care. *American Association of Occupational Health Nurses Journal* 36:174–77.

Pettigrew, D. January/February 1989. Investigating in mouth care. *Geriatric Nursing* 10:22–24.

Tolson, D. May 1–7, 1991. Making sense of . . . hearing aids. *Nursing Times* 87(18): 36–38.

Hair, Nail, and Foot Care

CONTENTS

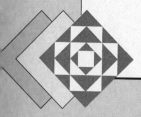

NURSING PROCESS GUIDE
HAIR, NAIL, AND FOOT CARE

HAIR CARE: ASSESSMENT

Determine

- History of the following conditions or therapies: recent chemotherapy, hypothyroidism, radiation of the head, unexplained hair loss, growth of excessive body hair
- Usual hair care practices
- Routinely used hair care products (e.g., hair spray, lubricant, shampoo, conditioners, hair dye, curling or straightening preparations)

Assess

- Evenness of hair growth over the scalp, in particular, any patchy loss of hair; hair texture, oiliness, thickness, or thinness; presence of lesions, infections, or infestations on the scalp; presence of hirsutism (see Chapter 11, page 212)
- Self-care abilities (e.g., any problems managing hair care)

RELATED DIAGNOSTIC CATEGORIES

- Self-care deficit: Grooming
- Impaired skin integrity
- High risk for Infection
- Body image disturbance

PLANNING

Client Goals
The client will

- Maintain or improve hair texture, growth, and cleanliness.
- Maintain or improve a sense of well-being.
- Prevent specific hair and scalp problems.

Outcome Criteria
The client

- Has resilient hair with a healthy sheen.
- Has reduced or absent scalp lesions or infestations.
- Describes contributing factors and interventions for dandruff (or other hair problem).
- Expresses positive statements about sense of well-being.

NAIL CARE: ASSESSMENT

Determine

- History of any problems associated with nails (e.g., inflammation of the tissue surrounding the nail, injury, prolonged exposure to water or chemicals, circulatory problems)
- Presence of circulatory impairments to the extremities
- Usual nail care practices

Assess

- Nail plate shape; angle between the nail and nail bed; nail texture; nail bed color; intactness of the tissues around the nails (see Chapter 11, page 213)
- Capillary refill (see Chapter 11, page 214)
- Self-care abilities (e.g., any problems managing nail care)

RELATED DIAGNOSTIC CATEGORIES

- Self-care deficit: Grooming
- High risk for Infection
- Knowledge deficit (nail care practices)

PLANNING

Client Goals
The client will

- Develop or maintain healthy nail care practices.
- Prevent infection, ingrown toenails, and injury to the tissues surrounding the nails.

Outcome Criteria
The client

- Has smooth, convex, clean nails.
- Has pink nail beds.
- Has intact cuticles and hydrated surrounding skin.
- Has quick return of nail bed color after the blanch test.
- Reports less or no pain and inflammation.
- Has short nails with smooth edges.
- Describes factors contributing to the nail problem.
- Describes preventive interventions for the specific nail problem.
- Demonstrates nail care as instructed.

Continued on page 424

Nursing Process Guide *CONTINUED*

FOOT CARE: ASSESSMENT

Determine

- History of any problems with foot odor; foot discomfort; foot mobility; circulatory problems (e.g., swelling, changes in skin color and/or temperature, and pain); structural problems (e.g., bunion, hammer toe, or overlapping digits)

- Usual foot care practices (e.g., frequency of washing feet and cutting nails, foot hygiene products used, how often socks are changed, whether the client ever goes barefoot)

Assess

- Skin surfaces for cleanliness, odor, and dryness

- Each foot and toe for shape, size, presence of lesions (e.g., corn, callus, wart, or rash), areas of tenderness, ankle edema (see Chapter 11, page 210)

- Skin temperatures of the two feet to assess circulatory status and the dorsalis pedis pulses

- Ability to stand, walk, and perform range-of-motion exercises with each ankle and set of toes

- Self-care abilities (e.g., any problems managing foot care)

RELATED DIAGNOSTIC CATEGORIES

- Self-care deficit: Bathing/hygiene

- Impaired skin integrity

- High risk for Impaired skin integrity

- High risk for Infection

- Impaired physical mobility

- Pain

- Knowledge deficit (foot care practices)

PLANNING

Client Goals
The client will

- Achieve or maintain healthy foot care practices.

- Prevent infection and injury to the feet.

Outcome Criteria
The client

- Has intact, pink, smooth, soft, and hydrated skin.

- Has warm skin.

- Reports less pain or discomfort.

- Has intact cuticles and skin surrounding nails.

- Has quick return of nail bed color after blanch test.

- Wears appropriate shoes and walks without discomfort.

- Describes hygiene practices and other interventions to maintain skin integrity and peripheral tissue perfusion.

- Describes interventions to prevent specific foot problems.

- Demonstrates correct foot and nail care practices.

- Performs self-care (foot hygiene) practices independently.

The Hair

Hair grows on the whole body surface except on the palms of the hands, the soles of the feet, the dorsal surfaces of terminal phalanges, and parts of the genitals (the inner surface of the labia and inner surface of the prepuce of the glans penis).

Surface hair is of two types: **vellus**, which is the fine, nonpigmented hair covering large areas of the body, and **terminal hair**, which is longer, coarser, and pigmented. Hair grows at varying rates and is shed at varying times.

The visible part of a hair is called the **hair shaft**. The root is in a tube known as a **hair follicle**. Muscles known as **arrector pili muscles** are attached to the hair follicles. When these contract, the skin assumes a gooseflesh appearance. Sebaceous glands, which secrete **sebum**, grow from the walls of hair follicles (Figure 17–1). Sebum is produced in greater quantities on the scalp and the face than elsewhere on the body.

Nutrients carried by the bloodstream to the skin and scalp move into the roots of the hair to nourish it. Protein is very important for healthy hair, and a deficiency can result in dullness, loss of color, and reduced growth.

Developmental Changes

Newborns may have **lanugo** (the fine hair on the body of the fetus, also referred to as *down* or *woolly hair*) over their shoulders, back, and sacrum. This gener-

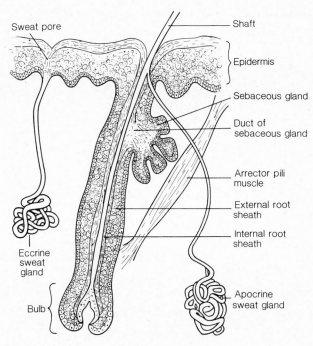

Sweat pore

Shaft

Epidermis

Sebaceous gland

Duct of sebaceous gland

Arrector pili muscle

External root sheath

Internal root sheath

Eccrine sweat gland

Apocrine sweat gland

Bulb

FIGURE 17–1   The anatomic parts of a hair follicle.

ally disappears, and the hair distribution becomes noticeable on the eyebrows, head, and eyelashes of young children. Some newborns have hair on their scalps; others are free of hair at birth but grow hair over the scalp during the first year of life.

Pubic hair usually appears in early puberty followed in about 6 months by the growth of axillary hair. Boys develop facial hair in later puberty.

In adolescence, the sebaceous glands increase in activity as a result of increased hormone levels. As a result, hair follicle openings enlarge to accommodate the increased amount of sebum, which can make the adolescent's hair more oily.

In elderly people, the hair is generally thinner, grows more slowly, and loses its color as a result of aging tissues and diminishing circulation. Men often lose their scalp hair and may become completely bald. This phenomenon may occur even when a man is relatively young. The older person's hair also tends to be drier than normal. With age, axillary and pubic hair becomes finer and scanter, in contrast to the eyebrows, which become bristly and coarse. Many women develop hair on their faces, which may be a problem to them.

Common Problems

Among the common problems of scalp hair are extreme dryness and coarseness due to the application of hair dyes, rinses, or curling or straightening preparations. Such products can also be allergens that

produce scalp itches and rashes. Other problems are dandruff, alopecia, lice, ticks, and hirsutism.

Dandruff appears as a diffuse scaling of the scalp often accompanied by itching. In severe cases, dandruff involves the auditory canals and the eyebrows. Infants during the first month of life may develop this crusting of the scalp, referred to as **cradle cap**.

Alopecia is a thinning of the hair or patchy loss due, for example, to a disease process, such as hypothyroidism, or to radiation and drug therapy for a malignancy.

Lice are parasitic insects that infest mammals. Hundreds of varieties of lice infest humans. Three that are particularly common are *Pediculus capitis* (the head louse), *Pediculus corporis* (the body louse), and *Pediculus pubis* (the crab louse). An infestation of lice is known as **pediculosis**.

Pediculus capitis is found on the scalp and tends to stay hidden by the hairs; similarly, *Pediculus pubis* stays in pubic hair. *Pediculus corporis* tends to cling to clothing, so that, when a client undresses, the lice may not be in evidence on the body; these lice suck blood from the person and lay their eggs (called *nits*) on the clothing. The nurse can suspect their presence in the clothing if (a) the person habitually scratches, (b) there are scratches on the skin, and (c) there are hemorrhagic spots on the skin where the lice have sucked blood.

Head and pubic lice lay their eggs on the hairs; the nits look like oval particles, similar to dandruff, clinging to the hair. Bites and pustular eruptions may also be noticed at the hair lines and behind the ears.

Lice are very small, grayish white, and difficult to see. The crab louse in the pubic area has red legs. Lice may be contracted from infested clothes and direct contact with an infected person.

Ticks are small parasites that bite into tissue and suck blood. They take many forms and can adapt to various conditions. They can attach to human beings and are found frequently in the hair. They can be as large as 1.3 cm (0.5 in) and appear gray-brown. They attach to a person with the apparatus by which they suck blood and should not be torn off, because the sucking apparatus will be left in the skin and become infected. Pouring oil on the tick deprives it of oxygen and causes it to lose its hold, and it withdraws its sucker.

Ticks transmit several diseases to people, in particular Rocky Mountain spotted fever, Lyme disease, and tularemia.

Scabies is a contagious skin infestation due to the itch mite. The characteristic lesion is the burrow produced by the female mite as it penetrates into the upper layers of the skin. Burrows are short, wavy, brown or black thread-like lesions most commonly observed between the webs of the fingers and the folds of the wrists and elbows. The mites cause intense itching that is more pronounced at night because the increased warmth of the skin has a stimulating effect on the parasites. Secondary lesions caused by scratching include vesicles, papules, pustules, excoriations, and crusts. Treatment involves thorough cleansing of the body with soap and water to remove scales and debris from crusts, and then an application of a scabicide lotion. All bed linens and clothing should be washed in very hot or boiling water.

Hirsutism is the growth of excessive body hair. The acceptance of body hair in the axillae and on the legs is largely dictated by culture. In North America, the well-groomed woman, as depicted in magazines, has no hair on her legs or under her axillae (although this idea is changing). In many European cultures, it is not customary for well-groomed women to remove this hair.

Excessive facial hair on a woman is thought unattractive in most Western and Asian cultures. For example, some Japanese brides follow the custom of shaving their faces the day before the wedding.

The cause of excessive body hair is not always known. Elderly women may have some on their faces, and women during menopause may also experience the growth of facial hair. These conditions may be due to the action of the endocrine system. It is also thought heredity influences both the pattern of hair distribution and the production of androgens by the adrenal glands.

Hair Care

Brushing and Combing the Hair

To be healthy, hair needs to be brushed daily. Brushing has three major functions: It stimulates the circulation of blood in the scalp, it distributes the oil along the hair shaft, and it helps to arrange the hair, although many people use a comb for that purpose.

Long hair may present a problem for hospitalized clients. A brush with stiff bristles provides the best stimulation to blood circulation in the scalp. The bristles should not be so sharp that they injure the client's scalp, however. To prevent hair from matting, the client or nurse needs to comb it at least daily. A comb with dull, even teeth is advisable. A comb with sharp teeth might injure the scalp; combs that are too fine can pull and break the hair. Some clients are pleased to have their hair tied neatly in the back or braided

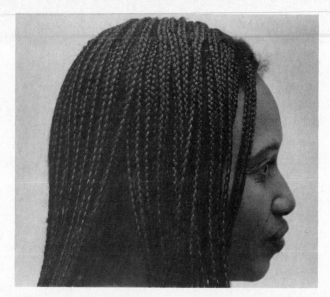

FIGURE 17–2 A black person's hair styled with cornrow braids.

until other assistance is available or until they feel better and can look after it. Others may consider such styles unattractive or juvenile. The nurse should work with the client to find an acceptable style.

Dark-skinned people often have thicker, drier, curlier hair than white-skinned people. Spiraled or very curly hair may stand out from the scalp. Although the shafts of spiraled hair look strong and wiry, they have less strength than straight hair shafts and can break easily.

Some blacks have their spiraled hair straightened. Even if straightened, the hair tends to tangle and mat easily, especially at the back and the sides if the client is confined to bed. Other blacks style their hair in cornrows (Figure 17–2). These cornrows do not have to be unbraided for shampooing and washing. The nurse should obtain the client's permission before any such unbraiding. Some black clients need to oil their hair daily because it tends to be dry. Oil also prevents the hair strands from breaking and the scalp from becoming too dry.

Neat, well-groomed hair usually gives clients a sense of well-being and improves their appearance. Appearance is often particularly important to clients when they have visitors. Technique 17–1 explains essential aspects of brushing and combing hair. Technique 17–2 describes how to provide hair care for black clients, and Technique 17–3 describes how to braid the hair.

17-1   **Brushing and Combing the Hair**

PURPOSES	• To stimulate the blood circulation to the scalp • To distribute hair oils and provide a healthy sheen • To increase the client's sense of well-being • To discover or monitor hair or scalp problems (e.g., matted hair or dandruff)
ASSESSMENT FOCUS	Usual hair care practices; routinely used hair care products; self-care abilities; any scalp problems.

EQUIPMENT

□ Clean brush with stiff bristles
□ Clean comb with dull, even teeth

□ Oil, e.g., mineral oil (optional)
□ Towel

INTERVENTION

1. Position and prepare the client appropriately.

• Assist the client who can sit to move to a chair. *Hair is more easily brushed and combed when the client is in a sitting position.* If health permits, assist a client confined to bed to a sitting position by raising the head of the bed. Otherwise, assist the client to alternate side-lying positions, and do one side of the head at a time.

• If the client remains in bed, place a clean towel over the pillow and the client's shoulders. Place it over the sitting client's shoulders. *The towel collects any hair, dirt, and scaly material removed from the head.*

• Remove any pins or ribbons in the hair.

2. Brush and comb the hair.

• For short hair, brush and comb one side at a time. Divide long hair into two sections by parting it down the middle from the front to the back (Figure 17–3). If the hair is very thick, divide each section into front and back subsections or into several layers (Figure 17–4).

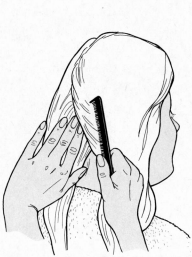

FIGURE 17–3 Dividing hair into two sections for thorough brushing.

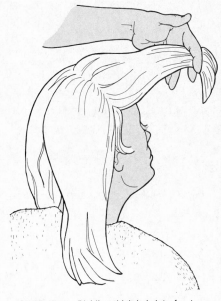

FIGURE 17–4 Dividing thick hair into front and back sections for thorough brushing.

• Holding one section at a time with one hand, brush from the scalp toward the ends. Rotate the wrist in such a way that the brush massages the scalp. Then comb that section of hair. *Massaging stimulates blood circulation in the scalp and thus nourishment of the hair.*

• Brush and comb each section, moving from one side of the head to the other.

3. Remove any mats or tangles gradually.

• Brush and comb each layer, working from the ends toward the scalp. Mats can usually be pulled apart with fingers or worked out with repeated brushings.

• If the hair is very tangled, rub alcohol or an oil, such as mineral oil, on the strands to help loosen the tangles. The hair may then

▶

▶ **Technique 17–1 Brushing and Combing the Hair** CONTINUED

need to be shampooed. See Techniques 17–4.

4. Arrange the hair as neatly and attractively as possible, according to the individual's desires.

• Braiding long hair helps prevent tangles. See Technique 17–3.

5. Document assessments and special nursing interventions.

• Daily combing and brushing of hair are not normally recorded.

• Record problems such as excessive dandruff, very dry or very oily hair, or the presence of lice.

EVALUATION FOCUS
Problems such as dandruff, alopecia, pediculosis, scalp lesions, excessive dryness, or excessive mats or tangles.

KEY ELEMENTS OF BRUSHING AND COMBING THE HAIR

• Report infestations promptly.

• Remove mats gradually, working from the ends toward the scalp.

17-2 Providing Hair Care for Black Clients

PURPOSES
• See Technique 17–1 on page 427.

ASSESSMENT FOCUS
Usual hair care practices; routinely used hair care products; self-care abilities; any scalp problems.

EQUIPMENT
☐ Large, open-toothed or long-toothed comb (a pic)
☐ Lubricant (optional)

INTERVENTION

1. Position and prepare the client appropriately.

• See Technique 17–1, step 1.

2. Comb the hair.

• Apply a lubricant as the client indicates or as needed.

• Using a large and open-toothed comb, start at the neckline and lift and fluff the hair outward, moving upward toward the forehead (Figure 17–5).

• Continue fluffing the hair outward and upward until all of the hair is combed on one half of the head. Repeat the procedure for the other half.

3. Remove tangles gradually.

• After the hair has been lubricated, weave and lift your opened fingers through the hair to ease the tangles free.

or

Support the hair securely at the base of the scalp, if possible, to prevent pulling and discomfort. Insert a long-toothed comb into the ends of the hair and carefully comb out the ends of the tangles (Figure 17–6).

▸ **Technique 17–2 Hair Care for Black Clients** *CONTINUED*

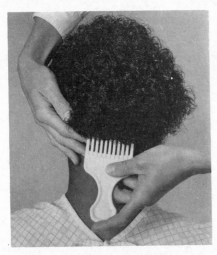

FIGURE 17–5 Using a large open-toothed comb to comb a black client's hair from the neckline upward toward the forehead.

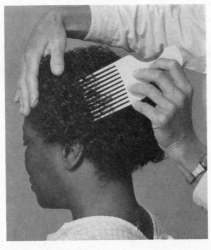

FIGURE 17–6 Removing tangles with a long-toothed comb.

- Repeat this step, each time working the comb farther up the hair shaft toward the scalp, until the hair is untangled.

4. Document assessments and special nursing interventions.

- See Technique 17–1, step 5.

EVALUATION FOCUS	Problems such as dandruff, alopecia, pediculosis, scalp lesions, or excessive dryness or mats.

KEY ELEMENTS OF PROVIDING HAIR CARE FOR BLACK CLIENTS

- Do not unbind cornrows without the client's permission.
- Lift and fluff the hair outward, starting at the nape of the neck and moving toward the forehead.

- For very dry hair, apply oil.

17-3 # Braiding the Hair

Braiding is a method of entwining hair. For young children who have long hair, two braids can provide a particularly neat and attractive appearance. Braids (except cornrows) need to be undone daily, and the hair needs to be brushed and combed.

PURPOSE	• To maintain a neat appearance

ASSESSMENT FOCUS	Does the client desire a braid or braids?

EQUIPMENT

- ☐ Towel
- ☐ Brush
- ☐ Comb

- ☐ Ribbon(s) or covered elastic band(s)

▸

▶ **Technique 17–3 Braiding the Hair** CONTINUED

INTERVENTION

1. Brush and comb the hair, and remove any tangles.

- See steps 2 and 3 in Technique 17–1.

2. Braid the hair.

- For one braid, divide the hair into three even sections (strands). For two braids, part the hair down the middle, and then divide each side into three strands. Two braids are usually more comfortable for clients lying in bed. *This avoids the need to lie on the bulk of one braid.*

- Hold the left strand in the left hand, the center strand by the second finger and thumb of the left hand, and the right strand in the right hand (Figure 17–7). Hold the strands firmly and tautly, but do not pull. *Pulling can damage the hair and cause pain.*

- Lay the right strand (3) over the middle strand (2). Transfer strand 3 to the left hand and strand 2 to the right hand (Figure 17–8). Strand 3 is now the middle strand, and strand 2 is the right strand.

- Still holding the strands of hair tautly, cross the left strand (1) over the middle strand (3) (Figure 17–9). Strand 1 is now the middle strand, and strand 3 is the left strand. The left hand holds strand 3, the right fingers hold strand 1, and the right hand holds strand 2.

- Cross the right strand (2) over the center strand (1) (Figure 17–10). Then cross the left strand (3) over the middle strand (2).

- Continue crossing the side strands over the center strand, alternating right and left sides until you reach the ends of the strands (Figure 17–11).

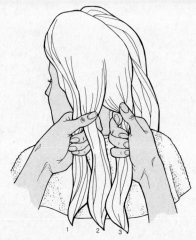

FIGURE 17–7 Beginning step for braiding hair: dividing the hair into three even strands.

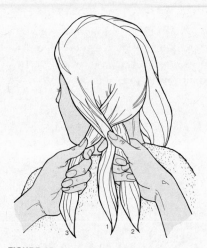

FIGURE 17–9 Crossing the left outside strand over the new middle strand.

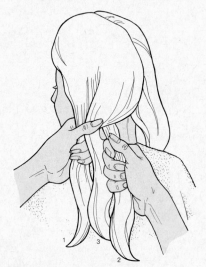

FIGURE 17–8 Crossing the right outside strand over the middle strand.

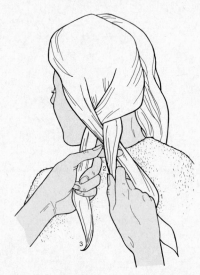

FIGURE 17–10 Continuing to cross alternate side strands over the center strand.

- When all the hair has been braided, firmly secure the end of the braid with a covered elastic band or a ribbon so that the strands cannot come undone.

- Braid the other side of the hair if a second braid is needed.

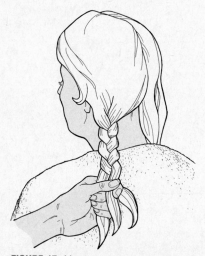

FIGURE 17–11 Appearance of braided hair.

Shampooing the Hair

When a client is hospitalized for extended periods or the hair becomes soiled, the nurse needs to help shampoo the client's hair. There are several ways to shampoo clients' hair, depending on their health, strength, and age. The client who is well enough to take a shower can shampoo while in the shower. The client who is unable to shower may be given a shampoo while sitting on a chair in front of a sink. The back-lying client who can move to a stretcher can be given a shampoo on a stretcher wheeled to a sink. The client who must remain in bed can be given a shampoo with water brought to the bedside. This method is the least convenient. Some hospitals have volunteer beauticians with portable shampoo chairs who assist with hair care.

Shampoo basins to catch the water and direct it to the washbasin or other receptacle are usually made of plastic or metal. If one is not available, a plastic drawsheet can be rolled up on three sides to make edges about 7 cm (3 in) high. These edges will guide the water to the receptacle, in which the unrolled fourth edge of the sheet is placed. A pail or large washbasin can be used as a receptacle for the shampoo water. If possible, the receptacle should be large enough to hold all the shampoo water so that it does not have to be emptied during the shampoo.

Water used for the shampoo should be 40.5 C (105 F) for an adult or child to be comfortable and not injure the scalp. Usually, the person will supply a liquid or cream shampoo. If the shampoo is being given to destroy lice, the physician will order the shampoo to be used. See Technique 17–5.

How often a person needs a shampoo is highly individual, depending to a large degree on the person's activities and the amount of sebum secreted by the scalp. Oily hair tends to look stringy and dirty, and it feels unclean to the person. Technique 17–4 explains how to provide a shampoo for a client confined to bed.

17-4 Shampooing the Hair of a Client Confined to Bed

PURPOSES
- To stimulate the blood circulation to the scalp through massage
- To clean the hair and increase the client's sense of well-being

ASSESSMENT FOCUS

Routinely used shampoo products; any scalp problems; activity tolerance of the client.

EQUIPMENT

- Comb and brush
- Plastic sheet or pad
- Two bath towels
- Shampoo basin
- Washcloth or pad

- Bath blanket
- Receptacle for the shampoo water
- Cotton fluffs (optional)

- Pitcher of water
- Bath thermometer
- Liquid or cream shampoo
- Hair dryer

INTERVENTION

1. Verify agency policy and the physician's order.

- Determine whether a physician's order is needed before a shampoo can be given. *Some hospitals require an order.*

- Determine the type of shampoo to be used, e.g., a medicated shampoo.

2. Prepare the client.

- Determine the best time of day for the shampoo. Discuss this with the client. A person who must remain in bed may find the shampoo tiring. Choose a time when the client is rested and can rest after the procedure.

- Assist the client to the side of the bed from which you will work.

- Remove pins and ribbons from the hair, and brush and comb it to remove any tangles.

3. Arrange the equipment.

- Put the plastic sheet or pad on the bed under the head. *The plastic keeps the bedding dry.*

▶

▶ **Technique 17–4 Shampooing the Hair** *CONTINUED*

- Remove the pillow from under the client's head, and place it under the shoulders. *This hyperextends the neck.*

- Tuck a bath towel around the client's shoulders. *This keeps the shoulders dry.*

- Place the shampoo basin under the head, putting a folded washcloth or pad where the client's neck rests on the edge of the basin. If the client is on a stretcher, the neck can rest on the edge of the sink with the washcloth as padding. *Padding supports the muscles of the neck and prevents undue strain and discomfort.*

- Fanfold the top bedding down to the waist, and cover the upper part of the client with the bath blanket. *The folded bedding will stay dry, and the bath blanket, which can be discarded after the shampoo, will keep the client warm.*

- Place the receiving receptacle on a table or chair at the bedside. Put the spout of the shampoo basin over the receptacle.

4. Protect the client's eyes and ears.

- Place a damp washcloth over the client's eyes (Figure 17–12). *The washcloth protects the eyes from soapy water. A damp washcloth will not slip.*

- Place cotton fluffs in the client's ears if indicated. *These keep water from collecting in the ear canals.*

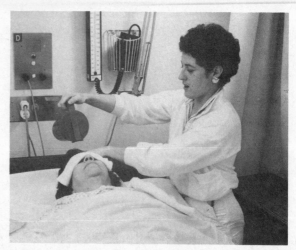

FIGURE 17–12 Protecting the eyes from soapy water with a damp washcloth.

5. Shampoo the hair.

- Wet the hair thoroughly with the water.

- Apply shampoo to the scalp. Make a good lather with the shampoo while massaging the scalp with the pads of your fingertips. Massage all areas of the scalp systematically, e.g., starting at the front and working toward the back of the head. *Massaging stimulates the blood circulation in the scalp. The pads of the fingers are used so that the fingernails will not scratch the scalp.*

- Rinse the hair briefly, and apply shampoo again.

- Make a good lather and massage the scalp as before.

- Rinse the hair thoroughly this time to remove all the shampoo. *Shampoo remaining in the hair may dry and irritate the hair and scalp.*

- Squeeze as much water as possible out of the hair with your hands.

6. Dry the hair thoroughly.

- Rub the client's hair with a heavy towel.

- Dry the hair with the dryer. Set the temperature at "warm."

- Continually move the dryer to prevent burning the client's scalp.

7. Ensure client comfort.

- Assist the person confined to bed to a comfortable position.

- Arrange the hair using a clean brush and comb.

8. Document the shampoo and any assessments.

- Report problems noted to the nurse in charge.

EVALUATION FOCUS

Any scalp problems or intolerance to procedure.

SAMPLE RECORDING

Date	Time	Notes
6/2/93	1300	Shampoo given. Abrasion 2.5 cm long on right occipital area. Area appears pink with some bluish discoloration surrounding it. White scaly area on left temporal area 4 cm in diameter. Dr King notified. —— Kim L. Krueger, SN

► **Technique 17–4** *CONTINUED*

KEY ELEMENTS OF SHAMPOOING THE HAIR OF A CLIENT CONFINED TO BED

- Assess the client's hair and scalp.
- Obtain a physician's order as required.
- Protect the client's eyes and support the neck as required.

- Apply shampoo to wet hair.
- Use the pads of the fingers to massage the scalp.
- Rinse all shampoo from the hair.

Pediculosis

Because lice live and feed from the skin and clothing, prompt elimination of the lice and their eggs is essential. Lice infestations may involve the total body, the hair, and the pubic region; they are spread through infested clothing, bed linen, shared use of combs and other personal items, and close contact with infected persons. Pubic lice are spread primarily through sexual contacts. Technique 17–5 explains the care of clients with pediculosis.

Clients who treat themselves at home need to be instructed to follow the manufacturer's directions carefully and to launder used linens, towels, and infested clothes in very hot water and detergent, separate from other laundry items. Clothing may also be dry-cleaned or pressed with a hot iron to help kill lice.

Other family members and close contacts should be inspected and, if infested, advised about treatment as above.

17-5

Care of the Client with Pediculosis

PURPOSE
- To destroy and remove lice

ASSESSMENT FOCUS

> Presence of skin abrasions from scratching; location of lice (head, body, or pubic area); presence of lice on other family members or other close contacts.

EQUIPMENT

For Head Lice
- ☐ Shampoo containing gamma benzene hexachloride (or lindane) or similar acting medications, e.g., Kwell, GBH, Scabine
- ☐ Fine-toothed comb and brush

For Body and Pubic Lice
- ☐ Cream, lotion, or powder containing a medication, e.g., Kwell
- ☐ Topical ointment for the skin as ordered, e.g., antibiotic, antipruritic, or steroid cream

For All Types
- ☐ Gown and gloves
- ☐ Surgical cap (as recommended by agency)
- ☐ Bath towels
- ☐ Impervious isolation bag
- ☐ Clean gown and bed linens

INTERVENTION

1. Remove head lice.

- Don gown, gloves, and (if agency recommends) surgical cap before the procedure. *These prevent spread to the nurse's clothing and skin and subsequent transmission to others.*

- Place a small damp or dry washcloth over the client's eyes to protect them from the shampoo. *The medication in the shampoo is irritating to the eyes.*

- Apply the medicated shampoo according to the manufacturer's

directions. Some shampoos may be left in place for 5 minutes.

- Shampoo the hair and scalp thoroughly. Be careful to keep the medicated shampoo out of the client's eyes.

►

▶ **Technique 17–5 Care of the Client with Pediculosis** *CONTINUED*

- Rinse the hair and scalp thoroughly. *Thorough rinsing removes dead lice and the medicated shampoo and prevents scalp irritation.*

- If necessary, remove dead lice and nits with a fine-toothed comb or brush dipped in hot vinegar (optional). *A comb or brush dipped in hot vinegar tends to loosen nit cement and facilitates removal of nits.*

- Disinfect the comb and brush with the medicated shampoo. Repeat the shampoo if indicated.

2. Remove body and pubic lice.

- Have the client bathe in soap and water.

- Don gown and gloves.

- Apply medicated topical cream or lotion to infested areas—e.g., axillae, chest, and pubic areas—and allow it to remain for the prescribed time period, according to the manufacturer's directions.

- Clean the treated areas with soap and water to remove dead lice and medication and prevent skin irritation.

- If eyelashes are involved, use a prescribed ophthalmic ointment as ordered and directed. Remove nits manually.

3. Dispose of linens and clothing appropriately.

- Place any used towels and the client's soiled gown and bed linen into a labeled isolation bag.

- Provide a clean gown and bed linens for the client.

- Dispose of your gown and gloves appropriately, and wash your hands.

4. Document any pertinent information.

- Include the date and time of treatment, area of the body treated, and all nursing assessments and interventions.

EVALUATION FOCUS	Client's knowledge of preventive and control measures and presence of pediculi.

SAMPLE RECORDING

Date	Time	Notes
11/9/93	1030	Hair shampooed with Kwell soap as ordered for pediculosis. Pustules present behind ears and at hairline. Instructed to shower and apply Kwell lotion. Infested clothing bagged for family to clean at home. ———————————— ———— Michelle M. Nutter, RN

KEY ELEMENTS OF CARE OF THE CLIENT WITH PEDICULOSIS

- Control and prevent transmission of infestation.
- Apply medication appropriately.
- Protect the client's eyes from the medication.

- Thoroughly clean treated areas after the medication has been applied for the prescribed time period.

Beard and Mustache Care

Beards and mustaches also require daily care. The most important aspect of the care is to keep them clean. Food particles tend to collect in beards and mustaches, and they need washing and combing periodically. Clients may also wish a beard or mustache trim to maintain a well-groomed appearance. A beard or mustache should not be shaved off without the client's consent.

Male clients often shave or are shaved after a bath. Frequently clients supply their own electric or safety razors. See the box on page 435 for the steps involved in shaving a beard with a safety razor.

The Nails

The fingernails and toenails are epidermal appendages. Like the hair, they are directly related to the epidermis; they are made of epidermal cells that have been changed to **keratin**, a type of protein. Today, the nails have little functional value except for cosmetic purposes. Nails usually grow regularly, about

---

Using a Safety Razor to Shave a Beard

- Apply shaving cream or shaving soap and water first to soften the bristles and make the skin more pliable.
- Hold the razor so that the blade is at a 45° angle to the skin, and shave in short, firm strokes in the direction of hair growth.
- Hold the skin taut, particularly around creases, to prevent cutting the skin.
- After shaving the entire area, wipe the client's face with a wet washcloth to remove any remaining shaving cream and hair.
- Dry the face well, then apply aftershave lotion or powder as the client prefers.
- To prevent irritating the skin, pat on the lotion with the fingers and avoid rubbing the face.

---

1 mm per week, but this growth may stop at times of severe stress or illness.

The nail itself is surrounded by **cuticle**, which tends to grow over the nail and thus regularly requires pushing back. A lost fingernail takes 3½ to 5½ months to regenerate, and a toenail takes 6 to 8 months.

Developmental Changes

Nails are normally present at birth. They continue to grow throughout life, and they change very little except to harden. As aging occurs, the nails tend to become tougher, more brittle, and in some cases thicker. The nails of an elderly person normally grow less quickly than those of a younger person, and they may be ridged and have grooves as a result of changes in circulatory status.

Common Problems

Common problems of nails are hangnails, paronychia, ingrown toenails, and broken nails. Regular nail care can help to prevent these problems. Other problems include changes in nail plate shape or curvature, changes in texture or thickness, and changes in color.

Hangnails are shreds of epidermal tissue at either side of the nail. A regular schedule of rubbing oil into the tissue around the nails will lubricate the tissue and prevent hangnails. When a hangnail develops and is not infected, it can be either carefully flattened and held in place with collodion or clipped off. Antiseptic should be applied to the area after clipping.

Paronychia is an inflammation of the tissue surrounding the nail. Acute paronychia is called **thecal whitlow**; it is a painful red swelling that develops quickly. It usually follows a hangnail or injury. This condition occurs most frequently in people who have their hands in water a great deal, and it is three times more common in clients who have diabetes. Careful manicuring that does not injure the adjacent soft tissue helps to prevent it.

Incurvated nails (ingrown toenails) are a relatively common condition. The lateral margin of the toenail grows into surrounding soft tissue and produces an inflammatory reaction of the lateral skin fold. The symptoms are pain with walking and when pressure is put on the nail, tenderness, and redness if inflammation has started in the soft tissues. The usual treatment is to remove the part of the nail that has curved into the tissue and to clear any debris and callus tissue in the area. The nail groove is then packed in such a way that the nail will grow forward rather than into the soft tissue. Any secondary infection is generally treated with an antibiotic ointment or powder.

Changes in thickness or texture include hypertrophy, atrophy, and Beau's line. **Nail hypertrophy** (increased thickness) may be associated with ischemia or chronic fungal infection. **Nail atrophy** (decreased thickness) is often associated with nutritional anemias. **Beau's line** is a transverse white line or groove on the nail that occurs as a result of severe stress or acute illness (Figure 11–16, page 213). Nail growth stops temporarily due to impaired keratin synthesis, and a deep line becomes visible across the nail.

Nail plate color changes may or may not be a problem. See Chapter 11, page 213, for normal nail bed colors. *Splinter hemorrhages* (red or brown longitudinal streaks in the nail) are generally insignificant and may occur with minor trauma or no apparent cause.

Beneath the translucent nail plate, the status of circulation to the extremities can be assessed in the nail bed. Nail bed color acquires a bluish tinge (cyanosis) with a lack of oxygen, instead of its normal pink. The nail beds are one of the first areas of the body where cyanosis is detected. The status of circulation to the extremities can also be determined by checking the rate of capillary refill. See the blanch test discussed in Chapter 11, page 214.

Nail Care

Daily nail care is part of the personal hygiene of most people. Nails are usually cleaned at the time of a bath and filed or cut when they become long. Most clients can attend to their own nail care, but the elderly, the very young, the confused, and the blind may require assistance. Often people enjoy nail care and feel better when it has been done. For cleaning and trimming nails, see Technique 17–6.

17-6 Cleaning and Trimming the Nails

Before cleaning and trimming the nails, determine (a) whether the client has impaired circulation to any extremities. Impaired circulation predisposes people to infections of the tissues surrounding the nails, and special precautions are indicated to prevent infection, and (b) agency policy regarding nail care for clients with impaired circulation to the extremities. Some agencies require a physician's order to cut the nails of these people.

PURPOSES

- To prevent infections around the nails
- To improve the client's appearance and sense of well-being

ASSESSMENT FOCUS

Inflammation of tissues around nails; broken areas in tissue or nails; nail abnormalities; routine nail care practices; self-care abilities.

EQUIPMENT

- Polish remover, if necessary
- Plastic sheet
- Bath blanket
- Washbasin and water at 40.5 C (105 F)
- Towel
- Nail cutter or pair of sharp scissors
- Nail file or emery board
- Orange stick
- Hand lotion, mineral oil, or petroleum jelly

INTERVENTION

1. Prepare the client.

- Assist the ambulatory client to a sitting position in a chair; assist the person confined to bed to a reclining position with the head of the bed elevated, if the client's health permits.

- Remove nail polish, if the person wishes. If the client is scheduled for anesthesia, remove colored nail polish. Some agencies permit clients to wear clear nail polish during surgery. *Colored nail polish obscures the view of the nail bed, and blood circulation to the extremities cannot be observed. Impaired oxygen in the body may be indicated by a bluish tinge in the nail beds. A pinkish tinge (or the person's normal color) indicates adequate oxygen.*

- If the toenails are to be soaked while the client is in bed, place a plastic sheet under the basin to catch any spills, and cover the client with a bath blanket.

- Soak the client's hands and/or feet in a basin of warm water if the nails are very thick and hard. Toenails can be soaked while attending to the fingernails.

- With a towel, dry the hand or the foot that has been soaking.

2. Trim or file each nail.

- Starting with the thumb or large toe, cut or file straight across the nail (Figure 17–13) beyond the end of the finger or toe. If the client has diabetes or circulatory problems, file the nails rather than cut them. *Trimming is done straight across, not down the sides, because of the danger of injuring the tissue around the nail. Filing further reduces the risk of tissue injury for susceptible clients.*

- Shape the fingernail with a file, rounding the corners. Toenails are not shaped. *Shaping the toe-*

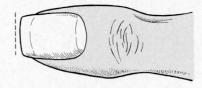
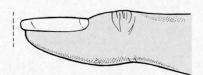

FIGURE 17–13 Trimming fingernails straight across.

nails may damage the tissues or cause a toenail to grow into the tissues.

- Clean under the nail, working from one side to the other, using the pointed end of the file or an orange stick.

- Proceed to the next finger or toe, and repeat the steps above for all nails.

▶ **Technique 17–6** *CONTINUED*

- Massage lotion onto the hands and feet, giving particular attention to the cuticles around the nails. *Lotion lubricates the cuticles and helps to prevent tearing.*

- Gently push the cuticle back around the base of the nail, using the orange stick or a special cuticle tool. Take care not to tear or injure the cuticle. *This could become the site of an infection.*

3. Document assessments.

- Include any problems, such as an infected cuticle or inflammation of the tissue around the nail. Nail care is not normally recorded.

EVALUATION FOCUS	Nail length and intactness; condition of cuticles and surrounding tissues.

SAMPLE RECORDING

Date	Time	Notes
1/14/93	0800	Toenails cut. Reddened, swollen area at base of nail on left 2d toe. States it is tender and feels hot. Dr Weil notified. ———————— Wendy J. Lum, SN

KEY ELEMENTS OF CLEANING AND TRIMMING THE NAILS

- Assess client for impaired circulation to the extremities.
- Determine agency policy regarding nail care for clients with impaired circulation to the extremities, e.g., those who have diabetes mellitus.

- Soak thick toenails before trimming or filing them.
- Trim nails straight across, and shape with a file when the client has impaired circulation.

The Feet

The feet are essential for ambulation and merit attention even when people are confined to bed. Each foot contains 26 bones, 107 ligaments, and 19 muscles. These structures function together for both standing and walking.

During childhood, the bones and small muscles of the feet are easily damaged by tight, binding stockings and ill-fitting shoes. For normal development, it is important that the arches be supported and that the bony structure and the feet grow with no external restrictions.

Development Changes

At birth a baby's foot is relatively unformed. The arches are supported by fatty pads and do not take their full shape until 5 to 6 years of age. Feet are not fully grown until about age 20. Healthy feet remain relatively unchanged during life. However, the elderly often require special attention for their feet. For

example, reduced blood supply and accompanying arteriosclerosis can make a foot prone to infection following trauma.

Common Problems

Foot problems that produce considerable discomfort are commonly observed. Among these are calluses, corns, unpleasant odors, plantar warts, fissures between the toes, and fungus infections, such as athlete's foot.

A **callus** is a thickened portion of epidermis, a mass of keratotic material. It is flat and usually found on the bottom or side of the foot over a bony prominence. Calluses are usually caused by pressure from shoes. They can be softened by soaking the area in warm water with Epsom salts and removed by an abrasive substance such as a pumice stone. Creams with lanolin can also be used to keep the skin soft and prevent the formation of calluses.

A **corn** is a keratosis caused by friction and pressure from a shoe. It commonly occurs on a toe, usually the fourth or fifth toe, and usually on a bony prominence such as a joint. Corns are usually conical (circular and raised). The base is the surface of the corn and the apex is in deeper tissues, sometimes even attached to bone. Corns are generally removed surgically. They are prevented from reforming by relieving the pressure on the area and massaging the tissue to promote circulation.

Unpleasant odors occur as a result of perspiration and its interaction with microorganisms. Regular and frequent washing of the feet and wearing clean hosiery help to minimize odor. Foot powders and deodorants also help to prevent this problem.

Plantar warts appear on the sole of the foot. These warts are caused by the virus *papovavirus hominis*. They are moderately contagious. The warts are frequently painful and often make walking difficult. The treatment ordered by a physician may be curettage, freezing with solid carbon dioxide several times, or repeated applications of salicylic acid.

Fissures between the toes occur frequently as a result of dryness and cracking of skin. The treatment of choice is good foot hygiene and application of an antiseptic to prevent infection. Often a small piece of gauze is inserted between the toes in applying the antiseptic and left in place to assist healing by allowing air to reach the area.

Athlete's foot, or **tinea pedis**, is caused by a fungus. The symptoms are scaling and cracking of the skin, particularly between the toes. Sometimes small blisters form, containing a thin fluid. In severe cases the lesions may also appear on other parts of the body, particularly the hands. Treatments vary from potassium permanganate soaks, using a 1:8000 solution, to commercial antifungal ointments or powders. Prevention is important. Common preventive measures are keeping the feet well ventilated, wearing clean socks or stockings, and not going barefoot in public showers.

Foot Hygiene

Foot hygiene is particularly important for clients who have an infection or abrasion, diabetes mellitus, or impaired circulation to the extremities. The latter two conditions predispose people to infections. These individuals need to learn proper foot care to prevent problems. Other clients normally care for their own feet. After determining a person's personal foot care practices, the nurse can identify the learning needs. Foot care is usually provided in conjunction with the bed bath but can be provided at any time. See Technique 17–7 for foot care.

17-7 Providing Foot Care

PURPOSES
- To maintain the skin integrity of the feet
- To prevent foot infections
- To prevent foot odors
- To maintain foot function

ASSESSMENT FOCUS
Skin surfaces; presence of edema or tenderness; circulatory status; usual foot care practices; self-care abilities.

EQUIPMENT
- Washbasin containing warm water
- Pillow
- Moisture-resistant disposable pad
- Towels
- Soap
- Washcloth
- Toenail cleaning and trimming equipment
- Lotion or foot powder

► **Technique 17–7** CONTINUED

INTERVENTION

1. Prepare the equipment and the client.

- Fill the washbasin with warm water at about 40 to 43 C (105 to 110 F). *Warm water promotes circulation, comforts, and refreshes.*

- Assist the ambulatory client to a sitting position in a chair, or the bed client to a supine or semi-Fowler's position.

- Place a pillow under the bed client's knees. *This provides support and prevents muscle fatigue.*

- Place the washbasin on the moisture-resistant pad at the foot of the bed for a bed client or on the floor in front of the chair for an ambulatory client.

- For a bed client, pad the rim of the washbasin with a towel. *This towel prevents undue pressure on the skin.*

2. Wash the foot, and soak it as required.

- Place one of the client's feet in the basin, and wash it with soap, paying particular attention to the interdigital areas.

- Rinse the foot well to remove soap. *Soap irritates the skin if not properly removed.*

- Rub callused areas of the foot with the washcloth. *This helps remove dead skin layers.*

- If the nails are brittle or thick and require trimming, replace the water and allow the foot to soak for 10 to 20 minutes. *Soaking softens the nails and loosens debris under them.*

- Clean the nails as required with an orange stick or the blunt end of a toothpick. *This removes excess debris that harbors microorganisms.*

- Remove the foot from the basin, and place it on the towel.

3. Dry the foot thoroughly, and apply lotion or foot powder.

- Blot the foot gently with the towel to dry it thoroughly, particularly between the toes. *Harsh rubbing can damage the skin. Thorough drying reduces the risk of infection.*

- Apply lotion or lanolin cream. *This lubricates dry skin.*
  or

Apply a foot powder containing a nonirritating deodorant if the feet tend to perspire excessively. *Foot powders have greater absorbent properties than regular bath powders; some also contain menthol, which makes the feet feel cool.*

4. If agency policy permits, trim the nails of the first foot while the second foot is soaking.

- See Technique 17–6 for the appropriate method to trim nails. Note that in many agencies toenail trimming is contraindicated for clients with diabetes mellitus, toe infections, and peripheral vascular disease, unless performed by a podiatrist or general practice physician.

5. Document any foot problems observed.

- Foot care is not generally recorded unless problems are noted.

- Record any signs of inflammation, infection, breaks in the skin, corns, troublesome calluses, bunions, and pressure areas. This is of particular importance for clients with peripheral vascular disease and diabetes.

EVALUATION FOCUS	Skin color and temperature; presence of foot odor; foot comfort; tenderness.

KEY ELEMENTS OF PROVIDING FOOT CARE

- Assess client for impaired circulation to the extremities.
- Assess integrity of the skin of the feet and any lesions.

- Determine agency policy about nail care for clients with circulatory impairment.
- Use the appropriate nail care technique for the client's health status.

Critical Thinking Challenge

Elena Rodriguez, a 26-year-old female, is admitted to the nursing unit following an auto accident in which she sustained a scalp laceration. Following treatment and suturing of the scalp laceration, you note that blood from the laceration has dried and matted in Ms Rodriguez' hair. Considering the injury, is it appropriate to shampoo Ms Rodriguez' hair? How would you remove the blood from her hair?

Related Research

Pierson, M. A. February 1991. Nurses' knowledge and perceptions related to foot care for older persons. *Journal of Nursing Education* 30:57–62.

References

Brodie, B. S. September/October 1989. Community health and foot health. *Canadian Journal of Public Health* 80: 331–36.

Edelstein, J. E. December 1988. Foot care for the aging. *Physical Therapy* 68:1882–86.

Evanski, P. M., and Reinherz, R. P. January 30, 1990. Easing the pain of common foot problems. *Patient Care* 25: 38–44, 47–50, 52–54.

Maier, T., and Pietrocarlo, T. March 1991. The foot and footwear. *Nursing Clinics of North America* 26: 223–31.

Marieb, E. N. 1989. *Human anatomy and physiology.* Redwood City, Calif.; Benjamin/Cummings.

Osterman H. M., and Stuck, R. M. November/December 1990. The aging foot. *Orthopedic Nursing* 9: 43–47, 76.

Parrott, T. E. September/October 1987. Care of long hair. *Associate Degree Nurse* 2:8–10.

Pelican, R.; Barbieri, E.; and Blair, S. December 1990. Toe the line: A nurse-run well foot care clinic. *Journal of Gerontological Nursing* 16: 6–10, 40–42.

Portnow, J., and Houtman, M. 1987. *Home care for the elderly.* New York: McGraw-Hill.

Thompson, J. February 1990. Foot and leg care. *Community outlook* 14: 16–17.

Wells, R., and Trostle, K. January 1984. Creative hairwashing techniques for immobilized patients. *Nursing 84* 14:47–51.

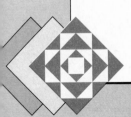

18

OBJECTIVES

- Identify reasons underlying select-ed steps of bed-making techniques

- Make closed, open, and occupied beds effectively

Bed-Making

CONTENTS

Bed Unit

Making Beds

Bed Unit

Hospital Beds

When people are ill, they can be confined to bed for days, weeks, or even months. The bed, then, becomes a very important piece of furniture; it becomes the client's territory. A bed at home is usually satisfactory if illness does not confine the person to bed for long periods of time. Hospital beds are often preferred by people who are ill for more than several weeks and are more convenient for nursing personnel because of the following characteristics:

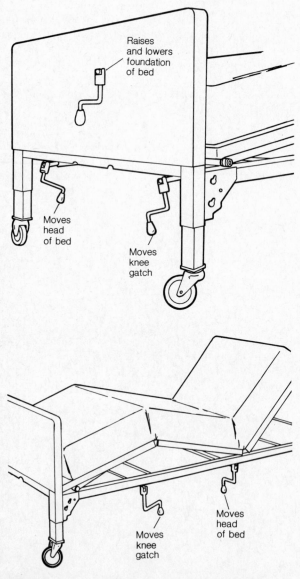

- Hospital beds can be adjusted to a variety of positions. Some hospitals have **gatch beds**. When the gatches, or joints, are flexed, the client is raised to a sitting position with the knees elevated. The cranks that operate the gatches are usually at the bottom or side of the bed (Figure 18–1). Manual cranks are left in the retracted position under the bed when they are not being used. Otherwise, people walking by the bed might easily hit their legs against the cranks. Many hospital beds have electric motors to operate the gatches. The motor is activated by pressing a button or moving a small lever, located either at the side of the bed or on a small panel separate from the bed but attached to it by a cable (Figure 18–2), which the client can readily use.

- Hospital beds are usually 66 cm (26 in) high. (Long-term care facilities for ambulatory clients usually have low beds to facilitate movement in and out of bed.) Some hospital beds have "high" and "low" positions that can be adjusted either mechanically by a crank at the center of the foot of the bed or electrically by a button or lever on the same panel as the gatch controls. The high position permits the nurse to reach the client without undue stretching or stooping. The low position allows the client to step easily to the floor.

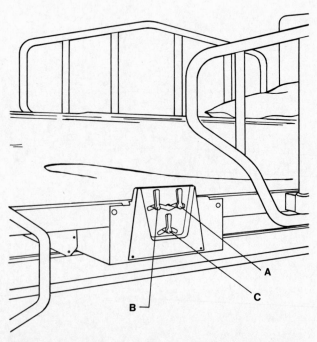

FIGURE 18–1 Cranks commonly used to change the position of a hospital bed.

FIGURE 18–2 Controls for a motor-operated hospital bed: *A*, Raises and lowers the backrest; *B*, raises and lowers the knee gatch; *C*, raises and lowers the foundation of the bed.

- A hospital bed is normally 0.9 m (3 ft) wide, which is narrower than the usual bed. This permits the nurse to reach the client from either side of the bed without undue stretching. The length is usually 1.9 m (6.5 ft). Some beds can be extended in length, if required.

- Most hospital beds have **casters** that permit people to move the bed easily and quietly.

Specialized Beds Whenever a client's body alignment must be strictly maintained, a specially designed bed that rotates on an axis turns the client from the supine to the prone position and vice versa. For additional information, see Chapter 45.

Cribs Infants and children under 3 feet tall should be placed in cribs covered with nets or domes See Figure 6–16, page 97. The crib's rails should be maintained in an elevated position, even when the crib is empty, so that the child cannot climb in and out of the crib (Whaley and Wong 1991).

Mattresses Most mattresses used in hospitals have innersprings, which give even support to the body. When changing a bed, nurses need to note any unevenness of the mattress surface, which might indicate a broken spring. Mattresses are usually covered with a water-repellent material that resists soiling and can be cleaned easily. Most mattresses have handles on the sides called lugs by which the mattress can be removed.

Foam rubber **egg crate mattresses** are also used in hospitals (Figure 18–3). They provide support and

have the advantage of relieving pressure on the body's bony prominences, such as the heels. Foam mattresses are particularly helpful for clients confined to bed for a long time. Another option is the air mattress (also called an **alternating pressure mattress**), which is attached to a motor that lowers or raises the air pressure inside the mattress. The **water mattress** is a plastic bag filled with water. This mattress employs the principle of weight displacement. If the body displaces 9 kg (20 lb) of water, there is 9 kg less pressure on the weight-bearing areas.

The surfaces of air and water mattresses must be intact so that the air or water will not escape. It is therefore inadvisable to use pins on the sheets covering these mattresses. Special mattresses are placed atop the standard bed mattress, although the water mattress may be placed on the base springs.

Side Rails **Side rails**, or safety sides, are used on both hospital beds and stretchers. They are of various shapes and sizes and are usually made of metal. Devices to raise and lower them differ. Often one or two knobs are pulled to release the side and permit it to be moved. When side rails are being used, it is important that the nurse *never* leave the bedside while the rail is lowered. Some side rails have two positions: up and down. Others have three: high, intermediate, and low. The down and low positions are employed when a side rail is not needed. With some models, the bed foundation (the mattress and frame supporting it) must be raised before the side rail can be put in the low position; otherwise, the side

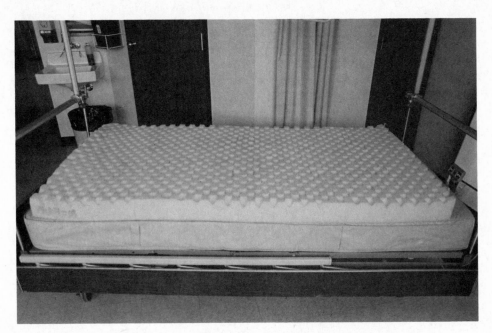

FIGURE 18–3 An egg crate mattress provides comfort and helps to distribute the body weight evenly, thus helping to reduce pressure on bony prominences.

rail might hit the floor and be damaged. The intermediate position is used when the bed is in the low position and the nurse is present. The up or high side rail position is used when a client is in bed and requires protection from falling. Some hospitals have a release form that the client can sign if the use of side rails is refused.

Footboards A **footboard** is a flat panel, often made of wood or plastic, placed at the foot of a bed. It serves three purposes:

1. To provide support for the client's feet and maintain a natural foot position while the client is in bed (Figure 18–4).

2. To keep the top bed covers off the client's feet, relieving the pressure of the weight of the covers.

3. To make the foot comfortable (for example, when a client has a painful foot).

Without the support of a footboard, a client's feet drop from their normal right angle to the legs and assume a plantar flexion position with the toes pointing toward the foot of the bed (Figure 18–5). Prolonged assumption of this position results in permanent shortening of the muscles and tendons at the back of the legs. When that happens, the client is unable to stand flat-footed on the floor, and walking is seriously impaired.

Footboards are often made in an L shape so that the base of the L fits under the foot of the mattress. Some footboards can be moved along the mattress to adjust to the client's height. If a board cannot be adjusted, sandbags and rolled pillows or blankets can be used to fill the space between the client's feet and the board.

Bed Cradles A **bed cradle**, sometimes called an Anderson frame, is a device designed to keep the top bedclothes off the feet, legs, and even abdomen of a client. The bedclothes are arranged over the device and may be pinned in place. There are several types of bed cradles. One of the most common is a curved metal rod that fits over the bed. Part of the cradle fits under the mattress, and small metal brackets press down on each side of the mattress to keep the cradle in place. The frame of some cradles extends over only half of a bed, above only one leg.

Bedside Tables

The bedside table is a small table placed beside the bed. It frequently has a drawer, in which a client can keep personal articles, and a cupboard beneath the drawer, containing a washbasin, soap dish and soap, mouthwash container, and emesis or kidney basin. Some bedside tables also have a place for a bedpan or urinal and a rod at the back for washcloths and towels.

Overbed Tables

The overbed table stands on the floor but fits over the client's bed. It is usually on casters, so it can be easily moved. It can be raised or lowered to suit the client, usually by turning a handle at the side. Some overbed tables have a mirror and a small compartment for personal articles beneath the table top. Overbed tables are often used for the client's meal tray. A person who can assume a sitting position in bed can eat from that table in relative comfort. Nurses also use these tables for supplies.

Chairs

Most hospital bed units have chairs for client and visitor use. Often one chair is without arms and is kept near the bed. There may also be an easy chair that is more comfortable to sit in for long periods.

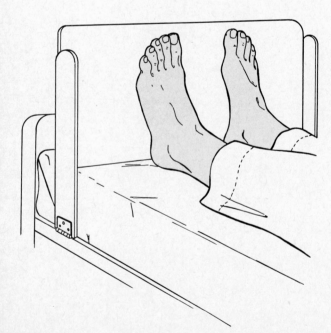

FIGURE 18–4 A footboard that can be adjusted to the client's height.

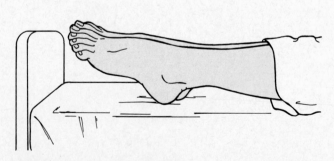

FIGURE 18–5 Feet in plantar flexion.

Clothing Storage Spaces

Hospital bed units generally contain a locker or closet for the storage of clothes. These facilities are usually larger in a long-term care unit than in an acute care setting. Some units also have a chest of drawers or other drawer space for clothing.

Lights

Each bed unit has one or more lights. Often a light at the head of the bed has an extendable neck that allows it to be moved. Some rooms have overhead lights as well. Most bed units also have a signal light. When a client pulls a switch or presses a button, a light goes on at a specific place in the hospital unit, such as the nurses' station or a service area. Clients generally turn on their signal lights when they require assistance. It is important for nurses to be aware of the signal light areas, so that they can note when a light goes on and answer quickly. Some acute care hospitals are equipped with intercoms that permit the nurse at the nursing station to talk with the client before going to the bedside. Intercom signal lights can also be turned off from the nurse's station. Nursing units generally have night lights, which provide subdued lighting during the night. Some also have emergency signal lights.

Other Equipment

Hospitals vary in the equipment provided as part of the bed unit. Long-term care facilities may have very little additional equipment, whereas an acute facility may have several commonly used devices built into each unit. Intravenous rods are often attached to the hospital beds. Some hospital units have overhead hanging rods on a track for IVs. Three types of equipment are often installed on the wall at the head of the bed: a suction outlet for several kinds of suction, an oxygen outlet for most oxygen equipment, and a sphygmomanometer to measure the client's blood pressure.

Some long-term care agencies also permit clients to have personal equipment, such as a television, a chair, and lamps, at the bedside.

Making Beds

Nurses need to be able to prepare hospital beds in different ways for specific purposes. In most instances, nurses make beds after the client receives certain care and when beds are unoccupied. At times, however, nurses need to make an occupied bed or prepare a bed for a client who is having surgery (an anesthetic, postoperative, or surgical bed). Regardless of what type of bed equipment is available, whether the bed is occupied or unoccupied, or the purpose for which the bed is being prepared, certain guidelines pertain to all bed-making.

CLINICAL GUIDELINES

Bed-Making

- Wash hands thoroughly after handling a client's bed linen. Linens and equipment that have been soiled with secretions and excretions harbor microorganisms that can be transmitted to others directly or by the nurse's hands or uniform. Note that some agencies recommend wearing gloves when making beds.

- Hold soiled linen away from your uniform.

- *Never* (even momentarily) place linen for one client on another client's bed.

- Place soiled linen directly in a portable linen hamper or tuck it into a pillowcase at the end of the bed before gathering it up for disposal in the linen hamper or linen chute.

- Never shake soiled linen in the air. Shaking can disseminate secretions and excretions and the microorganisms they contain.

- When stripping and making a bed, conserve time and energy by stripping and making up one side as completely as possible before working on the other side.

- To avoid unnecessary trips to the linen supply area, gather all needed linen before starting to strip a bed.

An **unoccupied bed** can be either closed or open. Generally, the top covers of an open bed are folded back (**open bed**) to make it easier for a client to get in. Open and closed beds are made the same way, except that the top sheet, blanket, and bedspread of a **closed bed** are drawn up to the top of the bed and under the pillows.

Hospital beds are often changed after bed baths. The linen can be collected before the bath. Nurses in some hospitals do not change all the linen unless it is soiled. Check the policy at each clinical agency. Unfitted sheets, blankets, and bedspreads are **mitered**, or folded at the corners of the bed. The purpose of mitering is to secure the bedclothes while the bed is occupied. Figure 18–6 on page 446 shows how to miter the corner of a bed. Clinical guidelines for bed-making are provided in the box above.

Technique 18–1 explains how to change an unoccupied bed.

A **surgical bed** is made for clients who are having surgical or diagnostic procedures that require use of an anesthetic agent. See Chapter 42, page 993, for information about how to prepare a surgical bed.

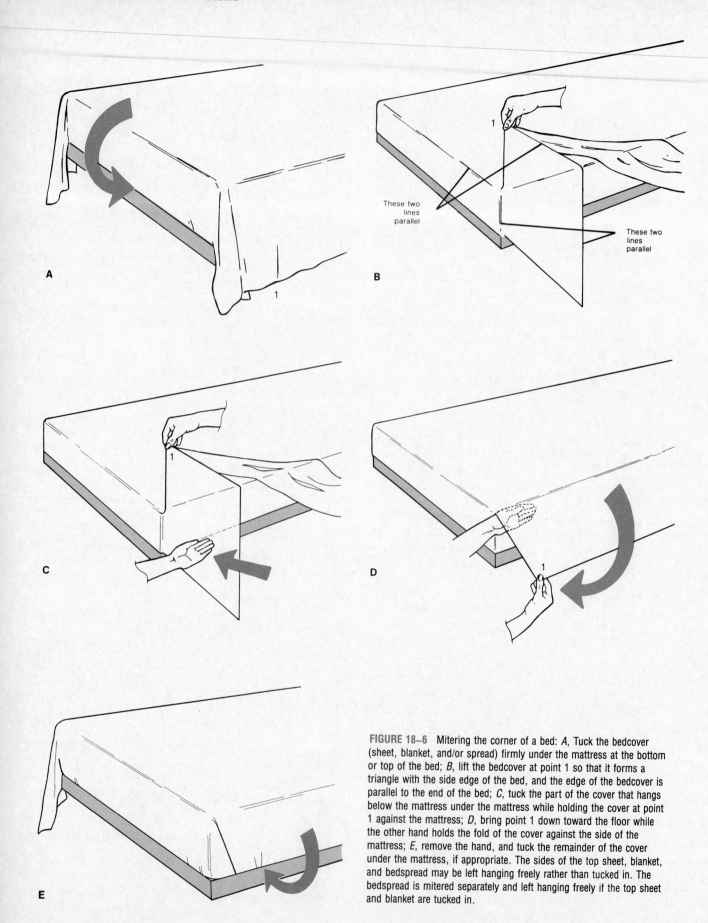

FIGURE 18–6 Mitering the corner of a bed: *A*, Tuck the bedcover (sheet, blanket, and/or spread) firmly under the mattress at the bottom or top of the bed; *B*, lift the bedcover at point 1 so that it forms a triangle with the side edge of the bed, and the edge of the bedcover is parallel to the end of the bed; *C*, tuck the part of the cover that hangs below the mattress under the mattress while holding the cover at point 1 against the mattress; *D*, bring point 1 down toward the floor while the other hand holds the fold of the cover against the side of the mattress; *E*, remove the hand, and tuck the remainder of the cover under the mattress, if appropriate. The sides of the top sheet, blanket, and bedspread may be left hanging freely rather than tucked in. The bedspread is mitered separately and left hanging freely if the top sheet and blanket are tucked in.

18-1 Changing an Unoccupied Bed

PURPOSES
- To promote the client's comfort
- To provide a clean, neat environment for the client
- To provide a smooth, wrinkle-free bed foundation, thus minimizing sources of skin irritation

EQUIPMENT
- Two large sheets
- Cloth drawsheet (optional)
- One blanket
- One bedspread
- Waterproof drawsheet or waterproof pads (optional)
- Pillowcase(s) for the head pillow(s)
- Portable linen hamper, if available

INTERVENTION

1. Place the fresh linen on the client's chair or overbed table; do not use another client's bed. *This prevents cross-contamination (the movement of microorganisms from one client to another) via soiled linen.*

2. Assess and assist the client out of bed.
- Make sure that this is an appropriate and convenient time for the client to be out of bed.
- Assess the client's health status to determine that the person can safely get out of bed. In some hospitals it is necessary to have a written order if the client has been in bed continuously.
- Assess the client's pulse and respirations if indicated.
- Assist the client to a comfortable chair.

3. Strip the bed.
- Check bed linens for any items belonging to the client, and detach the call bell or any drainage tubes from the bed linen.
- Loosen all bedding, starting at the head of the bed, moving down the bed, working around the foot, and moving up to the

other side of the head. *Moving around the bed systematically prevents stretching and reaching and possible muscle strain.*
- Remove the pillowcases, if soiled, and place the pillows on the bedside chair near the foot of the bed.
- Fold reusable linens, such as the bedspread and top sheet on the bed, into fourths. First, fold the linen in half by bringing the top edge even with the bottom edge, and then grasp it at the center of the middle fold and bottom edges (Figure 18–7). *Folding linens on the bed prevents strain on the nurse's arms and saves time and*

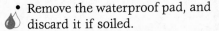
Head of bed

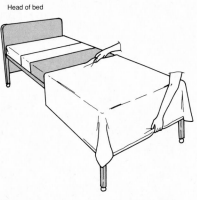
FIGURE 18–7 Folding reusable linens into fourths when removing them from the bed.

energy when reapplying the linens on the bed.
- Remove the waterproof pad, and discard it if soiled.
- Roll all soiled linen inside the bottom sheet, hold it away from your uniform, and place it directly in the linen hamper. *These actions are essential to prevent the transmission of microorganisms to yourself and others.*
- Grasp the mattress securely, using the lugs if present, and move the mattress up to the head of the bed.

4. Apply the bottom sheet and drawsheet.
- Place the folded bottom sheet with its center fold on the center of the bed. Make sure the sheet is hemside down for a smooth foundation. Spread the sheet out over the mattress, and allow a sufficient amount of sheet at the top to tuck under the mattress. *The top of the sheet needs to be well tucked under to remain securely in place, especially when the head of the bed is elevated.* Place the sheet along the edge of the mattress at the foot of the bed, and do not tuck it in (unless it is a contour sheet).

▶ **Technique 18–1 Changing an Unoccupied Bed** *CONTINUED*

• Miter the sheet at the top corner on the near side (Figure 18–6, earlier), and tuck the sheet under the mattress, working from the head of the bed to the foot.

• If a waterproof drawsheet is used, place it over the bottom sheet so that the center fold is at the center line of the bed and the top and bottom edges will extend from the middle of the client's back to the area of the midthigh or knee. Fanfold the uppermost half of the folded drawsheet at the center or far edge of the bed, and tuck in the near edge.

• Lay the cloth drawsheet over the waterproof sheet in the same manner described above.

• *Optional:* Before moving to the other side of the bed, place the top linens on the bed, hemside up, unfold them, tuck them in, and miter the bottom corners. *Completing the entire side of the bed saves time and energy.*

5. Move to the other side and secure the bottom linens.

• Tuck in the bottom sheet under the head of the mattress, pull the sheet firmly, and miter the corner of the sheet.

• Pull the remainder of the sheet firmly so that there are no wrinkles. *Wrinkles can cause discomfort for the client.* Tuck the sheet in at the side.

• Complete this same process for the drawsheet(s).

6. Apply or complete the top sheet, blanket, and spread.

• Place the top sheet, hemside up, on the bed so that its center fold is at the center of the bed and the top edge is even with the top edge of the mattress.

• Unfold the sheet over the bed.

• *Optional:* Make a vertical or a

horizontal toe pleat in the sheet to provide additional room for the client's feet.

a. *Vertical toe pleat:* Make a fold in the sheet 5 to 10 cm (2 to 4 in) perpendicular to the foot of the bed (Figure 18–8).

b. *Horizontal toe pleat:* Make a fold in the sheet 5 to 10 cm (2 to 4 in) across the bed near the foot (Figure 18–9).

Loosening the top covers around the feet after the client is in bed is another way to provide additional space.

• Follow the same procedure for the blanket and the spread, but place the top edges about 15 cm (6 in) from the head of the bed to allow a cuff of sheet to be folded over them.

• Tuck in the sheet, blanket, and

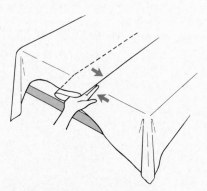

FIGURE 18–8 A vertical toe pleat.

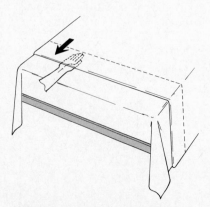

FIGURE 18–9 A horizontal toe pleat.

spread at the foot of the bed, and miter the corner, using all three layers of linen. Leave the sides of the top sheet, blanket, and spread hanging freely unless toe pleats were provided.

• Fold the top of the top sheet down over the spread, providing a cuff of about 15 cm (6 in). *The cuff of sheet makes it easier for the client to pull the covers up.*

• Move to the other side of the bed, and secure the top bedding in the same manner.

7. Put clean pillowcases on the pillows as required.

• Grasp the closed end of the pillowcase at the center with one hand.

• Gather up the sides of the pillowcase, and place them over the hand grasping the case. Then grasp the center of one short side of the pillow through the pillowcase (Figure 18–10).

• With the free hand, pull the pillowcase over the pillow.

• Adjust the pillowcase so that the pillow fits into the corners of the case and the seams are straight. *A smoothly fitting pillowcase is more comfortable than a wrinkled one.*

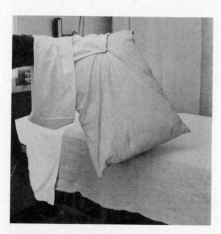

FIGURE 18–10 Method for putting a clean pillowcase on a pillow.

▶ **Technique 18–1** *CONTINUED*

- Align and place the pillows at the head of the bed in the center.

8. Provide for client comfort and safety.

- Attach the signal cord so that the client can conveniently use it. Some cords have clamps that attach to the sheet or pillowcase. Others are attached by a safety pin.

- If the bed is currently being used by a client, either fold back the top covers at one side or fanfold them down to the center of the bed. *This makes it easier for the client to get into the bed.*

- Place the bedside table and the overbed table so that they are available to the client.

- Leave the bed in the high position if the client is returning by stretcher, or place in the low position if the client is returning to bed after being up.

- After changing a crib, leave both side rails in the highest position.

9. Document and report pertinent data.

- Bed-making is not normally recorded.

- Record any nursing assessments such as the client's physical status and pulse and respiratory rates before and after being out of bed, as indicated.

KEY ELEMENTS OF CHANGING AN UNOCCUPIED BED

- Confirm that there is a physician's order allowing the client out of bed.
- Assess pulse, respirations, and physical status before getting the client out of bed if health status indicates.
- Use aseptic technique.
- Place the bed in the low position and make sure the wheels are locked before returning the client to bed.

- Make sure the signal cord is accessible to the client.
- Use only clean linen to change the bed.
- Foundation of bed should be smooth and without wrinkles.
- Allow sufficient toe room for the client.

Changing an Occupied Bed

Some clients may be too weak to get out of bed. Either the nature of their illness may contraindicate their sitting out of bed, or they may be restricted in bed by the presence of traction or other therapies. When changing an **occupied bed**, work quickly and disturb the client as little as possible to conserve the client's energy, using the following guidelines:

- Maintain the client in good body alignment. Never move or position a client in a manner that is contraindicated by the client's health. Obtain help if necessary to ensure safety.

- Move the client gently and smoothly. Rough handling can cause the client discomfort and abrade the skin.

- Throughout the procedure, explain what you plan to do before you do it. Use terms that the client can understand.

- Use the bed-making time, like the bed bath time, to assess and meet the client's needs.

Technique 18–2 describes how to change an occupied bed.

Changing An Occupied Bed

18-2

PURPOSES
- To conserve the client's energy and maintain current health status
- To promote client comfort
- To provide a clean, neat environment for the client
- To provide a smooth, wrinkle-free bed foundation, thus minimizing sources of skin irritation

ASSESSMENT FOCUS

Specific orders or precautions for moving and positioning the client; presence of incontinence or excessive drainage from other sources indicating the need for protective waterproof pads; skin condition and need for special mattress (e.g., egg crate), footboard, or heel protectors.

EQUIPMENT
- See Technique 18–1.

INTERVENTION

1. Remove the top bedding.

- Remove any equipment attached to the bed linen, such as a signal light.

- Loosen all the top linen at the foot of the bed, and remove the spread and the blanket.

- Leave the top sheet over the client (the top sheet can remain over the client if it is being changed and if it will provide sufficient warmth), *or* replace it with a bath blanket as follows:

  a. Spread the bath blanket over the top sheet.

  b. Ask the client to hold the top edge of the blanket.

  c. Reaching under the blanket from the side, grasp the top edge of the sheet and draw it down to the foot of the bed, leaving the blanket in place.

  d. Remove the sheet from the bed and place it in the soiled linen hamper.

2. Move the mattress up on the bed.

- Place the bed in the flat position

if the client's health permits.

- Grasp the mattress lugs, and, using good body mechanics, move the mattress up to the head of the bed. Ask the client to assist, if permitted, by grasping the head of the bed and pulling as you push. If the client is heavy, you may need help from another nurse.

3. Change the bottom sheet and drawsheet.

- Assist the client to turn on the

side facing away from the side where the clean linen is.

- Raise the side rail nearest the client. *This protects the client from falling.* If there is no side rail, have another nurse support the client at the edge of the bed.

- Loosen the foundation linen on the side of the bed near the linen supply.

- Fanfold the drawsheet and the bottom sheet at the center of the bed (Figure 18–11), as close to

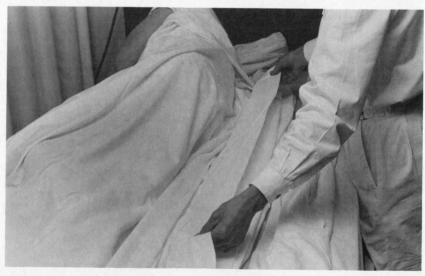

FIGURE 18–11 Fanfolding soiled linen as close to the client as possible.

► **Technique 18–2** *CONTINUED*

the client as possible. Doing this leaves the near half of the bed free to be changed.

- Place the new bottom sheet on the bed, and vertically fanfold the half to be used on the far side of the bed as close to the client as possible. Tuck the sheet under the near half of the bed, and miter the corner if a contour sheet is not being used.

- Place the clean drawsheet on the bed with the center fold at the center of the bed. Fanfold the uppermost half vertically at the center of the bed, and tuck the near side edge under the side of the mattress.

- Assist the client to roll over toward you onto the clean side of the bed. The client rolls over the fanfolded linen at the center of the bed.

- Move the pillows to the clean side for the client's use. Raise the side rail before leaving the side of the bed.

- Move to the other side of the bed, and lower the side rail.

- Remove the used linen, and place it in the portable hamper.

- Smooth out the mattress cover to remove any wrinkles. Unfold the fanfolded bottom sheet from the center of the bed.

- Facing the side of the bed, use both hands to pull the bottom sheet so that it is smooth, and tuck the excess under the side of the mattress.

- Unfold the drawsheet fanfolded at the center of the bed, and pull it tightly with both hands. Pull the sheet in three sections: (a) face the side of the bed to pull the middle section; (b) face the far top corner to pull the bottom section; and (c) face the far bottom corner to pull the top section.

- Tuck the excess drawsheet under the side of the mattress.

4. Reposition the client in the center of the bed.

- Reposition the pillows at the center of the bed.

- Assist the client to the center of the bed. Determine what position the client requires or prefers, and assist the client to that position.

5. Apply or complete the top bedding.

- Spread the top sheet over the client, and ask the client to hold the top edge of the sheet or tuck it under the shoulders. The sheet should remain over the client when the bath blanket or used sheet is removed.

- Complete the top of the bed.

6. Ensure continued safety of the client.

- Raise the side rails. Place the bed in the low position before leaving the bedside.

- Attach the signal cord to the bed linen within the client's reach.

- Put items used by the client within easy reach.

EVALUATION FOCUS | Client comfort and safety; patency of all drainage tubes; client's ability to summon help when needed.

KEY ELEMENTS OF CHANGING AN OCCUPIED BED

- Beforehand, determine positions that are contraindicated for the client.
- Assess the ease with which the client can turn from side to side or move to the edge of the bed.
- Use side rails to protect the client from falling.

- Change all soiled linens.
- Smooth the foundation of the bed.
- Allow sufficient toe room.
- Move client safely.

CRITICAL THINKING CHALLENGE

William Masters, a 52-year-old male, is assigned to your care. He is an ambulatory client, able to perform self care for bathing and toileting. He has completed his morning care and is resting in bed. When you ask to change his bed linens, he tells you not to bother and asks you to leave. What action will you take?

19

Body Mechanics and Moving Clients

OBJECTIVES

- Identify essential guidelines for safe and efficient body movements

- Use correct body mechanics when assisting clients to move

- Identify information required to assess a client's mobility status

- Describe essential steps of techniques to move and turn clients in bed and to transfer clients from bed to chair or stretchers

- Identify reasons underlying selected steps of each technique

- Move, turn, and transfer clients safely

CONTENTS

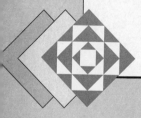

NURSING PROCESS GUIDE
MOVING CLIENTS

ASSESSMENT

Determine

- How the client's illness influences the ability to move and whether the client's health contraindicates any exertion, position, or movement.

- Assistive devices required, such as overhead trapeze, pull and/or turn sheet, roller bar, transfer or sliding bar, transfer belt.

- Encumbrances to movement, such as an IV in place or a heavy cast on one leg.

- Medications the client is receiving. Side effects of certain medications hamper movement or alertness.

- Your own skill and physical strength.

Assess the client's capabilities for movement. Specifically, observe the amount of assistance required for the following:

- Rising from a lying position to a sitting position on the edge of the bed. The client can normally rise without support from the arms; however, a client with muscle weakness may roll to the side and push with the arms or pull with the arms on side rails or nearby furniture to rise.

- Rising from a chair to a standing position. Normally this can be done without pushing with the arms; however, a person with weak muscles may use the arms to push upward and may thrust the upper body forward before rising.

- Moving in the bed. Specifically, observe the amount of assistance required for turning

  a. From a supine position to a lateral position.

  b. From a lateral position on one side to a lateral position on the other.

  c. From a supine position to a prone position.

  d. From a supine position to a sitting position in bed.

- Range of motion of joints needed to complete transfer movements. The nurse asks the client to perform range-of-motion exercises for the arms, ankles, knees, and hips. While the client performs the range-of-motion exercises, assess

  a. The degree of movement of the joint.

  b. Any discomfort experienced by the client.

  c. Any joint swelling or redness, which could indicate the presence of an injury or an inflammation.

  d. Any contractures.

- Mental alertness and ability to follow directions.

- Balance and coordination if the client is to be transferred from the bed.

- Presence of orthostatic hypotension before transfers. Specifically, determine increases in pulse rate, marked fall in blood pressure, dizziness, lightheadedness, and dimming of vision when the client moves from a supine to a vertical posture.

- Degree of comfort. People who have pain may not want to move and require an analgesic before they are moved.

- Weight. Moving obese people may require the assistance of another person or a hydraulic lifter.

RELATED DIAGNOSTIC CATEGORIES

- Activity intolerance

- High risk for Activity intolerance

- High risk for Disuse syndrome

- High risk for Injury

- Impaired physical mobility

- Fear (of falling)

PLANNING

Client Goals
The client will

- Maintain proper body alignment.

- Avoid injuries and falls.

Outcome Criteria
The client

- Demonstrates use of good body mechanics when lifting and pulling objects.

- Participates within capabilities when being moved.

Body Mechanics

Good **body mechanics** is the efficient, coordinated, and safe use of the body to produce motion and maintain balance during activity. Proper movement promotes body musculoskeletal functioning, reduces the energy required to move and maintain balance, therefore reducing fatigue and decreasing the risk of injury.

The major purpose of proper body mechanics is to facilitate safe and efficient use of appropriate groups of muscles. Good body mechanics is essential to both clients and nurses to prevent strain, injury, and fatigue.

Body mechanics involves three basic elements: Body alignment (posture), balance (stability), and coordinated body movement.

Body Alignment

Body alignment is the geometric arrangement of body parts in relation to each other. Good alignment promotes optimal balance and maximal body function in whatever position the client assumes: standing, sitting, or lying down. Good body alignment and good **posture** are synonymous terms. When the body is well aligned, it achieves balance without undue strain on the joints, muscles, tendons, or ligaments. Muscles are usually in a state of slight tension (**tonus**) when the body is healthy and well aligned. This state requires minimal muscular force and yet supports the internal framework and organs.

Proper body alignment enhances lung expansion and promotes efficient circulatory, renal, and gastrointestinal functions. Conversely, poor body alignment detracts from a pleasing appearance and affects an individual's health adversely. A person's posture is one criterion for assessing general health, physical fitness, and attractiveness. Posture reflects the mood, self-esteem, and personality of an individual.

Balance

Balance is a state of equipoise (equilibrium) in which opposing forces counteract each other. Good body alignment is essential to body balance. It is difficult to differentiate balance from body alignment, although balance is the result of proper alignment. A person maintains balance as long as the **line of gravity** (an imaginary vertical line drawn through an object's center of gravity) passes through the **center of gravity** (the point at which all of the mass of an object is centered) and the **base of support** (the foundation on which an object rests).

The center of gravity of a well-aligned standing adult is located slightly anterior to the upper part of

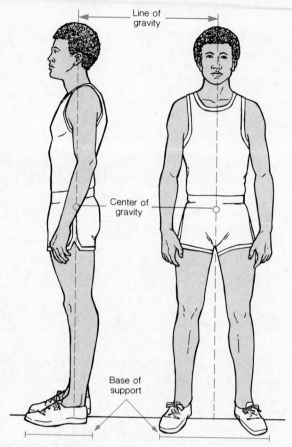

FIGURE 19–1 The center of gravity and the line of gravity influence standing alignment.

the sacrum (Figure 19–1). Standing posture can be unstable because of a narrow base of support, a high center of gravity, and a constantly shifting line of gravity. For greatest balance and stability, a standing adult must center body weight symmetrically along the line of gravity.

In a well-aligned standing person, the center of gravity remains fairly stable. When the person moves, however, the center of gravity shifts continuously in the direction of the moving body parts. Balance depends on the interrelationship of the center of gravity, the line of gravity, and the base of support. When a person moves, the closer the line of gravity is to the center of the base of support, the greater the person's stability (Figure 19–2, *A*). Conversely, the closer the line of gravity is to the edge of the base of support, the more precarious the balance (Figure 19–2, *B*). If the line of gravity falls outside the base of support, the person falls (Figure 19–2, *C*).

The broader the base of support and the lower the center of gravity, the greater the stability and balance. Body balance, therefore, can be greatly enhanced by (a) widening the base of support and

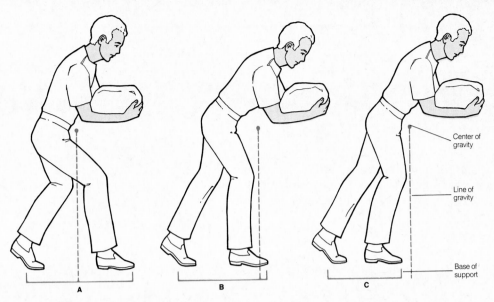

FIGURE 19–2 *A,* Balance is maintained when the line of gravity falls close to the center of the base of support. *B,* Balance is precarious when the line of gravity falls at the edge of the base of support. *C,* Balance cannot be maintained when the line of gravity falls outside the base of support.

(b) lowering the center of gravity, bringing it closer to the base of support. The base of support is easily widened by spreading the feet farther apart. The center of gravity is readily lowered by flexing the hips and knees until a squatting position is achieved. The importance of these alterations cannot be overemphasized for nurses.

When a person rests in a chair or bed, the feet of the chair or bed form a considerably wider base of support. The center of gravity is lower, and the line of gravity is less mobile. Thus, a person has greater stability and balance in a sitting or lying position than in a standing position.

Coordinated Body Movement

Body mechanics involves the integrated functioning of the musculoskeletal and nervous systems. Muscle tone, the neuromuscular reflexes (including the visual and proprioceptive reflexes), and the coordinated movements of opposing voluntary muscle groups (the antagonistic, synergistic, and antigravity muscles) play important roles in producing balanced, smooth, purposeful movement.

Principles of Body Mechanics

In addition to the concepts of center of gravity, line of gravity, and base of support, the nurse needs to consider the concepts of **leverage, force, friction,** and **inertia** when moving clients or objects. These concepts are defined and discussed in Tables 19–1 and 19–2.

The nurse should avoid two movements because of their potential for causing back injury: twisting (rotation) of the thoracolumbar spine and acute flexion of the back with hips and knees straight (stooping). Undesirable twisting of the back can be prevented by squarely facing the direction of movement, whether pushing, pulling, or sliding, and moving the object directly toward or away from one's center of gravity.

Lifting

When a person lifts or carries an object, the weight of the object becomes part of the person's body weight. This weight affects the location of the person's center of gravity, which is displaced in the direction of the added weight. To counteract this potential imbalance, body parts move in a direction away from

TABLE 19–1 CONCEPTS APPLICABLE TO MOVING CLIENTS

Concept	Definition
Friction	Force that opposes the motion of an object as it is slid across the surface of another object.
Force	The energy or power required to accomplish movement.
Inertia	The tendency of an object at rest to remain at rest and an object in motion to remain in motion.
Fulcrum	A fixed point (e.g., elbow) about which a lever moves.
Lever (first class)	A rigid piece that transmits or modifies motion or force. When force (energy) is applied to the rigid arm with a fixed point (fulcrum), an object at the other end of the rigid arm can be lifted more easily.

TABLE 19-2 SUMMARY OF PRINCIPLES AND GUIDELINES RELATED TO BODY MECHANICS

Principles	Guidelines
Balance is maintained and muscle strain is avoided as long as the line of gravity passes through the base of support.	Start any body movement with proper alignment.
	Stand as close as possible to the object to be moved.
	Avoid stretching, reaching, and twisting, which may place the line of gravity outside the base of support.
The wider the base of support and the lower the center of gravity, the greater the stability.	Before moving objects, increase your stability by widening your stance and flexing your knees, hips, and ankles.
Objects that are close to the center of gravity are moved with the least effort.	Adjust the working area to waist level, and keep the body close to the area.
	Elevate adjustable beds and overbed tables or lower the side rails of beds to prevent stretching and reaching.
Balance is maintained with minimal effort when the base of support is enlarged in the direction in which the movement will occur.	When *pushing* an object, enlarge the base of support by moving the front foot forward.
	When *pulling* an object, enlarge the base of support by either moving the rear leg back if facing the object or moving the front foot forward if facing away from the object.
The greater the preparatory isometric tensing, or contraction of muscles, before moving an object, the less the energy required to move it, and the less the likelihood of musculoskeletal strain and injury.	Before moving objects, contract your gluteal, abdominal, leg, and arm muscles to prepare them for action.
The synchronized use of as many large muscle groups as possible during an activity increases overall strength and prevents muscle fatigue and injury.	To move objects below your center of gravity, begin with the back and knees flexed. Use your gluteal and leg muscles rather than the sacrospinal muscles of your back to exert an upward thrust when lifting the weight.
	Distribute the work load between both arms and legs to prevent back strain.
	Always face the direction of the movement to prevent twisting of the spine and ineffective use of major muscle groups.
The closer the line of gravity to the *center* of the base of support, the greater the stability.	When moving or carrying objects, hold them as close as possible to your center of gravity.
	Pull an object toward you whenever possible rather than pushing it away to control its movement and keep it close to your center of gravity.
The greater the friction against the surface beneath an object, the greater the force required to move the object.	Provide a firm, smooth, dry bed foundation before moving a client in bed.
Pulling creates less friction than pushing.	Pull clients rather than push them whenever possible.
The heavier an object, the greater the force needed to move an object.	Encourage clients to assist as much as possible by pushing or pulling themselves to reduce your muscular effort.
	Use arms as levers whenever possible to increase lifting power.
	Use your own body weight to counteract the weight of the object. For example, lean forward when pushing an object, and rock your body weight backward when pulling an object or client toward you.
	Obtain the assistance of other persons or use mechanical devices to move objects that are too heavy.
Moving an object along a level surface requires less energy than moving an object up an inclined surface or lifting it against the force of gravity.	Avoid working against gravity.
	Pull, push, roll, or turn objects instead of lifting them.
	Lower the head of the client's bed before moving the client up in bed.
Continuous muscle exertion can result in muscle strain and injury.	Alternate rest periods with periods of muscle use to help prevent fatigue.

the weight. In this way, the center of gravity is maintained over the same point in the base of support (Figure 19–3). By holding the center of gravity of the lifted object as close as possible to the body's center of gravity, the lifter avoids undue displacement of the center of gravity and achieves greater stability.

Although there are three types of levers, the type nurses use most frequently in lifting is the third-class lever (Figure 19–4, *A*). In the body, the joints are the fulcrums and the bones of the skeleton act as levers. The force, or effort, provided by muscle contraction is applied where a muscle attaches to bone. When the nurse lifts objects, the resisting force or weight is held in the hands or on the forearms, the fulcrum is the elbow, and the force is applied by contraction of the flexor muscles of the forearm (Figure 19–4, *B*). The lifting power is increased when the elbow (fulcrum) is supported on a bed surface or a countertop. People can lift more weight when they use this lever than when they do not. Use of the arms as levers is often applied in clinical practice when the nurse needs to raise the head or buttocks of a client in bed, e.g., to assist the client onto a bedpan or to give back care to a client in traction (Figure 19–5 on page 458).

Because lifting involves movement against gravity, the nurse must use major muscle groups of the thighs, knees, upper and lower arms, abdomen, and pelvis to prevent back strain. The nurse can increase overall muscle strength by synchronized use of as many muscle groups as possible during an activity. For instance, when the arms are used in an activity, dividing the work between the arms and legs helps to prevent back strain. Lifting power is further enhanced by using the nurse's body weight to counteract the client's weight. The nurse increases hip and knee flexion to lower the center of gravity. As the nurse does so, the forearms and hands supporting the client automatically rise (Figure 19–5, *C* and *D*.)

Nursing personnel often lift objects from the floor and assume a bending position, e.g., when helping persons to put on slippers, placing foot pedals down on wheelchairs, picking up laundry and isolation bags, picking up toddlers, and lifting supplies from the bottom shelves of carts.

A lifting technique based on the principle of leverage is recommended (Owen 1980, p. 895). In this technique, the person flexes the back and knees until the load is at thigh level, at which point the person

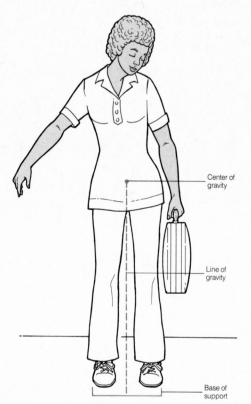

FIGURE 19–3 Body parts move in the direction opposite the weight to compensate for it and maintain the center of gravity over the base of support.

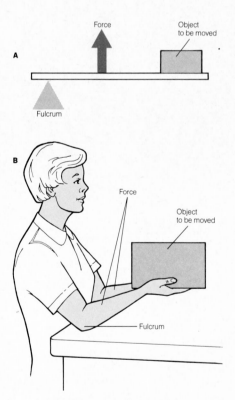

FIGURE 19–4 *A*, A third-class lever; *B*, using the arm as a lever.

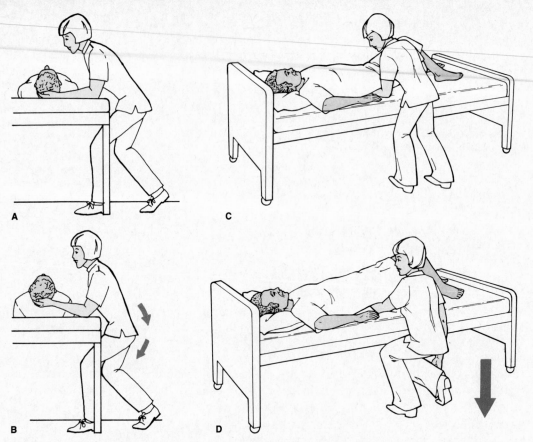

FIGURE 19-5 This nurse uses her arms as levers and employs her body weight to lift a client: *A*, position before lifting; *B*, position after lifting; *C* and *D*, Using positions *A* and *B* to lift a client's buttocks.

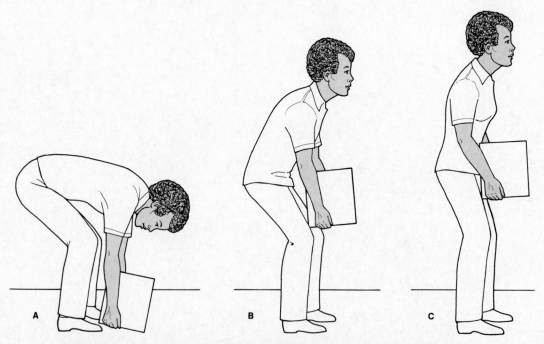

FIGURE 19-6 Stages in lifting an object to the waist: *A*, Move close to the object, and begin with the back and knees flexed to grasp the object. *B*, Start the lift by keeping the back flexed while the knees begin to straighten so that the leg muscles can exert an upward thrust. *C*, Keep the back and knees in a less flexed but not straight position (Owen 1980, p. 895).

flexes the knees more to provide thrust as the back begins to straighten (Figure 19–6). This technique provides for balance, leverage, and synchronized use of muscles, which help to avoid back pain and injury. When one lifts an object to knee level, the shoulder and arm muscles pull, the abdominal and lumbar muscles contract for leverage and pull, and the thigh and leg muscles exert the upward thrust to bring the object off the floor. When one lifts an object from mid-thigh to waist level, force is provided essentially by the leg and thigh muscle groups, but the back and lumbar muscles remain contracted.

In all positions, it is important to maintain a distance of at least 30 cm (12 in) between the feet and to keep the load close to the body, especially when it is at knee level (Owen 1985, p. 457). Before attempting the lift, the nurse must ensure that there are no hazards on the floor, that there is a clear path for moving the object, and that the nurse's base of support is secure.

Pulling and Pushing

 When pulling or pushing an object, a person maintains balance with least effort when the base of support is enlarged in the direction in which the movement is to be produced or opposed. For example, when pushing an object, a person can enlarge the base of support by moving the front foot forward. When pulling an object, a person can enlarge the base of support by (a) moving the rear leg back if the person is facing the object; or (b) moving the front foot forward if the person is facing away from the object. It is easier and safer to pull an object toward one's own center of gravity than to push it away, as the person can exert more control of the object's movement when pulling it.

Friction can be reduced by sliding the object on a smooth, lean, dry, firm surface, in contrast to a rough, wet, or soiled surface. To reduce friction when moving (sliding) a client up in bed, for example, the nurse provides a smooth, dry, firm bed foundation. It is preferable to pull rather than push a client along the surface of a bed because pushing compresses the client's vertebrae and creates discomfort. Also, pulling creates less friction than pushing, since the nurse must pull at an upward angle that reduces friction between the client and the bed. Friction can be further avoided by rolling, rather than pushing or pulling, the person. Because of inertia, the nurse must use more force to put an object into motion than to keep it in motion. The heavier the object, the greater the force required to put it into motion. To move an object efficiently, the nurse applies force directly toward or against the object's center of gravity and in the direction in which the movement is to occur. Use of the nurse's body weight in a rocking motion applies additional force or leverage. This counteracts the object's inertia and reduces the energy required to start the pulling, pushing, or lifting movement.

Proper use of body mechanics to pull objects is shown in Figure 19–7.

Pivoting

Pivoting is a technique in which the body is turned in a way that avoids twisting of the spine. To pivot, place one foot ahead of the other, raise the heels very

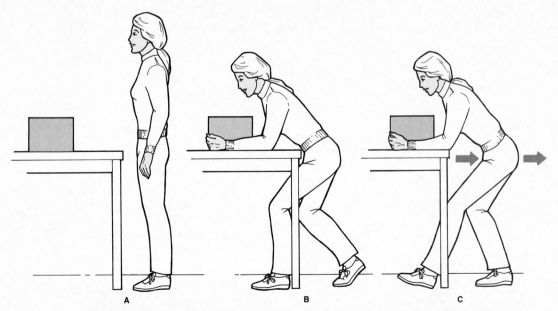

FIGURE 19–7 Schematic of proper body mechanics applied to pulling. *A,* The load to be pulled rests on a surface about as high as the person's center of gravity. *B,* The base of support is enlarged, the body is flexed, and the muscles are tensed for action. *C,* The weight is shifted toward the rear leg as the load is pulled toward the person.

slightly, and put the body weight on the balls of the feet. Taking the weight off the heels decreases the frictional surface and prevents the knees from twisting when the body turns. Keeping the body aligned, turn (pivot) about 90° in the desired direction. The foot that was forward will now be behind.

Moving and Turning Clients in Bed

Although healthy people usually take for granted that they can change body position and go from one place to another with little effort, ill people may have difficulty moving even in bed. How much assistance clients require depends on their own ability to move and their health status. In general, nurses should be sensitive to both the need of people to function independently and their need for assistance to move.

When assisting a person to move, the nurse needs to employ correct body mechanics to avoid injury. Actions and rationales common to the lifting and moving procedures that follow are outlined in the accompanying box. Correct body alignment for the client must also be maintained so that undue stress is not placed on the musculoskeletal system.

Summary of Actions and Rationales Applicable to Moving and Lifting Procedures

- Raise the height of the bed to bring the client close to your center of gravity.

- Lock the wheels on the bed, and raise the rail on the side of the bed opposite you to ensure client safety.

- Face the direction of the movement to prevent spinal twisting.

- Assume a broad stance to increase stability and provide balance.

- Incline your trunk forward, and flex your hips, knees, and ankles to lower your center of gravity, increase stability, and ensure use of large muscle groups during movements.

- Tighten your gluteal, abdominal, leg, and arm muscles to prepare them for action and prevent injury.

- Rock from the front leg to the back leg when pulling or from the back leg to the front leg when pushing to overcome inertia, counteract the client's weight, and help attain a balanced smooth motion.

◇ 19-1 ◇ Moving a Client Up in Bed

Clients who have slid down in bed from the Fowler's position or been pulled down by traction need assistance to move up in bed. The client should be encouraged to accomplish this movement independently whenever possible.

PURPOSES
- To maintain client comfort
- To restore proper body alignment
- To prevent muscle strain

ASSESSMENT FOCUS
Client's physical ability to assist; client's ability to comprehend instructions; client's degree of comfort; client's weight; your own strength and ability.

INTERVENTION

1. Adjust the bed and the client's position.

- Adjust the head of the bed to a flat position or as low as the client can tolerate. *Moving the client upward against gravity requires more force and can cause back strain.*

- Raise the bed to the height of your center of gravity.

- Lock the wheels on the bed and raise the rail on the side of the bed opposite you.

- Remove all pillows, then place one against the head of the bed.

This pillow protects the client's head from inadvertent injury against the top of the bed during the upward move.

2. Elicit the client's help in lessening your workload.

- Ask the client to flex the hips and

► **Technique 19–1** *CONTINUED*

knees and position the feet so that they can be used effectively for pushing. *Flexing the hips and knees keeps the entire lower leg off the bed surface, preventing friction during movement, and ensures use of the large muscle groups in the client's legs when pushing, thus increasing the force of movement.*

- Ask the client to

  a. Grasp the head of the bed with both hands and pull during the move, *or*

  b. Raise the upper part of the body on the elbows and push with the hands and forearms during the move, *or*

  c. Grasp the overhead trapeze with both hands and lift and pull during the move. *Client assistance provides additional power to overcome inertia and friction during the move. These actions also keep the client's arms partial-ly off the bed surface, reducing friction during movement, and make use of the large muscle groups of the client's arms to increase the force during movement.*

3. Position yourself appropriately, and move the client.

- Face the direction of the movement, and then assume a broad stance, with the foot nearest the bed behind the forward foot and weight on the forward foot. Incline your trunk forward from the hips. Flex hips, knees, and ankles.

- Place your near arm under the client's thighs. *This supports the heaviest part of the body (the buttocks). Push down on the mattress with the far arm (Figure 19–8). The far arm acts as a lever during the move.*

- Tighten your gluteal, abdominal, leg, and arm muscles, and rock from the back leg to the front leg and back again. *Then* shift the weight to the front leg as the client pushes with the heels and pulls with the arms, moving the client toward the head of the bed.

4. Ensure client comfort.

- Elevate the head of the bed and provide appropriate support devices for the client's new position.

- See the sections on positioning clients in Chapter 20.

VARIATION: A Client Who Has Limited Strength of the Upper Extremities

- Assist the client to flex the hips and knees as above. Place the client's arms across the chest. *This keeps them off the bed surface and minimizes friction during movement. Ask the client to flex the neck during the move and keep the head off the bed surface.*

- Position yourself properly (as above), and place one arm under the client's back and shoulders and the other arm under the client's thighs. *This placement of the arms distributes the client's weight and supports the heaviest part of the body (the buttocks). Shift your weight as above.*

VARIATION: Pulling a Client Up in Bed

This method emphasizes pulling the client up toward the head of the bed rather than lifting the client. It is designed to create less back strain for the nurse than a method that utilizes lifting. The steps are as follows:

- After lowering the head of the bed and removing all pillows, move the client to the edge of the bed closest to your body. (Technique 19–2 describes this action).

- Ask the client to assist (see step 2 above), or, if the client has limited strength of the upper extremities, place the client's arms

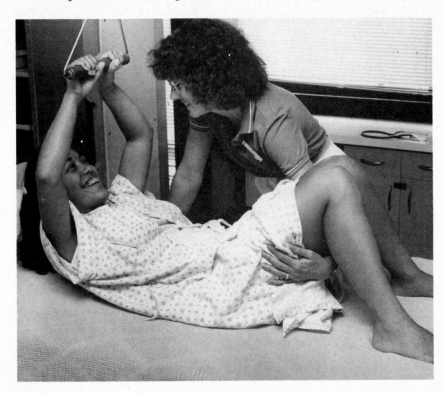

FIGURE 19–8   Moving a client up in bed.

▶ Technique 19–1 Moving a Client Up in Bed *CONTINUED*

across the chest and ask the client to flex the neck during the move.

- Stand toward the head of the bed, and face the foot of the bed. Position yourself appropriately, and place both hands together beneath the client's coccyx. Align your body so that it is directly in line with your hands. Your elbow closest to the client will be beneath the client's upper back. Both elbows should rest on the surface of the bed. *This placement of the arms, beneath the heaviest part of the client's body, allows you to pull the client directly toward your center of gravity, preventing spinal twisting. Pulling from the client's center of gravity directly toward your own center of gravity requires less force than lifting and allows greater control over the movement.*

- Coordinating your efforts with those of the client, rock backward and shift weight from the forward to the backward foot, pulling the client directly toward you while the client pushes with the heels and pulls with the arms. The hip closest to the bed

should slide along the side of the mattress. Your elbows should slide along the bed surface.

- ⚠️Ⓢ Raise the side rail and move to the opposite side of the bed. Move or pull the client as above, and move again to the opposite side of the bed. Move or pull the client back to the center of the bed. Raise the side rail.

VARIATION: Two Nurses Using a Hand-Forearm Interlock

Two people are required to move clients who are unable to assist because of their condition or weight. Using the technique described in step 3, with the second nurse on the opposite side of the bed, both of you interlock your forearms under the clients thighs and shoulders and lift the client up in bed (Figure 19–9).

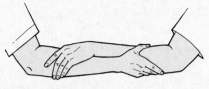

FIGURE 19–9 Two nurses using a hand-forearm interlock.

VARIATION: Two Nurses Using a Turn Sheet

Two nurses can use a turn sheet to move a client up in the bed. *A turn sheet distributes the client's weight more evenly, decreases friction, and exerts a more even force on the client during the move. In addition, it prevents injury of the client's skin, because the friction created between two sheets when one is moved is less than that created by the client's body moving over the sheet.*

- Place a drawsheet or a full sheet folded in half under the client, extending from the shoulders to the thighs. Each of you rolls up or fanfolds the turn sheet close to the client's body on either side.

- Both of you then grasp the sheet close to the shoulders and buttocks of the client. *This draws the weight closer to the nurses' center of gravity and increases the nurses' balance and stability, permitting a smoother movement.* Then follow the method of moving clients with limited upper extremity strength, described earlier.

EVALUATION FOCUS	Client comfort and body alignment; safety precautions required (e.g., side rails).

KEY ELEMENTS OF MOVING A CLIENT UP IN BED

- Assess the client's capabilities and limitations for movement.
- Assess your own skill and physical strength.
- Use correct body mechanics.
- Encourage the client to assist you as much as possible.
- Give explicit instructions to the client about what to do to help.

- Obtain the assistance of another health care worker to move helpless or heavy clients.
- Coordinate your efforts with those of the client and/or other health care worker(s).
- Use side rails as needed to prevent falls.

19-2 Moving a Client in Segments to the Side of the Bed

Whenever capable of assisting with this movement, the client lifts the body by holding onto the raised side rail or by using the overhead trapeze. In this movement, the nurse's weight is used to counteract the client's weight; the nurse's arms serve as connecting bars between the client and the nurse.

PURPOSE

• To position the client in preparation for moving the client onto a stretcher, in preparation for turning the client to the lateral (side-lying) position, or when changing the client's bed.

ASSESSMENT FOCUS

Client's physical ability to assist; client's ability to comprehend instructions; client's degree of comfort; client's weight; your own strength and ability.

INTERVENTION

1. Position yourself and the client appropriately before performing the move.

• Stand as close as possible at the side of the bed toward which the client will be moved and opposite the client's chest. *This position lessens the client's fear of falling and places your center of gravity close to the client's.*

• Place the client's near arm across the chest. *This avoids friction and resistance to movement and prevents injury to the arm.*

• Incline your trunk forward from the hips. Flex your hips, knees, and ankles. Assume a broad stance, with one foot forward and the weight placed upon this forward foot.

2. Move the client's head and trunk.

• Place your arms and hands with palms facing upward close together beneath the client's scapulae. *This focuses the force for movement under the heaviest part of the upper trunk. Placing the arms close together reduces the friction of the client's body against the bed, making the pull easier.*

• Flex your fingers around the client's far shoulder, and rest your elbows on the surface of the bed. *This prevents inadvertent lifting.*

• If the client cannot support the head during the movement, position your arm nearest the head of the bed so that it cradles the client's head.

• Tighten your gluteal, abdominal, leg, and arm muscles, rock backward, and shift your weight from the forward to the backward foot, while pulling the client's shoulders directly toward you.

3. Move the client's buttocks.

• Place your arms and hands close together beneath the client's buttocks, and pull the buttocks to the side of the bed as described above.

4. Move the client's legs and feet.

• Place your hands close together beneath the client's ankles, and repeat the steps above, pulling the client's legs and feet to the side of the bed.

• Elevate the side rail next to the client. *This prevents the client from falling off the bed.*

VARIATION: Using a Pull Sheet

Use a pull sheet beneath the client's trunk and thighs to pull the client to the side of the bed. Roll up the sheet as close as possible to the client's body, and pull the client's shoulders, then the buttocks, to the side of the bed. Move the legs and feet as described above.

EVALUATION FOCUS

Client safety.

KEY ELEMENTS OF MOVING A CLIENT IN SEGMENTS TO THE SIDE OF THE BED

See Key Elements for Technique 19–1.

19-3 Turning a Client to a Lateral or Prone Position in Bed

PURPOSES
- To relieve pressure areas and prevent decubitus ulcers
- To provide client comfort and prevent muscle strain
- To provide nursing care (e.g., to change the client's bed linen or to place a bedpan beneath the client)

ASSESSMENT FOCUS

See Technique 19–1.

INTERVENTION

1. Position yourself and the client appropriately before performing the move.

- Move the client closer to the side of the bed opposite the side the client will face when turned. See Technique 19–2. *This ensures that the client will be positioned safely in the center of the bed after turning.*

- While standing on the side of the bed nearest the client, place the client's near arm across the chest. Abduct the client's far shoulder slightly from the side of the body. *Pulling the one arm forward facilitates the turning motion. Pulling the other arm away from the body prevents that arm from being caught beneath the client's body during the roll.*

- Place the client's near ankle and foot across the far ankle and foot. *This facilitates the turning motion. Making these preparations on the side of the bed closest to the client helps the nurse prevent unnecessary reaching.*

- Raise the side rail next to the client before going to the other side of the bed. *This ensures that the client, who is close to the edge of the mattress, will not fall.*

- Position yourself on the side of the bed toward which the client will turn, directly in line with the client's waistline and as close to the bed as possible.

- Incline your trunk forward from the hips. Flex your hips, knees, and ankles. Assume a broad stance with one foot forward and the weight placed upon this forward foot.

2. Pull or roll the client to a lateral position.

- Place one hand on the client's far hip and the other hand on the client's far shoulder. (Figure 19–10, *A*). *This position of the hands supports the client at the two heaviest parts of the body, providing greater control in movement during the roll.*

- Tighten your gluteal, abdominal, leg, and arm muscles; rock backward, shifting your weight from the forward to the backward foot; and roll the client onto the side of the body to face you (Figure 19–10, *B*).

VARIATION: Turning the Client to a Prone Position

To turn a client to the prone position, follow all of the above steps, with two exceptions:

- Instead of abducting the far arm, keep the client's arm alongside the body for the client to roll

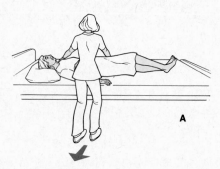

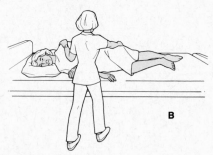

FIGURE 19–10 Moving a client to a lateral position.

over. *Keeping the arm alongside the body prevents it from being pinned under the client when the client is rolled.*

- Roll the client completely onto the abdomen. *It is essential to move the client as close as possible to the bed edge before the turn so that the client will be lying on the center of the bed after rolling. Never pull a client across the bed while the client is in the prone position. Doing so can injure a woman's breasts or a man's genitals.*

► **Technique 19–3** *CONTINUED*

| EVALUATION FOCUS | Client comfort and body alignment; safety precautions required (e.g., side rails). |

KEY ELEMENTS OF TURNING A CLIENT TO A LATERAL OR PRONE POSITION IN BED

See Key Elements for Technique 19–1. In addition:

• Turn a client in the prone position to the lateral or supine position before pulling the client across the bed.

19-4 Logrolling a Client

Logrolling is a technique used to turn a client whose body must be kept in straight alignment (like a log) at all times, e.g., the client with a spinal injury. Considerable care must be taken to prevent additional injury. This technique requires two nurses or, if the client is large, three nurses. *For the client who has a cervical injury, one nurse must maintain the client's head and neck alignment.*

PURPOSES
• To maintain the client's body alignment and prevent spinal injury
• To provide therapy (e.g., a bed linen change or backrub)
• To relieve skin pressure areas
• To provide client comfort

| ASSESSMENT FOCUS | Size of client to determine number of assistants required; presence of a cervical injury; client's ability to comprehend instructions; client's degree of comfort. |

INTERVENTION

1. Position yourselves and the client appropriately before the move.

• Stand on the same side of the bed, and assume a broad stance with one foot ahead of the other.

• Place the client's arms across the chest. *Doing so ensures that they will not be injured or become trapped under the body when the body is turned.*

• Incline your trunk, and flex your hips, knees, and ankles.

• Place your arms under the client as shown in Figure 19–11 or Figure 19–12, depending on the client's size. *Each nurse then has a major weight area of the client centered between the arms.*

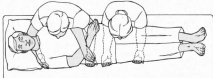

FIGURE 19–11 Proper arm placement for pulling the client to the side of the bed: two nurses.

• Tighten your gluteal, abdominal, leg, and arm muscles.

2. Pull the client to the side of the bed.

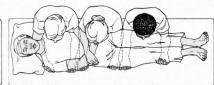

FIGURE 19–12 Proper arm placement for pulling the client to the side of the bed: three nurses.

▶ **Technique 19–4 Logrolling a Client** CONTINUED

- One nurse counts, "one, two, three, go." Then, at the same time, all nurses pull the client to the side of the bed by shifting weight to the back foot. *Moving the client in unison maintains the client's body alignment.*

- Ⓢ Elevate the side rail on this side of the bed. *This prevents the client from falling while lying so close to the edge of the bed.*

3. Move to the other side of the bed, and place supportive devices for the client when turned.

- Place a pillow where it will support the client's head after the turn. *The pillow prevents lateral flexion of the neck and ensures alignment of the cervical spine.*

- Place one or two pillows between the client's legs to support the upper leg when the client is turned. *This pillow prevents adduction of the upper leg and keeps the legs parallel and aligned.*

4. Roll and position the client in proper alignment.

- All nurses flex the hips, knees, and ankles and assume a broad stance with one foot forward.

- All nurses reach over the client and place hands as shown in Figure 19–13. *Doing so centers a ma-*

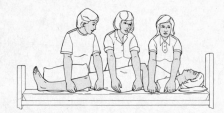

FIGURE 19–13 Proper hand placement in logrolling a client.

jor weight area of the client between each nurse's arms.

- One nurse counts, "one, two, three, go." Then, at the same time, all nurses roll the client to a lateral position.

- Place pillows to maintain the client's lateral position. See the discussion of the lateral position on page 492.

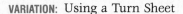

VARIATION: Using a Turn Sheet

- Use a turn sheet to facilitate logrolling. First, stand with another nurse on the same side of the bed. Assume a broad stance with one foot forward, and grasp half of the fanfolded or rolled edge of the turn sheet. On a signal, pull the client toward both of you (Figure 19–14).

- Before turning the client, place pillow supports for the head and legs, as described in step 3 above. This helps maintain the client's alignment when turning. Then go to the other side of the bed (farthest from the client), and assume a stable stance. Reaching over the client, grasp the far edges of the turn sheet, and roll the client toward you (Figure 19–15). The second nurse (behind the client) helps turn the client and provides pillow supports to ensure good alignment in the lateral position.

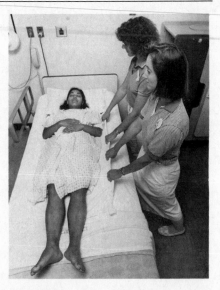

FIGURE 19–14 Using a turn sheet, the nurses pull the client toward them to the edge of the bed.

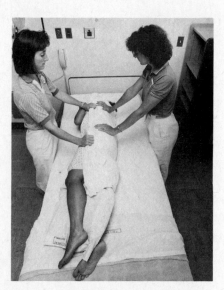

FIGURE 19–15 One nurse uses the far edge of the sheet to pull the client toward her, while the second nurse remains behind the client to assist.

KEY ELEMENTS OF LOGROLLING A CLIENT

See Key Elements for Technique 19–1. In addition: | • Maintain the client's spinal alignment.

19-5 Assisting a Client to a Sitting Position in Bed

A client may need assistance in raising the head and shoulders while the nurse rearranges pillows or provides back care. If the client needs to rise to a sitting position in bed, the easiest method is simply to raise the head of the bed to the desired height. If the hospital bed cannot be raised mechanically, the nurse may need to assist the client.

PURPOSES
- To provide comfort (e.g., to reposition pillows)
- To provide back care

ASSESSMENT FOCUS

Client's physical ability to assist; client's ability to comprehend instructions; client's degree of comfort or discomfort; client's weight; your own strength and ability.

INTERVENTION

1. Position yourself and the client appropriately before performing the move.

- Ask the client to place arms at the sides with the palms of the hands against the surface of the bed. *In this way, the client can push against the bed surface to provide additional power for the lift.*

- Face the head of the bed, and stand at the side of the bed beside the client's buttocks. Assume a broad stance with the foot farthest from the bed forward and body weight on this foot.

2. Lift the client to a sitting position.

- Ⓢ Place the hand nearest the client over the client's far shoulder to rest between the shoulder blades. *This hand position enables you to pull the client's upper body directly toward your center*

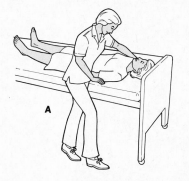 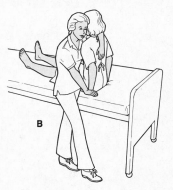

FIGURE 19–16 Assisting a client to a sitting position in bed.

of gravity and prevents spinal twisting.

- Place the hand of your free arm on the edge of the surface of the bed near the client's shoulder, and use it to push during the lift (Figure 19–16, A). *This provides balance and leverage.*

- Ⓢ Have the client lift with you simultaneously on your signal. Lift by pulling with the arm and hand

over the client's shoulder, pushing on the bed surface with the other hand, and shifting your weight from the forward to the back foot in a rocking motion (Figure 19–16, B). *Pushing with the muscles of one arm while pulling with the muscles of the other arm distributes the workload and increases lifting power.* The client simultaneously pushes with the hands and arms.

KEY ELEMENTS OF ASSISTING A CLIENT TO A SITTING POSITION IN BED

See Key Elements for Technique 19–1.

19-6 Moving a Client to a Sitting Position on the Edge of the Bed

PURPOSE
- To position the client in preparation for walking, moving to a chair or wheelchair, eating, or performing other activities

ASSESSMENT FOCUS

Client's physical ability to assist you and then maintain this position, ability to comprehend instructions, degree of discomfort when moving; vital signs before ambulating; presence of postural hypotension; your own strength and ability.

INTERVENTION

1. Position yourself and the client appropriately before performing the move.

- Assist the client to a lateral position facing you. See Technique 19–3.

- Raise the head of the bed slowly as high as it will go. *This decreases the distance that the client needs to move to sit up on the side of the bed.*

- Position the client's feet and lower legs just over the edge of the bed. *This enables the client's feet to move easily off the bed during the movement, and the client is aided by gravity into a sitting position.*

- Stand beside the client's hips and face the far corner of the bottom of the bed (the angle in which movement will occur). Assume a broad stance, placing the foot nearest the client forward. Incline your trunk forward from the hips. Flex your hips, knees, and ankles (Figure 19–17, *A*).

2. Move the client to a sitting position.

- Place one arm around the client's shoulders and the other arm beneath both of the client's thighs near the knees (Figure 19–17, *A*). *Supporting the client's shoulders prevents the client from falling backward during movement. Supporting the client's thighs reduces*

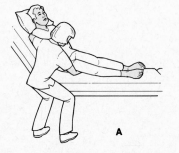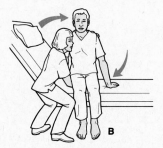

FIGURE 19–17 Assisting a client to a sitting position on the edge of the bed.

friction of the thighs against the bed surface during the move and increases the force of the movement.

- Tighten your gluteal, abdominal, leg, and arm muscles.

- Lift the client's thighs slightly. *This reduces the friction of the client's thighs and your arm against the bed surface.*

- Pivot on the balls of your feet in the desired direction facing the foot of the bed while pulling the client's feet and legs off the bed (Figure 19–17, *B*). *Pivoting prevents twisting of your spine. The weight of the client's legs swinging downward increases downward movement of the lower body and helps make the client's upper body vertical.*

- Keep supporting the client until the client is well balanced and comfortable. *This movement may cause some clients to faint.*

VARIATION: Teaching a Client How to Sit on the Side of the Bed Independently

A client who has had recent abdominal surgery or who is weak may have too much abdominal pain or too little strength to sit straight up in bed. This person can be taught to assume a "dangle" position without assistance. Instruct the client to

- Roll to the side and lift the far leg over the near leg (Figure 19–18, *A*).

- Grasp the mattress edge with the lower arm and push the fist of the upper arm into the mattress (Figure 19–18, *B*).

- Push up with the arms as the heels and legs slide over the mattress edge (Figure 19–18, *B*).

- Maintain the sitting position by pushing both fists into the mattress behind and to the sides of the buttocks.

▶ **Technique 19–6** *CONTINUED*

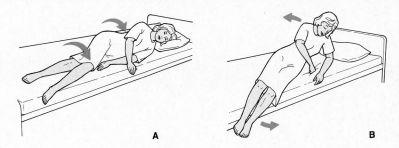

FIGURE 19–18 Moving to a sitting position independently.

EVALUATION FOCUS	Client's safety in this position (i.e., ability to maintain the position); status of vital signs, particularly if this is the first time up.

KEY ELEMENTS OF MOVING A CLIENT TO A SITTING POSITION ON THE EDGE OF THE BED

See Key Elements for Technique 19–1.

Transferring Clients

Many clients require some assistance in transferring between bed and chair or wheelchair, between wheelchair and toilet, and between bed and stretcher. Before transferring any client, however, the nurse must determine the client's physical and mental capabilities to participate in the transfer technique.

In addition, the nurse must mentally analyze and organize the activity. Generally guidelines for transfer techniques include the following:

- Planning what to do and how best to do it

- Obtaining essential equipment, e.g., transfer belt, sliding board, wheelchair, stretcher and checking them for function and safety

- Removing obstacles in the transfer area

- Informing the client about the transfer, enlisting the client's help, and explaining how the client can help

- Informing assistants of their roles and who will give directions (one person needs to be in charge)

- Always supporting or holding the client, not the equipment

- During the transfer, again informing the client step-by-step what the client is to do

- Making a written plan of the transfer so that all health care professionals can follow the same plan with the client (including how the client is to be returned to the original place)

Because wheelchairs and stretchers are unstable, they can predispose the client to falls and injury. Guidelines for the safe use of wheelchairs and stretchers are shown in the accompanying boxes.

CLINICAL GUIDELINES

Wheelchair Safety

- Always lock the brakes on both wheels of the wheelchair when the client transfers in or out of it.

- Raise the footplates before transferring the client into the wheelchair.

- Lower the footplates after the transfer, and place the client's feet on them.

- Ensure the client is positioned well back in the seat of the wheelchair.

- Use seat belts that fasten behind the wheelchair to protect confused clients from falls.

- Back the wheelchair into or out of an elevator, rear large wheels first.

- Place your body between the wheelchair and the bottom of an incline.

CLINICAL GUIDELINES

Safe Use of Stretchers

- Lock the wheels of the bed and stretcher before the client transfers in or out of them.

- Fasten safety straps across the client on a stretcher, and raise the side rails.

- Never leave a client unattended on a stretcher unless the wheels are locked and the side rails are raised on both sides and/or the safety straps are securely fastened across the client.

- Always push a stretcher from the end where the client's head is positioned. This position protects the client's head in the event of a collision.

- If the stretcher has two swivel wheels and two stationary wheels:

  - Always position the client's head at the end with the stationary wheels
    and

  - Push the stretcher from the end with the stationary wheels. The stretcher is maneuvered more easily when pushed from this end.

- Maneuver the stretcher when entering the elevator so that the client's head goes in first.

19-7 Transferring a Client Between a Bed and a Wheelchair

A client may need to be transferred between the bed and a wheelchair or chair, the bed and the commode, and a wheelchair and the toilet. There are numerous variations of this transfer technique; which variation the nurse selects depends on a number of factors (see Assessment Focus below). Transfer belts provide the greatest safety. This belt has a handle that allows the nurse to control movement of the client during the transfer (Figure 19–19). An increasing number of hospitals and nursing homes are requiring that personnel use the transfer belt to transfer clients.

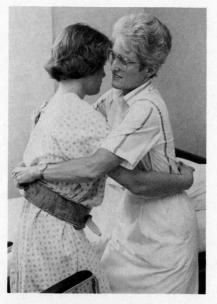

FIGURE 19–19   Using a transfer belt.

► **Technique 19–7** *CONTINUED*

ASSESSMENT FOCUS	The client's body size; ability to follow instructions; activity tolerance; muscle strength; joint mobility; presence of paralysis; level of comfort; presence of orthostatic hypotension; the technique with which the client is familiar; the space in which the transfer is maneuvered (bathrooms, for instance, are usually cramped); the number of assistants (1 or 2) needed to accomplish the transfer safely; and the skill and strength of the nurse(s).

INTERVENTION

1. Position the equipment appropriately.

- Lower the bed to its lowest position so that the client's feet will rest flat on the floor. Lock the wheels of the bed.

- Place the wheelchair parallel to the bed as close to the bed as possible (Figure 19–20). Lock the wheels of the wheelchair, and raise the footplate.

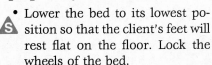

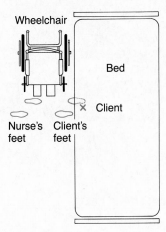

FIGURE 19–20 The wheelchair is placed parallel to the bed as close to the bed as possible. Note that the placement of the nurse's feet mirrors that of the client's feet.

2. Prepare and assess the client.

- Assist the client to a sitting position on the side of the bed. See Technique 19–6.

- Assess the client for orthostatic hypotension before moving the client from the bed.

- Assist the client in putting on a bathrobe and nonskid slippers or shoes.

- Place a transfer belt snugly around the client's waist. Check to be certain that the belt is securely fastened.

3. Give explicit instructions to the client. Ask the client to

- Move forward and sit on the edge of the bed. *This brings the client's center of gravity closer to yours.*

- Lean forward slightly from the hips. *This brings the client's center of gravity more directly over the base of support and positions the head and trunk in the direction of the movement.*

- Place the foot of the stronger leg beneath the edge of the bed and put the other foot forward. *In this way, the client can use the stronger leg muscles to stand and power the movement. A broader base of support makes the client more stable during the transfer.*

- Place the hands on the bed surface or on your shoulders so that the client can push while standing. *This provides additional force for the movement and reduces the potential for strain on your back. The client should not grasp your neck for support. Doing so can injure you.*

4. Position yourself appropriately.

- Stand directly in front of the client. Incline the trunk forward from the hips. Flex the hips, knees, and ankles. Assume a broad stance, placing one foot forward and one back. Mirror the placement of the client's feet, if possible (Figure 19–20). *This helps prevent loss of balance during the transfer.*

- Encircle the client's waist with your arms, and grasp the transfer belt at the client's back with thumbs pointing downward. *The belt provides a secure handle for holding onto the client and controlling the movement. Downward placement of the thumbs prevents potential wrist injury as you lift.* (Leinweber 1978). *By encircling the client in this manner, you keep the client from tilting backward during the transfer.*

- Tighten your gluteal, abdominal, leg, and arm muscles.

5. Assist the client to stand, and then move together toward the wheelchair.

- On the count of three:

   a. Ask the client to push with the back foot, rock to the forward foot, extend (straighten) the joints of the lower extremities, and push or pull up with the hands, while

   b. You push with the forward foot, rock to the back foot, extend the joints of the lower extremities, and pull the client (directly toward your center of gravity) into a standing position.

▶ **Technique 19–7 Transferring a Client Between a Bed and a Wheelchair** *CONTINUED*

• Support the client in an upright
Ⓢ standing position for a few moments. *This allows you and the client to extend the joints and provides you with an opportunity to ensure that the client is all right before moving away from the bed.*

• Together, pivot or take a few steps toward the wheelchair.

6. Assist the client to sit.

• Ask the client to

a. Back up to the wheelchair
Ⓢ and place the legs against the seat. *Having the client place the legs against the wheelchair seat minimizes the risk of the client's falling when sitting down.*

b. Place the foot of the stronger leg slightly behind the other. *This supports body weight during the movement.*

c. Keep the other foot forward. *This provides a broad base of support.*

d. Place both hands on the wheelchair arms or on your shoulders. *This increases stability and lessens the strain on you.*

• Stand directly in front of the client. Place one foot forward and one back.

• Tighten your grasp on the transfer belt, and tighten your gluteal, abdominal, leg, and arm muscles.

• On the count of three:

a. Have the client shift the body weight by rocking to the back foot, lower the body onto the edge of the wheelchair seat by flexing the joints of the legs and arms, and place some body weight on the arms, while

b. You shift your body weight by stepping back with the forward foot and pivoting toward the chair while lowering the client onto the wheelchair seat.

7. Ensure client safety.

• Ask the client to push back into
Ⓢ the wheelchair seat. *Sitting well back on the seat provides a broader base of support and greater stability and minimizes the risk of falling from the wheelchair. A wheelchair can topple forward when the client sits on the edge of the seat and leans far forward.*

• Lower the footplates, and place the client's feet on them.

• Apply a seat belt as required.

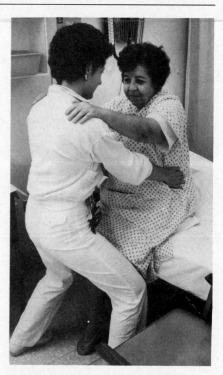

FIGURE 19–21 Transferring without a belt.

VARIATION: Angling the Wheelchair

For clients who have difficulty walking, place the wheelchair at a 45° angle to the bed. *This enables the client to pivot into the chair and lessens the amount of body rotation required.*

VARIATION: Transferring Without a Belt

• For clients who need minimal assistance, place the hands against the sides of the client's chest (not at the axillae) during the transfer (Figure 19–21). For clients who require more assistance, reach through the client's axillae, and place the hands on the client's scapulae during the transfer. Avoid placing hands or pressure on the axillae, especially for clients who have upper extremity paralysis or paresis.

• Follow the steps described previously.

VARIATION: Transferring with a Belt and Two Nurses

• When the client is able to stand, position yourselves on both sides of the client, facing the same direction as the client. Flex your hips, knees, and ankles; grasp the client's transfer belt with the hand closest to the client; and with the other hand support the client's elbows.

• Coordinating your efforts, all three of you stand simultaneously, pivot, and move to the wheelchair. Reverse the process to lower the client onto the wheelchair seat.

VARIATION: Transferring a Client with an Injured Lower Extremity

When the client has an injured lower extremity, movement should always occur toward the client's unaffected (strong) side. For example, if the client's right leg is injured and the client is sitting on the edge of the bed preparing to transfer to a wheelchair, position the wheelchair on the client's left side. *In this way, the client can use the unaffected leg most effectively and safely.*

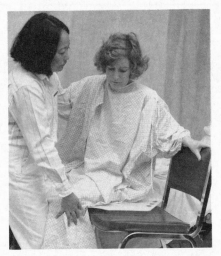

FIGURE 19–22 Using a sliding board.

VARIATION: Using a Sliding Board

Have a client who cannot stand use a sliding board to move without nursing assistance. This method not only promotes the client's sense of independence but preserves your energy (Figure 19–22).

EVALUATION FOCUS | Client comfort and safety after the transfer.

KEY ELEMENTS OF TRANSFERRING A CLIENT BETWEEN A BED AND A WHEELCHAIR

See Key Elements for Technique 19–1. In addition:
- Assess the client for orthostatic hypotension before the transfer.
- Lock the wheels of the bed and the wheelchair before the client transfers in or out of them.

- Use appropriate assistive devices such as a transfer belt and board.
- Apply a seat belt to the helpless client in a wheelchair.

19-8

Transferring a Client Between a Bed and a Stretcher

The stretcher, or gurney, is used to transfer supine clients from one location to another. Whenever the client is capable of accomplishing the transfer from bed to stretcher independently, either by lifting onto it or by rolling onto it, the client should be encouraged to do so. If the client cannot move onto the stretcher independently, at least two nurses are needed to assist with the transfer; more are needed if the client is totally helpless or heavy.

ASSESSMENT FOCUS | Ability to follow instructions; physical ability to assist with the transfer; degree of discomfort when moving.

▶ **Technique 19–8 Transferring Between a Bed and a Stretcher** CONTINUED

EQUIPMENT

☐ Stretcher
☐ Roller bar (optional)

INTERVENTION

1. Adjust the client's bed in preparation for the transfer.

- Lower the head of the bed until it is flat or as low as the client can tolerate.

- Raise the bed so that it is slightly higher than the surface of the stretcher. *It is easier and requires less effort for the client to move down an incline.*

- Ⓢ Ensure that the wheels on the bed are locked.

- Pull the drawsheet out from both sides of the bed.

2. Move the client to the edge of the bed, and position the stretcher.

- Roll the drawsheet as close to the client's side as possible.

- Pull the client to the edge of the bed, and cover the client with a sheet or bath blanket to maintain comfort.

- Ⓢ Place the stretcher parallel to the bed, next to the client, and lock its wheels.

- Fill the gap that exists between the bed and the stretcher loosely with bath blankets (optional).

3. Transfer the client securely to the stretcher.

- Ⓢ In unison with the other nurses, press your body tightly against the stretcher. *This prevents the stretcher from moving.*

- Roll the pull sheet tightly against the client. *This achieves better control over client movement.*

- Flex your hips, and pull the client on the pull sheet in unison directly toward you and onto the stretcher. *Pulling downward requires less force than pulling along a flat surface.*

- Ⓢ Ask the client to flex the neck during the move, if possible, and place arms across the chest. *This prevents injury to these body parts.*

4. Ensure client comfort and safety.

- Make the client comfortable, unlock the stretcher wheels, and move the stretcher away from the bed.

- Ⓢ Immediately raise the stretcher side rails and/or fasten the safety straps across the client. *Because the stretcher is high and narrow, the client is in danger of falling unless these safety precautions are taken.*

VARIATION: Using a Roller Bar During the Transfer

A roller bar is a metal frame covered with longitudinal rollers. Place the bar over the gap between the bed and the stretcher. Using a pull sheet, pull the client onto the roller bar, and roll the client easily onto the stretcher.

VARIATION: Using a Long Board

The long board, which may be referred to as the Smooth Mover or Easyglide, is a lacquered or smooth polyethylene board measuring 45–55 cm (18–22 in) by 182 cm (72 in) with handholds along its edges. This device may be used by one nurse alone or up to four nurses together. Turn the client to a lateral position away from you, position the board close to the client's back, and roll the client onto the board. Pull the client and board across the bed to the stretcher. Safety belts may be placed over the chest, abdomen, and legs.

EVALUATION FOCUS

Client safety and comfort.

KEY ELEMENTS OF TRANSFERRING A CLIENT BETWEEN A BED AND A STRETCHER

See Key Elements for Technique 19–1. In addition:

- Lock the wheels of the bed and the stretcher before the client transfers in or out of them.

- Fasten safety straps across the client on a stretcher and raise the side rails.

Hydraulic Lifts

Hydraulic lifts, such as the Hoyer Lift, are used primarily for clients who cannot help themselves or who are too heavy for others to lift safely. The lift can be used in transferring the client between the bed and a wheelchair, the bed and the bathtub, and the bed and a stretcher. The Hoyer lift consists of a base on casters, a hydraulic mechanical pump, a mast boom, and a sling (Figure 19–23). The sling may consist of a one-piece or two-piece canvas seat. The one-piece seat stretches from the client's head to the knees. The two-piece seat has one canvas strap to support the client's buttocks and thighs and a second strap extending up to the axillae to support the back. It is important to be familiar with the model used and the practices that accompany use. Before using the lift, ensure that it is in working order and that the hooks, chains, straps, and canvas seat are in good repair. *Most agencies recommend that two nurses operate a lift.* Check agency policy.

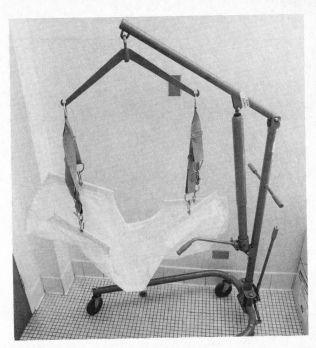

FIGURE 19–23 A one-piece seat hydraulic lift.

 19-9

Using a Hydraulic Lift

PURPOSE	• To facilitate transfer of a totally dependent client to and from bed, wheelchair, tub, or toilet, without strain on the nurse
ASSESSMENT FOCUS	Ability to comprehend instructions; degree of physical disability; weight of the client (to ensure that the lift can safely move the client); presence of orthostatic hypotension and pulse rate before transfer.

EQUIPMENT

☐ Hoyer lift with slings and canvas straps

INTERVENTION

1. Prepare the client.

• Explain the procedure, and demonstrate the lift. *Some clients are afraid of being lifted and will be reassured by a demonstration.*

2. Prepare the equipment.

• Lock the wheels of the client's bed.

• Raise the bed to the high position, and adjust the bed gatches so that the mattress is flat.

• Put up the side rail on the opposite side of the bed, and lower the side rail near you.

• Position the lift so that it is close to the client.

• Place the chair that is to receive the client beside the bed. Allow adequate space to maneuver the lift.

• Lock the wheels, if a chair with wheels is used.

3. Position the client on the sling.

• Roll the client away from you.

• Place the canvas seat or sling under the client, with the wide lower edge under the client's thighs to the knees and the more narrow upper edge up under the client's shoulders. *This places the sling under the client's center of gravity and greatest part of body weight. Correct placement permits*

▶

▶ Technique 19–9 Using a Hydraulic Lift CONTINUED

the client to be lifted evenly, with minimal shifting.

- ⑤ Raise the bed rail on your side of the bed, and go to the opposite side of the bed. Lower this side rail.

- Roll the client to the opposite side, and pull the canvas sling through.

- Roll the client to the supine position on top of the canvas sling.

4. Attach the sling to the swivel bar.

- Wheel the lift into position, with the footbars under the bed on the side where the chair is positioned. Lock the wheels of the ⑤ lifter.

- Lower the side rail.

- Lower the horizontal bar or mast boom to sling level by releasing the hydraulic valve. Lock the valve.

- Attach the lifter straps or hooks to the corresponding openings in the canvas seat. Check that the hooks are correctly placed and that matching straps or chains are of equal length.

5. Lift the client gradually.

- Elevate the head of the bed to place the client in a sitting position.

- Ask the client to remove eye-

glasses, and put them in a safe ⑤ place. *The swivel bar may come close to the face and cause breakage of eyeglasses.*

- Nurse 1: Close the pressure valve, and gradually pump the jack handle until the client is above the bed surface. *Gradual elevation of the lift is less frightening to the client than a rapid rise.*

- Nurse 2: Assume a broad stance, and guide the client with your hands as the client is lifted. *This prepares to hold the client and provide control during the movement.*

- ⑤ Check the placement of the sling before moving the client away from the bed.

6. Move the client over the chair.

- Nurse 1: With the pressure valve securely closed, slowly roll the lift until the client is over the chair. Use the steering handle to maneuver the lift.

- Nurse 2: Guide movement by hand until the client is directly over the chair (Figure 19–24). *Slow movement decreases swaying and is less frightening. Guidance also decreases swaying and gives a sense of security.*

7. Lower the client into the chair.

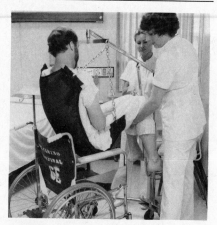

FIGURE 19–24 Moving the client with a hydraulic lift.

- Nurse 1: Release the pressure valve very gradually. *Gradual release is less frightening than a quick descent.*

- Nurse 2: Guide the client into the chair.

8. Ensure client comfort and safety.

- Remove the hooks from the canvas seat. Leave the seat in place. *The seat is left in place in preparation for the lift back to bed.*

- Align the client appropriately in a sitting position.

- Return the client's eyeglasses, if appropriate.

- ⑤ Apply a seatbelt or other restraint as needed.

- Place the call bell within reach.

EVALUATION FOCUS	Body alignment in sitting position; vital signs, especially pulse rate and blood pressure to determine response to the transfer; safety precautions required for clients after the transfer.

KEY ELEMENTS OF USING A HYDRAULIC LIFT

- Give explicit directions to the client about what to do to help.
- Follow the manufacturer's directions.
- Lock the wheels of the lift and the bed.

- Apply the canvas seat and straps appropriately and securely.
- Move the client slowly.
- Guide the client's movement.

CRITICAL THINKING CHALLENGE

After giving total care to an obese client, you note a pulling in your lower back and pain when twisting or bending. What action should you take? What actions might have prevented the injury?

RELATED RESEARCH

Goldberg, W. G., and Fitzpatrick, J. J. November/December 1980. Movement with the aged. *Nursing Research* 29:339–46.

Owen, B. D. November 1985. The lifting process and back injury in hospital nursing personnel. *Western Journal of Nursing Research* 7:445–59.

Snook, S. H.; Camponelli, R. A.; and Harsh, J. W. July 1978. A study of three preventive approaches to low back injury. *Journal of Occupational Health Medicine* 20:478–81.

REFERENCES

Davies, B. T. 1978. Training in manual handling and lifting. In Drury, C., editor, pp. 175–85. *Safety in manual material handling.* DHEW (NIOSH) Pub. no. 78–185, July. Cincinnati, Ohio: National Institute of Occupational Safety and Health.

Leinweber, E. December 1978. Belts to make moves smoother. *American Journal of Nursing* 78:2080–81.

Owen, B. D. May 1980. How to avoid that aching back. *American Journal of Nursing* 80:894–97.

———. November 1985. The lifting process and back injury in hospital nursing personnel. *Western Journal of Nursing Research* 7:445–59.

Swearingeu, P. L. 1992. *Photo Atlas of Nursing Procedures.* Redwood City, Calif.: Addison-Wesley Nursing.

Wightwick, S. June 1987. Canadian padded transfer board. *Physiotherapy* 73:309–10.

20

Client Positions

OBJECTIVES

- Describe positions that clients assume in bed

- Identify alignment problems in various positions

- Identify appropriate supportive devices that maintain correct body alignment

- Identify the pressure points created by various positions

- Identify information required to assess the client's need for supportive devices, strength to move, and pressure areas

- Effectively support clients in the various bed positions included in this chapter

- Explain reasons underlying selected steps of each technique

CONTENTS

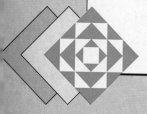

NURSING PROCESS GUIDE
POSITIONING CLIENTS

ASSESSMENT

Determine

- The client's need for supportive devices, such as pillows, rolled or folded towels, foam rubber supports, footboard, hand rolls, wrist splints, or sandbags by assessing the client's

  - *Adipose tissue.* A client who has ample adipose tissue generally requires less support and cushioning than the emaciated person while in a back-lying position, but greater support to maintain a lateral position.

  - *Skeletal structure.* Both the amount and the type of support needed vary according to the individual's skeletal structure. A person with a marked lumbar lordosis requires more lumbar support than one with a slight lumbar curvature.

  - *Health status.* A person who has flaccid or spastic paralysis requires supportive devices. The support differs with the client's specific health status.

  - *Discomfort.* A person who experiences pain during movement requires more support to prevent movement than one who can move without pain. A person who is unconscious is unable to indicate discomfort and will need appropriate support and change of position.

  - *Skin condition.* People who have nutrition problems and/or impaired circulation require more cushioning of the pressure points to prevent skin breakdown than do healthy people.

  - *Ability to move.* People who can move in bed can change position frequently. The client who is unable to move (e.g., the unconscious client) requires support so that muscles do not become strained.

  - *Hydration.* Dehydrated clients are at greater risk of decubitus ulcer formation than well-hydrated clients and therefore need more support under pressure areas.

Assess

- The client's strength and ability to move before the change of position, and obtain assistance as required. The risk of muscle strain and body injury, to both the client and nurse, is lowered when appropriate assistance is provided.

- Pressure areas of the body for any whitish or reddened spots. This discoloration can be caused by impaired blood circulation to the area. It should disappear in a few minutes when rubbing restores circulation.

- Pressure areas of the body for abrasions and excoriations. An abrasion (wearing away of the skin) can occur when skin rubs against a sheet, e.g., when the client is pulled. Excoriations (loss of superficial layers of the skin) can occur when the skin has prolonged contact with body secretions or excretions or with dampness in skinfolds.

- Stage of pressure sores, if present. Byrne and Feld (1984) describe four stages of superficial pressure sores:

  - Stage I: Pinkish-red mottled skin that does not return to normal color after the pressure is relieved

  - Stage II: Cracked, blistered, broken skin; shallow to full-thickness skin injury

  - Stage III: Broken skin with tissue involvement, exudate (usually), and a distinct ulcer

  - Stage IV: Extensive ulceration with penetration to the muscle and bone; necrotic tissue and profuse drainage usually present.

Palpate (with warm hands)

- The surface temperature of the skin over the pressure areas. Normally, the temperature is the same as that of the surrounding skin. Increased temperature is abnormal and may be due to inflammation or blood trapped in the area. A decreased temperature indicates impaired circulation.

- Over bony prominences and dependent body areas for the presence of edema. Edema will feel spongy upon palpation.

RELATED DIAGNOSTIC CATEGORIES

- Ineffective breathing pattern

- High risk for Disuse syndrome

- Impaired physical mobility

- Impaired skin integrity

- High risk for Impaired skin integrity

Continued on page 480

Nursing Process Guide CONTINUED

PLANNING

Client Goals
The client will

- Achieve or maintain proper body alignment.

- Avoid muscle shortening (contractures), reduced chest expansion, and other complications of poor alignment.

- Restore or maintain skin integrity, especially over bony prominences.

Outcome Criteria
The client

- Has intact, well-hydrated skin.

- Is free of pressure signs (pallor, redness, increased warmth or tenderness) over pressure areas.

- Experiences no muscle strain or shortening.

Positioning Clients

Positioning a bed-confined client in good body alignment and changing the position regularly and systematically are essential aspects of nursing practice. Clients who can move easily in bed automatically reposition themselves for comfort. Such people generally require minimal positioning assistance from nurses, other than guidance about ways to maintain body alignment and to exercise their joints. However, people who are weak, frail, in pain, paralyzed, or unconscious rely on nurses to provide or assist with position changes. For all clients, it is important to assess the skin and provide skin care before and after a position change.

Any position, correct or incorrect, can be detrimental if maintained for a prolonged period. Frequent change of position helps to prevent muscle discomfort, undue pressure resulting in **decubitus ulcers** (pressure sores), damage to superficial nerves and blood vessels, and **contractures** (permanent shortening of a muscle). Position changes also maintain muscle tone and stimulate postural reflexes.

 When the client is not able to move independently or assist with moving, the *preferred method is to use two or more nurses to move or turn the client.* Appropriate assistance reduces the risk of muscle strain and body injury to both the client and nurse.

When positioning clients in bed, the nurse can do a number of things to ensure proper alignment and promote client comfort and safety:

- Prior to placing the client in bed, make sure the mattress is firm and level yet has enough give to fill in and support natural body curvatures. A sagging mattress, a mattress that is too soft, or an underfilled water bed used over a prolonged period can contribute to the development of hip flexion contractures and low back strain and pain. Bed boards made of plywood and placed beneath

a sagging mattress are increasingly recommended for clients who have back problems or are prone to them. Some bed boards are hinged across the middle so that they will bend as the head of the bed is raised.

- Ensure that the bed is kept clean and dry. Wrinkled or damp sheets increase the risks of decubitus ulcer formation. Make sure extremities can move freely whenever possible. For example, the top bedclothes need to be loose enough for the client to move the feet.

- Place support devices (e.g., pillows, rolled towels, foam rubber supports) in specified areas according to the client's position. See Techniques 20–1 to 20–5. Use only those support devices needed to maintain alignment and to prevent stress on the client's muscles and joints. If the person is capable of movement, too many devices limit mobility and increase potential for muscle weakness and atrophy. Common alignment problems that can be corrected with support devices include the following:

  a. Flexion of the neck

  b. Internal rotation of the shoulder

  c. Adduction of the shoulder

  d. Flexion of the wrist

  e. Anterior convexity of the lumbar spine

  f. External rotation of the hips

  g. Hyperextension of the knees

  h. Plantar flexion of the ankle

- Avoid placing one body part, particularly one with bony prominences, directly on top of another body part. Excessive pressure can damage veins

Sample Schedule for Position Changes

Time		Position	Time		Position
10:00 A.M.	(1000 hr)	Left lateral	10:00 P.M.	(2200 hr)	Left Sims'
Noon	(1200 hr)	Fowler's or chair	Midnight	(2400 hr)	Supine
2:00 P.M.	(1400 hr)	Right lateral	2:00 A.M.	(0200 hr)	Right lateral
4:00 P.M.	(1600 hr)	Right Sims'	4:00 A.M.	(0400 hr)	Right Sims'
6:00 P.M.	(1800 hr)	Fowler's or chair	6:00 A.M.	(0600 hr)	Supine
8:00 P.M.	(2000 hr)	Left lateral	8:00 A.M.	(0800 hr)	Fowler's

and predispose the client to thrombus formation. Pressure against the popliteal space may damage nerves and blood vessels in this area.

• Plan a *systematic 24-hour schedule* for position changes. See the box above. Frequent position changes are essential to prevent decubitus ulcers in immobilized clients. Such clients should be repositioned every 2 hours throughout the day and night and more frequently when there is a risk for skin breakdown. This schedule is usually outlined on the client's nursing care plan. Schedule periods throughout the day during which the client assumes positions that provide full extension of the neck, hips, and knees to prevent flexion contractures of these joints.

• Always elicit information from the client to determine which position is most comfortable and appropriate. Seeking information from the client about what feels best is a useful guide when aligning persons and is an essential aspect of evaluating the effectiveness of an alignment intervention. Sometimes a person who appears well-aligned may be experiencing real discomfort. Both appearance, in relation to alignment criteria, and comfort are important in achieving effective alignment. To promote comfort, the nurse may administer prescribed analgesics approximately 30 minutes before moving or ambulating the client.

Pressure Sores

Pressure sores, also called decubitus ulcers, pressure ulcers, bedsores, or distortion sores, are reddened areas, sores, or ulcers of the skin occurring over bony prominences. See Figure 20–1. They are due to interruption of the blood circulation to the tissue, resulting in a localized ischemia. The tissue is caught between two hard surfaces, usually the surface of the bed and the bony skeleton. The localized

ischemia means that the cells are deprived of oxygen and nutrients, and the waste products of metabolism accumulate in the cells. The tissue dies because of the resulting anoxia. Prolonged, unrelieved pressure also damages the small blood vessels.

Causes of Pressure Sores

Shannon (1984) describes three causes of pressure sores: pressure, friction, and shearing force. Usually, two causes must be present before a pressure sore develops.

Pressure is the perpendicular force exerted on the skin by gravity. After the skin has been compressed, it appears white, as if the blood had been squeezed out of it. A white person's skin loses its pink color in the affected area, and a dark-skinned person's skin is also less pink, although the change is more difficult to see.

When pressure is relieved, the skin takes on a bright red flush, called **reactive hyperemia**, which

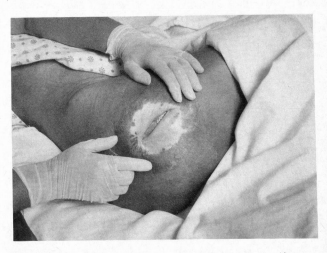

FIGURE 20–1 Decubitus ulcers most commonly form on the skin over bony prominences: shoulder blades, elbows, sacrum, hips (as in photo), knees, ankles, and heels.

is the body's mechanism for preventing pressure ulcers. The flush is due to vasodilation; extra blood floods to the area to compensate for the preceding period of impeded blood flow. The blood carries oxygen and removes the accumulated metabolic wastes. Reactive hyperemia usually lasts one half to three quarters as long as the duration of impeded blood flow to the area (Shannon and Miller 1988). If the redness disappears in that time, no tissue damage can be anticipated. If, however, the redness does not disappear, then tissue damage has occurred.

Friction is a force acting parallel to the skin. For example, when a client pulls up in bed, the skin rubbing against the sheet creates friction. Friction can abrade the skin, i.e., remove the superficial layers, making it more prone to breakdown.

Shearing force is a combination of friction and pressure. It occurs commonly when a client assumes a Fowler's position in bed. In this position, the body tends to slide downward toward the foot of the bed. This downward movement is transmitted to the sacral bone and the deep tissues. At the same time, the skin over the sacrum tends not to move because of the friction between the skin and the bedsheets. The skin and superficial tissues are thus relatively unmoving in relation to the bed surface, whereas the deeper tissues are firmly attached to the skeleton and move downward. This causes a shearing force in the area where the deeper tissues and the superficial tissues meet. The force damages the blood vessels and tissues in this area.

Six factors affect the formation of decubitus ulcers:

1. *Moisture.* Moisture due to urine, feces, drainage, and perspiration reduces the resistance of the skin to other forces, such as friction. The presence of moisture, e.g., due to incontinence, was found to be the single most reliable indicator of future development of a pressure sore (Exton-Smith et al. 1963).

2. *Hygiene.* Good hygiene reduces the number of microorganisms present on the skin. Bacteria localize in ischemic tissue, which is a good medium for their growth, and the presence of bacteria increases the severity of the sore and its rate of development.

3. *Nutrition.* Prolonged inadequate nutrition causes weight loss, muscle atrophy, and the loss of subcutaneous tissue. These three reduce the amount of padding between the skin and the bones, thus increasing the risk of pressure sore development.

4. *Body heat.* Body heat is a factor in the development of pressure sores. **Pyrexia** (elevated body temperature) increases the body's metabolic rate, thus increasing the need of the cells for oxygen. This increased need is reflected in the cells of the area

under pressure, which is already oxygen deficient. Therefore, severe infections with accompanying elevated body temperatures can affect the body's ability to deal with the effects of tissue compression.

5. *Anemia.* Anemia or anoxemia results in the decreased delivery of oxygen to the body cells. This is due to a decrease in the amount of hemoglobin present in the blood, because hemoglobin carries oxygen to the cells. Therefore, decreased hemoglobin exacerbates the oxygen deficiency already present in the tissues because of tissue compression.

6. *Mobility.* Normally, people move when they experience discomfort due to pressure on an area of the body. Healthy people rarely exceed their tolerance to pressure. However, paralysis, sensory disturbances, extreme weakness, apathy, and clouding of consciousness may diminish the ill person's response to tissue compression.

Other factors contributing to the formation of pressure sores are poor lifting techniques, incorrect positioning, repeated injections in the same area, hard support surfaces, and incorrect application of pressure-relieving devices. See Figure 20–2 for pressure areas in selected positions.

Preventing Pressure Sores

Preventive measures to reduce the risks of developing pressure sores include manipulation of the environment, ongoing assessment, proper positioning and nutrition, meticulous hygiene, and instruction in preventing pressure sores. The nurse manipulates the environment when making the client's bed, providing a smooth, firm, wrinkle-free foundation on which the client can lie. Some clients may require a special mattress, such as an alternating pressure, egg crate, or flotation mattress (available for beds and wheelchairs), to decrease pressure on body parts.

Using foam rubber pads and artificial sheepskins under pressure areas, such as the sacrum and heels, and elevating the heels above the bed surface decrease the likelihood that pressure sores will develop. Urine passes through artificial sheepskins, whereas real sheepskins retain urine. Thus, artificial sheepskins are preferred, especially for incontinent clients. Pressure-relieving equipment suggested for low-, medium-, and high-risk clients are shown in the box on page 484.

The nurse can reduce friction by applying a thin layer of cornstarch to the bedsheet or wheel chair seat cover. Shearing force can be reduced by elevating the head of the bed of bedfast clients no more than 30°, if this position is not contraindicated by the client's condition (e.g., clients with respiratory disorders may find it easier to breathe in a Fowler's position).

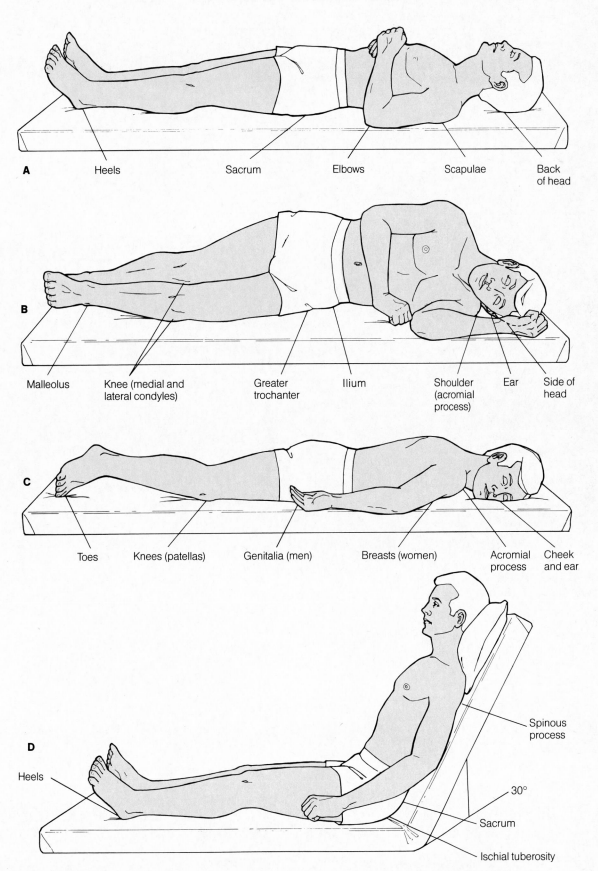

A   Heels   Sacrum   Elbows   Scapulae   Back of head

B   Malleolus   Knee (medial and lateral condyles)   Greater trochanter   Ilium   Shoulder (acromial process)   Ear   Side of head

C   Toes   Knees (patellas)   Genitalia (men)   Breasts (women)   Acromial process   Cheek and ear

D   Heels   Spinous process   30°   Sacrum   Ischial tuberosity

FIGURE 20–2   Body pressure areas in *A*, supine position; *B*, lateral position; *C*, prone position; *D*, Fowler's position.

Pressure-Relieving Equipment

Low-risk patients
- Sheepskins
- Hollow core fiber pads
- Bead overlays
- Foam overlays
- Gel pads

Medium-risk patients
- Foam overlays
- Foam replacement mattresses
- Combination foam/water mattresses
- Combination foam/gel mattresses
- Alternating air pads
- Water beds
- Double layer alternating air pads

High-risk patients
- Double layer alternating air pads
- Air flotation pads
- Dynamic air flotation mattress
- Air wave mattress
- Low air loss bed
- Air fluidized bed

Source: C. Dealy, How are you supporting your patients? A review of pressure relieving equipment, *Professional Nurse*, December 1990, 6: 134. Austen Cornish Publishers Ltd. Wallam Grove, London, England.

All clients at risk should have a systematic skin inspection at least once a day. The nurse needs to be alert to early symptoms of pressure sores, particularly over bony prominences.

The bedfast client's position should be changed at least every 15 minutes to 2 hours, depending on the client's need, even when a special support mattress is used, so that another body surface bears the weight. Six body positions can usually be used: prone, supine, right and left lateral (side-lying), and right and left Sims' positions. When the lateral position is used, avoid positioning the client directly on the trochanter. Position the client off the trochanter, on an angle. Good nutrition, particularly a diet high in protein and vitamin C, is an important preventive measure.

Meticulous nursing attention to client hygiene is another strategy for decreasing the incidence of pressure sores. The client's skin should be kept clean and dry. The nurse needs to protect the skin from irritation and maceration by urine, feces, sweat, incomplete drying after a bath, soap, and alcohol. When bathing the client, minimize the force and friction applied to the skin. Use mild cleansing agents that minimize irritation and dryness and that do not disrupt the skin's "natural barriers." Treat dry skin with moisturizers. Avoid the use of astringents. Apply powder, if used, sparingly because excessive accumulations may retain moisture, cause clumping, and aggravate the problem. Avoid massage over bony prominences because it may lead to deep tissue trauma.

Client teaching is another effective strategy in preventing pressure sores. The nurse teaches clients to be aware of discolored areas and of sensations such as tingling, which can indicate pressure, and to report changes in color or sensation promptly. The client needs to know that frequent shifts in position, even if only slight, effectively change the pressure point. The nurse encourages the client to shift weight every 15 to 30 minutes and, whenever possible, to exercise or ambulate to stimulate blood circulation.

Treating Pressure Sores

Pressure sores are a challenge for nurses because of the number of variables involved (e.g., risk factors, types of ulcers, and degrees of impairment) and the numerous treatment measures advocated. Existing and potential infections are the most serious complications of pressure sores. Suggested guidelines for treating existing pressure sores are included in the box on page 485.

Positioning Clients in Bed

Fowler's Position

Fowler's position, or semisitting position, is a bed position in which the head and trunk are raised 45° to 90° (Figure 20–3). In **low-Fowler's**, or **semi-Fowler's**, position, the head and trunk are raised 15° to 45°; in **high-Fowler's position**, the head and trunk are raised 90°. In this position, the knees may or may not be flexed. In some hospitals, *Fowler's position* refers to elevation of the upper part of the body without knee flexion, and the term *semi-Fowler's* is used to refer to the sitting position with knee flexion.

CLINICAL GUIDELINES

Treating Pressure Sores

- Clean the pressure sore daily, preferably in a whirlpool bath. The warmth and mechanical action of the whirlpool promotes circulation, decreases pressure on soft tissues, and helps debride the ulcer.

- Clean and dress the sore using surgical asepsis. Refrain from using antiseptics, such as alcohol, which are vasoconstrictors and reduce blood flow to the area.

- If the pressure sore **is not infected, cover it** with an occlusive dressing, e.g., Opsite, and leave the wound undisturbed for several days. Covering the sore with an occlusive dressing prevents microorganisms from entering it, and leaving the sore undisturbed promotes healing.

- If the pressure sore **is infected, obtain a sample** of the drainage for culture and sensitivity to antiseptic agents.

- Minimize direct pressure on the sore. Reposition the client at least every 2 hours. Make a schedule, and record position changes on the client's chart.

- Reduce friction by applying a small amount of cornstarch to the bedsheet.

- Reduce shearing force by keeping the head of the bed flat or elevated to a maximum of 30° unless contraindicated by the client's condition.

- If the client cannot keep weight off the pressure sore, **use a special mattress** or pad.

- Teach the client to move, if only slightly, to relieve pressure.

- Encourage ambulation or sitting in a wheelchair if the client's condition permits.

- Provide range-of-motion exercises as the client's condition permits.

Fowler's position is the position of choice for people who have difficulty breathing and for some people with heart problems. When the client is in this position, gravity pulls the diaphragm downward, allowing greater lung expansion. Clients who are confined to bed but are capable of eating, reading, watching television, or visiting find this position comfortable.

One of the devices nurses use to support clients in Fowler's position is the **trochanter roll**, a roll of cloth, frequently a towel, placed against the greater trochanter of the femur to prevent external rotation of the hip. The nurse palpates the greater trochanter and places the middle of the roll against it. Trochanter rolls need not extend more than 8 to 10 inches on either side of the trochanter, because leg rotation occurs at the hip joint. Firm support by the trochanter roll inhibits outward rotation. Trochanter rolls are made commercially or can be constructed as described in Figure 20–4. A commercial roll needs only to be covered before it is used. Covered sandbags are commonly used.

A common error nurses make when aligning clients in Fowler's position is placing an overly large pillow or more than one pillow behind the client's head. These errors promote the development of neck flexion contractures. If a client desires several head pillows, the nurse should encourage the client to rest without a pillow for several hours each day to extend the neck fully and counteract the effects of poor neck alignment.

An adaptation of high-Fowler's position is the **orthopneic position**. The client sits either in bed or on the side of the bed with an overbed table across the lap (Figure 20–5). This position facilitates respiration by allowing maximum chest expansion. It is particularly helpful to clients who have problems exhaling, because they can press the lower part of the chest against the overbed table.

Technique 20–1 describes how to support a client in Fowler's position.

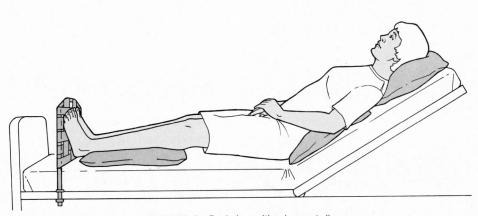

FIGURE 20–3 Fowler's position (supported).

A

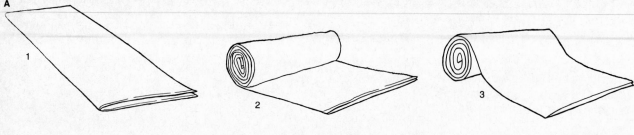

B

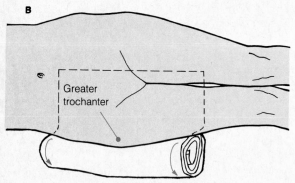

Greater
trochanter

FIGURE 20-4   *A,* Making a trochanter roll: (1) Fold the towel in half lengthwise; (2) roll the towel tightly, starting at one narrow edge and rolling within approximately 30 cm (1 ft) of the other edge; (3) invert the roll. *B,* Applying a trochanter roll: Place the flat part of the towel under the client's hip; turn the roll under, and position it tightly against the greater trochanter until the client's toes point directly upward, i.e., until the hip is neither externally nor internally rotated; repeat for the other leg if required.

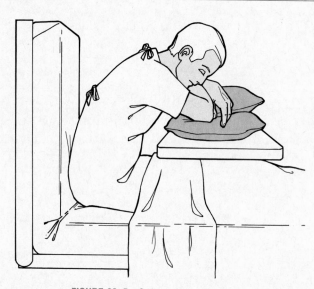

FIGURE 20-5   Orthopneic position.

20-1 Supporting a Client in Fowler's Position

PURPOSES

- To improve chest expansion and lung ventilation
- To provide increased comfort
- To facilitate performance of certain activities of daily living (e.g., eating, watching television)
- To reposition the client and help maintain intact skin

ASSESSMENT FOCUS

Presence of pressure areas of particular concern in Fowler's position (Figure 20-2, *D,* earlier), i.e., the heels, spinous process, sacrum, ischial tuberosities, and scapulae; breathing pattern, in particular, the presence of orthopnea.

► **Technique 20–1** *CONTINUED*

EQUIPMENT

☐ One to six small pillows, depending on client need

☐ One or two trochanter rolls (optional)

☐ Footboard

INTERVENTION

1. Position the client.

• Have the client flex the knees slightly before raising the head of the bed. *Slight knee flexion prevents the person from sliding toward the foot of the bed as the bed is raised.* Be certain the client's hips are positioned directly over the point where the bed will bend when the head is raised. *An appropriate hip position ensures that the client will be sitting on the ischial tuberosities when the head of the bed is raised.*

• Raise the head of the bed to 30°, 45°, or the angle required by or ordered for the client.

2. Provide supportive devices to align the client appropriately.

• Place a small pillow or roll under the lumbar region of the back if you feel a space in the lumbar curvature. *The pillow supports the natural lumbar curvature and prevents flexion of the lumbar spine.*

• Place a small pillow under the client's head. *The pillow supports the cervical curvature of the vertebral column.* Alternatively, have the client rest the head against the mattress. *Too many pillows beneath the head can cause neck flexion contracture.*

• Place one or two pillows under the lower legs from below the knees to the ankles. *The pillows provide a broad base of support that is soft and flexible, prevent uncomfortable hyperextension of the knees, and reduce pressure on the heels.* Make sure that no pressure is exerted on the popliteal space and that the knees are flexed. *Pressure against the popliteal space can damage nerves and vein walls, predisposing the client to thrombus formation. Keeping the knees slightly flexed also prevents the person from sliding down in the bed.*

• Avoid using the knee gatch of a hospital bed to flex the client's knees. *The position of the knee gatch rarely coincides with the position of the client's knees. Even when the knee gatch does bend at the client's knees, considerable pressure (due to the narrow base of support beneath the knees and the firm, unyielding mattress) can be exerted against the popliteal space and beneath the client's calves.*

• Put a trochanter roll lateral to each femur (optional). *This prevents external rotation of the hips.*

• Support the client's feet with a footboard. *This prevents plantar flexion.* The footboard should protrude several inches above the toes. *This protects the toes from pressure exerted by the top bedding.* The footboard should be placed 1 inch away from the heels. *This prevents undue pull on the Achilles tendon and discomfort.*

• Place pillows to support both arms and hands if the client does not have normal use of them. *These pillows prevent shoulder and muscle strain from the effects of downward gravitational pull, dislocation of the shoulder in paralyzed persons, edema of the hands and arms, and flexion contracture of the wrist.* Arrange the pillows to support only the forearms and hands, up to the elbow. In this way, the pillows support the shoulder girdle.

3. Document all relevant information.

• Record change of position according to agency protocol, any difficulty the client has with breathing, and any signs of pressure areas or contractures.

• Report problems promptly to the nurse in charge.

EVALUATION FOCUS

Malalignments associated with an *unsupported* Fowler's position (e.g., hyperextension or flexion of the neck, flexion of the lumbar curvature, hyperextension of the knees, external rotation of the legs, and plantar flexion); in clients who lack arm movement, shoulder muscle strain, edema of the hands and arms, and wrist flexion; pressure areas from previous position; ease of breathing; client comfort.

►

▶ **Technique 20–1 Supporting a Client in Fowler's Position** *CONTINUED*

KEY ELEMENTS OF SUPPORTING A CLIENT IN FOWLER'S POSITION

- Support the client appropriately to prevent the following:
  - Hyperextension or flexion of the neck
  - Flexion of the wrists
  - Flexion of the lumbar curvature
  - Hyperextension of the knees
  - External rotation of the hips
  - Plantar flexion

- Avoid using the knee gatch of a hospital bed.
- Avoid putting pressure on the popliteal space.
- Assess pressure areas of particular concern in Fowler's position:
  - Heels
  - Spinous processes
  - Sacrum
  - Ischial tuberosities
  - Scapulae

Dorsal Recumbent Position

In the **dorsal recumbent (back-lying) position**, the client's head and shoulders are slightly elevated on a small pillow (Figure 20–6). Although in some agencies the terms *dorsal recumbent* and *supine* are used interchangeably, strictly speaking, in the **supine,** or **dorsal, position**, the head and shoulders are not elevated. In both positions, the client's forearms may be elevated on pillows or placed at the client's sides. Supports are similar in both positions, except for the head pillow. Technique 20–2 describes how to support a client in the dorsal recumbent position.

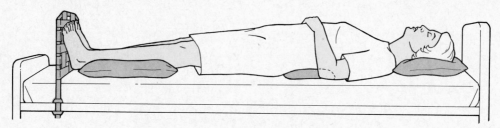

FIGURE 20–6 Dorsal recumbent position (supported).

20-2

Supporting a Client in the Dorsal Recumbent Position

PURPOSES
- To reposition the client and offset the possibility of skin breakdown
- To enhance client comfort

ASSESSMENT FOCUS

Presence of pressure areas of particular concern in the dorsal recumbent position (Figure 20–2, *A*, earlier), i.e., the heels, sacrum, elbows, scapulae, and back of the head.

▶ **Technique 20–2 Supporting a Client in Dorsal Recumbant Position** *CONTINUED*

EQUIPMENT

☐ Up to six small pillows, depending on client need
☐ Two trochanter rolls (optional)
☐ Footboard
☐ Handrolls or wrist splints, if needed

INTERVENTION

1. Assist the client to a supine position.

2. Provide supportive devices to align the client appropriately.

• Place a pillow of suitable thickness under the client's head and shoulders as needed. *This prevents hyperextension of the neck. Too many pillows beneath the head may cause or worsen neck flexion contracture.*

• Place a pillow under the lower legs from below the knees to the ankles. *This prevents hyperextension of the knees, keeps the heels off the bed, and reduces lumbar lordosis.*

• Place trochanter rolls laterally against the femurs (optional). *These prevent external rotation of the hips.*

• Place a rolled towel or small pillow under the lumbar curvature if you feel a space between the lumbar area and the bed. *This pillow supports the lumbar curvature and prevents flexion of the lumbar spine.*

• Put a footboard or rolled pillow on the bed to support the feet. *This prevents plantar flexion (foot drop).*

• If the client is unconscious or has paralysis of the upper extremities, elevate the forearms and hands (*not* the upper arm) on pillows. *This position promotes comfort and prevents edema. Pillows are not placed under the upper arms because they can cause shoulder flexion.*

• If the client has actual or potential finger and wrist flexion de-

formities, use handrolls or wrist/hand splints. *This prevents flexion contractures of the fingers.* Handrolls, having a circumference of 13 to 15 cm (5 to 6 in) exert even pressure over the entire flexor surface of the palm and fingers. Evidence suggests that a firm, unyielding handroll made of cardboard is more useful in preventing contractures than a soft, pliable roll (Dayhoff 1975, p. 1143).

3. Document all relevant information.

• Record change of position according to agency protocol and any signs of pressure areas or contractures.

• Report problems promptly to the nurse in charge.

EVALUATION FOCUS

Malalignment associated with an *unsupported* dorsal recumbent position (e.g., hyperextension or flexion of the neck, flexion of the lumbar curvature, external rotation of the legs, hyperextension of the knees, and plantar flexion); signs of pressure areas from previous position; client comfort.

KEY ELEMENTS OF SUPPORTING A CLIENT IN THE DORSAL RECUMBENT POSITION

• Support the client appropriately to prevent the following:
  • Hyperextension or flexion of the neck
  • Flexion of the lumbar curvature
  • External rotation of the legs
  • Hyperextension of the knees
  • Plantar flexion
• Avoid putting pressure on the popliteal space.

• Assess pressure areas of particular concern in the dorsal recumbent position:
  • Heels
  • Sacrum
  • Elbows
  • Scapulae
  • Back of head

Prone Position

In the **prone position**, the client lies on the abdomen with the head turned to one side. The hips are not flexed. Both children and adults sleep in this position, sometimes with one or both arms flexed over their heads (Figure 20–7). This position has several advantages. It is the only bed position that allows full extension of the hip and knee joints. When used periodically, the prone position helps to prevent flexion contractures of the hips and knees, thereby counteracting a problem caused by all other bed positions. The prone position also promotes drainage from the mouth and is especially useful for clients recovering from surgery of the mouth or throat.

The prone position also poses some distinct dis-

advantages. The pull of gravity on the trunk produces a marked lordosis in most persons, and the neck is rotated laterally to a significant degree. For this reason, physicians may not recommend this position, especially for persons with problems of the cervical or lumbar spine. This position also causes plantar flexion. Some clients with cardiac or respiratory problems find the prone position confining and suffocating, because chest expansion is inhibited during respirations. The prone position should be used only when the client's back is properly aligned, only for short periods, and only for persons with no evidence of spinal abnormalities. Technique 20–3 describes how to support a client in the prone position.

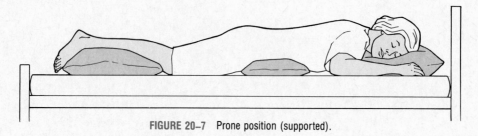

FIGURE 20–7   Prone position (supported).

 20-3

Supporting a Client in the Prone Position

PURPOSES
- To prevent flexion contractures of the knees and hips
- To promote drainage from the mouth
- To reposition the client and offset the possibility of skin breakdown

ASSESSMENT FOCUS

Presence of pressure areas of particular concern in the prone position (Figure 20–2, *C,* earlier), i.e., the toes, knees, genitals (men), breasts (women), acromial process of the shoulders, cheek, and ear; any tenderness or problems with the male genitals or female breasts; presence of any spinal, respiratory, or cardiac problems contraindicating this position.

EQUIPMENT
- Three pillows

► **Technique 20–3** *CONTINUED*

INTERVENTION

1. Assist the client to a prone position.

• See Technique 19–3 on page 464.

2. Provide supportive devices to position the client appropriately.

• Turn the client's head to one side, and either omit the pillow entirely if drainage from the mouth is being encouraged, or place a small pillow under the head to align the head with the trunk. *This prevents flexion of the neck laterally.* Avoid placing the pillow under the shoulders. *A pillow placed under the shoulders increases lumbar lordosis.*

• Place a small pillow or roll under the abdomen in the space between the diaphragm (or the breasts of a woman) and the iliac crests. *The pillow prevents hyperextension of the lumbar curvature, difficulty breathing, and, for some women, pressure on the breasts. Supports placed too low can increase lumbar lordosis and pressure on bony prominences.*

• Place a pillow under the lower legs from below the knees to just above the ankles. *This raises the toes off the bed surface and reduces plantar flexion. This pillow also flexes the knees slightly for comfort and prevents excessive pressure on the patellae.*

or

Position the client on the bed so that the feet are extended in a normal anatomic position over the lower edge of the mattress. There should be no pressure on the toes.

3. Document all relevant information.

• Record change of position according to agency protocol, any difficulty the client has with breathing, and any signs of pressure areas or contractures.

• Report problems promptly to the nurse in charge.

EVALUATION FOCUS

Malalignments and other problems associated with an *unsupported* prone position (e.g., acute flexion or hyperextension of the neck, hyperextension of the lumbar curvature, plantar flexion, pressure on a woman's breasts, and inhibited chest expansion causing breathing difficulties); signs of pressure areas from previous position; client comfort.

KEY ELEMENTS OF SUPPORTING A CLIENT IN THE PRONE POSITION

• Support the client appropriately to prevent the following:
  • Acute flexion or hyperextension of the neck
  • Hyperextension of the lumbar curvature
  • Pressure on a woman's breasts
  • Plantar flexion
• Omit the pillow under the head if drainage of mouth secretions is to be encouraged.
• Place abdominal supports at or below the level of the diaphragm to enable appropriate chest expansion.

• Assess pressure areas of particular concern in the prone position:
  • Toes
  • Knees
  • Genitals (men)
  • Breasts (women)
  • Acromial processes of shoulders
  • Cheek and ear

Lateral Position

In the **lateral** or **side-lying position**, the person lies on one side of the body (Figure 20–8). By having the client flex the top hip and knee and placing this leg in front of the body, a wider, triangular base of support is created, and greater stability is achieved. The greater the flexion on the top hip and knee, the greater the stability and balance in this position. This flexion reduces lordosis and promotes good back alignment. For this reason, the lateral position is good for resting and sleeping clients. The lateral position helps to relieve pressure on the sacrum and heels in persons who sit for much of the day or who are confined to bed and rest in Fowler's or dorsal recumbant positions much of the time. In the lateral position, most of the body's weight is borne by the lateral aspect of the lower scapula, the lateral aspect of the ilium, and the greater trochanter of the femur. Persons who have sensory or motor deficits on one side of the body usually find that lying on the uninvolved side is more comfortable.

Technique 20–4 describes how to support a client in the lateral position.

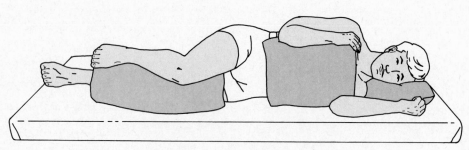

FIGURE 20–8 Lateral position (supported).

20-4 Supporting a Client in the Lateral Position

PURPOSES	• To promote client comfort and rest • To reposition the client and offset the possibility of skin breakdown
ASSESSMENT FOCUS	Presence of pressure areas of particular concern in the lateral position (Figure 20–2, *B,* earlier), i.e., the lateral malleolus of the lower ankle, medial malleolus of the upper ankle, medial condyle of the uppermost knee, lateral condyle of the lower knee, greater trochanter of the lower hip, ilium of the lower pelvis, acromial process of the lower clavicle, and lower ear and cheek; the client's preference for right or left side, if indicated.

EQUIPMENT

□ Up to five small pillows
□ Folded towel (optional)

▶ **Technique 20–4** *CONTINUED*

INTERVENTION

1. Assist the client to a lateral position.

- See Technique 19–3 on page 464.

2. Provide supportive devices to align the client appropriately.

- Place a pillow under the client's head so that the head and neck are aligned with the trunk. *The pillow prevents lateral flexion and discomfort of the major neck muscles, e.g., the sternocleidomastoid muscles.*

- Have the client flex the lower shoulder and position it forward so that the body does not rest on it. Rotate it into any position of comfort. *In this way, circulation is not disrupted.*

- Place a pillow under the upper arm. *This prevents internal rotation and adduction of the shoulder and downward pressure on the chest that could interfere with chest expansion during respiration.* If the client has respiratory

difficulty, increase the shoulder flexion and position the upper arm in front of the body off the chest.

- Place two or more pillows under the upper leg and thigh so that the extremity lies in a plane parallel to the surface of the bed. *A position parallel to the bed most closely approximates correct standing alignment and prevents internal rotation of the thigh and adduction of the leg. The pillow also prevents pressure caused by the weight of the top leg resting on the lower leg. Such pressure can damage the vein walls in the lower leg and predispose the client to thrombus formation.*

- Ensure that the two shoulders are aligned in the same plane as the two hips. If they are not, pull one shoulder or hip forward or backward until all four joints are aligned in the same plane. *Proper*

alignment prevents twisting of the spine.

- Place a folded towel under the natural hollow at the waistline (optional). *This prevents postural scoliosis of the lumbar spine.* Take care to fill in only the space at the waistline. *A towel support that extends too high or too low creates undue pressure against the rib cage or iliac crests.*

- Place a rolled pillow alongside the client's back to stabilize the position (optional). This pillow is not usually needed when the client's upper hip and knee are appropriately flexed.

3. Document all relevant information.

- Record change of position according to agency protocol and any signs of pressure areas or contractures.

- Report problems promptly to the nurse in charge.

EVALUATION FOCUS

Malalignment associated with the *unsupported* lateral position (e.g., lateral flexion of the neck, internal shoulder rotation/adduction of the upper arm, internal hip rotation/adduction of the upper leg, tendency for the spine to curve laterally toward the bed at the waist [postural scoliosis], twisting of the lumbar spine, and plantar flexion); signs of pressure areas from previous position; client comfort.

KEY ELEMENTS OF SUPPORTING A CLIENT IN THE LATERAL POSITION

- Support the client appropriately to prevent the following:
  - Lateral flexion of the neck
  - Internal rotation of the thigh and adduction of the upper leg
  - Internal rotation of the shoulder, adduction of the arm, and interference with chest expansion
  - Twisting of the spine

- Assess pressure areas of particular concern in the lateral position:
  - Lateral malleolus of lower ankle
  - Medial malleolus of upper ankle
  - Medial condyle of uppermost knee
  - Lateral condyle of lower knee
  - Greater trochanter of lower hip

Sims' Position

In **Sims'** or the **semiprone position**, the client assumes a posture halfway between the lateral and the prone positions (Figure 20–9). In Sims' position, the lower arm is positioned behind the client, and the upper arm is flexed at the shoulder and the elbow. Both legs are flexed in front of the client. The upper leg is more acutely flexed at both the hip and the knee than the lower one is.

Sims' position is occasionally used for unconscious clients because it facilitates drainage from the mouth. It is also used for paralyzed (paraplegic or hemiplegic) clients because it reduces pressure over the sacrum and greater trochanter of the hip. It is often used for clients receiving enemas and occasionally for clients undergoing examinations or treatments of the perineal area. Many people, especially pregnant women, find Sims' position comfortable for sleeping. Persons with sensory or motor deficits on one side of the body usually find that lying on the uninvolved side is more comfortable.

Technique 20–5 describes how to support a client in Sims' position.

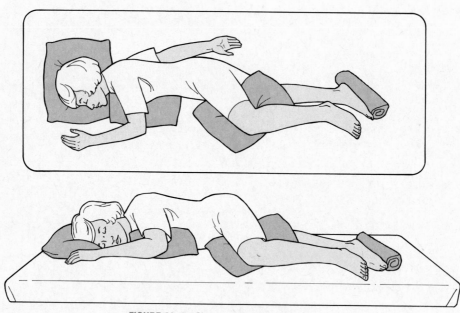

FIGURE 20–9 Sims' position (supported).

20-5 Supporting a Client in Sims' Position

PURPOSES

- To reposition the client and prevent skin breakdown
- To promote client comfort and rest
- To encourage drainage from the mouth and prevent aspiration

ASSESSMENT FOCUS

Presence of pressure areas of particular concern in this position, i.e., the side of the skull (temporal and parietal bones and the ear), acromial process of the lowermost clavicle, lowermost anterior superior iliac spine, lowermost greater trochanter of the femur, lateral aspect of the undermost knee, medial aspect of the uppermost knee, lateral malleolus of the undermost ankle, medial malleolus of the uppermost ankle, and medial aspect (epicondyle) of the uppermost elbow.

EQUIPMENT

☐ Three small pillows   ☐ Sandbag or rolled towel

► **Technique 20–5** *CONTINUED*

INTERVENTION

1. Turn the client as for a prone position.

2. Provide supportive devices to align the client appropriately.

- Place a small pillow under the client's head, unless drainage from the mouth is being encouraged. *The pillow prevents lateral flexion of the neck and cushions the cranial and facial bones and the ear.* It is contraindicated if drainage of mucus is required. *Too large a pillow produces an uncomfortable lateral flexion of the neck.*

- Place the lower arm behind and away from the client's body in a position that is comfortable and does not disrupt circulation. *This position prevents damage to the nerves and blood vessels in the axillae.*

- Position the upper shoulder so that it is abducted slightly from the body and the shoulder and elbow are flexed. Place a pillow in the space between the chest and abdomen and the upper arm and bed. *This position and support prevent internal shoulder rotation and adduction and maintain alignment of the upper trunk.*

- Place a pillow in the space between the abdomen and pelvis and the upper thigh and bed. *This position prevents internal rotation and adduction of the hip and also reduces lumbar lordosis.*

- Ensure that the two shoulders are aligned in the same plane as the two hips. If they are not, pull one shoulder or hip forward or backward until all four joints are aligned in the same plane. *This prevents twisting of the spine.*

- Place a support device, e.g., a sandbag or rolled towel, against the lower foot. *This device may prevent foot drop.* Efforts to correct plantar flexion in this position, however, are usually unsuccessful.

3. Document all relevant information.

- Record change of position according to agency protocol, any difficulty the client has with breathing, and any signs of pressure areas or contractures.

- Report problems promptly to the nurse in charge.

EVALUATION FOCUS

Malalignment associated with the *unsupported* Sims' position (e.g., lateral flexion of the neck, internal shoulder rotation and adduction of the upper arm, internal hip rotation and adduction of the upper leg, twisting of the thoracolumbar spine if the shoulders are rotated in one direction and the hips in another, lumbar lordosis, and plantar flexion); signs of pressure areas from previous position; client comfort.

KEY ELEMENTS OF SUPPORTING A CLIENT IN SIMS' POSITION

- Support the client appropriately to prevent the following:
  - Lateral flexion of the neck, unless drainage from the mouth is being encouraged
  - Disruption of circulation to the arm placed behind the body
  - Internal shoulder rotation and adduction of the upper arm
  - Internal rotation and adduction of the hip, and lumbar lordosis
  - Twisting of the spine
- Assess pressure areas of particular concern in Sims' position:
  - Side of the skull (temporal and parietal bone and the ear)
  - Acromial process of lowermost clavicle
  - Lowermost anterior superior iliac spine
  - Lowermost greater trochanter of the femur
  - Lateral aspect of undermost knee
  - Medial aspect of uppermost knee
  - Lateral malleolus of undermost ankle
  - Medial malleolus of uppermost ankle
  - Medial aspect (epicondyle) of uppermost elbow
- Omit the head pillow if drainage of mouth secretions is to be encouraged.
- Position the lower arm appropriately so that circulation is maintained.

CRITICAL THINKING CHALLENGE

Mildred Green is a frail elderly female who has been admitted to the nursing unit. During the admission assessment, you observe a reddened and edematous area on the sacrum approximately 2 inches in diameter. There is sloughing of some of the superficial skin tissue. What factors may have contributed to Ms Green's pressure sore? What actions should you take?

RELATED RESEARCH

Carlson, C. E., and King, R. B. 1990. Prevention of pressure sores. *Annual Review of Nursing Research* 8:35–56.

Meeham, M. November 1990. Multisite pressure ulcer prevalence survey. *Decubitus* 3:14–17.

Smith, A. M., and Malone, J. A. November 1990. Preventing pressure ulcers in institutionalized elders: Assessing the effects of small unscheduled shifts in body position. *Decubitus* 3:20–22, 24.

Stewart, T. P.; McKay, M. G.; and Magnano, S. November 1990. Pressure relief characteristics of an alternating pressure system. *Decubitus* 3:26–29.

Wardman, C. March 27–April 2, 1991. Norton vs Waterlow . . . tool for assessing pressure sore risks. *Nursing Times* 87:74, 76, 78.

REFERENCES

Agency for Health Care Policy and Research. July, 1992. Clinical guidelines: How to predict and prevent pressure ulcers. *American Journal of Nursing* 92:52–60.

Ahmed, M. C. December 1980. Special report: Choosing the best method to manage pressure ulcers. *Nurses' Drug Alert* 4(15):113–20.

Byrne, N., and Feld, M. April 1984. Preventing and treating decubitus ulcers. *Nursing 84* 14:55–57.

Colburn, L. December 1990. Preventing pressure ulcers: How to recognize and care for patients at risk. *Nursing* 20:60–63.

Collier, M. October 1990. A sore point . . . prevention of pressure sores. *Community Outlook* 29–30, 32.

Dayhoff, N. July 1975. Soft or hard devices to position hands? *American Journal of Nursing* 75:1142–44.

Dealy, C. December 1990. How are you supporting your patients? A review of pressure relieving equipment. *Professional Nurse* 6:134, 136, 138.

Exton-Smith, A. N., et al. 1963. A study of factors concerned in the production of pressure sores and their prevention. In *Investigation of geriatric nursing problems in hospitals.* London: The National Corporation for Care of Old People.

Green, E., and Katz, J. February 1991. Practice guidelines for management of pressure ulcers. *Decubitus* 4:36, 38, 40.

Kerr, J. C.; Stinson, S. M.; and Shannon, M. L. July/August 1981. Pressure sores: Distinguishing fact from fiction. *Canadian Nurse* 77:23–28.

Memmer, M. K. 1974. *Posture and alignment.* Los Angeles: The Intercampus Nursing Project, California State University and College System.

Murray, S. M., and Thompson, R. January 1991. We've organized our approach to pressure sores. *RN* 54:42–44.

Norton, D. February 13, 1975. Research and the problem of pressure sores. *Nursing Mirror* 140:65–67.

Shannon, M. L. October 1984. Five famous fallacies about pressure sores. *Nursing 84* 14:34–41.

Shannon, M. L., and Miller, B. M. May/June 1988. Pressure sore treatment: A case in point. *Geriatric Nursing* 9:154–57.

Waterlow, J. February 1991. A policy that protects: The Waterlow pressure sore prevention/treatment policy. *Professional Nurse* 6:258, 260, 262.

21

Exercise and Ambulation

OBJECTIVES

- Identify the effects of exercise

- Identify physiologic and psychologic responses to immobility

- Describe five major kinds of exercise

- Identify guidelines for providing passive exercises

- Describe exercises requisite to ambulation and using crutches

- Identify assessment data related to exercise and ambulation

- Explain the reasons underlying selected steps of the techniques in this chapter

- Adequately assess the client's muscle strength, body alignment and stance, gait, range of joint motion, and activity tolerance

- Help clients to ambulate safely with or without assistive devices

- Communicate and document relevant information about the client

CONTENTS

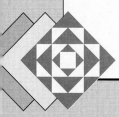

NURSING PROCESS GUIDE

EXERCISE AND AMBULATION

ASSESSMENT

Assess

- Length of time in bed.

- Visual acuity. Is it adequate to detect hazards and prevent falls?

- Mental alertness and ability to follow directions. Check medications the client is receiving that hinder the ability to walk safely (e.g., narcotics, sedatives, tranquilizers, and antihistamines cause drowsiness, dizziness, weakness, and orthostatic hypotension).

- Assistive devices used, such as a cane, walker, crutches, braces.

If the client is using assistive devices, determine the strength of the upper extremities:

- *Flexor muscles:* While the client fully extends each arm, ask the client to flex the arm while you attempt to hold it in extension.

- *Extensor muscles:* While the client flexes each arm, ask the client to extend the arm while you attempt to keep it flexed.

Determine strength in lower extremities by

- Inspecting the muscles of the thigh and calf for size. Compare the muscle on one side of the body to the same muscle on the other side. If there appears to be a discrepancy between the sides, measure the muscle with tape.

- Testing for muscle strength. Compare the right side with the left side. Note whether there is paralysis or normal movement against gravity and minimal or full resistance.

  a. *Hip muscles:* While the client is supine with both legs extended, ask the client to raise one leg at a time while you attempt to hold it down.

  b. *Hamstrings:* While the client is supine with both knees bent, ask the client to resist while you attempt to straighten them.

  c. *Quadriceps:* While the client is supine with knees partially extended, ask the client to resist while you attempt to flex the knee.

  d. *Muscles of the feet and ankles:* Ask the client to resist while you attempt to dorsiflex the foot and then plantar flex the foot.

Determine coordination and balance.

- Determine the client's abilities to hold the body erect, to bear weight and keep balance in a standing position on both legs or only one, to take steps, and to push off from a chair or bed.

Assess body alignment and stance. View the client from anterior, lateral, and posterior perspectives.

Assess gait. Ask the client to walk down a corridor and observe whether the client's

- Head is erect, and vertebral column is upright.

- Gaze is straight ahead.

- Toes point forward.

- Kneecaps point forward.

- Elbows are slightly flexed.

- Feet are dorsiflexed in swing phase.

- Arm opposite swing-through foot moves forward at same time.

- Legs follow through in the swing phase.

- Instep falls along the line of gravity or whether the feet are spread apart.

- Steps are appropriate or too small.

- Steps are smooth, coordinated, and rhythmic.

- Gait is free and easy or unsteady.

- Gait starts and stops with ease.

Assess **pace** (the number of steps taken per minute). A normal walking pace is 70 to 100 steps per minute.

Determine the range of motion of joints needed to ambulate. Ask the client to perform range-of-motion exercises for the ankles, knees, and hips. While the client performs the range-of-motion exercises, assess

- The degree of movement of the joint.

- Any discomfort experienced by the client.

- Any joint swelling or redness, which could indicate the presence of an injury or an inflammation.

- Any contractures.

Determine activity tolerance:

- Assess pulse, respiratory rate, and blood pressure before and after ambulation.

- Note facial color, shortness of breath, chest pain, profuse perspiration, feelings of dizziness, and weakness when ambulating.

Nursing Process Guide *CONTINUED*

RELATED DIAGNOSTIC CATEGORIES

- Activity intolerance
- High risk for Activity intolerance
- High risk for Disuse syndrome
- Fear (of falling)
- High risk for Injury
- Knowledge deficit
- Impaired physical mobility

PLANNING

Client Goals
The client will

- Restore or improve ambulatory capability.
- Develop an activity pattern supporting increased tolerance of activity.
- Not experience Disuse syndrome.
- Develop strategies to prevent injury and reduce fear of falling.
- Maintain normal musculoskeletal functioning.

Outcome Criteria
The client

- Stands erect when walking.
- Uses a walker to move independently from the bed to the nursing station three times a day.
- Demonstrates correct use of four-point (or three-point) crutch gait.
- Demonstrates correct methods of getting into and out of a chair and ascending and descending stairs with crutches.
- Performs active assistive exercises, as taught, to right arm three times a day.
- Identifies factors that may increase the potential of injury.
- Appropriately uses countermeasures to protect self from injury.
- Verbalizes signs of activity tolerance.
- Exhibits muscle size in legs and arms that is equal to baseline measurements.
- Exhibits joint range-of-motion that is equal to or better than baseline measurements.

◆ Mobility

The importance of movement to a person's health cannot be overemphasized. The overall benefits of exercise and the ability to carry out the activities of everyday life by walking and moving are often taken for granted by a healthy person. Being ill and confined to bed soon weakens the body and can result in serious impairments not only to movement but also to the functioning of other body systems.

A number of aspects of mobility are of particular relevance in health care: joint mobility, station and gait, activity tolerance, and exercise.

Joint Mobility

A joint, the functional unit of the musculoskeletal system, is where the bones of the skeleton articulate. Most of the skeletal muscles attach to the two bones at the joint. These muscles are categorized according to the type of joint movement they produce on **contraction**, the normal, active shortening or tensing of

a muscle. Muscles are therefore called flexors, extensors, internal rotators, and so on. The flexor muscles are stronger than the extensor muscles. Thus, when a person is inactive, the joints are pulled into a flexed (bent) position. If this is not counteracted with exercise and position changes, permanent shortening (**contracture**) of the muscles develops, and the joint becomes fixed in a flexed position.

The **range of motion** of a joint is the maximum movement that is possible for that joint. Not all people possess a similar range of motion. Each person's range is determined by genetic inheritance, developmental patterns, the presence or absence of disease, and the amount of physical activity the person normally does.

Each type of joint is capable of specific movements. These movements are described in relation to the anatomic body position and the three body planes: sagittal, transverse, coronal. The sagittal plane is a vertical line or plane dividing the body or its parts into right and left portions. The transverse plane is a horizontal line or plane dividing the body or its parts into superior and inferior portions. The frontal or coronal plane is any plane dividing the body into anterior (ventral) and posterior (dorsal) portions at right angles to the sagittal plane. For descriptions of the movements of joints, see Table 21–1. For normal ranges of joint movements, see Table 21–2.

Station and Gait

Station, or stance, is the way a person stands; **gait** is the way a person walks or ambulates. A desirable station for a person provides correct body alignment. However, an incorrect stance can develop because of postural habits or disease processes. Incorrect body alignment places undue strain on some of the muscles and bones of the body.

Activity Tolerance

Activity tolerance, or endurance, is the ability to withstand activity in terms of duration. It generally increases with repeated activity over a period of time. Tolerance is affected by a number of factors: pain, physical strength, cardiopulmonary status, age, lifestyle, and emotional state.

Exercise

Exercise has a number of purposes: (a) to restore, maintain, or increase the tone and strength of the muscles; (b) to maintain or increase the flexibility of the joints: (c) to maintain or promote the growth of bones through the application of physical stressors; and (d) to improve the functioning of other body systems, such as the cardiovascular and gastrointestinal systems. Further information on the effects and types of exercise is provided later in this chapter.

Effects of Exercise

Exercise and adequate movement of the joints have many positive effects on the body as a whole. Promoting exercise to maintain a client's muscle tone and joint mobility is one of the essential functions of nursing personnel.

Musculoskeletal System

The size, shape, tone, and strength of muscles (including the heart muscle) are maintained with mild exercise and increased with strenuous exercise. With strenuous exercise, muscles **hypertrophy** (enlarge), and the efficiency of muscular contraction increases. Hypertrophy is commonly seen in the arm muscles of a tennis player, the leg muscles of a skater, the arm and hand muscles of a carpenter, and the body muscles of weight lifters.

Exercise also helps maintain joint mobility. Moreover, bone density is maintained through weight-

TABLE 21–1   TYPES OF JOINT MOVEMENTS

Movement	Action
Flexion	Decreasing the angle of the joint (e.g., bending the elbow)
Extension	Increasing the angle of the joint (e.g., straightening the arm at the elbow)
Hyperextension	Further extension or straightening of a joint (e.g., bending the head backward)
Abduction	Movement of the bone away from the midline of the body
Adduction	Movement of the bone toward the midline of the body
Rotation	Movement of the bone around its central axis
Circumduction	Movement of the distal part of the bone in a circle while the proximal end remains fixed
Eversion	Turning the sole of the foot outward by moving the ankle joint
Inversion	Turning the sole of the foot inward by moving the ankle joint
Pronation	Moving the bones of the forearm so that the palm of the hand faces downward when held in front of the body
Supination	Moving the bones of the forearm so that the palm of the hand faces upward when held in front of the body
Protraction	Moving a part of the body forward in the same plane parallel to the ground
Retraction	Moving a part of the body backward in the same plane parallel to the ground

bearing. The stress of weight-bearing maintains a balance between *osteoblasts* (bone-building cells) and *osteoclasts* (bone-resorption and breakdown cells).

Cardiovascular System

With adequate exercise, the heart rate increases, arterial (systolic) blood pressure increases, and blood is shunted from the nonexercising tissues to the heart and the muscles. Cardiac output (the amount of blood pumped by the heart) increases due to the redirection of the blood flow. Exercise can increase cardiac output to 22 L/min in the average person (Guyton 1986, p. 283). Normal cardiac output is 5 to 7 L/min.

Respiratory System

Ventilation (the amount of air circulating into and out of the lungs) increases. In strenuous exercise, the intake of oxygen increases to as much as 20 times normal intake (Guyton 1986, p. 511). Normal ventilation is about 5 or 6 L/min. Adequate exercise also prevents pooling of secretions in the bronchi and bronchioles.

Text continues on page 507.

TABLE 21–2   RANGES OF JOINT MOVEMENTS

Movement	Major Muscle(s)	Normal Range	Illustration
TEMPROMANDIBULAR JOINT (TMJ)			
TMJ opening. Open mouth.		3 to 6 cm (1 to 2.3 in)	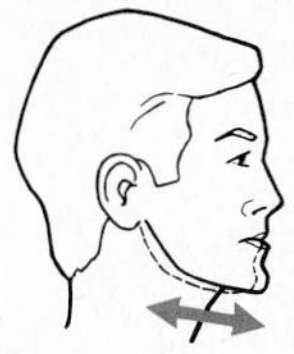
TMJ closure. Close mouth.	Masseter and temporalis	Complete closure	Figure 1
Protrusion. Jut chin out. See Figure 1.	Pterygoideus lateralis		
Retrusion. Tuck chin in. See Figure 1.			
Lateral motion. Move jaw from side to side. See Figure 2.	Pterygoideus lateralis and pterygoideus medialis	1 to 2 cm (0.3 to 0.7 in) from midline	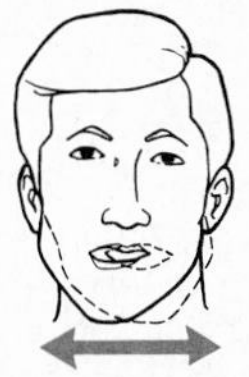 Figure 2
NECK—PIVOT JOINT			
Flexion. Move the head from the upright midline position forward, so that the chin rests on the chest. See Figure 3.	Sternocleidomastoideus	45° from midline	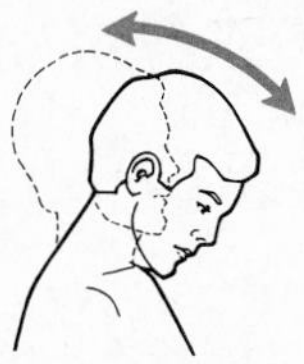 Figure 3
Extension. Move the head from the flexed position to the upright position. See Figure 3.	Trapezius	45° from midline	
Hyperextension. Move the head from the upright position back as far as possible.	Trapezius	10°	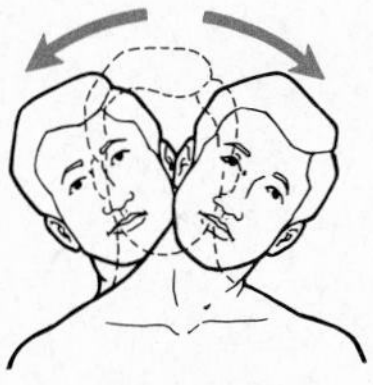 Figure 4
Lateral flexion. Move the head laterally to the right and left shoulders, while facing front. See Figure 4.	Sternocleidomastoideus	40° from midline	
Rotation. Turn the face as far as possible to the right and left. See Figure 5.	Sternocleidomastoideus and trapezius	70° from midline	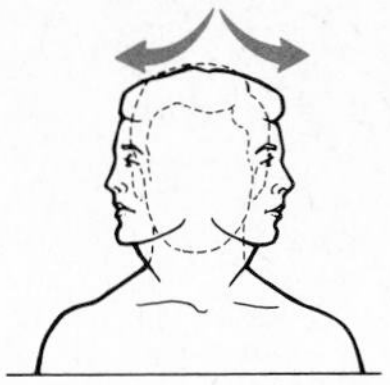 Figure 5
SHOULDER—BALL-AND-SOCKET JOINT			
Flexion. Raise each arm from a position by the side forward and upward to a position beside the head. See Figure 6.	Pectoralis major, coracobrachialis, and deltoideus	180° from the side	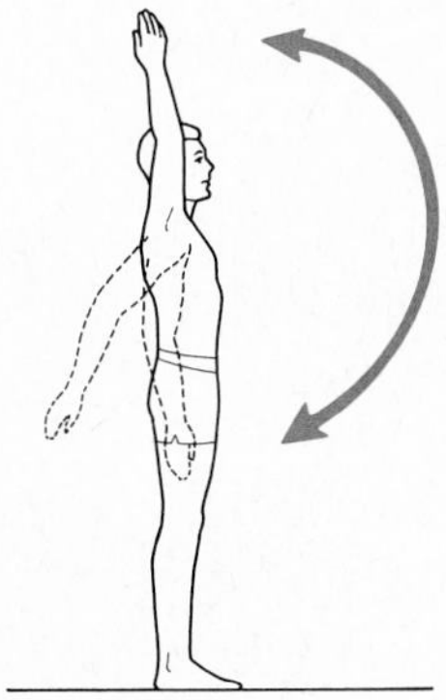
Extension. Move each arm from a vertical position beside the head forward and down to a resting position at the side of the body. See Figure 6.	Latissimus dorsi, deltoideus, and teres major	180° from vertical position beside the head	
Hyperextension. Move each arm from a resting side position to behind the body. See Figure 6.	Latissimus dorsi, deltoideus, and teres major	50° from side position	Figure 6

▶ **TABLE 21–2** RANGES OF JOINT MOVEMENTS *(continued)*

Movement	Major Muscle(s)	Normal Range	Illustration
SHOULDER—BALL-AND-SOCKET JOINT *(continued)*			
Abduction. Move each arm laterally from a resting position at the sides to a side position above the head, palm of the hand away from the head. See Figure 7.	Deltoideus and supraspinatus	180°	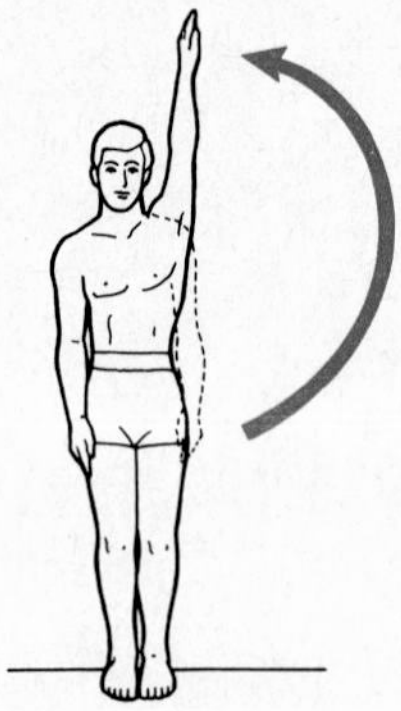 Figure 7
Adduction (anterior). Move each arm from a position beside the head downward laterally and across the front of the body as far as possible. See Figure 8.	Pectoralis major and teres major	230°	
Adduction (posterior). Move each arm from a position beside the head downward laterally and across behind the body as far as possible.	Latissimus dorsi and teres major	230°	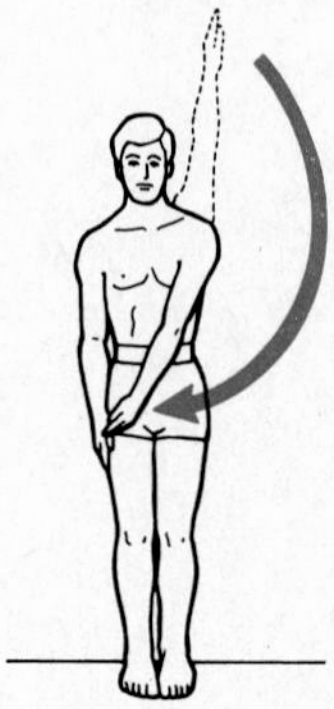 Figure 8
Horizontal flexion. Extend each arm laterally at shoulder height, and move it through a horizontal plane across the front of the body as far as possible. See Figure 9.	Pectoralis major and coracobrachialis	130° to 135°	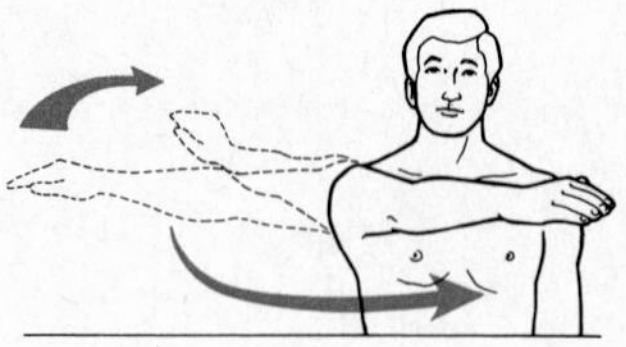
Horizontal extension. Extend each arm laterally at shoulder height, and move it through a horizontal plane as far behind the body as possible. See Figure 9.	Latissimus dorsi, teres major, and deltoideus	45°	Figure 9
Circumduction. Move each arm forward, up, back, and down in a full circle. See Figure 10.	Deltoideus, coracobrachialis, latissimus dorsi, and teres major	360°	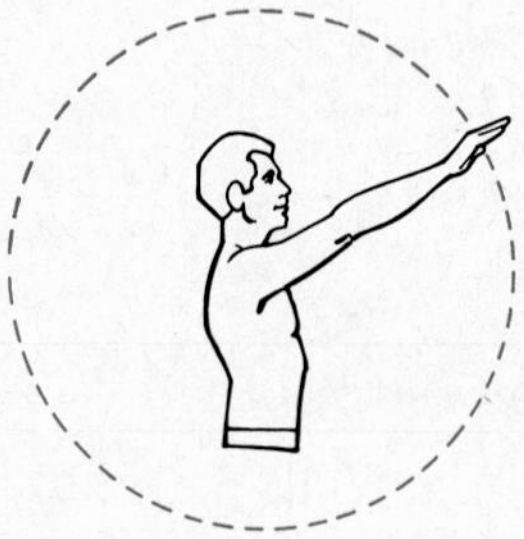
External rotation. With each arm held out to the side to the shoulder level and the elbow bent to a right angle, fingers pointing down, move the arm upward so that the fingers point up. See Figure 11.	Infraspinatus and teres minor	90°	Figure 10
Internal rotation. With each arm held out to the side at shoulder level and the elbow bent to a right angle, fingers pointing up, bring the arm forward and down so that the fingers point down. See Figure 11.	Subscapularis, pectoralis major, latissimus dorsi, and teres major	90°	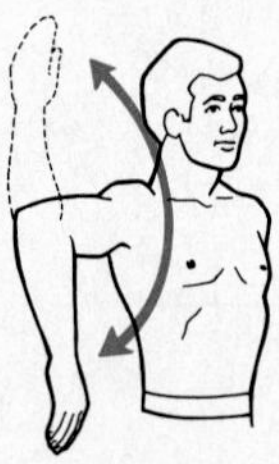 Figure 11

TABLE 21–2 *(continued)*

Movement	Major Muscle(s)	Normal Range	Illustration
ELBOW—HINGE JOINT			
Flexion. Bring each lower arm forward and upward so that the hand is at the shoulder. See Figure 12.	Biceps brachii, brachialis, and brachioradialis	150°	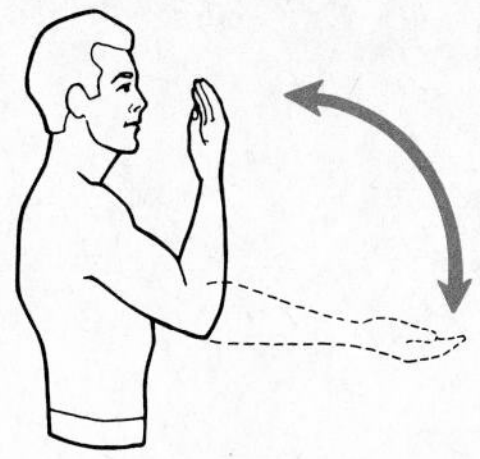
Extension. Bring each lower arm forward and downward, straightening the arm. See Figure 12.	Triceps brachii	150°	Figure 12
Rotation for supination. Turn each hand and forearm so that the palm is facing upward. See Figure 13.	Biceps brachii and supinator	70° to 90°	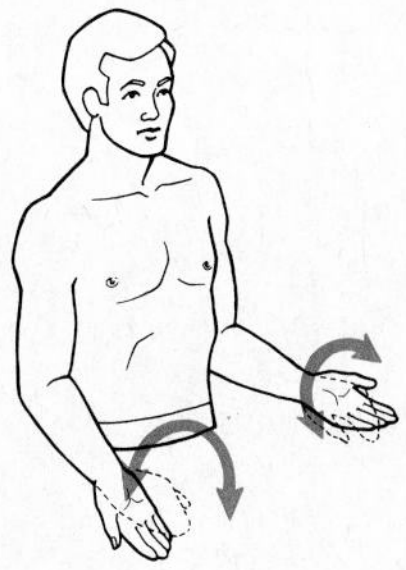
Rotation for pronation. Turn each hand and forearm so that the palm is facing downward. See Figure 13.	Pronator teres and pronator quadratus	70° to 90°	Figure 13
WRIST—CONDYLOID JOINT			
Flexion. Bring the fingers of each hand toward the inner aspect of the forearm. See Figure 14.	Flexor carpi radialis and flexor carpi ulnaris	80° to 90°	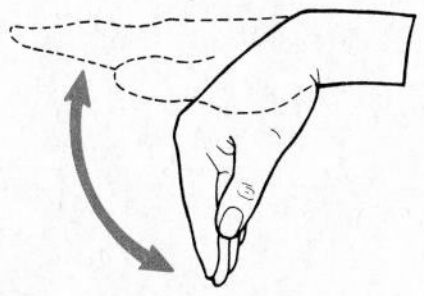 Figure 14
Extension. Straighten each hand to the same plane as the arm. See Figure 14.	Extensor carpi radialis longus	80° to 90°	
Hyperextension. Bend each hand back as far as possible. See Figure 15.	Extensor carpi radialis longus extensor, carpi radialis brevis, and extensor carpi ulnaris	70° to 90°	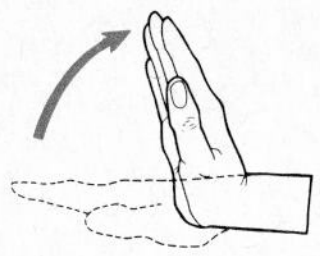 Figure 15
Radial flexion (abduction). Bend each wrist laterally toward the thumb side with hand supinated. See Figure 16.	Extensor carpi radialis longus	0 to 20°	
Ulnar flexion (adduction). Bend each wrist laterally toward the fifth finger with the hand supinated.	Extensor carpi ulnaris	30° to 50°	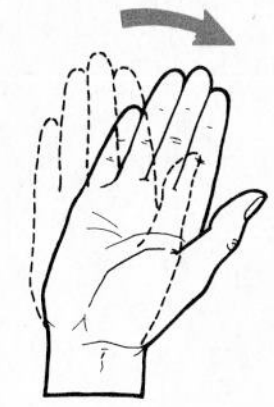 Figure 16
HAND AND FINGERS: METACARPOPHALANGEAL JOINTS—CONDYLOID; INTERPHALANGEAL JOINTS—HINGE			
Flexion. Make a fist with each hand. See Figure 17.	Interossei dorsales manus and flexor digitorum superficialis	90°	
Extension. Straighten the fingers of each hand. See Figure 17.	Extensor indicis and extensor digiti minimi	90°	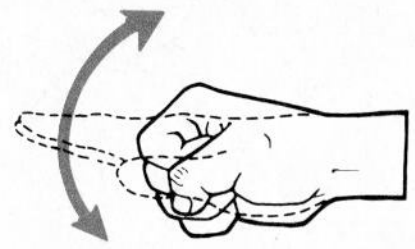 Figure 17
Hyperextension. Bend the fingers of each hand back as far as possible.	Extensor indicis and extensor digiti minimi	30°	

▶ **TABLE 21–2** RANGES OF JOINT MOVEMENTS *(continued)*

Movement	Major Muscle(s)	Normal Range	Illustration
HANDS AND FINGERS *(continued)*			
Abduction. Spread the fingers of each hand apart. See Figure 18.	Interossei dorsales manus, abductor digiti minimi manus, and opponens digiti minimi	20°	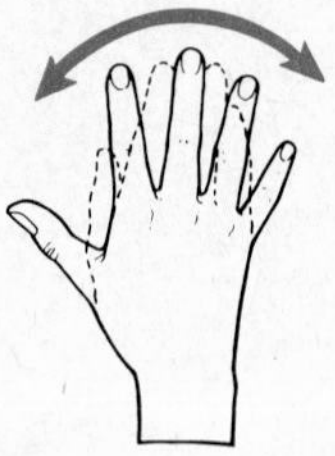 Figure 18
Adduction. Bring the fingers of each hand together. See Figure 18.	Interrossei palmares	20°	
			Figure 19
THUMB—SADDLE JOINT			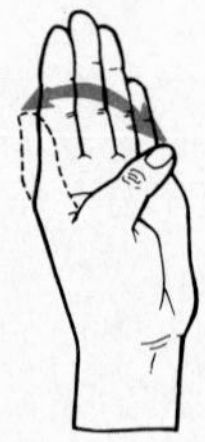
Flexion. Move each thumb across the palmar surface of the hand toward the fifth finger. See Figure 19.	Flexor pollicis brevis and opponens pollicis	90°	
Extension. Move each thumb away from the hand.	Extensor pollicis brevis and extensor pollicis longus	90°	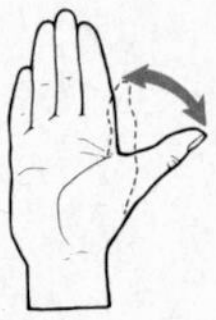 Figure 20
Abduction. Extend each thumb laterally. See Figure 20.	Abductor pollicis brevis and abductor pollicis longus	30°	
Adduction. Move each thumb back to the hand. See Figure 20.	Adductor pollicis	30°	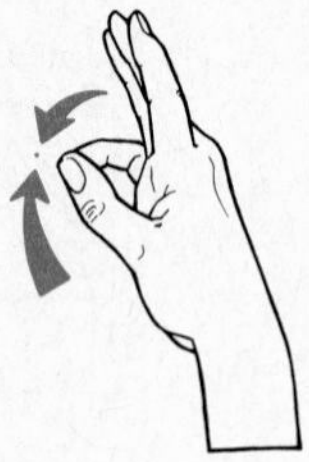
Opposition. Touch each thumb to the tip of each finger of the same hand. The thumb joint movements involved are abduction, rotation, and flexion. See Figure 21.	Opponens pollicis and flexor pollicis brevis		Figure 21
			Figure 22
HIP—BALL-AND-SOCKET JOINT			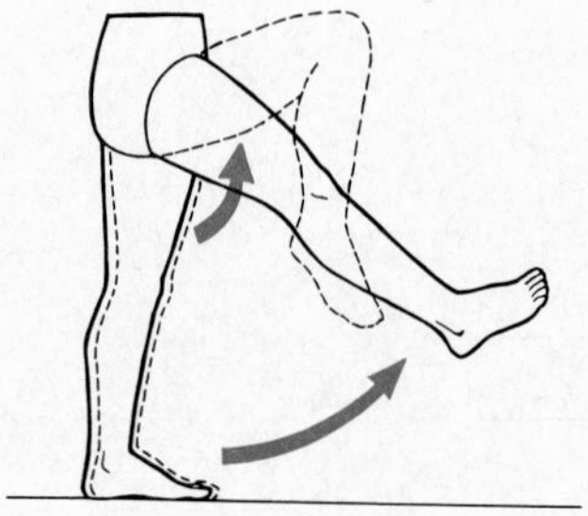
Flexion. Move each leg forward and upward. The knee may be extended or flexed. See Figure 22.	Psoas major and iliacus	Knee extended, 90°; knee flexed, 120°	
Extension. Move each leg back beside the other leg. See Figure 23.	Gluteus maximus, adductor magnus, semitendinosus, and semimembranosus	90° to 120°	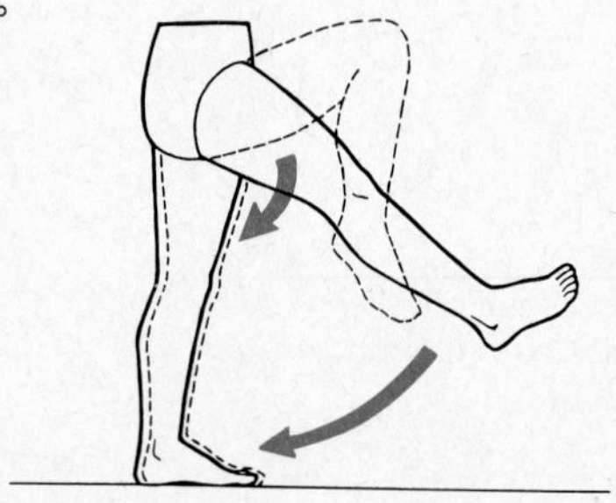
Hyperextension. Move each leg back behind the body.	Gluteus maximus semitendinosus, and semimembranosus	30° to 50°	Figure 23

TABLE 21–2 *(continued)*

Movement	Major Muscle(s)	Normal Range	Illustration
Abduction. Move each leg out to the side. See Figure 24.	Gluteus medius and gluteus minimus	45° to 50°	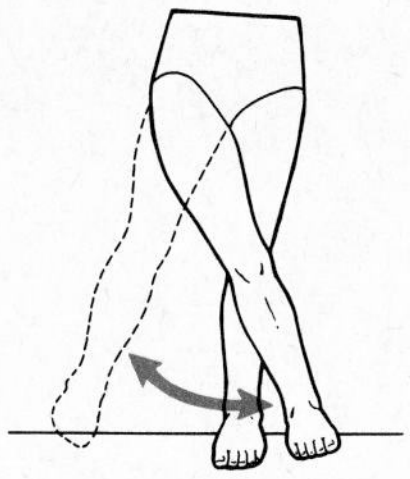
Adduction. Move each leg back to the other leg and beyond in front of it. See Figure 24.	Adductor magnus, adductor brevis, and adductor longus	20° to 30° beyond other leg	Figure 24
Circumduction. Move each leg backward, up, to the side, and down in a circle. See Figure 25.	Psoas major, gluteus maximus, gluteus medius, and adductor magnus	360°	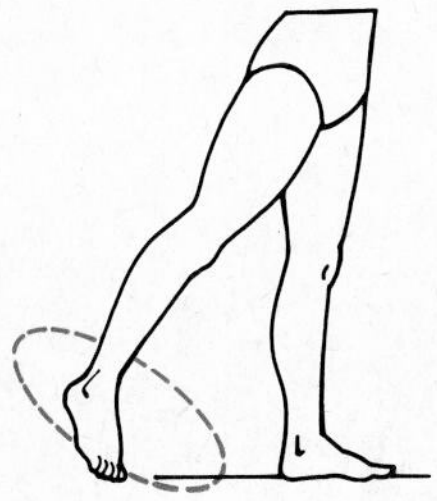 Figure 25
Internal rotation. Turn each foot and leg inward so that the toes point as far as possible toward the other leg. See Figure 26.	Gluteus minimus and tensor fasciae latae	90°	
External rotation. Turn each foot and leg outward so that the toes point as far as possible away from the other leg. See Figure 26.	Obturator externus, obturator internus, and quadratus femoris	90°	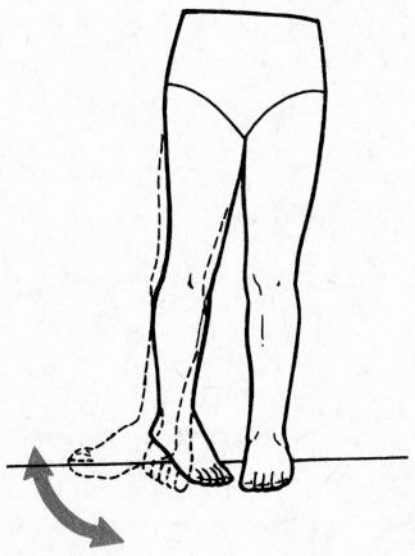 Figure 26
KNEE—HINGE JOINT			
Flexion. Bend each leg bringing the heel toward the back of the thigh. See Figure 27.	Biceps femoris, semitendinosus, and semimembranosus	120° to 130°	
Extension. Straighten each leg, returning the foot to its position beside the other foot. See Figure 27.	Rectus femoris, vastus lateralis, vastus medialis, and vastus intermedius	120° to 130°	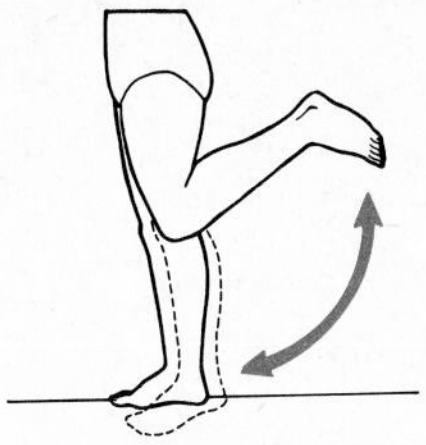 Figure 27
ANKLE—HINGE JOINT			
Extension (plantar flexion). Point the toes of each foot downward. See Figure 28.	Gastrocnemius and soleus	45° to 50°	
Flexion (dorsiflexion). Point the toes of each foot upward. See Figure 28.	Peroneus tertius and tibialis anterior	20°	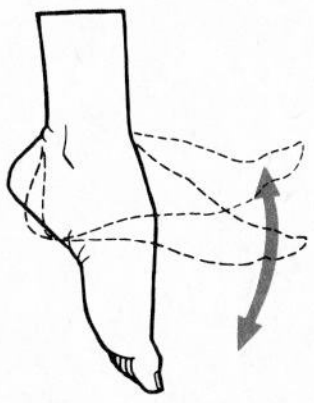 Figure 28
FOOT AND TOES: INTERPHALANGEAL JOINT—HINGE; METATARSOPHALANGEAL JOINT—HINGE; INTERTARSAL JOINT—GLIDING			
Eversion. Turn the sole of each foot laterally. See Figure 29.	Peroneus longus and peroneus brevis	5°	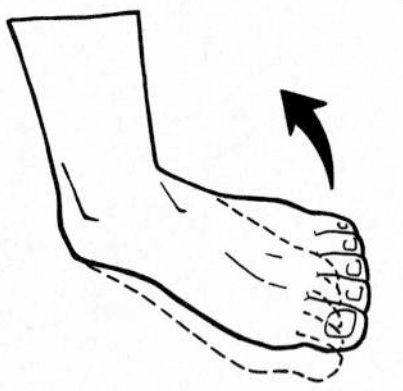
Inversion. Turn the sole of each foot medially.	Tibialis posterior and tibialis anterior	5°	Figure 29

▶ **TABLE 21-2**   RANGES OF JOINT MOVEMENTS *(continued)*

Movement	Major Muscle(s)	Normal Range	Illustration
FOOT AND TOES *(continued)*			
Flexion. Curve the toe joints of each foot downward. See Figure 30.	Flexor hallucis brevis, lumbricales pedias, and flexor digitorum brevis	35° to 60°	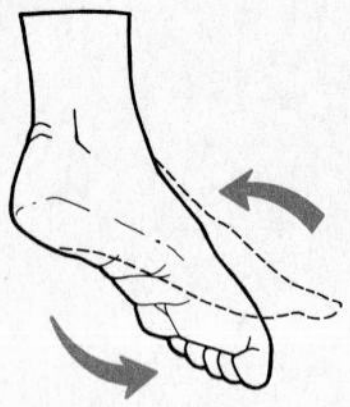 Figure 30
Extension. Straighten the toes of each foot. See Figure 30.	Extensor digitorum longus, extensor digitorum brevis and extensor hallucis longus	35° to 60°	
Abduction. Spread the toes of each foot apart.	Interossei dorsales pedis and abductor hallucis	0° to 15°	
Adduction. Bring the toes of each foot together.	Adductor hallucis and interossei plantares	0° to 15°	
TRUNK—GLIDING POINT			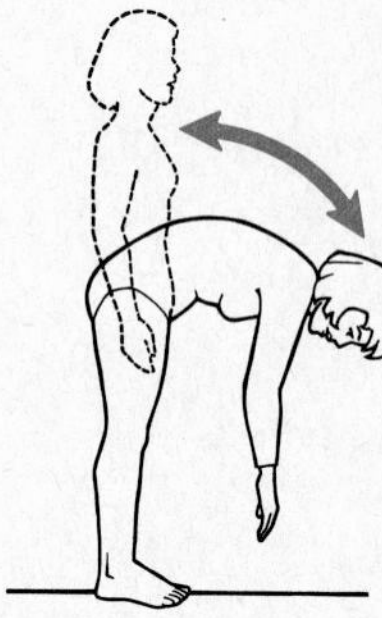
Flexion. Bend the trunk toward the toes. See Figure 31.	Rectus abdominis, psoas major, and psoas minor	70° to 90°	Figure 31
Extension. Straighten the trunk from a flexed position. See Figure 31.	Longissimus thoracis, iliocostalis thoracis, iliocostalis lumborum, erector spinae, and longissimus cervicis	70° to 90°	
Hyperextension. Bend the trunk backward.	Longissimus thoracis, iliocostalis thoracis, iliocostalis lumborum, erector spinae, and longissimus cervicis	20° to 30°	
Lateral flexion. Bend the trunk to the right and to the left. See Figure 32.	Quadratus lumborum	35° on each side	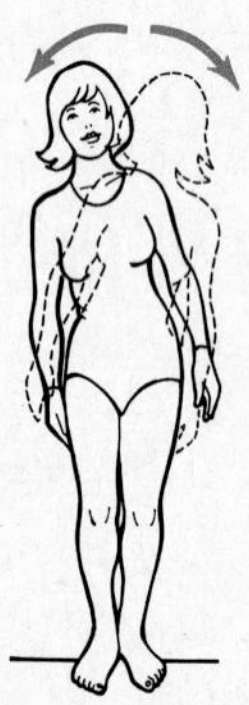 Figure 32
Rotation. Turn the upper part of the body from side to side. See Figure 33.	Erector spinae	30° to 45°	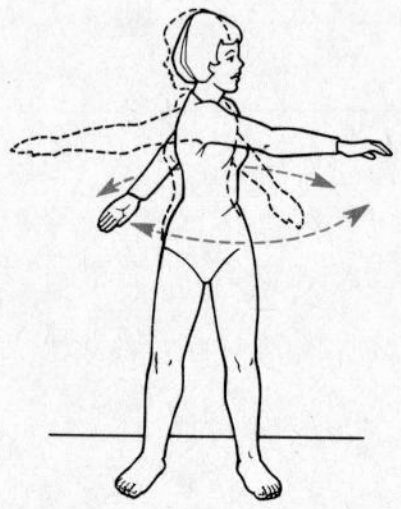 Figure 33

Gastrointestinal System

Adequate exercise improves the appetite and increases gastrointestinal tract tone, improving digestion and elimination.

Urinary System

Because adequate exercise promotes efficient blood flow, the body excretes wastes more effectively. Also, stasis (stagnation) of urine in the bladder is prevented.

Metabolism

Metabolism refers to all physical and chemical processes of the body. *Basal metabolism* is the minimal energy expended for the maintenance of these processes. The metabolic rate is the rate of basal metabolism expressed in calories per hour per square meter of body surface. During very strenuous exercise, the metabolic rate can increase to as much as 20 times the normal rate. Lying in bed and eating an average diet utilizes 1,850 calories per day (Guyton 1986, p. 845).

Psychoneurologic System

Exercise produces a sense of relaxation and restores well-being.

Effects of Immobility

Although the term *immobility* denotes complete lack of movement, it is frequently used in nursing to refer to a decrease in activity from a person's normal level. Immobility brings about several psychologic and physical problems.

Psychologic and Social Problems.

People who are unable to carry out the usual activities related to their roles (e.g., as breadwinner, husband, mother, or athlete) become aware of an increased dependence on others. These factors lower the person's self-esteem. Frustration and the decrease in self-esteem may in turn provoke exaggerated emotional reactions. Emotional reactions vary considerably. Some individuals become apathetic and withdrawn; some regress; and some become angry and aggressive.

Because the immobilized person's participation in life becomes much narrower and the variety of stimuli decreases, the person's perception of time intervals deteriorates. Problem-solving and decision-making abilities often deteriorate as a result of lack of intellectual stimulation and the stress of the illness and immobility. In addition, the loss of control over events can cause anxiety.

Immobility can impair the social and motor development of young children.

Musculoskeletal Problems

- *Disuse osteoporosis.* Without the stress of weight-bearing activity, the bones demineralize. They are depleted chiefly of calcium, which gives the bones strength and density. Regardless of the amount of calcium in a person's diet, the demineralization process, known as **osteoporosis**, continues with immobility. The bones become spongy and may gradually deform and fracture easily.

- *Disuse atrophy.* Unused muscles **atrophy** (decrease in size), losing most of their strength and normal function.

- *Contractures.* When the muscle fibers are no longer able to shorten and lengthen, contractures limit joint mobility. This process eventually involves the tendons, ligaments, and joint capsules; it is irreversible except by surgical intervention. Joint deformities such as foot drop occur when a stronger muscle dominates the opposite muscle.

- *Stiffness and pain in the joints.* Without movement, the collagen (connective) tissues at the joint become **ankylosed** (permanently immobile). In addition, as the bones demineralize, excess calcium may be deposited in the joints, contributing to stiffness and pain.

Cardiovascular Problems

- *Diminished cardiac reserve.* Prolonged immobility weakens the cardiovascular system, which cannot fully meet the demands placed on it. Decreased mobility creates an imbalance in the autonomic nervous system, resulting in a preponderance of sympathetic activity over cholinergic activity that increases heart rate. Resting heart rate increases approximately 0.5 beats/minute per each day of immobilization (Kottke and Lehmann 1990, p. 1124).

  In a mobile, active person with a slow heart rate, the diastolic phase of the cardiac cycle is longer than the systolic phase. Since blood flow through coronary vessels occurs primarily during the diastolic phase, there is sufficient time for adequate blood flow through the coronary arteries. During immobility, however, the rapid heart rate reduces diastolic pressure, coronary blood flow, and the capacity of the heart to respond to any metabolic demands above the basal levels. Because of this diminished cardiac reserve, the immobilized person may experience tachycardia and angina with even minimal exertion.

- *Increased use of the Valsalva maneuver.* The *Valsalva maneuver* refers to holding the breath and straining against a closed glottis while moving. For example, clients tend to hold their breath when attempting to move up in a bed or sit on a bedpan. This builds up sufficient pressure on the large veins in the thorax to interfere with the return blood flow to the heart and coronary arteries. When the client exhales and the glottis again opens, pressure is suddenly released, and a surge of blood flows to the heart. Tachycardia and cardiac arrhythmias can result, if the client has cardiac pathology.

• *Orthostatic (postural) hypotension.* Orthostatic hypotension is a common sequel of immobilization. Under normal conditions, sympathetic nervous system activity causes automatic vasoconstriction in the blood vessels in the lower half of the body when a mobile person changes from a horizontal to a vertical posture. Vasoconstriction prevents pooling of the blood in the legs and effectively maintains central blood pressure to ensure adequate perfusion of the heart and brain. During any prolonged immobility, this reflex becomes dormant. When the immobolized person attempts to sit or stand, this reconstricting mechanism fails to function properly in spite of increased adrenalin output. The blood pools in the lower extremities, and central blood pressure drops. Cerebral perfusion is seriously compromised, and the person feels dizzy or lightheaded and may even faint. This sequence is usually accompanied by a sudden and marked increase in heart rate, the body's effort to protect the brain from an inadequate blood supply.

• *Venous vasodilation and stasis.* The skeletal muscles of an active person contract with each movement, compressing the blood vessels in those muscles and helping to pump the blood back to the heart against gravity. The tiny valves in the leg veins, which remain constricted, aid in venous return to the heart by preventing backward flow of blood and pooling. In an immobilized person, the skeletal muscles do not contract sufficiently, and the muscles atrophy. The skeletal muscles can no longer assist in pumping blood back to the heart against gravity. Blood pools in the leg veins, causing vasodilation and engorgement. The valves in the veins can no longer work effectively to prevent backward flow of blood and pooling (Figure 21–1). This phenomenon is known as *incompetent valves.* As the blood continues to pool in the veins, its greater volume increases venous blood pressure, which can become much higher than that exerted by the tissues surrounding the vessel.

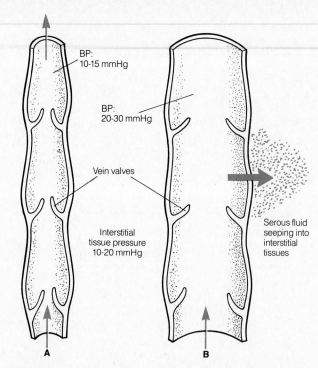

FIGURE 21–1   Leg veins: *A*, in a mobile person; *B*, in an immobilized person.

• *Dependent edema.* When the venous pressure is sufficiently great, some of the serous part of the blood is forced out of the blood vessel into the interstitial spaces surrounding the vessel, causing edema. Edema is most common in parts of the body positioned below heart level and maintained in that position. Dependent edema is most likely to occur around the sacrum or heels of a client who sits up in bed or in the feet and lower legs of a client who sits on the side of the bed. Edema further impedes venous return of blood to the heart, causing more pooling and more edema. Edematous tissue is uncomfortable and more susceptible to injury than normal tissue.

• *Thrombus formation.* Three factors, known as *Virchow's triad*, collectively predispose a client to the formation of a *thrombophlebitis* (a clot that is loosely attached to an inflamed vein wall). These are impaired venous return to the heart, hypercoagulability of the blood, and injury to a vessel wall.

A thrombus is particularly dangerous if it breaks loose from the vein wall to enter the general circulation as an *embolus* (a clot that has moved from its place of origin causing obstruction to circulation elsewhere). At least 15% of deep vein thrombi do migrate (Fahey 1984, p. 36). Large emboli that enter the pulmonary circulation may occlude the vessels that nourish the lungs to cause an infarcted (dead) area of the lung. If the infarcted area is large, pulmonary function may be seriously compromised, or death may ensue. Emboli traveling to the coronary vessels or brain can produce a similarly dangerous outcome.

Respiratory Problems

- *Decreased respiratory movement*. In a recumbent, immobilized client, ventilation of the lungs is passively altered. The rigid bed presses against the body and curtails chest movement. The abdominal organs push against the diaphragm, further restricting chest movement and making it difficult to expand the lungs fully. An immobilized, recumbent person rarely sighs, partly because overall muscle atrophy also affects the respiratory muscles and partly because there is no need to do so without the stimulus of activity. Without these periodic stretching movements, the cartilaginous intercostal joints may become fixed in an expiratory phase of respiration, further restricting the potential for maximal ventilation. These changes produce shallow respirations and reduce vital capacity significantly. **Vital capacity** is the maximum amount of air that can be exhaled after a maximum inhalation. An immobilized, paralyzed client can lose as much as 25% to 50% of normal vital capacity (Kottke and Lehmann 1990, p. 1128).

- *Pooling of respiratory secretions*. Secretions of the respiratory tract are normally expelled by changing positions or posture and by coughing. Inactivity allows secretions to pool by gravity (Figure 21–2), interfering with the normal diffusion of oxygen and carbon dioxide in the alveoli. The ability to cough up secretions may also be hindered by loss of respiratory muscle tone, dehydration (which thickens secretions), or sedatives that depress the cough reflex. Poor oxygenation and retention of carbon dioxide in the blood can, if allowed to continue, predispose the person to respiratory acidosis, a potentially lethal disorder.

- *Atelectasis*. When ventilation is decreased, pooled secretions may accumulate in a dependent area of a bronchiole and effectively block it. Due to changes in regional blood flow, bed rest decreases the amount of surfactants produced. (Surfactants enable the alveoli to remain open.) The combination of decreased surfactants and blockage of a bronchiole with mucus can cause atelectasis (the collapse of a lobe or of an entire lung) distal to the mucous blockage. Immobilized, elderly,

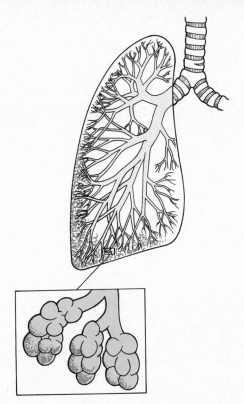

FIGURE 21–2 Pooling of secretions in the lungs of an immobilized person.

postoperative clients are at greatest risk of atelectasis.

- *Hypostatic pneumonia*. Pooled (hypostatic) secretions provide excellent media for bacterial growth. Under these conditions, a minor upper respiratory infection can evolve rapidly into a severe infection of the lower respiratory tract. Hypostatic pneumonia caused by static respiratory secretions can severely impair oxygen-carbon dioxide exchange in the alveoli and is a fairly common cause of death among weakened, immobilized individuals, especially those who are heavy smokers.

Metabolic and Nutritional Problems

- *Decreased metabolic rate*. In immobilized clients, the basal metabolic rate decreases as the energy requirements of the body decrease. Gastrointestinal motility and secretions of various digestive glands are also reduced.

- *Negative nitrogen balance*. In an active person, there is a balance between protein synthesis (*anabolism*) and protein breakdown (*catabolism*). Immobility creates a marked imbalance, and the catabolic processes exceed the anabolic processes. Over time, more nitrogen is excreted than is ingested, producing a negative nitrogen balance. Catabolized muscle mass is the source of this excreted nitrogen. Excessive amounts are excreted in the urine, reaching peak levels at about the sixth to tenth day of immobilization (Kottke and Lehmann 1990, p. 1125). The negative nitrogen balance represents a depletion of protein stores that are essential for building muscle tissue and for wound healing.

• *Anorexia*. Loss of appetite (anorexia) occurs as a result of the decreased metabolic rate and the increased catabolism that accompany immobility. Reduced caloric intake is usually a response to the decreased energy requirements of the inactive person. If protein intake is reduced, the nitrogen imbalance may become more pronounced, sometimes so severely that malnutrition ensues.

• *Negative calcium balance*. A negative calcium balance occurs as a direct result of immobility. Greater amounts of calcium are extracted from bone than can be replaced. The absence of weight-bearing and of stress on the musculoskeletal structures is the direct cause of the calcium loss from bones. Weight-bearing and stress, absent during immobility, are also required for calcium to be replaced in bone. A similar process

occurs with the body's stores of phosphate to cause a negative phosphate balance to develop during immobility.

Urinary Problems

• *Urinary stasis*. Gravity plays an important role in the emptying of the kidneys and the bladder in mobile persons. The shape and position of the kidneys and active kidney contractions are important in completely emptying the urine from the calyces, renal pelvis, and ureters (Figure 21–3, *A*). The shape and position of the urinary bladder (the detrusor muscle) and active bladder contractions are also important in achieving complete emptying (Figure 21–4, *A*).

When the person remains in a horizontal position, gravity impedes the emptying of urine from the kidneys and the urinary bladder. To urinate, the person who is supine (in a back-lying

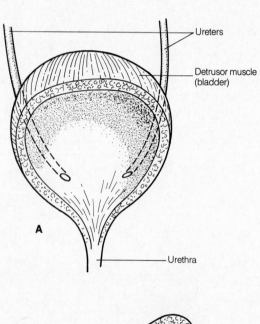

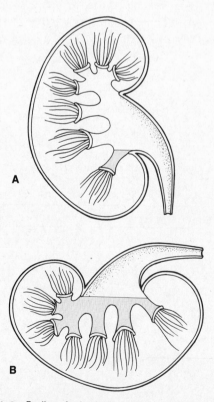

FIGURE 21–3 Pooling of urine in the kidney: *A*, when the client is in an upright position; *B*, when the client is in a back-lying position.

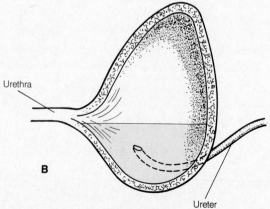

FIGURE 21–4 Pooling of urine in the urinary bladder: *A*, when the client is in an upright position; *B*, when the client is in a back-lying position.

position) must push upward, against gravity (Figures 21–3, *B* and 21–4, *B*). The renal pelvis may fill with urine before it is pushed into the ureters. Emptying is not as complete, and urinary stasis occurs after a few days of bed rest. Due to the overall decrease in muscle tone during immobilization, including the tone of the detrusor muscle, bladder emptying is further compromised.

- *Renal calculi.* In a mobile person, calcium in the urine remains dissolved because calcium and citric acid are balanced in an appropriately acid urine. With immobility and the resulting excessive amounts of calcium (and phosphate) in the urine, this balance is no longer maintained. The urine becomes more alkaline, and the calcium salts precipitate out as crystals to form renal calculi (stones). In an immobile person in a horizontal position, the renal pelvis filled with stagnant, alkaline urine is an ideal location for calculi to form. The stones usually develop in the renal pelvis and pass through the ureters into the bladder. As the stones pass along the long, narrow ureters, they cause extreme pain and bleeding and can sometimes obstruct the urinary tract.

- *Urinary retention.* The immobile person may suffer from urinary retention, bladder distention, and occasionally urinary *incontinence* (involuntary urination). The decreased muscle tone of the urinary bladder inhibits its ability to empty completely, and the immobilized person is unable to relax the perineal muscles sufficiently to urinate. The discomfort of using a bedpan or urinal, the embarrassment and lack of privacy associated with this function, and the unnatural position for urination combine to make it difficult for the client to relax the perineal muscles sufficiently to urinate while lying in bed.

  When urination is not possible, the bladder gradually becomes distended with urine. The bladder may stretch excessively, eventually inhibiting the urge to void. When bladder distention is considerable, some involuntary urinary "dribbling" may occur (*retention with overflow*). This does not relieve the urinary distention, because most of the stagnant urine remains in the bladder.

- *Urinary infection.* Static urine provides an excellent medium for bacterial growth. The flushing action of normal, frequent urination is absent, and urinary distention often causes minute tears in the bladder mucosa, allowing infectious organisms to enter. The increased alkalinity of the urine caused by the hypercalcuria supports bacterial growth. The organism most commonly causing urinary tract infections is *Escherichia coli*, which normally resides in the colon. The normally sterile urinary tract may be contaminated by improper perineal care, the use of an indwelling urinary catheter, or occasionally *urinary reflux* (backward flow). During reflux, contaminated urine from an overly distended bladder backs up into the renal pelvis to contaminate the kidney pelvis as well.

Fecal Elimination Problems

Constipation is a frequent problem for immobilized persons. Due to increased adrenalin production, peristalsis and colon motility are decreased, and the sphincters are more tightly constricted (Kottke and Lehmann 1990, p. 1128). The overall skeletal muscle weakness affects the abdominal and perineal muscles used in defecation. When the stool becomes very hard, more strength is required to expel it. The immobilized person may lack this strength.

The bedfast person's unnatural and uncomfortable position on the bedpan does not facilitate elimination. The backward-leaning posture does not promote effective use of the muscles used in defecation. Some persons are reluctant to use the bedpan in the presence of others. The embarrassment, lack of privacy, dependence on others to assist with the bedpan, and disruption of normal bowel habits may cause the individual to postpone or ignore the urge for elimination. Repeated postponement eventually suppresses the urge and weakens the defecation reflex.

Some persons may make excessive use of the Valsalva maneuver by straining at stool in an attempt to expel the hard stool. This effort dangerously increases intra-abdominal and intrathoracic pressures and places undue stress on the heart and circulatory system.

Integumentary Problems

- *Reduced skin turgor.* The skin can atrophy as a result of prolonged immobility. Shifts in body fluids between the fluid compartments can affect the consistency and health of the dermis and subcutaneous tissues in dependent parts of the body, eventually causing a gradual loss in skin turgor (elasticity).

- *Skin breakdown.* Normal blood circulation relies on muscle activity. Immobility impedes circulation and diminishes the supply of nutrients to specific areas. As a result, skin breakdown and formation of decubitus ulcers can occur. See Chapter 20.

Types of Exercise

Five major kinds of exercise may be chosen according to the person's health and strength: isotonic, isometric, active range-of-motion (ROM), passive ROM, and active-assistive ROM.

Isotonic (dynamic) **exercises** are those in which muscle tension is constant and the muscle shortens to produce muscle contraction and movement. Because the muscles contract, the size, shape, and strength of the muscles, and joint mobility are maintained. Most physical conditioning exercises—running, walking, swimming, cycling, and other such activities—are isotonic, as are ADLs and active ROM exercises. Examples of isotonic bed exercises are pushing or pulling against a stationary object, pressing the feet against a footboard, using a trapeze to lift the body off the bed, lifting the buttocks off the bed by pushing with the hands against the mattress, and pushing the body to a sitting position.

Isotonic exercises increase muscle strength and endurance and can improve cardiorespiratory function. During isotonic exercise, both heart rate and cardiac output quicken to increase blood flow to all parts of the body. Little or no change in blood pressure occurs.

Isometric (static or setting) **exercises** are those in which there is a change in muscle tension but no change in muscle length. No muscle or joint movement occurs. These exercises are useful for strengthening abdominal, gluteal, and quadriceps muscles used in ambulation but are not useful in preventing joint contracture, because joint movement is absent. When an immobilized client's leg is confined in a cast or traction, isometric exercises may help maintain muscle strength in the affected limb. Isometric exercises may be useful for strengthening arm muscles in preparation for crutch-walking. These exercises are most effective in increasing muscle strength when five maximal tensions are achieved in succession, each lasting 5 seconds with 2 minutes rest in between (Brower and Hicks 1972, p. 1252).

Isometric exercises produce a moderate increase in heart rate and cardiac output, but no appreciable increase in blood flow to other parts of the body. A marked increase in blood pressure occurs with isometric exercise, and use of the Valsalva maneuver is essentially unavoidable. This combination can pose real danger for any cardiac client, who should be taught to *exhale* when performing these exercises.

Active ROM exercises are isotonic exercises in which the client moves each joint in the body through its complete range of movement, maximally stretching all muscle groups within each plane, over the joint. These exercises maintain or increase muscle strength and endurance and help to maintain cardiorespiratory function in an immobilized client.

CLIENT TEACHING

Active ROM Exercises

- Perform each ROM exercise as taught to the point of slight resistance, but not beyond, and never to the point of discomfort.
- Perform the movements systematically, using the same sequence during each session.
- Perform each exercise three times.
- Perform each series of exercises twice daily.

They also prevent deterioration of joint capsules, ankylosis, and contractures.

Full ROM does not occur spontaneously in the immobilized individual who independently achieves ADLs, independently moves about in bed, independently transfers between bed and wheelchair or chair, or independently ambulates a short distance, because only a few muscle groups are maximally stretched during these activities. Although the client may successfully achieve some active ROM movements of the upper extremities while combing the hair, bathing, and dressing, the immobilized client is very unlikely to achieve any active ROM movements of the lower extremities when these are not used in their normal functions of standing and walking about. For this reason, most wheelchair and many ambulatory clients need active ROM exercises until they regain their normal activity levels.

A physician's order for ROM exercises is usually required if a client has an abnormal or injured musculoskeletal part or if the client's overall condition could be compromised by exercise. A nursing order to carry out preventive exercises is expected for the client whose musculoskeletal system is otherwise normal but who is suffering from the consequences of immobility. Instructions for the client performing active ROM exercises are shown in the box above. At first, the nurse may need to help the client perform the needed ROM exercises; eventually, the client may be able to accomplish these independently, with only periodic guidance from the nurse.

During **passive ROM exercises**, another person moves each of the client's joints through their complete range of movement, maximally stretching all muscle groups within each plane over each joint. Since the client does not contract the muscle, passive ROM exercises are of no value in maintaining muscle strength but are useful in maintaining joint flexibility. For this reason, passive ROM exercises should be performed only when the client is unable to accomplish the movements actively.

Passive ROM exercises should be accomplished for each movement of the arms, legs, and neck *that the client is unable to achieve actively.* As with active ROM exercises, passive ROM exercises should be accomplished to the point of slight resistance, but not beyond, and never to the point of discomfort. The movements should be systematic, and the same sequence should be followed during each exercise session. Each exercise should consist of three repetitions, and the series of exercises should be done twice daily (Kottke and Lehmann 1990, p. 444). Per-forming one series of exercises along with the bath is helpful. Passive ROM exercises are accomplished most effectively when the client lies supine in bed.

For elderly clients, it is not essential to achieve full range of motion in all joints. Instead, emphasize achieving a sufficient range of motion to carry out ADLs such as walking, dressing, combing hair, show-ering, and preparing a meal.

General guidelines for providing passive exer-cises are shown in the box below. Technique 21–1 explains how to perform the exercises.

CLINICAL GUIDELINES

Guidelines for Providing Passive Exercises

- Ensure that the client understands the reason for doing ROM exercises.

- If there is a possibility of hand swelling, make sure rings are removed.

- Clothe the client in a loose gown, and cover the body with a bath blanket.

- Use correct body mechanics when providing ROM exercises to avoid muscle strain or injury to both your-self and the client.

- Position the bed at an appropriate height.

- Expose only the limb being exercised to avoid embar-assing the client.

- Support the client's limbs above and below the joint as needed to prevent muscle strain or injury (Figure 21–5). This may also be done by cupping joints in the palm of the hand or cradling limbs along the nurse's forearm (Figure 21–6). If a joint is painful (e.g., arthritic), support the limb in the muscular areas above and below the joint).

- Use a firm, comfortable grip when handling the limb.

- Move the body parts smoothly, slowly, and rhythmically. Jerky movements cause discomfort and, possibly, injury. Fast movements can cause *spasticity* (sudden, prolonged involuntary muscle contraction) or *rigidity* (stiffness or inflexibility).

- Avoid moving or forcing a body part beyond the existing range of motion. Muscle strain, pain, and injury can result. This is particularly important for people with flac-cid (limp) paralysis, whose muscles can be stretched and joints dislocated without their awareness.

- If muscle spasticity occurs during movement, stop the movement temporarily, but continue to apply slow, gen-tle pressure on the part until the muscle relaxes; then proceed with the motion.

- If a contracture is present, apply slow firm pressure without causing pain, to stretch the muscle fibers.

- If rigidity occurs, apply pressure against the rigidity, and continue the exercise slowly.

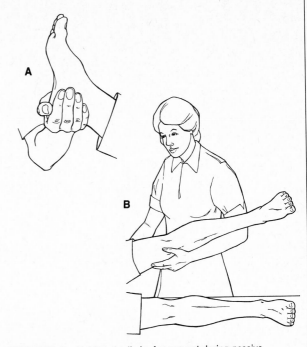

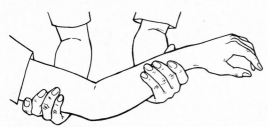

FIGURE 21–5 Supporting a limb above and below the joint for passive exercise.

FIGURE 21–6 Holding the limbs for support during passive exercise: *A,* cupping; *B,* cradling.

During **active-assistive ROM exercises,** the client uses a stronger, opposite arm or leg to move each of the joints of a limb incapable of active motion. The client learns to support and move the weak arm or leg with the strong arm or leg as far as possible. Then the nurse continues the movement passively to its maximal degree. This activity increases active movement on the strong side of the client's body and maintains joint flexibility on the weak side. Such exercise is especially useful for stroke victims who are hemiplegic (paralyzed on one half of the body). Some clients who begin with passive ROM exercises after a disability progressively improve to use active-assistive ROM exercises, and finally active ROM exercises.

Resistive exercises are a form of either isotonic or isometric exercise during which the client moves (isotonic) or tenses (isometric) against resistance. Resistive exercise is used in physical conditioning. Helping clients to push their feet against a footboard placed in the bed, lift weights, or use an overhead trapeze to lift themselves up toward the head of the bed are examples.

21-1 Providing Passive Range-of-Motion Exercises

PURPOSES
- To maintain joint flexibility for effective daily functioning
- To prevent joint stiffness

ASSESSMENT FOCUS
Degree of range-of-motion of joints needed to ambulate or perform essential ADLs; presence of contractures, joint swelling, redness, or pain.

INTERVENTION

1. Before beginning the exercises, obtain the physician's or physiotherapist's order.

2. Assist the client to a supine position near you, and expose the body parts requiring exercise.

- Place the client's feet together, place the arms at the sides, and leave space around the head and the feet. *Positioning the client close to you prevents excessive reaching.*

3. Return to the starting position after each motion. Repeat each motion three times on the affected limb.

Shoulder and Elbow Movement
Begin each exercise with the client's arm at the client's side. Grasp the arm beneath the elbow with one hand and beneath the wrist with the other hand, unless otherwise indicated (Figure 21–7).

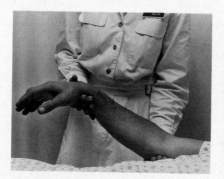

FIGURE 21–7 Supporting the client's arm.

4. Flex, externally rotate, and extend the shoulder.

- Move the arm up to the ceiling and toward the head of the bed (Figure 21–8). The elbow may need to be flexed if the headboard is in the way.

5. Abduct and externally rotate the shoulder.

- Move the arm away from the body (Figure 21–9) and toward the client's head until the hand is under the head (Figure 21–10).

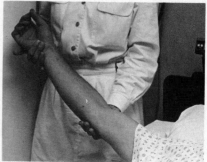

FIGURE 21–8 Flexing and extending the shoulder.

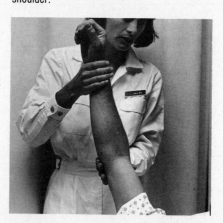

FIGURE 21–9 Abducting the shoulder.

▸ **Technique 21–1** *CONTINUED*

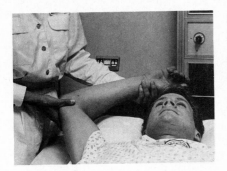

FIGURE 21–10   Externally rotating the shoulder.

6. Adduct the shoulder.

- Move the arm over the body (Figure 21–11) until the hand touches the client's other hand.

7. Rotate the shoulder internally and externally.

- Place the arm out to the side at shoulder level (90° abduction), and bend the elbow so that the forearm is at a right angle to the mattress (Figure 21–12).

- Move the forearm down until the palm touches the mattress (Figure 21–13) and then up until the

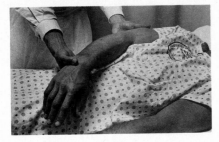

FIGURE 21–11   Adducting the shoulder.

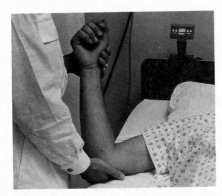

FIGURE 21–12   Position before rotating the shoulder.

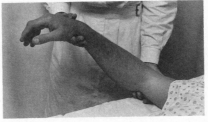

FIGURE 21–13   Rotating the shoulder.

back of the hand touches the bed.

8. Flex and extend the elbow.

- Bend the elbow until the fingers touch the chin, then straighten the arm (Figure 21–14).

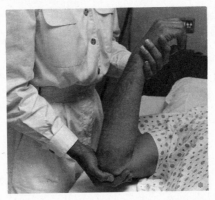

FIGURE 21–14   Flexing and extending the elbow.

9. Pronate and supinate the forearm.

- Grasp the client's hand as for a handshake, and turn the palm downward (Figure 21–15) and upward (Figure 21–16), ensuring that only the forearm (not the shoulder) moves.

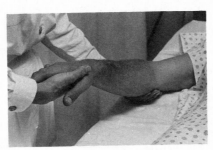

FIGURE 21–15   Pronating the forearm.

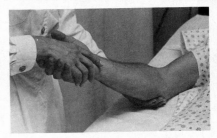

FIGURE 21–16   Supinating the forearm.

Wrist and Hand Movement

For wrist and hand exercises, flex the client's arm at the elbow until the forearm is at a right angle to the mattress. Support the wrist joint with one hand while your other hand manipulates the joint and the fingers (Figure 21–17).

10. Hyperextend the wrist, and flex the fingers.

- Bend the wrist backward, and at the same time flex the fingers, moving the tips of the fingers to the palm of the hand (Figure 21–18).

- Align the wrist in a straight line with the arm, and place your fingers over the client's fingers to make a fist.

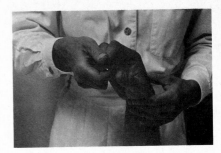

FIGURE 21–17   Position for wrist and hand movements.

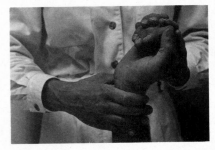

FIGURE 21–18   Hyperextending the wrist and flexing the fingers.

▸

► **Technique 21-1 Providing Passive Range-of-Motion Exercises** CONTINUED

11. Flex the wrist, and extend the fingers.

- Bend the wrist forward, and at the same time extend the fingers (Figure 21-19).

12. Abduct and oppose the thumb.

- Move the thumb away from the fingers and then across the hand toward the base of the little finger (Figure 21-20).

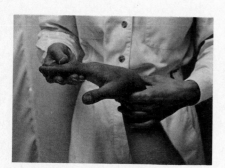

FIGURE 21-19 Flexing the wrist and extending the fingers.

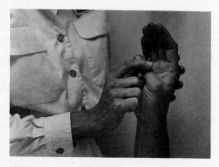

FIGURE 21-20 Abducting the thumb.

Leg and Hip Movement

To carry out leg and hip exercises, place one hand under the client's knee and the other under the ankle (Figure 21-21).

13. Flex and extend the knee and hip.

- Lift the leg and bend the knee, moving the knee up toward the chest as far as possible. Bring the leg down, straighten the knee, and lower the leg to the bed (Figure 21-22).

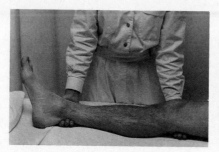

FIGURE 21-21 Position for knee and hip movements.

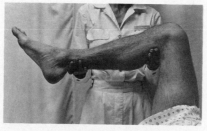

FIGURE 21-22 Flexing the knee and the hip.

14. Abduct and adduct the leg.

- Move the leg to the side, away from the client (Figure 21-23) and back across in front of the other leg (Figure 21-24).

15. Rotate the hip internally and externally.

- Roll the leg inward (Figure 21-25), then outward (Figure 21-26).

Ankle and Foot Movement

For ankle and foot exercises, place your hands in the positions described, depending on the motion to be achieved.

16. Dorsiflex the foot and stretch the Achilles tendon (heel cord).

- Place one hand under the client's heel, resting your inner forearm against the bottom of the client's foot.

- Place the other hand under the knee to support it.

- Press your forearm against the foot to move it upward toward the leg (Figure 21-27).

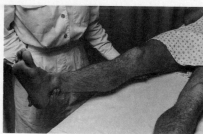

FIGURE 21-23 Abducting the leg.

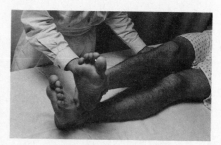

FIGURE 21-24 Adducting the leg.

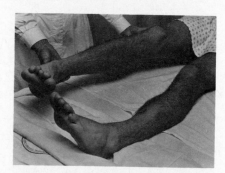

FIGURE 21-25 Internally rotating the hip.

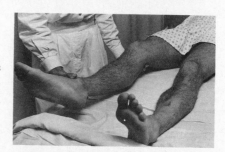

FIGURE 21-26 Externally rotating the hip.

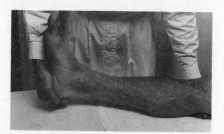

FIGURE 21-27 Dorsiflexing the foot.

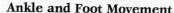

▶ **Technique 21–1** *CONTINUED*

17. Invert and evert the foot.

- Place one hand under the client's ankle and the other over the arch of the foot.

- Turn the whole foot inward (Figure 21–28), then turn it outward (Figure 21–29).

18. Plantar flex the foot, and extend and flex the toes.

- Place one hand over the arch of the foot to push the foot away from the leg.

- Place the fingers of the other hand under the toes, to bend the toes upward (Figure 21–30), and

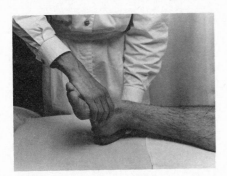

FIGURE 21–28 Inverting the foot.

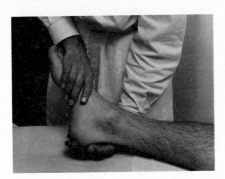

FIGURE 21–29 Everting the foot.

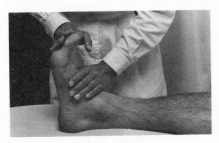

FIGURE 21–30 Extending the toes.

then over the toes, to push the toes downward (Figure 21–31).

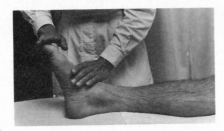

FIGURE 21–31 Plantar flexing the foot and flexing the toes.

Neck Movement
Remove the client's pillow.

19. Flex and extend the neck.

- Place the palm of one hand under the client's head and the palm of the other hand on the client's chin.

- Move the head forward until the chin rests on the chest, then back to the resting supine position without the head pillow (Figure 21–32).

20. Laterally flex the neck.

- Place the heels of the hands on each side of the client's cheeks.

- Move the top of the head to the right and to the left (Figure 21–33).

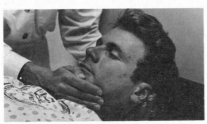

FIGURE 21–32 Flexing the neck.

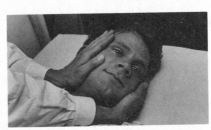

FIGURE 21–33 Laterally flexing the neck.

Hyperextension Movements

21. Assist the client to a prone or lateral position on the side of the bed nearest you but facing away from you.

22. Hyperextend the shoulder.

- Place one hand on the shoulder to keep it from lifting off the bed and the other under the client's elbow.

- Pull the upper arm up and backward (Figure 21–34).

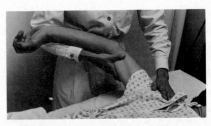

FIGURE 21–34 Hyperextending the shoulder.

23. Hyperextend the hip.

- Place one hand on the hip to stabilize it and keep it from lifting off the bed. With the other arm and hand, cradle the lower leg in the forearm, and cup the knee joint with the hand.

- Move the leg backward from the hip joint (Figure 21–35).

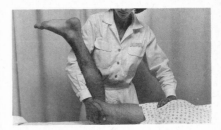

FIGURE 21–35 Hyperextending the hip.

24. Hyperextend the neck.

- Remove the pillow. With the client's face down, place one hand on the forehead and the other on the back of the skull.

- Move the head backward (Figure 21–36).

▶ **Technique 21–1 Providing Passive Range-of-Motion Exercises** *CONTINUED*

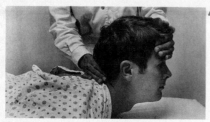

FIGURE 21–36   Hyperextending the neck.

⚠ Avoid hyperextending the neck of the immobilized elderly client, because such movements can cause painful nerve damage (Hogan and Beland 1976, p. 1106).

Following the Exercise

25. Assess the client's pulse and endurance of the exercise.

26. Report to the nurse in charge any unexpected problems or notable changes in the client's movements, e.g., rigidity or contractures.

27. Document the exercises and your assessments.

EVALUATION FOCUS	Ability to tolerate the exercise; range of motion of the joint; any discomfort during the exercises.

SAMPLE RECORDING

Date	Time	Notes
06/14/93	1100	Passive exercises provided to R leg and foot for 5 minutes with no pain. Full ROM in hip, knee, and ankle. ——————— Sally S. Ames, SN

KEY ELEMENTS OF PROVIDING PASSIVE RANGE-OF-MOTION EXERCISES

- Obtain the physician's or physiotherapist's order before beginning an exercise program.
- Support the client's joints and limbs appropriately during the exercises.

- Move body parts smoothly, slowly, and rhythmically up to the client's existing or normal range of motion.

Continuous Passive Motion (CPM) Devices

The continuous passive motion (CPM) machine is most frequently used on clients undergoing total knee replacement (Figure 21–37). CPM devices can also provide continuous passive motion to the hip, ankle, shoulder, wrist, and fingers. The machine flexes and extends the limb continuously—usually 12 to 14 hours a day.

CPM machines consist of either a metal or vinyl durable motorized base with a nonslip surface and a movable metal cradle that guides the extremity through the prescribed range of motion. A control device attached to the base gives the operator or client access to an on/off switch. Three adjustable controls set the degree of joint flexion, the degree of joint extension, and the speed of movement stated in the physician's orders. Many CPMs have attachments that affix them to the bed, and a supportive sling pads the metal cradle.

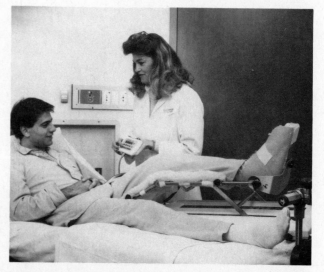

FIGURE 21–37   A continuous passive motion machine for the knee.

Technique 21–2 explains the steps involved in applying a continuous passive motion device.

Applying a Continuous Passive Motion Device to the Knee

PURPOSES
- To prevent contractures, muscle atrophy, venous stasis, and thromboembolism
- To increase the joint range of motion
- To reduce joint swelling

ASSESSMENT FOCUS

Complaints of discomfort; appearance of joint (i.e., size and color); character and amount of drainage.

EQUIPMENT
- ☐ Continuous passive motion device
- ☐ Padding for the cradle
- ☐ Restraining straps
- ☐ Goniometer

INTERVENTION

1. Check the safety test date.
- Note the date the machine was tested for electrical safety, and ensure that it is within the guidelines established at the agency.

2. Verify the physician's orders and agency protocol.
- Determine the degrees of flexion, extension, and speed initially prescribed.
- Check agency protocol and physician's orders about increases in degrees and speed for subsequent treatments.

3. Set up the machine.
- Place the machine on the bed. Remove an egg crate mattress, if indicated. *This provides a stable surface.*
- Apply a supportive sling to the movable metal cradle.
- Attach the machine to a Balkan frame using traction equipment.
- Connect the control box to the machine.

4. Set the prescribed levels of flexion and extension and speed.
- Most postoperative clients are started on 10° to 45° of flexion and 0° to 10° of extension (Maier 1986, p. 47).
- Flexion is usually increased to 5° to 10° per shift or 20° in 24 hours if tolerated (Maier 1986, p. 47).
- Adjust the speed control to the slow to moderate range for the first postoperative day, and then increase the speed as ordered and tolerated.
- Check that the machine is functioning properly by running it through a complete cycle.

5. Position the client, and place the leg in the machine.
- Place the client in a supine position, with the head of the bed slightly elevated.
- Support the leg and, with the client's help, lift the leg and place it in the padded cradle.
- Lengthen or shorten appropriate sections of the frame to fit the machine to the client. The knee and hip should be at the hinged joints of the machine.
- Adjust the footplate so that the foot is supported in a neutral position or slight dorsiflexion (e.g., 20°). Check agency protocol.

- Ensure that the leg is neither internally nor externally rotated.
- Apply restraining straps around the thigh and top of the foot and cradle, allowing enough space to fit several fingers under it.

6. Start the machine.
- Ensure the controls are set at the prescribed levels.
- Turn the on/off switch to the "on" position, and press the start button.
- (S) When the machine reaches the fully flexed position, stop the machine, and verify the degree of flexion with a goniometer.
- Restart the machine, and observe a few cycles of flexion and extension to ensure proper functioning.

7. Ensure continued client safety and comfort.
- Make sure that the client is comfortable.
- (S) Raise the side rails to keep the machine and client contained.
- (S) Stay with a confused or sedated client while the machine is on.

▶ **Technique 21–2 Applying a Continuous Passive Motion Device** *CONTINUED*

- Instruct a mentally alert client how to operate the on/off switch.

- Loosen the straps, and check the client's skin at least twice per shift.

- Wash the perineal area at least once per shift, and keep it dry.

- Drape a towel over the groin of a male client. *This prevents scrotal irritation by contact with the machine.*

8. Document all relevant information.

- Record the procedure, the degree of flexion, the degree of extension, the speed, and the duration of the therapy.

EVALUATION FOCUS

Response to therapy; increase in tolerance and range of motion; degree of discomfort; skin integrity of feet, elbow, sacrum, and groin.

SAMPLE RECORDING

Date	Time	Notes
07/11/93	0900	Continuous passive motion machine applied to knee as ordered for 30 minutes. Flexion control set at 80°; extension at 0°. Procedure tolerated well. — Michaela Nichols, RN

KEY ELEMENTS OF APPLYING A CONTINUOUS PASSIVE MOTION DEVICE TO THE KNEE

- Ensure the machine is electrically safe.
- Verify orders about the prescribed degrees of flexion, extension, and speed.
- Ensure the machine is stabilized on the bed.
- Ensure the client's knee is placed at the hinged joint of the machine and the foot is supported correctly.

- After starting the machine, use a goniometer to verify the degree of flexion.
- Ensure client safety by raising the side rails and remaining with a confused or sedated client.
- Inspect the client's skin at least twice per shift, keep the perineal area clean and dry, and prevent scrotal irritation in a male client.

Ambulation

Ambulation (the act of walking) is a function that most people take for granted. However, when people are ill they are often confined to bed and are thus nonambulatory. The longer clients are in bed the more difficulty they have walking.

Even 1 or 2 days of bed rest can make a person feel weak, unsteady, and shaky when first getting out of bed. A client who has had surgery, is elderly, or has been immobilized for a longer time will feel more pronounced weakness. The potential problems of immobility are far less likely to occur when clients become ambulatory as soon as possible. The nurse can assist clients to prepare for ambulation by helping them become as independent as possible while in bed. Nurses should encourage clients to perform ADLs, maintain good body alignment, and carry out active range-of-motion exercises to the maximum degree possible yet within the limitations imposed by their illness and recovery program.

Common Problems

Common problems that affect walking include pathology of the muscles, disease or injury of the bones of the lower extremities, and impaired balance—e.g., as a result of an inner ear infection or a cerebrovascular accident (CVA) that produces **hemiplegia** (loss of movement on one side of the body). Other diseases, such as multiple sclerosis and Parkinson's disease, affect walking through impairment of muscle function. A less serious and more common problem is muscle weakness. When muscles are not used for as short a period as 24 hours, they can weaken, and the joints can stiffen. Clients with a prolonged acute illness can become considerably weakened.

Nurses frequently need to assist clients in walking, and a variety of such devices as canes, walkers, and crutches can assist people to walk safely.

Preambulatory Exercises

Clients who have been in bed for long periods often

need a plan of muscle tone exercises to strengthen the muscles used for walking before attempting to walk. One of the most important muscle groups is the quadriceps femoris, which extends the knee and flexes the thigh. This group is also important for elevating the legs, e.g., for walking upstairs. To strengthen these muscles, the client consciously tenses them, drawing the kneecap upward and inward. The client pushes the popliteal space of the knee against the bed surface, relaxing the heels on the bed surface (Figure 21–38). On the count of 1, the muscles are tensed; they are held during the counts of 2, 3, 4; and they are relaxed at the count of 5. The exercise should be done within the client's tolerance, i.e., without fatiguing the muscles. Carried out several times an hour during waking hours, this simple exercise significantly strengthens the muscles used for walking.

Assisting Clients to Ambulate

Clients who have been immobilized for even a few days may require assistance with ambulation. The amount of assistance will depend on the client's condition, e.g., age, health status, and length of inactivity. Assistance may mean walking alongside the client while providing physical support (see Technique 21–3) or providing instruction to the client about the use of assistive devices such as a cane, walker, or crutches (See Teaching Clients to Use Mechanical Aids for Walking, later in this chapter).

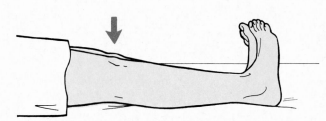

FIGURE 21–38   Tensing the quadriceps femoris muscles before ambulation.

 **21-3**   # Assisting a Client to Walk

A physician's order for ambulation is usually required, especially if the client has been immobilized in bed for any length of time.

PURPOSES	• To increase muscle strength and joint mobility
	• To prevent some potential problems of immobility
	• To increase the client's sense of independence and self-esteem

ASSESSMENT FOCUS

Length of time in bed and time up previously; pulse rate, respiratory rate, and blood pressure for baseline data before walking, especially if this is the client's first time up; range-of-motion of joints needed for ambulating (e.g., hips, knees, ankles); muscle strength of lower extremities; need for ambulation aids (e.g., cane, walker, crutches); client's intake of medications (e.g., narcotics, sedatives, tranquilizers, and antihistamines) that may cause drowsiness, dizziness, weakness, and orthostatic hypotension and seriously hinder the client's ability to walk safely; presence of joint inflammation, fractures, muscle weakness, or other conditions that impair physical mobility; ability to understand directions; need for the assistance of another nurse.

EQUIPMENT

□ Walking belt (optional)

▶

▶ **Technique 21–3 Assisting a Client to Walk** CONTINUED

INTERVENTION

1. Prepare the client for ambulation.

- Apply elastic (antiemboli) stockings as required. See Technique 42–3 on page 991.

- Assist the client to sit on the edge of the bed.

- ⑤ Assess the client carefully for signs and symptoms of orthostatic hypotension (dizziness, lightheadedness, or a sudden increase in heart rate) prior to leaving the bedside.

- ⑤ Ensure that the client is appropriately dressed to walk and wears shoes or slippers with non-skid soles. *Proper attire and footwear prevent chilling and falling.*

- Assist the client to stand by the side of the bed until the client feels secure.

- Plan the length of the walk with the client, in light of the nursing or physician's orders. Be prepared to shorten the walk according to the person's activity tolerance.

One Nurse

2. Ensure client safety while assisting the client to ambulate. ⑤

- Encourge the client to ambulate independently if the client is able, but walk beside the client.

- Remain physically close to the client in case assistance is needed at any point.

- Use a transfer or walking belt if the client is slightly weak and unstable. Make sure the belt is pulled snugly around the client's waist and fastened securely. Grasp the belt at the client's back, and walk behind and slightly to one side of the client (Figure 21–39).

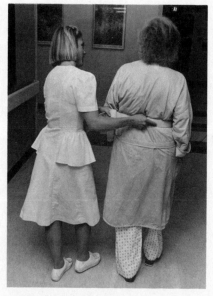

FIGURE 21–39 A walking belt.

- If it is the client's first time out of bed following surgery, injury, or an extended period of immobility, or if the client is quite weak or unstable, have an assistant follow you and the client with a wheelchair in the event that it is needed quickly.

- If the client is moderately weak and unstable, interlock your forearm with the client's closest forearm, and walk on the client's weaker side. Encourage the client to press the forearm against your hip or waist for stability if desired. In addition, have the client wear a transfer or walking belt so that you can quickly grab the belt and prevent a fall if the client feels faint.

- If the client is very weak and unstable, place your near arm around the client's waist, and with your other arm support the client's near arm at the elbow. Walk on the client's stronger side. Again, have the client wear a transfer or walking belt in case of an emergency.

- Encourage the client to assume a normal walking stance and gait as much as possible.

3. Protect the client who begins to fall while ambulating.

- ⑤ If a client begins to experience the signs and symptoms of orthostatic hypotension or extreme weakness, quickly assist the client into a nearby wheelchair or other chair, and help the client to lower the head between the knees. *Lowering the head facilitates blood flow to the brain.*

- Stay with the client. *A client who faints while in this position could fall, head first, out of the chair.*

- When the weakness subsides, assist the client back to bed.

- If a chair is not close by, assist the client to a horizontal position on the floor before fainting occurs (Figure 21–40). *A vertical position may increase feelings of faintness.*

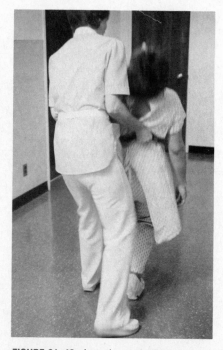

FIGURE 21–40 Lowering to the floor a client who has fainted.

▶ **Technique 21–3** *CONTINUED*

a. Assume a broad stance with one foot in front of the other. *A broad stance widens your base of support for stability. Placing one foot behind the other allows you to rock backward and use the femoral muscles when supporting the client's weight and lowering the center of gravity (see the next step), thus preventing back strain.*

b. Bring the client backward so that your body supports the person. *Clients who do faint or start to fall and cannot regain their strength or balance usually drop straight downward or pitch slightly forward because of the momentum of ambulating; thus, their head, hips, and knees are most vulnerable to injury. Bringing the client's weight backward against your body allows gradual movement to the floor without injury to the client.*

c. Allow the client to slide down your leg, and lower the person gently to the floor, making sure the client's head does not hit any objects.

Two Nurses

4. Prepare the client.

• See step 1 above.

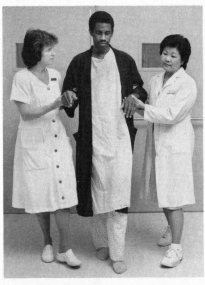

FIGURE 21–41 Two nurses assisting a client to ambulate by grasping the client's upper arm with one hand and the hand or forearm with the other hand.

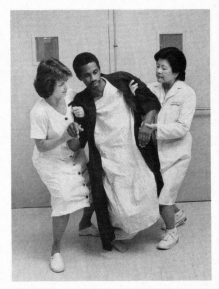

FIGURE 21–42 Two nurses lowering the client to the floor.

5. Ensure client safety.

Ⓢ • After the client stands, assume a position with one nurse at either side. Grasp the inferior aspect of the client's upper arm with your nearest hand and the client's lower arm or hand with your other hand (Figure 21–41). *This provides a secure grip for each nurse.*

• *Optional:* Place a walking belt around the client's waist. Each nurse grasps the side handle with the near hand and the lower aspect of the client's upper arm with the other hand.

• Walk in unison with the client, using a smooth, even gait, at the same speed and with steps the same size as the client's. *This*

gives the client a greater feeling of security.

• If the client starts to fall and cannot regain strength or balance, slip your arms under the client's axillae, grasp the client's hands, and lower the person gently to the floor or to a nearby chair (Figure 21–42). *Placing the nurse's arms under the client's axillae evenly balances the client's weight between the two nurses, preventing injury to both the nurses and the client.*

6. Document all relevant information.

• Document the time of the walk, the distance walked or time taken, and all nursing assessments.

EVALUATION FOCUS

The client's gait (including body alignment) when walking; the client's pace; activity tolerance when walking (e.g., pulse rate, facial color, any shortness of breath, feelings of dizziness, or weakness); distance walked and degree of support required; pulse rate, respiratory rate, and blood pressure after an initial ambulation to compare with baseline data.

▶ **Technique 21–3 Assisting a Client to Walk** *CONTINUED*

KEY ELEMENTS OF ASSISTING A CLIENT TO WALK

- Assess the client's (a) medication intake and (b) pulse, respirations, and blood pressure before and after walking if the client has not walked regularly.
- Schedule and implement muscle tone exercises before ambulating clients who have been immobilized for long periods of time.

- Obtain a physician's or primary nurse's order before ambulating clients who have been confined to bed.
- Make sure the client wears nonskid footwear.
- Use a walking belt for unsteady clients.

Teaching Clients to Use Mechanical Aids for Walking

Canes

Three types of canes are used today: the standard straight-legged cane; the tripod or crab cane, which has three feet; and the quad cane, which has four feet and provides the most support (Figure 21–43). Cane tips should have rubber caps to improve traction and prevent slipping. The standard cane is 91 cm (36 in) long; some aluminum canes can be adjusted from 56 to 97 cm (22 to 38 inches). The length should permit the elbow to be slightly flexed. Clients may use either one or two canes, depending on how much support they require. Technique 21–4 explains how to assist a client to use a cane.

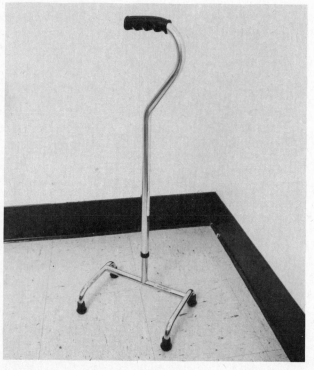

FIGURE 21–43 A quad cane.

21-4 Assisting a Client to Use a Cane

PURPOSES
- To enhance the client's balance and gait alignment
- To provide additional support (e.g., when the client has weakness on one side of the body) even though weight-bearing is possible

ASSESSMENT FOCUS

Client's abilities to walk with a cane (i.e., physical strength of the lower extremities and arm and hand holding the cane); ability to bear body weight; ability to keep balance in a standing position on one or both legs; ability to hold the body erect.

EQUIPMENT

☐ Cane of the correct length with rubber tip

INTERVENTION

1. Prepare the client for walking.

• Ask the client to hold the cane on the *stronger* side of the body. *This provides maximum support and appropriate body alignment when walking. The arm opposite the advancing foot normally swings forward when walking, so the hand holding the cane will come forward and the cane will support the weaker leg.*

• Position the tip of a standard cane (and the nearest tip of other canes) about 15 cm (6 in) to the side and 15 cm (6 in) in front of the near foot, so that the elbow is slightly flexed. *This provides the best balance and prevents the person from leaning on the cane. In this position the client stands erect, with the center of gravity within the base of support.*

• Ensure that the client has balance and feels well enough to walk.

2. When maximum support is required, instruct the client to move as follows:

• Move the cane forward about 30 cm (1 ft), or a distance that is comfortable while the body weight is borne by both legs (Figure 21–44, *A*).

• Then, move the affected (weak) leg forward to the cane while the weight is borne by the cane and stronger leg (Figure 21–44, *B*).

• Next, move the unaffected (stronger) leg forward ahead of

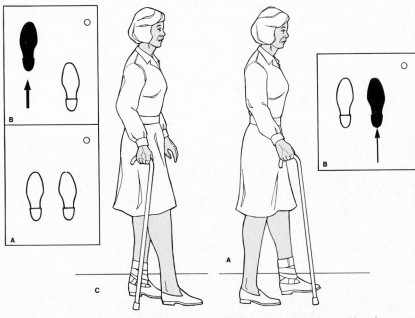

FIGURE 21–44 Steps involved in using a cane to provide maximum support.

FIGURE 21–45 Steps involved in using a cane when less than maximum support is required.

the cane and weak leg while the weight is borne by the cane and weak leg (Figure 21–44, *C*).

• Repeat the above three steps. This pattern of moving provides at least two points of support on the floor at all times.

3. When the client becomes stronger and requires less support, instruct the client to follow these steps:

• Move the cane and weak leg forward at the same time, while the weight is borne by the stronger leg (Figure 21–45, *A*).

• Move the stronger leg forward while the weight is borne by the

cane and the weak leg (Figure 21–45, *B*).

4. Ensure client safety.

• Walk beside the client on the affected side. *The client is most likely to fall toward the affected side.*

• Walk the client for the time or distance indicated on the nursing care plan.

• If the client loses balance or strength and is unable to regain it, slide your hand up to the client's axilla, and take a broad stance to provide a base of support. Have the client rest against your hip until assistance arrives, or gently lower yourself and the client to the floor.

EVALUATION FOCUS

Body alignment standing and walking with a cane; gait when walking with the cane (see Nursing Process Guide on page 498).

► **Technique 21–4 Assisting a Client to Use a Cane** CONTINUED

> ## KEY ELEMENTS OF ASSISTING A CLIENT TO USE A CANE
>
> - Assess the client's abilities to use a cane, i.e., assess physical strength and balance.
> - Select an appropriate cane if balance is poor, or use a walker.
> - Make sure the cane has a rubber cap on the tip(s) and is of the appropriate length or height.
>
> - Instruct the client to hold the cane on the appropriate side of the body.
> - Walk beside the client on the affected side.

Walkers

Walkers are mechanical devices for ambulatory clients who need more support than a cane provides. There are many types of walkers of different shapes and sizes, with devices suited to individual needs. The standard type is made of polished aluminum. It has four legs with rubber tips and plastic hand grips (Figure 21–46). Many walkers have adjustable legs.

The standard walker needs to be picked up to be used. The client therefore requires partial strength in both hands and wrists; strong elbow extensors, such as the triceps brachii; and strong shoulder depressors, such as the pectoralis minor. The client also needs the ability to bear at least partial weight on both legs.

Four-wheeled models of walkers (roller walkers) do not need to be picked up to be moved, but they are less stable than the standard walker. They are used by clients who are too weak or unstable to pick up and move the walker with each step. Some roller walkers have a seat at the back so the client can sit down to rest when desired. An adaptation of the standard and four-wheeled walker is one that has two tips and two wheels. This type provides more stability than the four-wheeled model yet still permits the client to keep the walker in contact with the ground all the time. The client tilts the walker toward the body, lifting the tips while the wheels remain on the ground, then pushes the walker forward.

The nurse may need to adjust the height of a client's walker so that the hand bar is just below the client's waist and the client's elbows are slightly flexed. This position helps the client assume a more normal stance. A walker that is too low causes the client to stoop; one that is too high makes the client stretch and reach. Instructions for using walkers are provided in the accompanying box.

Crutches

Crutches may be a temporary need for some people and a permanent one for others. Crutches should

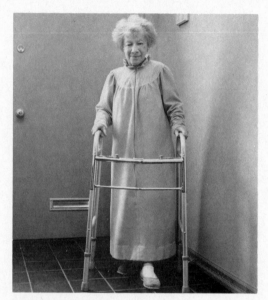

FIGURE 21–46 A standard walker.

 ## CLIENT TEACHING

Using Walkers

When Maximum Support Is Required

- Move the walker ahead about 15 cm (6 in) while your body weight is borne by both legs.
- Then, move the right foot up to the walker while your body weight is borne by the left leg and both arms.
- Next, move the left foot up to the right foot while your body weight is borne by the right leg and both arms.

If One Leg Is Weaker Than the Other

- Move the walker and the weak leg ahead together about 15 cm (6 in) while your weight is borne by the stronger leg.
- Then, move the stronger leg ahead while your weight is borne by the affected leg and both arms.

enable a person to ambulate independently; therefore, it is important to learn to use them properly. Sometimes clients are discouraged when they attempt crutch walking. Clients confined to bed are often unaware of weakness that becomes apparent when they try to stand or walk. Clients realize that they can no longer take balance for granted when they must cope with the weight of a heavy cast or a paralyzed limb. Frequently, progress may be slower than the client anticipated. Encouragement from the nurse and the setting of realistic goals are especially important.

There are several kinds of crutches. The most frequently used are the underarm crutch, or *axillary crutch* with hand bars, and the *Lofstrand crutch*, which extends only to the forearm. The underarm crutch can be extended. It has double uprights, an underarm bar, and a hand bar (Figure 21–47, *A*). The Lofstrand crutch is a single adjustable tube of aluminum to which are attached a curved piece of steel, a rubber-covered hand bar, and a metal forearm cuff (Figure 21–47, *B*). This type of crutch is most useful

as a substitute for a cane. The metal cuff around the forearm and the metal bar stabilize the wrists and thus make walking safer and easier. The person can release the hand bar to use his or her hand, and the metal cuff will hold the crutch in place, while a cane would fall.

The *Canadian*, or *elbow extensor crutch*, like the Lofstrand, is made of a single tube of aluminum with lateral attachments, a hand bar, and a cuff for the forearm, but it also has a cuff for the upper arm (Figure 21–47, *C*). This crutch is usually used by clients who require support for weak extensor muscles of the arm (e. g., weak triceps brachii).

All crutches require suction tips, usually made of rubber, which help to prevent the crutches from slipping on a floor surface. Suggested client instructions for using crutches are provided in the accompanying box.

Exercises for Crutch Walking
In crutch walking, the client's weight is borne by the muscles of the shoulder girdle and the upper extrem-

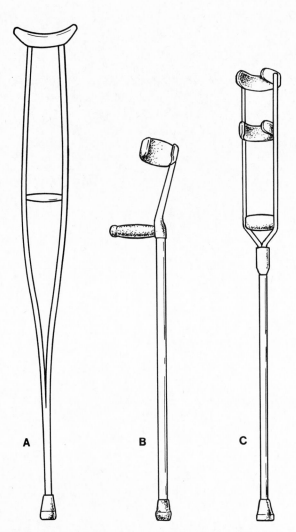

FIGURE 21–47 Three types of crutches: *A*, axillary crutch; *B*, Lofstrand crutch; *C*, Canadian, or elbow extensor, crutch.

CLIENT TEACHING

Using Crutches
- Follow the plan of exercises developed for you to strengthen your arm muscles before beginning crutch walking.
- Have a health care professional establish the correct length for your crutches and the correct placement of the handpieces. Crutches that are too long force your shoulders upward and make it difficult for you to push your body off the ground. Crutches that are too short will make you hunch over and develop an improper body stance.
- The weight of your body should be borne by the arms rather than the axillae (armpits). Continual pressure on the axillae can injure the radial nerve and eventually cause **crutch palsy**, a weakness of the muscles of the forearm, wrist, and hand.
- Maintain an erect posture as much as possible to prevent strain on muscles and joints and to maintain balance.
- Each step taken with crutches should be a comfortable distance for you. It is wise to start with a small rather than large step.
- Inspect the crutch tips regularly, and replace them if worn.
- Keep the crutch tips dry to maintain their surface friction. If the tips become wet, dry them well before use.

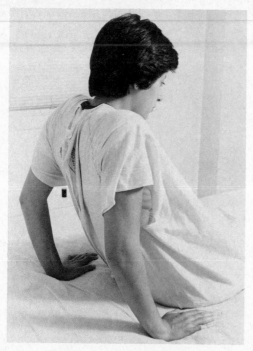

FIGURE 21–48 Strengthening the flexor and extensor muscles of the arms and the muscles that dorsiflex the wrists.

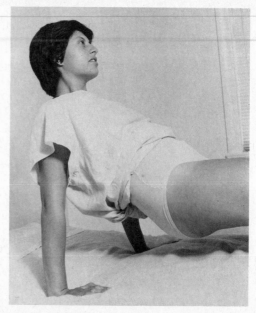

FIGURE 21–49 Strengthening the extensor muscles of the arms in preparation for crutch walking.

ities. Before beginning crutch walking, the following exercises are recommended:

- Flexing and extending the arms in several directions.

- Moving from a supine position to a sitting position by flexing the elbows and pushing the hands against the bed surface (Figure 21–48). This exercise strengthens the flexor and extensor muscles of the arms and the muscles that dorsiflex the wrists.

- Lifting the body off the bed surface by pushing down with the hands and extending the elbows (Figure 21–49). This exercise is particularly use-

ful in strengthening the extensor muscles of the arms.

- Squeezing a rubber ball or a gripper with the hands. This exercise strengthens the flexor muscles of the fingers.

Measuring Clients for Crutches
When nurses measure clients for axillary crutches, it is most important to obtain the correct length for the crutches and the correct placement of the hand piece. There are two methods of measuring crutch length:

1. The client lies in a supine position, and the nurse measures from the anterior fold of the axilla to a point 10 cm (4 in) lateral from the heel of the foot (Figure 21–50).

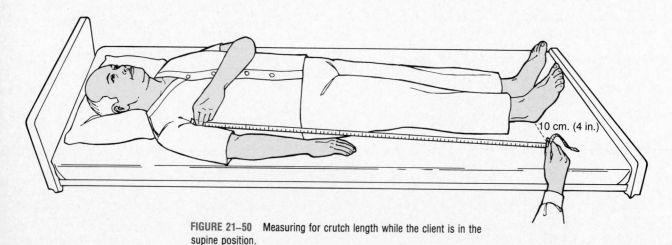

10 cm. (4 in.)

FIGURE 21–50 Measuring for crutch length while the client is in the supine position.

2. The client stands erect and positions the crutch tips 5 cm (2 in) in front of and 15 cm (6 in) to the side of the feet (Figure 21–51). The nurse makes sure the shoulder rest of the crutch is at least 3 finger widths, i.e., 2.5 to 5 cm (1 to 2 in), below the axilla.

To determine the correct placement of the hand bar:

1. The client stands upright and supports the body weight by the hand grips of the crutches.

2. The nurse measures the angle of elbow flexion. It should be about 30°. A goniometer (Figure 11–91, page 269) may be used to verify the correct angle.

Crutch Gaits

The crutch gait is the gait a person assumes on crutches by alternating body weight on one or both legs and the crutches. Five standard crutch gaits are the four-point gait, three-point gait, two-point gait, swing-to gait, and swing-through gait. The gait used depends on the following individual factors: (a) the ability to take steps, (b) the ability to bear weight and keep balance in a standing position on both legs or only one, and (c) the ability to hold the body erect.

A physiotherapist or a physician usually decides which crutch gait is best for a particular client. Nurses are increasingly involved in these decisions, however. Often, a physiotherapist teaches the crutch gait initially, but nurses give follow-through lessons. In some instances, nurses alone teach the client the technique.

Clients also need instruction about how to get into and out of chairs and go up and down stairs safely. All of these crutch skills are best taught before the client is discharged and preferably before the client has surgery. Technique 21–5 explains how to assist clients to use various crutch gaits, get into and out of chairs, and go up and down stairs safely.

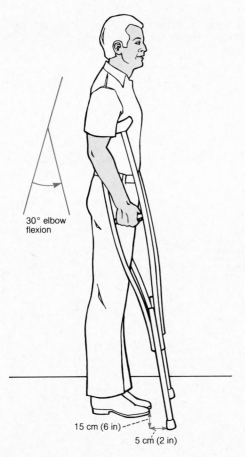

FIGURE 21–51 The standing position for measuring the correct length of crutches.

21-5 Assisting a Client to Use Crutches

PURPOSES	• To increase the client's sense of independence • To help the client walk and move with crutches safely and with minimum expenditure of energy
ASSESSMENT FOCUS	Leg or foot disability (i.e., whether the client can bear weight on one leg only or partially on the affected leg or foot; ability to maintain balance in an erect standing position; muscle strength, particularly in the arms and unaffected leg; previous experience with crutches; learning needs.

EQUIPMENT

□ Crutches with suction tips, hand bars, and axillary pads

□ Walking belt (optional)

▶ Technique 21–5 Assisting a Client to Use Crutches CONTINUED

INTERVENTION

1. Prepare the client.

- Verify the correct length for the crutches and the correct placement of the handpieces. (See Measuring Clients for Crutches, on page 528).

- Ensure that the client is wearing supportive, nonskid shoes with **S** laces or Velcro.

2. Assist the client to assume the tripod (triangle) position, the basic crutch stance used before crutch walking.

- Ask the client to stand and place the tips of the crutches 15 cm (6 in) in front of the feet and out laterally about 15 cm (6 in). See Figure 21–52. *The tripod position provides a wide base of support and enhances both stability and balance.*

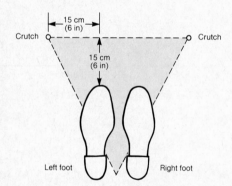

FIGURE 21–52 The tripod position.

- Make sure the feet are slightly apart. A tall person requires a wider base than a short person.

- Ensure that posture is erect; i.e., the hips and knees are extended, the back is straight, and the head is held straight and high. There should be no hunch to the shoulders and thus no weight borne by the axillae. The elbows should be extended sufficiently to allow weight-bearing on the hands.

- Stand slightly behind and on the client's affected side. *By standing behind the client and toward the*

affected side, the nurse can provide support if the client loses balance.

- If the client is unsteady, place a walking belt around the client's waist, and grasp the belt from above, not from below. *A fall can be prevented more effectively if the belt is held from above.*

3. Teach the client the appropriate crutch gait.

Four-Point Alternate Gait

This is the most elementary and safest gait, providing at least three points of support at all times, but it requires coordination. It can be used when walking in crowds because it does not require much space. To use this gait, the client has to be able to bear some weight on both legs (Figure 21–53, read-

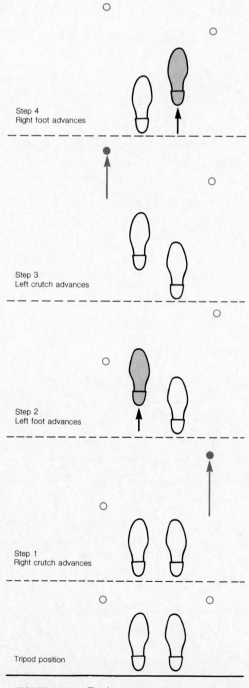

FIGURE 21–53 The four-point alternate crutch gait.

Technique 21–5 CONTINUED

ing from bottom to top). Ask the client to

• Move the right crutch ahead a suitable distance, e.g., 10 to 15 cm (4 to 6 in).

• Move the left foot forward, preferably to the level of the crutch.

• Move the left crutch forward.

• Move the right foot forward.

Three-Point Gait

To use this gait, the person must be able to bear entire body weight on the unaffected leg. The two crutches and the unaffected leg bear weight alternately (Figure 21–54, reading from bottom to top). Ask the client to

• Move both crutches and the weaker leg forward.

• Move the stronger leg forward.

Two-Point Alternate Gait

This gait is faster than the four-point gait. It requires more balance, because only two points support

the body at one time; it also requires at least partial weight bearing on each foot. In this gait, arm movements with the crutches are similar to the arm movements during normal walking (Figure 21–55, reading from bottom to top). Ask the client to

• Move the left crutch and the right foot forward together.

• Move the right crutch and the left foot ahead together.

Swing-To Gait

The swing gaits are used by people with paralysis of the legs and hips. Prolonged use of these gaits results in atrophy of the unused muscles. The swing-to gait is the easier of these two gaits (Figure 21–56). Ask the client to

• Move both crutches ahead together.

• Lift body weight by the arms and swing *to* the crutches.

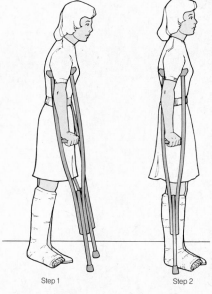

FIGURE 21–56 The swing-to crutch gait.

Swing-Through Gait

This gait requires considerable client skill, strength, and coordination (Figure 21–57). Ask the client to

• Move both crutches forward together.

• Lift body weight by the arms and swing *through and beyond* the crutches.

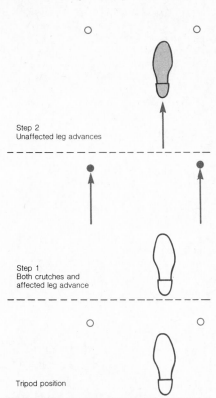

FIGURE 21–54 The three-point crutch gait.

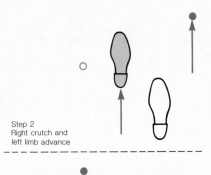
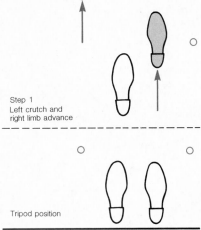

FIGURE 21–55 The two-point alternate crutch gait.

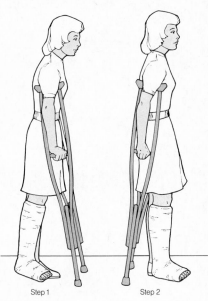

FIGURE 21–57 The swing-through crutch gait.

► **Technique 21–5 Assisting a Client to Use Crutches** *CONTINUED*

4. Teach the client to get into and out of a chair.

Getting Into a Chair

- Ensure that the chair has armrests and is secure or braced against a wall.

- Instruct the client to

  a. Stand with the back of the unaffected leg centered against the chair. *The chair helps support the client during the next steps.*

  b. Transfer the crutches to the hand on the affected side, hold the crutches by the hand bars, and then grasp the arm of the chair with the hand on the unaffected side (Figure 21–58). *This allows the client to support the body weight on the arms and the unaffected leg.*

  c. Lean forward, flex the knees and hips, and lower into the chair.

Getting Out of a Chair

- Instruct the client to

  a. Move forward to the edge of the chair and place the unaffected leg slightly under or at the edge of the chair. *This position helps the client stand up from the chair and achieve balance, because the unaffected leg is supported against the edge of the chair.*

  b. Grasp the crutches by the hand bars in the hand on the affected side, and grasp the arm of the chair by the hand on the unaffected side. *The body weight is placed on the crutches and the hand on the armrest to support the unaffected leg when the client rises to stand.*

  c. Push down on the crutches and the chair armrest while elevating the body out of the chair.

  d. Assume the tripod position before moving.

5. Teach the client to go up and down stairs.

Going Up Stairs

- Stand behind the client and slightly to the affected side.

- Ask the client to

  a. Assume the tripod position at the bottom of the stairs.

  b. Transfer the body weight to the crutches and move the unaffected leg onto the step (Figure 21–59).

  c. Transfer the body weight to the unaffected leg on the step and move the crutches and affected leg up to the step. *The affected leg is always supported by the crutches.*

- Repeat steps b and c until the top of the stairs is reached.

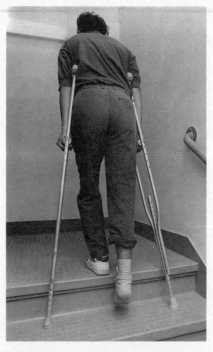

FIGURE 21–59 Climbing stairs: placing weight on the crutches while first moving the unaffected leg onto a step.

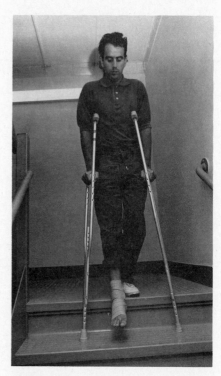

FIGURE 21–60 Descending stairs: moving the crutches and affected leg first down to the next step.

Going Down Stairs

- Stand one step below the person on the affected side.

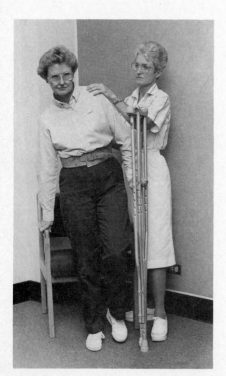

FIGURE 21–58 A client with crutches getting into a chair.

▶ **Technique 21–5** *CONTINUED*

• Ask the client to

   a. Assume the tripod position at the top of the stairs.

   b. Shift the body weight to the unaffected leg, and move the crutches and affected leg down onto the next step (Figure 21–60).

   c. Transfer the body weight to the crutches, and move the unaffected leg to that step. *The affected leg is always supported by the crutches.*

   d. Repeat steps b and c until the bottom of the stairs is reached.

   or

• Ask the client to

   a. Hold both crutches in the outside hand and grasp the hand rail with the other hand for support.

   b. Move as in steps b and c, above.

6. Document teaching and all assessments.

EVALUATION FOCUS

How well the client achieves stability in gait without falling; correct use of crutch gait taught; ability to get into and out of chairs as taught; ability to go up and down stairs as taught.

KEY ELEMENTS OF ASSISTING A CLIENT TO USE CRUTCHES

• Assess strength of the client's upper extremities, ability to bear weight, and balance.

• Develop an appropriate muscle-strengthening exercise program before crutch walking if the client needs one.

• Make sure the crutches are equipped with rubber suction tips, are of the appropriate length, and the hand bars are placed appropriately.

• Instruct the client to bear the weight of the body by the arms rather than the axillae.

• Make sure the client has learned appropriate crutch skills before discharge.

CRITICAL THINKING CHALLENGE

Harold Knowles, an 84-year-old-male, is recovering from a mild stroke (cerebral vascular accident). Although he has been receiving daily physical therapy, some residual left-sided weakness is still present. The physician has ordered that Mr. Knowles be ambulated in the hall three times a day. Mr. Knowles states that he feels dizzy when he stands and is fearful that he will fall. What do you think is causing his dizziness? What factors must be considered before the walk? What precautions should you take?

RELATED RESEARCH

Bhambhani, Y. N.; Clarkson, H. M.; and Gomes, P. S. June 1990. Axillary crutch walking: Effects of three training programs. *Archives of Physical Medicine and Rehabilitation* 71:484–8.

Gehlsen, G. M., and Whaley, M. H. September 1990. Falls in the elderly: Balance, strength, and flexibility. Part 2. *Archives of Physical Medicine and Rehabilitation* 71:739–41.

Gillis, A. J. 1989. The effect of play on immobilized children in hospital. *International Journal of Nursing Studies* 26(3): 261–69.

Goldberg, W. G., and Fitzpatrick, J. J. November/December 1980. Movement with the aged. *Nursing Research* 29:339–46.

Sandler, R. B. December 1989. Muscle strength assessments and the prevention of osteoporosis: A hypothesis. *Journal of American Geriatrics Society* 37:1192–97.

REFERENCES

Angelucci, D.; Todaro, A.; and Reno, A. March 1991. When our patients get up is our decision . . . physicians authorize us to write activity orders. *RN* 54:19–20.

Brower, P., and Hicks, D. July 1972. Maintaining muscle function in patients on bedrest. *American Journal of Nursing* 72:1250–53.

Clarkson, H., and Bhambhani, Y. Summer 1990. Complications from using axillary crutches. *Canadian Journal of Rehabilitation* 3:233–39.

Corwin, D., and Miller, C. A. November 1990. Get your patient off on the right foot. *RN* 53:44–46.

Davis, K. May/June 1991. Toward greater mobility. *Clinical Management* 11:24–30.

Elia, E. A. January 1991. Exercise and the elderly. *Clinics in Sports Medicine* 10:141–55.

Fahey, V. March 1984. An in-depth look at deep-vein thrombosis. *Nursing 84* 14:35–41.

Freed, M. M.; Hofkosh, J.; Kaplan, L. I., and Neuhauser, C. October 1987a. Choosing ambulatory aids. *Patient Care* 21:20–23, 26–27, 30–32.

———. October 1987b. Using ambulatory aids. *Patient Care* 21:36–40, 42, 45–47.

Guyton, A. C. 1986. *Textbook of medical physiology.* 7th ed. Philadelphia: W. B. Saunders Co.

Hall, J., and Clarke, A. K. May 1990. Open-cuff crutches. *Physiotherapy* 76:271.

Hogan, L., and Beland, I. July 1976. Cervical neck syndrome. *American Journal of Nursing* 76:1104–7.

Joyce, B. M., and Kirby, R. L. February 1991. Canes, crutches and walkers. *American Family Physician* 43:535–42.

Kottke, F. J., and Lehmann, J. F., editors. 1990. *Krusen's handbook of physical medicine and rehabilitation.* 4th ed. Philadelphia: W. B. Saunders Co.

Lane, P. L., and Leblanc, R. September 1990. Crutch walking. *Orthopaedic Nursing* 9:31–38.

Maier, P. September 1986. Take the work out of range-of-motion exercises with continuous passive motion machine. *RN* 49:46–49.

Oka, R. K. November/December 1990. Cardiovascular response to exercise. *Cardiovascular Nursing* 26:31–36.

Olson, E. V.; Johnson, B. J.; and Thompson, L. F. March 1990. The hazards of immobility. *American Journal of Nursing* 43–44, 46–48.

Rickert, L. October/December 1989. Benefits of exercise. *Journal of Urological Nursing* 8(4):758–59.

Smith, J. E. May/June 1990. Applying the continuous passive motion device. *Orthopaedic Nursing* 9:54–56.

Nutrition

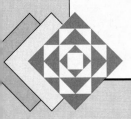

NURSING PROCESS GUIDE

NUTRITION

ASSESSMENT

Follow the "ABCD" approach:

- *(A) anthropometric measurements:* Anthropometric measurements are measurements of the size and composition of the body. See page 541 and Technique 22–1.

- *(B) biochemical data:* Some of the most common laboratory studies to detect subclinical malnutrition involve the following:

  - *Hemoglobin and red blood cell indices.* Low levels provide evidence of iron deficiency.

  - *Hematocrit (Hct), or packed cell volume.* An elevated level is evidence of dehydration.

  - *Serum albumin concentration.* A concentration of less than 1500 suggests prolonged protein depletion.

  - *Transferrin levels.* High levels indicate low iron stores; low levels indicate excessive iron stores. *Transferrin* is a blood protein that binds with iron and transports it throughout the body. The transferrin level is considered a more sensitive indicator of protein malnutrition than albumin level because transferrin responds more promptly to changes in protein intake and has a smaller body pool.

  - *Total lymphocyte count.* Certain nutrient deficiencies and forms of **PCM** (protein-calorie malnutrition) can depress the immune system. The total number of lymphocytes decreases as protein depletion occurs.

  - *Blood urea nitrogen (BUN).* A low BUN level suggests inadequate protein intake. Elevated BUN levels may occur with starvation or with severe dehydration.

  - *Urine creatinine levels.* Decreased levels can suggest malnutrition resulting from skeletal muscle atrophy.

- *(C) Clinical signs:* Examples indicating poor nutrition status include the following:

  - *Hair:* Dry, dull, patchy in growth

  - *Skin:* Dry, broken out in rash, scaly, rough, bruised

  - *Eyes:* Dry, reddened

  - *Tongue:* Reddened in patches, swollen

  - *Mucous membranes:* Reddened, dry, cracked

  - *Cardiovascular system:* Rapid heart rate, elevated blood pressure, irregular heart rhythm

  - *Muscles:* Poor in tone, soft, underdeveloped

  - *Gastrointestinal system:* Manifesting anorexia, indigestion, diarrhea, constipation

  - *Neurologic system:* Irritable, inattentive, confused, emotionally labile, reflexes decreased

  - *Vitality:* Lacking energy, tired, apathetic, sleeping poorly

  - *Weight:* Overweight, underweight

- *(D) Dietary history:* A dietary history generally includes data about the usual eating patterns and habits, food preferences and restrictions, allergies, daily fluid intake, use of vitamin or mineral supplements, any dietary problems (such as difficulty chewing or swallowing), physical activity, health history, and concerns related to food buying and preparation.

Identify clients at risk for nutritional problems:

- Chewing or swallowing difficulties (including ill-fitting dentures, dental caries, and missing teeth)

- Inadequate food intake

- Restricted or fad diets

- No intake for 10 or more days

- Intravenous fluids (other than total parenteral nutrition for 10 or more days)

- Inadequate food budget

- Inadequate food preparation facilities

- Inadequate food storage facilities

- Physical disabilities

- Elderly living and eating alone

RELATED DIAGNOSTIC CATEGORIES

- Altered nutrition: Less than body requirements

- Altered nutrition: More than body requirements

- Altered nutrition: High risk for more than body requirements

- Self-care deficit: Feeding

PLANNING

Client Goals
The client will

- Achieve or maintain optimal nutritional status.

- Avoid nutritional problems.

Nursing Process Guide *CONTINUED*

Outcome Criteria
The client

- Identifies factors contributing to inadequate (or excessive) nutritional intake.

- Explains any necessary dietary alterations (foods to include and avoid).

- Keeps a log of foods ingested in a 7-day period.

- Has a triceps skinfold measurement, arm muscle circumference (AMC) and body mass index (BMI) within predetermined ranges.

- Has a stable daily weight, or weight increase of 2 kg/week, or decrease of 1.5 kg/week.

- Feeds self independently using self-feeding aid.

- Plans a balanced meal using the diet information provided.

- Identifies foods high in specific nutrients (e.g., calcium, iron, potassium).

- Reports decrease (or absence of) signs of malnutrition cited in the defining characteristics.

- Demonstrates life-style changes to regain or maintain weight at satisfactory level for height and body build.

Nutrition and Metabolism

Nutrition is the sum of all the interactions between an organism and the food it consumes (Christian and Greger 1988, p. 4). In other words, nutrition is what a person eats and how the body uses it. People require food or essential nutrients for the growth and maintenance of all body tissues and the normal functioning of all body processes. **Nutrients** are the organic and inorganic chemicals found in foods and required for proper body functioning. *Organic* substances are those containing carbon and are derived from living organisms. *Inorganic* substances are not derived from hydrocarbons and are not of organic origin.

The amount of energy that nutrients or foods supply to the body is their **caloric value.** A **calorie** is a unit of heat energy. A **small calorie** is the amount of heat required to raise the temperature of 1 g of water 1 degree C. A **large calorie (Calorie, kilocalorie [kcal])** is the amount of heat required to raise the temperature of 1 kg of water 1 degree C and is the unit used in nutrition.

Metabolism refers to all cellular chemical reactions that make it possible for body cells to continue living (Guyton 1986, p. 844). The energy in food maintains the basal metabolic rate of the body and provides energy for activities such as running and walking. Metabolic rate is normally expressed in terms of the rate of heat liberated during chemical reactions. The **basic metabolic rate (BMR)** is the rate at which the body metabolizes food to maintain the energy requirements of a person who is awake and at rest.

Basic Four Food Guide

The Basic Four Food Guide is based on four basic food groups: milk and milk products; meats and alternates; breads and cereals; and fruits and vegetables. Foods selected from the guide generally supply 1000 to 1400 kcal daily. Numbers and sizes of servings are listed for each group. See Table 22–1 on page 538.

Because individual needs vary with age, sex, and activity, additional calories to meet energy requirements can be obtained by increasing the number and size of servings from the various food groups and/or by adding other foods that are not listed in the food groups. Table 22–2 provides a food guide for children and adolescents. In addition, daily intake of 4 to 6 cups or more of liquid from any source is recommended. Iodized salt should be used. Unless there is an adequate supply in drinking water, fluoride, too, should be supplemented. Also, a person can follow this guide and still eat insufficient fiber, which is found in raw fruits, vegetables, and whole grains.

Modified Diets

Hospitals supply a variety of diets for clients.

Regular Diet

Clients who do not have special needs eat the regular or general diet, whose quantity and content are designed to meet the needs of most people. Some hospitals provide a daily menu from which to select food for the next day. Other hospitals provide standard meals to each client on a general diet. Certain

TABLE 22–1 BASIC FOUR FOOD GUIDE

Food Groups and Servings	Foods and Sizes of Servings	Major Nutrients
DAIRY GROUP Child under 9: 2 to 3	One serving = 8 oz fluid milk: whole, low-fat, skim, buttermilk, or reconstituted dry milk or evaporated milk; 1 ⅓ oz hard cheese, 1⅓ cups cottage cheese, 1⅔ cups ice cream, 1 cup yogurt	Protein; fat; vitamins A and D; riboflavin; B_{12}; calcium; phosphorus
Child 9 to 12: 3 or more Teenager: 4 or more Adult: 2 or more Pregnant: 3 or more Lactating: 4 or more		
PROTEIN GROUP 2 or more servings	One serving = 2 to 3 oz beef, pork, lamb, veal, poultry, or fish. Substitutes for ½ serving of meat: 1 egg, ½ cup cooked dry beans or peas, or 2 tbsp peanut butter	Protein; carbohydrate in plant alternatives; fat, except in legumes; B_{12} in meat, fish, and poultry; niacin; iron; zinc
VEGETABLE-FRUIT GROUP 4 or more servings, including:	One serving = ½ cup vegetable or fruit or one piece fresh fruit	Carbohydrate; vitamin C in citrus fruits and tomatoes; vitamin A in dark green or deep yellow vegetables; folacin; iron; calcium; fiber
1 or 2 servings of good sources of vitamin C	Grapefruit or grapefruit juice, orange or orange juice, cantaloupe, raw strawberries, broccoli, Brussel sprouts, green pepper. Fair sources include melons, tangerines, asparagus, cabbage, cauliflower, collards, potatoes, spinach, tomatoes	
1 good source of vitamin A at least every other day	Apricots, broccoli, cantaloupe, carrots, chard, collards, kale, pumpkin, spinach, sweet potatoes, turnip greens, winter squash	
GRAIN GROUP 4 or more servings	One serving = 1 slice whole grain or enriched bread, 1 oz ready-to-eat cereal, ½ cup of the following: cooked cereal, cornmeal, grits, spaghetti, macaroni, noodles, or rice	Carbohydrate; some protein; thiamine; niacin; iron; fiber
OTHER FOODS Sweets, oil, butter, salad dressings, condiments, alcohol	Used to round out meals, provide flavor, and meet energy requirements	Fat; carbohydrate

Sources: Adapted from S. G. Dudek, *Nutrition handbook for nursing practice* (Philadelphia: J. B. Lippincott Co., 1987), pp. 177–78; D. E. Scholl, *Nutrition and diet therapy: A handbook for nurses* (Oradell, N. J.: Medical Economics Books, 1986), pp. 4–6; and Minister of Health and Welfare, Department of Health and Welfare, *Canada's food guide* (Ottawa: Department of Health and Welfare, 1983).

foods (e.g., cabbage, which tends to produce flatus, and highly seasoned and fried foods, which are difficult for some people to digest) are usually omitted from the regular diet.

Light Diet

A variation of the regular diet is the light diet, designed for postoperative and other clients who are not ready for the regular diet. Foods in the light diet are plainly cooked. Foods containing large amounts of fat are usually omitted, as are bran and foods containing a great deal of fiber. Not all agencies provide a light diet.

Soft Diet

A soft diet is easily chewed and digested. It is often ordered for clients who have difficulty chewing and swallowing (dysphagia). A soft diet is a lightly seasoned, low-residue (low-fiber) diet. The *pureed diet* is a modification of the soft diet. Liquid may be added to the food, which is then blended to a semisoft consistency.

Full Liquid Diet

A full liquid diet contains only liquids or foods that turn to liquid at room temperature, such as ice cream. Full liquid diets are provided to clients who have gas-

TABLE 22–2   THE BASIC FOUR FOOD GUIDE FOR CHILDREN AND ADOLESCENTS

Food Group	Recommended Servings*
Milk and milk products	Children up to 9 years: 2–3 servings
	Children 9 to 12 years: 3 or more servings
	Adolescents: 4 or more cups
Meats and alternates	All ages: 2 or more servings
Grain Products	All ages: 4 or more servings
Fruits and vegetables	All ages: 4 or more servings

*Serving sizes and foods are shown in Table 22–1.

Sources: J. L. Christian and J. L. Greger, *Nutrition for living* (Menlo Park, Calif.: The Benjamin/Cummings Publishing Co., 1988), p. 48; and S. Williams, *Nutrition and diet therapy*, 4th ed. (St. Louis: C. V. Mosby Co., 1984).

trointestinal disturbances or are otherwise unable to tolerate solid food.

Clear Liquid Diet

The clear liquid diet is often limited to water, tea, coffee, clear broths, ginger ale or other carbonated beverages, apple juice, and plain gelatin. It does not permit milk. This diet provides the client with fluid and carbohydrate (in the form of sugar), but it does not supply adequate protein, fat, vitamins, and minerals. It is usually a short-term diet for clients who are seriously ill or is given immediately after certain surgeries.

Other Special Diets

Some special diets are therapeutic, devised especially for individual clients. These frequently prescribe the kind and amount of food as well as the frequency of eating:

- A *reducing diet* provides a limited number of calories so that the person will lose weight.

- A *diabetic diet* provides protein, fat, and carbohydrate in accordance with the individual's ability to produce insulin.

- A *low-salt* (NaCl) or *sodium-restricted diet* is designed to limit the sodium (Na) intake. Some low-salt diets merely limit the salt added to food during cooking or eating. Others restrict certain foods because they are naturally high in sodium. These diets are usually prescribed for clients with certain cardiovascular diseases.

- *Allergy diets* omit the particular foods to which a client is allergic. Some foods that commonly produce allergic reactions are cow's milk, wheat, and eggs.

Personal Diets

Diets also vary according to an individual's personal sociocultural beliefs. Some people are vegetarians. There are two basic vegetarian diets: those that permit only plant foods and those that include milk, eggs, and dairy products. Some people eat fish and poultry but not beef, lamb, or pork; others eat plant foods and dairy products but not eggs.

Ethnicity and religion may also influence a person's eating habits. Traditional foods, such as rice for Asians and pasta for Italians, often are eaten long after other ethnic customs are abandoned.

Age-Related Dietary Changes

Infants

Full-term newborns are able to digest and absorb simple carbohydrates, proteins, and moderate amounts of fat. Simple carbohydrates are required because the starch-splitting enzyme amylase is not present at birth. The newborn's diet must be balanced and supply all essential nutrients discussed earlier to meet the energy requirements of rapid growth. Caloric requirements are about 110 to 120 kcal/kg/day. Water requirements are high (140 to 160 ml/kg/day) because of the infant's inability to concentrate urine. Fluids must be increased in hot weather or if the infant is ill. Essential amino acids are required for body tissue growth and maintenance. Carbohydrates provide quick energy, spare protein for building and repair, and help burn body fat. Adequate vitamins and minerals are also needed to prevent deficiency states. Iron intake is affected by the amount of iron stored during fetal life and by the mother's iron intake during pregnancy and when nursing.

Because milk is the infant's major or only food during the first 6 months, it must be appropriate for the infant's needs. Breast milk, commercial formulas (cow's-milk-based and soy-based), and evaporated milk formula all meet the infant's needs. Hypoallergenic and premature infant formulas are also available to meet special needs. Breast milk and all standard infant formulas have an appropriate balance of protein, fat, and carbohydrate. Pasteurized milk (whole, 2%, or skim), however, has too much protein for infants and, with the exception of whole milk, too little fat. Although whole milk contains sufficient fat, the infant has difficulty digesting and absorbing the fat in whole milk.

Because breast milk has some characteristics that cannot be duplicated by even the most sophisticated formula, some authorities consider breast-feeding better than infant formula for most babies. Formula feeding, however, is a highly acceptable substitute.

Toddlers and Preschoolers

More teeth erupt during the infant's second and third year of life. By age 3, when most of the deciduous teeth have emerged, the child is able to bite and chew adult table foods well. Manipulative skills are sufficiently developed for self-feeding, although the child still needs some adult assistance and small utensils. Children should be taught table manners only after they master manipulative skills. The average toddler or preschooler generally requires the following:

* The milk group: two to three servings per day (one serving equals ½ to ¾ cup)

* The meat group: two or more servings per day (one serving equals 3 to 4 Tbsp)

* Cereals and breads: four or more servings per day (one serving equals ½ to 1 slice of bread or ½ to ¾ cup of dried or cooked cereal)

* Vegetables and fruits: four or more servings per day, to include at least one or more servings of citrus fruit and one or more servings of green or yellow vegetables (one serving equals 3 to 4 Tbsp)

School-Age Children

Children of school age need the same number of servings per day of the four basic food groups as preschoolers do, but in larger amounts to meet growth needs. For example, one serving of milk is 1 cup; one serving of meat is 6 to 8 Tbsp; one serving of vegetable or fruit is ⅓ to ½ cup; and one serving of bread and cereal equals 1 to 2 slices or ½ to 1 cup.

Adolescents

Teenage boys and girls have high energy requirements because of their rapid growth and need a diet plentiful in milk, meats, and green and yellow vegetables. Adults should encourage teenagers to eat nutritious snacks, e.g., fresh fruit and vegetables. Food fads are common among teenagers, some of which may be extreme and cause for concern.

Pregnant adolescents may need to learn to eat regular, well-balanced meals. Their energy requirements are usually very high because of their own growth needs as well as those of the fetus. They also need extra protein, iron, and calcium.

Young Adults

Young adults require balanced diets and caloric intakes appropriate to their energy output. Of special consideration, however, is the pregnant and lactating woman. In addition to the basic diet for an adult, the pregnant woman needs the following:

* Increased protein because of the growth of the fetus and accessory tissues of the woman

* Double the usual calcium and phosphorus requirements

* An additional 150 mg of magnesium daily

* Iron to build sufficient hemoglobin and provide iron for the fetus

* Iodine (175 mg), found commonly in iodized salt, seafood, and milk

* Zinc (5 mg above the normal daily requirement) to meet the needs of newly forming maternal and fetal tissue

Some physicians also recommend folic acid supplements; however, the need for general vitamin supplements is questionable unless the woman is at nutritional risk.

Middle-Aged Adults

Both men and women in the middle years need to reduce their caloric intakes primarily because metabolic rates decrease, growth is complete, and activity slackens. Therefore, middle-aged adults need to eat less or increase activity to prevent obesity.

People in their middle years need to choose their foods from the four food groups and at the same time adhere to a prudent diet. The latter includes more low-fat milk products, poultry, fish, and beans and limits eggs to three times per week. Vegetables, fruit, cereals, and whole-grain breads are recommended for their fiber and protein content.

Elderly Adults

Metabolic rates decrease with age, and physical activity usually slackens; therefore, elderly people require fewer calories then they required formerly. Some may have an increased need for carbohydrates for fiber and bulk, but most nutrient requirements remain relatively unchanged. Such physical changes as tooth loss and impaired sense of taste and smell may also affect eating habits. See the box on page 541 for specific suggestions for the elderly person's nutrition.

Nutrition for Older Adults

- Reduce fat consumption by drinking low-fat milk, eating more poultry and fish rather than red meats, limiting meat portions to 4 to 6 oz per day, and limiting the intake of added fats, e.g., butter, margarine, and oil-based salad dressings.

- Consume desserts such as fresh or canned fruit and puddings made with low-fat milk rather than pies, cookies, cakes, or ice cream.

- Make sure that intake of meat, poultry, fish, eggs, and cheese is sufficient, because intakes of these foods are often decreased in the older population.

- Because of a lowered glucose tolerance, consume more complex carbohydrates, e.g., breads, cereals, rice, pasta, potatoes, and legumes, rather than sugar-rich foods.

- Ensure an intake of at least 800 mg of calcium to prevent bone loss. Milk and milk products, e.g., cheese, yogurt, cream soups, milk puddings, and frozen milk products are principal sources of calcium.

- Make sure that intake of vitamin D is sufficient. Vitamin D is essential to maintain calcium homeostasis. To meet vitamin D requirements, include some milk in the diet, since such dairy products as cheese, cottage cheese, and yogurt are not usually fortified with vitamin D. If milk or milk products cannot be tolerated because of a lactose deficiency, supplements should be taken.

- Because sodium may be restricted for older adults who have hypertension or other cardiac problems, avoid such foods as canned soups; ketchup; mustard; and salted, smoked, cured, and pickled meats, poultry, and fish. No salt should be added during the cooking of foods.

- Because of the increased incidence of gastrointestinal disturbances and chronic diarrhea, the regular aspirin use among some elderly women, and the possible reduction in meat intake, the need for iron may be increased.

- Difficulties with chewing raw fruits and vegetables may lead to a deficiency in vitamins A and C, minerals, and fiber. Adaptations in food preparation may be necessary. Chop fruits and vegetables finely, shred green leafy vegetables, and select ground meat, poultry, or fish rather than foods that are more difficult to chew.

- Consume fiber-rich foods to prevent constipation and minimize use of laxatives. Fiber-rich foods also provide bulk and a feeling of fullness. They are therefore useful in helping people control their appetites and lose weight.

- Mealtime is commonly a social activity. When possible, make arrangements to promote appropriate social interaction at meals.

- Eat essential foods first, and follow with limited foods in moderation afterward.

- Having the major meal at noon may decrease difficulty sleeping at night after a heavy meal. Avoid tea, coffee, or other stimulants in the evening.

Anthropometric Measurements

Anthropometric measurements include measurements of height, weight, body mass index, skinfolds (fat folds), and arm muscle circumference. Anthropometric measurements reflect the client's caloric-energy expenditure balance, muscle mass, body fat, and protein reserves.

Assessment of height and weight is discussed in Chapter 11. Ideal body weight (IBW) ranges by age, sex, and frame for adults are given in Table 11–5, page 208. An inadequately nourished person can be underweight, overweight, or obese: In every case, caloric intake is not in balance with the expenditure of energy. Clients whose weight is 20% greater than ideal or 10% less than ideal and those who have had an unintentional weight gain or loss of 10% are considered at risk for poor nutritional status.

The **body mass index (BMI)** indicates whether weight is appropriate for the person's height. To calculate the BMI, see Technique 22–1, step 5. A **skinfold measurement** indicates the amount of body fat, the main form of stored energy. The fold of skin includes the subcutaneous tissue but not the underlying muscle. This measurement can be considered an index of the body's energy stores. The triceps, subscapular, biceps, and suprailiac skinfolds can be measured with special calipers. The site most commonly used is the triceps fold. Technique 22–1, step 2 describes only the triceps and subscapular skinfold measurements.

Because muscle serves as the major protein reserve of the body, the **arm muscle circumference (AMC)** can be considered an index of the body's protein reserves. The arm muscle circumference is calculated from the triceps skinfold and mid-upper-arm circumference (MUAC). See Technique 22–1, step 4.

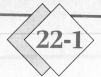

22-1 Taking Anthropometric Measurements

PURPOSES

- To assess the client's balance of caloric intake and energy expenditure
- To determine the body's energy stores or body fat (skinfold measurements)
- To obtain information about the individual's muscle mass and protein reserves (MUAC and AMC)
- To determine whether weight is appropriate for the client's height (BMI)

EQUIPMENT

- ☐ Flexible steel tape measure calibrated in millimeters
- ☐ Calipers

INTERVENTION

1. Prepare the client.

- Assist the client to a comfortable sitting position.
- Remove all the person's upper clothing so that the upper non-dominant arm and the subscapular area are exposed.

2. Measure the skinfolds.

Triceps Skinfold (TSF)

- Locate the midpoint of the upper arm.
- Grasp the skin on the back of the upper arm along the long axis of the humerus (Figure 22-1).
- Placing the calipers 1 cm (0.4 in)

below your fingers, measure the thickness of the fold to the nearest millimeter. The fold of skin includes the subcutaneous tissue but not the underlying muscle.

Subscapular Skinfold

- Pick up the skin below the scapula. Three fingers should be on top of the fold just below the scapula, the thumb below the fold and the forefinger at the lower tip of the scapula. The skinfold should be angled about 45° from the horizontal plane, upward medially and downward laterally (Figure 22-2).
- Placing the calipers about 1 cm (0.4 in) above or below your fingers, measure the skin fold.

3. Measure the mid-upper-arm circumference (MUAC).

- Make sure the upper arm hangs freely in a dependent position and the forearm is positioned horizontally.
- Locate the midpoint of the upper arm, that is, halfway between the acromial process and the olecranon process (Figure 22-3).
- Use the tape measure to measure the circumference of the arm at the midpoint to the nearest millimeter. Maintain the tape in a horizontal plane and avoid distortion of the skin surface.

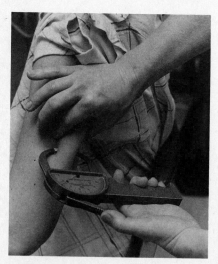

FIGURE 22-1 Measuring the triceps skinfold.

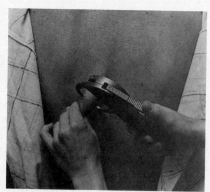

FIGURE 22-2 Measuring the subscapular skinfold.

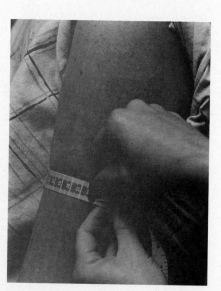

FIGURE 22-3 Measuring the mid-upper-arm circumference.

▶ **Technique 22–1** *CONTINUED*

4. Calculate the arm muscle circumference (AMC).

- Calculate the AMC in millimeters, using the following formula:
  AMC = MUAC (mm) − [3.14 × triceps skin fold (mm)]
  or
  Use available tables.

5. Calculate the body mass index (BMI).

- To calculate the BMI, measure the height in meters and the weight in kilograms (e.g., 5 feet, 7 inches is equal to 1.7 meters, and 153 pounds is equal to 69 kilograms). Then multiply the height by itself (1.7 multiplied by 1.7 is 2.89), and divide the weight by this total to obtain the BMI (69 divided by 2.89 is 24).

6. Record all measurements on the appropriate records.

EVALUATION FOCUS

Comparison of all measurements with average ranges (all figures cited are average ranges for white adults over 25 years of age): TSF of 10 to 12 mm in men and 21 to 25 mm in women (however, wide variations occur [National Center for Health Statistics]); MUAC of 319 to 322 mm in men and 277 to 299 in women (National Center for Health Statistics); AMC of 279 to 281 mm in men and 212 to 290 mm in women; BMI of 20 to 27 (generally considered healthy, although the risk of health problems, e.g., heart disease increases with an index over 25).

KEY ELEMENTS OF TAKING ANTHROPOMETRIC MEASUREMENTS

- Measure the triceps skinfold on the upper back of the arm along the long axis of the humerus.
- Measure the scapular skinfold at an angle of about 45° from the horizontal plane, upward medially and downward laterally.
- When measuring the MUAC, make sure that the upper arm hangs freely and the forearm is positioned horizontally.
- Use the appropriate formula to calculate the AMC, or use available tables.
- To calculate the BMI, measure the height in meters and the weight in kilograms; then multiply the height by itself, and divide the weight by this total.

Assisting Adults with Meals

Some people who are ill require assistance eating. The amount and type of assistance needed depend on the physical and mental limitations of the person. Two groups of people frequently require help: the elderly, who are weakened and quickly fatigued when they are ill; and the handicapped (e. g., blind people), those who must remain in a back-lying position, or those who do not have use of their hands. The client's nursing care plan will indicate that assistance is required with meals.

Because adults are normally able to eat independently, they may find assistance of any kind embarrassing and difficult to accept. Often clients become depressed because they require help and because they believe they are burdensome to busy nursing personnel. It is very important not to convey either verbally or nonverbally impatience or annoyance while assisting people to eat. Rather, appear unhurried, and convey that you have ample time.

Because clients are frequently confined to their beds, particularly in acute care settings, most hospitals must have meals brought to the client. Often the client receives a tray that has been assembled in a central hospital kitchen or a kitchen adjacent to the nursing unit. Nursing personnel may be responsible for giving out and collecting the trays; in some settings, this is done by special dietary personnel. Some hospitals serve meals to ambulatory clients in a special dining area, and the clients are expected to go there to eat. Other agencies, e.g., day-care centers, have a coffee shop for food or machines from which clients can obtain sandwiches and beverages.

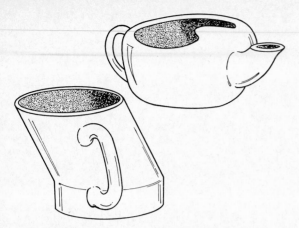

FIGURE 22–4   Two types of special drinking cups.

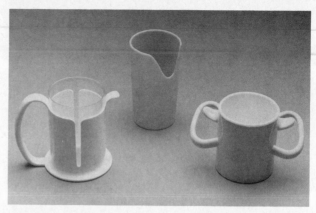

FIGURE 22–5   Left to right: glass holder; cup with hole for nose; two-handled cup with thumb tabs.

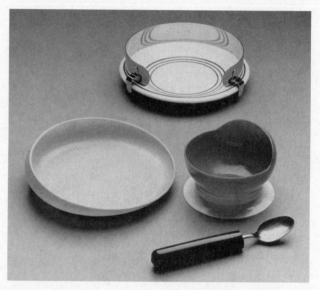

FIGURE 22–6   Clockwise from top: dinner plate with guard attached; bowl with stable base and lip; wide-handled spoon; lipped plate.

Although normal utensils should be used whenever possible, the nurse may need to use special utensils to assist a client to eat. Straws help many people who have difficulty drinking from a cup or glass. Straws often permit clients to obtain liquids with less effort and with less spillage, which can be embarrassing to many clients. Special drinking cups are also available. One model has a spout; another is specially designed to permit drinking with less tipping of the cup than is normally required (Figure 22–4).

Many adaptive feeding aids are available to help clients maintain independence. A standard eating utensil with a built-up or widened handle helps clients who cannot grasp objects easily. Utensils with wide handles can be purchased, or a regular eating utensil can be modified by taping foam around the handle. The foam increases friction and thus steadies the client's grasp. Handles may be bent or angled to compensate for limited motion. Collars or bands that prevent the utensil from being dropped can be attached to the end of the handle and fit over the client's hand.

Plates with rims and plastic or metal plate guards enable the client to pick up the food by first pushing it against this raised edge. A suction cup or damp sponge or cloth may be placed under the dish to keep it from moving while the client is eating. No-spill mugs and two-handled drinking cups are especially useful for persons with impaired hand coordination. Stretch terry cloth and knitted or crocheted glass covers enable the client to keep a secure grasp on a glass. Lidded tip-proof glasses are also available. Figures 22–5 and 22–6 show some of these eating aids.

Technique 22–2 explains the steps involved in assisting clients with meals.

22-2   Assisting an Adult to Eat

PURPOSES
- To maintain the client's nutritional status
- To teach the client required eating skills

ASSESSMENT FOCUS

Self-care abilities for eating and assistance required (note hand coordination, level of consciousness, and visual acuity); appetite for and tolerance of food and fluid; difficulty swallowing; anthropometric measurements for baseline data as required; any need for a special diet; any food allergies and food likes and dislikes.

EQUIPMENT
- Meal tray with the correct food and fluids
- Extra napkin or small towel
- Straw, special drinking cup, weighted glass, or other adaptive feeding aid as required

INTERVENTION

1. Confirm the client's diet order.

- Check the client's chart or Kardex for the diet order and to determine whether the client is fasting for laboratory tests or surgery or whether the physician has ordered "nothing by mouth" (NPO). For clients who are fasting or on NPO, ensure that the appropriate signs are placed on either the room door or the client's bed, according to agency practice.

- If there is a change in the type of food the client is to receive, notify the dietary staff.

2. Prepare the client and overbed table.

- Assist the client to the bathroom or onto a bedpan or commode if the client needs to urinate.

- Offer the client assistance in washing the hands prior to a meal. If the client has problems with oral hygiene, brushing the teeth or using a mouthwash can improve the taste in the mouth and hence the appetite.

- Clear the overbed table so that there is space for the tray. If the

client must remain in a lying position in bed, arrange the overbed table close to the bedside so that the client can see the food.

3. Position the client and yourself appropriately.

- Assist the client to a comfortable position for eating. Most people sit during a meal; if it is permitted, assist the client to sit in bed (Figure 22–7) or in a chair, whichever is appropriate.
  or
  If the client is unable to sit, assist the client to a lateral position. *People will swallow more easily in*

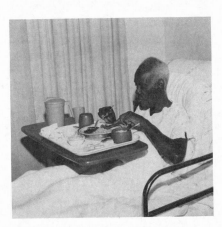

FIGURE 22–7   A supported sitting position contributes to a client's comfort while eating.

these positions than in a back-lying position.

- If the client requires assistance with feeding, assume a sitting position, if possible, beside the client. *This position conveys a more relaxed presence, which is more conducive to the client's eating an adequate meal.*

4. Assist the client as required.

- Check each tray for the client's name, the type of diet, and completeness. If the diet does not seem to be correct, check it against the client's chart. Confirm the client's name by checking the wristband before leaving the tray. Do *not* leave an incorrect diet for a client to eat.

- Encourage the client to eat independently, assisting as needed. Do not take over the feeding process. *Participation by the client enhances feelings of independence.*

- Remove the food covers, butter the bread, pour the tea, and cut the meat, if needed.

- For a blind person, identify the placement of the food as you

► **Technique 22–2 Assisting an Adult to Eat** *CONTINUED*

would describe the time on a clock. For instance, say, "The potatoes are at eight o'clock; the beef steak at 12 o'clock; and the green beans at 4 o'clock." (Figure 22–8).

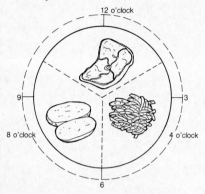

FIGURE 22–8 The clock system used to describe the location of food on the plate for a blind client.

- If assistance with feeding is required,

  a. Ask in which order the client desires to eat the food.

  b. Use normal utensils whenever possible. *Using ordinary utensils enhances self-esteem.*

See also the discussion of adaptive feeding aids on page 544.

c. If the client cannot see, tell which food you are giving.

d. Warn the client if the food is hot or cold.

e. Allow ample time for the client to chew and swallow the food before offering more.

f. Provide fluids as requested, or, if the client is unable to tell you, offer fluids after every three or four mouthfuls of solid food.

g. Use a straw or special drinking cup for fluids that would spill from normal containers.

h. Make the time a pleasant one, choosing topics of conversation that are of interest to the client, if the person wants to talk.

5. After the meal, ensure client comfort.

- Assist the client to clean the mouth and hands.

- Reposition the client.

- Replace the food covers, and remove the food tray from the bedside.

6. Document all relevant information.

- Note how much and what the client has eaten and the amount of fluid taken. Record fluid intake and calorie count as required.

- If the client is on a special diet or is having problems eating, record the amount of food eaten and any pain, fatigue, or nausea experienced.

- If the client is not eating, notify the nurse in charge so that the diet can be changed or other nursing measures can be taken, e.g., rescheduling the meals, providing smaller, more frequent meals, or obtaining special self-feeding aids.

EVALUATION FOCUS

Appetite; tolerance of food and fluids taken; amount of fluid intake, if being measured; calorie count, if required; any chewing or swallowing difficulties and the need for any adjustments in food consistency (e.g., minced or pureed foods, need for special feeding aids); comparison of anthropometric measurements to baseline data, as required.

SAMPLE RECORDING

Date	Time	Notes
05/13/93	0800	Refused all solid food. Ingested 120 ml milk. Nauseated. Dull crampy pain persists in epigastric region. —————— Wendy B. Low, SN

KEY ELEMENTS OF ASSISTING AN ADULT TO EAT

- Assess clinical signs of nutrition status for baseline data.
- Determine how much and what kind of assistance is needed for meals.
- Position the client appropriately for meals.

- Encourage as much independence as possible.
- Observe the client's food intake.
- Document any assessments and specific interventions.

Breast-Feeding

Three types of breast milk are produced: (a) colostrum, (b) transitional milk, and (c) mature milk. **Colostrum** is a yellowish or creamy fluid that is thicker than later milk and contains more protein, fat-soluble vitamins, and minerals. It also contains high levels of immunoglobulins, which may be a source of immunity for the newborn. Colostrum production may last for several days after birth. **Transitional milk** is produced from 2 to 4 days after delivery until approximately 2 weeks postpartum. This milk contains higher levels of fat, lactose, water-soluble vitamins, and calories than colostrum does. **Mature milk** has a high percentage of water, and although it appears similar to skim milk it has more calories: 20 calories per ounce, whereas skim milk provides only 10 calories per ounce.

Breast-feeding is advantageous to both the mother and the baby for these reasons:

- Suckling stimulates the release of oxytocin in the mother so that uterine involution (retrogression) occurs more quickly after delivery.
- It is convenient and economical, negating the need to purchase and prepare formula.
- It fosters psychologic closeness between the mother and the baby.

Within a breast-feeding period, the composition of the mother's milk changes somewhat. Initially, the water content of milk is high, and the milk appears thin and bluish. Thus, the infant gets relatively dilute milk at the beginning of the feeding, when the infant is very thirsty. As feeding progresses, the fat content increases, and the milk is more concentrated. Most of the fat is produced in the last minute of nursing. The infant then stops nursing and resumes feeding only if the lower fat milk from the other breast is offered. General instructions about breast-feeding are shown in the box on page 548.

22-3   Assisting a Mother to Breast-Feed

PURPOSES

- To provide essential nourishment for the infant's physical growth and development
- To provide protective immunoglobulins for the infant
- To enhance mother/infant attachment

ASSESSMENT FOCUS

Infant: general nutritional status; weight gain or loss; eagerness to nurse or fatigue; ability to suck, or conditions that affect ability to suck (e.g., age, neurologic deficit, or other physiologic stressors); urinary output. *Mother:* soreness or cracking of the nipples; breast engorgement; signs of **mastitis** (red, tender, or warm breasts and fever); elevated temperature or other signs of infection; ingestion of medications that might transfer to breast milk; pleasure or problems from the feeding relationship; mother's attitude about breast-feeding; influence of the father's attitude about breast-feeding.

EQUIPMENT

- ☐ Nursing or support bra
- ☐ Pillows
- ☐ Towel or other protective pillow cover (optional)
- ☐ Water-based cream or hydrous lanolin (optional)
- ☐ Breast pads (optional)

INTERVENTION

1. Ensure infant and mother comfort before the feeding.

- Check whether the infant needs a diaper change. If so, change the diaper, and wash your hands. *A clean diaper is conducive to a pleasurable feeding period.*
- Make sure that the mother voids

immediately before the feeding. *This will prevent discomfort during or disruption of the feeding.*

2. Help the mother to assume a ▶

General Instructions About Breast-Feeding

- Newborns are generally put to the breast as soon as possible after birth. Although some infants are not interested this soon, the experience can be soothing to those who are and provides the mother with psychologic and physiologic benefits.

- Colostrum has sufficient nutrients to satisfy the infant until milk is established. (However, some cultures, e.g., Mexican-American, Navajo, Filipino, and Vietnamese, do not offer colostrum to the newborn. In these cultures, breast-feeding begins when the milk flow is established, several days after delivery.)

- Establishment of lactation depends on the frequency of nursing and the strength of the infant's sucking.

- Breast milk is more easily digested than formula, so breast-fed infants become hungry sooner and feed more frequently.

- Fatigue or excitement may decrease the milk supply temporarily, but increasing the frequency of feeding will alleviate this problem.

- The infant will probably demand more frequent feedings during growth spurts: at 10 to 14 days, 5 to 6 weeks, and 3 months.

- Infants routinely lose several ounces during their first few days of life. This weight loss is no cause for alarm.

- The mother can expect some cramping of the uterus during breast-feeding until it returns to its original size. The release of oxytocin, which contracts the muscles of the uterus and initiates the *letdown reflex* (milk ejection reflex) causes this cramping.

- Relaxation promotes the letdown reflex, which may take 3 minutes to activate. When this reflex occurs, the mother may feel a tingling sensation, and milk may spray or drip from her nipples.

- Developing a breast-feeding routine takes time. There is no standard schedule.

- Adequacy of intake is difficult to determine with breast-fed babies, since there is no visual assurance of the amounts consumed. Intake is adequate if the baby gains weight and wets six or more diapers a day. The mother can also listen for and hear the sounds of the baby swallowing during nursing.

- Supplementary feedings, such as glucose and water, are unnecessary for breast-fed infants. Frequent supplemental bottle feedings often confuse the infant and weaken the sucking reflex; the infant may also become used to the artificial nipple and reject the mother's breast. If an infant fails to nurse sufficiently, it is preferable to express milk manually and offer it through a small syringe or medicine dropper.

- Manual expression of milk may be necessary if the mother will be absent for a scheduled feeding or if she is advised to forego a feeding because of breast discomfort. The milk is manually expressed by squeezing the nipple between the thumb and index finger. Because milk supply decreases if the breasts are not emptied regularly, manual expression of milk maintains the milk supply. Manually expressed milk can be frozen in a plastic bottle for a future feeding. Use of glass bottles is discouraged because antibodies in milk adhere to the sides of glass bottles, thus depleting the milk of some of its benefits.

- Some nipple soreness is to be expected initially with breast-feeding. It is most pronounced during the first few minutes until the letdown reflex is established. Nipple soreness can be relieved by having the infant change feeding positions, from the cradle hold to side-lying positions. In the side-lying position, the infant can be positioned with either the feet toward or away from the mother's head (see Figure 23–10). Nipple trauma and soreness can also be decreased if the mother nurses more frequently and for less lengthy periods.

- Breast engorgement (breasts that are hard, painful, warm to the touch, and taut and shiny in appearance) may occur when the milk initially comes in. Engorgement is initially caused by venous congestion due to the increased vascularity in the breasts. The problem is compounded by the pressure of accumulating milk. Comfort and corrective measures include application of hot compresses to the breasts, massage of the breasts, wearing a supportive nursing bra, frequent nursing if possible, manual expression of milk, use of a nontraumatic breast pump to initiate milk flow, and judicious use of analgesics. Engorgement is generally relieved in 12 to 24 hours.

- The mother should be encouraged to take a nap every day, especially for the first few weeks after delivery.

- The mother needs to eat a balanced diet and drink plenty of fluids (8 glasses per day) while breast-feeding.

- The mother should avoid taking medications that can be secreted in milk, e.g., aspirin, antibiotics, alcohol, addicting drugs, and cathartics. If the mother requires medical treatment, her physician should be informed that she is nursing.

▶ **Technique 22–3 Assisting a Mother to Breast-Feed** *CONTINUED*

comfortable feeding position. *A comfortable position aids the letdown reflex.*

- The *madonna* or *cradle position* (Figure 22–9) for breast-feeding is usually preferred.

    a. The mother sits comfortably in a chair or in bed with the infant.

    b. She supports the infant on her lap and her forearm on the side of the exposed breast.

    c. The infant's neck rests on the antecubital space of her arm.

    d. She supports her forearm with a pillow (optional). *The madonna position allows the mother a free hand to manipulate her breast and thus facilitate breast-feeding.*

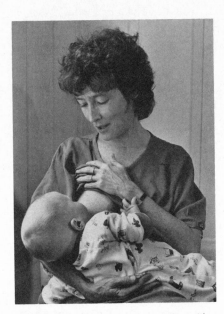

FIGURE 22–9 The madonna or cradle position for breast-feeding.

- The *side-lying position* (Figure 22–10) is particularly useful for a mother who has had a cesarean section and cannot tolerate having the infant rest against her abdomen for long periods or for a mother who has had an episiot-

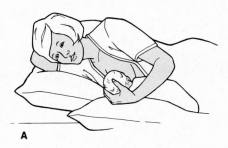

A

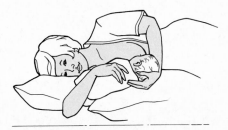

B

FIGURE 22–10 The side-lying position for breast feeding: *A,* infant positioned with feet away from the mother's head; *B,* infant positioned with feet toward the mother's head.

omy and cannot sit comfortably for long periods.

    a. The mother lies on her side.

    b. She raises her lower arm and flexes it beneath her head on a pillow.

    c. The infant is positioned with the feet either away from the mother's head (Figure 22–10, *A*) or toward her head (Figure 22–10, *B*).

    d. The mother feeds the infant on either breast.

3. Help the mother expose her breast and insert the nipple into the infant's mouth.

- Instruct her to position the infant so that the child's entire body is turned toward her and the mouth is adjacent to the nipple. *This prevents the mother from having to lift her shoulder or breast when directing the nipple into the mouth and ensures the comfort of both mother and infant during the feeding.*

- Instruct her to place her thumb

above the nipple on the areolar tissue and two fingers below the nipple, or place her index finger above and middle finger below the nipple to guide the nipple into the infant's mouth.

- Have her stroke the infant's cheek closest to the breast with the nipple. She should avoid touching the other cheek or both cheeks together. *Touching the cheek nearest the breast stimulates the rooting reflex. Touching the other cheek may make the infant turn away from the breast. Touching both cheeks confuses the infant.*

- As the infant is rooting for the nipple, instruct her to insert the nipple, including as much areolar tissue as possible, into the baby's mouth. Direct the nipple straight into the mouth, not toward the tongue or palate. *As much areolar tissue as possible is inserted so that as the baby sucks, sufficient pressure is exerted by the lips, gums, and cheek muscles to compress the milk sinuses directly beneath the areola.*

- Have the mother check for occlusion of the infant's nostrils while nursing. If they are occluded, have her press her finger on the breast below the infant's nostrils. *This pushes the breast away to make breathing room for the infant.*

- If the infant is either too sleepy or too active to suck and feed, have the mother rub the infant's feet, change the diaper, loosen the clothing, and/or change her position or the infant's. *Stimulation and activity will arouse the sleepy infant. These activities may also assist an active newborn to calm down.*

- If the infant is initially reluctant to nurse or uninterested in

► **Technique 22–3 Assisting a Mother to Breast-Feed** *CONTINUED*

breast-feeding, the nurse should instruct the mother

a. That it may take several days for the infant to adjust.

b. To express a small amount of milk and then encourage the infant to suck. *Already flowing milk encourages some infants to suck eagerly.*

4. Instruct the mother to nurse from both breasts at each feeding.

- Advise her to begin with 5 minutes on each side and progress to 7 minutes and then 10 minutes on each side within 3 days. *A 10- to 15-minute period usually empties the breast.*

- Advise the mother to alternate breasts at each feeding, i.e., start with the breast used last at the previous feeding. *Alternating breasts during and between feeding facilitates access to mature milk from each breast and may decrease breast soreness.*

- Advise her to fasten a small safety pin to the bra cup on the side used last for nursing. *The safety pin reminds her to start nursing on that side at the next feeding.*

5. Remove the infant from the breast, and burp the infant.

- To remove the infant from the breast, instruct the mother to insert a finger into the side of the infant's mouth. *Inserting a finger breaks the suction seal and allows the nipple to be removed without trauma.*

- Have the mother burp the infant

before feeding on the other breast and at the end of the feeding. See Technique 22–4, page 553, for burping techniques. *Burping helps the infant expel swallowed air and therefore consume maximum amounts of milk.*

- If the infant has been crying, burp the infant before the feeding begins.

6. Encourage actions that enhance attachment/bonding.

- If the infant remains awake and the mother wishes, allow the mother to nurse the infant longer than ten minutes. *This satisfies the infant's need to suck and promotes bonding.*

- When the mother has finished nursing, encourage her to hold the infant if desired.

7. Ensure infant safety after nursing.

- Place the infant in the lateral position, with a roll at the back for support, or in the prone position. *These positions prevent aspiration of vomitus should regurgitation occur.*

8. Provide instructions about nipple care.

- Have the mother air dry her nipples for at least 15 minutes and apply lanolin or cream, if desires. *These measures prevent nipple irritation and cracking or relieve existing irritation.*

- Although there is no need to remove the lanolin or cream before the next feeding, the infant may

object to the taste of the substance. If so, have the mother wash her nipples with water. Avoid use of soap and a washcloth. *Soap and washcloths may remove the natural oils and keratin layer buildup on the aerolar tissue.*

9. Provide instructions about leakage of milk between feedings. Instruct the mother

- To insert absorbent breast pads in her bra. Avoid the use of plastic-lined breast pads. *Plastic liners interfere with air circulation and may cause nipple irritation. Breast pads without plastic liners absorb secretions.*

- To change the breast pads frequently. *Moist pads can contribute to nipple irritation or nipple infection.*

- To apply direct pressure to the breast with her fingers, hand, or forearm. *Pressure to the breast stops the leaking.*

- That milk leakage will cease when the supply of milk meets the demands of the infant. Initially more milk is being produced than the infant requires.

10. Recognize and support the mother's breast-feeding efforts.

11. Document relevant information.

- Record the teaching provided and any problems experienced by mother or baby.

- Adjust the client's nursing care plan to include areas in which she needs further assistance.

EVALUATION FOCUS

Infant: weight gain; interest in and effectiveness of nursing; adequacy of urine output (i.e., six or more wet diapers daily). *Mother:* nipple status; feelings when nursing; presence of breast engorgement or milk leakage.

▶ **Technique 22–3** *CONTINUED*

Date	Time	Notes
05/12/93	1100	Assisted with breast feeding. Mother relaxed when nursing and infant eager to nurse. Routine instructions about breast feeding provided. (See agency pamphlet). Infant weight—3.6 kg. Mother's nipples intact; some milk leakage. Nipples air-dried × 15 min. after nursing. Absorbent breast pads applied. ——————————————— Sheila A. Whyte, SN

KEY ELEMENTS OF ASSISTING A MOTHER TO BREAST-FEED

- Change the infant's diaper, and ensure that the mother's bladder is empty before the feeding.
- Make sure that the mother assumes a comfortable feeding position with the infant.
- Teach the mother
  a. How to guide her nipple into the infant's mouth.
  b. How to stimulate the rooting reflex.
  c. How to prevent occlusion of the infant's nose while nursing.
  d. How to stimulate a sleepy infant.
  e. Length of time to nurse each breast and to alternate breasts at each feeding.
  f. How to remove the infant from the breast.
  g. Burping techniques.
  h. Actions that enhance bonding.
  i. Proper positions of the infant after feeding.
  j. Nipple care.
- Assess infant weight gains or losses and the mother's physical and psychologic comfort with breast-feeding.

Formula (Bottle) Feeding

Several types of infant milk feedings are available: cow's milk formulas, soy formulas, and predigested formulas. These products are designed to resemble human milk as closely as possible but have different types and amounts of protein, fats, and carbohydrates. Many are fortified with vitamins A and D. If there is a family history of allergy, cow's milk formula (or other nonhuman formulas) may trigger an allergic reaction and should be introduced with care.

Cow's Milk Formulas

Most formulas are made from modified cow's milk. The major protein in cow's milk—casein—produces a tough curd in the stomach and is difficult for the infant to digest; thus, most milk-based formulas are heat-treated to make the casein easier to digest. The butterfat is replaced by more readily absorbed polyunsaturated vegetable oils. Additional lactose or other carbohydrate is included, and vitamins and most minerals are added in amounts resembling those in human milk. Because there is some debate about the infant's need for iron, most infant formula producers make two products—one fortified with iron and one not fortified. Some experts believe that the healthy newborn has sufficient iron stores in the liver to last for about 6 months; others believe that infants who receive an iron-supplemented formula will not deplete their own stores. The new mother needs to be advised to seek her pediatrician's advice when deciding which product to choose. Most formulas are available as a powder, a liquid concentrate, or a ready-to-use product. Before use, powders and liquid concentrates, including evaporated milk, require reconstitution with water.

Soy Formulas

Soy formulas are made from the protein of soybeans. These formulas may be recommended for infants who are potentially allergic to cow's milk protein. Because infant's can also be allergic to soy protein, it is not recommended for infants who have already shown signs of an allergy. Infants may be allergic to both types of protein.

Predigested Formulas

In predigested formulas, the protein, fat, or carbohydrate, or all three, are modified to suit the infant with allergies or digestive problems. They are based on a nonallergic and highly digestible protein. Examples are Pregestimil and Nutramigen.

22-4 Bottle-Feeding an Infant

PURPOSES
- To provide the nutrients required for normal growth and life
- To provide feelings of love and security to the infant for sound psychologic development

ASSESSMENT FOCUS

The infant's general nutritional status; weight gain or loss; development of suck reflex; eagerness to take fluids; family history of allergy. The mother's education level or ability to understand feeding instructions; previous experience with infant feeding.

EQUIPMENT

- Sterile bottle
- Sterile nipple
- Sterile formula
- Bib or clean cloth

INTERVENTION

1. Obtain essential information before the feeding:

- The type of formula recommended by the physician

- The amount per feeding, e.g., 4 to 5 oz

- The type of bottle and nipple used

- The frequency of feeding, e.g., every 4 hours, and the specific times of day

- How the formula is prepared, i.e., at what dilution

- What other fluids, e.g., water or apple juice, are given at scheduled times per day and the amounts

2. Prepare the bottle, nipple, and formula.

- If the formula is refrigerated, warm it to room temperature. The formula should feel lukewarm to the inner wrist when a few drops are shaken onto it. *Babies digest formula at room temperature more quickly than cold formula and are less likely to develop abdominal cramps.*

- Test the size of the nipple holes by turning the bottle upside down. If a drop of milk appears

at the tip of the nipple, the holes are the correct size. If no milk appears or if milk flows out freely, the nipple needs to be changed. *The nipple holes need to be large enough to allow the baby to get formula with normal sucking but not large enough to allow milk to flow freely, which can cause choking and regurgitation. Nipple holes that are too small require too much energy to suck, and too much air is sucked with them.*

3. Ensure infant comfort.

- Check whether the infant needs a diaper change. If so, change the diaper. Handle the infant calmly, gently, and unhurriedly. *A clean, dry diaper is conducive to pleasurable feeding. Calm, gentle handling soothes the infant.*

- Arrange a quiet, comfortable environment in which to feed the infant. *A calm environment is conducive to successful feeding.*

- Carry the infant, using the football hold, to the feeding chair (see Figure 15–7, page 390). *The football hold supports the infant's head and back yet frees one of the nurse's hands to carry the bib and formula.*

- Sit comfortably in the chair, and

relax. *Discomfort and tension can be transmitted to the infant and can interfere with feeding and digestion.*

- Tuck the bib or clean cloth under the infant's chin.

4. Position the infant appropriately.

- Cradle the baby in your arms, with the head slightly elevated. Support the head and neck in the bend of your elbow while the buttocks rest on your lap. *Elevating the head facilitates swallowing. Infants need to be held while being fed to feel warm and loved.*

- If the baby cannot be removed from an isolette or crib because of therapy (e.g., an oxygenated croupette or traction), provide as much hand contact as possible, and stay with the infant during the feeding.

- Never leave an infant with a propped bottle. *The infant can suck in excessive air or ingest the formula too quickly. Both circumstances induce regurgitation and possible aspiration of fluid into the lungs, which can cause pneumonia in the baby.*

5. Insert the nipple, and feed the infant.

▶ **Technique 22–4** *CONTINUED*

- Insert the nipple gently along the infant's tongue and hold the bottle at about a 45° angle so that the nipple is filled with formula and not air (Figure 22–11). *Excessive swallowed air causes gas, abdominal distention, discomfort, and possible regurgitation.*

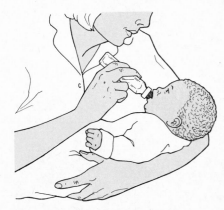

FIGURE 22–11 Position of infant and bottle when bottle-feeding an infant.

6. Remove the bottle periodically and burp (bubble) the baby.

- Small infants may need to be burped after every ounce or at least at the middle and end of the feeding. With some collapsible feeding bottles, infants suck in very little air and may need to be burped only at the end of the feeding. The infant who was crying before the feeding may have swallowed air and may need to be burped before the feeding begins or after taking just enough formula to calm down. *Periodic burping helps the infant expel the swallowed air and therefore consume the maximum amount of formula.*

- Place the baby either

  a. Over your shoulder (Figure 22–12).

  b. In a supported sitting position on your lap (Figure 22–13). *This position is often preferred because the infant's responses can be observed continuously.*

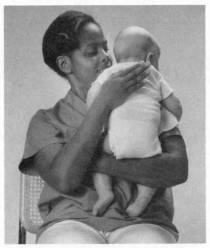

FIGURE 22–12 Burping an infant over the shoulder.

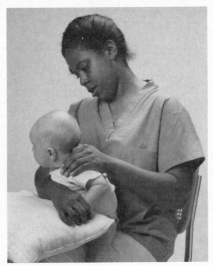

FIGURE 22–13 Burping an infant in a supported sitting position.

  c. In a prone position over your lap (Figure 22–14).

- Place the bib where it will protect your clothing. *Newborns frequently regurgitate small amounts of feedings. This normal occurrence may be due initially to excessive mucus and gastric irritation from foreign substances in the stomach from birth. Later, regurgitation may occur when the infant feeds too rapidly and swallows air or when the infant is overfed and the cardiac sphincter*

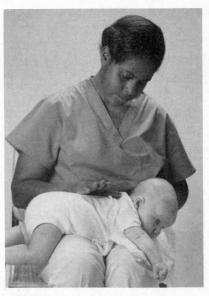

FIGURE 22–14 Burping an infant in a prone position.

allows the excess to be regurgitated.

- Rub or pat the infant's back gently. *Patting encourages relaxation of the cardiac sphincter of the stomach and the expulsion of air.*

7. Continue with the feeding until the formula is finished and/or the baby is satisfied.

- An infant feeding generally takes about 30 minutes. *Prolonged feeding times tend to foster lazy eating habits.*

- For newborns who need encouragement to continue sucking during initial feedings, provide gentle tactile stimulation to the feet and hands. *Stimulation helps maintain sucking for a sufficient time to complete a feeding.*

- Once feedings are established, encourage the infant to set the pace.

- Avoid overfeeding or feeding every time the infant cries. *Overfeeding results in infant obesity. A fat baby is not necessarily healthy.*

▶

Technique 22–4 Bottle-Feeding an Infant *CONTINUED*

8. Ensure infant safety and comfort after the feeding.

- Return the infant to the crib or isolette.

- Check whether the diaper needs changing, and change it if necessary. *Smaller infants commonly move their bowels while feeding because of the gastrocolic reflex.*

- Position the infant on the side or on the abdomen with the head to one side. *In these positions, the infant is less likely to aspirate any fluid that may be regurgitated. For infants in whom regurgitation is a problem, a right side-lying position tends to facilitate the expulsion of air without regurgitation, since the cardiac sphincter is on the left side of the stomach.*

- Ensure that the crib sides are elevated before leaving the infant.

- Assess the infant for signs of allergic reaction, particularly with initial formula usage or when formula type is changed.

9. Document all relevant information.

- Record the type and the amount of the feeding taken and all assessments.

EVALUATION FOCUS

Responses of the infant (e.g., amount and frequency of regurgitation, whether the infant seems satisfied after the feeding and rests quietly, any allergy), weight gain or loss; color and characteristics of the feces or urine.

SAMPLE RECORDING

Date	Time	Notes
06/06/93	0700	5 oz Similac taken well. Regurgitated small amount formula × 1. Resting quietly on right side. ——————————— Sally R. Duprez, SN

KEY ELEMENTS OF BOTTLE-FEEDING AN INFANT

- Use sterile equipment and formula.
- Warm a refrigerated formula to room temperature before the feeding.
- Test the size of the nipple holes.
- Change the infant's diaper before the feeding.
- Handle the infant calmly and gently.
- Cradle the infant with its head slightly elevated.

- Hold the bottle at a 45° angle so that the nipple is filled with formula, not air.
- Never leave an infant with a propped bottle.
- Burp the infant periodically.
- Monitor infant for signs of allergic reaction to formula.
- Ensure infant safety and comfort after the feeding.

Introduction of Solid Foods

The introduction of solid foods to an infant's diet is based on (a) the infant's need for nutrients that solid foods provide and (b) developmental stage or readiness to handle solid foods. Both of these phenomena occur at about the same time—4 to 7 months of age. See the box on page 555 for an infant's developmental abilities relative to feeding.

At 4 to 6 months, infants begin to lose their iron stores if they have not received iron supplements. In addition, the rapid growth of the infant demands foods that provide more energy than breast milk or formula. Iron-fortified infant rice cereal mixed with breast milk or formula is usually introduced as the first solid food. It provides iron and has a smooth, semiliquid texture that the infant can readily handle. As the child develops oral skills and is able to eat foods of thicker consistency, less milk is added to the cereal. The next addition recommended at 6 to 8 months is mashed or chopped cooked or soft fruits and vegetables. These foods provide vitamins A and

C and have lumpier texture that encourages more chewing and tongue movements. At this time, other cereals and "finger" breads, which provide B vitamins and iron, can also be added since the infant's palmar and pincer grasp begins to develop. When the infant is about 7 to 10 months old, minced or finely cut meat casseroles and table foods can be added. The infant who is able to sit in a high chair at this age should be encouraged to adhere to the family eating schedule. At 10 months, the infant begins to handle a cup and manipulate a spoon. Children do not learn to master a spoon until they are 15 to 16 months old. The final transition is a change from breast milk or formula to whole pasteurized milk. This change occurs when the child is about 1 year old, gets a good assortment of foods from the basic four food groups, and eats three meals a day.

New foods are introduced one at a time and in small amounts to permit recognition of allergies. The adult places 2 ml (1/4 tsp) of food well back on the infant's tongue without exerting pressure that would cause the infant to gag. New foods are offered when the infant is hungry and before the formula or food to which the baby is accustomed. No sweetener or medications should be added. Initially, the foods need to be soft and smooth (strained or pureed) and at moderate temperatures. When their teeth begin to erupt (at 6 months of age), infants prefer foods that they can chew, e.g., teething biscuits or chopped cooked vegetables. The shift from pureed to chopped foods needs to be gradual.

At about 7 months of age or later, the infant can be introduced to using a cup at meals. Some infants begin self-feeding with a cup at 9 to 10 months of age, when they are also beginning to manipulate a spoon. By the end of the transition period, all of the infant's nutritional requirements can be met by a mixed diet of table foods.

Infants may be fed solids while being held in the arms, as for bottle-feeding, or while seated and

The Infant's Developmental Abilities in Relation to Feeding

- The extrusion reflex is normally present for the first 4 months. This reflex causes young infants to spit out solids rather than swallow them. At 4 months, because infants can reach their mouths with their hands, the hands may get in the way during feeding.

- Between 4 and 6 months of age, the infant learns to transfer soft foods from the front of the tongue to the back.

- By 5 to 6 months, infants can sit with support, can grasp objects in a mittenlike fashion, can bring their lips to the rim of a cup and begin drinking, and can begin to chew.

- At 7 months, infants can feed themselves a biscuit, like to play with food and smear it, bang cups and objects on the table, and enjoy finger foods (e.g., pieces of banana).

- At 9 months, infants can hold their bottles, sit erect unsupported in a highchair, and develop finger-to-thumb (pincer) movements to pick up food.

- At 10 months, infants poke at food with their index fingers, reach for food and utensils, and like to hold a spoon and push objects with it.

- Beyond 10 months, infants show an increased desire to feed themselves. They begin to use a spoon and to hold a cup with both hands, but frequency spill food. Between 2 and 3 years of age, self-feeding is completed with only occasional spilling.

restrained in an infant seat. When old enough to sit unsupported, the infant can sit on the nurse's or another person's lap rather than in an infant seat. Young children progress to a highchair.

22-5 Feeding Solid Foods to an Infant

PURPOSES
- To provide nutrients and calories to meet the infant's needs
- To promote muscular development of the mouth and tongue

ASSESSMENT FOCUS
Developmental status (e.g., extrusion reflex); appetite; food likes and dislikes; food allergies.

▶ Technique 22–5 Feeding Solid Foods to an Infant CONTINUED

EQUIPMENT

- ☐ Small feeding spoon and unbreakable dishes
- ☐ Proper food (e.g., pureed or diced) at room temperature
- ☐ Bib
- ☐ Infant seat or high chair, if required

INTERVENTION

1. Prepare the infant and yourself for the meal.

- Change the diaper if damp or soiled.

- Wash hands.

- Approach the infant in a pleasant, relaxed manner, and provide a calm environment. *An infant old enough to eat solids will be well aware of this, because interest in the surroundings is increasing.*

- Put the bib on the infant, and place the infant on your lap or in the infant seat or highchair.

- Seat yourself comfortably, and relax. *Feeding times need to be unhurried and relaxed to promote good eating habits and good digestion.*

2. Promote acceptance and digestion of the food.

- Control the infant's hands with your free hand by giving something to hold or by gently holding the arms (Figure 22–15). *Holding the arms prevents young infants from smearing their food.*

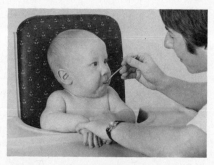

FIGURE 22–15 Controlling an infant's hands when feeding the infant in a highchair.

- Offer plain foods before sweet ones, e.g., cereal and vegetables before fruits. *Infants may reject plain foods after eating the sweeter tasting ones.*

- Place small spoonfuls of food well back on the infant's tongue. *Putting food well back in the mouth overcomes the extrusion reflex, if it is present.*

- Scrape up any food that is pushed back out of the mouth, and refeed it.

- Continue to feed at a pace appropriate for the infant until the infant is satisfied. Hungry infants tend to eat quickly and show frustration if the food is given too slowly.

- Talk to the infant throughout the meal. *Friendly talk at mealtimes is conducive to digestion and socialization.*

3. Provide follow-up care as needed.

- Wash and dry the infant's face and hands.

- Feed a young infant the recommended formula.

- Change the diaper, if required.

- Place the infant in a safe position in the crib. (See Technique 22–4, step 8.) Encourage the child to nap or rest. Ensure that the crib sides are elevated before leaving the infant.

4. Document all relevant information.

- Record assessments, the type and amount of feeding taken, and the infant's responses.

EVALUATION FOCUS	Type and amount of food ingested; weight gain or loss; specific food likes and dislikes.

KEY ELEMENTS OF FEEDING SOLID FOODS TO AN INFANT

- Change a soiled diaper before the feeding.
- Provide a calm, relaxed environment.
- Control the infant's hands during feeding.
- Introduce new foods one at a time, and watch for allergic reactions.

- Offer plain foods before sweet ones.
- Place food well back on the tongue.
- Ensure infant comfort and safety following the meal.

CRITICAL THINKING CHALLENGE

Maria Gonzalez is a 42-year-old female who is being treated as an outpatient for gall bladder disease. Her physician has ordered a low fat diet and has given her a diet instruction sheet. After reviewing the instruction sheet, Ms Gonzalez confides in the nurse that she doesn't see any foods she likes, and asks if she can eat her usual foods. What should the nurse say and do?

RELATED RESEARCH

Carr, E. K., and Mitchell, J. R. A. 1991. A comparison of the mealtime care giver to patients by nursing using two different meal delivery systems. *International Journal of Nursing Studies* 28:19–25.

Dimant, J., and Solow, B. A. Summer 1988. Nutritional assessment in nursing home patients: Improving nutritional status. *The Journal of Long Term Care Administration* 16:7–9.

Hill, P. D. March 1988. Maternal attitudes and infant feeding among low-income mothers. *Journal of Human Lactation* 4:7–11.

Ott, F.; Readman, T.; and Backman, C. April 1991. Mealtimes of the institutionalized elderly: A quality of life issue. *Canadian Journal of Occupational Therapy* 58:7–16.

REFERENCES

Chernoff, R. February 1990. Physiologic aging and nutritional status. *Nutrition in Clinical Practice* 5:8–13.

Christian, J. L., and Greger, J. L. 1988. *Nutrition for living.* 2d ed. Menlo Park, Calif.: Benjamin/Cummings.

Curtas, S.; Chapman, G.; and Meguid, M. M. June 1989. Evaluation of nutritional status. *Nursing Clinics of North America* 24:301–13.

Dimico, G. May 1991. Teaching breast feeding to working mothers. *International Journal of Childbirth Education* 6:20–21.

Drapo, P. J. 1991. Selecting age-related foods. In Smith, D. P., editor. pp. 371–79. *Comprehensive Child and Family Nursing Skills.* St. Louis: C. V. Mosby Co.

Grant, J. A., and Kennedy-Caldwell, C. 1988. *Nutritional support in nursing.* New York: Grune and Stratton.

Guyton, A. C. 1986. *Textbook of medical physiology.* 7th ed. Philadelphia: W. B. Saunders Co.

Iverson-Carpenter, M. S.; Haskin, D.; Maas, M.; Hardy, M.; and Button, M. April 1988. Fulfilling nutritional requirements. *Journal of Gerontological Nursing* 14:16–24, 46–47.

Kolodny, V., and Malek, A. June 1991. Improving feeding skills. *Journal of Gerontological Nursing* 17:20–24.

Minister of Health and Welfare, Department of Health and Welfare. 1983. *Canada's food guide.* Ottawa: Department of Health and Welfare.

National Center for Health Statistics. *Health and Nutrition Examination Survey of 1971 to 1974,* DHEW Pub. No. (PHS) 79–1310.

Olds, S. B.; London, M. L.; and Ladewig, P. W. 1992. *Maternal-newborn nursing: A family-centered approach.* 4th ed. Redwood City, Calif.: Addison-Wesley Nursing.

Scholl, D. E. 1986. *Nutrition and diet therapy: A handbook for nurses.* Oradell, N.J.: Medical Economics Books.

Williams, S. 1984. *Nutrition and diet therapy.* 4th ed. St. Louis: C. V. Mosby Co.

Williams, S. R.; Worthington-Roberts, B. S.; Schlenker, E. D.; Pipes, P.; Rees, J. M.; and Mahan, L. K., editors. 1988. *Nutrition throughout the life cycle.* St. Louis: Times Mirror/Mosby College Publishing.

23

Gastric and Jejunal Feedings

Contents

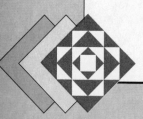

NURSING PROCESS GUIDE

GASTRIC AND JEJUNAL FEEDINGS

ASSESSMENT

Assess

- Allergies to any food in the feeding. Commonly included foods are milk, sugar, water, eggs, and vegetable oil.

- Bowel sounds to determine intestinal activity.

- Abdominal distention at least daily. Measure the client's abdominal girth at the umbilicus. A distended abdomen may indicate intolerance to a previous feeding.

- Correct placement of the tube before feedings (see page 560).

- Presence of regurgitation and feelings of fullness after feedings.

- Dumping syndrome. Jejunostomy clients may experience nausea, vomiting, diarrhea, cramps, pallor, sweating, heart palpitations, increased pulse rate, and fainting after a feeding. These are signs of dumping syndrome, which results when hypertonic foods and liquids suddenly distend the jejunum. To make the intestinal contents isotonic, body fluids shift rapidly from the client's vascular system. Smaller, more frequent feedings, slower feedings, and a longer adjustment period may relieve dumping.

- Presence of diarrhea, constipation, or flatulence. The lack of bulk in liquid feedings may cause constipation. The presence of concentrated ingredients may cause diarrhea and flatulence.

- Urine for sugar and acetone. Monitor the client's urine every 4 to 6 hours for the first 48 hours after initial feedings are begun.

- Hydration status. Measure the client's fluid intake and output, and note any complaints of thirst. Additional water may need to be instilled between feedings.

- Changes in anthropometric measurements, i.e., weight, triceps skin fold, and arm muscle circumferences. See Chapter 22.

- Blood glucose, electrolytes, blood urea nitrogen, creatinine, transferrin, albumin, total protein, cholesterol levels, complete blood count, and liver function. All or some of the above tests may be ordered weekly or monthly.

Identify factors that may increase the risk for inadvertent respiratory placement of feeding tubes:

- Inability of the client to cooperate during tube insertion (e.g., inability to swallow on command)

- Absent or diminished reflexes to protect the airway (e.g., impaired cough reflex, impaired gag reflex)

- Decreased mental status

- Neurologic impairment

- Advanced age and debilitation

- Critical illness

- Use of neuromuscular blocking agents

- Presence of endotracheal tube with low-pressure cuff or tracheostomy

- Nasopharyngeal or gastroesophageal surgery, trauma, or congenital malformation

RELATED DIAGNOSTIC CATEGORIES

- High risk for Aspiration

- Fluid volume deficit

- High risk for Fluid volume deficit

- Altered nutrition: Less than body requirements

- Self-care deficit: Feeding

PLANNING

Client Goals
The client will

- Achieve or maintain hydration and nutritional status.

- Avoid problems associated with tube feedings.

Outcome Criteria
The client

- Has a triceps skinfold measurement, AMC, and BMI within predetermined ranges.

- Has a stable daily weight, weight increase of 2 kg/week, or appropriate weight gain for age.

- Verbalizes feelings of comfort after the feeding.

- Has normal bowel sounds following the feeding.

- Has no abdominal distention or constipation.

- Has normal blood and urine glucose.

Enteral Nutrition

Enteral nutrition or feeding is the administration of nutrients directly through the gastrointestinal tract. Although the most desirable method of providing nutrients is by the independent oral route, this method is not always possible. Tube feedings, administered directly into the stomach or the jejunum, are alternate methods commonly used to maintain or restore the client's nutritional status. To be effective, tube feedings rely upon a functional gastrointestinal tract.

Nasogastric/Nasointestinal Feedings

A **nasogastric feeding (gastric gavage)** or small intestine tube feeding is the instillation of specially prepared nutrients into the digestive tract through a tube that is inserted through one of the nostrils, down the nasopharynx, and into the alimentary tract. In some instances, the tube is passed through the mouth and pharynx, although this route may be more uncomfortable for the adult client and cause gagging. This approach is often used for infants who are obligatory nose breathers (who must breathe through the nose) and premature infants who have no gag reflex.

Traditional firm *large-bore* nasogastric tubes (i.e., those larger than 12 Fr. in diameter) are placed in the stomach. Examples are the *Levin tube*, a flexible, rubber or plastic, single-lumen tube with holes near the tip, or the *Salem-sump tube*, with a double lumen. The larger tube of the Salem sump tube drains gastric contents; the smaller tube allows for an inflow of atmospheric air, which prevents a vacuum if the gastric tube adheres to the wall of the stomach. Irritation of the gastric mucosa is thereby avoided. Newer, softer, more flexible and less irritating *small-bore* tubes (smaller than 12 Fr. in diameter) can be placed in either the stomach or the upper small intestine (i.e., duodenum or jejunum). Clients at risk for pulmonary aspiration (e.g., those with altered pharyngeal reflexes and/or unconsciousness) should be fed via the small intestine rather than the stomach (Metheny 1988, p. 324).

Generally, the position of small-bore pliable tubes is confirmed by radiography before introducing feedings. A major responsibility of the nurse, however, is to verify tube placement (i.e., gastrointestinal placement versus respiratory placement) before each intermittent feeding and at regular intervals (e.g., at least once per shift) when continuous feedings are being administered. Traditionally, placement of large-bore tubes has been verified by the following methods, none of which alone is any guarantee that the tube is correctly positioned. In addition, many methods do not apply to small-bore tubes.

- *Aspirate gastrointestinal secretions.* Gastrointestinal secretions are aspirated more readily through large-bore tubes than through small-bore tubes. Failure to obtain aspirate even with large-bore tubes may or may not indicate that the tube is malpositioned. For example, the tubing parts may be obstructed by the stomach mucosa. Failure to obtain fluid from a small-bore tube may indicate that the walls of the tube collapsed on syringe application.

- *Measure the pH of aspirated fluid.* An acidic pH generally indicates gastric fluid. Values within the acidic range may be as low as 0.8 (with hydrochloric acid secretion) and as high as 5 (Guyton 1986, p. 774). If the client is taking medication altering the pH, some secretions may even become alkaline. Intestinal fluids have a slightly alkaline pH in the range of 7.5 to 8.0 (Guyton 1986, p. 784). Because normal pleural fluid has a pH of 7.4 (Byrne, Saxton, Pelikan, and Nugent 1986, p. 468), this test to determine placement of small-bore intestinal tubes is not effective in differentiating intestinal from pleural fluid. However, it is usually effective in differentiating gastric from intestinal or pleural fluid.

- *Inject 5 to 20 ml of air through the feeding tube while auscultating the epigastrium or left upper abdominal quadrant and listening for a whooshing, gurgling, or bubbling sound.* For infants and small children, inject 0.5 to 5 ml of air to prevent gastric distention with excessive air. Because of the difficulty encountered in aspirating gastrointestinal secretions through small-bore tubes, many nurses in practice prefer and use this method to test tube placement. Air injected in the stomach should be heard immediately. However, it is difficult to differentiate esophageal, gastric, distal duodenal, and proximal jejunal tube placement because of the proximity of these sites. Several authors also report "pseudoconfirmatory gurgling" sounds heard when the tube is malpositioned in the pharynx, esophagus, and respiratory tract (Hand, Kempster, Levy, Rogol, and Spirn 1984; Miller, Tomlinson, and Sahn 1985;

and Metheny, Spies, and Eisenberg 1988). Further research may indicate more precise differentiation of these sounds using a Doppler stethoscope.

- *Ask the client to speak or hum.* It is generally assumed that large-bore tubes placed in the trachea will interfere with the client's ability to speak. However, clients with small-bore tubes may be able to speak, because the vocal cords may not be sufficiently separated to affect phonation.

- *Observe the client for coughing and choking.* Coughing and choking are likely to occur when large-bore tubes enter the respiratory tract but are less likely to occur with the use of small-bore tubes. These responses, however, may be absent with either type of tube in clients with decreased tracheal irritability and an altered level of consciousness.

Currently, the most effective method appears to be radiographic verification of tube placement. Repeated X rays, however, are not feasible in terms of cost and radiation risk. More research is required to devise effective alternatives, especially for placement of small-bore tubes. In the meantime, nurses should (a) ensure initial radiographic verification of small-bore tubes, (b) aspirate contents when possible and check their acidity, (c) auscultate air insufflation, (d) closely observe the client for signs of obvious distress, and (e) suspect tube dislodgement after episodes of coughing, sneezing, and vomiting.

Tube Feedings

Tube feedings are indicated for clients who cannot eat by mouth or swallow a sufficient diet without aspirating food or fluid into the lungs. Feedings may be given continuously over a 24-hour period or at prescribed intervals, e.g., four times per day. Liquid feeding mixtures are available commercially or may be prepared by the dietary department in accordance with the physician's orders. A standard formula provides 1 kcal per milliliter of solution with protein, fat, carbohydrate, minerals, and vitamins in specified proportions. The frequency of feedings and amounts to be administered are ordered by the physician. An adult often requires 300 to 500 ml of mixture per feeding.

Before administering a tube feeding, the nurse must determine any food allergies of the client and assess tolerance to previous feedings. The nurse checks the expiration date on a commercially prepared formula or the preparation date and time of agency-prepared solution, discarding any formula that has passed the expiration date or solution more than 24 hours old.

Feedings are usually adminstered at room temperature unless the order specifies otherwise. The specified amount of solution is warmed in a basin of warm water or left to stand for a while until it reaches room temperature. Continuous feeding should be kept cold; excessive heat coagulates feedings of milk and egg, and hot liquids can irritate the mucous membranes. However, excessively cold feedings can reduce the flow of digestive juices by causing vasoconstriction and may cause cramps. Commercially prepared feedings are available in cans or bottles ready for administration. Some containers are designed so that ice chips can be placed in an outer section to keep the formula cooled.

A feeding pump can be used with a prefilled tube-feeding set to regulate the exact amount of feeding for the client (Figure 23–1). The pump is often used to administer the feeding in instances when smaller-bore gastric tubes are used or when gravity flow is insufficient to instill the feeding. Because the feeding is administered over a long time period, a formula that is warmed can grow microorganisms. It should not hang longer than the manufacturer recommends, e.g., 3 to 4 hours. If it will hang longer, it should be kept cool with ice chips.

Techniques 23–1, 23–2, and 23–3 describe how to insert a nasogastric tube, administer a feeding through an established tube, and remove a nasogastric tube, respectively.

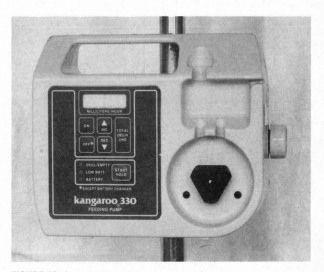

FIGURE 23–1 A feeding pump.

23-1   Inserting a Nasogastric Tube

Before inserting a nasogastric tube determine the size of tube to be inserted and whether or not the tube is to be attached to a suction.

PURPOSES

- To administer tube feedings and medications to clients unable to eat by mouth or swallow a sufficient diet without aspirating food or fluids into the lungs
- To establish a means for suctioning stomach contents to prevent gastric distention, nausea, and vomiting
- To remove stomach contents for laboratory analysis
- To **lavage** (wash) the stomach in case of poisoning or overdose of medications

ASSESSMENT FOCUS

Patency of nares and intactness of nasal tissues (note especially history of nasal surgery or deviated septum); presence of gag reflex; mental status or ability to cooperate with procedure.

EQUIPMENT

- Large- or small-bore tube (plastic or rubber)
- Solution basin filled with warm water (if a plastic tube is being used) or ice (if a rubber tube is being used)
- Nonallergenic adhesive tape, 2.5 cm (1 in) wide
- Disposable gloves

- Water-soluble lubricant
- Facial tissues
- Glass of water and drinking straw or medicine cup with water
- 20- to 50-ml syringe with an adapter
- Basin
- Stethoscope

- Clamp (optional)
- Suction apparatus if required
- Gauze square or plastic specimen bag and elastic band
- Safety pin and elastic band
- Infant seat, towel, or pillow
- Restraint or hand mitts (for infants or small children)
- 5-ml or 12-ml syringe

INTERVENTION

1. Prepare the client.

- Explain to the client what you plan to do. The passage of a gastric tube is not painful, but it is unpleasant because the gag reflex is activated during insertion.

- Assist the client to a high-Fowler's position if health permits, and support the head on a pillow. *It is often easier to swallow in this position, and gravity helps the passage of the tube.*

- Place the infant in an infant seat, or position the infant with a rolled towel or pillow under the head and shoulders.

- Place the towel across the chest. A bib or diaper can be used for an infant.

2. Assess the client's nares.

- Ask the client to hyperextend the head, and, using a flashlight, observe the intactness of the tissues of the nostrils, including any irritations or abrasions.

- Examine the nares for any obstructions or deformities by asking the client to breathe through one nostril while occluding the other.

- Select the nostril that has the greater airflow.

- Obstruct one of the infant's nares, and feel for air passage from the other.

3. Prepare the tube.

- If a rubber tube is being used,

place it on ice. *This stiffens the tube, facilitating insertion.* If a plastic tube is being used, place it in warm water. *This makes the tube more flexible, facilitating insertion.*

4. Determine how far to insert the tube.

- Use the tube to mark off the distance from the tip of the client's nose to the tip of the earlobe and then from the tip of the earlobe to the tip of the sternum (Figure 23–2). *This length approximates the distance from the nares to the stomach. This distance varies among individuals.*

- Measure from the edge of the nares to the tip of the earlobe and then from the tip of the earlobe

▶ **Technique 23–1** *CONTINUED*

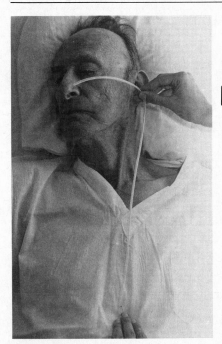

FIGURE 23–2 Measuring the appropriate length to insert a nasogastric tube.

to the point midway between the umbilicus and the xiphoid process (Whaley and Wong 1990).

- Mark this length with adhesive tape if the tube does not have markings.

- For tubes that are to be placed into the duodenum or jejunum, add an additional 20 to 30 cm (Grant and Kennedy-Caldwell 1988, p. 126).

5. Insert the tube.

- Don gloves.

- Lubricate the tip of the tube well with water-soluble lubricant or water to ease insertion. *A water-soluble lubricant dissolves if the tube accidentally enters the lungs. An oil-based lubricant, such as petroleum jelly, will not dissolve and could cause respiratory complications if it enters the lungs.*

- Insert the tube, with its natural curve toward the client, into the selected nostril. Ask the client to hyperextend the neck, and gently

advance the tube toward the nasopharynx. *Hyperextension of the neck reduces the curvature of the nasopharyngeal junction.*

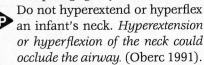 Do not hyperextend or hyperflex an infant's neck. *Hyperextension or hyperflexion of the neck could occlude the airway.* (Oberc 1991).

- Direct the tube along the floor of the nostril and toward the ear on that side. *Directing the tube along the floor avoids the projections (turbinates) along the lateral wall.*

- Slight pressure is sometimes required to pass the tube into the nasopharynx, and some clients' eyes may water at this point. Tears are a natural body response. Provide the client with tissues as needed.

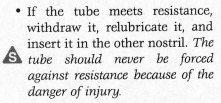 If the tube meets resistance, withdraw it, relubricate it, and insert it in the other nostril. *The tube should never be forced against resistance because of the danger of injury.*

- Once the tube reaches the oropharynx (throat) the client will feel the tube in the throat and may gag and retch. Ask the client to tilt the head forward, and encourage the client to drink and swallow. *Tilting the head forward facilitates passage of the tube into the posterior pharynx and esophagus rather than into the larynx; swallowing moves the epiglottis over the opening to the larynx* (Figure 23–3).

- If the client gags, stop passing the tube momentarily. Have the client rest, take a few breaths, and take sips of water to calm the gag reflex.

- In cooperation with the client, pass the tube 5 to 10 cm (2 to 4 in) with each swallow, until the indicated length is inserted.

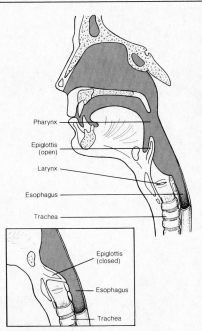

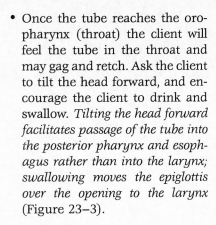

FIGURE 23–3 Swallowing closes the epiglottis.

- If the client continues to gag and the tube does not advance with each swallow, withdraw it slightly, and inspect the throat by looking through the mouth. *The tube may be coiled in the throat.* If so, withdraw it until it is straight, and try again to insert it.

6. Ascertain correct placement of the tube.

- Aspirate stomach contents, and check their acidity.

- Auscultate air insufflation.

- Use other methods in accordance with agency protocol (see page 560).

- If the signs do not indicate placement in the stomach, advance the tube 5 cm (2 in), and repeat the tests.

7. Secure the tube by taping it to the bridge of the client's nose.

- If the client has oily skin, wipe the nose first with alcohol.

- Cut 7.5 cm (3 in) of tape, and

Technique 23–1 Inserting a Nasogastric Tube *CONTINUED*

split it lengthwise at one end, leaving a 2.5-cm (1-in) tab at the end.

- Place the tape over the bridge of the client's nose, and bring the split ends under the tubing and back up over the nose (Figure 23–4). *Taping in this manner prevents the tube from pressing against and irritating the edge of the nostril.* For infants or small children, tape the tube to the area between the end of the nares and the upper lip, as well as to the cheek.

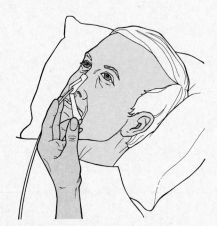

FIGURE 23–4 Taping a nasogastric tube to the bridge of the nose.

8. Attach the tube to a suction source or feeding apparatus as ordered, or clamp the end of the tubing.

- The tube, if inserted preoperatively, is usually clamped, or it may be covered with a gauze square or plastic specimen bag and an elastic band.

9. Secure the tube to the client's gown.

- Loop an elastic band around the end of the tubing, and attach the elastic band to the gown with a safety pin.
or
Attach a piece of adhesive tape to the tube, and pin the tape to the gown. *The tube is attached to prevent it from dangling and pulling.*

- For infants and young children, restraints may be necessary during tube insertion and throughout therapy. *Restraints will prevent accidental dislodging of the tube.*

10. Document relevant information.

- Document the insertion of the tube, means by which correct placement was determined, and assessments (e.g., discomfort or abdominal distention). See sample recording below.

11. Establish a plan for providing daily nasogastric tube care.

- Inspect the nostril for discharge and irritation.

- Clean the nostril and tube with moistened, cotton-tipped applicators.

- Apply water-soluble lubricant to the nostril if it appears dry or encrusted.

- Change the adhesive tape as required.

- Give frequent mouth care. *The client may breathe through the mouth and cannot drink.*

12. If suction is applied, ensure that the patency of both the nasogastric and suction tubes is maintained.

- Irrigations of the tube with 30 ml of normal saline may be required at regular intervals. For infants or small children, use 1 to 10 ml of saline. In some agencies, irrigations must be ordered by the physician. Managing gastrointestinal suction and irrigating a nasogastric tube are discussed in Technique 42–5, page 995.

- Keep accurate records of the client's fluid intake and output, and record the amount and characteristics of the drainage.

VARIATION: Inserting an Orogastric Tube

If the nasal passageway is very small or is obstructed, an **orogastric** tube may be more appropriate.

- Measure from the corner of the mouth to the tip of the earlobe.

- Open the mouth of an infant or comatose client, or ask an older child or adult to open the mouth wide.

- Advance the tube to the back of the throat along the side of the tongue. Withdraw the tube if the client gags.

- Stimulate swallowing with sips of water, and advance the tube with each swallow.

- Check tube placement.

- Tape tubing to the cheek.

EVALUATION FOCUS	Degree of client comfort; client tolerance of tube; correct placement of nasogastric tube in stomach; client understanding of restrictions; color and amount of gastric contents, if attached to suction or contents aspirated.

► **Technique 23–1** *CONTINUED*

SAMPLE RECORDING

Date	Time	Notes
12/09/93	0900	Small bore tube #10 inserted into left nares. No obstruction or difficulty encountered with insertion. Gurgling audible during insertion of air and straw-colored clear fluid with pH of 4 aspirated. Placement confirmed by radiography ———————————————— Colin Nicholson, SN

KEY ELEMENTS OF INSERTING A NASOGASTRIC TUBE

- Minimize discomfort by positioning the client appropriately, lubricating the tube, and working cooperatively with the client.
- Never force the tube against resistance.

- Confirm correct placement of the tube.
- Secure the tube appropriately to the client's nose or nose and cheek.

23-2 Administering a Tube Feeding Through an Established Feeding Tube

Before commencing a nasogastric or orogastric feeding determine the type, amount, and frequency of feedings and tolerance of previous feedings.

PURPOSES
- To restore or maintain nutritional status
- To administer medications

ASSESSMENT FOCUS

Clinical signs of malnutrition or dehydration (see Chapters 22 and 24, pages 536 and 574); allergies to any food in the feeding; presence of bowel sounds; any problems that suggest lack of tolerance of previous feedings, e.g., abdominal distention, dumping syndrome, constipation, or dehydration.

EQUIPMENT

- Correct amount of feeding solution
- Pacifier
- 20- to 50-ml syringe with an adapter
- Emesis basin
- Bulb syringe (for an intermittent feeding)
  or

- Calibrated plastic feeding bag and a drip chamber, which can be attached to the tubing
  or
- Prefilled bottle with a drip chamber, tubing, and a flow-regulator clamp

- Measuring container from which to pour the feeding (if using bulb syringe)
- Water (60 ml unless otherwise specified) at room temperature
- Feeding pump (optional)

►

▶ **Technique 23–2 Administering a Tube Feeding** *CONTINUED*

INTERVENTION

1. Prepare the client and the feeding.

- Explain to the client that the feeding should not cause any discomfort but may cause a feeling of fullness. For an adult, the usual intermittent feeding will take about 30 minutes; the exact length of time depends largely on the volume of the feeding.

- Provide privacy for this procedure if the client desires it. *Nasogastric feedings are embarrassing to some people.*

- Assist the client to a Fowler's position in bed or a sitting position in a chair, the normal position for eating. If a sitting position is contraindicated, a slightly elevated right side-lying position is acceptable. *These positions enhance the gravitational flow of the solution and prevent aspiration of fluid into the lungs.*

P - Position a small child or infant in your lap, and provide a pacifier during feeding. *This promotes comfort, supports the normal sucking instinct of the infant, and facilitates digestion.*

2. Assess tube placement.

- Attach the syringe to the open end of the tube, aspirate alimentary secretions. Check the pH. See page 560 for other methods.

3. Assess residual feeding contents.

- Aspirate all the stomach contents, and measure the amount prior to administering the feeding. *This is done to evaluate absorption of the last feeding, i.e., whether undigested formula from a previous feeding remains.*

P - If 50 ml or more of undigested formula is withdrawn in adults, or 10 ml or more in infants,

check with the nurse in charge before proceeding. The precise amount is usually determined by the physician's order or by agency policy. *At some agencies a feeding is withheld when the specified amount or more of formula remains in the stomach. In other agencies, the amount withdrawn is subtracted from the total feeding and that volume (less the undigested portion) is administered slowly.*
or
Reinstill the gastric contents into the stomach if this is the agency or physician's practice. Remove the syringe bulb or plunger, and pour the gastric contents via the syringe into the nasogastric tube. *Removal of the contents could disturb the client's electrolyte balance.*

4. Administer the feeding.

- Before administering the feeding:

  a. Check the expiration date of the feeding.

  b. Warm the feeding to room temperature. *An excessively cold feeding may cause cramps.*

Bulb Syringe

- Remove the bulb from the syringe, and connect the syringe to a pinched or clamped nasogastric tube. *Pinching or clamping the tube prevents excess air from entering the stomach and causing distention.*

- Add the feeding to the syringe barrel (Figure 23–5).

- Permit the feeding to flow in slowly. Raise or lower the syringe to adjust the flow as needed. Pinch or clamp the tubing to stop the flow for a minute if the client experiences discomfort. *Quicky*

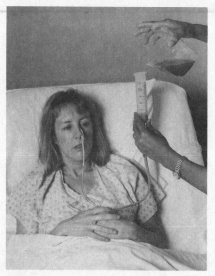

FIGURE 23–5 Using a bulb syringe to administer a tube feeding.

administered feedings can cause flatus, crampy pain, and/or reflux vomiting.

Feeding Bag

- Hang the bag from an infusion pole about 30 cm (12 in) above the tube's point of insertion into the client.

- Clamp the tubing, and add the formula to the bag, if it is not prefilled.

- Open the clamp, run the formula through the tubing, and reclamp the tube. *The formula will displace the air in the tubing, thus preventing the instillation of excess air into the client's stomach or intestine.*

- Attach the bag to the nasogastric tube (Figure 23–6), and regulate the drip by adjusting the clamp to drop factor on bag, e.g., 20 drops/cc.

Prefilled Bottle with Drip Chamber

- Remove the sealed cap from the container, and replace it with the screw-on cap to which the drip

▶ **Technique 23–2** *CONTINUED*

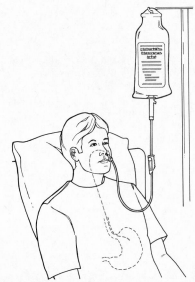

FIGURE 23–6 Using a calibrated plastic bag to administer a tube feeding.

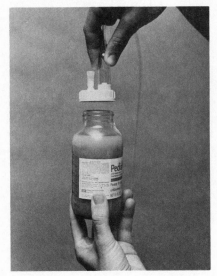

FIGURE 23–7 A prefilled bottle with drip chamber.

chamber and tubing are attached (Figure 23–7).

- Close the clamp on the tubing.

- Hang the container on an intravenous pole about 30 cm (12 in) above the tube's insertion point into the client. *At this height the formula should run at a safe rate into the stomach or intestine.*

- Squeeze the drip chamber to fill it to one-third to one-half of its capacity.

- Open the tubing clamp, run the formula through the tubing, and reclamp the tube. *The formula will displace the air in the tubing, thus preventing the installation of excess air.*

- Attach the feeding set tubing to the feeding tube, and regulate the drip rate to deliver the feeding over the desired length of time. Some prefilled tube-feeding sets can be attached to a feeding pump.

5. Rinse the feeding tube immediately before all of the formula has run through the tubing.

- Instill 60 ml of water through the feeding tube. *Water cleans the lumen of the tube, preventing future blockage by sticky formula.*

- Be sure to add the water before the feeding solution has drained from the neck of a bulb syringe or from the tubing of an administration set. Before adding water to a feeding bag or prefilled tubing set, first clamp and disconnect both feeding and administration tubes. *Adding the water before the syringe or tubing is empty prevents the instillation of air into the stomach or intestine and thus prevents unnecessary distention.*

6. Clamp and cover the feeding tube.

- Clamp the feeding tube before all of the water is instilled. *Clamping prevents leakage and air from entering the tube if done before water is instilled.*

- Cover the end of the feeding tube with gauze held by an elastic band. *Covering the tube end prevents leakage from it.*

7. Ensure client comfort and safety.

Ⓢ• Pin the tubing to the client's

gown. *This minimizes pulling of the tube, thus preventing discomfort and dislodgement.*

- Ask the client to remain sitting upright in Fowler's position or in a slightly elevated right lateral position for at least 30 minutes. *These positions facilitate digestion* Ⓢ *and movement of the feeding from the stomach along the alimentary tract, and prevent potential aspiration of the feeding into the lungs.*

- Check the agency's policy on the frequency of changing the nasogastric tube and the use of smaller-lumen tubes if a large-bore tube is in place. *These measures prevent irritation and erosion of the pharyngeal and esophageal mucous membranes.*

8. Dispose of equipment appropriately.

- If the equipment is to be reused, wash it thoroughly with soap and water so that it is ready for reuse.

- Change the equipment every 24 hours or according to agency policy.

9. Document all relevant information.

- Document the feeding, including the amount and kind of solution taken, duration of the feeding, and assessments of the client. See sample below.

- Record the volume of the feeding and water administered on the client's intake and output record.

10. Monitor the client for possible problems.

- Carefully assess clients receiving tube feedings for possible problems.

- To prevent dehydration, give the client supplemental water in addition to the prescribed tube feeding as ordered.

▶

► **Technique 23–2 Administering a Tube Feeding** *CONTINUED*

VARIATION: Continuous-Drip Feeding

If the feeding is a continuous-drip tube feeding, discontinue the feeding at least every 6 hours, or as in- dicated by agency policy, and as- pirate and measure the gastric contents. Then flush the tubing with 30 to 50 ml of water. Small- bore tubes should be flushed but not aspirated. *This ensures adequate absorption and verifies correct place- ment of the tube. If placement of a small bore tube is questionable, a re- peat X ray should be done.*

EVALUATION FOCUS	Tolerance of feeding; weight gain or loss; fecal elimination pattern; skin turgor; urine output.

SAMPLE RECORDING

Date	Time	Notes
06/09/93	1210	2 ml of straw colored fluid withdrawn. pH 4. 350 ml Meritene feeding administered via NG tube in 30 min. Eructed small amount of flatus. Tolerated feeding s̄ emesis. No discomfort noted. ———— Juan S. Ramirez, SN

KEY ELEMENTS OF ADMINISTERING A NASOGASTRIC OR OROGASTRIC FEEDING

Before Administering the Feeding

- Assess the client for feelings of abdominal dis- tention, belching, loose stools, flatus, or pain; bowel sounds; and allergies to foods in the feeding.
- Check the expiration date of the feeding.
- Warm the feeding to room temperature.
- Confirm correct placement of the tube.
- Aspirate residual stomach contents, measure the amount, and check about reinstilling it or con- tinuing the feeding.
- Remove air from the feeding tubes of burette and prefilled bottles with drip chambers.

- Deliver the feeding over the desired length of time.

During the Feeding

- Hold and cuddle an infant, and provide a pacifier.

After the Feeding

- Rinse the nasogastric tube with water.
- Clamp the nasogastric tube before all of the rinse solution has run through.
- Have the client remain in a Fowler's or slightly elevated right lateral position for at least 30 minutes.

23-3 **Removing a Nasogastric Tube**

ASSESSMENT FOCUS	Presence of bowel sounds; absence of nausea or vomiting when tube is clamped.

EQUIPMENT

- Disposable pad
- Tissues
- Clean disposable gloves

- 50-ml syringe (optional)
- Plastic disposable bag

► **Technique 23–3** *CONTINUED*

INTERVENTION

1. Confirm the physician's order to remove the tube.

2. Prepare the client.

- Explain that the procedure will cause no discomfort.

- Assist the client to a sitting position if health permits.

- Place the disposable pad across the client's chest to collect any spillage of mucous and gastric secretions from the tube.

- Provide tissues to the client to wipe the nose and mouth after tube removal.

3. Detach the tube.

- Disconnect the nasogastric tube from the suction apparatus, if present.

- Unpin the tube from the client's gown.

- Remove the adhesive tape securing the tube to the nose.

4. Remove the tube.

- Put on disposable gloves.

- (Optional). Instill 50 ml of air into the tube. *This clears the tube of any contents such as feeding or gastric drainage.*

- Ask the client to take a deep breath and to hold it. *This closes the glottis, thereby preventing accidental aspiration of any gastric contents.*

- Pinch the tube with the gloved hand. *Pinching the tube prevents any contents inside the tube from draining into the client's throat.*

- Quickly and smoothly withdraw the tube.

- Place the tube in the plastic bag. *Placing the tube immediately into the bag prevents the transference of microorganisms from the tube to other articles or people.*

- Observe the intactness of the tube.

5. Ensure client comfort.

- Provide mouthwash if desired.

- Assist the client as required to blow the nose. *Excessive secretions may have accumulated in the nasal passages.*

6. Dispose of the equipment appropriately.

- Place the pad, bag with tube, and gloves in the receptacle designated by the agency. *Correct disposal prevents the transmission of microorganisms.*

7. Assess the nasogastric drainage if suction was used.

- Measure the amount of gastric drainage, and record it on the client's fluid output record.

- Inspect the drainage for appearance and consistency.

8. Document all relevant information.

- Record the removal of the tube, the amount and appearance of any drainage if connected to suction, and any relevant assessments of the client.

EVALUATION FOCUS	Presence of bowel sounds; absence of nausea or vomiting when tube is removed; intactness of tissues of the nares.

SAMPLE RECORDING

Date	Time	Notes
02/06/93	1800	Active bowel sounds present. Sips of water tolerated without nausea. NG tube removed as ordered. Nares tissues intact. Tube intact. Mouth care given. — Jody Collins, SN

KEY ELEMENTS OF REMOVING A NASOGASTRIC TUBE

- Turn off the suction, and disconnect the tube from suction.
- Clamp the tubing before removal.

- Don disposable gloves.
- Withdraw the tubing while the client holds the breath.

Gastrostomy or Jejunostomy Feeding

A **gastrostomy feeding** is the instillation of liquid nourishment through a tube that enters a surgical opening (called a gastrostomy) through the abdominal wall into the stomach. A **jejunostomy feeding** is the instillation of liquid nourishment through a tube that enters a surgical opening (a jejunostomy) through the abdominal wall into the jejunum.

Gastrostomy and jejunostomy feedings allow clients greater mobility than gastric or duodenal tube feedings and enable clients to feed themselves. Similar principles for administration and assessment are appropriate. The amount of solution is gradually increased with each feeding, from 200 to 800 ml. Commercially prepared formulas that are past the manufacturer's expiration date and agency-prepared solutions older than 24 hours must be discarded. See Technique 23–4.

23-4

Administering a Gastrostomy or Jejunostomy Feeding

Before commencing a gastrostomy or jejunostomy feeding determine the type and amount of feeding to be instilled and frequency of feedings, and any pertinent information about previous feedings, e.g., the position in which the client best tolerates the feeding.

PURPOSES
- To improve or maintain nutritional status
- To administer medications

ASSESSMENT FOCUS

See Technique 23–2 on page 565.

EQUIPMENT

- Correct amount of feeding solution
- Graduated container to hold the feeding
- Large bulb syringe
- Graduated container with 60 ml of water to flush the tubing
- Graduated container to measure residual formula
- Pacifier

For a Tube Sutured in Place
- 4 × 4 gauze squares to cover the end of the tube
- Elastic band

For Tube Insertion
- Clean disposable gloves
- Moistureproof bag
- Water-soluble lubricant
- #18 Fr. whistle-tip catheter or other feeding tube
- Tubing clamp

For Cleaning the Peristomal Skin and Dressing the Stoma
- Mild soap and water
- Petrolatum, zinc oxide ointment, or other skin protectant
- Precut 4 × 4 gauze squares
- Uncut 4 × 4 gauze squares
- Abdominal pads
- Abdominal binder or Montgomery straps

INTERVENTION

1. Assess and prepare the client.
- See Technique 23–1.

2. Insert a feeding tube, if one is not already in place.
- Wearing gloves, remove the os-

tomy dressing. Then discard the dressing and gloves in the moistureproof bag.

- Lubricate the end of the tube, and insert it into the ostomy opening 10 to 15 cm (4 to 6 in).

3. Check the patency of a tube sutured in place.
- Determine placement of the tube. See page 560.
- Pour 15 to 30 ml of water into the syringe, remove the tube clamp,

▶ **Technique 23–4** *CONTINUED*

and allow the water to flow into the tube. *This determines the patency of the tube. If water flows freely, the tube is patent.*

- If the water does not flow freely, notify the nurse in charge and/or physician.

4. Check for residual formula.

- Attach the bulb to the syringe, and compress the bulb. *Compressing the bulb before the syringe is attached to the feeding tube prevents the instillation of air into the stomach or jejunum.*

- Attach the syringe to the end of the feeding tube, and withdraw and measure the stomach or jejunal contents.

- Follow agency practice if there is no more than 50 ml of undigested formula. Hold the feeding if there is more than 150 ml, and recheck in 3 to 4 hours. Notify the physician if a large residual remains at that time.

- For continuous feedings, check the residual every 4 to 6 hours, and hold feedings if there is a 2-hour volume. Then recheck in 2 hours, and restart unless the residual remains large; the physician should be notified if a large residual persists.

5. Administer the feeding.

- Position infant comfortably in your lap, and provide a pacifier.

- Hold the syringe 7 to 15 cm (3 to 6 in) above the ostomy opening.

- Slowly pour the solution into the syringe, and allow it to flow through the tube by gravity.

- Just before all the formula has run through and the syringe is empty, add 30 ml of water. *Water rinses the tube and preserves its patency.*

- If the tube is sutured in place, hold it upright, remove the syringe, and then clamp the tube to prevent leakage. Cover the end of the tube with a 4 × 4 gauze, and secure the gauze with a rubber band.

- If a catheter was inserted for the feeding, remove it.

6. Ensure client comfort and safety.

- After the feeding, ask the client to remain in the sitting position or a slightly elevated right lateral position for at least 30 minutes. *This minimizes the risk of aspiration.*

- Assess status of peristomal skin. *Gastric or jejunal drainage contains digestive enzymes that can irritate the skin.* Document any

redness and broken skin areas.

- Check orders about cleaning the peristomal skin, applying a skin protectant, and applying appropriate dressings. Generally, the peristomal skin is washed with mild soap and water at least once daily. Petrolatum, zinc oxide ointment, or other skin protectant may be applied around the stoma, and precut 4 × 4 gauze squares may be placed around the tube. The precut squares are then covered with regular 4 × 4 gauze squares, and the tube is coiled over them. The coiled tube is covered with abdominal pads and secured with either an abdominal binder or Montgomery straps.

- Observe for common complications of enteral feedings: aspiration, hyperglycemia, abdominal distention, diarrhea, and fecal impaction. Report findings to physician. Often a change in formula or rate of administration can correct problems.

- When appropriate, teach the client how to administer feedings and when to notify the physician or nurse practitioner concerning problems.

7. Document all assessments and interventions.

EVALUATION FOCUS	See Technique 23–2, page 568.

SAMPLE RECORDING

Date	Time	Notes
06/09/93	1210	Gastrostomy tube patent. 40 ml residual stomach contents aspirated. 350 ml Sustagen feeding administered. No discomfort verbalized. Bowel sounds normal. ——————————————— Joan S. Cortez, SN

► **Technique 23–4 Administering a Gastrostomy or Jejunostomy Feeding** *CONTINUED*

KEY ELEMENTS OF ADMINISTERING A GASTROSTOMY OR JEJUNOSTOMY FEEDING

Before the Feeding

- Confirm whether the feeding is to be withheld if more than 50 ml of stomach or jejunal contents are aspirated.
- Position the client appropriately.
- Lubricate tubes before inserting them into stomas.
- Aspirate, measure, and reinstill (if indicated) stomach or jejunal contents.

After the Feeding

- Rinse the tube with water.
- Position the client appropriately for at least 30 minutes.
- Clean the peristomal skin and inspect it for irritation.
- Apply peristomal skin protectants and appropriate dressings.

CRITICAL THINKING CHALLENGE

Marianne Jordan is a 26-year-old who has had a gastrostomy tube inserted for long-term feedings. When receiving nursing care Ms Jordan refuses to look at the ostomy tube and states she doesn't want any visitors. She refuses to learn self-care of the tube. What will you say and do?

RELATED RESEARCH

Fawcett, H., and Yeoman, C. March 1991. A tube to suit all NG needs? Evaluation of fine bore nasogastric tubes. *Professional Nurse* 6:324, 326–27, 329.

Metheny, N.; McSweeney, M.; Wehrle, M. A.; and Wiersema, L. September/October 1990. Effectiveness of the auscultatory method in predicting feeding tube location. *Nursing Research* 39:262–67.

REFERENCES

Byrne, C. J.; Saxton, D. F.; Pelikan, P. K.; and Nugent, P. M. 1986. *Laboratory tests: Implications for nursing care.* 2d ed. Menlo Park, Calif.: Addison-Wesley Publishing Co.

Grant, J. A., and Kennedy-Caldwell, C. 1988. *Nutritional support in nursing.* New York: Grune and Stratton.

Guyton, A. C. 1986. *Textbook of medical physiology.* 7th ed. Philadelphia: W. B. Saunders Co.

Hand, R.; Kempster, M.; Levy, J.; Rogol, R.; and Spirn, P. 1984. Inadvertent transbronchial insertion of narrow-bore feeding tubes. *Journal of the American Medical Association* 251:2396–97.

Kohn, C. L., and Keithley, J. K. June 1989. Enteral nutrition: Potential complications and patient monitoring. *Nursing Clinics of North America* 24:339–53.

Konstantinides, N. N., and Shronts, E. September 1983. Tube feeding: Managing the basics. *American Journal of Nursing* 83:1312–18.

Metheny, M. M. January 1985. 20 ways to prevent tube-feeding complications. *Nursing 85* 15:47–50.

Metheny, N. November/December 1988. Measures to test placement of nasogastric and nasointestinal feeding tubes: A review. *Nursing Research* 37:324–29.

Metheny, N.; Dettenmeier, P.; Hampton, K.; Wiersema, L.; and Williams, P. November 1990. Detection of inadvertent respiratory placement of small-bore feeding tubes: A report of 10 cases. *Heart and Lung* 19:631–38.

Metheny, N. A.; Spies, M. A.; and Eisenberg, P. August 1988. Measures to test placement of nasoenteral feeding tubes. *Western Journal of Nursing Research* 10:367–83.

Miller, K.; Tomlinson, J.; and Sahn, S. August 1985. Pleuropulmonary complications of enteral tube feeding. *Chest* 88:230–33.

Oberc, M. C. 1991. Inserting and maintaining a gastric or jejunal tube. In Smith, D. A., editor. pp. 418–28. *Comprehensive child and family nursing skills.* St. Louis: C. V. Mosby Co.

Whaley, L. F., and Wong, D. L. 1990. *Nursing care of infants and children.* 4th ed. St. Louis: C. V. Mosby Co.

24

Fluids and Electrolytes

OBJECTIVES

- Describe the body's two major fluid reservoirs

- Describe factors affecting the proportion of the body weight that is fluid

- Identify the major electrolytes of the intracellular and extracellular fluid compartments and body secretions

- Describe three major sources of fluids and electrolytes

- Describe four sources of fluid output

- Identify unusual sources of fluid intake and output during illness

- Identify normal daily fluid intakes and outputs

- List factors that influence fluid and electrolyte balance

- Recognize clinical signs and laboratory findings of selected fluid and electrolyte imbalances

- Describe four primary acid-base disturbances

- Identify data required to assess the client's fluid and electrolyte status

- Monitor a client's fluid intake and output

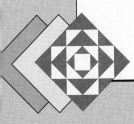

NURSING PROCESS GUIDE

FLUID & ELECTROLYTE BALANCE

ASSESSMENT

Determine

- The usual amount and type of fluids ingested each day.

- Foods rich in protein, sodium, potassium, and calcium eaten each day.

- Any recent changes in food or fluid intake and reason (e.g., presence of nausea, pain, **anorexia**, or **dysphagia**).

- Any recent changes in frequency or amount of urine output.

- Major losses of body fluid through vomiting, diarrhea, excessive perspiration, or other route (e.g., drainage from gastrointestinal function, ileostomy, colostomy, or burn sites).

- History of any long-term or recent disease processes that might disrupt fluid, electrolyte, and acid-base balance: kidney disease, heart disease, high blood pressure, diabetes mellitus, diabetes insipidus, thyroid or parathyroid disorders, asthma, emphysema, severe trauma, or other chronic disease states (e.g., cancer, colitis, ileitis).

- Medication therapy that could affect fluid and electrolyte balance: diuretics, steroids, potassium supplements, aldosterone inhibitor agents.

- Recent treatments such as dialysis, total parenteral nutrition, tube drainages (e.g., nasogastric or intestinal suction), or tube feedings.

Assess the client for

- Signs that indicate too little hydration: excessive thirst, dry skin and mucous membranes, concentrated urine, reduced urine output, poor tissue turgor, depressed periorbital spaces.

- Signs indicating too much hydration: swollen ankles, difficulty breathing, sudden weight gain, ascites, moist crackles (rales) in lungs.

- Signs that might indicate an electrolyte or acid-base imbalance: loss of mental alertness; disorientation; faintness; muscle weakness, twitching, cramps, fatigue, pain, or spasm; abnormal sensations (e.g., burning, prickling, tingling); abdominal cramps or distention; heart palpitations.

Obtain clinical measurements:

- Baseline and daily weight. Rapid losses or gains of 5% to 8% of total body weight indicate moderate to severe fluid volume deficit or excesses.

- Vital signs. An increased *body temperature* may indicate hypernatremic dehydration; a decreased body temperature may result from hypovolemia. An increased *pulse* rate and a weak, thready pulse may occur with fluid volume deficit or potassium deficit; a decreased pulse rate may indicate potassium excess. An increased rate and depth of *respiration* may cause carbonic acid deficit (respiratory alkalosis); shallow respirations may create a carbonic acid excess (respiratory acidosis). Either may be a compensatory mechanism for metabolic acid-base imbalances. An elevated systolic *blood pressure* may indicate a fluid volume excess; a decreased systolic pressure exceeding 10 mm Hg usually indicates a fluid volume deficit.

- 24-hour fluid intake and output (see Technique 24–1 on page 584).

Review results of laboratory tests:

- Serum electrolyte levels

- Hematocrit

- Urine pH

- Urine specific gravity

- Arterial blood gases (ABGs)

Identify clients at risk for fluid and electrolyte imbalances:

- Postoperative clients

- Clients with severe trauma or burns

- Clients with chronic diseases, such as congestive heart failure, diabetes, chronic obstructive lung disease, and cancer

- Clients who are permitted nothing by mouth (NPO)

- Clients with intravenous infusions

- Clients with retention catheters and urinary drainage systems

- Clients with special drainages or suctions, such as a nasogastric suction

- Clients receiving diuretics

- Clients experiencing excessive fluid losses and requiring increased intake

- Clients who retain fluids

- Clients with fluid restrictions

Nursing Process Guide *CONTINUED*

- Elderly clients who may not be taking in the fluids they need

- Clients unable to respond to the thirst sensation, e.g., comatose clients

- Clients receiving electrolyte therapy, i.e., K^+ supplements

- Clients unable to communicate desire for fluid, i.e., very young clients

- Clients with very high or very low total body water

RELATED DIAGNOSTIC CATEGORIES

- Fluid volume deficit

- High risk for Fluid volume deficit

- Fluid volume excess

- Impaired gas exchange

PLANNING

Client Goal
The client will regain or maintain adequate fluid and electrolyte balance.

Outcome Criteria
The client with **Fluid volume deficit** or with **High risk for Fluid volume deficit**

- Has a balanced fluid intake and output (average of 2500 ml per day) for 3 days.

- Has good skin turgor.

- Has moist mucous membranes.

- Is free of thirst.

- Is free of vomiting and diarrhea.

- Has a normal urine specific gravity (1.010 to 1.025).

- Has normal vital signs for age, sex, and health status.

- Explains reasons for fluid/electrolyte imbalance.

- Explains purposes and side-effects of ordered medications.

- Identifies amounts and types of foods and fluids to consume to prevent recurrence.

The client with **Fluid volume excess** in addition:

- Is gradually free of edema, i.e., able to wear shoes again.

- Has intact skin.

- Is free of dyspnea and able to breathe in the supine position.

- Loses __kg body weight within 1 week and then maintains stable body weight.

Body Fluid

Fluids and electrolytes are necessary to maintain good health, and their relative amounts in the body must be maintained within a narrow range. The balance of fluids and electrolytes in the body is a part of physiologic homeostasis.

Distribution

The body's fluid is divided into two major reservoirs, intracellular and extracellular. The **intracellular fluid (ICF)**, also referred to as the **cellular fluid**, is found within the cells of the body. It constitutes two-thirds to three-quarters of the total body fluid. The **extracellular fluid (ECF)** is found outside the cells; it is subdivided into two compartments, **intravascular** (plasma) and **interstitial**. **Plasma** is fluid found within the vascular system; **interstitial fluid** is fluid that surrounds the cells, and it includes **lymph**, the transparent, slightly yellow fluid found within the lymphatic vessels. Extracellular fluids constitute one-third to one-fourth of the total body fluid. Normal body functioning requires that the volume of each fluid compartment remain relatively constant.

Proportions

The proportion of fluid in the human body varies with age, body fat, and sex. As age increases, the proportion of body water decreases. For example, whereas 77% of a newborn's body weight is fluid, only 55% of an adult female's body weight is fluid. See Table 24–1. Because body fat is essentially free of fluid, the amount of fat substantially alters the total volume of fluid in proportion to a person's weight.

TABLE 24–1 FLUID PERCENTAGE OF BODY WEIGHT, BY AGE*

Developmental Stage	Percentage of Water (Approximate)
Newborn infant	75
Adult male	57
Adult female	55
Elderly adult	45

*Note: As age increases, proportion of body water decreases.

For example, an obese person's body may have only 50% fluid in relation to weight while a thin person's may have 60% fluid. This variable of body fat also accounts for the difference in total body fluid between the sexes. Adult females have a higher proportion of body fat than adult males, and thus less fluid.

Composition

All body fluids contain important substances, such as salts, oxygen from the lungs, dissolved nutrients (glucose, fatty acids, and amino acids) from the digestive tract, and waste products of metabolism (e.g., carbon dioxide).

The salts in solution break into one or more electrically charged particles called **ions** or **electrolytes**. For example, sodium chloride breaks into one ion of sodium (Na) and one ion of chloride (Cl). Ions that carry a positive charge are called *cations*, and those carrying a negative charge are called *anions*. Examples are the following:

Cations	*Anions*
Sodium (Na^+)	Chloride (Cl^-)
Potassium (K^+)	Bicarbonate (HCO_3^-)
Calcium (Ca^{2+})	Phosphate (HPO_4^{2-})
Magnesium (Mg^{2+})	Sulfate (SO_4^{2-})

In solution, positive and negative ions are attracted to one another until a balance is attained.

The electrolyte composition of the fluid compartments varies from one to another. For example, the principal ions of the extracellular compartment are sodium and chloride, while the principal ions of the intracellular compartment are potassium and phosphate. Just as the fluid volumes within the compartments must be maintained, so must the electrolyte compositions of the various compartments. Although the specific numbers of cations and anions may differ in the fluid compartments, in a state of homeostasis the total number of cations equals the total of anions within each compartment.

Sources of Fluids and Electrolytes

The healthy person obtains fluids and electrolytes from three major sources:

1. Solid foods account for about half the fluid requirement of the average adult (750 ml). The water content of fresh vegetables is approximately 90% and of fresh fruits about 85%. Electrolytes are also found in foods. Table 24–2 shows the chief sources of some of the major electrolytes needed by the body.

2. Ingested fluids, such as water and juices, account for most of the other half of fluid requirements. The needed intake varies with the age and health of the individual.

3. Oxidation of food within the body also produces water. *Oxidation* is a chemical process by which a substance combines with oxygen; energy is released, and other substances are formed.

Table 24–3 shows the sources of a healthy adult's average daily fluid intake (2500 to 2600 ml). Note the 4:2:1 ratio, which assists recall.

The ill person, who cannot ingest food or fluids, may receive fluids through unusual routes: (a) intravenous fluids (see Chapter 25); (b) nasogastric tube feedings (see Technique 23–2); and (c) gastrostomy or jejunostomy feedings (see Technique 23–4).

TABLE 24–2 MAJOR FOOD SOURCES OF SELECTED ELECTROLYTES

Electrolyte	Sources
Sodium (Na)	Table salt, cheese, ham, processed meats, canned foods, fish
Potassium (K)	Dark leafy greens, bananas, oranges, nuts, meat, fish, liver
Calcium (Ca)	Milk, cheese, yogurt
Magnesium (Mg)	Nuts, peanut butter, whole grains
Phosphorus (P)	Milk, poultry, fish, cereals

TABLE 24–3 SOURCES OF ADULT AVERAGE DAILY FLUID INTAKE

Source	Amount (ml)	Ratio
Water consumed as fluids	1500	4
Water present in food	750	2
Water produced by oxidation	350	1
Total	2600	

Maintaining Fluid Volume

In a healthy person, the fluid volume and chemical composition of the fluid compartments stay within narrow, safe limits. Normally, a person's fluid intake is counterbalanced by fluid loss. Illness can upset this balance, so that the body has too little or too much fluid.

Fluid Intake

During periods of moderate activity at moderate temperature, the average adult drinks about 1500 ml per day but needs 2500 ml per day, an additional 1000 ml. This added volume is acquired from foods (referred to as *preformed water*) and from the oxidation of these foods during metabolic processes. Interestingly, the water content of food is relatively large, contributing about 750 ml per day. The water content of fresh vegetables is approximately 90%, of fresh fruits about 85%, and of lean meats around 60%. See Table 24–4 for average fluid requirements.

Fluid Output

Fluid losses counterbalance the adult's 2500-ml daily intake of water. The main channel of excretion is the kidneys, which are responsible for an output of about 1500 ml per day in the adult. This approximates the amount of fluid an adult drinks per day. Oral intake and kidney output are frequently and easily measured in nursing practice.

The following are three other routes of fluid output:

1. Insensible loss through the skin as perspiration and through the lungs as water vapor in the expired air

2. Noticeable loss through the skin as sweat

3. Loss through the intestines in feces

See Table 24–5 for the average daily fluid output for an adult. The normal loss from skin and lungs accounts for about two-thirds of the urinary loss, whereas loss in the feces is minimal. It is important to remember that daily intake equals daily output.

Obligatory loss is the essential fluid loss required to maintain body functioning. Water lost as vapor in expired air and as vapor from the skin, a minimum volume of about 500 ml from the kidneys, and the fluid required to excrete the solid metabolic wastes produced daily are the obligatory losses, totaling about 1300 ml per day.

Because the vaporized losses are not readily measured, the measured obligatory kidney loss becomes of prime importance in critical illness. An adult hourly urine volume of less than 30 ml or daily volume under 500 ml is serious. Clients with inadequate output require immediate attention, and such a finding by the nurse must therefore be reported promptly. Although losses from the skin, lungs, and intestines in health account for approximately half of the daily loss, they can account for a much larger percentage of loss from a client who has a fever or accelerated respiration. Increases in respiratory rate, fever, **diaphoresis** (sweating), and diarrhea can magnify fluid loss from the normal routes immensely. Other routes of loss, such as from the stomach through emesis or suction or from abnormal body openings such as fistulas or surgically implanted drainage tubes, often account for significant losses, all of which require intake replacements.

In healthy clients, the output volumes shown in Table 24–5 vary noticeably from day to day and throughout the day. For example, sweat gland activity can increase when the environmental temperature increases. Urinary volume automatically increases as the amount of fluids ingested increases, e.g., on a hot summer day. If fluid loss from the skin is large, however, the urinary volume may decrease to maintain

TABLE 24–4 AVERAGE DAILY FLUID REQUIREMENTS, BY AGE AND WEIGHT

Age	Approximate Body Weight (kg)	ml/24 hours
3 days	3.3	300
1 year	10.0	1000
3 years	15.0	1250
5 years	20.0	1500
8 years	30.0	1750
13 years	60.0	2050
Adult	65.0	2500

Sources: Adapted from S. R. James and S. R. Mott, *Child health nursing: Essential care of children and families* (Menlo Park, Calif.: Addison-Wesley Publishing Co., 1988), p. 638; M. F. Hazinski, Nursing care of the critically ill child: A seven-point check. *Pediatric Nursing*, November/December 1985, 11:460; and John Plonk, M.D., chief pediatric resident, Vanderbilt University Hospital, December 1984.

TABLE 24–5 AVERAGE DAILY FLUID OUTPUT FOR AN ADULT

Route	Amount (ml)
Urine	1400 to 1500
Insensible losses	
Lungs	350 to 400
Skin	350 to 400
Sweat	100
Feces	100 to 200
Total	2300 to 2600

the fluid volumes in the body. Balance is maintained between the intake and output by the homeostatic mechanisms in the body.

Factors Affecting Fluid and Electrolyte Balance

Age

Fluid intake requirements vary with age. Intake requirements have been determined for various ages in relation to body surface area, metabolic requirements, and body weight.

Infants and growing children have much greater fluid turnover than adults, i.e., greater water needs and greater water losses. This is due to their greater metabolic rate, which increases fluid loss through the kidneys. Because immature kidneys are less efficient than adult kidneys, infants lose more fluid through the kidneys. Infant losses from both the lungs and the skin are also greater in proportion to body weight, essentially because respirations are more rapid and the body surface area is proportionately greater. The more rapid turnover of fluid plus the losses produced by disease can create critical fluid imbalances in children much more rapidly than in adults. See Table 24–4 for approximate fluid requirements at different ages according to body weight.

In elderly people, fluid and electrolyte imbalances are often associated with kidney or cardiac problems. Because the kidneys are less able to concentrate urine, elderly persons may need to take in additional fluid to meet their fluid needs.

Environmental Temperature

Excessive heat stimulates the sympathetic nervous system and causes the person to sweat. When the person is not acclimatized to the heat, the sweat glands are strongly stimulated, and as much as 700 ml to 2 liters per hour can be lost through sweating. The sodium chloride (NaCl) in the sweat is also lost.

Diet

A person's diet obviously affects the intake of fluids and electrolytes. When nutritional intake is inadequate or unbalanced, the body tries to preserve stored protein by breaking down glycogen and fat. Once these resources are gone, the body draws on protein stores, and the serum albumin level decreases.

Stress

Stress affects a person's fluid and electrolyte balance. Stress can increase cellular metabolism, blood glucose concentration, and muscle glycolysis. These mechanisms can lead to sodium and water retention. In addition, stress can increase production of the antidiuretic hormone, which in turn decreases urine production. The overall response of the body to stress is to increase the blood volume. See Chapter 37 for additional information.

Illness

Extensive surgical procedures can change a person's fluid and electrolyte balance through a number of mechanisms. The stress response and tissue trauma can cause the loss of fluid and electrolytes from within the damaged cells. An example of such trauma is severe burns.

Cardiac and renal disorders also affect the body's fluid and electrolyte balance. For example, impaired heart function can decrease blood flow to the kidneys and thus hinder the elimination of the waste products of metabolism. When urine output decreases, the body retains sodium, and circulatory overload (hypervolemia) can result. Fluid retention can also lead to pulmonary edema (fluid in the lungs).

Disturbances in Fluid and Electrolyte Balance

Extracellular Fluid (ECF) Deficit

An extracellular fluid deficit is also called a **fluid volume deficit (FVD)**, **hypovolemia**, or **dehydration**.

ECF deficit can occur because of an abrupt decrease in fluid intake or a marked increase in fluid output, i.e., an acute loss as in hemorrhage. The body's initial reponse to a fluid deficit is depletion of the intravascular compartment. Then fluid is drawn from the interstitial compartment into the intravascular compartment, depleting the interstitial compartment. To compensate for the decreased interstitial volume, the body then draws intracellular fluid out of the cells. See the box in the left column of page 579 for clinical signs of ECF deficit.

Extracellular Fluid (ECF) Excess

An excess of extracellular fluid, also called *fluid volume excess* (FVE), can lead to (a) **hypervolemia** (increased blood volume or **circulatory overload**) and (b) **edema** (excess fluid in the interstitial compartment). **Overhydration** is another term sometimes used synonymously with ECF excess. When the interstitial spaces are filled with fluid and the extracellular osmotic pressure increases, fluid is pulled from within the cells, resulting in edema. Edema is most frequently observed around eyes, and in the feet and hands. **Dependent edema** is found in the lowest body parts, e.g., in the feet and legs or in the sacrum of the sitting client. A common cause of ECF excess is decreased renal function and/or iatrogenic causes such as the administration of IV fluids at too rapid a rate. See the box in the right column of page 579 for the clinical signs of ECF excess.

Clinical Signs of ECF Deficit

Observations

- Postural hypotension
- Weight loss
- Dryness of mucous membranes
- Decreased tissue turgor
- Weak, thready, rapid pulse
- Sunken eyeballs
- Oliguria—i.e., less than 30ml/hr
- Skin pale

Laboratory Findings

- Increased specific gravity of urine
- Elevated hematocrit
- Decreased central venous pressure (CVP)

Clinical Signs of ECF Excess

Observations

- Peripheral edema (face, hands, feet or dependent areas)
- Weight gain
  a. Mild: 2% in an adult
  b. Moderate: 5% in an adult
  c. Severe: 8% in an adult
- Distended neck veins when sitting at 45°
- Moist crackles in lungs
- Distended peripheral veins
- Ascites
- Bounding full pulse

Laboratory Findings

- Decreased hematocrit due to plasma dilution
- Decreased BUN due to plasma dilution

Sodium (Na$^+$)

Hyponatremia is a sodium deficit in the blood plasma. It is the result of

- *Net gain of water.* The intake of water exceeds the corresponding intake of sodium, e.g., drinking excessive quantities of water or administering excessive amounts of 5% dextrose in water (D5W) intravenously.

- *Loss of sodium-rich fluids that are replaced only by water.* Excessive sodium loss can be the result of excessive sweating or the prolonged use of strong diuretics. Also, clients can lose abnormally large amounts of sodium through the gastrointestinal tract. The sodium content of pancreatic secretions and gastric mucus is especially high. Severe, prolonged diarrhea or a draining pancreatic fistula can result in abnormally high sodium loss. Gastric suction, which withdraws gastric mucus along with other gastric fluids, can also be the cause.

Hypernatremia is sodium excess in the blood plasma. Hypernatremia is the result of

- *Net loss of water.* Body water loss exceeds sodium loss in situations of water deprivation (dehydration). Also, clients may lose more water than sodium through a draining intestinal wound or through untreated watery diarrhea. A client who is not treated for watery diarrhea may experience

hypernatremia on about the fifth or sixth day after onset.

- *Excessive sodium intake.* Sodium intake rarely exceeds water intake but may occur when a person, for example, mistakenly ingests a large number of sodium chloride tablets or is given a hypertonic saline solution intravenously, e.g., 3% or 5% normal saline solution.

The clinical signs of hyponatremia and hypernatremia are shown in Table 24–6 on page 580.

Potassium (K$^+$)

Potassium is the major cation of intracellular fluid. Potassium balance is regulated in the kidneys by two mechanisms: exchange with sodium ions in the kidney tubules and secretion of aldosterone. Aldosterone is extremely important in controlling potassium concentrations in extracellular fluids.

Potassium affects the functions of most body systems, including the cardiovascular system, the gastrointestinal system, the neuromuscular system, and the respiratory system. Most of the body's potassium is found inside the cells. A small amount is found in the plasma and interstitial fluids. See Table 24–6 for additional information about potassium.

Hypokalemia is a potassium deficit in the blood plasma. Leading causes of potassium deficit are the use of powerful **diuretics** (agents that increase urine production) and decreased dietary intake. **Hyperkalemia** is a potassium excess in the blood plasma.

TABLE 24–6   FLUID AND ELECTROLYTE DATA

Clinical Factor (Normal)	Food Sources	Clinical Signs	Nursing Intervention
Extracellular fluid (infant: 29% of body weight; adult: 15% of body weight)	Oral fluids, fruits, vegetables	*ECF deficit* See page 579	*Deficit:* Give oral fluids as permitted. Administer and monitor IV fluids as ordered. Monitor fluid intake and output. Assess for signs of dehydration. Monitor vital signs.
		ECF excess See page 579	*Excess:* Assist adherence to sodium-restricted diet as ordered. Monitor response to diuretics, weigh daily. Monitor intake, output, and vital signs. Restrict fluids as ordered.
Sodium (Na$^+$) (135–45 mEq/L [serum])	Table salt (NaCl), cheese, pork, salted meats, canned vegetables, potato chips	*Hyponatremia* Feelings of apprehension Lethargy Muscle cramps Anorexia, nausea, vomiting Postural hypotension Seizures, coma	Monitor fluid intake and output. Assess for presence of symptoms such as anorexia, nausea, vomiting. Assist with intake of foods and fluids containing sodium.
		Hypernatremia Extreme thirst Dry, sticky mucous membranes Tongue red, dry, swollen Elevated body temperature	Monitor fluid intake and output. Monitor for presence of symptoms. Assist with fluid intake. Advise regarding low-sodium foods and fluids as ordered.
		Severe Hypernatremia Agitated behavior Fatigue Restlessness	
Potassium (K$^+$) (3.6–5.0 mEq/L [serum])	Bananas, broccoli, cantaloupe, citrus fruits, potatoes, nuts, fish	*Hypokalemia* Muscle weakness, leg cramps Fatigue Anorexia, nausea, vomiting Decreased bowel sounds Weak, irregular pulse Electrocardiogram may show flattening of the T waves and depression of the ST segment	Monitor cardiac changes. Administer potassium as ordered. Teach client about food sources high in potassium. Monitor for presence of symptoms. Monitor intake and output.
		Hyperkalemia Gastrointestinal hyperactivity, diarrhea Irritability, apathy, confusion Cardiac arrhythmia, bradycardia, cardiac arrest Muscle weakness, numbness, areflexia (absence of reflexes)	Monitor cardiac function for irregular pulse rate and bradycardia. Restrict potassium in diet. Monitor serum potassium.
Calcium (Ca^{2+}) (4.3–5.3 mEq/L [serum])	Milk, milk products, grains, cereals, fruits, nuts, greens	*Hypocalcemia* Numbness, tingling of the extremities Muscle tremors, cramps Altered blood clotting causing bleeding Cardiac dysrhythmias Anxiety, irritability Positive **Trousseau's** and **Chvostek's signs**	Administer calcium supplement as needed. Advise to adjust the regular dietary calcium as required. Initiate seizure precautions. Monitor serum calcium. Assess client for signs of hypocalcemia.
		Hypercalcemia Deep bone pain Flank pain secondary to urinary calculi Lethargy, weakness Reduced muscle tone Anorexia, nausea, vomiting	Monitor serum calcium. Assess client for signs of hypercalcemia. Inspect urine for calculi.

▶ **TABLE 24–6** *CONTINUED*

Clinical Factor (Normal)	Food Sources	Clinical Signs	Nursing Intervention
Magnesium (Mg^{2+}) (1.5–2.5 mEq/L [serum])	Whole grains, green leafy vegetables	*Hypomagnesemia* Neuromuscular irritability with tremors Increased reflexes, tremors, convulsions Positive Chvostek's and Trousseau's signs Tachycardia Disorientation and confusion	Monitor breathing. Employ safety precautions if confusion or seizures are anticipated. Assist with magnesium replacement as ordered.
		Hypermagnesemia Lethargy, drowsiness Coma Impaired respirations Nausea, vomiting Muscle weakness, paralysis Hypotension	Monitor vital signs. Monitor level of consciousness.
Chloride (Cl^-) (98–108 mEq/L [serum])	Table salt, dairy products	*Hypochloremia* Usually associated with hyponatremia (see sodium above)	Monitor serum sodium and chloride.
		Hyperchloremia Usually associated with hypernatremia (see sodium, above)	See above for hypernatremia.
Phosphate (PO_4^-) (1.2–3.0 mEq/L [serum])	Milk, cheese, fish, poultry, milk products, whole grains	*Acute hypophosphatemia* Confusion, seizures, coma Muscle pain Decreased muscle strength	Monitor serum phosphate levels. Assess neurologic signs and orientation. Administer IV phosphate as ordered. Teach client about food sources high in phosphorus.
		Chronic hypophosphatemia Memory loss Fatigue Bone pain and joint stiffness	
		Hyperphosphatemia Anorexia, nausea, and vomiting Hyperreflexia, tetany Tachycardia	Administer magnesium or calcium or antacids as ordered. Assist with diet low in phosphorus.

Hyperkalemia is most often caused by a decreased urinary excretion of potassium, leakage of potassium from the body's cells, e.g., after severe burns, or by excessive ingestion of potassium, e.g., the intravenous administration of excessive amounts of potassium when kidney function is impaired. The clinical signs of hypokalemia and hyperkalemia are shown in Table 24–6.

Calcium (Ca^{2+})

The richest sources of calcium are milk and milk products. Drinking water in some parts of the country also contains an absorbable calcium. Calcium functions in bone formation and in the transmission of nerve impulses, muscle contraction, blood coagulation, and activation of certain enzymes, e.g., pancreatic lipase and phospholipase.

Hypocalcemia is a calcium deficit in the blood plasma. Two causes of hypocalcemia are hypoparathyroidism and excessive loss of intestinal secretions, which contain a great deal of calcium. Severe depletion can cause **tetany** (muscle spasms, sharp flexion of the wrists and ankles, cramps), which can lead to convulsions. **Hypercalcemia** is an excess of calcium in the blood plasma. It can be due to prolonged immobilization, hyperparathyroidism, or a tumor of the parathyroid glands. The clinical signs of hypocalcemia and hypercalcemia are given in Table 24–6.

Magnesium (Mg^{2+})

Magnesium, the fourth most abundant cation in the body, is important for maintaining neuromuscular activity within the body. Like calcium, magnesium is regulated by the parathyroid glands. Increased extracellular magnesium levels (**hypermagnesemia**) depress nervous system activity and skeletal muscle contractions. Low concentrations of magnesium (**hypomagnesemia**), by contrast, cause increased irritability of the nervous system, peripheral vasodilation, and cardiac arrhythmias (Guyton 1986, p.

872). For clinical signs of hypomagnesemia and hypermagnesemia, see Table 24–6.

Chloride (Cl⁻)

Chloride is the major anion of extracellular fluid. Chloride is found in blood, interstitial fluid, and lymph. A very small amount is found in intracellular fluid. It functions as sodium does to maintain the osmotic pressure of the blood. **Hypochloremia** (a deficit in serum chloride) and **hyperchloremia** (an excess in serum chloride) usually develop along with sodium disturbances. See Table 24–6 for clinical signs.

Phosphate (PO₄⁻)

The phosphate anion is found both in intracellular and extracellular fluid. Most of the phosphorus (P^+) in the body exists as PO_4^-. Together with calcium, phosphate is involved in bone and tooth formation. It is also involved in many chemical actions of the cells. Phosphate is absorbed exceedingly well from the intestine, and it is excreted in the urine. See Table 24–6 for clinical signs of **hypophosphatemia** (phosphate deficit) and **hyperphosphatemia** (phosphate excess).

Acid-Base Balance

The body's cellular activity requires an alkaline medium. Alkalinity and its opposite, acidity, are measured in terms of hydrogen ion concentration, expressed on a scale called **pH**. Body fluids are normally maintained at a pH of about 7.4. Alterations of pH of even a few tenths can be incompatible with cellular activity. The normal pH range of extracellular fluid is 7.35 to 7.45 (Figure 24–1). This precise balance is maintained as long as the ratio of 1 carbonic acid molecule to 20 bicarbonate ions is maintained in the extracellular fluid. The ratio, rather than the specific amount of each, is important.

Opposing the body's alkalinity are cellular chemical processes that are constantly producing large amounts of acid as by-products of metabolism. Fortunately, precise control mechanisms maintain the pH of body fluids within a very narrow range. The pH is controlled by buffer systems in all body fluids and by respiratory and kidney regulatory systems.

Buffer Systems

A *buffer system* resists change in the pH of a fluid by chemically binding excess hydrogen ions to prevent an increase in pH or by releasing hydrogen ions to prevent a decrease in the pH. Buffers do not neutralize; acid-base buffers decrease the effect of strong acids and strong bases, so that the pH of a body fluid falls or rises only slightly.

There are three main buffer systems in the body: the bicarbonate buffer, the phosphate buffer, and the protein buffer.

Bicarbonate Buffer System The bicarbonate (HCO_3^-) buffer system is important in controlling the pH of *extracellular* fluids of the body. It consists of sodium bicarbonate ($NaHCO_3$) or potassium bicarbonate ($KHCO_3$) and carbonic acid (H_2CO_3) in the same solution.

Although the bicarbonate buffer system is not the strongest buffer system in the body (the most powerful and plentiful one consists of the proteins of plasma and cells), it is important, because the concentration of sodium bicarbonate is regulated by the kidneys and the concentration of carbonic acid by the respiratory system.

Phosphate Buffer System The phosphate buffer system is an important *intracellular* buffer system. Phosphate ions (HPO_4^{2-}), like bicarbonate ions and ammonia ions, are present in the urine. The phosphate buffer system is composed of two elements, $H_2PO_4^-$ and HPO_4^{2-}. This phosphate buffer system is particularly important in buffering the fluids in the kidney tubules and the fluid inside the cells.

Protein Buffer System The protein buffer system is the largest buffer system in the body. The buffers are the proteins of the cells and of the plasma. It has been shown that about three-fourths of all chemical buffering in the body takes place inside the cells and results from intracellular proteins.

Respiratory Regulation

Elimination of carbon dioxide by the lungs also regulates acid-base balance. The carbon dioxide that a person exhales comes from carbonic acid as follows:

$$H_2CO_3 \rightarrow CO_2 + H_2O$$

The more CO_2 exhaled, the more H_2CO_3 is removed from the blood, thus elevating the blood pH to a more

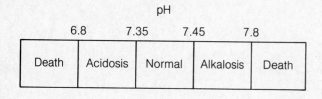

pH

	6.8		7.35		7.45		7.8	
Death		Acidosis		Normal		Alkalosis		Death

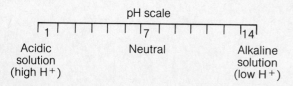

pH scale

1 ——————— 7 ——————— 14

Acidic solution (high H⁺)   Neutral   Alkaline solution (low H⁺)

FIGURE 24–1 Body fluids are normally slightly alkaline, between a pH of 7.35 and 7.45.

alkaline level. Increasing the ventilation rate raises the pH. By contrast, holding one's breath, or hypoventilating, causes the body to retain CO_2, which is then available to form carbonic acid, reducing the pH and acidifying body fluids.

Renal Regulation

The kidney's role in maintaining acid-base balance is complex. A simplified account of the process follows. The kidneys excrete hydrogen ions and form bicarbonate ions in specific amounts as indicated by the pH of the blood. When the plasma pH drops (becomes more acidic), hydrogen ions (acid) are excreted, and bicarbonate ions (base) are formed and retained. Conversely, when the plasma pH rises (becomes more alkaline), hydrogen ions are retained in the body, and bicarbonate ions are excreted.

Primary Acid-Base Imbalances

Imbalances in pH can result in either acidosis or alkalosis. **Acidosis** (blood pH below 7.35) occurs with increases in blood carbonic acid or with decreases in blood bicarbonate. It is also referred to as **acidemia**. **Alkalosis** (blood pH above 7.45) occurs with increases in blood bicarbonate or decreases in blood carbonic acid. It is also referred to as **alkalemia**. A client will not become acidotic or alkalotic, however, unless the normal ratio of 1 carbonic acid molecule to 20 bicarbonate ions is altered.

The primary general cause or origin of a pH imbalance is indicated by the terms *metabolic* or *respiratory*. Metabolic acidosis and metabolic alkalosis are imbalances brought about by changes in bicarbonate levels as a result of metabolic alterations. Respiratory acidosis and respiratory alkalosis are imbalances brought about by changes in carbonic acid levels as a result of respiratory alterations.

In all acid-base imbalances, there is a corrective body response by both the kidneys and the lungs called **compensation**. Any given acid-base imbalance can be described as compensated until body reserves are used up. Then the condition is described as uncompensated. In compensated acidosis or alkalosis, the kidneys and lungs are able to restore the altered ratio of 1 carbonic acid molecule to 20 bicarbonate ions, thereby maintaining a normal pH. For example in (compensated) respiratory acidosis, the plasma pH is maintained at normal even though there is an increase in the carbonic acid because the kidneys retain bicarbonate.

Respiratory Acidosis (Carbonic Acid Excess) Respiratory acidosis occurs when exhalation of carbon dioxide is inhibited, creating a carbonic acid excess in the body. Hypoventilation is its general cause.

Respiratory Alkalosis (Carbonic Acid Deficit) Respiratory alkalosis occurs when exhalation of carbon dioxide is excessive, resulting in a carbonic acid deficit. Its root cause is hyperventilation, which can be due to fever, anxiety, or pulmonary infections.

Metabolic Acidosis (Base Bicarbonate Deficit) Metabolic acidosis occurs when levels of base bicarbonate are low in relation to carbonic acid blood levels. The kidneys normally retain bicarbonate (HCO_3^-) or excrete hydrogen ions (H^+) in response to altered blood pH. Starvation, renal impairment, and diabetes mellitus are among the conditions that deluge the plasma with acid metabolites.

Metabolic Alkalosis (Base Bicarbonate Excess) Metabolic alkalosis occurs when the level of base bicarbonate is high. Metabolic alkalosis may be due to excess intake of baking soda and other alkalis, prolonged vomiting, and other conditions that flood plasma with the bicarbonate anion.

Monitoring Fluid Intake and Output

The nurse or physician may order the monitoring (measurement) of a client's fluid intake and output (I & O) for a variety of reasons. It is commonly measured for clients at risk of developing fluid imbalances (see Assessment in the Nursing Process Guide on page 574).

Most agencies have two forms for recording I & O: (a) a bedside worksheet record for all items measured and their quantities per shift (Figure 24–2) and

BEDSIDE INTAKE-OUTPUT RECORD

Name: Mary Brown   Room No.: 747-2   Date: 7/11

	INTAKE		OUTPUT		
Time	Liquids	Intravenous	Urine	Emesis	Drainage etc.
8-4	0900 Juice 120 Coffee 180 Cream 90 0930 Water 90 1200 Tea 180 Cream 90 Jello 50 1400 Juice 180		0700 - 250 1100 - 400 1500 - 350		
Total	980		1000		
4-12					
Total					
12-8					
Total					

FIGURE 24–2 A sample bedside fluid intake and output record.

(b) a 24-hour permanent record on the client's chart, noting the totals for an 8-hour or 24-hour period (see Figure 3–5 on page 51). Some agencies have another form to record the specifics of intravenous fluids, such as the type of solution, additives, time started, amounts absorbed, and amounts remaining per shift. However, the total amounts for a specific period (e.g., per shift) are then recorded on the permanent I & O record.

The unit used to measure intake and output is the milliliter (ml) or cubic centimeter (cc); these are equivalent metric units of measurement. In household measures, 30 ml is roughly equivalent to 1 fluid ounce, 500 ml is about 1 pint, and 1000 ml is about 1 quart. To measure fluid intake, the capacity of household containers, such as a glass, cup, or soup bowl, need to be converted to metric units. Most agencies provide conversion tables, because the sizes of dishes vary from agency to agency. A table is often provided on or with the bedside I & O record. Examples of equivalents follow:

Water glass	200 ml
Juice glass	120 ml
Cup	180 ml
Soup bowl	
Adult	180 ml
Child	100 ml
Teapot	240 ml
Creamer	
Large	90 ml
Small	30 ml
Water pitcher	1000 ml
Jello, custard dish	100 ml
Ice cream dish	120 ml
Paper cup	
Large	200 ml
Small	120 ml

24-1 Monitoring Fluid Intake and Output

PURPOSES
- To assess the body's fluid balance
- To determine whether a client is taking adequate fluids to meet normal requirements
- To verify an increased fluid intake
- To verify a restricted fluid intake
- To determine voiding patterns and urinary function
- To assess the effectiveness of a medication, such as a diuretic, that increases urinary output

ASSESSMENT FOCUS

Clinical signs of fluid imbalances; body weight (weigh the client daily at the same time and with the same clothing); urine pH and specific gravity; presence and degree of edema (to assess ankle edema daily, measure the ankle circumference with a measuring tape); fluid likes and dislikes, particularly if the client is on forced fluids; any problems with voiding or ingesting fluids.

EQUIPMENT
- Bedside I & O form and a pencil or pen
- Bedside bedpan, commode, or urinal
- Calibrated container to measure intake and a separate container to measure output

▶ **Technique 24–1** *CONTINUED*

INTERVENTION

1. Prepare the client.

- Explain to the client that an accurate measurement of fluid intake and output is required, the reason for it, and the need to use a bedpan or urinal (unless a urinary drainage system is in place). Many people wish to be involved in recording these measurements and need to be given further information about how to compute the values and what foods are considered fluids.

- Establish with the client a regular plan for ingesting the required amount of fluid. Generally, one half the total volume is ingested on the day shift, and the other half is divided between the evening and night shifts, with the majority on the evening shift.

2. Measure the client's fluid intake.

- Following meals, record on the bedside I & O form the amount of each fluid item taken, if the client has not already done so. Specify the kind of fluid and the time. Measure all obvious fluids, such as water, milk, juice, soft drinks, coffee, tea, cream, soup, sherry, and wine. Also include such foods as ice cream, sherbet, custard, and gelatin (Jell-O), i.e., any food that turns to liquid at room temperature. Do not measure foods that are pureed. *Pureed foods are simply solid foods prepared in a different form.*

- Determine whether the client had taken any other fluids ingested between meals, and add the amounts to the form. Include water that is taken with medications. To assess the amount of water used from a water pitcher, measure what remains, and subtract this amount from the full amount of the pitcher. Then refill the pitcher.

- Include the total volumes of intravenous fluids, including blood transfusions and any intravenous piggyback medications.

3. Measure the client's fluid output.

- Following each voiding, pour the urine into the measuring container, observe the amount, and record it and the time of voiding on the bedside I & O form. Clean the bedpan and measuring container, and return the bedpan to the client.

- For clients with retention catheters, note and then record the amount of urine at the end of the shift, and then empty the drainage bag. The drainage bag usually has markings that indicate the amount of urine. If there is any doubt about the amount in the drainage bag, empty it first into an accurate measuring container.

- Record any other output, such as emesis, liquid feces, and other drainage. Specify the type of fluid and the time.

- If the client is incontinent of urine or is extremely diaphoretic, estimate and record these "outputs." For example, of an incontinent client you might record "Incontinent × 3," or "Drawsheet soaked in 12-in diameter." Of a diaphoretic client you might record: "Perspiring profusely [or +++]. Gown and drawsheet changed × 2." Follow agency practices in this regard.

4. Total the measurements at the end of the shift, i.e., every 8 or 12 hours (Figure 24–2).

- Include the total volumes of intravenous fluids, including blood transfusions.

- *Note:* in some critical care units, you may need to total the fluid measurements hourly.

5. Communicate pertinent information.

- Document pertinent assessment data and the totals of the client's I & O on the permanent record.

- Report to the nurse in charge inadequate intakes and outputs. An adult intake of less than 1000 ml in 24 hours is considered inadequate. An adult urine output of less than 500 ml in 24 hours or less than 30 ml per hour is considered inadequate.

- Adjust the nursing care plan as needed to ensure appropriate fluid intake for the client and appropriate measurement of I & O.

EVALUATION FOCUS

Comparison of the total fluid output measurement with the total fluid intake measurement and comparison of both measurements to previous measurements (this determines whether the fluid output reflects the fluid intake and any changes in fluid balance); changes in clinical signs of fluid imbalance.

▶

▶ **Technique 24–1 Monitoring Fluid Intake and Output** *CONTINUED*

KEY ELEMENTS OF MONITORING FLUID INTAKE AND OUTPUT

- Determine the client's intake and output (fluid balance), and observe the client for signs of dehydration or overhydration.
- Monitor I & O for all clients who have (a) insufficient fluid intake by mouth, (b) excessive fluid losses via normal or abnormal routes, (c) fluid retention, or (d) medications prescribed that alter fluid output.
- Weigh clients who have fluid retention or who are receiving diuretics daily.

CRITICAL THINKING CHALLENGE

Catherine Sullivan is a 72-year-old female who was admitted to the nursing unit with severe dehydration. She has been ordered a fluid intake of 1500 ml per day, with continuous assessment of her fluid balance and state of hydration. When adding her oral fluid intake, you note that she is not drinking enough fluids. When you ask, Ms Sullivan states that she "hates water and has never drunk much of it." How would you interpret what Ms Sullivan is saying? How will you respond? What factors should you consider to promote her fluid intake? How will you assess her state of hydration?

RELATED RESEARCH

Mountain, R. D.; Heffner, J. E.; Brackett, N. C.; Sahm, S. A.; September 1990. Acid-base disturbances in acute asthma. *Chest* 98:651–55.

REFERENCES

Brenner, M., and Welliver, J. December 1990. Pulmonary and acid-base assessment. *Nursing Clinics of North America* 25:761–70.

Byrne, C. J.; Saxton, D. F.; Pelikan, P. K.; and Nugent, P. M. 1986. *Laboratory tests: Implications for nursing care.* 2d ed. Menlo Park, Calif.: Addison-Wesley Publishing Co.

Carpenito, L. J. 1989. *Nursing diagnosis: Application to clinical practice.* 3d ed. Philadelphia: J. B. Lippincott Co.

Chenevey, B. December 1987. Overview of fluids and electrolytes. *Nursing Clinics of North America* 22:749–59.

Finberg, L. April 30, 1991. Clinical cues to dehydration. *Patient Care* 25:45–48, 51.

Gaspar, P. M. July/August 1988. What determines how much patients drink? *Geriatric Nursing* 9:221–24.

Graves, L., III. November 1990. Disorder of calcium, phosphorus, and magnesium. *Critical Care Nursing Quarterly* 13:3–13.

Guyton, A. C. 1986. *Textbook of medical physiology.* 7th ed. Philadelphia: W. B. Saunders Co.

Hazinski, M. F. November/December 1985. Nursing care of the critically ill child: A seven-point check. *Pediatric Nursing* 11:460.

Heitkemper, M. M., and Bond, E. January/February 1988. Fluid and electrolytes: Assessment and interventions. *Journal of Enterostomal Therapy* 15:18–23.

James, S. R., and Mott, S. R. 1988. *Child health nursing: Essential care of children and families.* Menlo Park, Calif.: Addison-Wesley Publishing Co.

Janusek, L. W. July 1990. Metabolic acidosis: Pathophysiology, signs and symptoms. *Nursing 90* 20:52–53.

Kim, M. J.; McFarland, G. K.; and McLane, A. M. 1989. *Pocket guide to nursing diagnoses.* 3d ed. St. Louis: C. V. Mosby Co.

Lancaster, L. E. December 1987. Renal and endocrine regulation of water and electrolyte balance. *Nursing Clinics of North America* 22:761–72.

Mims, B. C. March 1991. Interpreting ABGs . . . arterial blood gas. *RN* 54:42–47.

Terry, J. May/June 1991. The other electrolytes: Magnesium, calcium, and phosphorous. *Journal of Intravenous Nursing* 14:167–76.

Toto, R. D. August 1991. Acid-base balance in the CCU patient. *Hospital Medicine* 27:103–5, 108, 111.

The ups and downs of pH. July 1990. *Nursing* 20:32H.

Yarnell, R. P. July 1991. Detecting hypomagnesemia: The most overlooked electrolyte imbalance. *Nursing* 21:55–57.

Intravenous Therapy

CONTENTS

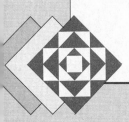

NURSING PROCESS GUIDE
INTRAVENOUS THERAPY

ASSESSMENT

Assess

- Vital signs (pulse, respirations, and blood pressure) for baseline data, if not already available. Because fluid is instilled directly into the circulatory system, problems such as fluid excess can be reflected in the vital signs.

- Fluid balance. Determine oral fluid intake, amount of urine output and its specific gravity, and amount and routes of other fluid losses (see also Chapter 24, page 587).

- Electrolyte balance, e.g., sodium and potassium levels. Refer to data in laboratory records.

- Skin turgor. Lift the skin over the anterior chest with two fingers. An inverted V, called *tenting*, that remains after the skin is released indicates decreased turgor and possible fluid deficit.

- Allergy to tape or iodine.

- Tendency to bleed easily. Such clients require special observation after venipuncture.

- Disease or injury to extremities. Intravenous therapy is contraindicated in affected limbs of clients who have had cerebrovascular accidents, axillary lymph nodes removed (e.g., during mastectomies), arteriovenous fistulas, or any circulatory impairment.

- Any abrasions in the skin area chosen for the venipuncture. If an abraded area must be used, record the abrasions.

- Veins that would be satisfactory venipuncture sites. Veins that are continually distended with blood, that have been damaged because of previous venipunctures, or that have become knotted and tortuous are normally not used. Veins that are easily palpated are often easier to enter than veins that are highly visible or deeply buried under adipose tissue. Highly visible veins tend to roll away from the needle.

- Intravenous fluid infiltration, phlebitis, circulatory overload, and bleeding at the intravenous site during infusions. See pages 601–603.

RELATED DIAGNOSTIC CATEGORIES

- Fluid volume deficit
- High risk for Fluid volume deficit
- Fluid volume excess

PLANNING

Client Goals
The client will

- Regain or maintain adequate fluid and electrolyte balance.

- Avoid complications associated with intravenous therapy.

Outcome Criteria
See Chapter 24, page 575.

Intravenous Infusions

An **intravenous (IV) infusion** is the installation into a vein of fluid and sometimes electrolytes or nutrient substances. It is given to clients who require extra fluid or who cannot take fluids and/or nutrients orally. A physician is responsible for ordering the type of solution to be administered, the amount to be given, and the rate at which it is to be infused.

Intravenous therapy can be prescribed for these reasons:

- To supply fluid when clients are unable to take in an adequate volume of fluids by mouth

- To provide salts needed to maintain electrolyte balance

- To provide glucose (dextrose), the main fuel for metabolism.

- To provide water-soluble vitamins and medications

- To establish a lifeline for rapidly needed medications

Common Types of Solutions
Common solutions administered intravenously include nutrient solutions, electrolyte solutions, alkalizing and acidifying solutions, and blood volume expanders. *Nutrient solutions* contain some form of carbohydrate (e.g., dextrose, glucose, or levulose) and water. Water is supplied for fluid requirements and carbohydrate for calories and energy. For example, 1

liter of 5% dextrose provides 170 calories. Nutrient solutions are useful in preventing dehydration and ketosis but do not provide sufficient calories to promote wound healing, weight gain, or normal growth in children. Common nutrient solutions are 5% dextrose in water (D5W) and 5% dextrose in 0.45% sodium chloride (dextrose in half-strength saline).

Electrolyte solutions contain varying amounts of cations and anions. Commonly used solutions are normal saline (0.9% sodium chloride solution), Ringer's solution (which contains sodium, chloride, potassium, and calcium), and lactated Ringer's solution (which contains sodium, chloride, potassium, calcium, and lactate). Lactate is a salt of lactic acid that is metabolized in the liver to form bicarbonate (HCO_3^-). Saline solutions are frequently used as initial hydrating solutions. Multiple electrolyte solutions approximate the ionic profile of plasma and are used to prevent dehydration or to restore or correct fluid and electrolyte imbalances.

Alkalizing solutions are administered to counteract metabolic acidosis. One commonly used solution is lactated Ringer's solution. *Acidifying solutions*, in contrast, are administered to counteract metabolic alkalosis. Examples of acidifying solutions are 5% dextrose in 0.45% sodium chloride and 0.9% sodium chloride solution.

Blood volume expanders are used to increase the volume of blood following severe loss of blood (e.g., from hemorrhage) or plasma (e.g., from severe burns, which draw large amounts of plasma from the bloodstream to the burn site). Common blood volume expanders are dextran, plasma, and human serum albumin.

Peripheral Venipuncture Sites

The site chosen for venipuncture varies with the client's age, the infusion time, the type of solution used, and the condition of veins. For adults, veins in the arm are commonly used; for infants, veins in the scalp are used. The larger veins of the forearm are preferred to the metacarpal veins of the hand for infusions that need to be given rapidly and for solutions that are hypertonic, are highly acidic or alkaline, or contain irritating medications.

The most convenient veins for venipuncture in the adult are the basilic and median cubital veins in the crease of the elbow, i.e., the antecubital space (Figure 25–1, *A*). Laboratory technicians often withdraw blood for examination from these large superficial veins. Unfortunately, use of these veins for prolonged infusions limits arm mobility, because a splint is needed to stabilize the elbow joint. For prolonged therapy, veins on the back of the hand and on the forearm are preferred. The metacarpal, basilic, and cephalic veins are commonly used (Figure 25–1, *B*). The ulna and radius act as natural splints at these sites, and the client has greater freedom of arm movements for activities such as eating. If an infusion is to be maintained for a long period, veins in the back of the hand or the dorsum of the foot are used (Figure 25–1, *C*).

Because infants do not have large veins in the antecubital fossa, blood specimens for examination are usually taken from the external jugular vein and femoral veins. Common sites for infusions in infants and children are shown in Figure 25–2 on page 590.

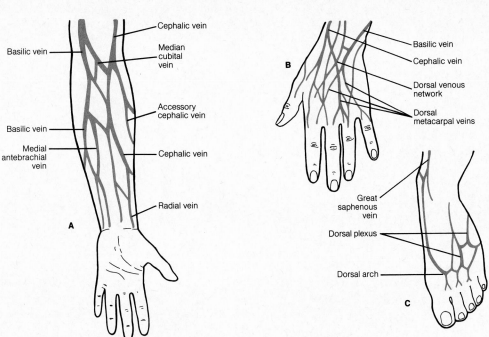

FIGURE 25–1 Commonly used venipuncture sites of the *A*, arm; *B*, hand; *C*, foot.

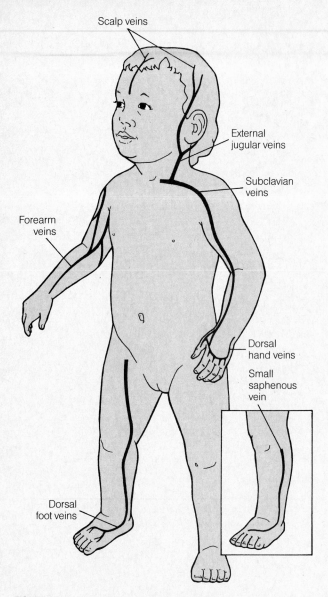

Scalp veins

External jugular veins

Subclavian veins

Forearm veins

Dorsal hand veins

Small saphenous vein

Dorsal foot veins

FIGURE 25–2 Venipuncture sites used in children.

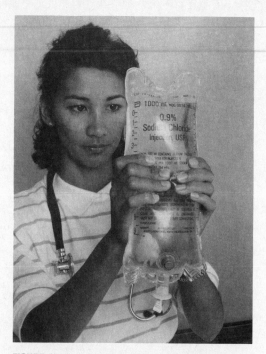

FIGURE 25–3 A plastic intravenous fluid container.

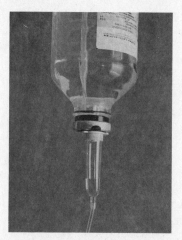

FIGURE 25–4 An intravenous container with an inside air vent.

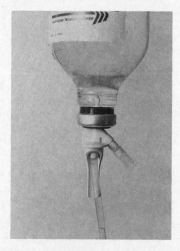

FIGURE 25–5 A nonvented intravenous container. Note the air vent on administration tubing.

Equipment

Because equipment varies according to the manufacturer, the nurse must become familiar with the equipment used in each particular agency.

Solution containers are available in various sizes (50, 100, 250, 500, or 1000 ml); the smaller containers are often used to administer medications. Most solutions are currently dispensed in plastic bags (Figure 25–3). However, glass bottles may need to be used if the administered medications are incompatible with plastic. Some glass solution bottles have a tube inside the bottle that serves as an air vent, so that air replaces the solution as it runs out of the bottle (Figure 25–4). Containers without air vents require a vent on the administration set (Figure 25–5). Air vents usually have filters to remove any contamination from the air that enters the container. Air vents are not required for plastic solution containers, because plas-

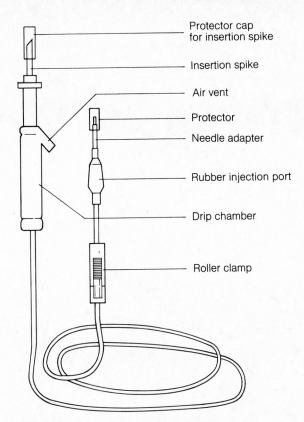

- Protector cap for insertion spike
- Insertion spike
- Air vent
- Protector
- Needle adapter
- Rubber injection port
- Drip chamber
- Roller clamp

FIGURE 25–6 Schematic of a standard vented administration set.

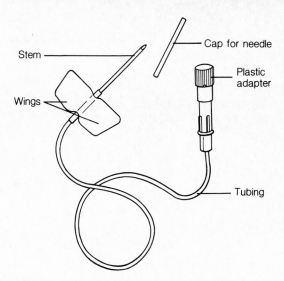

- Stem
- Wings
- Cap for needle
- Plastic adapter
- Tubing

FIGURE 25–7 Schematic of a butterfly needle with adapter.

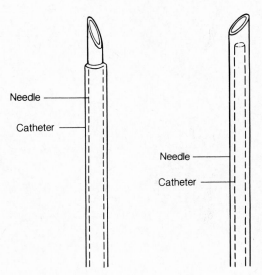

- Needle
- Catheter
- Needle
- Catheter

FIGURE 25–8 Schematic of an over-the-needle catheter and an inside-the-needle catheter.

tic bags collapse under atmospheric pressure when the solution enters the client's vein.

Administration sets consist of an insertion spike, a drip chamber, a roller valve or screw clamp, tubing, and a protective cap over the needle adapter (Figure 25–6). The insertion spike is kept sterile and inserted into the solution container when the equipment is set up and ready to start. The drip chamber permits a predictable amount of fluid to be delivered. A commonly used drip chamber is the macrodrip, which delivers 10 to 20 drops per milliliter of solution. This information is found on the package. There are also microdrip sets, which deliver 60 drops per milliliter of solution. The roller valve or screw clamp, which compresses the lumen of the tubing, controls the rate of the flow. The protective cap over the needle adapter maintains the sterility of the end of the tubing so that it can be attached to a sterile needle inserted in the client's vein.

IV poles (rods) are needed to hang the solution container. Some poles are attached to hospital beds; others stand on the floor or hang from the ceiling. Still others are floor models with casters that can be pushed along when a client is up and walking. The height of most poles is adjustable. The higher the solution container, the greater the force of the solution as it enters the client and the faster the rate of flow.

Many kinds of needles and catheters are commonly used for intravenous infusions. *Butterfly* or *wing-tipped needles* with plastic flaps attached to the shaft are shown in Figure 25–7. The flaps are held tightly together to hold the needle securely as it is inserted; after insertion, they are flattened against the skin and secured with tape. They vary in length from 1.5 to 3 cm (½ to 1¼ in), and from #25 to #17 gauge in diameter. The larger the gauge number, the smaller the diameter of the shaft. Needles of #20 to #22 gauge and short lengths are commonly used for adults. A *catheter or angiocatheter* is a plastic tube inserted into the vein. Some catheters fit over a needle during insertion, whereas others fit inside a needle (Figure 25–8). An angiocatheter has a metal stylet (needle), which is used to pierce the skin and vein and is then withdrawn, leaving the catheter in place.

IV filters are increasingly being used to remove air, particulate matter, and microbes from intravenous infusions and to reduce the risk of contamination and complications (e.g., infusion-related phlebitis) associated with routine intravenous therapies. In addition, most agencies advise use of a filter if the infusion contains KCl or if the site is to be used for medication administration. Although all clients may benefit from the use of filters, the National Intravenous Therapy Association (NITA) recommends them for clients at risk (e.g., those receiving long-term infusion therapy, total parenteral nutrition (discussed later in Chapter 26), and intra-arterial infusion chemotherapy. Further research to prove the value of filters in preventing clinical infection is needed.

Most IV filters in current use consist of a membrane (pore size of 0.22 μm, although sizes vary). Ideally, the filter should be located within the intra-venous line as close to the venipuncture site as possible (Crow 1987, p. 101). Some problems associated with filters include (a) clogging of the filter surface, which may stop or slow the flow rate when debris accumulates, and (b) drug binding of some drugs (e.g., insulin and amphotericin B) to the surface of the filter. When using filters, the nurse should remember that the filter should never be considered a substitute for quality care and meticulous aseptic technique.

Variations from the Standard Infusion

When more than one solution needs to be infused at the same time, *secondary sets* are used. Two set-ups are used for this purpose: the tandem setup and the piggyback set up. In a *tandem setup*, a second container is attached to the line of the first container at the lower, secondary port (Figure 25–9, *A*). It permits

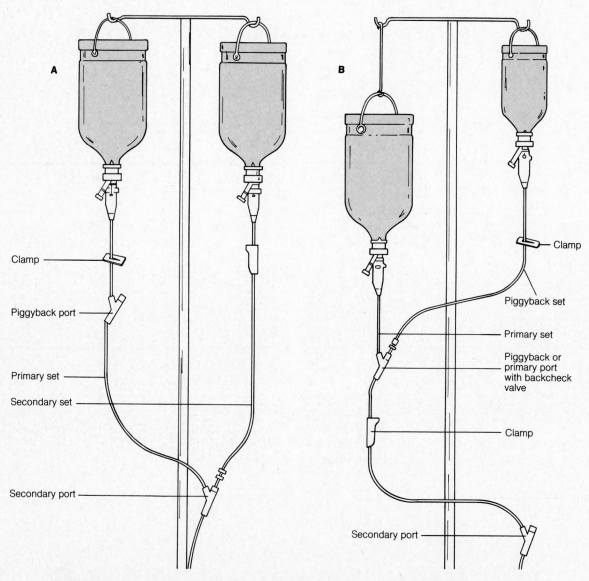

FIGURE 25–9 Secondary intravenous lines: *A*, a tandem intravenous alignment; *B*, a piggyback intravenous alignment.

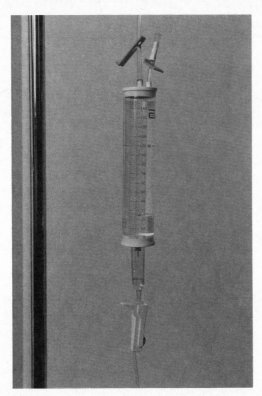

FIGURE 25–10 A volume-control set above the drip chamber of an intravenous infusion.

medications to be administered intermittently or simultaneously with the first solution.

In the *piggyback alignment*, a second set connects the second container to the tubing of the first at the upper port (Figure 25–9, *B*). This setup is used solely for intermittent drug administration. Various manufacturers describe these sets differently, so the nurse must check the manufacturer's labeling and directions carefully.

Another variation is a *volume-control set*, which is used if the volume of fluid administered is to be carefully controlled. The set is attached below the solution container, and the drip chamber is placed below the set (Figure 25–10). Volume-control sets are frequently used in pediatric settings, where the volume administered is critical.

Pumps and Controllers

A number of kinds of electronic pumps and controllers are available to control intravenous flow rates more precisely than the standard IV system. For further information, see page 611.

Sterile Injection Cap (Heparin or Saline Lock)

This device may be attached to an existing intravenous catheter to keep the route of venous access available for the administration of intermittent or emergency medications. The device is commonly

referred to as a *heparin* or *saline lock* because periodic injection with heparin or saline is used to keep blood from coagulating within the tubing. The lock consists of small plastic tubing with one self-sealing end into which medications can be injected (see Figure 36–41, on page 887.) The other end is inserted into the intravenous catheter.

Implantable Venous Access Devices (IVAD)

Recently developed implantable venous access devices or ports (IVAD) are used in the management of clients with chronic illness who require long-term intravenous therapy, e.g., intermittent medications, continuous infusions of fluid, blood, or parenteral nutrition fluids, and frequent blood samples (Figure 25–11). For further information, see Technique 25–9 on page 615.

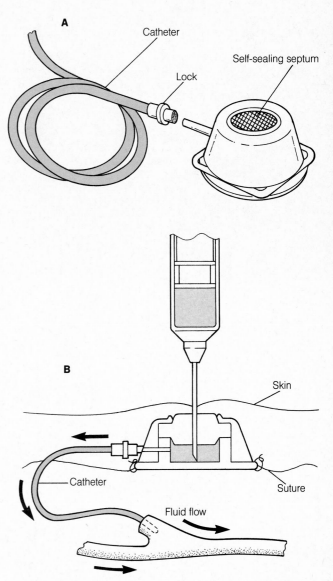

FIGURE 25–11 An implantable venous access device (IVAD): *A*, components; *B*, the device in place.

Preparing for an Intravenous Infusion

An intravenous infusion is set up before venipuncture so that the infusion can be quickly attached to the needle or catheter immediately after it is inserted. Before preparing the infusion, the nurse first verifies the physician's order indicating the type of solution, the amount to be administered, and the rate of flow of the infusion.

When selecting containers, the nurse should avoid using containers with greater volumes than ordered. For example, if 750 ml D5NS (750 ml of 5% dextrose in normal saline) has been ordered, obtain one 500-ml container and one 250-ml container, which total 750 ml. Do not obtain a 1000-ml container with the intention of stopping the solution after 750 ml has been administered. Too often, the incorrect amount can be instilled. If a 1000-ml solution container *must* be used, remove 250 ml before starting the infusion. Note that some agencies use abbreviations to describe commonly used solutions, e.g., DW (distilled water), NS (normal saline), D5W (5% dextrose in water), D5NS (5% dextrose in normal saline). The nurse should therefore become familiar with the abbreviations used by the agency.

It is essential that the solution be sterile and in

 good condition, i.e., clear. Cloudiness, evidence that the container has been opened previously, or leaks indicate possible contamination. The nurse should also check the expiration date on the label and squeeze and inspect plastic solution bags for leaks or hairline cracks. The nurse must return any unsatisfactory container to the central supply or distributing department, indicating the reason for the return.

Selection of an appropriate administration set depends on several factors:

- *Vents.* Tubing appropriate for either the rigid or flexible container should be selected.

- *Drop size.* For accurate regulation, a *microdrip* set is usually required if the fluid is to be administered at a rate of 50 to 75 ml/hr or less; a *macrodrip* should be selected when large quantities of solution or fast rates are required.

- *IV ports.* Ports are required to administer secondary infusions and medications.

- *Volumetric chamber.* This will be required if small doses of medication or fluid are to be delivered over an extended period of time.

To set up the intravenous infusion, see Technique 25–1.

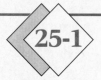 **25-1**   # Setting Up an Intravenous Infusion

PURPOSES   See page 588.

EQUIPMENT

- Appropriate administration set
- Correct container(s) of sterile intravenous solution
- IV pole

- Medication and timing labels for the infusion container, if required
- Label for the IV tubing

- IV filter, according to agency policy
- Infusion control pump (optional)

INTERVENTION

1. Open and prepare the administration set.

- Remove tubing from the container, and straighten it out.

- Slide the tubing clamp along the tubing until it is just below the drip chamber to facilitate its access.

- Close the clamp.

- Leave the ends of the tubing covered with the plastic caps until the infusion is started. *This will maintain the sterility of the ends of the tubing.*

2. Spike the solution container.

For a Bottle with a Rubber Stopper

- Remove the metal disc while

maintaining the sterility of the stopper. If the stopper becomes contaminated while you are removing the metal disc, swab it with disinfectant.

- Remove the cap from the tubing, and insert the spike firmly through the rubber stopper into the port, maintaining sterile technique.

▶ **Technique 25–1** *CONTINUED*

For a Bottle with an Indwelling Vent

- Remove the metal disc and the rubber diaphragm, keeping the stopper sterile, and listen for a hissing sound as the air rushes into the bottle. If there is no hissing sound, discard the container. *This indicates that the container was probably not sealed.*

- Insert the spike into the larger hole (the one without the vent).

For Spiking a Plastic Bag

- Remove the protective cover from the entry site, and insert the spike (Figure 25–12).

3. Hang the solution container on the pole.

- Adjust the pole so that the container is suspended about 1 m (3 ft) above the client's head. *This height is needed to enable gravity to overcome venous pressure and facilitate flow of the solution into the vein.*

4. Partially fill the drip chamber with solution.

For a Flexible Drip Chamber

- Squeeze the chamber gently until it is half full of solution (Figure 25–13).

For a Firm Drip Chamber

- The chamber will usually fill automatically. *The drip chamber is partly filled with solution to prevent air from moving down the tubing.*

5. Prime the tubing.

For Protective Caps without Air Vents

- Remove the protective cap, and hold the tubing over a cup or basin. Maintain the sterility of the end of the tubing and the cap.

- Release the clamp, and let the fluid run through the tubing until all bubbles are removed. Tap the tubing if necessary with your fingers to help the bubbles move. *The tubing is primed to prevent the introduction of air into the client. Air bubbles in large amounts (e.g., 10 ml) can act as emboli in the bloodstream. Air bubbles smaller than 0.5 ml usually do not cause problems in peripheral lines* (Millam 1991, p. 75).

- Reclamp the tubing, and replace the tubing cap, maintaining sterile technique.

For Caps with Air Vents

- Do not remove the cap when priming this tubing. The flow of solution through the tubing will cease when the cap is moist with one drop of solution.

- If an infusion control pump or controller is being used, follow the manufacturer's directions for inserting the tubing and setting the infusion rate.

6. Apply a medication label to the solution container, according to agency policy.

- In many agencies, medications and labels are applied in the pharmacy; if they are not, apply the label upside down on the container (see Figure 36–35 on page 880). *The label is applied upside down so it can be read easily when the container is hanging up.*

7. Label the IV tubing.

- Label tubing with date, time of attachment, and initials (Figure 25–14). This labeling may also be done at the time the infusion is started. *The tubing is labeled to ensure that it is changed at regular intervals* (i.e., every 24 to 72 hours according to agency policy).

8. Apply a timing label on the solution container.

- The timing label may be applied at the time the infusion is started. Follow agency practice. See discussion of regulating infusion flow rates, Figure 25–21 on page 600.

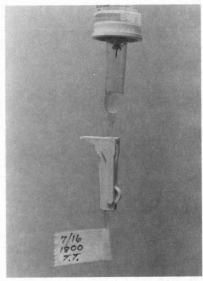

FIGURE 25–14 Tubing labeled with the date, time of attachment, and nurse's initials.

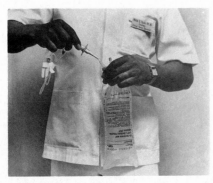

FIGURE 25–12 Inserting the spike.

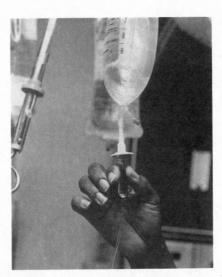

FIGURE 25–13 Squeezing the drip chamber.

▶ **Technique 25–1 Setting Up an Intravenous Infusion** CONTINUED

KEY ELEMENTS OF SETTING UP AN INTRAVENOUS INFUSION

- Maintain asepsis.
- Select the correct solution.
- Prime the tubing.

- Label the container appropriately.
- Label the IV tubing with the date and time of attachment.

Selecting a Venipuncture Site

As a general rule, the nurse should use the distal veins of the hands and arms when initiating intravenous therapy. Guidelines for vein selection are shown in the accompanying box. The nurse must observe and palpate the extremity before choosing a vein.

Starting an Intravenous Infusion

Agency practices vary about which nurses perform venipunctures and start intravenous infusions. In many settings, nurses must be supervised and certified before they are permitted to start infusions on their own. Some agencies have teams of specially prepared nurses who initiate all intravenous infusions. Before starting an infusion, the nurse must determine the following:

- The physician's exact orders.
- Whether the client has any allergies, e.g., to tape or povidone-iodine.
- The agency policy about shaving the area before a venipuncture. Some agencies advise against shaving because of the possibility of nicking the skin and subsequent infection.

To perform venipuncture and start an intravenous infusion, see Technique 25–2.

Guidelines for Vein Selection

- Use distal veins of the arm first.
- Use the nondominant arm of the client whenever possible.
- Use veins in the feet and legs only when arm veins are inaccessible, because they are more prone to thrombus formation and subsequent emboli.
- Select a vein that
  a. Is easily palpated and feels soft and full.
  b. Is naturally splinted by bone.
  c. Is large enough to allow adequate circulation around the catheter.

Avoid using the following veins:
- Those in areas of flexion (e.g., the antecubital fossa)
- Those that are highly visible, because they tend to roll away from the needle
- Those damaged by previous use, phlebitis, infiltration, or sclerosis
- Those continually distended with blood or that have become knotted or tortuous
- Veins of a surgically compromised or injured extremity (e.g., following a mastectomy) because of possible impaired circulation and discomfort for the client.

25-2 Starting an Intravenous Infusion Using a Butterfly Needle or an Angiocatheter

Before commencing an intravenous infusion determine any client allergies, e.g., to tape or povidone-iodine.

PURPOSES   See page 588.

ASSESSMENT FOCUS

Vital signs (pulse, respiratory rate, and blood pressure) for baseline data; skin turgor; allergy to tape or iodine; bleeding tendencies; disease or injury to extremities and status of veins to determine appropriate venipuncture site.

▶ **Technique 25–2** CONTINUED

EQUIPMENT

- Restraints for pediatric or confused clients.
- Intravenous administration set
- Container of sterile parenteral solution
- Intravenous stand (pole)
- Adhesive or nonallergenic tape
- Skin preparation materials, if the skin at the site will be shaved
- Gloves
- Tourniquet (rubber band or

blood pressure cuff may be used for infants)
- Antiseptic swabs
- Antiseptic ointment, e.g., povidone-iodine (Betadine)
- Sterile butterfly (wing-tipped) needle (a 2.5-cm (1-in) needle, #21 or #23 gauge, is used for most infusions; a #19 needle for whole blood; and a #24 gauge for infants)

or

- Angiocatheter of suitable size, e.g., #22 gauge for clear liquid infusions, #20 gauge for infusing drug boluses or peripheral fat solutions
- Gauze squares or other appropriate dressings
- Arm splint, if required
- Towel or pad
- Receptacle for discarded fluid

INTERVENTION

1. Prepare the client.

- Explain the procedure to the client. A venipuncture can cause discomfort for a few seconds, but there should be no discomfort while the solution is flowing. Use a doll to demonstrate for children and explain the procedure to the parents. Clients often want to know how long the process will last. The physician's order may specify the length of time of the infusion, e.g., 3000 ml over 24 hours.

- Provide any scheduled care before establishing the infusion to minimize movement of the affected limb during the procedure. *Moving the limb after the infusion has been established could dislodge the needle.*

- Make sure that the client's gown can be removed over the IV apparatus if necessary. Some agencies provide special gowns that open over the shoulder and down the sleeve for easy removal.

- Seek assistance from another health care worker to restrain the child during the procedure. *This prevents injury due to excessive movement.*

- Apply wrist restraints or hand mitts bilaterally, after explaining the need for them to the child and parent. *Restraints prevent accidental or intentional removal of*

the catheter, or injury by IV needle due to sudden movement during the insertion.

- Wash hands

2. Set up the infusion equipment if not already prepared.

- See Technique 25–1 on page 594.

- Prepare strips of adhesive tape to stabilize the needle once it is inserted.

3. Select and prepare the venipuncture site.

- Starting at the distal end of the vein, select a site by palpating accessible veins. Veins can become sclerotic from irritation by the infusion or the needle. Sclerosis may then interfere with venous flow. If so, use more proximal parts of the veins.

- If necessary, shave the skin where adhesive tape will be applied (about a 2-inch area around the intended site). Check agency policy.

4. Dilate the vein.

- Place the extremity in a dependent position (lower than the client's heart). *Gravity slows venous return and distends the veins. Distending the veins makes it easier to insert the needle properly.*

- Apply a tourniquet firmly 15 to

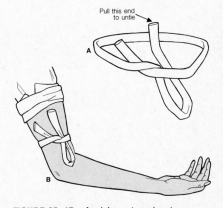

FIGURE 25–15 Applying a tourniquet.

20 cm (6 to 8 in) above the venipuncture site (Figure 25–15). For children, explain that the tourniquet will feel tight. The tourniquet must be tight enough to obstruct venous flow but not so tight that it occludes arterial flow. *Obstructing arterial flow inhibits venous filling.* If a radial pulse can be palpated, the arterial flow is not obstructed.

- If the vein is not sufficiently dilated,

  a. Massage or stroke the vein distal to the site and in the direction of venous flow toward the heart. *This action helps fill the vein.*

  b. Encourage the client to clench and unclench the fist rapidly. *Contracting the muscles compresses the distal veins, forcing blood along the veins and distending them.*

► **Technique 25–2 Starting an Intravenous Infusion** CONTINUED

c. Lightly tap the vein with your fingertips. *Tapping may distend the vein.*

- If the above steps fail to distend the vein so that it is palpable, remove the tourniquet, and apply heat to the entire extremity for 10 to 15 minutes. *Heat dilates superficial blood vessels, causing them to fill.* Then repeat the steps above.

5. Don gloves, and clean the venipuncture site. *Gloves protect the nurse from contamination by the client's blood.*

- Clean the skin at the site of entry with a topical antiseptic swab, e.g., alcohol, and then an anti-infective solution e.g., povidone-iodine (Betadine).

- Use a circular motion, moving from the center outwards for several inches. *This motion carries microorganisms away from the site of entry.*

6. Insert the needle or angio-catheter, and initiate the infusion.

- Use one thumb to pull the skin taut below the entry site. *This stabilizes the vein and makes the skin taut for needle entry. It can also make initial tissue penetration less painful.*

For a Butterfly Needle

- Hold the needle, pointed in the direction of the blood flow, at a 30° angle, with the bevel up, and pierce the skin beside the vein about 1 cm (½ in) below the site planned for piercing the vein (Figure 25–16).

- Once the needle is through the skin, lower the needle so that it is almost parallel with the skin. *Lowering the needle reduces the chances of puncturing both sides of the vein.* Follow the course of

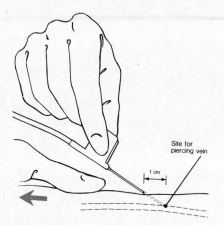

FIGURE 25–16 Inserting a butterfly needle.

the vein, and pierce one side of the vein.

- When blood flows back into the needle tubing, insert the needle farther up the vein 2 to 2.5 cm. (¾ to 1 in) or to the hub of the butterfly needle. Sudden lack of resistance can be felt as blood enters the needle.

- Release the tourniquet, attach the infusion, and initiate flow as quickly as possible. *Attaching the tubing quickly prevents blood from clotting and obstructing the needle.*

For an Angiocatheter

- Insert the catheter by the direct or indirect method. The direct method is preferred for large veins and the indirect method for smaller veins (Peck 1985, p. 40). For the *direct method,* hold the catheter with bevel up, at a 15° to 20° angle, and insert the catheter through the skin and into the vein in one thrust. For the *indirect method,* first pierce the skin, then reduce the angle and advance the catheter into the vein. Sudden lack of resistance is felt as the catheter enters the vein.

- Once blood appears in the catheter or you feel the lack of resis-

tance, lower the catheter so that it is almost parallel with the skin, then advance it another 0.6 cm (¼ in). *The catheter is advanced to ensure that it, and not just the metal needle, is in the vein.*

- Release the tourniquet.

- Remove the protective cap from the distal end of the tubing, and hold it ready to attach to the catheter, maintaining the sterility of the end.

- Grasp the hub of the catheter with your thumb and index finger, and withdraw the needle (Figure 25–17).

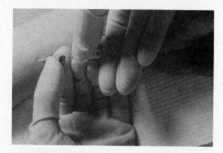

FIGURE 25–17 Withdrawing the needle from an angiocatheter.

- Advance the catheter up to the hub or until you feel resistance.

- Attach the end of the infusion tubing to the catheter hub. Initiate the infusion.

7. Secure the needle or catheter with tape.

- Tape the butterfly needle securely by the H method (Figure 25–18) or crisscross (chevron)

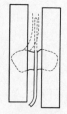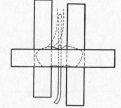

FIGURE 25–18 Taping the butterfly needle by the H method.

▶ **Technique 25–2** CONTINUED

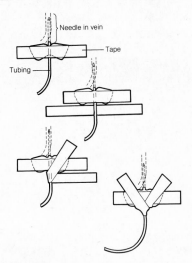

FIGURE 25–19 Taping the butterfly needle by the crisscross (chevron) method.

method (Figure 25–19). Place a cotton ball or small gauze square under the needle, if required. *The gauze keeps the needle in position in the vein.*

• Tape the catheter:

a. Place the first tape, sticky side up, under the catheter hub, and fold the sticky sides down on the skin along each side of the catheter distal to the insertion point.

b. Place the second strip, sticky side down, across the catheter hub.

c. Place the third strip, sticky side up, under the catheter hub distal to the second strip, and fold each side diagonally across the catheter.

8. Dress and label the venipuncture site according to agency policy.

• In some agencies, the nurse puts a small amount of antiseptic ointment, e.g., povidone-iodine, over the venipuncture site, then a gauze square. In other agencies, a sterile transparent occlusive dressing is applied. This permits assessment of the site without disturbing the dressing. This type of dressing can be left on for 72 hours, unless there are complications (Peck 1985, p. 32).

• Loop the tubing, and secure it to the dressing with tape. *Looping and securing the tubing prevent the weight of the tubing or any movement from pulling on the needle or catheter.*

• Label a piece of tape with the date and time of insertion, type and gauge of needle or catheter used, and your initials. Apply the tape label over the venipuncture dressing (Figure 25–20).

9. Ensure appropriate infusion flow.

• Apply a padded arm board (fold-

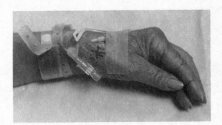

FIGURE 25–20 Properly labeled tape over venipuncture dressing.

ed towel on a board) to splint the elbow or wrist joint, if needed.

• Apply restraints to the infusion site to immobilize the site if a child is agitated or very active, or to any extremity that might be used to dislodge the catheter.

• Adjust the infusion rate of flow according to the order.

10. Document relevant data, including assessments.

• Record the start of the infusion on the client's chart. Some agencies provide a special form for this purpose. Include the date and time of the venipuncture; amount and type of solution used, including any additives (e.g., kind and amount of medications); absorption time; container number; drip rate, type and gauge of the needle or catheter; venipuncture site; and client's general response.

EVALUATION FOCUS

Skin status at IV site (warm temperature and absence of pain, redness, and swelling); dressing clean and dry; IV flow rate consistent with that ordered; ability to perform self-care activities; understanding of any mobility limitations; vital signs at baseline level.

SAMPLE RECORDING

Date	Time	Notes
06/08/93	1800	IV #1–1000 ml D5W started in the right basilic vein. BF needle #21G inserted. Drip rate 125 ml/hr. Completion time 0200 hours. IV running at prescribed rate s̄ signs of infiltration. No discomfort voiced. Dino C. Anastasio, NS

▶ **Technique 25–2 Starting an Intravenous Infusion** CONTINUED

KEY ELEMENTS OF STARTING AN INTRAVENOUS INFUSION USING A BUTTERFLY NEEDLE OR AN ANGIOCATHETER

See also Key Elements for Technique 25–1.
- Select an appropriate gauge needle (catheter).
- Determine allergies to tape or to iodine.
- Wear gloves.
- Select the most distal vein site possible.
- Dilate the vein before venipuncture.

- Insert the needle or catheter correctly.
- Ensure that IV flow is established.
- Secure the IV needle or catheter securely.
- Dress the venipuncture site, and label the dressing appropriately.

Regulating Intravenous Flow Rates

An important nursing function is to regulate the flow rate of an intravenous infusion. The physician usually describes in the order how long an infusion should last, e.g., 3000 ml over 24 hours. It is then a nursing responsibility to calculate the correct flow rate and regulate the infusion. Problems that can result from incorrectly regulated infusions include hypervolemia and hypovolemia. Unless a regulating device (i.e., a controller, infusion pump, or in-line manual adjuster) is being used, the nurse administering the intravenous solution must regulate the drops per minute manually by using the roller clamp to ensure that the prescribed amount of solution will be infused in the correct time span.

There are a number of commercially prepared infusion sets, each with its own type of drip chamber; so, it is important to know the number of drops per milliliter of solution for a particular drip chamber before calculating a drip rate. This rate, called the **drop** or **drip factor**, is printed on most commercially prepared packages. Common drop factors are 10, 15, and 20 for macrodrips (regular infusion sets) and 60 for microdrips (minidrip infusion sets).

To calculate flow rates, the nurse must know the volume of fluid to be infused and the specific time for the infusion. Two commonly used methods of indicating flow rates are designating the number of milliliters to be administered in 1 hour (ml/hr) and the number of drops to be given in 1 minute (gtt/min). Since 1 milliliter of fluid displaces 1 cubic centimeter of space, the volume to be infused in the first method may also be designated as cubic centimeters per hour (cc/hr).

Milliliters per Hour

Hourly rates of infusion can be calculated by dividing the total infusion volume by the total infusion time in hours. For example, if 3000 ml is infused in 24 hours, the number of milliliters per hour is

$$\frac{3000 \text{ ml (total infusion volume)}}{24 \text{ hr (total infusion time)}} = 125 \text{ ml/hr}$$

Nurses need to check infusions at least every hour to ensure that the indicated milliliters per hour have infused. A strip of adhesive marking the exact time and/or amount to be infused may be taped to the solution bottle. Some agencies make premarked labels available (Figure 25–21).

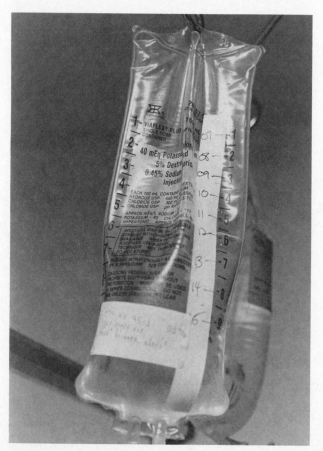

FIGURE 25–21 Timing label on an intravenous container.

Drops per Minute

The nurse who begins an infusion must regulate the drops per minute to ensure that the prescribed amount of solution will infuse. Drops per minute are calculated by the following formula:

Drops per minute =
$$\frac{\text{Total infusion volume} \times \text{drops/ml (or drop factor)}}{\text{Total time of infusion in } \textit{minutes}}$$

If the requirements are 1000 ml in 8 hours (480 minutes) and the drip factor is 20 drops/ml, the drops per minute should be

$$\frac{1000 \text{ ml} \times 20 \text{ drops/ml}}{480 \text{ min}} = 41 \text{ drops/min}$$

Approximating this rate as 40 drops/min, the nurse must then regulate the drops per minute by tightening or releasing the intravenous tubing clamp and counting the drops the same way a pulse is counted. Devices such as battery-operated rate meters and infusion pumps with alarm systems facilitate a regulated flow. See pages 607 to 614 for infusion flow devices, e.g., volume control devices, Dial-A-Flo inline device, and pumps and controllers.

Monitoring an Intravenous Infusion

An important nursing responsibility is to monitor an intravenous infusion so that the flow of the correct solution is maintained at the correct rate. The nurse needs to assess the whole infusion system at least every hour to identify problems. Common problems are fluid infiltration, phlebitis, circulatory overload, bleeding at the venipuncture site, and blockage of the infusion flow.

Monitoring and Maintaining an Intravenous Infusion

PURPOSES	• To maintain the prescribed flow rate • To prevent complications associated with IV therapy
ASSESSMENT FOCUS	Appearance of infusion site; patency of system; type of fluid being infused and rate of flow; any adverse response of the client.

INTERVENTION

1. Gather pertinent data.

• From the physician's order, determine the type and sequence of solutions to be infused.

• Determine the rate of flow and infusion schedule.

2. Ensure that the correct solution is being infused.

• If the solution is incorrect, slow the rate of flow to a minimum to maintain the patency of the catheter. *If the infusion is terminated, the client will have to have another venipuncture before the new solution is administered.*

• Report the error to the nurse in charge, and change the solution to the correct one. Note that agencies have different policies about how and to whom to report an incident.

3. Observe the rate of flow every hour.

• Compare the rate of flow regularly, e.g., every hour, against the infusion schedule. *Infusions that are off schedule can be harmful to a client.*

• If the rate is *too fast*, slow it so that the infusion will be completed at the planned time. *Solution administered too quickly may cause a significant increase in circulating blood volume (which is about 6 liters in an adult). Hypervolemia may result in pulmonary edema and cardiac failure.* The clinical signs of cardiac failure are dyspnea, reduced urine output, edema, weak and rapid pulse, and shallow, rapid respirations. The clinical signs of pulmonary edema are dyspnea, coughing, frothy sputum, and rales on lung ascultation.

• If the rate is *too slow*, check agency practice. Some agencies permit nursing personnel to adjust a rate of flow 3 ml/min or less. Adjustments above 3 ml/min may require a physician's order. *Solution that is administered too slowly can supply insufficient fluid, electrolytes, or medication for a client's needs.*

• If the rate of flow is 150 ml/hr or

▶ **Technique 25–3 Monitoring an Intravenous Infusion** CONTINUED

S more, check the rate of flow more frequently, e.g., every 15 to 30 minutes.

4. Inspect the patency of the IV tubing and needle.

- Inspect the tubing for pinches or kinks or obstructions to flow. Arrange the tubing so that it is lightly coiled and under no pressure. Sometimes the tubing becomes caught under the client's arm and the weight of the arm blocks the flow.

- Observe the position of the tubing. If it is dangling below the venipuncture, coil it carefully on the surface of the bed. *The solution cannot flow upward into the vein against the force of gravity.*

- Open the drip regulator, and observe for a rapid flow of fluid from the solution container into the drip chamber. Then partially close the drip chamber to reestablish the prescribed rate of flow. *Rapid flow of fluid into the drip chamber indicates patency of the IV line. Closing the drip chamber to the prescribed rate of flow prevents fluid overload.*

- Lower the solution container below the level of the infusion site, and observe for a return flow of blood from the vein. *A return flow of blood indicates that the needle is patent and in the vein. Blood returns in this instance because venous pressure is greater than the fluid pressure in the IV tubing. Absence of blood return may indicate that the needle is no longer in the vein.*

- Observe the position of the solution container. If it is less than 1 m (3 ft) above the IV site, readjust it to the correct height of the pole. *If the container is too low, the solution may not flow into the vein because there is insufficient gravitational pressure to*

overcome the pressure of the blood within the vein.

- Observe the drip chamber. If it is less than half full, squeeze the chamber to allow the correct amount of fluid to flow in (Figure 25–13, earlier).

- Determine whether the bevel of the catheter is blocked against the wall of the vein. If it is blocked, pull back gently, turn it slightly, or carefully raise or lower the angle of insertion slightly, using a sterile gauze pad underneath to protect the skin and change the position of the catheter bevel.

- If there is leakage, locate the source. If the leak is at the catheter connection, tighten the tubing into the catheter. If the leak cannot be stopped, slow the infusion as much as possible without stopping it, and replace the tubing with a new sterile set. Estimate the amount of solution lost, if it was substantial.

5. Inspect the infusion site for fluid infiltration.

- The escape of intravenous fluid into the interstitial tissues, usually near the intravenous site, often causes swelling. In such a case the needle becomes dislodged from the vein, and the intravenous fluid flows into the subcutaneous tissue. The clinical signs are swelling, coolness, pain, pallor at the site, and discomfort.

- To ascertain the presence of infiltration:

  a. Palpate the surrounding tissue for edema.

  b. Feel the surrounding skin for changes in temperature.

6. If infiltration is not evident but the infusion is not flowing,

determine whether the needle is dislodged from the vein.

- Gently pinch the IV tubing adjacent to the needle site. *This will cause blood to flow (flash back) into the tubing if the needle is in the vein.*

- Use a sterile syringe of saline to withdraw fluid from the rubber at the end of the tubing near the venipuncture site. If blood does not return, discontinue the intravenous infusion.

- Try to stop the flow by applying a tourniquet 10 to 15 cm (4 to 6 in) above the insertion site and opening the roller clamp wide. *If the infusion continues to flow slowly, the needle is in subcutaneous tissue (it has infiltrated). If the infusion has infiltrated, immediately discontinue the infusion. See Technique 25–5 on page 605.*

7. Inspect the infusion site for phlebitis (inflammation of a vein).

- Inspect and palpate the site every 8 hours (Lonsway 1987, p. 107). Phlebitis can occur as a result of injury to a vein, e.g., because of mechanical trauma or chemical irritation. Chemical injury to a vein can occur from intravenous electrolytes (especially potassium and magnesium) and medications. The clinical signs are redness, warmth, and swelling at the intravenous site and burning pain along the course of a vein.

- If phlebitis is detected, discontinue the infusion, and apply warm compresses to the venipuncture site. Do not use this injured vein for further infusions.

8. Inspect the intravenous site for bleeding.

- Oozing or bleeding into the sur-

▶ **Technique 25–3** *CONTINUED*

rounding tissues can occur while the infusion is freely flowing but is more likely to occur after the needle has been removed from the vein.

- Observation of the venipuncture site is extremely important for clients who bleed readily, e.g., clients receiving anticoagulants.

9. Teach the client ways to maintain the infusion system. Instruct the client to:

- Call for assistance if the solution stops dripping or the venipuncture site becomes swollen.
- Avoid sudden twisting or turning movements of the arm with the needle or catheter.
- Avoid stretching or placing tension on the tubing.
- Try to keep the tubing from dangling below the level of the needle.

- Notify a nurse if:

  a. There is a sudden change in the flow rate or if the solution stops dripping.

  b. The solution container is nearly empty.

  c. There is blood in the IV tubing.

  d. Discomfort or swelling is experienced at the IV site.

EVALUATION FOCUS	Amount of fluid infused according to the schedule; intactness of IV system; appearance of IV site (e.g., dry, tissue infiltration, discomfort); urinary output compared to urinary intake; tissue turgor; specific gravity of urine; vital signs compared to baseline data.

KEY ELEMENTS OF MONITORING AND MAINTAINING AN INTRAVENOUS INFUSION

- Maintain asepsis.
- Ensure that the correct type and amount of fluid is infused within the specified time period.

- Prevent or identify early fluid infiltration, phlebitis, and signs of circulatory overload.

Changing Intravenous Containers and Tubing

Intravenous solution containers are changed when only a small amount of fluid remains in the neck of the container and fluid still remains in the drip chamber. The Centers for Disease Control (CDC) (1982) recommend that tubing be changed every 48 hours to decrease the incidence of phlebitis and infection. However, recent studies indicate that 72-hour intervals may be appropriate (Josephson et al. 1985, p. 367; Snydman et al. 1987, p. 116). Tubing is changed most easily when a new container is added. Technique 25–4 provides guidelines for changing an intravenous container and tubing.

Changing an Intravenous Container and Tubing

PURPOSES	• To maintain the flow of required fluids • To maintain sterility of the IV system and decrease the incidence of phlebitis and infection • To maintain patency of the IV tubing

▶

► **Technique 25–4 Changing an IV Container and Tubing** *CONTINUED*

ASSESSMENT FOCUS	Presence of fluid infiltration, bleeding, or phlebitis at IV site; allergy to tape or iodine; infusion rate and amount absorbed; blockages in IV system.

EQUIPMENT

- Container with the correct kind and amount of sterile solution
- Administration set, including sterile tubing and drip chamber
- Timing label
- Gloves
- Sterile swabs
- Receptacle (e.g., a basin) for discarded fluid
- Antiseptic solution and/or ointment for cleaning the site. Check agency practice.
- Tape
- Sterile gauze square for positioning the needle

INTERVENTION

1. Obtain the correct solution container.

- Verify the physician's order.

- Compare the number on the new container against the number on the used container.

- Read the label of the new container.

2. Set up the intravenous equipment with the new container, and label them.

- See Technique 25–1, earlier.

- Apply a timing label to the container.

- Prime the tubing.

- Label the tubing as shown in Figure 25–14, earlier.

3. Remove the venipuncture dressing to expose the needle or catheter hub.

- Loosen the tape at the venipuncture site.

- Don gloves to prevent exposure to the client's secretions.

- Remove the tape and the dressing from around the needle or catheter, taking care not to dislodge the needle or catheter from the vein.

4. Disconnect the used tubing.

- Place a sterile swab under the hub of the catheter. *This absorbs any leakage that might occur when the tubing is disconnected.*

- Holding the hub of the needle with the nondominant hand, loosen the tubing with the dominant hand, using a twisting, pulling motion. *Holding the needle firmly but gently maintains its position in the vein.*

- Clamp and remove the used IV tubing.

- Place the end of the tubing in the basin or other receptacle.

5. Connect the new tubing, and reestablish the infusion.

- Continue to hold the needle, and grasp the new tubing with the dominant hand.

- Remove the protective tubing cap, and, maintaining sterility, insert the tubing end securely into the needle hub. Twist it to secure it.

- Open the clamp to start the solution flowing.

6. Clean the venipuncture site, and apply a sterile dressing with label.

- Clean the venipuncture site, working from the insertion point outward in a circular manner. Iodine or ethyl alcohol is frequently used. Some agencies also place water-soluble iodine ointment, e.g., Betadine, at the site.

- Tape the needle in place. See Technique 25–2.

- Apply a sterile dressing over the site.

- Remove gloves.

- Apply a labeled tape over the dressing. The label should include (a) the date and time the dressing is applied; (b) the original date and time of the venipuncture; (c) the size of the catheter or needle; and (d) your initials, as the nurse who changed the dressing.

7. Regulate the rate of flow of the solution according to the order on the chart.

8. Document all relevant information.

- Record the change of the solution container and/or tubing in the appropriate place on the client's chart. Also record the fluid intake according to agency practice. Record the number of the container if the containers are numbered at the agency. Also record your assessments.

▶ **Technique 25–4** *CONTINUED*

EVALUATION FOCUS	Skin integrity around IV insertion site; absence of signs of infection, circulatory overload, infiltration, or phlebitis.

SAMPLE RECORDING

Date	Time	Notes
09/06/93	1100	1000 ml of D₅W added to IV. Tubing changed and labelled. Flow adjusted to 125 ml/hr. Insertion site care provided. Site appears clean. No inflammation or signs of infiltration present.————————— Don Rasowski, SN

KEY ELEMENTS OF CHANGING AN INTRAVENOUS CONTAINER AND TUBING

- Determine allergies to tape or iodine.
- Select the correct solution.
- Maintain asepsis.
- Prime the tubing before attaching it to the IV needle.
- Wear gloves when there is the possibility of contact with body secretions.
- Prevent needle dislodgement when disconnecting and connecting the IV tubing and when cleaning the venipuncture site.

- Make sure the IV system is intact and the correct flow rate is established.
- Inspect and clean the venipuncture site appropriately.
- Secure the needle appropriately with tape, and apply an appropriate dressing.
- Label the container, tubing, and dressing appropriately.

Discontinuing an Intravenous Infusion

Discontinuing an infusion is not uncomfortable; in fact, it is usually a relief for the client and takes only a couple of minutes. Infusions are usually discontinued for one of three reasons:

1. The client's oral fluid intake and hydration status are satisfactory, so that no further intravenous solutions are ordered.

2. There is a problem with the infusion that cannot be fixed. The nurse must consult with the nurse in charge before discontinuing an IV because of such a difficulty.

3. The medications administered by the intravenous route (e.g., antibiotics) are no longer required.

Before removing a catheter or needle from the vein, the nurse must determine whether a sterile injection cap (heparin lock) should be attached to the catheter so that intravenous medications can be administered intermittently.

 25-5

Discontinuing an Intravenous Infusion

ASSESSMENT FOCUS	Appearance of the venipuncture site; any bleeding from the infusion site; amount of fluid infused.

EQUIPMENT
- Gloves

- Dry or antiseptic-soaked swabs, according to agency practice

- Small sterile dressing and tape

▶

▶ **Technique 25–5 Discontinuing an IV Infusion** *CONTINUED*

INTERVENTION

1. Prepare the equipment.

- Clamp the infusion tubing. *Clamping the tubing will prevent the fluid from flowing out of the needle onto the client or bed.*

- Loosen the tape at the venipuncture site while holding the needle firmly and applying countertraction to the skin. *Movement of the needle can injure the vein and cause discomfort to the client. Countertraction prevents pulling the skin and causing discomfort.*

- Don gloves, and hold a swab above the venipuncture site. *Gloves prevent direct contact with the client's blood.*

2. Withdraw the needle or catheter from the vein.

- Withdraw the needle or catheter by pulling it out along the line of the vein. *Pulling out in line with the vein avoids injury to the vein.*

- Immediately apply firm pressure to the site, using the swab, for 2 to 3 minutes. *Pressure helps stop the bleeding and prevents hematoma formation.*

- Hold the client's arm or leg above the body if any bleeding persists. *Raising the limb decreases blood flow to the area.*

3. Examine a catheter removed from the client.

- Check the catheter to make sure it is intact. *If a piece of tubing remains in the client's vein it could move centrally (toward the heart or lungs) and cause serious problems.*

- Report a broken catheter to the nurse in charge immediately.

- If the broken piece can be palpated, apply a tourniquet above the insertion site. *Application of a tourniquet decreases the possibility of the piece moving until a physician is notified.*

4. Cover the open wound.

- Apply the sterile dressing. *The dressing continues the pressure and covers the open area in the skin, preventing infection.*

- Discard the IV solution container, if infusions are being discontinued, and discard the used supplies appropriately.

5. Document all relevant information.

- Record the amount of fluid infused on the intake and output record and on the chart, according to agency practice. Include the container number, type of solution used, time of discontinuing the infusion, and the client's response.

EVALUATION FOCUS	Appearance of the venipuncture site; the pulse, respirations, skin color, edema, sputum, cough, and urine output; and how the person feels physically and psychologically.

SAMPLE RECORDING

Date	Time	Notes
06/09/93	0600	IV #3 1000 ml D5W infused and discontinued. Catheter removed intact. Venipuncture site dry. Dry dressing applied ———— Serena Lam, RN

KEY ELEMENTS OF DISCONTINUING AN INTRAVENOUS INFUSION

- Maintain asepsis.
- Prevent discomfort to the client.
- Prevent bleeding and hematoma formation.

- Make sure a catheter is removed intact.
- Wear gloves to prevent contamination by the client's body secretions.

The Dial-A-Flo In-Line Device

The Dial-A-Flo in-line device is equipped with a dial regulator that calibrates the desired volume of fluid to be infused (Figure 25–22). It can be attached during the initial venipuncture procedure or during an IV tubing change. Technique 25–6 describes how to use a Dial-A-Flo in-line device.

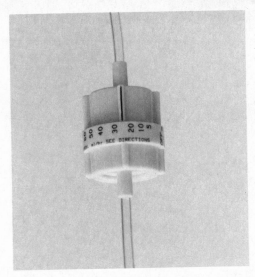

FIGURE 25–22 The Dial-A-Flo in-line device.

25-6 Using a Dial-A-Flo In-Line Device

PURPOSE	• To regulate delivery of the correct amount of intravenous fluid
ASSESSMENT FOCUS	Patency of existing IV line; amount of solution prescribed.

EQUIPMENT
- Dial-A-Flo in-line device
- Equipment for an intravenous

infusion. See Technique 25–1, page 594.

INTERVENTION

1. Attach the Dial-A-Flo device appropriately.

- Connect the Dial-A-Flo device to the end of the IV tubing.

- Connect the insertion spike of the IV tubing to the solution container.

2. Prime the tubing.

- Adjust the regulator on the Dial-A-Flow to the open position.

- Open all clamps and infusion flow regulators on the IV tubing.

- Remove the protective cap at the end of the tubing, and allow the fluid to run through the tubing.

- Reclamp the tubing to prevent continued flow of fluid.

3. Establish the infusion.

- Attach the primed tubing to the

venipuncture needle or catheter hub.

- Open the IV tubing flow regulator.

- Align the Dial-A-Flo regulator to the arrow indicating the desired volume of fluid to infuse over 1 hour.

4. Confirm the appropriate drip rate.

► **Technique 25–6 Using a Dial-A-Flow In-Line Device** CONTINUED

- Count the drip rate for 15 seconds, and multiply by 4. *This ensures that the rate coincides with the calculated drip rate.*

- Recheck the drip rate after 5 minutes and again after 15 minutes. *This detects potential changes in the rate resulting from expansion or contraction of the tubing.*

- If the drip rate does not coincide with that calculated, it may be necessary to adjust the height of the IV pole. *Elevation of the IV pole facilitates flow by gravity.*

5. Monitor the infusion flow.

- Check the volume of fluid infused at least every hour, and compare it with the time tape on the IV container.

6. Document all relevant information.

- Record the date and time of starting the infusion, the type and amount of fluid infused, the rate at which the IV is being infused, the infusion device used, the status of the IV insertion site, and any adverse responses of the client.

EVALUATION FOCUS

Amount of fluid infused in designated time period; status of IV insertion site; any adverse responses of client.

SAMPLE RECORDING

Date	Time	Notes
12/03/93	1500	1000 ml IV D$_5$W started at 125 ml/hour using Dial-A-Flo. Venipuncture site dry and clean c̄ no signs of infiltration or infection.—— Carola Brown, SN

KEY ELEMENTS OF USING A DIAL-A-FLO IN-LINE DEVICE

- Maintain asepsis of the IV system.
- Make sure the infusion rate is correctly set and the Dial-A-Flo regulator is operating accurately.

- Confirm the appropriate drip rate by counting the drops per minute after 5 minutes and again in 15 minutes.
- Monitor the infusion flow at least hourly, and compare the volume of fluid infused with the time tape on the IV container.

Volume Control Devices

A variety of types of volume control sets (also referred to as *burettes*) are available. All have a limited capacity (100 to 150 ml in size) to minimize the possibility of overloading the circulation, especially in children, and to facilitate the administration of medications (such as some antibiotics) that do not remain stable for the length of time it takes an entire solution container to infuse. When using these devices, the nurse must ensure that the tubing between the bottle and the chamber is firmly clamped to prevent additional fluid from flowing into the chamber.

Volume control sets are designed to deliver a reduced drop size (60 drops/ml). These microdroppers facilitate the calculation of flow rates. Since there are 60 minutes in an hour, the number of drops per minute equals the number of milliliters to be delivered per hour. For example, if the solution is to be infused at a rate of 40 ml per hour, the nurse regulates the infusion to deliver 40 drops per minute.

Some volume control sets have a stationary filter; others have a floating valve filter at the base of the chamber (Figure 25–23). These designs necessitate different methods for filling the drip chamber. See Technique 25–7.

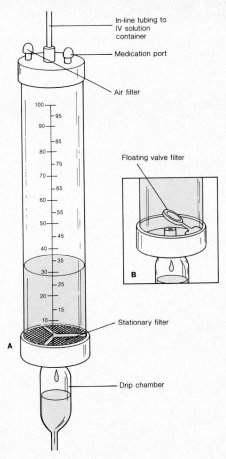

FIGURE 25–23 A volume-control intravenous infusion set: *A*, with a stationary filter; *B*, with a floating valve filter.

25-7

Using a Volume Control Device

PURPOSES	• To prevent fluid overflow • To administer intravenous medications (see Technique 36–8).
ASSESSMENT FOCUS	Amount of solution prescribed; patency of existing IV line and needle (see page 602).

EQUIPMENT

- □ Volume control set (e.g., Buretrol, Soluset, Volutrol, Pediatrol)
- □ IV solution
- □ IV medication, if ordered
- □ IV pole
- □ IV administration set with compatible IV tubing
- □ Alcohol swabs and tape

INTERVENTION

1. Inspect the patency of the IV tubing and needle.

- See Technique 25–3, step 4, on page 602.

2. Attach the volume control set between the intravenous solution container and the insertion spike of the IV tubing (Figure 25–10, earlier).

- Close the clamps above and below the volume control chamber.
- Open the air vent on top of the volume chamber.

▶

► **Technique 25–7 Using a Volume Control Device** *CONTINUED*

- Insert the spike of the volume control set into the solution container, and hang the container on the pole.

- Insert the IV tubing into the volume control set.

3. Fill the volume control drip chamber, and prime the tubing.

For a Set with a Stationary Membrane Filter

- Open the upper clamp, and allow the fluid chamber to fill with about 30 ml of solution or until about one-third full.

- Close the upper clamp and ensure that the air vent of the volume control device is open. *Fluid will not flow if the air vent is closed.*

- Open the lower clamp, and flatten the drip chamber with two fingers and the thumb of your opposite hand. *The membrane filter can be damaged if the drip chamber is squeezed while the lower clamp is closed.*

- While keeping the drip chamber flattened, close the lower clamp. *These actions create a vacuum, so that solution from the fluid chamber will then flow into the drip chamber.*

- Release your pressure on the drip chamber, and reshape it until it becomes full or only about half full if an IV medication is to be added.

- Repeat the above steps as necessary.

- Open the lower clamp, prime the tubing, and close the clamp.

For a Set with a Floating Valve Filter

- Open the upper clamp, and squeeze the fluid chamber until it is filled with about 30 ml of solution.

- Close the clamp, and again gently squeeze the drip chamber until it is filled to the desired volume.

- Open the lower clamp, prime the tubing, and close the clamp.

4. Fill the volume control drip chamber.

- Add the prescribed medication, if ordered. See Technique 36–8, page 884.

- Add fluid to a maximum of 2 hours' worth of fluid into the chamber. *This amount prevents the possibility of fluid overload if there is an inadvertent increase in the drip rate.*

- Close the upper clamp. *This prevents more fluid from entering the volume control chamber and subsequent fluid overload.*

5. Initiate, regulate, and monitor the infusion flow.

- Perform a venipuncture, or connect the tubing to the primary IV tubing or catheter. Don gloves before performing a venipuncture.

- Open the lower clamp, and adjust the drip rate to the desired rate of administration.

- Check the volume control chamber at least hourly, and add more fluid to the device when needed. *Periodic monitoring of the apparatus ensures that the desired rate and infusion flow is maintained.*

6. Ensure client comfort and safety.

- Position the client appropriately.

- Place the call light within easy reach.

7. Document all relevant information.

- Record the type and amount of solution, medication if administered, and times of starting and completing the infusion.

- Record fluid volume on the intake and output record.

VARIATION: Ensuring a More Precise Flow Rate

To facilitate a more precise flow rate, attach a Dial-A-Flo regulator, infusion pump, or syringe pump to the volume control system. See Techniques 25–6 and 25–8.

EVALUATION FOCUS	Patency of IV system; IV flow rate; amount of fluid infused in specified time; clinical signs of fluid deficit or excess.

SAMPLE RECORDING

Date	Time	Notes
02/26/93	1900	500 ml D$_5$W IV with Pediatrol started using 23g butterfly needle in R forearm vein. Extremity restrained.————————— Rosana Ruiz, SN

▶ **Technique 25–7** *CONTINUED*

KEY ELEMENTS OF USING A VOLUME CONTROL DEVICE

- Maintain asepsis.
- Ensure the patency of an existing IV system before attaching the volume control sets.
- Attach the volume control set between the IV solution container and the insertion spike of the IV tubing.
- Make sure that the air vent on the volume control device is open on top of the volume chamber when filling the drip chamber.

- After filling the volume control chamber, close the upper clamp to prevent fluid overload.
- Prime the tubing before attaching it to the IV tubing.
- Ensure that the correct type and amount of fluid and medication, if ordered, are infused within the specified period.

Pumps and Controllers

An infusion *pump* (Figure 25–24) delivers fluids intravenously by exerting positive pressure on the tubing or on the fluid. In situations where the fluid flow is unrestricted, the pump pressure is comparable to that of gravity flow. However, if restrictions develop (increased venous resistance), the pump can main-

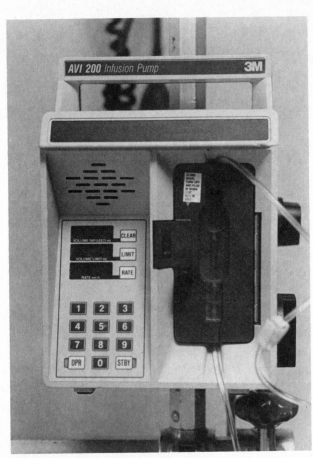

FIGURE 25–24 An intravenous infusion pump.

tain the fluid flow by increasing the pressure applied to the fluid.

A *controller*, by contrast, operates solely by gravitational force. The delivery pressure depends on the height of the container in relation to the venipuncture site. The container must be at least 76 cm (30 in) above the venipuncture site for a controller to work. A controller does not have the ability to add pressure to the line and to overcome resistances to fluid flow.

Resistance may develop (a) when a large catheter is used in a small vein, (b) when the fluid being administered is viscous, or (c) when the venous pressure is increased or the height of the fluid container is decreased. Such resistance can cause the flow rate to decrease and the controller alarm to sound.

Controllers are often the preferred choice in situations requiring close monitoring of fluid or medication administration because drugs or solutions delivered under high pressure by a pump can contribute to infiltration at the IV site or to vein irritation.

Two types of delivery systems are provided: drops per minute and milliliters per hour. The drops-per-minute models, also referred to as *rate consistent devices*, are useful when fluid needs to be delivered at a constant and consistent rate to maintain a specific drug level in the client's blood or to achieve a desired client response. The milliliters-per-hour system, or *volumetric device*, is useful when a specific volume of fluid is to be delivered over a unit of time, e.g., 500 ml in 2 hours. Newborns, burn victims, and clients with renal or congestive heart failure usually require volumetric accuracy.

Some or all of the following special features may be included on pumps and controllers (Wittig and Semmler-Bertanzi 1983, p. 1023):

- *Alarms.* Both visible and audible alarms are usually available. In controllers, the alarm is triggered when the infusion flow cannot be maintained by gravity at the selected rate. In pumps, an occlusion alarm sounds when a restriction to flow cannot be overcome as the pump increases its pressure. When an alarm is activated, some devices automatically stop; others maintain a low flow rate (e.g., 1 to 4 ml/hour) to keep the vein open. Some devices may also be equipped to trigger a remote alarm at the nurse-call system. The nurse needs to explain and demonstrate the alarm to clients so that they will know what to expect when it comes on later.

- *Meters.* Some meters indicate the amount of fluid that has been delivered; others indicate the amount of fluid to be delivered.

- *Flow rate settings.* On most models, the flow rate setting is simply set to the desired rate, i.e., in either drops/minute or milliliters/hour.

- *Drop sensor.* The drop sensor is a photoelectric device placed on the drip chamber. It detects drops as they form and activates the alarm when no drops are formed (e.g., when the solution container is empty or when the tubing is occluded).

- *Air detector.* Some models activate an alarm when air is in the tubing.

- *Infiltration detector.* This flat rubber pad containing two temperature sensors is taped to the skin at the venipuncture site. The two temperature sensors compare skin temperature at separate points. When fluid that is relatively cool compared to skin temperature infiltrates the tissues, the detector activates an alarm.

- *Occlusion detector.* The pump sensor activates an alarm when back pressure becomes greater than the pump's preset limit (e.g., 10 or 15 psi). Most pumps have a psi rating that describes the maximum pressure at which the pump will trigger an occlusion alarm. This pressure rating differs from the actual pressure of fluid delivery. Excessive back pressure may be caused by kinked or pinched tubing, an unopened tubing clamp, or an obstructed in-line filter or bottle airway. The nurse can ensure accurate functioning of the occlusion alarm by pinching or clamping the tubing once or twice each shift.

- *Battery.* To allow client mobility, most models are equipped with a rechargeable battery that operates the device from 1 to 4 hours.

Technique 25–8 describes how to use an infusion controller or pump.

25-8   Using an Infusion Controller or Pump

PURPOSES	• To maintain the prescribed fluid infusion rate • To prevent fluid overload
ASSESSMENT FOCUS	Amount and type of IV fluid prescribed; flow rate.

EQUIPMENT

- Infusion controller or pump
- The IV solution or medication
- A volume control chamber (Buretrol or Solu-set) for pediatric clients
- An IV pole
- An IV administration set with compatible IV tubing
- Sterile peristaltic tubing or a cassette if required
- Alcohol swabs and tape

INTERVENTION

Infusion Controller

1. Attach the controller to the IV pole.

- Attach the controller to the IV pole so that it will be below and in line with the IV container.

- Plug the machine into the electric outlet, unless battery power is used.

2. Set up the IV infusion.

- Open the IV container, maintaining the sterility of the port, and

spike the container with the administration set.

- Place the IV container on the IV pole, and position the drip chamber 76 cm (30 in) above the venipuncture site. *This provides*

▶ **Technique 25–8** *CONTINUED*

sufficient gravitational pressure for the fluid to flow into the client.

- Fill the drip chamber of the IV tubing one-third full. *If the drip chamber is filled more than halfway, the drops may be miscounted.*

- Rotate the drip chamber. *This removes vapor that could make the drop count inaccurate.*

- Prime the tubing, and close the clamp. Nonvolumetric controllers (regulators that measure the infusion in drops/minute) use standard tubing that is gravity-primed. *Priming expels all the air from the tubing.*

3. Attach the IV drop sensor, and insert the IV tubing into the controller.

- Attach the IV drop sensor (electronic eye) to the drip chamber so that it is below the drip orifice and above the fluid level in the drip chamber. *This placement ensures an accurate drop count. If the sensor is placed too high, it can miss drops; if placed too low it may mistake splashes for drops.*

- Make sure the sensor is plugged into the controller.

- Insert the tubing into the controller according to the manufacturer's instructions.

4. Initiate the infusion.

- Perform a venipuncture or connect the tubing to the primary IV tubing or catheter. Don gloves before performing a venipuncture.

- Open the IV control clamp completely.

5. Set volume dials for the appropriate volume per hour.

- Close the door to the controller, and ensure that all tubing clamps are wide open. *This enables the controller to regulate the fluid flow.*

- Set the dials on the front of the controller to the appropriate infusion rate and volume. Set the volume at 50 ml less than the required amount, if the controller counts the volume infused. *This will give you time to attach a new container before the present one runs out completely.*

- Press the power button and the start button.

- Count the drops for 15 seconds, and multiply the result by 4. *This verifies that the rate has been correctly set and the controller is operating accurately.*

- Some nurses recommend that all connections be taped. Count the drop rate again after the taping. *Taping could change the drop rate.*

6. Set the alarm (optional). *The alarm notifies the nurse when a set volume of fluid has been infused or indicates malfunctioning of the equipment.*

7. Monitor the infusion.

- Check the volume of fluid infused at least every hour, and compare it with the time tape on the IV container. *This confirms the actual volume of fluid infused.*

- If the volume infused does not coincide with the time tape or the alarm sounds, check that:

  a. The time tape is accurate.

  b. The rate/volume settings are accurate.

  c. The drip chamber is correctly filled.

  d. The IV tubing clamp is fully open.

  e. The container still has solution.

  f. The drop sensor is correctly placed.

  g. The IV container is correctly placed.

  h. The tubing is not pinched or kinked.

Infusion Pump

8. Attach the pump to the IV pole.

- Attach the pump at eye level on the IV pole. *Because the pump does not depend on gravity pressure, it can be placed at any level. Eye level is convenient for checking its functioning.*

- Plug the machine into the electric outlet, unless battery power is used.

9. Set up the infusion.

- Check the manufacturer's directions before using an IV filter or before infusing blood. *Infusion pump pressures may damage filters or cause rate inaccuracies. Certain models may also cause hemolysis of red blood cells.*

- Open the IV container, maintaining the sterility of the port, and spike the container with the administration set.

- Place the IV container on the IV pole above the pump.

- Fill the drip chamber, and rotate it as described in step 2 above.

- Prime the tubing, and close the clamp. Most volumetric chamber pumps, i.e., pumps calibrated to infuse a specific volume of fluid at a specific rate (ml/hour), have a cassette that must also be primed. Manufacturers give instructions for doing this. Often the cassette must be inverted or tilted to be filled with fluid. Some volumetric pumps use special tubing that is gravity-primed.

10. Attach the IV drop sensor, and insert the IV tubing into the pump.

- Position the drop sensor, if required, on the drip chamber. See step 3.

▶ **Technique 25–8 Using an Infusion Controller or Pump** CONTINUED

- Load the machine according to the manufacturer's instructions.

- Ensure the correct pressure is set.

11. Initiate the infusion.

- See step 4.

12. Set dials for the required drops per minute or milliliters per hour.

- Close the door to the pump, and ensure that the IV tubing clamps are open.

- Press the power button to the "on" position, and press the start button.

13. Set the alarm, and monitor the infusion.

- See steps 6 and 7.

- If the tubing does not contain a regular cassette, slightly change the sections of tubing placed inside the infusion clamp. *This prevents tubing collapse from continual squeezing by the pump.*

14. Document relevant information.

- Record the date and time of starting the infusion, the type and amount of fluid being infused, the rate at which it is being infused, the infusion device used, the status of the IV insertion site, and any adverse responses of the client.

EVALUATION FOCUS

Amount of fluid infused in designated time period; status of IV insertion site, especially the presence of infiltration.

SAMPLE RECORDING

Date	Time	Notes
02/12/93	0900	1000 ml IV D$_5$W started at 125 ml/hour using controller. Venipuncture site clean and dry with no signs of infiltration or infection. Rodney Stewart, SN

KEY ELEMENTS OF USING AN INFUSION CONTROLLER OR PUMP

- Explain and demonstrate the alarm system to the client.

- If a controller is used, make sure the IV container is placed at the appropriate height.

- Maintain asepsis.

- Make sure the infusion rate is correctly set and the pump or controller is operating accurately.

- Confirm the appropriate drip rate by counting the drops per minute after 5 minutes and again in 15 minutes.

- Monitor the infusion flow at least hourly, and compare the volume of fluid infused with the time tape on the IV container.

Implantable Venous Access Device (IVAD)

The implantable venous access device (IVAD) is designated to provide repeated access to the central venous system, hence avoiding the trauma and complications of multiple venipunctures.

The device consists of two parts: a radiopaque silicone catheter and a plastic or stainless steel injection chamber with a self-sealing silicone-rubber septum measuring 1 to 1½ inches (Figure 25–11, earlier). Current brand names of the implantable ports are Port-a-Cath, Infuse-A-Port, Mediport, and Chemo-Port. Manufacturers guarantee the septum for a specific number of punctures (e.g., 1000 to 2000).

Implantable ports are surgically placed into a small subcutaneous pocket, using local anesthesia, usually over the third or fourth rib lateral to the sternum. The distal end of the catheter is inserted into the desired central venous blood vessel (see the discussion of central venous sites in Chapter 26); the proximal end is routed through a subcutaneous tunnel to the injection portal. These ports can be used immediately after placement. However, a special *Huber needle* must be used to access the port. The delivery opening of this needle is on the side rather than the tip. The needle is inserted at a 90° angle. The site of the port is located by palpation and observation. Externally the IVAD is visible as a small bump on the chest. Agency protocol must be followed when accessing these devices. Before use, aseptic skin preparation is required; after every use, the port must be flushed with heparinized saline to maintain catheter patency.

The IVAD provides several advantages:

- It is easily palpable.

- It can be used immediately after insertion.

- It can be punctured up to 2000 times before replacement is necessary.

- It minimizes the likelihood of infection.

- The client's activity is not limited.

- Maintenance involves flushing only every 28 days or every 5 days if it is not accessed at least once per month.

- It needs to be surgically changed only every 2 or 3 years.

The major disadvantages of the IVAD are (a) a needle puncture is required with each access, and (b) the implant can be used for only one infusion at a time (some dual IVADs are available to overcome this latter problem), and (c) removal requires minor surgery. Technique 25–9 describes how to use an IVAD.

25-9 Using an Implantable Venous Access Device (IVAD)

PURPOSES
- To administer intravenous infusions, or medications
- To administer blood and blood products
- To obtain blood samples for laboratory analysis

ASSESSMENT FOCUS
Client's understanding and response to the system; type of therapy prescribed.

EQUIPMENT

- Priming solution of bacteriostatic saline
- IV solution container and administration set
  or
- Blood or blood product with transfusion set
  or

- Blood specimen tubes and syringe and needle
- Sterile gloves
- 5 ml syringes of normal saline flush and heparinized saline (100 μ/ml of heparin)
- 2% lidocaine with subcutaneous syringe and needle (optional)

- Povidone-iodine and alcohol solution and swabs
- #22-gauge Huber needle
- Adhesive or nonallergenic tape
- Occlusive dressing materials
- Povidone or antibiotic ointment

INTERVENTION

1. Assemble the equipment.

- Attach the IV tubing to the infusion or transfusion container.

- Prime the infusion tubing with saline.

- Prepare syringes of normal saline and heparinized saline. Currently, saline is used to flush the device either before and after medications or just periodically (once per day or per shift—check agency policy) followed by heparinized saline each time.

Heparinized saline helps prevent clotting.

2. Position the client appropriately, and locate the implant port.

- Position the client in either a supine or sitting position.

- Locate the IVAD device, and grasp it between two fingers of your nondominant hand to stabilize it. Palpate and locate the septum, the rubber disc at the center of the port where the needle will be inserted.

3. Prepare the site.

- Wash hands, and put on sterile gloves.

- *Optional:* Insert 2 percent lidocaine subcutaneously in the injection site. *This anesthetizes the area for injection.* It may be ordered during the first few weeks after the implant surgery, when the area is tender and swollen and more pain from the needle puncture is felt.

- Prepare the skin in accordance with agency policy and let the

▶

► **Technique 25–9 Using an Implantable Venous Access Device** *CONTINUED*

area dry after applying such solutions as povidone-iodine and alcohol.

4. Insert the Huber needle.

• Grasp the device, and again palpate the septum for injection.

• Insert the needle at a 90° angle to the septum, and push it firmly through the skin and septum until it contacts the base of the IVAD chamber.

• Avoid tilting or moving the needle when the septum is punctured. *Needle movement can damage the septum and cause fluid leakage.*

5. Secure the needle, and ensure proper placement of the IVAD catheter.

• Aspirate blood when the needle contacts the base of the septum.

• Support the Huber needle with 2×2 dressings and Steristrips.

• Infuse the saline flush and priming solution. There should be no

sign of subcutaneous infiltration after infusion of the saline fluid and priming solution.

6. After use, flush the system with heparinized saline.

• When flushing, maintain a positive pressure, and clamp the tubing as soon as the flush is finished. *These actions avoid reflux of the heparinized saline.*

7. Attach a "hep-lock" to the Huber needle.

• A Huber needle with a "hep-lock" can remain in place for one week before it needs to be changed. *The "hep-lock" allows for infusion of medications or fluid without continuous puncturing of the skin covering the IVAD.*

8. Prevent manipulation or dislodgement of the needle.

• Apply occlusive transparent dressings to the needle site.

• Apply povidone or antibiotic ointment to the site before dress-

ings are applied as agency protocol dictates.

9. Document all relevant information.

• Record the procedure performed and all nursing assessments.

VARIATION: Obtaining a Blood Specimen

To obtain a blood specimen:

• Withdraw 10 ml of blood and discard it. *This initial specimen may be diluted with saline and heparin from previous flushes.*

• Draw up the required amount of blood and transfer it to the appropriate containers (see Technique 25–12).

• *Slowly* instill 20 ml of normal saline over a 5-minute period (Holder and Alexander 1990, p. 45). *This thoroughly flushes the catheter and avoids excess pressure.*

• Inject 5 ml of heparin (100 μ/ml) to prevent clotting.

EVALUATION FOCUS

Infusion or transfusion rate; appearance of IVAD site; clinical signs indicating venous thrombosis (pain in the neck, arm, and/or shoulder on the side of the insertion site; neck and/or supraclavicular swelling); infection (redness and swelling at the site); and dislodgement of the needle or catheter (shortness of breath, chest pain, coolness in the chest).

KEY ELEMENTS OF USING AN IMPLANTABLE VENOUS ACCESS DEVICE

• Prime the administration tubing before infusing the fluid.

• Wear gloves.

• Prepare the site in accordance with agency protocol.

• Stabilize the IVAD before inserting the Huber needle.

• Insert the needle at a 90° angle.

• Avoid tilting or moving the needle when the septum is punctured.

• Before administering fluid or medication, ensure proper placement of the catheter by aspirating blood.

• Secure the needle appropriately as agency protocol dictates.

• After IVAD use, flush the system with heparinized saline.

Blood Transfusions

A **blood transfusion** is the introduction of whole blood or components of the blood (e.g., plasma or erythrocytes) into the venous circulation.

Blood Groups

Human blood is classified into four main groups (A, B, AB, and O) on the basis of polysaccharide antigens on the erythrocyte surface. These antigens, type A and type B, commonly cause antibody reactions and are called **agglutinogens**. In other words, group A blood contains type A agglutinogen, group B blood contains type B agglutinogen, group AB blood contains both A and B agglutinogens, and group O blood contains neither agglutinogen.

In addition to agglutinogens on the erythrocytes, **agglutinins** (antibodies) are present in the blood plasma. No individual can have agglutinins and agglutinogens of the same type; that person's system would attack its own cells. Thus, group A blood does not contain agglutinin A but does contain agglutinin B. Group B blood does not contain agglutinin B but does contain agglutinin A. Group AB blood contains neither agglutinin, and Group O contains both anti-A and anti-B agglutinins. Blood transfusions must be matched to the client's blood type in terms of compatible agglutinogens. Mismatched blood will cause a hemolytic reaction.

Rhesus (Rh) and other factors Rh antigens, also on the surface of erythrocytes, are present in about 85% of the population and can be a major cause of hemolytic reactions. Persons who possess the **Rh factor** are referred to as *Rh positive*; those who do not are referred to as *Rh negative*. Some other blood factors are the M, N, S, s, P, Kell, Lewis, Duffy, Kidd, Diego, and Lutheran factors (Guyton 1986, p. 73). These rarely cause major reactions because their antigenic properties are poor.

Unlike the A and B agglutinogens, the Rh factor cannot cause a hemolytic reaction on the first exposure to mismatched blood, because the Rh antibody is *not* normally present in the plasma of Rh-negative persons.

Transfusion Reactions

Transfusion reactions can be categorized as hemolytic, febrile, and allergic. The nurse must assess a client closely for reactions. Signs of an acute reaction include sudden chills or fever, low back pain, a drop in blood pressure, nausea, flushing, agitation or respiratory disorders. Signs of less severe allergic reactions include hives and itching but no fever.

Blood Administration

Blood is usually provided in plastic bags by the blood bank. One unit of whole blood is 500 ml of blood in a container. No more than one blood component or unit is obtained for the client at a time.

There are two types of blood administration sets: the straight line and the Y-set. The Y-set is preferred because the vein can be kept open with saline if any adverse effects arise from the transfusion (Figure 25–25). In many instances, however, the tubing must also be changed. The infusion tubing has a filter inside the drip chamber. The tubing clamp should be just under the drip chamber. A Y-set can also be used when a saline solution is needed to run with the blood (e.g., when giving packed cells) or to flush the line before the blood enters the tubing (e.g., when running an intravenous infusion that is not saline). Some agencies recommend that saline be run through the tubing before and after a blood transfusion. Saline is used because it simulates plasma isotonicity.

Blood transfusions are administered through a #18 needle or catheter. When blood is to be administered quickly, a #15 needle or large catheter, e.g., #14, is often used. Large-gauge needles prevent damage to red blood cells (RBCs).

To start, maintain, and terminate a blood transfusion, see Technique 25–10.

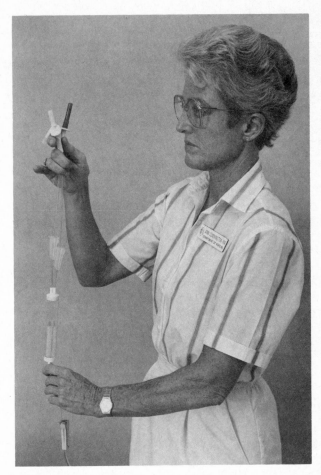

FIGURE 25–25 A Y-set for blood administration.

25-10

Initiating, Maintaining, and Terminating a Blood Transfusion

Before commencing a blood transfusion determine:
- Baseline data regarding blood pressure, temperature, pulse, and respirations;
- Any previous reactions to a blood transfusion;
- The appropriate consent form has been completed.

PURPOSES
- To restore blood volume after severe hemorrhage
- To restore the capacity of the blood to carry oxygen
- To provide plasma factors, e.g., antihemophilic factor (AHF) or factor VIII, or platelet concentrates, which prevent or treat bleeding

ASSESSMENT FOCUS

Clinical signs of a reaction (e.g., sudden chills, nausea, itching, rash, dyspnea); status of infusion site; any unusual symptoms.

EQUIPMENT

- Unit of whole blood
- Blood administration set, either a straight line or a Y-set (the Y-set is preferred)
- Container of 250 ml of normal saline solution
- IV pole

- Venipuncture set containing a #18 needle or catheter (if one is not already in place) or, if blood is to be administered quickly, a #15, needle or a larger catheter (e.g., #14)

- Alcohol swabs
- Tape
- Disposable gloves

INTERVENTION

1. Obtain client consent and baseline data before the transfusion.

- Obtain signed consent form if required.

- Assess vital signs for baseline data.

- Determine any known allergies or previous adverse reactions to blood.

- Note specific signs related to the client's pathology and reason for transfusion. For example, for an anemic client, note the hemoglobin level.

2. Prepare the client.

- Explain the procedure and its purpose to the client. Instruct the client to report promptly any sudden chills, nausea, itching, rash, dyspnea, or other unusual symptoms.

- If the client has an intravenous solution infusing, check whether the needle and solution are appropriate to administer blood. The needle should be #18 gauge or larger, and the solution must be saline. If the infusing solution is not compatible, remove it and dispose of it according to agency policy. Dextrose, which causes lysis of RBCs, Ringer's solution, medications and other additives, and hyperalimentation solutions are incompatible.

- If the client does not have an intravenous solution infusing, check agency policies. In some agencies an infusion must be running before the blood is obtained from the blood bank. In this case, you will need to perform a venipuncture on a suitable vein (see Technique 25–2) and start an IV infusion of normal saline.

3. Obtain the correct blood component for the client.

- Check the physician's order with the requisition.

- Check the requisition form and the blood bag label with a laboratory technician or according to agency policy. Specifically check the client's name, identification number, blood type (A, B, AB, or O) and Rh group, the blood donor number, and the expiration date of the blood.

- With another nurse (the agency may require an RN), compare the laboratory blood type record with

   a. The client's name and identification number. Ask the client to state the full name as a double check.

   b. The number on the blood bag label.

▶ **Technique 25–10** *CONTINUED*

c. The ABO group and Rh type on the blood bag label.

- Sign the appropriate form with the other nurse according to agency policy.

- ⒮ Make sure that the blood is left at room temperature for no more than 30 minutes before starting the transfusion. *RBCs deteriorate and lose their effectiveness after 2 hours at room temperature.* Agencies may designate different times at which the blood must be returned to the blood bank if it has not been started. *As blood components warm, the risk of bacterial growth also increases.*

4. Verify the client's identity.

- Ask the client's full name.

- ⒮ Check the client's arm band. Do not administer blood to a client without an arm band.

5. Set up the infusion equipment.

- Ensure that the blood filter inside the drip chamber is suitable for whole blood or the blood components to be transfused. Blood filters have a surface area large enough to allow the blood components through easily but are designed also to trap clots.

- Close all the clamps on the Y-set: the main flow rate clamp and both Y-line clamps.

- Spike a container of 0.9% saline solution with the Y-set spike containing the vented tubing.

- Insert the remaining Y-set spike into the blood bag.

- Hang the saline solution and blood with the Y-set attached on an IV pole about 1 m (36 in) above the planned venipuncture site.

6. Prime the tubing with saline solution.

- Open the clamp on the normal saline tubing, and squeeze the drip chamber until it is one-third full.

- Remove the IV tubing needle adapter cover, open the main flow rate clamp, and prime the tubing. Close both clamps, and replace the needle adapter cover.

7. Perform venipuncture, if required.

- See Technique 25–2.

8. Establish the saline infusion.

- Connect the primed tubing to the IV needle or catheter.

- Tape the tubing to the IV needle securely.

- Open the saline solution clamp and the main roller clamp.

- Close the saline solution clamp and the main flow clamp.

9. Establish the blood transfusion.

- ⒮ Invert the blood bag gently several times to mix the cells with the plasma. *Rough handling can damage the cells.*

- Expose the port on the blood bag by pulling back the tabs (Figure 25–26).

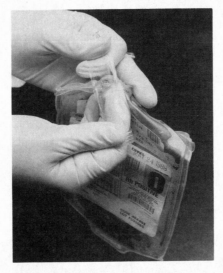

FIGURE 25–26 Exposing the port on the blood bag by pulling back the tabs.

- Open the blood line clamp.

- Squeeze the blood drip chamber until the filter is completely immersed in blood.

- Open the main flow rate clamp, and regulate the blood's flow rate.

10. Observe the client closely for the first 5 to 10 minutes.

- Run the blood for the first 15 minutes at 20 drops per minute.

- ⒮ Note adverse reactions, such as chilling, nausea, vomiting, skin rash, or tachycardia. *The earlier a transfusion reaction occurs, the more severe it tends to be. Identifying such reactions promptly helps to minimize the consequences.*

- Remind the client to call you immediately if any unusual symptoms are felt during the transfusion.

- If any of these reactions occur, report these to the nurse in charge, and take appropriate nursing action.

11. Document relevant data.

- Record starting the blood, including vital signs, type of blood, blood unit number, sequence number (e.g., #1 of three ordered units), site of the venipuncture, size of the needle, and drip rate.

12. Monitor the client.

- Fifteen minutes after initiating the transfusion, check the vital signs of the client. If there are no signs of a reaction, establish the required flow rate. Most adults can tolerate receiving one unit of blood in 1½ to 2 hours.

- Assess the client every 30 minutes or more often, depending on the health status, including vital signs.

13. Terminate the transfusion.

▶

▶ **Technique 25–10 Initiating, Maintaining, and Terminating a Blood Transfusion** CONTINUED

- Don gloves.

- If no infusion is to follow, clamp the blood tubing and remove the needle.

- If the primary IV is to be continued, flush the line with saline solution, attach the primary IV container, and adjust the drip to the desired rate. *Often a normal saline or other solution is kept running in case of a delayed reaction to the blood.*

- Discard the administration set according to agency practice. Needles should be placed in a la-

beled, puncture-resistant container designed for such disposal. Blood bags and administration sets should be bagged and labeled before being sent for decontamination and processing. See agency policy.

- Remove gloves.

- Again monitor vital signs.

14. Follow agency protocol for appropriate disposition of the blood bag.

- On the requisition attached to the blood unit, fill in the time the

transfusion was completed and the amount transfused.

- Attach one copy of the requisition to the client's record and another to the empty blood bag.

- Return the blood bag and requisition to the blood bank.

15. Document relevant data.

- Record completion of the transfusion, the amount of blood absorbed, the blood unit number, and the vital signs. If the primary intravenous infusion was continued, record connecting it.

EVALUATION FOCUS	Changes in vital signs or health status; presence of chills, nausea, vomiting, or skin rash.

SAMPLE RECORDING

Date	Time	Notes
12/12/93	1100	1 unit whole blood administered. No adverse reactions. BP stable at 120/70, TPR 37, 88, 14. 500 ml saline started at 10 gtt/min. ———— Selina L. Ward, SN

KEY ELEMENTS OF INITIATING, MAINTAINING, AND TERMINATING A BLOOD TRANSFUSION

- Confirm that there is an order and a signed consent from the client.

- Have two health care professionals confirm that the client name and ID number, blood type, and product unit numbers are correct. Check also the expiration date.

- Make sure the transfusion is started within 30 minutes of arrival at the bedside.

- Maintain asepsis.

- Use the appropriate blood filter.

- Flush the tubing first with normal saline.

- Mix the blood cells with plasma gently to maintain their integrity.

- Wear gloves before performing venipuncture, transfusing the blood, and when terminating blood and disposing of equipment.

- Assess the client closely for reactions to the transfusion.

Blood Specimens

Blood specimens are taken for a number of reasons and by different members of the health team, including nurses. It is important, however, for nurses to be familiar with the nurse practice acts in their jurisdictions and with the policies of agencies about LVNs, LPNs, and RNs performing venipunctures and obtain-

ing blood specimens. In some instances, students are expected only to assist another health professional.

Three types of blood specimens are taken: capillary, venous, and arterial. Capillary and venous specimens are taken most frequently. Arterial blood specimens are generally taken only in special acute care facilities to measure arterial blood gases. Some tests require whole blood; others require clotted blood (serum) or blood plasma, which is unclotted blood. Different containers are usually required for each type of specimen.

Capillary Blood Specimens

A capillary blood specimen is often taken to measure blood glucose and hemoglobin levels when frequent tests are required or when a venipuncture cannot be performed. This technique is less painful than a venipuncture and easily performed. Hence, clients can perform this technique on themselves.

The development of home glucose test kits and reagent strips has simplified the testing of blood glucose and greatly facilitated the management of home care by diabetic clients. A number of manufacturers have developed blood glucose meters (Figure 25–27). Most permit measurements between 20 and 800 mg

per 100 ml of blood. These meters use either a dry wipe or wet wash method of testing. The dry wipe method requires that the nurse or client wipe off excessive blood on the reagent strip with a dry cotton ball before making the reading. For the wet wash method, the reagent strip is flushed with water before it is inserted into the meter.

Capillary blood specimens are the major method of blood collection in children, infants, and neonates. Venipuncture in neonates, in particular, is technically difficult. Specimens are usually obtained from the side of the finger, earlobe, or outer aspect of the heel (Figure 25–28). The use of special lancet injectors (e.g., Monojector) for finger and heel sticks enable the nurse to control the depth of the puncture more precisely than the use of regular lancets.

Technique 25–11 describes how to obtain a capillary blood specimen and measure blood glucose.

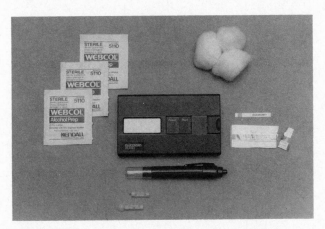

FIGURE 25–27 Equipment to measure capillary blood glucose. Clockwise around the glucose meter, from top left: antiseptic swabs, cotton balls, reagent strips, lancet.

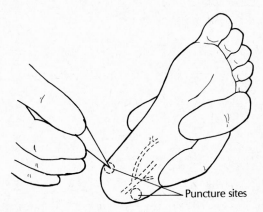

FIGURE 25–28 Puncture sites for a heel stick.

◆ 25-11 ◆

Obtaining a Capillary Blood Specimen and Measuring Blood Glucose

Before obtaining a capillary blood specimen, determine the frequency and type of testing, the client's understanding of the procedure, and the client's response to previous testing.

PURPOSES

- To determine or monitor blood glucose levels of clients at risk for hyperglycemia or hypoglycemia
- To promote blood glucose regulation by the client
- To evaluate the effectiveness of insulin administration

ASSESSMENT FOCUS

Client's learning needs.

▶ Technique 25–11 Obtaining a Capillary Blood Specimen *CONTINUED*

EQUIPMENT

- ▢ Blood glucose meter
- ▢ Blood glucose reagent strip compatible with the meter
- ▢ Paper towel
- ▢ Warm cloth or other warming
- device (optional)
- ▢ Antiseptic swab
- ▢ Disposable gloves
- ▢ Sterile lancet or #19 or #21-gauge needle
- ▢ Lancet injector (optional)
- ▢ Cotton ball to wipe the glucose reagent strip (dry wipe method)

INTERVENTION

1. Prepare the equipment.

- Obtain a reagent strip from the container.

- Insert the strip into the meter according to the manufacturer's instructions, and make any required adjustments. *Some meters require calibration or the adjustment of the timer.*

- Remove the reagent strip from the meter, and place it on a clean, dry paper towel. *Moisture can change the strip, thereby altering the test results.*

2. Select and prepare the vascular puncture site.

- Choose a vascular puncture site, e.g., the side of an adult's finger or the heel, finger, or earlobe of an infant or child. Avoid sites beside bone.

- If either the heel or the finger is used, wrap it first in a warm cloth for 30 to 60 seconds (optional), *or* hold a finger in a dependent position and massage it toward the site. If the earlobe is used, rub it gently with a small piece of gauze. *These actions increase the blood flow to the area, ensure an adequate specimen, and reduce the need for a repeat puncture.*

- Clean the site with the antiseptic swab, and permit it to dry.

3. Obtain the blood specimen.

- Don gloves.

- Place the injector, if used, against

the site, and release the needle, thus permitting it to pierce the skin. Make sure the lancet is perpendicular to the site. *The lancet is designed to pierce the skin at a specific depth when it is in a perpendicular position relative to the skin.*

or

Prick the site with a lancet or needle, using a darting motion.

- Wipe away the first drop of blood with a cotton ball. *The first blood usually contains a greater proportion of serous fluid, which can alter test results.*

- Gently squeeze the site until a large drop of blood forms.

- Hold the reagent strip under the puncture site until enough blood covers the indicator squares. The pad will absorb the blood, and a chemical reaction will occur. Do not smear the blood. *This will cause an inaccurate reading.*

- Ask the client to apply pressure to the skin puncture site with a cotton ball. *Pressure will assist hemostasis.*

4. Expose the blood to the test strip for the period specified by the manufacturer.

- As soon as the blood is placed on the test strip:

  a. Press the timer on the glucose meter, and monitor the time as indicated by the

manufacturer, e.g., 60 seconds. *The blood must remain in contact with the chemical for a prescribed time for accurate results.*

  b. Lay the glucose strip on a paper towel or on the side of the timer. *The strip should be kept flat so that blood will not pool on only one part of the pad.*

- When the timer displays the time indicated by the manufacturer, no blood should remain on the test pad. Wipe excessive blood from the test pad using a cotton ball (dry wipe method), or flush it away with water (wet wash method). *The strip must be free of excessive blood for the meter to measure the glucose level accurately.*

5. Measure and document the blood glucose.

- Place the strip into the meter according to the manufacturer's instructions.

- At the designated time, e.g., another 60 seconds, activate the meter to display the glucose reading. *Correct timing ensures accurate results.*

- Turn off the meter, and discard the test strip and cotton balls.

- Document the method of testing and results on the client's record.

- Report results to the physician.

▶ **Technique 25–11** *CONTINUED*

EVALUATION FOCUS	Comparison of glucose meter reading with normal blood glucose levels; status of puncture site; motivation of client to perform the test independently.

SAMPLE RECORDING

Date	Time	Notes
12/04/93	0700	Skin puncture performed on right index finger for blood glucose. Results 82 by glucometer. Dr. Warren notified.————— Selenie Daznard, RN

KEY ELEMENTS OF OBTAINING A CAPILLARY BLOOD SPECIMEN AND MEASURING BLOOD GLUCOSE

- Wear gloves, and use aseptic technique.
- Read and follow the manufacturer's directions.
- Keep the reagent strip dry before use.
- Avoid puncture sites beside bone.

- Increase blood supply to the puncture site before the test.
- Discard the first drop of blood after puncture.

Venous Blood Specimens

Venous blood specimens are usually taken from the veins in the antecubital fossa (see Figure 25–1, *A*, earlier) in adult clients or older children and adolescents. For younger children, the femoral or external jugular veins may be used. The jugular site is advantageous in that the vein is large and becomes prominent when the child cries. However, the jugular site can be particularly frightening, because the child must extend the neck and turn the head to the side to expose the vein adequately. Younger children will need to be appropriately restrained during the procedure so that they remain as still as possible and avoid inadvertent injury.

To obtain a venous blood specimen, the nurse may use either a needle and syringe or a special vacucontainer that allows the withdrawal of multiple blood samples (Figure 25–29). Technique 25–12 describes how to obtain a venous blood specimen from an adult by venipuncture.

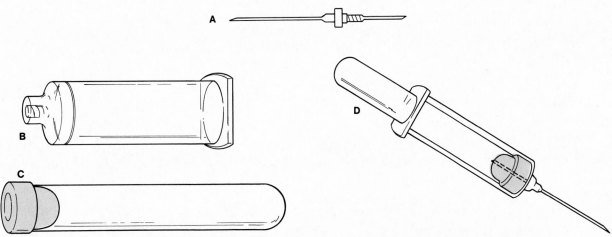

FIGURE 25–29   A vacucontainer set used to obtain specimens of blood: *A*, a double-pointed needle; *B*, a plastic adapter; *C*, a sealed vacuum tube; *D*, the assembled vacucontainer set, in which the vacuum tube is placed inside the plastic adapter with the top of the tube piercing the short needle.

25-12 Obtaining a Venous Blood Specimen from an Adult by Venipuncture

Before obtaining a venous blood specimen determine specific conditions to be met before obtaining the blood; previous disease, injury, or therapy that places client at risk for a venipuncture, e.g., bleeding disorder, anticoagulant therapy; presence of IV infusion that can alter test results; client's ability to cooperate with procedure.

PURPOSES
- To assess specific elements or constituents of venous blood (e.g., red or white blood cell count, differential white blood cell count, glucose, electrolytes, drugs, bacteria)
- To determine an individual's blood type
- To monitor a client's response to specific therapies

ASSESSMENT FOCUS
Condition of veins and surrounding skin for selected site.

EQUIPMENT

- Correct test tubes for the tests (Vacuum specimen tubes are required for the vacucontainer method)
- Disposable gloves
- Topical antiseptic swab
- Tourniquet
- Sterile 1-inch needles, usually #19 or #21 gauge for adults

or
- Vacucontainer and sterile double-ended needles that screw into the adaptor
- Sterile syringe of appropriate size for the amount of blood required (sizes 5 to 10 ml are frequently used)

- 2 × 2 gauze pad
- Dry sterile sponges
- Band-Aid
- Completed labels for each container
- Completed requisition

INTERVENTION

1. Verify the physician's orders for the tests to be obtained, and obtain the correct test tubes specific for the test ordered.

2. Identify the client appropriately.

- Check the client's wristband, and compare the name with the name on the requisition and chart.

3. Don gloves, and perform venipuncture.

- See steps 3 through 6 in Technique 25–2, page 597.

4. Obtain the specimen.

Using Sterile Syringe and Needle

- When the needle is in the vein, gently pull back on the syringe plunger until the appropriate amount of blood is obtained (usually about 5 ml).

- Remove the tourniquet when sufficient blood is obtained, and remove the needle from the vein. Withdraw the needle in line with the vein while placing a 2 × 2 gauze pad over the site without applying pressure. *Removing the tourniquet and applying the gauze pad minimizes bleeding at the site when the needle is withdrawn. Careful removal of the needle reduces vein trauma and client discomfort.*

- Cover the venipuncture site with a sterile gauze, and ask the client to hold it firmly in place for 2 to 3 minutes, if able. *This facilitates clotting and minimizes bleeding from the site.*

- Transfer the specimens to the tubes:

    a. Remove the top from the

laboratory test tube. Avoid touching the inside of the tube or spilling the contents. *This maintains asepsis of the test tube and contents.*

b. Remove the needle from the blood-filled syringe, and gently insert the blood down one side of the tube. *Careful ejection of the blood sample is essential to prevent damage to the erythrocytes.*

c. Replace the test tube lid or stopper.
or
Insert the needle directly through the stopper of the blood tube, and allow the vacuum to fill the tube with blood (Figure 25–30). Some nurses change the needle to a sterile #18-gauge needle to

▶ **Technique 25–12** *CONTINUED*

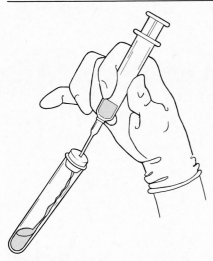

FIGURE 25–30 Inserting a blood specimen directly through the stopper of the blood tube.

facilitate transfer of the blood by this method.

- For all blood tubes containing additives, gently rotate or invert the test tube several times. *This mixes the blood with the tube contents. Shaking is contraindicated because it can cause the erythrocytes to rupture.*

Using a Vacucontainer System

- Do not advance the venipuncture needle of a vacucontainer into the vein after the venipuncture.

- As soon as the venipuncture needle is positioned in the vein, hold the plastic adapter securely, and press the vacuum tube firmly into the short needle until it pierces the top of the tube. Blood will then spurt rapidly into the tube.

- Fill the vacucontainer with blood, release it, and set it aside.

- Insert another vacucontainer if more blood is required.

- Release the tourniquet, and remove the needle from the vein as described above.

- Cover the venipuncture site with a sterile gauze as above.

5. Ensure client comfort and safety.

- Assess the client's venipuncture site for oozing. This is especially important for clients who have prolonged blood coagulation times.

- If clots have not begun to form at the site, continue to apply pressure until bleeding has stopped.

- When bleeding is minimized, apply a Band-Aid over the site.

6. Label the test tubes appropriately, and send them to the laboratory.

- Attach labels to all test tubes. Ensure that the information on each label and the laboratory requisition is completely correct. *Inappropriate identification of specimens can lead to errors of diagnosis or therapy for the client.*

- Arrange for the specimen to be taken to the laboratory or stored appropriately, e.g., in a refrigerator. Blood obtained for culture should be transported immediately and should not be refrigerated. See Variation, next.

7. Document and report relevant information.

- Record the date and time blood is withdrawn, the test(s) to be performed, description of the venipuncture site after specimen collection.

- Report "stat" or any abnormal test results to the physician.

VARIATION: Collecting a Blood Specimen For Culture

In addition to blood withdrawal equipment, two sets of paired culture media bottles (Figure 25–31), a povidone-iodine or alcohol swab, and additional needles are required for this specimen collection.

- Prepare the venipuncture site

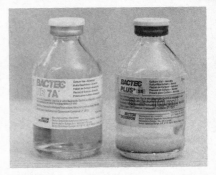

FIGURE 25–31 Culture bottle set for blood cultures.

with povidone-iodine. Use alcohol if the client is allergic to iodine.

- Collect 5 ml of blood from a vein that does *not* have an IV running into it. *A specimen drawn through an intravenous infusion site will alter the test results.*

- Remove the venipuncture needle, and replace it with a sterile needle. *The needle used to puncture the skin may contaminate the specimen and affect culture results.*

- Swab the top(s) of the blood culture blood bottle(s). Insert the needle through the tops, and carefully inject 2½ to 5 ml of blood into one or both bottles, according to agency protocol.

- Use a new sterile needle when puncturing each bottle top. *This will avoid transmitting microorganisms to the blood from the bottle top.*

- Collect the second specimen after 15 minutes or according to agency protocol. Prepare the skin again with povidone-iodine or alcohol solution.

- Place this second sample in a set of paired culture bottles as above and according to the practice at your agency.

- Remove gloves.

- Label the bottles, and transport the specimen to the laboratory *immediately.*

▶

► **Technique 25–12 Obtaining a Venous Blood Specimen** CONTINUED

EVALUATION FOCUS	Appearance of the venipuncture site after venipuncture; results of the laboratory tests.

SAMPLE RECORDING

Date	Time	Notes
12/22/93	0700	Venipuncture performed in antecubital vein. Specimen for complete blood count and electrolytes sent to laboratory. Venipuncture site has minimal bleeding. No evidence of hematoma.————————— George Sawyers, RN

KEY ELEMENTS OF OBTAINING A VENOUS BLOOD SPECIMEN FROM AN ADULT BY VENIPUNCTURE

- Obtain the correct specimen tubes.
- Wear gloves, and use aseptic technique.
- Avoid performing venipuncture on areas of the body that have recently been injured or on extremities that have had associated lymph nodes removed or have an intravenous infusion.
- Use the distal aspect of the vein first.
- Distend the veins before implementing venipuncture.
- Release the tourniquet when blood is obtained.

- Apply pressure to the needle site following venipuncture.
- Handle blood specimens appropriately to prevent damage to the erythrocytes.
- Use a new sterile needle when transferring blood for culture into the specimen tube.
- Immediately transport blood specimens for culture to the laboratory.

CRITICAL THINKING CHALLENGE

The physician has ordered 2000 ml D5W to be administered over 24 hours to a client who has a history of circulatory overload during intravenous therapy. Calculate the drip rate using the following drop factors: 10 gtts/ml, 15 gtts/ml, 20 gtts/ml, and 60 gtts/ml. What is the relationship between the drop factor and the flow rate? What is the relationship between the drop factor and the size of the intravenous needle or catheter? What implications does this have for selecting an administration set appropriate to the solution being administered and the needs of the client? Is the amount of fluid appropriate for this client? Why?

RELATED RESEARCH

Ahrens, T.; Wiersema, L.; and Weilitz, P. B. March/April 1991. Differences in pain perception associated with intravenous catheter insertion. *Journal of Intravenous Nursing* 14:85–89.

Bostrom-Ezrati, J.; Dibble, S.; and Rizzuto, C. November 1990. Intravenous therapy management: Who will develop insertion site symptoms? *Applied Nursing Research* 3:146–52.

Maki, D. G.; Botticelli, J. T.; Leroy, M. L.; et al. October/December 1990. Prospective study of replacing administration sets for intravenous therapy at 48- vs 72-hour intervals—72 hours is safe and cost effective. *Canadian Intravenous Nurses Association Journal* 6:12–16.

REFERENCES

Boykoff, S. L.; Boxwell, A. O.; and Boxwell, J. J. February 1988. Six ways to clear air from an IV line. *Nursing 88:* 46–48.

Bryan, C. S. June 1987. "CDC says . . .": The case of IV tubing replacement, *Infection Control* 8:255–56.

Campbell, L. S., and Jackson, K. June 1991. Starting intravenous lines in children: Tips for success. *Journal of Emergency Nursing* 17:177–78.

Centers for Disease Control. 1982. Guidelines for prevention of intravascular infections. *Infection Control* 3:61–72.

Crow, S. March/April 1987. Infection risks in IV therapy. *Journal of the National Intravenous Therapy Association* 10:101–5.

Guyton, A. C. 1986. *Textbook of medical physiology*. 7th ed. Philadelphia: W. B. Saunders Co.

Holder, G., Alexander, J. February 1990. A new and improved guide to I.V. therapy . . . protocols for intravenous therapy. *American Journal of Nursing* 90:43–47.

Josephson, A.; Gombert, M. E.; Sierra, M. F.; Karanfil, L. V.; and Tansino, G. F. September 1985. The relationship between intravenous fluid contamination and the frequency of tubing replacement. *Infection Control* 6:367–70.

Knox, L. S. January/February 1987. Implantable venous access devices. *Critical Care Nursing* 7:70–73.

LaRocca, J. C., and Otto, S. E. 1989. *Pocket guide to intravenous therapy*. St. Louis: C. V. Mosby Co.

Lenox, A. C. March 1990. I.V. Therapy: Reducing the risk of infection. *Nursing 90* 20:60–61.

Millam, D. A. May/June 1991. Initiating intravenous therapy. *Advancing Clinical Care* 6:21–23.

Lonsway, R. A. March/April 1987. Research, standards, and infection control: The impact of I.V. nursing. *Journal of the National Intravenous Therapy Association* 10:106–9.

Metheny, N. M. June 1990. Why worry about I.V. fluids? *American Journal of Nursing* 90:50–57.

Millam, D. A. May 1991. Myths and facts . . . about IV therapy. *Nursing* 21:75–76.

Peck, N. May, June, and July 1985. Perfecting your IV therapy techniques. 3 parts. *Nursing 85* 15:38–43; 48–51; 32–35.

Schoenike, S., and Brown, S. October/December 1990. A practical review: Ambulatory infusion devices. *Canadian Intravenous Nursing Association Journal* 6:7–9.

Snydman, D. R.; Donnelly-Reidy, M.; Perry, L. K.; and Martin, W. J. March 1987. Intravenous tubing containing burettes can be safely changed at 72-hour intervals. *Infection Control* 8:113–16.

Weinstein, S. May 1987. Intravenous filters. *Infection Control* 8:113–16.

Wilkinson, R. April 3–9, 1991. The challenge of intravenous therapy. *Nursing Standards* 5:24–27.

Wittig, P., and Semmler-Bertanzi, D. J. July 1983. Pumps and controllers: A nurse's assessment guide. *American Journal of Nursing* 83:1022–25.

26

Central Venous Lines

CONTENTS

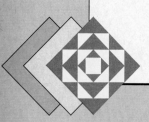

NURSING PROCESS GUIDE
CENTRAL VENOUS LINES

ASSESSMENT

Assess

- Hydration and electrolyte status for baseline data. See assessment guide for Chapter 24, page 574. Refer also to data in laboratory records.

- Nutritional status for baseline data, e.g., weight, anthropometric measurements, calorie intake (optional). See assessment guide for Chapter 22 on page 536.

- Vital signs for baseline data. Sudden unexpected changes in vital signs may occur during infusion of hyperosmolar solutions, and a body temperature increase may signal an infectious process.

- Allergy to tape, iodine, or components of fluids infused.

- Any bleeding tendency. Such clients, especially those receiving anticoagulants, require special observation after catheter insertion.

- Client's ability to understand instructions during the procedure and ability to perform Valsalva's maneuver.

- Signs of complications associated with central venous catheters and TPN and Intralipid therapy:

  a. Pneumothorax (may occur during insertion).
  b. Air embolism (must be monitored throughout therapy; see Table 26–1 on page 632 for clinical signs).
  c. Infection (see Table 26–1 on page 632 for clinical signs).
  d. Hyperglycemia (see Table 26–3 on page 648 for clinical signs).
  e. Hypoglycemia (see Table 26–3 on page 648 for clinical signs).

- Presence of factors or conditions that contraindicate the administration of TPN or Intralipid solutions, e.g., impaired pancreatic, pulmonary, liver, or kidney function; coagulation disorder.

RELATED DIAGNOSTIC CATEGORIES

- Fluid volume deficit

- High risk for Fluid volume deficit

- Altered nutrition: Less than body requirements

PLANNING

Client Goals
The client will

- Regain or maintain adequate fluid and electrolyte balance.

- Regain or maintain nutritional status.

- Avoid complications associated with a central venous catheter, TPN therapy, and Intralipid therapy.

Outcome Criteria
The client

- Experiences no untoward effects or complications as a result of the procedure.

- Has a balanced fluid intake and output.

- Has good skin turgor.

- Has moist mucous membranes.

- Has a normal urine specific gravity and fingerstick blood glucose.

- Has vital signs normal for age, sex, and health status.

- Has a triceps skinfold measurement, upper arm circumference, and body mass index within predetermined ranges.

- Has a stable daily weight.
  or

- Gains ____kg body weight within 1 week.

Central Venous Lines

A **central venous line** is a catheter inserted into a large vein located centrally in the body. The tip of the catheter may terminate in the vein, e.g., the superior vena cava, or in the right atrium of the heart. The catheters are radiopaque so that they will show up on fluoroscopy or X-ray films. Correct placement of the catheter is confirmed by X-ray film.

Central venous lines are usually inserted by phy-

sicians, although some nurses who are specially prepared may insert them.

Central venous lines are inserted primarily for the following reasons:

- To spare the client numerous venipunctures associated with short-term peripheral IV catheters

- To administer nutritional solutions that are highly irritating to smaller veins

- To administer irritating medications, antibiotic therapy for more than 1 week, continuous narcotic infusions, or chemotherapy

- To monitor central venous pressure (CVP)

Types of Central Venous Lines

Standard central venous lines are catheters of variable length that are inserted in a nonsurgical procedure. They are usually made of polyethylene or silicone rubber. Sizes range from #23 to #16 gauge and from 40 to 60 cm (16 to 24 in) in length. A #16 gauge catheter is frequently used. Short lines are used when the tip is inserted to the superior vena cava or subclavian vein; longer lines are used when the tip is inserted to the right atrium of the heart. A **peripherally inserted central catheter** (**PIC catheter**, or **PICC**) is a long venous catheter; two kinds are the *Intrasil catheter* and the *Drum catheter.*

Multilumen catheters are designed with #18 gauge proximal and middle lumens and a #16 gauge larger distal lumen. Each lumen has a separate port. Most nurses use the distal lumen for total parenteral nutrition (TPN) therapy, but the manufacturer may recommend using the middle lumen and reserving the distal lumen for central venous pressure readings or for infusing blood. The proximal lumen is used for other IV solutions or for drawing blood. Dente-Cassidy (1991, p. 30) emphasizes that the nurse should be consistent and always use the same port for the same purpose.

Catheters are also inserted surgically. Because these catheters are implanted through a subcutaneous tunnel they are often referred to as central venous tunneled catheters (CVTCs). Examples are the *Hickman catheter* and the *Broviac catheter.* The Hickman is a single- or double-lumen catheter, with a 1.6-mm internal diameter of the lumen. It is therefore large enough for the passage of nutritional substances, blood, and antibiotics. The drawbacks of the single-lumen Hickman catheter are that the administration of nutritional substances must be interrupted if the catheter needs to be used for measuring central venous pressure or to administer blood, and the risk of infection is increased. For this reason, a double Hickman catheter, the fusion of two Hickman catheters or a Hickman and a Broviac catheter, is used. The Broviac line has an internal diameter of 1.0 mm, narrower than the Hickman but still large enough to administer nutritional substances. With the double-luman catheter, the administration of TPN can be continued through the smaller lumen while antibiotics, for example, can be administered through the larger lumen. The Broviac catheter used alone is like a single Hickman catheter. However, because its

lumen is narrower, blood cannot be withdrawn through it. There are also catheters with three and four separate lumens, which can be used for blood, medications, and TPN solution, for example. These surgically inserted lines are intended for use over an extended period.

Nonsurgical Insertion

In the nonsurgical procedure, three insertion sites may be used: The subclavian vein, the internal jugular vein, or a peripheral vein.

Subclavian Vein Two approaches may be used.

1. The *infraclavicular approach* (below the clavicle), in which the catheter is inserted into the right or left subclavian vein. The tip of the catheter remains in the subclavian vein or the superior vena cava (Figure 26-1, *A*), i.e., a short line is used; it can also be extended into the atrium of the heart (Figure 26-1, *B*), i.e., a long line can be used. This site permits

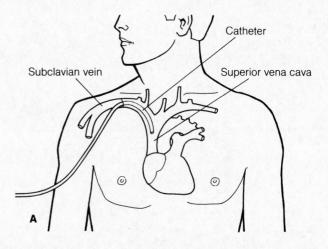

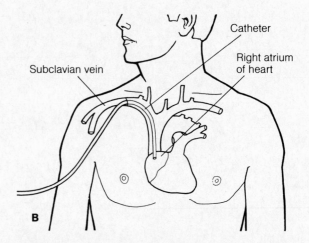

FIGURE 26-1 A central venous line with the exit site on the chest below the clavicle: *A*, the tip of the catheter is in the superior vena cava; *B*, the tip of the catheter is in the right atrium.

freedom of movement for ambulation, but a pneumothorax can occur during insertion. Clinical signs include sudden, sharp chest pain; cough; sudden shortness of breath; hypotension; weak, rapid pulse; pallor or cyanosis; and anxiety.

2. The *supraclavicular approach* (above the clavicle), in which the catheter also enters the subclavian vein.

Internal Jugular Vein The right or left internal jugular vein may be approached anteriorly, posteriorly, or between the heads of the sternocleidomastoid muscles. This site hinders head and neck movement somewhat but provides a straight line to the subclavian vein (and superior vena cava; Figure 26–2). This site is also difficult to dress and tape securely.

Peripheral Vein In the peripheral approach, the catheter is inserted in the basilic or cephalic veins at the antecubital fossa of the right arm. The tip of the catheter may be placed in either the brachiocephalic vein or the superior vena cava. The median basilic vein is the preferred site because the basilic vein offers the most direct route to the central venous system (Figure 26–3). The exit of this catheter (at the antecubital fossa) looks like that of an intravenous line. It is important for nurses to know that the catheter extends farther into the vein and that its purpose and care differ.

When the infra- and supraclavicular approaches are used, a local anesthetic is usually applied to the site prior to the catheter insertion. While the physician is inserting the catheter, the nurse monitors the client's pulse rate. The onset of arrhythmia may indicate that the catheter tip is irritating the heart and placement requires adjustment.

Surgical Insertion

The surgical insertion of a central venous catheter involves an incision into the tissues of the chest. The catheter is inserted under the subcutaneous tissue to a centrally located vein, e.g., the subclavian vein. It is then inserted into the vein and extended into the atrium of the heart (Figure 26–4). These catheters usually have Dacron cuffs that promote growth of the subcutaneous tissue around the catheter, thus helping to prevent infection. With this type of insertion, the exit site of the catheter is on the chest, usually between the clavicle and the nipple. In some instances, the surgeon may attach an implantable venous access device to the catheter. See the discussion of implantable venous access devices in Chapter 25, page 593.

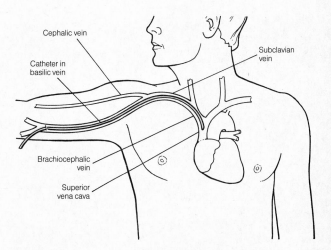

FIGURE 26–3 A central venous line (PIC catheter) inserted peripherally in the basilic or cephalic veins at the antecubital fossa of the right arm. The tip of the catheter is placed in the superior vena cava.

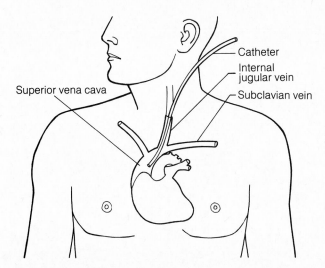

FIGURE 26–2 A central venous line inserted into the left jugular vein with the tip of the catheter in the superior vena cava.

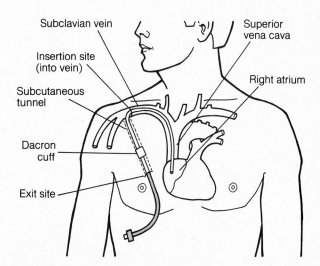

FIGURE 26–4 A central catheter surgically inserted into the chest wall, entering the subclavian vein, and extending into the right atrium.

Complications Associated with Central Venous Lines

Many of the sepsis problems associated with conventional IV therapy are also associated with central venous lines. Moreover, the problems are magnified because (a) clients with central venous lines are often critically ill, may be malnourished, and are sometimes immunosuppressed; (b) the catheters are left in place for long periods of time; and (c) the intralipids used in TPN therapy support the growth of a wide variety of microorganisms. Infection control is therefore of utmost importance during central venous catheter (CVC) therapy.

A potentially lethal complication associated with central venous lines is air embolism. Nurses caring for clients with central venous lines must therefore be aware of the potential danger and implement precautions to prevent its occurrence.

Table 26–1 describes the signs and symptoms of these complications, preventive actions, and immediate actions to implement should they occur.

Inserting a Central Venous Catheter

For a central vein insertion (subclavian or internal jugular), the physician uses a large needle and syringe to penetrate the vein. Once the vein is entered and the needle placed correctly, the physician removes the syringe, advances the catheter through the needle to the desired length, and sutures it in place. When the catheter is in place, the physician then withdraws the stylet or obturator, if used, and removes the needle.

To maintain patency of a newly established central venous system, a small IV solution container of 5% dextrose in water or normal saline is used until appropriate placement of the catheter tip is confirmed by X-ray film.

When setting up the infusion administration set, the nurse can attach an air-eliminating cellulose membrane filter to the distal end of the tubing to reduce the risk of air embolism (Figure 26–5). Technique 26–1 describes how to assist with the insertion of a central venous catheter. Technique 26–2 explains how to maintain and monitor a CVC system.

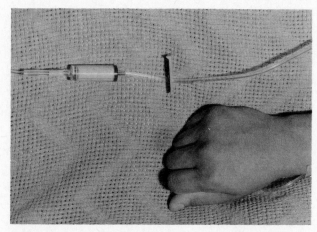

FIGURE 26–5 An air-eliminating filter on a central venous line.

TABLE 26–1 COMPLICATIONS ASSOCIATED WITH CENTRAL VENOUS LINES

Problem	Signs and Symptoms	Preventive Actions	Immediate Actions
Infection	Redness, swelling, pain or purulent drainage at insertion site; abrupt rise in temperature; presence of chills diaphoresis; general malaise	Use aseptic technique.	Inform physician.
Air embolism	Shortness of breath; cough; tachycardia; hypotension; pallor; cyanosis; substernal chest pain; change in mental alertness	Tape all tubing junctions. Have the client perform Valsalva's maneuver during insertion and removal of the catheter and during tubing changes.	Clamp the catheter. Position the client in left lateral Trendelenburg's position. Administer 100% oxygen by mask. Notify physician.

26-1   Assisting with the Insertion of a Central Venous Catheter

PURPOSE
- To administer nutritional fluids and medications that cannot be given by a peripheral route or when peripheral routes cannot be obtained

ASSESSMENT FOCUS

> Baseline vital signs; actual and desired mobility status of the client, which may affect the approach used (supraclavicular or infraclavicular); exit sites for skin integrity and signs of infection; status of antecubital veins if PIC is to be inserted; client's ability to hold breath, maintain the required position, and not move when requested; agency protocol regarding care of central lines and sites.

EQUIPMENT

For insertion

- Sterile gloves for the physician and the nurse (2 pairs for the nurse)
- Skin preparation set, if the area needs to be shaved, or soap, water, a washcloth, and a towel
- Povidone-iodine sponges and ointment, or, if the client is allergic to iodine, 70% alcohol with sterile gauze squares and a combination of antifungal and antimicrobial ointment
- Masks for the nurse and the physician (in some agencies the client is also required to wear a mask)
- Bath blanket (if subclavian or jugular insertion is used)

- Sterile or clean gown for the physician (check agency policy)
- Subclavian insertion tray
- Cut-down tray
- Sterile 3-ml syringe with a 1-in #25 gauge needle
- Skin anesthetic (e.g., lidocaine 1 or 2% without epinephrine)
- Radiopaque subclavian catheter of suitable size and length
- Sterile 4 × 4 gauze squares
- Moistureproof sterile dressing material
- Adhesive tape

For establishing the infusion

- Small IV solution container of normal saline or 5% dextrose in water

- Sterile TPN tubing or IV administration set with drip chamber and tubing (microdrip tubing is used when less than 100 ml/hour is administered; macrodrip tubing is used when more than 100 ml/hour is given)
- Extension tubing (30 in)
- *Optional:* A 0.22-micron cellulose membrane air-eliminating filter
- Tape to secure the tubing connections if Luer-Lok connections are not available
- IV pole
- Soft-tipped clamp without teeth to clamp tubing if problems arise

INTERVENTION

1. Prepare the client.

- Describe the procedure, and explain the purpose of the catheter and the procedures involved in care and maintenance of the line.

- Before commencing, ensure that the client has given an informed consent.

- Instruct the client on how to perform Valsalva's maneuver (forced expiration against a closed glottis), i.e., to take a breath, close the mouth, breathe out, and bear down. Encourage the client to practice this maneuver before the procedure, unless contraindicated by the client's condition.

- If the client is unable to perform Valsalva's maneuver

  a. Ask the client to hold the breath at the end of a deep inspiration or during the expiratory phase of the respiratory cycle and/or

  b. Have an assistant compress the client's abdomen with both hands.

2. Prepare the IV infusion equipment for attachment to the catheter.

- Connect in sequence:

  a. The infusion tubing spike into the port of the normal saline or 5% dextrose in water solution container, using surgical aseptic technique.

  b. The filter.

▶ **Technique 26–1 Assisting with the Insertion of a Central Venous Catheter** CONTINUED

c. The extension tubing. Place the filter between the infusion tubing and the extension tubing to avoid subsequently disrupting the dressing.

• Tape the tubing connections. *This will prevent inadvertent separation, which can lead to air embolism, leakage, and contamination.* For easy reopening, double-tabbed tapes are available.

• Start the flow of solution, and prime the tubing to remove air. *This dislodges air bubbles and prevents air embolism.*

• Stop the flow of solution, place the tubing protector cap on the end of the tubing, and hang the tubing on the IV pole. *The protector cap maintains the sterility of the open-ended tubing.*

3. Position the client appropriately.

• Assist the client to a Trendelenburg position (approximately a 15° to 30° angle). If the client cannot tolerate this position, use a supine position and modified Trendelenburg position with only the feet elevated 45° to 60°. *In Trendelenburg's position, the veins will dilate, and the risk of an air embolism is reduced because slight positive pressure is induced in the central veins.*

• For *subclavian insertion*, place a rolled bath blanket under the client's back between the shoulders. *In this position, venous distention is increased.*
or
For *jugular insertion:*

a. Place a rolled bath blanket under the opposite shoulder. *The blanket will extend the neck, making anatomic structures more visible for selecting the site.*

b. Turn the client's head to the opposite side. *This position makes the site more visible and reduces the chance of contamination from microorganisms in the client's respiratory tract.*
or

For a *peripheral vein insertion* in the brachiocephalic vein or the superior vena cava, place the client supine with the dominant arm at a 90° angle to the trunk. *This arm position provides the straightest, most direct route to the central venous system. The dominant arm is often used because movement accelerates blood flow and decreases the risk of dependent edema.*

4. Clean and shave the insertion area.

• Open skin preparation equipment and don gloves.

• Wash and dry the insertion site with soap and water. *Washing will remove dirt and reduce the number of microorganisms present.*

• Shave the client's neck and upper thorax *if ordered.*

• Discard the gloves.

• Don a mask and sterile gloves.

• Clean the site with povidone-iodine sponges for 2 minutes or, if using 70% alcohol, for 10 minutes or according to agency protocol. Use a circular motion, working outward. *This reduces the number of microorganisms. Working outward prevents reintroducing microorganisms to the site.*

5. Support and monitor the client.

• Explain to the client what is going on, and provide support.

• Maintain the client in position.

• Monitor the client for signs of respiratory distress, complaints of chest pain, tachycardia, pallor, and cyanosis. *These observations facilitate early detection of pneumothorax and air embolism. An improperly placed catheter may cause pneumothorax, resulting in chest pain and labored breathing. Signs of air embolism are shown in Table 26–1.*

6. Attach the primed IV tubing to the catheter.

• While the physician removes the stylet from the catheter, quickly attach the IV tubing to the catheter, and simultaneously ask the client to perform Valsalva's maneuver as practiced. *Valsalva's maneuver increases intrathoracic pressure, creating more pressure on the large veins entering the heart and reducing the return of blood to the heart. It therefore reduces the risk of air entering the large heart vein via the opened catheter and the risk of subsequent air embolism.*

7. After the infusion is attached, apply a temporary dressing to the site.

• Put on the second pair of sterile gloves.

• Apply povidone-iodine ointment to the site if agency protocol dictates. Many agencies no longer use ointment, believing it causes skin maceration.

• Apply a 4 × 4 sterile gauze dressing or a transparent occlusive dressing according to agency protocol.

8. After X-ray examination or fluoroscopy confirms the position of the catheter, secure the dressing with tape.

• See Technique 26–3.

► **Technique 26–1** *CONTINUED*

- Tape the IV tubing to the catheter. *Taping prevents inadvertent separation of parts, leakage, and potential infection.*
- Label the dressing with the date and time of insertion and the length of the catheter, if it is not indicated on the catheter.

9. Establish the appropriate infusion.

- See Technique 26–2.

10. Document all relevant information.

- Document the time of insertion, the size and length of the catheter, the site of insertion, the name of the physician, the time of the X-ray examination and the results, the kind of infusion, the rate of flow, and all nursing assessments and interventions.

| | EVALUATION FOCUS | Clinical signs of sepsis and air embolism (see Table 26–1) and pneumothorax (see page 631). |

SAMPLE RECORDING

Date	Time	Notes
12/12/93	1900	18-cm subclavian catheter inserted by Dr. R. Sullivan. 1,000 ml D5W started at 36 ml/hr. Placement confirmed by fluoroscopy at 1850 hr. Vital signs stable. Slight pallor. ———————————— Naomi Treasure, NS

KEY ELEMENTS OF INSERTING A CENTRAL VENOUS CATHETER

- Check allergy to iodine and tape.
- Maintain strict asepsis.
- Wear masks and gloves during the procedure.
- Make sure the client understands the procedure.
- Prime the IV tubing before attachment.
- Tape all tubing connections.

- Instruct the client to perform Valsalva's maneuver while the stylet is removed from the catheter and while the IV tubing is attached to the catheter.
- Apply an occlusive dressing.
- Assess client for air embolism, pneumothorax, and sepsis.

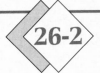

26-2

Maintaining and Monitoring a CVC System

Before monitoring a CVC system, determine agency policy about central line care, the type of catheter (single- or multiple-lumen) used, and the type and sequence of solutions to be infused.

| | PURPOSES | • To maintain the prescribed infusion flow rate
• To maintain patency of the central venous system
• To prevent complications associated with central venous lines |

| | ASSESSMENT FOCUS | Appearance of catheter site; rate of flow; any adverse response of the client. |

►

▶ **Technique 26–2 Maintaining and Monitoring a CVC System** CONTINUED

EQUIPMENT

- □ Tape
- □ Items for tubing change and dressing change (see Technique 26–3)
- □ #21 gauge 1-in needles

- □ Luer-Lok adapters
- □ Soft-tipped clamp without teeth
- □ Alcohol or povidone-iodine wipes
- □ 10-ml syringe

- □ Sterile normal saline
- □ 3-ml syringe
- □ Heparin flush solution (e.g., 100 units heparin per 1 ml of saline)

INTERVENTION

1. Label each lumen of multilumen catheters.

- Mark each lumen or port of the tubing with a description of its purpose (e.g., the distal lumen for CVP monitoring and infusing blood; the middle lumen for TPN; and the proximal lumen for other IV solutions or for blood samples.
  or
  Use a color code established by the agency to label the proximal, middle, and distal lumens. *Labeling prevents mixing of incompatible medications or infusions and reserves each lumen for specific therapies.*

2. Monitor tubing connections.

- Ensure that all tubing connections are taped or secured according to agency protocol.
- Check the connections every 2 hours.
- Tape cap ends if agency protocol indicates.

3. Change tubing according to agency policy.

- See Technique 26–3.
- Some agencies advocate changing TPN tubing every 24 hours and tubing for other infusions every 48 to 72 hours.

4. Change the catheter site dressing according to agency policy.

- See Technique 26–3.
- Most agencies recommend that the dressing be changed every 48 to 72 hours.

5. Administer all infusions as ordered.

- Use a controller or pump for all fluids (see Technique 25–8 on page 612).
- Prime all tubing to remove air.
- Maintain the fluid flow at the prescribed rate.
- *Optional:* If a *nonviscous* or *intermittent* solution is used, attach a #21 gauge short needle to the infusion tubing, and insert it through a clean Luer-Lok adapter cap. Tape this connection.
- If a *viscous* solution is to be infused, remove the Luer-Lok adapter, and apply the infusion tubing directly to the port or lumen.
- Whenever the line is interrupted for any reason, instruct the client to perform Valsalva's maneuver. If the client is unable to perform Valsalva's maneuver, place the client in a supine position, and clamp the lumen of the catheter with a soft-tipped clamp. Place a strip of tape (about 3 in from the end) over the catheter before applying the clamp. *The clamp is placed over the taped area to prevent damage to the tubing. A clamp without teeth prevents piercing.*

6. Cap lumens without continuous infusions, and flush them regularly.

- Cap ports not in use with an intermittent infusion (IIP) cap to seal the end of a catheter.
- Clean the adapter caps with al-

cohol or povidone-iodine swab before penetration.

- Flush noninfusing tubings with 1 or 2 ml of heparin flush solution every 8 hours or according to agency protocol. *Flushing prevents obstruction of the catheter by a blood clot.*
- Always aspirate for blood before flushing tubings (or infusing medications). *This validates that the catheter is appropriately placed in the vein.*
- Use a #25 gauge 5/8-in needle to penetrate the adapter cap when flushing the catheter. *A small gauge needle minimizes the possibility of leakage through the adapter plug, and a short needle minimizes the possibility of damaging the catheter.*

7. Administer medications as ordered.

- If a capped port is used for medications, first flush the line with 5 or 10 ml of normal saline according to agency protocol. *Many medications are incompatible with heparin.*
- After the medication is instilled through the port, inject normal saline first and then the heparin flush solution according to agency protocol. *The saline solution flushes the line of the medication. The heparin maintains the patency of the catheter by preventing blood clotting.*

8. Monitor the client for complications.

- At least every 4 hours, assess the client's vital signs, skin color,

► **Technique 26–2** *CONTINUED*

mental alertness, appearance of the catheter site, and presence of adverse symptoms. (See Table 26–1 on page 632.)

- If air embolism is suspected, give the client 100% oxygen by mask, place the person in a left Trendelenburg position (Durant maneuver), and notify the physician. *Lowering the head increases intrathoracic pressure, decreasing the flow of air into the vein during* *inhalation. A left side-lying position helps prevent the air from moving to the pulmonary artery.*

- If sepsis is suspected, replace a TPN, blood, or other infusion with 5% or 10% dextrose solution, change the IV tubing and dressing, save the remaining solution for lab analysis, record the lot number of the solution and any additives, and notify the physician immediately. When changing the dressing, take a cul-

ture of the catheter site as ordered by the physician or according to agency protocol.

9. Document all relevant information.

- Record the date and time of any infusion started; type of solution, drip rate, and number of milliliters infusing per hour; dressing or tubing changes; appearance of insertion site; and all other nursing assessments.

EVALUATION FOCUS	Rate of infusion flow; appearance of catheter site; any adverse response of the client.

SAMPLE RECORDING

Date	Time	Notes
12/02/93	1410	Bag #6 of hyperalimentation infusion started and running at 80 ml per hour per infusion pump. Catheter insertion site clean without inflammation or tenderness. ———————————————————— Carolyn Churchill, RN

KEY ELEMENTS OF MAINTAINING AND MONITORING A CVC SYSTEM

- Use sterile aseptic technique when changing solutions, tubing, filters, and dressings.
- Label each lumen of multilumen catheters.
- Ensure that all tubing junctions are securely taped.
- Change tubing and catheter site dressings at least every 48 to 72 hours.
- Prime all tubing before attachment to the central catheter.
- Always have the client perform Valsalva's maneu-

ver whenever the line is interrupted, and use a soft-tipped clamp to close the line.
- Cap lumens without continuous infusions, and flush them regularly with heparin flush solution to maintain their patency.
- Always aspirate for blood before flushing tubings or administering medications.
- Use small gauge, short needles whenever penetrating an adapter cap.
- Monitor the client closely for signs of air embolism and infection.

Changing CVC Tubing and Dressings

The CDC recommends that TPN tubing be changed at least once every 24 to 48 hours (CDC Simmons 1981, p. 72). Some experts advise that it be changed every 24 hours. This procedure is best carried out when the solution container is being changed. CVC dressings should be changed every 48 to 72 hours (CDC Simmons 1981, p. 72) and more frequently if a dressing becomes wet or loose. The Intravenous

Nurses Society recommends changing dressings every 48 hours (Camp-Sorrell 1990, p. 361). The high glucose concentration of the TPN solution makes the hyperalimentation insertion site very vulnerable to infection. Meticulous asepsis is essential to prevent infection. The nurse needs to change an intermittent infusion port (IIP) cap, using sterile technique, every 48 hours or as agency protocol dictates.

Technique 26–3 describes how to change a CVC tubing and dressing.

26-3 Changing a CVC Tubing and Dressing

PURPOSES
- To prevent excessive growth of microorganisms and infection
- To inspect the catheter insertion site
- To maintain the flow of required fluids

ASSESSMENT FOCUS
Allergy to tape or iodine; infusion rate and amount absorbed; patency of IV system; presence of infiltration at catheter site.

EQUIPMENT

For tubing change
- New solution container and administration set (tubing)
- Sterile gloves
- Mask (especially if the client is immunocompromised)
- Sterile 2 × 2 gauze squares
- Antiseptic
- Tape

For dressing change
- Central catheter dressing set
  or

- Two face masks (one for the nurse and one for the client)
- 70% isopropyl alcohol
- Gloves (2 pairs)
- 4 × 4 gauze sponges
- Antiseptic swabs (e.g., 10% acetone and 1% iodine tincture or povidone-iodine solutions or, if client is allergic to iodine, 70% alcohol)

- Povidone-iodine ointment or, if client is allergic to iodine, a combination of antimicrobial and antifungal agents (optional)
- Precut sterile drain gauze or 2 × 2 gauze and sterile scissors
- Tincture of benzoin
- Elastoplast tape or transparent occlusive dressing such as Op-Site
- Nonallergenic 2.5-cm (1-in) tape

INTERVENTION

Tubing Change

1. Prepare the client.

- Assist the client to the supine position. *This lowers the negative pressure in the vena cava, thus decreasing the risk of air embolism when the catheter is opened.*

2. Prepare the equipment.

- Prepare the solution container, attach the new IV tubing, and prime the tubing as you would for a conventional IV. See Technique 25–1 on page 594.

- Remove the tape securing the tubing to the dressing and the catheter hub connection.

- Don sterile gloves and mask.

- Place the sterile gauze underneath the connection site of the catheter and tubing. Clean the junction of the catheter and tubing with the antiseptic, if required by agency protocol. *This*

prevents the transfer of microorganisms from the client's skin to the open CVC catheter tip when it is detached; it also decreases the number of microorganisms at the catheter-tubing junction.

3. Change the tubing.

- Ask the client to perform Valsalva's maneuver (that is, to take a deep breath and bear down) and to turn the head away while you detach the IV tubing by rotating it out of the hub. *Performance of Valsalva's maneuver reduces the risk of air embolism, and turning the head to the side reduces the chances of contaminating the equipment.*
  or
  Use the soft-tipped clamp to close the line.

- Quickly attach the new primed IV tubing to the TPN catheter, ensuring a tight seal. *The tubing must be attached quickly while the*

client is performing Valsalva's maneuver.

- Release the soft-tipped clamp, if used.

- Open the clamp on the new tubing, and adjust the flow to the rate ordered.

- Secure the tubing to the catheter with tape if a Leur-Lok connection is not present. *This prevents accidental separation of the tubes and contamination of the system.*

- Loop and tape the tubing over the dressing. *This prevents tension on the catheter and inadvertent separation of the tubing and the catheter.*

4. Label the tubing, and document the tubing change.

- Mark the date and time of the tubing change on the new IV tubing or drip chamber.

- Document the tubing change and all assessments.

▶ **Technique 26–3** *CONTINUED*

Dressing Change

5. Prepare the client.

- Assist the client to a supine or a semi-Fowler's position.

Ⓢ • Don a mask, and have the client don a mask (if tolerated or as agency protocol indicates), and/ or ask the client to turn the head away from the insertion site. *This helps protect the insertion site from the nurse's and client's nasal and oral microorganisms. Turning the client's head also makes the site more accessible.*

6. Prepare the equipment.

- Wash hands before handling sterile supplies and, if agency policy indicates, apply alcohol, and allow the hands to air dry.

- Open the sterile supplies.

7. Change the dressing.

- Remove the soiled dressing by pulling the tape slowly and gently from the skin. *This prevents catheter displacement and skin irritation.*

- Inspect the skin for signs of irritation or infection. Inspect the catheter for signs of leakage or other problems. If infection is suspected, take a swab of the drainage for culture, label it, send it to the laboratory, and notify the physician.

💧 • Don sterile gloves.

- Clean the catheter insertion site with sterile gauze sponges soaked in a solvent such as 10% acetone. Clean in a circular motion, moving from the insertion site outward to the edge of the adhesive border. Take care not to jostle or get acetone on the catheter. Take a new sponge for each wipe. Repeat until the sponge is unstained after use. *Acetone defats the skin, destroys bacterial cell walls, and removes old adhesive tape, which could irritate the skin. Cleaning from the insertion*

site outward and discarding the sponges after each wipe avoids introducing contaminants from the uncleaned area to the site. Jostling the catheter can cause discomfort to the client and could dislodge the catheter. Acetone is kept off the catheter because it could damage the catheter.

- Using the method described above, clean the insertion site with povidone-iodine solution. If using 70% alcohol as a substitute for iodine, clean the area for 5 minutes. *The iodine solution is an antiseptic with antimicrobial properties that last a long time, even after drying.* Some agencies require cleansing with alcohol before applying povidone-iodine solution, and some require cleansing with alcohol afterward to remove the povidone-iodine solution, which can burn some people's skin.

- Optional. Apply the povidone-iodine ointment to the insertion site and to the catheter hub. Check agency policy.

- Apply a precut sterile drain gauze around the catheter (Figure 26–6). (If precut gauze is not available, cut a 2 × 2 sterile gauze square, using the sterile scissors.) Apply sufficient sterile gauze dressings to cover the catheter and skin. *This protects*

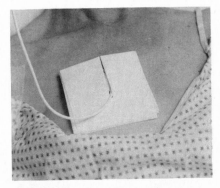

FIGURE 26–6 A precut sterile gauze placed around a central venous catheter over the insertion site.

the catheter and skin surrounding the insertion site from airborne contaminants.
or
If using Elastoplast dressing, apply tincture of benzoin to the skin surrounding the dressing gauzes, and allow it to air dry about 1 minute. *This protects the skin when adhesive tape or Elastoplast is applied and promotes adhesion of the cover dressing. Appropriate drying time is essential to prevent skin breakdown when the dressing is removed.*

- Remove your gloves.

8. Secure the dressing and the tubing.

Ⓢ • Ask the client to abduct the arm and turn the head away from the dressing site. Tape the dressing securely to the skin with transparent occlusive dressing or Elastoplast. Make sure that the adhesive covering is occlusive. *Arm abduction and head rotation ensure that the client's range of motion is not limited by the dressing and decreases the potential for skin abrasion caused by movement of the adhesive.*

- Loop and tape the IV tubing (not the filter) over the occlusive dressing. *Looping prevents tension on the catheter and its inadvertent detachment if the tubing is pulled.*

- Label the dressing with the date, time, and your initials.

- See Technique 25–2, step 8 on page 599.

9. Document the tubing and the dressing change, including all nursing assessments.

VARIATION: Changing a Dressing for a Surgically Inserted Central Venous Line

The distal end of a surgically inserted central venous catheter lies

▶

▶ **Technique 26–3 Changing a CVC Tubing and Dressing** *CONTINUED*

on the chest somewhere between the nipple and the sternum. The proximal tip lies in the right atrium of the heart. When the catheter is newly inserted, two sites require dressing: the insertion site, where the catheter enters the vein, and the exit site, where the catheter leaves the chest. Once the insertion site incision has healed, only the catheter exit site requires care.

The distal end of the catheter is threaded and has a male Luer-Lok cap. In some agencies, the Luer-Lok cap is replaced with a special cap that has an injection port, which is also threaded. The cap is screwed onto the catheter securely. Some authorities also recommend that the cap be taped to prevent it from dislodging or allowing an air embolus to enter. Some authorities suggest that the catheter should have a smooth clamp in place continuously. The clamp must not have teeth, because they could damage the catheter. It is normally placed over tape on the line as an added precaution against severing the catheter. The clamp is closed when the catheter is not being used.

Nurses clean the insertion site for the catheter as they would any surgical incision until it heals. See Technique 39–2. The frequency of dressing changes varies among agencies; however, once every 24 or 48 hours is not unusual.

The nurse also cleans the exit site and changes the dressing until the site heals completely. At that point, practices vary at different agencies. At some, the healed exit site is left exposed to the air and cleaned with hydrogen perioxide only when it is soiled. Agencies also vary in choice of dressing materials and cleansing solutions.

EVALUATION FOCUS	Appearance of catheter insertion site; presence of drainage, patency of tubing, infusion rate.

SAMPLE RECORDING

Date	Time	Notes
12/12/93	1805	CVC container and tubing changed. D5W infusing via IVAC pump at 60 ml/hr. Dressing changed at right subclavian triple-lumen catheter site using aseptic technique. No redness, edema or drainage. Povidone-iodine ointment applied. ——————————————————— Evylin Loo, RN

KEY ELEMENTS OF CHANGING A CVC TUBING AND DRESSING

CVC Tubing

- Wear gloves.
- Maintain asepsis to prevent infection.
- Prime the IV tubing.
- Instruct clients to perform Valsalva's maneuver and/or close the line with a soft-tipped clamp while attaching the new tubing.
- Tape the catheter to the tubing.
- Mark the date and time of the tubing change on the tubing.

CVC Dressing

- Wear gloves.
- Maintain asepsis.
- Wear masks (client and nurse).
- Prevent catheter displacement and damage.
- Make sure the adhesive covering of the dressing is occlusive and does not limit the client's arm abduction and head rotation.
- Label the dressing with date, time, and your initials.

Drawing Blood from a Central Venous Catheter

Procedures for drawing blood vary according to whether the cap on the catheter is to be removed or left in place. The nurse may withdraw specimens directly through the cap of a capped catheter port using a syringe and needle or by clamping the catheter, removing the cap on the end of the port, and attaching the syringe tip directly to the catheter hub. See Technique 26–4 on page 641.

To prevent air embolism, the nurse must ensure that the central catheter is clamped whenever detaching it from an infusion or removing the cap. To avoid unnecessary blood loss and frequent use of heparin, coordination of blood sampling tests is essential.

Drawing Blood From a Central Venous Catheter

Before drawing blood from a CVC determine the types of blood samples to be drawn to obtain the correct blood specimen tubes; the amount of blood to be drawn for the specified tests; the type of CV catheter (if triple-lumen catheter is used, determine appropriate port for drawing the blood sample); agency policy about the amount of saline and heparin flush solutions to use.

PURPOSE

- To avoid repeated venipuncture of the client for drawing blood samples

ASSESSMENT FOCUS

Patency of IV system; appearance of catheter site (note the presence of infiltration or infection at the catheter site).

EQUIPMENT

- □ Sterile gloves
- □ Sterile drape
- □ Sterile syringes (10- and 20-ml)
- □ Sterile needles (#20 to #22 gauge)

- □ Plastic or soft-tipped clamp for catheter
- □ Sterile #18 gauge needle to transfer blood specimen (optional)
- □ Povidone-iodine or alcohol wipes

- □ Blood tubes, labels, and requisitions
- □ Saline solution
- □ Heparin flush solution (optional)

INTERVENTION

1. Prepare the equipment.

- Prepare the saline and heparin flush syringes as required.

- Some agencies recommend stopping the infusions in all ports of the line for 1 minute before blood sampling.

- Clamp the catheter using the plastic or soft-tipped clamp. *If the cap is removed, the catheter must be clamped to prevent the entrance of air.*

- Don gloves.

- Place the sterile drape under the catheter hub.

- Remove the catheter cap (Figure 26–7), and, if agency policy dictates, clean the catheter hub with a povidone-iodine or alcohol wipe. Avoid contaminating the catheter lumen.

2. Withdraw initial blood, and discard this aspirate.

- Using aseptic technique, place

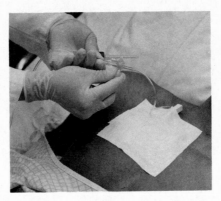

FIGURE 26–7 Removing the cap from the end of a central venous catheter.

the tip of a 10-ml syringe into the catheter.

- Unclamp the catheter.

- Withdraw 3 to 5 ml of blood from the catheter, and again clamp the catheter.

- Set this syringe aside, and discard it later in the appropriate place designated by agency policy. *This aspirate is discarded because it may be diluted with in-*

fusion fluid.

3. Obtain the blood specimen.

- Attach a second 10-ml syringe (or a larger one of a size equal to the volume of blood to be withdrawn) to the exposed catheter hub.

- Unclamp the catheter, and withdraw the necessary blood for the samples required. *Blood required for the samples is collected all at once to minimize the time that the catheter is open.*

- Clamp the catheter, and withdraw the syringe.

- Transfer the blood into the laboratory tubes (see Technique 25–12, step 4, on page 624).

4. Flush the catheter with saline.

- Attach the syringe with the saline flush solution to the catheter. *Blood precipitates with most fluids other than normal saline.*

- Unclamp the catheter, and gently ▶

▶ **Technique 26–4 Drawing Blood from a CVC** CONTINUED

infuse the solution. *This clears the catheter of all blood that may clog the lumen.*

• Clamp the catheter, and withdraw the syringe.

5. Optional: If there is no infusion to be attached to the catheter port, heparinize the catheter, and replace the cap.

• Check agency policy about the amount of heparin to use or whether to use a heparin/saline flush solution.

• Connect the heparin flush syringe to the catheter hub, release the clamp, flush, and reclamp the catheter as in step 4.

6. If an intravenous infusion is to be attached, establish the infusion.

• Connect the primed intravenous tubing to the catheter.

• Release the soft-tipped clamp.

• Regulate the infusion as ordered.

7. Ensure client safety.

• Tape all tubing connections.

• Coil and pin the tubing to the client's gown as agency policy dictates.

8. Document all relevant information.

• Record the date and time of procedure, volume of blood aspirat-

ed, port used for taking blood sample (if a double or multilumen catheter is in place), and any adverse response on the part of the client.

VARIATION: Drawing Blood from a CV Catheter When the Catheter Cap Is Not to Be Removed

Clean the injection cap with a povidone-iodine or alcohol wipe. Insert the needle of the syringe containing 10 ml of normal saline, and gently inject the saline. *Flushing with saline ensures patency of the catheter.* Then follow steps 2 to 4 to obtain the blood specimen.

EVALUATION FOCUS

Any difficulties encountered in obtaining blood specimen; any adverse response of the client.

SAMPLE RECORDING

Date	Time	Notes
02/17/93	0800	Blood specimens for serum electrolytes taken from proximal lumen of CV catheter. Specimens labelled and sent to lab. ———— Lawrence Lewis, RN

KEY ELEMENTS OF DRAWING BLOOD FROM A CENTRAL VENOUS CATHETER

• Use aseptic technique.
• Discard the first 3 to 5 ml of blood drawn.
• If the cap is to be removed, always clamp the catheter before attaching the syringe to an exposed catheter hub.
• Clean the injection cap with an antiseptic wipe before inserting a needle through it.

• Flush the catheter with saline before withdrawing blood.
• Flush the catheter with saline flush solution before reestablishing an infusion, or heparinize the catheter if there is no infusion to be attached.

Removing a Central Venous Catheter

It is essential that the nurse employ precautions that minimize the risk of air embolism when removing a subclavian line. Preventive measures include (a) positioning the client appropriately before and after the

procedure, (b) increasing intrathoracic pressure during removal to prevent air entry into the subclavian vein, and (c) applying an occlusive barrier after removal to block air entry at the exit site. Technique 26–5 describes how to remove a central venous catheter.

26-5 Removing a Central Venous Catheter

ASSESSMENT FOCUS

Exit site of CV catheter for skin integrity and signs of infection; baseline vital signs.

EQUIPMENT

- Sterile suture removal set
- Sterile drape
- Alcohol sponges
- Povidone-iodine ointment and 4 × 4 sterile gauze squares, or
- Vaseline gauze
- Mask for the nurse; one for the client if an infection is suspected
- Sterile gloves
- Sterile moistureproof dressing materials

INTERVENTION

1. Prepare the equipment.

- Open a sterile suture removal set, and establish a sterile field.

- Open the sterile packages, i.e., sterile gauze squares and alcohol sponges.

- Place some povidone-iodine ointment on one of the sterile gauze squares if this ointment is to be used. Check agency protocol.

- Don a mask, and put one on the client if necessary.

- Close the clamp on the infusion.

2. Position the client appropriately.

- Place the client in a supine or slight Trendelenburg position. *These positions distend the central veins with blood, increase intrathoracic pressure, and limit air entry into the central vein.*

- Loosen and remove the dressing.

- Don sterile gloves.

- Remove any sutures that secure the catheter.

3. Remove the catheter.

- Ask the client to perform Valsalva's maneuver during removal. *This maneuver also raises intrathoracic pressure and prevents air entry into the central vein.*

- Grasp the catheter hub or needle, and carefully withdraw it,

maintaining the direction of the vein.

- Inspect the catheter to make sure it is intact. If it is not, immediately place the client in a left lateral Trendelenburg position and notify the nurse in charge or physician immediately. *A piece of the catheter in a vein could cause an embolus.*

4. Immediately after catheter removal, apply pressure with an air-occlusive dressing over the subclavian site.

- Use an air-occlusive dressing, such as Vaseline gauze or Telfa covered with antibiotic ointment or plain sterile gauze (check agency policy). *Manual pressure and the occlusive dressing force the tissues together and seal off an air entry path.*

- When bleeding is controlled, replace the gauze dressing with an air-occlusive dressing while the client again performs Valsalva's maneuver.

- Completely cover the insertion site with povidone-iodine ointment, if used, sterile gauze pads, and moistureproof tape. *Nonporous tape helps to ensure impermeability to air.*
  or
  If agency protocol indicates, use a sterile transparent air-occlusive dressing. *A transparent*

dressing allows direct observation of the puncture site for signs of infection and bleeding.

- Leave the air-occlusive dressing in place for 24 to 72 hours or the length of time agency protocol recommends. *The longer the duration of the catheter, the more time required for the subclavian tunnel to seal.*

5. Ensure client safety.

- Ask the client to remain flat and supine for a short time after the subclavian catheter is removed. *This position helps to maintain a positive intrathoracic pressure and allows the tissue tract to begin sealing.*

- Observe the client for signs of air embolism (see page 631).

- If an air embolism is suspected, immediately place the client in a left lateral Trendelenburg position, and administer 100% oxygen by face mask. *The left lateral Trendelenburg position increases intrathoracic pressure, preventing air entry, and oxygen by mask provides oxygen to poorly perfused tissues.*

6. Document all pertinent information.

- Document the time of removal; the size, length, and condition of the catheter; and all nursing assessments and interventions.

▶ **Technique 26–5 Removing a Central Venous Catheter** CONTINUED

EVALUATION FOCUS	Appearance of exit site for catheter; comparison of vital signs to baseline data; presence of signs of air embolism.

SAMPLE RECORDING

Date	Time	Notes
01/06/93	1100	18-cm subclavian catheter removed intact. Transparent air occlusive dressing applied. BP 150/90, P 62 and regular, R 15. —— Rosanna Rodrigues, NS

KEY ELEMENTS OF REMOVING A CENTRAL VENOUS CATHETER

- Maintain asepsis.
- Remove any sutures that secure the catheter before removing the catheter.
- Place the client in a Trendelenburg position during removal.

- Have the client perform Valsalva's maneuver during removal of the catheter.
- Make sure the catheter is intact.
- Cover the insertion site with an air-occlusive dressing.

Central Venous Pressure (CVP)

Measurement of the **central venous pressure (CVP)** determines the pressure of blood in the right atrium (right atrial blood pressure), which reflects the right ventricular blood pressure. A CVP determines the blood volume and the capacity of the right side of the heart to receive and eject blood. The CVP can be measured with a manometer attached to an IV apparatus and a central catheter that terminates in the right atrium or in the superior vena cava. Computerized systems are also available for use in many critical care settings.

Normally the CVP ranges from 6 to 12 cm H_2O in the vena cava and 0 to 4 cm H_2O in the right atrium. Variations occur from person to person and within the same client as a result of changes in position and hydration status or blood volume. Manometer readings are usually intermittent, and intravenous fluid is infused through the central catheter at other times.

The IV tubing must not have an in-line filter, which distorts CVP readings. Some agencies use a separate line and normal saline solution for CVP measurements if the primary IV solution contains dextrose. Dextrose solutions tend to be sticky and interfere with the movement of the manometer ball and flow of solution in the manometer. The separate line with normal saline may be set up in tandem with the primary IV line. Determine agency protocol.

There are several kinds of CVP manometers. One type is a disposable one-piece apparatus (Figure 26–8); other kinds have two parts: a disposable length

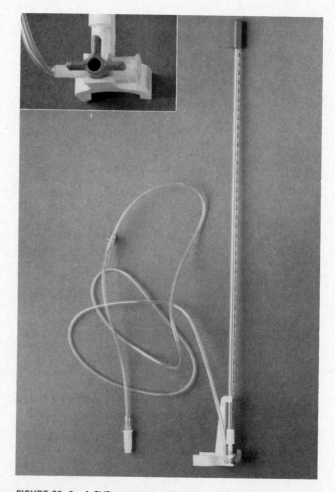

FIGURE 26–8 A CVP manometer. Note the enlargement of the stopcock in the upper-left corner.

of tubing attached to a stopcock and a reusable metal measuring scale. The measuring scale usually ranges from 0 to 30 cm of water.

Stopcocks can be a source of contamination if the ports are not covered when not in use. Individually packaged stopcocks have protective covers on all three ends, which protect the stopcock from contamination when it is removed from the package. Aseptic handling of these covers is important when they are temporarily removed.

Measuring Central Venous Pressure

PURPOSES
- To assess hydration status
- To monitor fluid replacement and determine specific fluid requirements
- To evaluate blood volume, e.g., to monitor the degree of hemorrhage in a postoperative client

ASSESSMENT FOCUS

Patency of CVC line; presence of infection or air embolism; central venous pressure.

EQUIPMENT

- Intravenous tubing
- Manometer set, including stopcock
- A leveling device, if available
- Nonallergenic tape or an indelible marker
- Masks
- Sterile gloves

INTERVENTION

1. Prepare the client.

- Place the client in a supine position without a pillow unless this position is contraindicated. If the client feels breathless, elevate the head of the bed slightly; note the exact position, because it must be used for all subsequent CVP readings, and the manometer level must be adjusted accordingly. *The client must always be in the same position to ensure reliable comparative CVP readings.*

- Locate the level of the client's right atrium at the 4th intercostal space on the midaxillary line.

- Mark this site with indelible pen or piece of nonallergenic tape.

2. Prepare the equipment.

- Prepare the IV tubing and infusion, prime the tubing, and then close the clamp on the tubing.

- If you are using a separate manometer and stopcock, attach the manometer to the stopcock. The manometer is attached to the vertical arm of the stopcock (Figure 26–8, earlier).

- If you are using a one-piece manometer and stopcock, attach these to the IV pole.

- Attach the IV tubing to the left side of the three-way stopcock.

3. Flush the manometer and stopcock.

- Do *not* attach the stopcock to the client's catheter until it is flushed free of air. *Air in the line will interfere with the CVP reading and could cause an air embolism.*

- Turn the stopcock to the IV-container-to-manometer position (Figure 26–9, *A*).

- Open the IV tubing clamp and fill the manometer with the IV so-

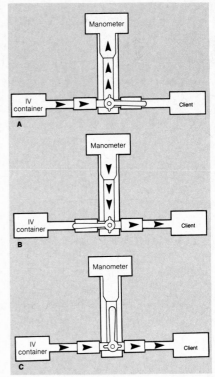

FIGURE 26–9 Positions of a stopcock; *A*, IV container to manometer; *B*, Manometer to client; *C*, IV container to client.

▶ Technique 26–6 Measuring Central Venous Pressure CONTINUED

lution to a level of about 18 to 20 cm.

- Close the IV tubing clamp.

- Turn the stopcock to the IV-container-to-client position (Figure 26–9, C) and flush the stopcock.

- Close the IV tubing clamp.

4. Attach the manometer to the central catheter.

- Place sterile 4 × 4 gauze under the catheter hub.

- Ask the client to perform Valsalva's maneuver (take a deep breath and bear down) and to turn the head away while you quickly attach the manometer tubing to the catheter. *Performing Valsalva's maneuver reduces risk of air embolism, and turning the head reduces the chance of contaminating the equipment.*

- Turn the stopcock so that the IV runs into the client. (Figure 26–9, C) and open the IV clamp.

5. Measure the central venous pressure.

- Check that the level of the client's right atrium (zero reference point) is aligned with the zero point on the manometer scale. To align them, use the leveling rod on the manometer or a yardstick with a level attached (Figure 26–10). When the rod is horizontal (i.e., aligned with the client's right atrium), a bubble appears between two lines in the viewing window of the leveling device. If an adjustment is required, first raise or lower the bed, and second readjust the manometer on the IV pole. *To ensure an accurate reading, the zero mark of the manometer must correspond with the level of the client's right atrium, and the manometer must be vertical.*

- Adjust the stopcock to the manometer-to-client setting (Figure 26–9, B).

- Observe the fall in fluid level in the manometer tube. Note also the slight fluctuations in the fluid level with the client's inspiration and expiration. If the fluid level does not fluctuate, ask the client to cough. *The fluid level falls with inspiration because of a decrease in intrathoracic pressure. It rises with expiration because of an increase in intrathoracic pressure. No fluctuation may indicate that the CVP catheter is lodged against the vein wall. Coughing can change the catheter position.*

- Lightly tap the manometer tube with your index finger when the fluid level stabilizes. *This dislodges air bubbles that can distort the reading.*

- Take a reading at the end of an expiration or according to agency protocol. Inspect the column at eye level, and take the CVP reading from the base of the meniscus. If the manometer tube contains a small floating ball, take the reading from its midline.

- Refill the manometer, and take another reading of the CVP. *A repeat measurement ensures accuracy.*

- Readjust the stopcock to the IV-container-to-client position (see Figure 26–9, C) and adjust the infusion to the ordered rate of flow.

6. Return the client to a comfortable position.

7. Document CVP.

- Include the date and time of the CVP reading, the condition and rate of infusion flow, and all assessments.

- Report the changes in CVP as ordered. In many instances a 🔺 change of 5 cm or more is reported immediately.

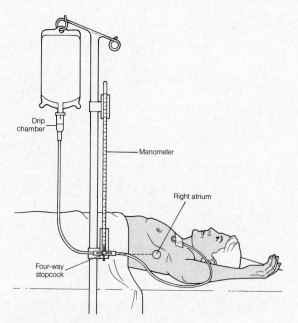

FIGURE 26–10 The zero point on the manometer scale must be at the level of the client's right atrium.

Drip chamber

Manometer

Right atrium

Four-way stopcock

▶ **Technique 26–6** *CONTINUED*

<table>
<tr><td align="right">EVALUATION
FOCUS</td><td>Central venous pressure; degree of fluctuation of pressure.</td></tr>
</table>

SAMPLE RECORDING

Date	Time	Notes
06/06/93	1500	CVP 9. Skin warm and moist. Central line dressing dry. Fluid infusing at 40 ml/hr. ———————————————————— Roberta Smith, SN

KEY ELEMENTS OF MEASURING CENTRAL VENOUS PRESSURE

- Maintain asepsis.
- Determine the patency of the catheter.
- Have the client assume a position used for previous readings.
- Align the right atrium of heart with the zero point on the manometer scale.

- Take a reading at the end of the expiration or according to agency protocol.
- Take a reading at eye level and at the base of the meniscus or the middle of the ball.

Total Parenteral Nutrition

Total parenteral nutrition (TPN), also referred to as **hyperalimentation**, is the intravenous infusion of water, protein, carbohydrates, electrolytes, minerals, and vitamins through a central vein. A description of the components of parenteral nutrition is provided in Table 26–2. TPN formulas provide all of the known essential nutrients in quantities that promote weight gain, wound healing, anabolism, and, in children, growth. The proportion of nutrients and total calories delivered vary with the individual's nutritional needs. Thus, a thorough nutritional assessment is required to determine the appropriate TPN regimen.

Traditionally, the dextrose, amino acids, electrolytes, vitamins, and minerals are mixed together in one container and infused as the primary solution. Lipid emulsions containing primarily essential fatty acids are administered from a separate container through a Y connector into the TPN intravenous line. See Intralipid Therapy on page 651. Solution stability problems occur when lipids are mixed with the other components of the parenteral nutrition solution.

TABLE 26–2 COMPONENTS OF PARENTERAL NUTRITION

Component	Description
Protein	Supplied as crystalline synthetic amino acids; contains essential and nonessential amino acids (4 calories/gram of protein; 1 gram nitrogen/6 grams protein)
Carbohydrate	Supplied as dextrose at 3.4 calories/gram. Peripheral administration 0% to 10% dextrose; central administration up to 50%, although usual is 20% to 25%
Electrolytes	Added to formula; can include sodium, potassium, chloride, acetate, calcium, phosphorus, magnesium; administered according to need
Minerals	Added to formula; can include zinc, chromium, manganese, and copper; administered according to need
Vitamins	Recommended allowances of vitamins A, thiamin, riboflavin, B_6, B_{12}, C, D, E, folic acid, niacin, biotin, and pantothenic acid*
Fat	Contains primarily essential fatty acids; requires separate container due to stability problems

*10 ml of MVI-12 (USV Labs) provides 100 mg ascorbic acid, 3300 IU vitamin A, 200 IU vitamin D, 10 IU vitamin E, 3 mg vitamin B_1, 3.6 mg vitamin B_2, 4 mg vitamin B_6, 40 mg niacinamide, 15 mg pantothenic acid, 60 mg biotin, 400 mg folic acid, and 5 mg vitamin B_{12}.

Source: C. R. Kneisl and S. W. Ames. *Adult health nursing: A biopsychosocial approach.* Addison-Wesley Publishing Co. Redwood City, Calif. 1986, p. 204.

Because of the high volume of blood flow in the central veins, higher concentrations of dextrose can be given, allowing for a greater carbohydrate caloric intake, i.e., up to 50%.

TPN is indicated for the following clients:

- Those, who for prolonged periods, are unable to ingest food because of trauma, a comatose state, or a disease process

- Those who are unable to absorb food via the gastrointestinal tract, e.g., a client with paralytic ileus

- Those who are malnourished or at risk for malnutrition and who will need the parenteral nutrition for longer than 5 days

- Those in whom the bowel or other organs need to rest, such as those with inflammatory bowel disease or pancreatitis

The client receiving TPN is at risk for the same complications as are clients with a CVC: i.e., catheter misplacement and pneumothorax, air embolism, systemic infection, or infection at the infusion site. In addition, metabolic complications are possible. Significant changes occur in the client's fluid, electrolyte, glucose, amino acid, vitamin, and mineral levels. Hyperglycemia, hypoglycemia (see Table 26–3), acidosis, and electrolyte deficiency or excesses such as hyperkalemia, hyponatremia, and hypocalcemia, are potential complications that require meticulous monitoring during therapy.

The nurse must therefore monitor the client's fluid balance and weight daily. Initial weight gain is common because of the fluid intake. Electrolyte balance is best assessed by monitoring serum levels. Because of the dextrose concentration, parenteral nutrition is administered by an infusion pump. The pump precisely regulates the rate of infusion, controlling the rate of dextrose administration. The proper rate of intravenous dextrose infusion helps regulate glucose homeostatis and causes an appropriate insulin response. The nurse also monitors blood glucose levels to assess for blood glucose imbalances.

As with any central venous catheter, strict aseptic technique is essential during TPN therapy. The nurse must implement aseptic measures to prevent contamination of the parenteral nutrition solution and the infusion catheter. Fungi grow readily in the parenteral solution and bacteria in the fat emulsion. The nurse should handle solutions and infusion tubing carefully, especially when setting up or changing the tubing. An in-line filter, connected at the end of the parenteral nutrition tubing, can be used to collect small organisms that enter the system. In-line filters are contraindicated, however, for fat emulsion infusions (see Technique 26–8). Aseptic technique is also essential during tubing and dressing changes (see Technique 26–3, earlier).

Because TPN solutions are high in glucose content, infusions are started gradually to prevent hyperglycemia. The client needs to adapt to TPN therapy by increasing insulin output from the pancreas. For example, an adult client may be given 1 liter/day (40 ml/hour) of TPN solution the first day, if the infusion

---

TABLE 26–3   MAJOR COMPLICATIONS ASSOCIATED WITH TOTAL PARENTERAL NUTRITION

Problem/Cause	Signs and Symptoms	Preventive Actions	Immediate Actions
Hyperglycemia: May occur if hypertonic glucose infusion is too fast or if there is too little insulin in the solution.	Presence of sugar in the urine (glucosuria); high blood sugar; excessive thirst (polydipsia); excessive urination (polyuria); excessive hunger (polyphagia)	Administer concentrated glucose solutions *very slowly* via infusion pump. Monitor blood glucose levels. If infusion rate slows, maintain prescribed drip rate; never increase the infusion rate.	Decrease infusion rate if too fast; notify physician, who may order that insulin be added to the infusion.
Hypoglycemia: May occur if infusion flow stops abruptly or if there is too much insulin in the solution.	Blood glucose level below 60 mg/dl; diaphoresis; tachycardia; anxiety; trembling; hunger; dizziness; personality change; unconsciousness	Use an infusion pump to administer the infusion, and maintain prescribed flow rate. Monitor blood glucose levels.	Adjust infusion rate, or decrease insulin in infusion.

is tolerated; the amount may be increased 20 to 40 ml per hour each day. When TPN therapy is to be discontinued, the TPN infusion rates are decreased slowly to prevent hyperinsulinemia and hypoglycemia. Weaning a person from TPN traditionally took 48 hours, but it is now considered safer to taper the TPN for 1 to 2 hours before terminating therapy (Worthington and Wagner 1989, p. 369).

Technique 26–7 describes how to initiate and monitor TPN through an established CVC.

26-7 Initiating and Monitoring TPN through an Established Central Venous Catheter

PURPOSES
- To maintain or improve the client's nutritional status
- To produce a positive nitrogen balance
- To increase or maintain the client's weight

ASSESSMENT FOCUS

Vital signs, including recent body temperature; client's weight; daily caloric intake and fluid balance; urine for specific gravity; fingerstick blood glucose measurements; any allergy to contents of the TPN solution.

EQUIPMENT

- TPN solution ordered
- Timing tape
- Infusion pump
- Tubing with filter

INTERVENTION

1. Inspect and prepare the solution.

- Remove the ordered TPN solution from the refrigerator 1 hour before use, and check each ingredient and the proposed rate against the order on the chart. *Infusion of a cold solution can cause pain, hypothermia, and venous spasm and constriction.*

- Inspect the solution for cloudiness or presence of particles, and ensure that the container is free from cracks.

- Before administering any TPN solution, check its expiration date. Most solutions must be used within 24 hours of preparation, unless they are refrigerated.

- Apply a timing tape on the solution container.

2. Change the solution contain-

er from the normal saline or dextrose solution to the TPN solution ordered.

- First ensure that correct placement of the TPN catheter has been confirmed by X-ray examination.

- Ensure that the tubing has an in-line filter connected at the end of the TPN tubing. *The filter traps bacteria and particles.*

- Attach and connect the tubing to an infusion pump, if not present. See Technique 25–8 on page 612. *A pump eliminates the changes in flow rate that occur with alterations in the client's activity and position.*

- Clamp the intravenous tubing, and attach the TPN solution to the IV administration tubing. If a double- or triple-lumen tube is in place, attach the infusion to the appropriate lumen.

3. Regulate and monitor the flow rate.

- Establish the prescribed rate of flow, i.e., set dials on the infusion pump for the required drips per minute or milliliters per hour.

- Set the pump alarm, and monitor the infusion at least every 30 minutes. Compare the amount of fluid infused against the timing label.

- Never accelerate an infusion that has fallen behind schedule. *Wide fluctuations in blood glucose can occur if the rate of TPN infusion is irregular.*

- Never interrupt or discontinue the infusion abruptly. If TPN solution is temporarily unavailable, infuse a solution containing at least 5% dextrose. *This prevents rebound hypoglycemia.*

4. Monitor and maintain the pa-

▶ **Technique 26–7 Initiating and Monitoring TPN** *CONTINUED*

tency of the central vein infusion.

- See Technique 26–2, page 635.

- Change the administration set and filter every 24 hours.

5. **Monitor the client for complications.**

- Monitor the vital signs every 4 hours. If fever or abnormal vital signs occur, notify the physician. *An elevated temperature is one of the earliest indications of catheter-related sepsis.*

- Collect double-voided urine specimens at least every 6 hours or in accordance with agency policy, and test the urine for specific gravity. If the specific gravity is abnormal, notify the physician, who may alter the constituents of the TPN solution.

- Assess fingerstick blood glucose levels every 2 to 4 hours according to agency protocol. *Blood glu-*

cose is tested to make certain the infusion is not running too rapidly for the body to metabolize glucose or too slowly for caloric needs to be met.

- Notify the physician of abnormal glucose levels. For hyperglycemia, supplementary insulin may be ordered and given subcutaneously or added directly to the TPN solution by pharmacy personnel. For hypoglycemia the infusion rate may need to be increased.

- Measure the daily fluid intake and output and calorie intake. *Precise replacement for fluid and electrolyte deficits can then be more readily determined.*

- Monitor the results of laboratory tests (e.g., serum electrolytes and blood urea nitrogen) and report abnormal findings to the physician.

- Monitor the client for air embolism. See Table 26–1 and Technique 26–2, step 8, page 636.

6. **Assess weight and anthropometric measurements.**

- Weigh the client daily, at the same time and in the same garments. A gain of more than 0.5 kg (1.1 lb) per day indicates fluid excess and should be reported.

- Measure arm circumference and triceps skinfold thickness weekly or in accordance with agency protocol to assess the physical changes.

7. **Document all relevent information.**

- Record the type and amount of infusion, rate of infusion, vital signs q4h, fingertsick blood glucose levels as ordered, client's weight daily, and anthropometric measurements.

EVALUATION FOCUS	Client's response to TPN (e.g., appearance, color, mood, and orientation); vital signs and blood glucose level; weight gain or loss.

SAMPLE RECORDING

Date	Time	Notes
02/27/93	0800	1000 ml 20% Dextrose solution with 10 ml MV1-12 added started at 40 ml per hour. Blood sugar 100 mg/dl at 0730. Weight 52kg. Afebrile, vital signs stable. T-37.2, P-88, R-16, B.P. 124/85. Lungs clear to auscultation. —————— Laureen Bruce, RN

KEY ELEMENTS OF INITIATING AND MONITORING TPN

- Check the expiration date of the TPN solution, and ensure that it is free of particulate matter and not cloudy.
- Confirm correct placement of the central venous catheter before initiating TPN.
- Allow the TPN solution to reach room temperature before infusion.
- Use aseptic technique when adding solution containers.

- Use an infusion pump to regulate the flow.
- Assess the client's vital signs and fingersticks for blood glucose as frequently as agency policy dictates.
- Weigh the client daily.
- Be alert for signs of air embolism.

Peripheral Parenteral Nutrition

Parenteral nutrition can also be administered through a peripheral vein. In **peripheral parenteral nutrition (PPN)**, isotonic lipid emulsions are used as the main source of nonprotein calories because concentrations of dextrose higher than 10% irritate peripheral veins. For example, a 20% lipid emulsion can provide nearly 2000 kilocalories (Kcal) per day by a peripheral vein. PPN is considered to be a safe and convenient form of therapy over central venous TPN. It does not have the metabolic problems associated with highly concentrated dextrose solutions nor the septic complications associated with CVCs. One major disadvantage, however, is the frequent incidence of phlebitis associated with PPN.

PPN is administered to clients whose needs for intravenous nutrition will last only a short time or in whom placement of a CVC is contraindicated. It is a form of therapy used more frequently to *prevent* nutritional deficits than to correct them.

Total Nutrient Admixture (TNA)

A new TPN preparation called **total nutrient admixture (TNA)** has come into use within the last decade. It is often referred to as "3 in 1" because it combines dextrose, amino acids, and lipids, along with vitamins and minerals, in a single container. It is administered to the client over a 24-hour period. Because mixing lipids with dextrose, amino acids, and other additives creates an emulsion that can become unstable, the use of TNA in North America has lagged behind that in Europe.

Separation of the solution ("cracking") can lead to possible fat embolism or lipid deposits in the lungs, spleen and reticuloendothelial system (Geels and Bowens 1989, p. 78). When administering TNA it is therefore essential that the nurse check the container and avoid using any emulsion that does not appear to be completely homogeneous.

TNA has some advantages over conventional TPN therapy (Geels and Bowens 1989, p. 78).

- There is a smaller risk of line contamination, because the closed system used in TNA is interrupted only once a day.

- The client can be more mobile without the additional pump, bottle, and tubing of TPN therapy.

- It saves both money and the nurse's time, because only one container per day is required.

However, TNA also has some disadvantages:

- An in-line filter cannot be used.

- Inspection for particulate matter in the solution is difficult because the solution is opaque.

- A client's needs may not conform to the current pretested combinations of carbohydrates, protein, and fat in the TNA.

- TNA systems may support more bacterial growth than the conventional systems.

Intralipid Therapy

Intralipid therapy is the infusion of essential fatty acids or fat emulsions. The emulsions are usually 10% to 20% solutions and are often administered piggyback through a central venous line. Because fat emulsions are too thick to go through an in-line filter, they are piggybacked to the tubing beyond the filter. The solution contains large fat globules and is therefore administered through macrodrip tubing or tubing designated by the manufacturer, because the solution may be incompatible with certain types of plastic.

Intralipid solutions are usually administered at room temperature over 12 hours (500 ml). During the initial stage of the infusion (i.e., the first hour), the nurse closely monitors the client's vital signs, as well as signs of any side-effects, e.g., fever, flushing, diaphoresis, dyspnea, cyanosis, headache, nausea, or vomiting. Four hours after the infusion, serum lipids may be monitored and liver function tests may be carried out.

Fat emulsions, such as Intralipid 10% with soybean oil or Liposyn 10% with safflower oil, are often administered via piggyback system attached to a main line. Alternatively, the emulsion may be mixed with a central vein solution in one container to infuse over a 24-hour period. In the latter instance, the admixed solution is administered in the same manner as other TPN solutions (see Technique 26–7). Fat emulsions are contraindicated for clients who are unable to metabolize fat, e.g., those with acute pancreatitis or jaundice. Caution is also necessary for clients who have a predisposition to the formation of fat emboli, e.g., those with anemia, coagulation disorders, or abnormal liver or pulmonary function. Because additives such as vitamins, minerals, or medications may be incompatible with fat emulsions, putting additives into the IV bottle is contraindicated.

Technique 26–8 explains how to administer a fat emulsion by piggyback system.

26-8

Administering a Fat Emulsion by Piggyback System

PURPOSES

- To maintain or improve nutritional staus
- To correct essential fatty acid deficiency

ASSESSMENT FOCUS

Baseline vital signs before the procedure; status of IV site (note presence of erythema or edema); clinical signs of essential fatty acid deficit (e.g., rash or dry, scaly skin; sparse hair growth; impaired wound healing); presence of predisposing factors that could promote fat emboli.

EQUIPMENT

- □ Fat emulsion from pharmacy
- □ Antiseptic sponges (e.g., iodophor, povidone-iodine, alcohol)
- □ Macrodrip tubing without a filter or the manufacturer's suggested tubing

- □ #18 or #20 gauge needle or small gauge needle if piggybacking into dual injection site (optional)

- □ Tape
- □ Infusion pump
- □ Syringe with normal saline

INTERVENTION

1. Inspect and prepare the solution.

- Follow directions for administration temperature; e.g., remove Intralipid from the refrigerator 1 hour before administration to warm it to room temperature. *A cold fat emulsion is uncomfortable to receive.*
  or
  Obtain Liposyn (nonrefrigerated) from the pharmacy.

- Observe the solution for complete emulsion, i.e., consistency in texture and color. Discard the solution if there is an accumulation of fat globules or froth.

- Avoid shaking the bottle excessively. *This disrupts the physical stability of the fat globules.*

- Label the bottle with the client's name, room number, date, time, flow rate, bottle number, and start and stop times.

2. Attach the piggyback tubing to the solution container.

- Swab the stopper on the IV bottle with an antiseptic sponge, and allow it to dry.

- Spike the solution bottle with the piggyback tubing, and hang the container on the IV pole. Twist the spike. *Twisting the spike prevents particles from the stopper falling into the emulsion.*

- Prime the drip chamber until it is one-half to two-thirds full.

- Slowly prime the tubing. *All tubing must be purged with fluid to prevent air from entering the vascular system. Priming at a slow rate reduces the chance of air bubbles entering this solution.*

- Clamp the tubing.

3. Attach the primed piggyback tubing to the mainline IV tubing.

- Clean the appropriate mainline tubing injection port beyond the in-line filter with a povidone-iodine or alcohol swab. *Cleaning removes surface microorganisms at the injection site and prevents* *them from entering the circulatory system. The injection port beyond the filter is used because fat emulsions are thick and would clog an in-line filter.*

- Attach the primed tubing either directly to the correct injection port of the primary IV line or via a needle attached to the fat emulsion tubing.

- Tape this connection site. *Taping prevents the connection from becoming dislodged.*

4. Regulate and monitor the flow rate.

- Start the infusion very slowly according to the physician's orders, the manufacturer's directions, and agency policy. The following schedule is commonly used for a 10% emulsion in adults:

First 5 minutes — 10 gtts/min or 1 ml/min
Next 25 minutes — 40 gtts/min
Thereafter — 60 gtts/min

► **Technique 26–8** *CONTINUED*

The client's tolerance must be assessed.

- Set the infusion pump dials accordingly.

 5. Ensure client safety.

- Monitor the client's vital signs every 10 minutes for 1 hour and hourly thereafter *or* in accordance with agency policy.

- Observe for side-effects (see Evaluation Focus). If side-effects occur, stop the infusion, and notify the physician.

6. Discontinue the procedure.

- Clamp and remove the infusion

when the fat emulsion is absorbed.

- Flush the tubing with normal saline.

- Recap or tape the infusion port.

- Reregulate the primary IV infusion.

7. Document all relevant information.

- Record the date and time the infusion began; name, type, and amount of infusion; rate of infusion flow; vital signs before and after the procedure; and any

untoward reactions to the infusion.

8. Implement follow-up care.

- Obtain serum lipids and liver function tests as ordered, usually 4 to 6 hours after the infusion. *If blood is drawn too soon after the infusion, incorrect blood values may result. Liver function tests determine the client's ability to metabolize the lipids.*

- Record the client's intake and output every shift.

- Record the client's temperature every shift.

EVALUATION FOCUS	Clinical signs of side-effects to the solution, e.g., chills, fever, flushing, cyanosis, diaphoresis, dyspnea, headache, vertigo, and back pain; vital signs to compare to baseline data; results of serum lipids and liver function studies when obtained.

SAMPLE RECORDING

Date	Time	Notes
07/28/93	1130	Intralipid 10% solution infused via piggyback system at 10 gtts per minute first 5 minutes and 40 gtt per min. for next 25 minutes. BP, P, and R checked q10 min. and stable at 128/78, 84, 14. No complaints. Skin color good. – Rosemarie Robinson, RN

KEY ELEMENTS OF ADMINISTERING A FAT EMULSION

- Administer the solution at the appropriate temperature.
- Use correct tubing without filter.
- Prime the tubing before attaching it to the primary line.
- Use an infusion pump to regulate the flow.

- Maintain asepsis.
- Use the injection port beyond the filter closest to the insertion site.
- Tape the injection site.
- Monitor vital signs closely during the infusion.
- Observe the client for possible side-effects.

CRITICAL THINKING CHALLENGE

Kevin Hardy is a 19-year-old who has been admitted to the surgical intensive care unit with multiple injuries following an auto accident. As part of his therapy, a triple-lumen central venous line has been inserted to allow monitoring of central venous pressure and to facilitate the administration of antibiotics. When assessing the flow rate, you note that it is not dripping properly. What is the most likely cause of this problem? What action will you take?

RELATED RESEARCH

Weybright, D.; Sahnd, S.; and Hamilton, C. February 1991. Heparin locks for emergency department patients. *Journal of Emergency Nursing* 17:11–14.

REFERENCES

Ashton, J.; Gibson, V.; and Summers, S. November 1990. Effects of heparin versus saline solution on intermittent infusion device irrigation. *Heart and Lung* 19:608–12.

Brosnan, K. M.; Parham, A. M.; Rutledge, B.; Baker, D. J.; and Redding, J. S. March 1988. Stopcock contamination. *American Journal of Nursing* 88:320–23.

Camp-Sorrell, D. November/December 1990. Advanced central venous access: Selection, catheters, devices and nursing management. *Journal of Intravenous Nursing* 13:361–70.

Dente-Cassidy, A. M. July 1991. Myths and facts . . . about central venous catheters. *Nursing* 21:30.

Geels, W., and Bowens, B. April 1989. T.P.N. alternative: Nutrition that is "3 in 1". *Nursing* 19:78.

Jordan, L. April 1991. Should saline solution be used to maintain heparin locks? *Focus on Critical Care* 18:144–45, 147–48, 150–51.

Kandt, K. A. March/April 1991. An implantable venous access device for children. *American Journal of Maternal Child Nursing* 16:88–91.

Newman, L. N. June 1989. A side-by-side look at two venous access devices. *American Journal of Nursing* 89:826–33.

Oellrich, R. G.; Murphy, M. R.; Goldberg, L. A.; et al. March/April 1991. The percutaneous central venous catheter for small or ill infants. *American Journal of Maternal Child Nursing* 16:92–96.

Pauly-O'Neill, S. January 1991. Questioning the use of invasive technology . . . pulmonary artery (PA) catheter. *American Journal of Nursing* 91:19–20.

Simmons, B. P. October 1981. Centers for Disease Control: Guidelines for prevention of intravascular infections. *Infection Control* 4:61–72.

The PIC catheter: A different approach. August 1991. *American Journal of Nursing* 91:22–28.

Thielen, J. B., and Nyquist, J. March/April 1991. Subclavian catheter removal: Nursing implications to prevent air emboli. *Journal of Intravenous Nursing* 14:114–18.

Worthington, P. H., and Wagner, B. A. June 1989. Total parenteral nutrition. *Nursing Clinics of North America* 24:355–71.

27

Fecal Elimination

CONTENTS

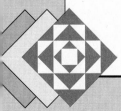

NURSING PROCESS GUIDE
FECAL ELIMINATION

ASSESSMENT

Determine

- Defecation pattern: The frequency and time of day of the client's defecation. Has this pattern changed recently? Does it ever change? If so, does the client know what factors affect it?

- Behavioral patterns: The use of laxatives, fluids, and the like to maintain the normal defecation pattern. What routines does the client follow to maintain the usual defecation pattern (e.g., a glass of hot lemon juice with breakfast or a long walk before breakfast)?

- Diet: What foods does the client believe affect defecation? What foods does the client typically eat? What food does the client always avoid? Are meals taken at a regular time?

- Fluid intake: What amount and kind of fluid does the client take each day (e.g., six glasses of water, five cups of coffee)?

- Exercise: What is the client's usual daily exercise pattern? Obtain specifics about exercise rather than asking whether it is sufficient or not, since people have different ideas of what is sufficient.

- Use of elimination aids: What routines does the client follow to maintain usual defecation pattern? Does the client use natural aids, such as specific foods or fluids, laxatives, or enemas to maintain elimination?

- Medications: Has the client taken any medications that could affect the gastrointestinal tract (e.g., iron in multivitamin supplements, antihistamines in cold preparations, antacids, narcotic analgesics)?

- Pertinent illness or surgery: Has the client had any surgery or illness that affects the intestinal tract? The presence of any ostomies must be explored (e.g., a colostomy or ileostomy).

Assess

- Vital signs: (pulse, respirations, and blood pressure) for baseline data, particularly before administering commercial enemas and digital removal of a fecal impaction.

- Abdominal distention: Distention will appear as an overall outward protuberance of the abdomen, with the skin appearing tight and tense. When palpated, the abdomen feels firm. Measure a distended abdomen at the level of the umbilicus by placing a tape measure around the body. Repeated measurements will indicate whether the distention is increasing or decreasing.

- Bowel sounds: Auscultate all four abdominal quadrants for 5 to 15 seconds to determine the degree of activity or frequency of sounds.

- Consistency and color of feces: Normal feces are brown and formed but soft and moist. Note abnormal colors. For example, black, tarry feces may indicate the presence of blood from the stomach or small intestine; *acholic* feces usually indicate the absence of bile; and green or orange stools may indicate the presence of an intestinal infection. Food may also affect the color of feces; e.g., beets can color stool red or sometimes green. Medications, too, can alter the color of feces; iron, for example, can make stool black.

- Presence of constipation, diarrhea, or fecal incontinence.

- Perianal region and anus: Inspect these areas for discolorations, inflammations, scars, lesions, fissures, fistulas, or hemorrhoids. The color, size, location, and consistency of any lesion is noted.

- Presence of abdominal or rectal pain.

- Presence of flatulence and signs associated with flatulence, such as eructations and their frequency and the passage of flatus by the rectum. Also assess respiratory rate. Flatulence can cause pressure on the diaphragm, resulting in difficult respirations.

Identify clients at risk for developing fecal elimination problems:

- Clients who have insufficient fluid or roughage in the diet.

- Clients who do not exercise sufficiently.

- Individuals who use constipating medications.

- Persons who ingest excessive gas-forming foods.

RELATED DIAGNOSTIC CATEGORIES

- Bowel incontinence

- Colonic constipation

- Perceived constipation

- Diarrhea

- Knowledge deficit

- High risk for Impaired skin integrity (if intestinal contents threaten skin integrity)

- High risk for Fluid volume deficit (if diarrhea is severe)

Nursing Process Guide *CONTINUED*

PLANNING

Client Goals
The client will

- Restore or maintain a regular elimination pattern.
- Maintain fluid balance (if the client has had prolonged diarrhea).

Outcome Criteria
The client with **Constipation**

- Experiences regular soft brown bowel movements that are symmetric in contour.
- Resumes previously identified "normal" elimination schedule (e.g., every 1 to 3 days).
- Reports absence of distention, flatus, or feeling of rectal fullness before defecation.
- Reports absence of discomfort or straining during defecation.
- Establishes a regular time for defecation.
- Verbalizes satisfaction with present bowel habits.
- Consumes a well-balanced diet that includes fiber and eight to ten glasses of fluid daily.
- Names five foods high in fiber.
- Incorporates daily exercise (minimum of a 15-minute walk per day) into life-style.

- Attends to defecation urge when it arises.
- Takes oral laxative as prescribed and understands its desired effects.
- Takes over-the-counter laxatives rarely.

The client with **Diarrhea**

- Has no more than two bowel movements per day.
- Defecates formed stool.
- Demonstrates signs of adequate hydration, e.g., well-hydrated skin and a urine output of 60 ml per hour.
- Is free of abdominal pain or discomfort, urgency, and perianal skin irritation.
- Alters contributing factors associated with diarrhea (e.g., avoids certain foods, implements stress-management techniques).
- States action and side-effects of prescribed medications.

The client with **Bowel incontinence**

- Establishes a regular defecation pattern.
- Experiences fewer episodes of incontinence.
- Is free of perianal irritation and odor.
- Participates actively in bowel-training program.
- Resumes previous patterns of social interaction.

Defecation

The frequency of defecation is highly individual, varying from several times per day to two or three times per week. The amount defecated also varies from person to person. When peristaltic waves move the feces into the sigmoid colon and the rectum, the sensory nerves in the rectum are stimulated, and the individual becomes aware of the need to defecate. The internal anal sphincter relaxes, and feces move into the anal canal. After the individual is seated on a toilet or bedpan, the external anal sphincter is relaxed voluntarily. Expulsion of the feces is assisted by contraction of the abdominal muscles and the diaphragm, which increases abdominal pressure, and by contraction of the levator ani muscles of the pelvic floor, which moves the feces through the anal canal

(Figure 27–1 on page 658). The feces are then expelled through the anus.

Normal defecation is facilitated by (a) thigh flexion, which increases the pressure within the abdomen, and (b) a sitting position, which increases the downward pressure on the rectum.

If the defecation reflex is ignored or if defecation is consciously inhibited by contracting the external sphincter muscle, the urge to defecte normally disappears for a few hours before occurring again. Repeated inhibition of the urge to defecate can result in expansion of the rectum to accommodate accumulated feces and eventual loss of sensitivity to the need to defecate. Constipation can be the ultimate result.

Normal feces are made of about 75% water and 25% solid materials. They are soft but formed. If the

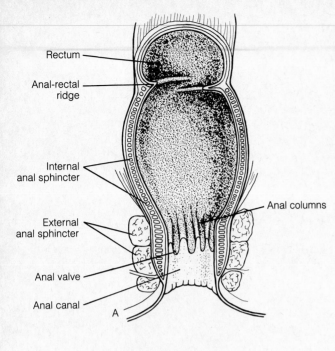

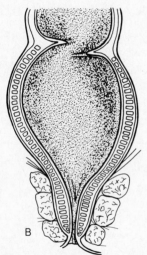

FIGURE 27–1 The rectum, anal canal, and anal sphincters: *A*, open; *B*, closed.

feces are propelled very quickly along the large intestine, so that there is not time for most of the water in the chyme to be reabsorbed, the feces will be more fluid, perhaps containing 95% water. Normal feces require a normal fluid intake; feces that contain less water may be hard and difficult to expel.

Feces are normally brown, chiefly due to the presence of stercobilin and urobilin, which are derived from bilirubin (a red pigment in bile). Another factor that affects fecal color is the action of bacteria such as *Escherichia coli* or *staphylococci*, which are normally present in the large intestine. The action of microorganisms on the chyme is also responsible for the odor of feces. See Table 27–1 for characteristics of normal and abnormal feces.

An adult usually forms 7 to 10 liters of flatus (air or gas) in the large intestine every 24 hours. The gases include carbon dioxide, methane, hydrogen, oxygen, and nitrogen. Some are swallowed with food and fluids taken by mouth, and others are formed through the action of bacteria on the chyme in the large intestine (Guyton 1986, p. 805).

Factors That Affect Defecation

Age and Development
Age affects not only the character of fecal elimination but also its control. See the next section, Developmental Changes.

Diet
Sufficient bulk (cellulose, fiber) in the diet is necessary to provide fecal volume. Certain foods are difficult or impossible for some people to digest. This inability results in digestive upsets and, in some instances, the passage of watery stools. Irregular eating can also impair regular defecation. Individuals who eat at the same times every day have a regularly timed, physiologic response to the food intake and a regular pattern of peristaltic activity in the colon. Spicy foods can produce diarrhea and flatus in some individuals.

Fluid
When fluid intake is inadequate or output (urine or vomitus, for example) is excessive for some reason, the body continues to reabsorb fluid from the chyme as it passes along the colon. Healthy fecal elimination usually requires a daily fluid intake of 2000 to 3000 ml. If chyme moves abnormally quickly through the large intestine, however, there is less time for fluid to be absorbed into the blood; as a result, the feces are soft or even watery.

Activity
Activity also stimulates peristalsis, thus facilitating the movement of chyme along the colon. Weak abdominal and pelvic muscles are often ineffective in increasing the intra-abdominal pressure during defecation or in controlling defecation.

Psychologic Factors
Certain diseases that involve severe diarrhea, such as ulcerative colitis, may have a psychologic component. It is also known that some people who are anxious or angry experience increased peristaltic activity and subsequent diarrhea. In addition, people who are depressed may experience slower intestinal motility, resulting in constipation.

Life-Style
Early bowel training may establish the habit of defecating at regular times, such as daily after breakfast,

TABLE 27–1 CHARACTERISTICS OF NORMAL AND ABNORMAL FECES

Characteristic	Normal	Deviations from Normal	Possible Reason
Color	Adult: brown Infant: yellow	Clay or white	Absence of bile pigment (bile obstruction); diagnostic study using barium
		Black or tarry	Drug (e.g., iron); bleeding from upper gastrointestinal tract (e.g., stomach, small intestine); diet high in red meat and dark green vegetables (e.g., spinach)
		Red	Bleeding from lower gastrointestinal tract (e.g., rectum); some foods (e.g., beets)
		Pale	Malabsorption of fats; diet high in milk and milk products and low in meat
		Orange or green	Intestinal infection
Consistency	Formed, soft, semisolid, moist	Hard, dry, constipated stool	Dehydration; decreased intestinal motility resulting from lack of fiber in diet, lack of exercise, emotional upset, laxative abuse
		Diarrhea	Increased intestinal motility (e.g., irritation of the colon by bacteria)
Shape	Cylindrical (contour of rectum) about 2.5 cm (1 in) in diameter in adults	Narrow, pencil-shaped, or stringlike stool	Obstructive condition of the rectum
Amount	Varies with diet (about 100 to 400 g per day)		
Odor	Aromatic: affected by ingested food and person's own bacterial flora	Pungent	Infection, blood
Constituents	Small amounts of undigested roughage; sloughed dead bacteria and epithelial cells; fat; protein; dried constituents of digestive juices (e.g., bile pigments); inorganic matter (calcium, phosphates)	Pus	Bacterial infection
		Mucus	Inflammatory condition
		Parasites	
		Blood	Gastrointestinal bleeding
		Large quantities of fat	Malabsorption
		Foreign objects	Accidental ingestion

or it may lead to an irregular pattern of defecation. The availability of toilet facilities, embarrassment about odors, and the need for privacy also affect fecal elimination patterns. A client who shares a room in a hospital may be unwilling to use a bedpan because of the lack of privacy and embarrassment about odors.

Medications
Some drugs have side-effects that can interfere with normal elimination. Some cause diarrhea; others, such as large doses of certain tranquilizers and repeated administration of morphine and codeine, cause constipation.

Some medications directly affect elimination. **Laxatives** are medications that stimulate bowel activity and so assist fecal elimination. There are

medications that soften stool, facilitating defecation. Certain medications, such as dicyclomine hydrochloride (Bentyl), suppress peristaltic activity and sometimes are used to treat diarrhea.

Diagnostic Procedures
Before certain diagnostic procedures, such as visualization of the sigmoid colon (sigmoidoscopy), the client is allowed no food or fluid after midnight preceding the examination. Often the client is given a cleansing enema prior to the examination. In these instances the client will not usually defecate normally until eating has been resumed.

Barium (used in radiologic exams) presents a further problem. It hardens if allowed to remain in the colon, producing constipation and sometimes an impaction.

Anesthesia and Surgery

General anesthetics cause the normal colonic movements to cease or slow down by blocking parasympathetic stimulation to the muscles of the colon. Clients who have regional or spinal anesthesia are less likely to experience this problem.

Surgery that involves direct handling of the intestines can cause temporary cessation of intestinal movement. This is called *paralytic ileus*, a condition that usually lasts 24 to 48 hours. Listening for bowel sounds that reflect intestinal motility is an important nursing assessment following surgery.

Pathologic Conditions

Spinal cord injuries and head injuries, for example, can decrease the sensory stimulation for defecation. Impaired mobility may limit the client's ability to respond to the urge to defecate when the client is unable to reach a toilet or summon assistance. As a result, the client may experience constipation. Or a client may experience fecal incontinence because of poorly functioning anal sphincters (see the discussion of fecal incontinence, later in the chapter).

Irritants

Spicy foods, bacterial toxins, and poisons can irritate the intestinal tract and produce diarrhea and often large amounts of flatus.

Pain

Clients who experience discomfort when defecating, e.g., following hemorrhoid surgery, will often suppress the urge to defecate to avoid the pain. Such clients can experience constipation as a result.

Developmental Changes

 Some control of defecation starts at 1½ to 2 years of age. By this time, children have learned to walk, and the nervous and muscular systems are sufficiently well developed to permit bowel control. A desire to control daytime bowel movements and to use the toilet generally starts when the child becomes aware of (a) the discomfort caused by a soiled diaper and (b) the sensation that indicates the need for a bowel movement. Daytime control is normally attained by age 2½, after a process of toilet training.

Nurses may become directly or indirectly involved in the bowel training of children. Direct involvement may occur when a young child is admitted to a health care agency and the staff continues a bowel training program established at home. In this situation, it is important for nurses to know what words and gestures the child uses to indicate a need and the child's usual routine for defecation. Indirect involvement often includes providing information to parents about ways to facilitate the toilet training pro-

cess. The following measures are helpful to assist a child with toilet training:

- Provide clothing that the child can remove independently.

- Give the child a personal toilet seat—either a portable toilet or a special seat for the regular toilet. In the latter instance, provide a step so that the toddler can reach the toilet.

- Allow sufficient time, and provide a consistent, relaxed routine.

- Offer praise for successful behavior, but avoid excessive praise.

- Avoid punishment or disapproval when the child is unsuccessful. Children generally wish to please adults but cannot always be successful.

- Initiate toilet training during nonstressful periods of the child's life. For example, avoid beginning at the time a move to a new house is occurring or on admission to a hospital.

The elderly also experience changes that can affect bowel evacuation. Two of these are **atony** (lack of normal muscle tone) of the smooth muscle of the colon, which can result in a slower peristalsis and thus hardened (drier) feces, and decreased tone of the abdominal muscles, which also decreases the pressure that can be exerted during bowel evacuation. Some elderly people also have decreased control of the anal sphincter muscles, which can result in an urgency to defecate.

Common Problems

Common problems associated with bowel elimination are constipation, fecal impaction, diarrhea, incontinence, flatulence leading to bowel distension, and the presence of parasitic worms.

Constipation refers to the passage of small, dry, hard stool or the passage of no stool for a period of time. It occurs when the movement of feces through the large intestine is slow, thus allowing time for additional reabsorption of fluid from the large intestine. Associated with constipation are difficult evacuation of stool and increased effort or straining of the voluntary muscles of defecation. It is important to define constipation in relation to the person's regular elimination pattern. Some people normally defecate only a few times a week and therefore are not necessarily constipated when they fail to defecate every day. Other people defecate more than once a day; to them, a movement only once a day can indicate constipation. Careful assessment of the person's habits is necessary before a diagnosis of constipation is made. A number of factors contribute to constipation, including irregular defecation habits, overuse of laxatives, and a low intake of fiber in the diet.

Fecal impaction is a mass or collection of hardened, puttylike feces in the folds of the rectum. Impaction results from prolonged retention and accumulation of fecal material. In severe impactions, the feces accumulate and extend well up into the sigmoid colon and beyond. Fecal impaction is recognized by the passage of liquid fecal seepage (diarrhea) and no normal stool. The liquid portion of the feces seeps out around the impacted mass (Figure 27–2).

Along with fecal seepage and constipation, symptoms include frequent but nonproductive desire to defecate and rectal pain. A generalized feeling of illness results; the client becomes anorexic, the abdomen becomes distended, and nausea and vomiting may occur.

Impaction can also be assessed by digital examination of the rectum, during which the hardened mass can often be palpated. Digital examination of the impaction through the rectum should be done gently and carefully, because stimulation of the vagus nerve in the rectal wall can slow the client's heart. Some nurses advise against digital rectal examination without a physician's order.

Although fecal impaction can generally be prevented, digital removal of impacted feces is sometimes necessary. When fecal impaction is suspected, the client is often given an oil retention enema, a cleansing enema 2 to 4 hours later, and daily addi-

tional cleansing enemas, suppositories, or stool softeners. If these measures fail, manual removal is often necessary. See Technique 27–6.

Diarrhea refers to the passage of liquid feces and an increased frequency of defecation. It is the opposite of constipation and results from rapid movement of fecal contents through the large intestine. Rapid passage of chyme reduces the time available for the large intestine to reabsorb water and electrolytes. Some people pass stool with increased frequency, but diarrhea is not present unless the stool is relatively unformed and excessively liquid. The person with diarrhea finds it difficult or impossible to control the urge to defecate for very long. Diarrhea and the threat of incontinence are sources of concern and embarrassment. Often, spasmodic and piercing abdominal cramps are associated with diarrhea. Sometimes the client passes blood and excessive mucus; nausea and vomiting may also occur. With persistent diarrhea, irritation of the anal region extending to the perineum and buttocks generally results. The skin should be kept clean, washed with a mild soap, rinsed, and dried when soiled, and protective ointments such as zinc oxide or petrolatum applied to protect the skin. Fatigue, weakness, malaise, and emaciation are the results of prolonged diarrhea.

Fecal incontinence refers to loss of voluntary ability to control fecal and gaseous discharges through the anal sphincter. The incontinence may occur at specific times, such as after meals, or it may occur irregularly. Two types of fecal incontinence are described: partial and major. *Partial incontinence* is the inability to control flatus or to prevent minor soiling. *Major incontinence* is the inability to control feces of normal consistency (Hanauer 1988, p. 107).

Fecal incontinence is generally associated with impaired functioning of the anal sphincter or its nerve supply, such as in some neuromuscular diseases, spinal cord trauma, and tumors of the external anal sphincter muscle. It is estimated that 60% of the elderly may be affected by fecal incontinence at some time (Hanauer 1988, p. 105).

Flatulence is the presence of excessive flatus and leads to stretching and inflation of the intestines (*intestinal distention*). This condition is also referred to as **tympanites**. Large amounts of air and other gases can accumulate in the stomach, resulting in gastric distention, considerable abdominal discomfort, and pressure on the diaphragm, resulting in difficult respirations.

Most gases that are swallowed are expelled through the mouth by **eructation** (belching). The gases formed in the large intestine are chiefly absorbed, through the intestinal capillaries, into the circulation. Flatulence can occur in the colon, however, from a variety of causes, such as abdominal surgery, anesthetics, or narcotics. If this gas cannot

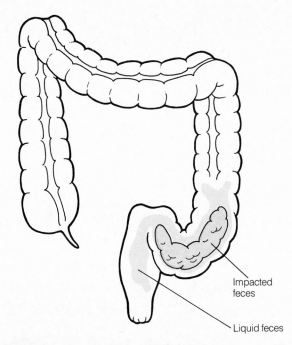

FIGURE 27–2 A fecal impaction with liquid feces passing around the impaction.

be expelled through the anus, it may be necessary to insert a rectal tube or provide a return flow enema to remove it. See Techniques 27–3 and 27–5.

Common *parasitic worms* (helminths) that infest the intestine in North America are the hookworm, roundworm, pinworm, and tapeworm. They cause faulty digestion, intestinal inflammation, intestinal obstruction, and anemia. Medications used against worms are called *anthelmintics. Hookworms* are transmitted by soil contaminated with the larvae that comes in contact with the skin (e.g., when a person is walking barefoot), or by contaminated food or water that is ingested. They are small, less than 1 cm (0.3 in) long, but they have teeth that hook the head into the mucosa and enable it to gain nourishment from the blood. *Roundworms* are larger in length, 25 cm (10 in), and round in the body section. They also enter the body by means of contaminated food or drink. *Pinworms,* which are 1.2 cm (0.5 in) long, are the most common worm parasites in North America, generally infesting children. The female pinworm moves through the anal opening at night and deposits ova in the surrounding area, causing the anal region to itch. This leads to scratching, contamination of the fingernails, and ultimately reinfection by mouth. *Tapeworms* are flat, segmented, large worms, up to 10 m (30 ft) long, with small heads that are equipped with suckers. The suckers embed the head into the intestinal mucosa. Common tapeworms are those transmitted by uncooked beef or pork.

Bedpans and Urinals

Although the focus of this chapter is fecal elimination, both bedpans and urinals are discussed in this section and in Technique 27–1.

There are two main types of bedpans: the regular, or high-back, pan (Figure 27–3, *A*) and the slipper, or fracture, pan (Figure 27–3, *B*). The slipper pan has a low back and is used for people who are unable to elevate their buttocks because of physical problems or therapy that contraindicates such movement.

A urinal is a receptacle for urine only. Several designs are available: one is used for males (Figure 27–4, *A*) and one for females (Figure 27–4, *B*). Female clients often use a bedpan for both urine and feces, while male clients generally use a urinal for urine and a bedpan for feces.

A commode is sometimes used instead of a bedpan when a person can get out of bed but is unable to go to a bathroom. A commode is like an armchair with an open seat (like a toilet seat) with a receptacle under it to receive the urine and feces. The receptacle may be a special one that fits the commode or simply

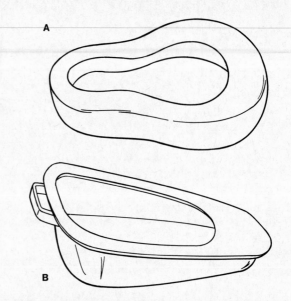

FIGURE 27–3 Two types of bedpans: *A*, the high-back, or regular, pan; *B*, the slipper, or fracture, pan.

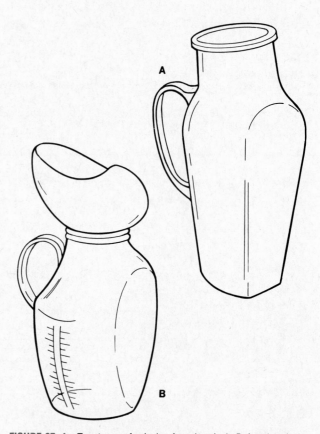

FIGURE 27–4 Two types of urinals: *A*, male urinal; *B*, female urinal.

a bedpan that fits under the toiletlike seat. A commode may or may not be on wheels and freely movable. Some commodes have a plain seat as well, thus doubling as regular chairs.

Guidelines for the care of bedpans and urinals: The care of bedpans and urinals relates largely to preventing the transmission of microorganisms and to the feelings people attach to elimination.

- To maintain medical asepsis, each client in a hospital is provided with a separate bedpan or urinal.

- Bedpans and urinals are stored in an appropriate place out of sight. Bedside units are often designed to provide a specific place for bedpans and urinals that is not visible to others and is separate from the client's personal possessions. It is usually also separated from other equipment used for hygienic care. Medical aseptic practice prohibits the placing of a bedpan on the floor under the bed or overbed tables. Some bedside tables have a hook on which the urinal can hang so that it is accessible to the client.

- A clean bedpan cover is placed over the bedpan after use and for transporting it to and from the bedside. Covers are also available for covering and transporting urinals.

- Bedpans and urinals should always be handled from the outside. Urinals and the slipper (fracture) pan have handles that the nurse can use to carry them. The high-back bedpan needs to be supported with both hands on its base for transport.

- Elimination equipment is thoroughly cleaned and dried after use. Disposable equipment is discarded. Rinsing devices, cleaning brushes, and disinfectant solutions are generally located in the bathrooms or unit utility rooms. Bedpans and urinals periodically need to be recycled through a central supply area for comprehensive cleaning, which includes resterilization.

Many people confined to bed are able to use a bedpan or urinal independently, provided the equipment is placed within safe and easy reach. Some, however, require varying degrees of assistance from a nurse. The nurse has to determine the individual's needs and provide the appropriate assistance.

Using a bedpan or urinal can be embarrassing to many people. For the elderly, physically impaired, or critically ill people, it can also be a tiring procedure. Most male clients will be familiar with a male urinal. Some female clients, however, may not be familiar with female urinals and may require instruction about their use. Note that some female clients find it easier to void using a bedpan rather than a urinal.

27-1 Giving and Removing a Bedpan and Urinal

PURPOSES
- To provide a receptacle for elimination of waste material for clients confined to bed
- To obtain a specimen of urine or stool for laboratory examination
- To obtain an accurate measurement or assessment of the client's urine or stool

ASSESSMENT FOCUS

Color, odor, amount, clarity, and consistency of urine; color, odor, amount, and consistency of feces; redness or excoriation of the perineal area; method client uses to indicate need to defecate or urinate.

EQUIPMENT

- Clean bedpan or urinal and cover
- Toilet tissue
- Basin of water, soap, washcloth, and towel
- Aerosol freshener (optional)
- Equipment for a specimen as required (see Technique 27–2)
- Disposable gloves (optional)

► **Technique 27–1 Giving and Removing a Bedpan** CONTINUED

INTERVENTION

Giving a Bedpan

1. Prepare the equipment.

• Tuck the bedpan cover under the mattress at the side of the bed. Warm the bedpan by running water inside the rim of the pan or over the pan. Dry the outside of the pan, and place it on the foot of the bed or on an adjacent chair. *A cold bedpan may make a person tense and thus hinder elimination. When warming a metal pan, which retains heat, take care not to burn the client.*

2. Prepare the client.

• For clients who can assist by raising their buttocks, fold down the top bed linen on the near side to expose the hip, and adjust the gown so that it will not fall into the bedpan. *A pie fold of the top bedclothes exposes the client minimally and facilitates placement of the bedpan.*

• For helpless clients who cannot raise their buttocks onto and off a bedpan, fold the top bedclothes down to the hips.

3. Give the bedpan.

• For the client who can assist,

  a. Ask the client to flex the knees, rest the weight on the back and the heels, and then raise the buttocks. Assist the client to lift the buttocks by placing the hand nearest the person's head palm up under the lower back, resting the elbow on the mattress, and using the forearm as a lever (Figure 27–5). *Use of appropriate body mechanics by both client and nurse prevents unnecessary muscle strain and exertion.*

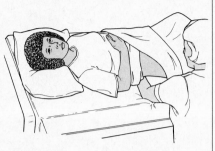

FIGURE 27–5 Assisting a client to raise the hips.

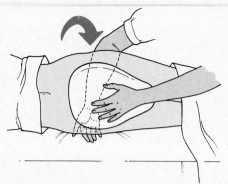

FIGURE 27–6 Placing the bedpan against the buttocks.

  b. Place a regular bedpan under the buttocks with the narrow end toward the foot of the bed and the buttocks resting on the smooth, rounded rim. Place a slipper (fracture) pan with the flat end under the client's buttocks. *Improper placement of the bedpan can cause skin abrasion to the sacral area and spillage of the bedpan's contents.*

  c. Replace the top bed linen and the side rail as needed.

  d. Provide the client with toilet tissue, and ensure that the call light is readily accessible. Ask the client to signal when finished. Leave only when, in your judgment, it is safe to do so. *Having necessary items within reach prevents falls.*

• For the helpless client,

  a. Assist the person to a side-lying position with the back toward you.

  b. Place the bedpan against the buttocks with the open rim toward the foot of the bed.

  c. Hold the far hip with one hand and the bedpan with the other. Smoothly roll the client toward you and onto

the back with the bedpan in place (Figure 27–6). Assume a wide stance, and move weight from the front leg to the back leg when moving the client. *Use of appropriate body mechanics prevents undue muscle exertion and strain.*

  d. Elevate the head of the bed to a semi-Fowler's position. *This position relieves strain on the client's back and permits a more normal position for elimination.*

  e. If the person is unable to assume a semi-Fowler's position, place a small pillow under the back, or help the client to another comfortable position.

  f. Ensure that the call light is within reach.

Removing a Bedpan

3. Position the bed for the client who can help.

• Elevate the bed to the high position, and then remove the bedpan by again pie-folding the top linen back and asking the client to raise the buttocks.

• Cover the bedpan, and place it on an adjacent chair or at the foot of the bed. *Covering the bed-*

Technique 27–1 CONTINUED

pan reduces offensive odors and reduces the client's embarrassment.

4. Assist the client with any needed hygienic measures.

- Wrap toilet tissue several times around the hand, and wipe the person from the pubic area to the anal area, using one stroke for each piece of tissue. *Cleaning in this direction—from the less soiled area to the more soiled area—helps prevent the spread of microorganisms.*

- Turn the client on the side, spread the buttocks, and clean the anal area in the same manner as above.

- Place the soiled tissue in the bedpan.

- Wash the anal area with soap and water as indicated, and thoroughly dry the area. *Adequate washing and drying prevents skin abrasion and excessive accumulation of microorganisms.*

- Replace the drawsheet if it is soiled.

- Offer the client materials to wash and dry the hands. *Hand washing following elimination is a practice that helps prevent the spread of microorganisms.*

5. Position the bed for the helpless client.

- Return the bed to the flat position if health permits.

- Fold the top bed linen down to the thighs.

- Gently roll the client to a side-lying position facing either toward or away from you while holding the bedpan securely with one hand. If you are alone, it is safer and easier to roll the client toward you rather than away

from you. If you are planning to turn the client away from you, raise the side rail on the far side, or have another nurse present to prevent a fall.

- Remove and cover the bedpan, and place it safely on an adjacent chair or at the foot of the bed.

- Clean the perineal area as described above.

- Offer the client materials to wash and dry the hands.

6. Attend to any unpleasant odors in the environment.

- Spray the air with an air freshener unless contraindicated because of respiratory problems or because it is offensive. *Elimination odor can be embarrassing to clients and visitors alike. However, sprays may be harmful to people with respiratory problems, and some perfume sprays are offensive to some people.*

7. Attend to the used bedpan.

- Acquire a specimen if required. Place it in the appropriately labeled container.

- Empty and clean the bedpan. Provide a clean bedpan cover, if necessary, before returning it to the client's unit.

- Go to step 12.

Giving a Urinal

8. Assist the client to an appropriate position.

- Both males and females confined to bed may prefer a semi-Fowler's position, or the male may prefer a standing position at the side of the bed if health permits.

9. Assist the client with using the urinal.

- Offer the urinal so that the client can position it independently.

or
Place the urinal between the client's legs with the handle uppermost so that urine will flow into it.

- Tuck the urinal cover under the mattress at the side of the bed.

- Leave the signal cord within reach of the person. *The client can then call for assistance if required.*

- Leave for 2 to 3 minutes or until the client signals.
or
Remain if the client needs support to stand at the bedside or other assistance.

Removing the Urinal

10. Assist the client as needed.

- Remove and cover the urinal, or place it in a urinal bag.

- If wet, wipe the area around the urethral orifice with a tissue.

- Make sure the perineum is dry.

- Offer a dampened washcloth or water, soap, and a towel to wash and dry hands.

- Change the drawsheet if it is wet.

11. Attend to the urine as required.

- Measure the urine if the client is on monitored intake and output, and provide a specimen if required.

- Empty and rinse out the urinal, and return it to the bedside unit.

12. Document all assessments.

- Record the defecation results and all assessments.

- Record the amount of urine, if it was measured, and all assessment data, e.g., cloudy urine, reddened perineum.

▶ **Technique 27–1 Giving and Removing a Bedpan** *CONTINUED*

EVALUATION FOCUS	Urine: amount, color, clarity, and odor; presence of abnormal constituents. Feces: amount, color, consistency, and odor; presence of abnormalities. Urine and feces: condition of perineum.

SAMPLE RECORDINGS

Date	Time	Notes
04/23/93	1300	Large, dark brown, liquid stool. Complained of cramplike pain in lower abdomen before defecation. Pain relieved on defecation. ———————— ———————————————————————————— Annette S. Cohen, NS

Date	Time	Notes
08/15/93	0900	Voided 275 ml (9 fl oz) of cloudy dark orange urine. Arnold S. Shaw, NS

KEY ELEMENTS OF GIVING AND REMOVING A BEDPAN AND URINAL

- Assess how much assistance the client requires.
- For incontinent clients, establish a regular schedule for using the bedpan or urinal.
- Determine whether a specimen is required for testing or whether urine output is to be measured.
- Maintain medical asepsis.
- Warm a bedpan before use.

- Position the bedpan and client appropriately.
- Make sure the call light is readily accessible.
- After elimination, clean and dry the perineal area of dependent clients, and replace the drawsheet if it is soiled.
- Assess the amount, color, and consistency of feces and urine eliminated.

Fecal Specimens and Tests

Specimens of feces are collected for a variety of tests. Often, the specimen is sent to the laboratory. However, the nurse can perform the test for **occult** blood (blood that is not visible). Some of the reasons for testing feces are the following:

- To detect the presence of occult blood. In this case, only a small sample (about 1 tbsp) of stool is required, and it need not be kept warm or examined immediately. The client is sometimes placed on a diet free of red meat for 3 days before specimen collection, because meat ingestion can create falsely positive results. The presence of blood in the stool may indicate bleeding from a duodenal ulcer or from other lesions elsewhere in the intestine. Oral iron preparations may also be discontinued because undigested portions of them may mask the presence of occult blood in the stool.

- To analyze for dietary products and digestive secretions, e.g., fat content or bile. For these kinds of tests, the nurse needs to collect and send the total quantity of stool expelled at one time instead of a small sample. An excessive amount of fat in the stool (steatorrhea) can indicate faulty absorption of fat from the small intestine. A decreased amount of bile can indicate obstruction of bile flow from the liver and gallbladder into the intestine.

- To detect the presence of parasites, such as amebae, worms, or their eggs. The stools of clients with diarrhea or dysentery are commonly analyzed for parasites. To test for parasites, the specimen must be sent to the laboratory while it is still warm.

- To detect the presence of bacteria or viruses. Only a small amount of feces (1 gram) is required for this type of analysis, because the specimen will be cultured. With diarrheal stools a large sterile cotton swab may be dipped into the specimen and the swab taken to the laboratory in a sterile test tube. Stools need to be sent to the laboratory immediately for viral or bacterial cultures. Because clients receiving antibiotics or sulfonamides may produce falsely negative cultures, the nurse needs to note these medications on the requisition for the stool specimen.

Technique 27–2 describes how to obtain and test a specimen of feces. When obtaining stool samples, i.e., when handling the client's bedpan, when transferring the stool sample to a specimen container, and when disposing of the bedpan contents, the nurse follows medical aseptic technique meticulously.

To secure a stool specimen from a baby or young child who is not toilet trained, the nurse obtains newly passed feces from the diaper.

27-2 Obtaining and Testing a Specimen of Feces

Before obtaining a specimen, determine the reason for collecting the stool specimen and the correct method of obtaining and handling it (i.e., how much stool to obtain, whether a preservative needs to be added to the stool, and whether it needs to be sent immediately to the laboratory). It may be necessary to confirm this information by checking with the agency laboratory. In many situations, only a single specimen is required; in others, timed specimens are necessary, and every stool passed is collected within a designated time period.

PURPOSE

- To determine the presence of occult blood, parasites, bacteria, viruses, or other abnormal constituents in the stool

ASSESSMENT FOCUS

Client's need for assistance to defecate or use a bedpan; any abdominal discomfort before, during, or after defecation; status of perianal skin for any irritation, especially if the client defecates frequently and has liquid stools; any interventions related to the specimen collection, e.g., dietary or medication orders; presence of hemorrhoids that may bleed (particularly important for clients who are constipated, because constipated stool can aggravate existing hemorrhoids; any bleeding can affect test results); any interventions (e.g., medication) ordered to follow a defecation.

EQUIPMENT
Collecting a Specimen of Feces

- Clean or sterile bedpan or bedside commode (for an infant, the stool is scraped from the diaper)
- Disposable gloves
- Cardboard or plastic specimen container (labeled) with a lid

or, for stool culture, a sterile swab in a test tube, as policy dictates
- Two tongue blades
- Paper towel
- Completed laboratory requisition
- Air freshener

Testing for Occult Blood in the Feces

- Clean bedpan or bedside commode
- Disposable gloves
- Two tongue blades
- Paper towel
- Test product

INTERVENTION

1. Give ambulatory clients the following information and instructions.

- The purpose of the stool specimen and how the client can assist in collecting it.

- Defecate in a clean or sterile bedpan or bedside commode.

▶ **Technique 27–2 Obtaining and Testing a Specimen of Feces** CONTINUED

- Do not contaminate the specimen, if possible, by urine or menstrual discharge. Void before the specimen collection.

- Do not place toilet tissue in the bedpan after defecation, because contents of the paper can affect the laboratory analysis.

- Notify the nurse as soon as possible after defecation, particularly for specimens that need to be sent to the laboratory immediately after collection.

2. **Assist clients who need help.**

- Assist the client to a bedside commode or a bedpan placed on a bedside chair or under the toilet seat in the bathroom.

- After the client has defecated, cover the bedpan or commode. *Covering the bedpan reduces odor and embarrassment to the client.*

- Put on gloves to prevent hand contamination, and clean the client as required. Inspect the skin around the anus for any irritation, especially if the client defecates frequently and has liquid stools.

3. **Transfer the required amount of stool to the stool specimen container.**

- Use one or two tongue blades to transfer some or all of the stool to the specimen container, taking care not to contaminate the outside of the container. The amount of stool to be sent depends on the purpose for which the specimen is collected. Usually 2.5 cm (1 in) of formed stool or 15 to 30 ml of liquid stool is adequate. For some timed specimens, however, the entire stool passed may need to be sent. Visible pus, mucus, or blood should

be included in the sample.
or
For a culture, dip a sterile swab into the specimen, preferably where purulent fecal matter is present in the feces. Place the swab in a sterile test tube using sterile technique.
or
For an occult blood test, see step 5 below.

- Wrap the used tongue blades in a paper towel before disposing of them in a waste container. *Wrapping the used tongue blades prevents the spread of microorganisms by contact with other articles.*

- Place the lid on the container as soon as the specimen is in the container. *Putting the lid on immediately prevents the spread of microorganisms.*

4. **Ensure client comfort.**

- Empty and clean the bedpan or commode, and return it to its place.

- Remove gloves.

- Provide an air freshener for any odors unless contraindicated by the client; e.g., a spray may increase dyspnea.

5. **Label and send the specimen to the laboratory.**

- Ensure that the specimen label and the laboratory requisition have the correct information on them and are securely attached on the specimen container. *Inappropriate identification of the specimen can lead to errors of diagnosis or therapy for the client.*

- Arrange for the specimen to be taken to the laboratory. Specimens to be cultured or tested for parasites need to be sent im-

mediately. If this is not possible, follow the directions on the specimen container. In some instances refrigeration is indicated because bacteriologic changes take place in stool specimens left at room temperature.
or

Test the stool for occult blood.

- Select a test product.

- Put on gloves.

- Follow the manufacturer's directions. For example:

   a. For a Guaiac test, smear a thin layer of feces on a paper towel or filter paper with a tongue blade, and drop reagents onto the smear as directed.

   b. For a Hematest, smear a thin layer of feces on filter paper, place a tablet in the middle of the specimen, and add two drops of water as directed.

   c. For a Hemoccult slide, smear a thin layer of feces over the circle inside the envelope, and drop reagent solution onto the smear.

- Note the reaction. For all tests, a blue color indicates a positive result, i.e., the presence of occult blood.

6. **Document all relevant information.**

- Record the collection of the specimen on the client's chart and on the nursing care plan. Include in the recording the date and time of the collection and all nursing assessments. See Evaluation Focus.

- For an occult blood test, record the type of test product used and the reaction.

► **Technique 27–2** *CONTINUED*

EVALUATION FOCUS	Color, odor, consistency, and amount of feces; presence of abnormal constituents, e.g., blood or mucus; results of test for occult blood if obtained; discomfort during or after defecation; status of perianal skin; any bleeding from the anus after defecation.

SAMPLE RECORDING

Date	Time	Notes
08/12/93	0830	Stool specimen obtained for parasites and sent to laboratory. Stool is light brown, soft and without form. No evidence of blood or mucus. Perianal skin intact. ———————————————————— Stacey McNamara, RN *or* Guaiac test performed for occult blood. Results positive. ———————————————————— Stacey McNamara, RN

KEY ELEMENTS OF OBTAINING AND TESTING A SPECIMEN OF FECES

- Provide the client with appropriate instructions to collect the specimens.
- Wear disposable gloves, and use aseptic technique.
- Prevent contamination of the specimen by urine or menstrual discharge.
- Ensure that the appropriate amount of stool is collected for ordered tests.
- Check whether the client needs to be placed on a diet free of red meat and whether to discontinue oral iron preparations before an occult blood test.
- Send stool specimens collected for the assessment of parasites, bacteria, or viruses *immediately* to the laboratory.
- Document medications on the laboratory requisition that accompanies specimens taken for culture and sensitivity.

Administering Enemas

An **enema** is a solution introduced into the rectum and sigmoid colon. Its function is to remove feces and/or flatus. Enemas are classified into four groups, according to their action: cleansing, carminative, retention, or return flow. A *cleansing enema* stimulates peristalsis by irritating the colon and rectum and/or by distending the intestine with the volume of fluid introduced. Two kinds of cleansing enemas are the high enema and the low enema. The *high enema* is given to clean as much of the colon as possible. It is often used before diagnostic studies. Often about 1000 ml (1 liter) of solution is administered to an adult. The client changes from the left lateral to the dorsal recumbent position and then to the right lateral position during the administration so that the fluid can follow the large intestine. The fluid is administered at a higher pressure than for a low enema; that is, the container of solution is held higher. Cleansing enemas are most effective if held for 5 to 10 minutes. The *low enema* is used to clean the rectum and sigmoid colon only. About 500 ml (0.5 liter) of solution is administered to an adult, and the client maintains the left side-lying position during its administration.

A *carminative enema* is given primarily to expel flatus. The solution instilled into the rectum releases gas, which in turn distends the rectum and the colon, thus stimulating peristalsis. For an adult, 60 to 180 ml of fluid is instilled.

A *retention enema* introduces oil into the rectum and sigmoid colon. The oil is retained for a relatively long period of time (e.g., ½ to 1 hour). It acts to soften the feces and to lubricate the rectum and anal canal, thus facilitating passage of the feces.

A *return flow enema*, sometimes referred to as the *Harris flush* or *colonic irrigation*, is used to expel flatus. Alternating flow of 100 to 200 ml of fluid into and out of the large intestine stimulates peristalsis and the expulsion of feces.

Various solutions are used for enemas. The specific solution may be ordered by the physician or indicated by agency protocol. Table 27–2 lists some of these solutions, giving the quantity and proportions frequently used.

An enema is a relatively safe procedure for the client. The chief dangers are irritation of the rectal mucosa by too much soap or an irritating soap and negative effects of a *hypertonic solution* (possessing a greater tonicity than blood) or *hypotonic solution* (possessing a lesser tonicity than blood) on the body fluid and electrolytes. A hypertonic solution, such as the phosphate solutions of some commercially prepared enemas, is slightly irritating to the mucous membrane and causes fluid to be drawn into the colon from the surrounding tissues. The process by which this happens is called *osmosis*. Because only a small amount of fluid is normally administered, the advantages of comfort, retention for only 5 to 7 minutes, and convenience generally outweigh these disadvantages.

The repeated administration of hypotonic solutions, such as tap water enemas, can result in absorption of the water from the colon into the bloodstream. This increases the blood volume and can produce water intoxication. For this reason, some health agencies limit to three the number of tap water enemas given consecutively. This is of particular concern when the order is "enemas until returns are clear"— for example, prior to a visual examination of the large intestine. Hypotonic solutions can also be unsafe for clients, particularly elderly clients with decreased kidney function or acute heart failure.

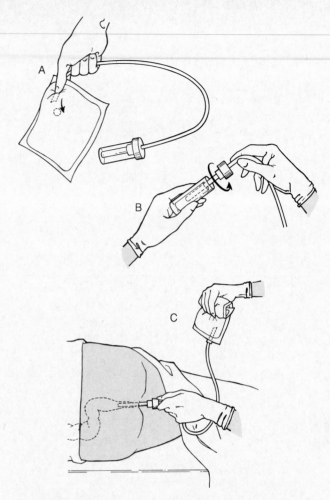

FIGURE 27–7 One type of commercially prepared disposable enema: *A,* The bead that seals the tube is expelled from the tube into the bag so that the solution can flow through the tubing; *B,* the protector cover of the insertion tip is rotated to distribute the lubricant on the tip before the cover is removed; *C,* after the tube has been inserted, the bag is inverted and compressed.

Some agencies use commercially prepared disposable enemas (Figure 27–7). It is important that the nurse be aware that prepackaged enemas have their own instructions, which should be followed unless there are other instructions from the physician or the agency.

Guidelines for Administering Enemas

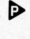Enemas for adults are usually given at 40 to 43 C (105 to 110 F); those for children are given at 37.7 C (100 F), unless otherwise specified. Some oil retention enemas are given at 33 C (91 F). High temperatures can be injurious to the bowel mucosa; cold temperatures are uncomfortable for the client and may trigger a spasm of the sphincter muscles.

The amount of solution to be administered depends on the kind of enema, the age of the person, and the person's ability to retain the solution. The following are approximate amounts:

TABLE 27–2 TYPES OF ENEMAS COMMONLY USED FOR ADULTS

Name	Constituents
Commercially prepared enema	90 to 120 ml of a hypertonic solution, such as sodium phosphate (see directions on the package)
Saline	9 ml of sodium chloride to 1000 ml of water
Tap water	500 to 1000 ml of tap water
Soap	20 ml of castile soap in 500 to 1000 ml of water
Oil, e.g., olive oil	90 to 120 ml of oil (commercially prepared): mineral, olive, or cottonseed

Age	Volume
18 months	50 to 200 ml
18 months to 5 years	200 to 300 ml
5 to 12 years	300 to 500 ml
12 years and older	500 to 800 ml
Adult	750 to 1000 ml

The rectal tube needs to be of an appropriate size:

Age	Size
Infant/small child	#10 to 12 Fr.
Toddler	#14 to 16 Fr.
School-age child	#16 to 18 Fr.
Adults	#22 to 30 Fr.

The force of flow of the solution is governed by the (a) height of the solution container, (b) size of the tubing, (c) viscosity of the fluid, and (d) resistance of the rectum. The higher the solution container is held above the rectum, the faster the flow and the greater the force (pressure) in the rectum. During most adult enemas, the solution container should be no higher than 30 cm (12 in) above the rectum. During a high cleansing enema, the solution container is usually held 30 to 45 cm (12 to 18 in) above the rectum, because the fluid is instilled farther to clean the entire bowel. For an infant, the solution container is held no more than 7.5 cm (3 in) above the rectum.

The time it takes to administer an enema largely depends on the amount of fluid to be instilled and the client's tolerance. Large volumes, such as 1000 ml, may take 10 to 15 minutes to instill; small volumes require less time.

The amount of time the client retains the enema solution depends on the purpose of the enema and the client's ability to contract the external sphincter to retain the solution. Oil retention enemas are usually retained 2 to 3 hours. Other enemas are normally retained 5 to 10 minutes.

Many children require an enema prior to undergoing gastrointestinal procedures; the procedure for giving an enema to an infant or child is similar to that for an adult. The enema solution should be isotonic (usually normal saline). If prepared saline is not available, the nurse can prepare it by mixing one teaspoon of table salt in 500 ml of tap water. Plain water is hypotonic and can therefore create a rapid fluid shift and fluid overload. Some hypertonic commercial solutions (e.g., Fleet enema) can lead to hypovolemia and electrolyte imbalances. In addition, the osmotic effect of the Fleet enema may produce diarrhea and subsequent metabolic acidosis.

Infants and small children do not exhibit sphincter control and need to be assisted in retaining the enema. The nurse administers the enema while the infant or child is lying with the buttocks over the bedpan (See Technique 27–3), and the nurse firmly presses the buttocks together to prevent the immediate expulsion of the solution. Older children can usually hold the solution if they understand what to do and are not required to hold it for too long a period. It may be necessary to ensure that the bathroom is available for an ambulatory child before starting the procedure or to have a bedpan ready.

Technique 27–3 describes how to administer an enema; Technique 27–4 describes how to siphon an enema. For an explanation of how to insert a rectal tube to relieve flatulence and how to remove a fecal impaction digitally, see Techniques 27–5 and 27–6, respectively.

27-3 Administering an Enema

Before administering an enema, determine whether a physician's order is required. At some agencies, a physician must order the kind of enema and the time to give it, e.g., the evening before surgery or the morning of the examination. When the client has rectal pathology, the physician may also specify the size of the rectal tube to use. At other agencies, enemas are given at the nurses' discretion, i.e., as necessary on a prn order. In addition, determine the presence of kidney or cardiac disease that contraindicates the use of a hypotonic solution.

PURPOSES
- To stimulate peristalsis and remove feces or flatus
- To soften feces and lubricate the rectum and colon
- To clean the rectum and colon in preparation for an examination
- To remove feces prior to a surgical procedure or a delivery, thereby preventing inadvertent defecation and subsequent contamination

▶ **Technique 27–3 Administering an Enema** *CONTINUED*

ASSESSMENT FOCUS	When the client last had a bowel movement and the amount, color, and consistency of the feces; presence of abdominal distention (the distended abdomen appears swollen and feels firm rather than soft when palpated); whether the client has sphincter control; whether the client can use a toilet or commode or must remain in bed and use a bedpan.

EQUIPMENT

- ▢ Moistureproof absorbent pad
- ▢ Bath blanket
- ▢ Bedpan or commode if the client is unable to reach the bathroom
- ▢ Disposable enema unit with instructions for use (Figure 27–7)

or

- ▢ Enema set containing:
  - a. Container to hold the solution
  - b. Tubing
  - c. Clamp
  - d. Rectal tube of the correct size

- ▢ Lubricant
- ▢ Thermometer to measure temperature of solution
- ▢ Prescribed amount of solution at the correct temperature
- ▢ Disposable gloves
- ▢ Disposable towel

INTERVENTION

1. Prepare the client.

- Explain the procedure to the client. Indicate that the client may experience a feeling of fullness while the solution is being administered. Careful explanation is especially important for the preschool child. *An enema is an intrusive procedure and therefore threatening.*

- Assist the adult client to a left lateral position, with the right leg as acutely flexed as possible (Figure 27–8). *This position facilitates the flow of solution by gravity into the sigmoid and descending colon, which are on the left side. Having the right leg acutely flexed provides for adequate exposure of the anus.*

- During a high cleansing enema, have the client change position from left lateral to dorsal recumbent and then to right lateral. *In this way the entire colon is reached by the fluid.*

- For infants and small children, the dorsal recumbent position is frequently used. Position them on a small padded bedpan with support for the back and head. Secure the legs by placing a diaper under the bedpan and then over and around the thighs (Figure 27–9).

- Place the waterproof pad under the client's buttocks to protect the bed linen, and drape the client with the bath blanket.

2. Prepare the equipment.

- Lubricate about 5 cm (2 in) of the rectal tube (some commercially prepared enema sets already have lubricated nozzles). *Lubrication facilitates insertion through the sphincters and minimizes trauma.*

- Open the clamp, and run some solution through the connecting tubing and the rectal tube to expel any air in the tubing; then close the clamp. *Air instilled into the rectum, although not harmful, causes unnecessary distention.*

💧 3. Don gloves, and insert the rectal tube.

- For clients in the left lateral position, lift the upper buttock to ensure good visualization of the anus.

- Insert the tube smoothly and slowly into the rectum, directing it toward the umbilicus (Figure 27–10). *This angle follows the*

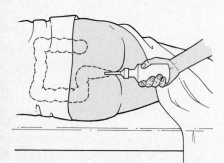

FIGURE 27–8 Assuming a left lateral position for an enema. Note the commercially prepared enema.

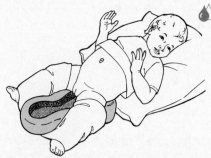

FIGURE 27–9 Immobilizing an infant's legs for an enema by placing a diaper under the bedpan and over the thighs.

► **Technique 27–3** CONTINUED

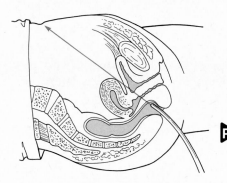

FIGURE 27–10   Inserting the rectal tube following the direction of the rectum.

normal contour of the rectum. Slow insertion prevents spasm of the sphincter.

- Insert the tube 7 to 10 cm (3 to 4 in) in an adult. *Since the anal canal is about 2.5 to 5 cm (1 to 2 in) long in the adult, insertion to this point places the tip of the tube beyond the anal sphincter into the rectum.* Insert the tube 5 to 7.5 cm (2 to 3 in) in the child and only 2.5 to 3.75 cm (1 to 1.5 in) in the infant.

- If resistance is encountered at the internal sphincter, ask the client to take a deep breath, then run a small amount of solution through the tube to relax the internal anal sphincter.

- Never force tube entry. If resistance persists, withdraw the tube, and report the resistance to the nurse in charge.

4. Slowly administer the enema solution.

- Raise the solution container, and open the clamp to allow fluid flow.
  or
  Compress a pliable container by hand.

- During most adult enemas, hold the solution container no higher than 30 cm (12 in) above the rectum. *The higher the solution container is held above the rectum, the faster the flow and the greater the*

force (pressure) in the rectum. Damage to the mucosal lining may result if the container is held higher than 30 cm. During a high enema, hold the solution container a little higher, e.g., 4 to 6 inches. *The fluid must be instilled farther to clean the entire bowel.* For children, lower the height of the solution container appropriately for the age of the child. See the guidelines on page 671.

- Administer the fluid slowly. If the client complains of fullness or pain, use the clamp to stop the flow for 30 seconds, and then restart the flow at a slower rate. *Administering the enema slowly and stopping the flow momentarily decrease the likelihood of intestinal spasm and premature ejection of the solution.*

- If you are using a plastic commercial container, roll it up as the fluid is instilled. *This prevents subsequent suctioning of the solution.*

- After all of the solution has been instilled or when the client cannot hold any more and wants to defecate (the urge to defecate usually indicates that sufficient fluid has been administered), close the clamp, and remove the rectal tube from the anus.

- Place the rectal tube in a disposable towel as you withdraw it.

5. Encourage the client to retain the enema.

- Ask the client to remain lying down. *It is easier for the client to retain the enema when lying down than when sitting or standing because gravity promotes drainage and peristalsis.*

- To assist a small child in retaining the solution, apply firm pressure over the anus with tissue wipes, or firmly press the buttocks together.

- Ensure that the client retains the solution for the appropriate amount of time, e.g., 5 to 10 minutes for a cleansing enema or at least 30 minutes for a retention enema.

6. Assist the client to defecate.

- Assist the client to a sitting position on the bedpan, commode, or toilet. *A sitting position facilitates the act of defecation.*

- Ask the client who is using the toilet not to flush it. *The nurse needs to observe the feces.*

- If a specimen of feces is required, ask the client to use a bedpan or commode.

7. Record and report relevant data.

- Record administration of the enema; the amount, color, and consistency of the returns; and the relief of flatus and abdominal distention.

VARIATION: Administering an Enema to an Incontinent Client

Occasionally a nurse needs to administer an enema to a client who is unable to control the external sphincter muscle and thus cannot retain the enema solution for even a few minutes. In that case the client assumes a supine position on a bedpan. The head of the bed can be elevated slightly, e.g., to 30° if necessary, and the client's head and back are supported by pillows. Pressing the buttocks together may help the client to retain the solution. The nurse wears gloves to prevent direct contact with the solution and feces that are expelled over the hand into the bedpan during the administration of the enema.

VARIATION: Administering a Return Flow Enema

Administering the return flow enema (the Harris flush, or colonic

▶ **Technique 27–3 Administering an Enema** *CONTINUED*

irrigation) is similar to administering and siphoning an enema. Initially, the solution (100 to 200 ml for an adult) is instilled into the client's rectum and sigmoid colon. Then the solution container is lowered so that the fluid flows back out through the rectal tube into the container. The inflow-outflow process is repeated five or six times (to stimulate peristalsis and the expulsion of flatus), and the solution is replaced several times during the procedure as it becomes thick with feces. A total of about 1000 ml of solution is usually used for an adult.

EVALUATION FOCUS
> Amount, color, and consistency of returns; relief of flatus or abdominal distention; any problems encountered, e.g., resistance at the external or internal sphincter when inserting the rectal tube.

SAMPLE RECORDING

Date	Time	Notes
06/29/93	2100	1,000 ml saline enema given. Returned large amount of hard, white stool and large amount of flatus. Abdomen soft and less distended. P72. — Roxy-Ann B. Stanley, NS

KEY ELEMENTS OF ADMINISTERING AN ENEMA

All enemas
- Determine the type and purpose of the enema and whether a physician's order is required.
- Position the client appropriately.
- Assess the returns.
- Wear gloves.

Cleansing enema
- Use the correct type, amount, and temperature of solution.
- Flush the tubing before administering the enema to remove air.
- Lubricate the rectal tube before insertion.

- Direct the insertion tube toward the client's umbilicus.
- Ask the client to take a deep breath during tube insertion.
- Hold the solution container at the correct height.
- Administer the solution slowly, and start and stop the flow of solution temporarily when indicated.

Commercial enema
- Follow the manufacturer's instructions.

Retention enema
- Instruct client to retain the enema at least 30 minutes.

27-4   Siphoning an Enema

In some instances, a client may be unable to expel the solution after the administration of an enema. The solution must then be siphoned off. In siphoning, the nurse uses the force of gravity to draw the fluid out of the rectum and colon. Siphoning an enema may require a physician's order.

PURPOSE
- To remove retained enema solution

ASSESSMENT FOCUS
> Amount of enema solution instilled, presence of abdominal distention, abdominal pain or feeling of fullness; rate and quality of respirations.

▶ **Technique 27–4 Siphoning an Enema** *CONTINUED*

EQUIPMENT

- ☐ Bedpan
- ☐ Rectal tube
- ☐ Lubricant
- ☐ Container of water at 40 C (105 F)
- ☐ Disposable large plastic volume enema container

INTERVENTION

1. Position the client appropriately.

- Assist the client to a *right* side-lying position. *In this position, the sigmoid colon is uppermost, thus facilitating drainage of the solution from the rectum and colon by gravity.*

- Ensure that the client's hips are close to the side of the bed. *This placement prevents undue stretching and reaching by the nurse and facilitates siphoning into the container and bedpan.*

2. Prepare the equipment.

- Place the bedpan on a chair at the side of the bed near the client's hips. The chair must be lower than the client's hips.

- Attach the open end of the rectal tube to the partially filled enema set.

- Lubricate the rectal tube.

3. Siphon the enema solution.

- Fill the tube with solution, then pinch it and gently insert it into the rectum as for an enema.

- Hold the enema container about 10 cm (4 in) above the anus, release the pinched rectal tube, and quickly lower the enema container. *This action should draw the fluid from the colon and rectum, permitting it to flow through the rectal tube into the solution container.*

4. Document all relevant information.

- Record the amount of fluid siphoned off as well as the characteristics of the returns.

EVALUATION FOCUS

Amount of fluid returns; color, odor, and presence of any feces; abnormal constituents, e.g., blood or mucus.

SAMPLE RECORDING

Date	Time	Notes
12/13/93	1030	700 ml enema fluid siphoned through anal canal. Returns tinged with mucus and dark brown hard stool. Respirations 16 and shallow. C/O abdominal pain. — Ned Zabirski, RN

KEY ELEMENTS OF SIPHONING AN ENEMA

- Position the client in a right side-lying position close to the edge of the bed.
- Ensure that the bedpan on the chair is lower than the client's hips.
- Fill the enema tube with solution, and lubricate it before inserting it into the rectum.
- Immediately after inserting the unclamped rectal tube, quickly lower the enema container.
- Assess the returns for amount, color, and consistency.

27-5 Inserting a Rectal Tube to Relieve Flatulence

Rectal tubes are left in the rectum for varying lengths of time. Generally, it is recommended that a tube remain in the rectum for no longer than 30 minutes to prevent undue irritation of the rectal lining. The nurse then reinserts the tube as needed every 2 to 3 hours.

PURPOSE
- To relieve abdominal distention

ASSESSMENT FOCUS

> Presence of abdominal discomfort or rectal pain; flatulence and signs associated with flatulence, e.g., eructations and their frequency and the passage of flatus by the rectum; respiratory rate; degree of abdominal distention; bowel sounds.

EQUIPMENT

- Rectal tube (#22 to #30 Fr. for adults)
- Lubricant
- Paper towel
- Tape to attach the rectal tube to the buttock (optional)
- Either a moistureproof absorbent pad to wrap around

the open end of the rectal tube, or a connecting tube and a receptacle containing water

INTERVENTION

1. Prepare the client.

- Assist the client to a left lateral position, and fold back the bedclothes to expose the anus.

2. Prepare the equipment.

- Lubricate the insertion tip of the rectal tube liberally for 5 cm (2 in). *Lubrication reduces resistance to passage of the tube through the anal sphincters.*

3. Introduce the rectal tube.

- Gently insert the rectal tube into the rectum 10 to 15 cm (4 to 6 in) for an adult. *The rectal tube can be inserted farther for this procedure than is recommended for an enema because fluid will not be administered.*

- Tape the rectal tube to the buttock if it is not likely to be retained otherwise. *Taping prevents the tube from dislodging.*

- Place the open end of the rectal tube in a folded absorbent pad. *The folded absorbent pad will catch any liquid fecal material that seeps through the tube.*
  or
  Some nurses advocate attaching the open end of the rectal tube to a connecting tube and a drainage receptacle filled with water. If this process is implemented, place the distal end of the tubing below the level of the water in the collecting receptacle. *Gas bubbles can be noted only if the tubing is below the water level.*

- Leave the client in a comfortable lateral position.

- After 30 minutes, remove the rectal tube.

4. Determine the effectiveness of the treatment.

- Ask the client whether the flatus was expelled and whether dis-

comfort has been alleviated.

- Palpate the abdomen for any change in the degree of firmness and distention, and auscultate bowel sounds.

5. Teach the client measures that will prevent flatulence and distention.

- These measures depend on the cause. For example, an anxious person who is hyperventilating and swallowing large amounts of air may need to learn appropriate breathing patterns and ways to relax. Others may need to reduce their ingestion of carbonated beverages. Most people will achieve more effective elimination of flatus with increased ambulation.

6. Document the insertion and removal of the rectal tube and all assessments.

EVALUATION FOCUS

> Change in abdominal distention; bowel sounds; presence of discomfort.

▶ **Technique 27–5** *CONTINUED*

SAMPLE RECORDING

Date	Time	Notes
08/02/93	1310	Rectal tube 22 Fr. inserted for flatulence and abdominal distention. P82, R24. —————— Sarah P. Stein, NS
	1340	Rectal tube removed. States feels some relief; much flatus expelled. P82, R20. —————— Sarah P. Stein, NS

KEY ELEMENTS OF INSERTING A RECTAL TUBE TO RELIEVE FLATULENCE

- Assess abdominal firmness and distention and bowel sounds before and after the technique.
- Lubricate the tube before insertion.

- Insert the tube 4 to 6 inches.
- Leave the rectal tube in place no more than 30 minutes.

27-6 Removing a Fecal Impaction Digitally

Digital removal involves breaking up the fecal mass digitally and removing it in portions. Because the bowel mucosa can be injured during this procedure, some agencies restrict and specify the personnel permitted to conduct digital disimpactions. Rectal stimulation is also contraindicated for some people because it may cause an excessive vagal response resulting in cardiac arrhythmia. After a disimpaction, the nurse can use various interventions to remove remaining feces, e.g., a cleansing enema or the insertion of a suppository.

PURPOSES
- To relieve pain and discomfort caused by blockage of impacted feces
- To reestablish normal defecation

ASSESSMENT FOCUS

Pattern of defecation; presence of an impaction confirmed by digital examination; presence of nausea, headache, abdominal pain, malaise, or abdominal distention.

EQUIPMENT

- ☐ Bath blanket
- ☐ Moisture-resistant bedpan
- ☐ Bedpan and cover
- ☐ Toilet tissue
- ☐ Disposable gloves
- ☐ Lubricant
- ☐ Soap, water, and towel

INTERVENTION

1. Prepare the client.

- Explain to the client what you plan to do and why. This procedure is distressing, tiring, and uncomfortable, so the person may desire the presence of another nurse or support person.

- Assist the client to a right lateral or Sims' position with the back toward you. *When the person lies on the right side, the sigmoid colon is uppermost; thus, gravity can aid removal of the feces.*

- Cover the client with the bath blanket.

2. Prepare the equipment.

- Place the disposable bedpan under the client's hips, and arrange the top bedclothing so that it falls obliquely over the hips, exposing only the buttocks.

- Place the bedpan and toilet tissue nearby on the bed or a bedside chair.

▶

► **Technique 27–6 Removing a Fecal Impaction** *CONTINUED*

 • Put on the gloves.

• Lubricate the gloved index finger. *Lubricant reduces resistance by the anal sphincter as the finger is inserted.*

3. Remove the impaction.

• Gently insert the index finger into the rectum, moving toward the umbilicus.

• Gently massage around the stool. *Gentle action prevents damage to the rectal mucosa. A circular motion around the rectum dislodges the stool, stimulates peristalsis, and relaxes the anal sphincter.*

• Work the finger into the hardened mass of stool to break it up.

If you cannot break up the impaction with one finger, insert two fingers and try to break up the impaction scissor style.

• Work the stool down to the anus, remove it in small pieces, and place them in the bedpan.

• Carefully continue to remove as much fecal material as possible; at the same time, assess the client for signs of pallor, feelings of faintness, shortness of breath, and perspiration. Terminate the procedure if these occur. *Manual stimulation could result in excessive vagal nerve stimulation and subsequent cardiac arrhythmia.*

• Assist the client to a position on a clean bedpan, commode, or toilet. *Digital stimulation of the rectum may induce the urge to defecate.*

4. Assist the client with hygienic measures as needed.

• Wash the rectal area with soap and water and dry gently.

• Remove the gloves.

5. If appropriate, teach the client measures to promote normal elimination. Alterations in diet and fluid intake and the use of stool softeners may be necessary.

6. Document the technique and all assessments.

EVALUATION FOCUS

Color, consistency, odor, and amount of feces; presence of abnormal constituents; passage of flatus; client comfort; vital signs; abdominal distention.

SAMPLE RECORDING

Date	Time	Notes
09/28/93	1000	Rectal examination for fecal impaction. Moderate amount dark brown feces removed digitally. Vital signs stable. Unable to defecate following procedure. — Bruce L. Ching, NS

KEY ELEMENTS OF REMOVING A FECAL IMPACTION DIGITALLY

• Assess vital signs before and after the procedure.

• Position the client in the right lateral position.

• Wear gloves.

• Lubricate your gloved fingers before insertion.

• Break up the stool very gently, avoiding excessive rectal stimulation.

CRITICAL THINKING CHALLENGE

Eleanor Richey is an 82-year-old female who has a fecal impaction in the lower bowel. The physician has ordered a soap suds enema to cleanse her bowel. While you are administering the enema, Ms Richey becomes anxious because she is unable to retain the solution. What will you say? What action will you take?

RELATED RESEARCH

Battle, E., and Hanna, C. September 1980. Evaluation of a dietary regimen for chronic constipation: Report of a pilot study. *Journal of Gerontological Nursing* 6:527–32.

McKeever, M. P. October 1990. An investigation of recognized incontinence within a health authority. *Journal of Advanced Nursing* 15:1197–1207.

CHAPTER 27 FECAL ELIMINATION **679**

REFERENCES

Doughty, D. May/June 1991. Maintaining normal bowel function in the patient with cancer. *Journal of Enterostomal Nursing* 18:90–94.

Ellickson, E. B. January 1988. Bowel management plan for the homebound elderly. *Journal of Gerontological Nursing* 14:16–19.

Evans, K. November/December 1990. Pediatric management problems . . . chronic constipation. *Pediatric Nursing* 16:590–91.

Field, M. Y. July 1991. Relieving constipation and pain in the terminally ill. *American Journal of Nursing* 91:18–19.

Hanauer, S. B. March 30, 1988. Fecal incontinence in the elderly. *Hospital Practice* 23:105–8.

Hill, P. April 3–9, 1991. Assessing fecal soiling in children. *Nursing Times* 87:61–62, 64.

McShane, R. E., and McLane, A. M. April 1988. Constipation: Impact of etiological factors. *Journal of Gerontological Nursing* 14:31–34.

Mowlam, V.; North, K.; and Myers, C. November 26–December 2, 1986. Continence: Managing fecal incontinence. *Nursing Times* 82:55, 57, 59.

Resnick, B. July/August 1985. Constipation: Common but preventable. *Geriatric Nursing* 6:213–15.

Wadle, K. R. December 1990. Diarrhea. *Nursing Clinics of North America* 25:901–8.

Whaley, L. F., and Wong, D. L. 1989. *Essentials of pediatric nursing.* 3d ed. St. Louis: C. V. Mosby Co.

Urinary Elimination

CONTENTS

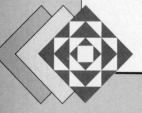

NURSING PROCESS GUIDE
URINARY ELIMINATION

ASSESSMENT

Determine the client's usual patterns and frequency of urination. Ask the client the approximate times that voiding occurs each day.

Determine any recent alterations in voiding in regard to

- Passage of large amounts of urine.

- Passage of small amounts of urine.

- Voiding at more frequent intervals.

- Trouble getting to the bathroom in time or feeling of urgency to void.

- Painful voiding.

- Difficulty starting urine stream.

- Frequent dribbling of urine or feeling of bladder fullness associated with voiding small amounts of urine.

- Reduced force of stream.

- Accidental leakage of urine. If so, when this occurs (e.g., when coughing, laughing, or sneezing; at night; during the day).

Obtain the medical history of elimination problems and urinary tract disease or surgery and other diseases that may affect urinary elimination problems, including

- Urinary tract infections of the kidney, bladder, or urethra.

- Urinary calculi.

- Urinary tract surgery, such as kidney surgery, bladder surgery, prostate removal, or other surgical procedures that alter urinary routes, e.g., ureterostomy.

- Cardiovascular disease, such as hypertension or heart disease.

- Chronic diseases that alter urinary characteristics or impair urinary function, such as diabetes mellitus, neurologic disease (e.g., multiple sclerosis), and cancer.

Assess the volume and characteristics of the client's urine:

- When the client last voided and the amount. Volumes of less than 30 ml or more than 500 ml per hour must be reported immediately.

- Dark, cloudy, or discolored urine.

- Presence of mucous plugs.

- Offensive odor.

Determine any factors influencing urinary elimination:

- Medications: Any medications that could increase urinary output (e.g., diuretic) or cause retention of urine (e.g., anticholinergic-antispasmodic, antidepressant-antipsychotic, anti-parkinsonism drugs, antihistamines, antihypertensives) or that may discolor urine (e.g., Azogantricin, multivitamins, Elavil). Note specific medication and dosage.

- Fluid intake: Amount and kind of fluid taken each day (e.g., six glasses of water, five cups of coffee, three cola drinks with or without caffeine).

- Environmental factors: Any problems with toileting (mobility, dexterity with clothing, toilet seat too low, facility without grab bar).

- Presence of long-term catheter: How the client cares for the catheter, any discomfort with it or other problems, and how the nurse can help to manage it.

- Disease: Any illnesses other than urinary tract disease that may affect urinary function, such as hypertension, heart disease, neurologic disease (e.g., multiple sclerosis), cancer, prostatic enlargement, diabetes mellitus, or diabetes insipidus.

- Diagnostic procedures: Recent procedures such as a cystoscopy or spinal anesthetic.

Determine the presence of pain:

- Bladder pain. Pain over the suprapubic region.

- Kidney or flank pain. Pain between ribs and ileum which may spread to the abdomen and be associated with nausea and vomiting
    or
  Pain at costovertebral angle, which may radiate to the umbilicus.

- Ureteral pain. Pain in back which may radiate to abdomen, upper thigh, testes, or labia.

Review of data from diagnostic tests and examinations:

- pH under 4.5 or over 8.

- Specific gravity under 1.010 or over 1.025.

- Presence of glucose or acetone.

- Presence of occult or visible blood.

- Presence of protein, urobilinogen, or nitrite.

- Presence of microorganisms.

- Presence of obstructions.

- Blood serum: blood urea nitrogen (BUN), creatinine, sodium, potassium.

Nursing Process Guide *CONTINUED*

RELATED DIAGNOSTIC CATEGORIES

- Functional urinary incontinence
- Reflex urinary incontinence
- Stress urinary incontinence
- Total urinary incontinence
- Urge urinary incontinence
- Altered pattern of urinary elimination
- Urinary retention
- Self-care deficit: Toileting
- Pain
- Knowledge deficit
- Self-esteem disturbance (if incontinent)
- High risk for Infection
- High risk for Impaired skin integrity (if incontinent)

PLANNING

Client Goals
The client will

- Restore or maintain usual elimination pattern.
- Avoid associated risks, such as infection, skin breakdown, and lowered self-esteem.

Outcome Criteria
The client with **Urinary incontinence**

- Identifies interventions to prevent incontinence.
- Alters environment and clothing to accommodate needs.
- Attempts voiding every 2 hours and gradually increases to every 3 or 4 hours.
- Experiences a gradual decrease in episodes of incontinence to less than three times a week.

- Has intact skin around the urinary meatus and perineum (or under condom or urinary diversion stoma appliance).
- Establishes bladder conditioning regimen.
- Demonstrates techniques to strengthen pelvic floor muscles.
- Performs pelvic floor strengthening exercises three times a day for 4 months.
- Remains continent even with increased intra-abdominal pressure (stress incontinence).
- Manages incontinence sufficiently to maintain social functioning.
- Reports increased time interval between urge and involuntary loss of urine.
- Manages care of catheter or urinary diversion stoma appropriately.

The client with **Urinary retention**

- Voids sufficient amounts with no palpable bladder distention.
- Has a postvoid residual urine of less than 50 ml.
- Is free of overflow dribbling.

The client with **Altered pattern of urinary elimination** has

- Normal color, odor, and consistency of urine.
- A urinary output in balance with fluid intake.
- A negative urine culture.
- No dysuria or frequency.
- Urinary pH of less than 5.5.
- Urinary output of at least 1500 ml/day.
- Fluid intake of at least 2500 ml/day.

The Urinary System

Urine is formed in the kidneys, which are situated in the retroperitoneal space within the body. The kidneys filter from the blood products for which the body has no use. Once urine is formed within the kidney, it is carried into the kidney pelvis, a funnel-shaped tube, and the ureter. The ureters of an adult are about 25 cm (10 in) long. They extend from the kidneys to the urinary bladder and enter the bladder on the posterior aspect of the base.

The urinary bladder, a hollow, muscular organ, lies behind the symphysis pubis. In the male, it lies in front of the rectum and above the prostate gland (Figure 28–1); in the female, it lies in front of the uterus and vagina (Figure 28–2). The urethra of the adult female is approximately 4 cm (1.5 in) in length. In the adult male, it is about 20 cm (8 in) long. The urethra extends from the bladder to the external surface of the body. This external opening is called the *urinary meatus.* In the female, it is located between the labia minora, in front of the vagina and below the

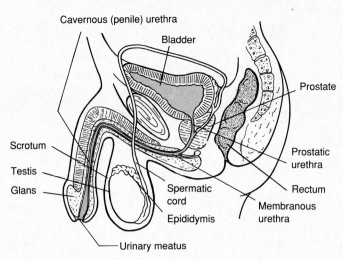

FIGURE 28-1 The male urogenital system.

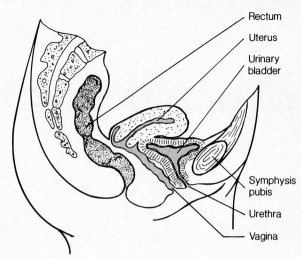

FIGURE 28-2 The female urinary system.

clitoris (Figure 28–3); in the male, it is located at the distal end of the penis (Figure 28–1).

The urethra, in both males and females, has a continuous mucous membrane lining with the bladder and the ureters. Thus, an infection of the urethra can readily extend through the urinary tract to the kidneys.

Micturition, voiding, and **urination** all refer to the process of emptying the urinary bladder. Urine collects in the bladder until pressure stimulates special sensory nerve endings in the bladder wall called stretch receptors. This occurs when the adult bladder contains between 250 and 450 ml of urine. In children, a considerably smaller volume, 50 to 200 ml, stimulates these nerves. Babies have no conscious control, and the urine is released after a small amount accumulates in the bladder.

Once excited, the stretch receptors transmit impulses to the spinal cord, specifically to the voiding reflex center at the level of the second to fourth sacral vertebrae. Some impulses continue up the spinal cord to the voiding control center in the cerebral cortex. If the time is appropriate to void, the brain then sends impulses through the spinal cord to the motor neurons in the sacral area, causing stimulation of the parasympathetic nerves. The parasympathetic nervous system innervates the detrusor muscle and the internal urethral sphincter muscle, producing (a) contraction of the detrusor muscle and (b) relaxation of the internal sphincter muscle. As a result, urine can be released from the bladder, but it is still impeded by the external urinary sphincter. If the time and place are appropriate for urination, the conscious portion of the brain relaxes the external urethral sphincter muscle, and urination takes place. If the time and place are inappropriate, the micturition reflex usually subsides until the bladder becomes more filled and the reflex is stimulated again. In the

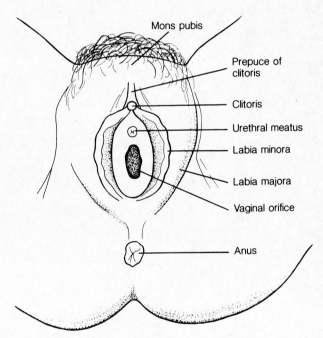

FIGURE 28-3 Location of the female urinary meatus in relation to surrounding structures.

female the external urethral sphincter is situated at about the midpoint of the urethra; in the male, it is distal to the prostatic portion of the urethra.

The sympathetic nervous system also innervates the bladder, causing it to relax. However, the nerves do not normally enter into micturition control.

Voluntary control of micturition is possible only if the nerves supplying the bladder and urethra, the cortico-regulatory tracts of the cord and brain, and the motor area of the cerebrum are all intact. Injury to any of these parts of the nervous system—by, e.g., a cerebral hemorrhage or spinal cord injury above the level of the sacral region—results in intermittent involuntary emptying of the bladder.

TABLE 28–1 CHANGES IN URINARY ELIMINATION THROUGH THE LIFE CYCLE

Stage	Variations
Fetus	The fetal kidney begins to excrete urine between the 11th and 12th week of development.
	Fetal urine is hypotonic to plasma.
	The placenta serves as a pseudo-kidney in regulating fetal fluid and electrolyte balance.
	The kidney does not function independently until after birth.
Infant	Ability to concentrate urine is minimal; therefore, urine appears light yellow.
	Voluntary urinary control is absent.
Children	Kidney function reaches maturity between the first and second year of life; urine is concentrated effectively and appears a normal amber color.
	Voluntary control of urine begins at 18 to 24 months of age, when the child starts to recognize bladder fullness, holds urine beyond the urge to void, and warns parents of the urge to void.
	Full urinary control is not gained until age 4 or 5 years; daytime control is usually achieved by age 2 years.
	Boys are slower than girls in gaining control.
	The kidneys grow in proportion to overall body growth.
Adults	The kidneys reach maximum size between 35 and 40 years of age.
	After age 50 the kidneys begin to diminish in size and function. Most shrinkage occurs in the cortex of the kidney, due primarily to the loss of glomeruli.
Elderly adults	There is an estimated 30% loss of glomeruli by age 80 (Richard 1986, p. 38).
	Renal blood flow decreases because of vascular changes and a decrease in cardiac output.
	Urine concentratability declines.
	Excessive urination at night and increased frequency of urination occur because of loss of concentratability and diminished bladder muscle tone.
	Residual urine may increase because of diminished bladder muscle tone and contractability, which increases the risk of bacterial growth and infection.
	Urinary incontinence may occur due to mobility problems or neurologic impairments.

Developmental Changes

Only with maturation of the central nervous system and the body muscles can urinary control be established. This normally takes place between 2 and 4½ years of age. Boys are usually slower than girls in developing this control. Once individuals develop control, they normally maintain it through life unless disease processes occur. See Table 28–1.

The volume of urine output in a 24-hour period normally increases from the time of birth to adulthood. The output of an elderly person, however, may decrease from that of the normal adult. This can be due to the deterioration of the kidneys that comes with age. See Table 28–2.

Common Problems

Urinary retention is the accumulation of urine in the bladder and inability of the bladder to empty itself. Because urine production continues, retention results in distention of the bladder. An adult urinary

TABLE 28–2 AVERAGE DAILY EXCRETION OF URINE BY AGE

Age	Amount (ml)
1–2 days	15–60
3–10 days	100–300
10 days–2 months	250–450
2 months–1 year	400–500
1–3 years	500–600
3–5 years	600–700
5–8 years	700–1000
8–14 years	800–1400
14 years through adulthood	1500
Older adulthood	1500 or less

bladder normally holds 250 to 450 ml of urine when the micturition reflex is initiated. With urinary retention, some adult bladders may distend to hold 3000 to 4000 ml of urine.

Occasionally, a person will have urinary retention with overflow. In this situation the bladder is holding urine, and only the overflow urine is excreted when the pressure of the urine becomes too great for sphincter control. The client then voids small amounts of urine frequently or dribbles urine, while the bladder remains distended.

Retention can be identified by several clinical signs: discomfort in the pubic area, bladder distention, inability to void or frequent voiding of small volumes (25 to 50 ml), a disproportionately small amount of fluid output in relation to intake, and increasing restlessness and need to void. Bladder distention can be assessed by palpation and percussion above the symphysis pubis.

Urinary incontinence is a temporary or permanent inability of the external sphincter muscles to control the flow of urine from the bladder. It is the opposite of retention. Complete emptying of the bladder during episodes of incontinence is referred to as *complete incontinence;* incomplete emptying of the bladder during these episodes (e.g., dribbling) is referred to as *partial incontinence.*

Incontinence is seen in clients who have enlarged prostate glands, spinal cord injuries, urinary tract infections, bladder spasms, or loss of consciousness or people who are taking medications that interfere with sphincter control, e.g., narcotics and sedatives.

Five kinds of incontinence are often distinguished: *Stress incontinence* is the inability to control urine flow at a time when the intraabdominal pressure increases, e.g., when coughing, sneezing, or even laughing. *Total incontinence* is a continuous and unpredictable loss of urine. Common causes are injury to the external urinary sphincter in the male, injury to the perineal musculature or a fistula between the bladder and vagina in the female, and congenital or acquired neurogenic disease. *Urge incontinence* follows a sudden strong desire to urinate and is due to involuntary detrusor contraction. It is also sometimes referred to as *unstable bladder,* because the detrusor contractions are unreliable and bladder emptying cannot be controlled. The client is unable to stop urine flow when it starts and often fails to get to the bathroom in time. *Functional incontinence* is the involuntary, unpredictable passage of urine. Functional incontinence is also defined as incontinence that persists because of a physical or mental disorder or some environmental factor that prevents the client from reaching the bathroom. *Reflex incontinence* is an involuntary loss of urine occurring at somewhat predictable intervals when a specific bladder volume is reached. The client has no awareness of bladder filling.

▶ **Enuresis** (bedwetting) occurs most often in children. When wetting occurs in a child over the age of 4 or 5, it generally occurs at night and is referred to as *nocturnal enuresis.* It may happen once or several times during the night.

Frequency is generally considered voiding at frequent intervals, that is, more often than usual. The frequency of voiding normally increases with an increase in fluids. Frequency without an increase in fluid intake may be the result of *cystitis* (an acutely inflamed bladder), stress, or pressure on the bladder, e.g., due to pregnancy. The total amount of urine voided may be normal, because the amounts voided each time are small, such as 50 to 100 ml.

Nocturia, or **nycturia**, is increased frequency at night that is not a result of increased fluid intake. Like frequency, it is usually expressed in number of times the person voids, for example, "nocturia × 4."

Urgency is the feeling that the person *must* void. There may or may not be a great deal of urine in the bladder, but the person feels a need to void immediately.

Dysuria is either painful or difficult voiding. It can accompany a *stricture* (decrease in caliber) of the urethra, urinary infections, and injury to the bladder and/or urethra. Often people will describe a need to push to void or that burning accompanies or follows voiding. Burning during micturition is often due to an irritated urethra; burning following urination may be the result of a bladder infection when the irritated rugae (ridges) of the *trigone* rub together. The burning may be described as severe, like a hot poker, or more subdued, like a sunburn.

Polyuria, or **diuresis**, is the production of abnormally large amounts of urine by the kidneys, such as 2500 ml/day, without an increased fluid intake. This can happen as a result of diabetes mellitus, hormone imbalances (e.g., deficiency of antidiuretic hormone), or chronic kidney disease.

Oliguria refers to voiding scant amounts of urine, such as 100 to 500 ml/day. The average amount of urine excreted per day in a healthy adult is 1400 to 1500 ml/day. **Anuria** refers to voiding less than 100 ml/day. The terms *complete kidney shutdown, renal failure,* and *urinary suppression* have the same meaning. Oliguria may result from an extremely low fluid intake but may also follow disease. Both anuria and oliguria can result from kidney disease, severe heart failure, burns, and shock. These clinical signs can be fatal if some other means—such as an artificial kidney—is not used to remove body wastes. Oliguria may also normally accompany fever and heavy perspiration. Because of excessive fluid losses via the skin, urine production is decreased.

Collecting Urine Specimens

The nurse is responsible for collecting urine specimens for a number of tests: clean voided specimens for routine urinalysis, *clean-catch* or *midstream urine specimens* for urine culture, and timed urine specimens for a variety of tests that depend on the client's specific health problem. A clear voided specimen is usually adequate for routine examination; a clear-catch specimen is needed for bacteriologic culture.

Clean-catch or midstream specimens must be as free as possible from external contamination by microorganisms near the urethral opening. Sterile specimen containers and lids are used for those specimens. Commercially prepared disposable clean-catch kits are available (Figure 28–4).

Several urine tests require timed specimens. Urine specimens are collected at timed intervals, for short periods (1 to 2 hours) or long periods (12 to 24 hours). All timed urine specimens should be refrigerated to prevent bacterial growth and decomposition of the urine components, unless a special preservative has been added. Each voiding of urine is collected in a small, clean container and then emptied immediately into the large refrigerated bottle or carton. Some of the tests performed on timed urine specimens include the following:

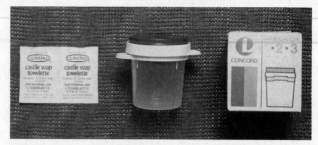

FIGURE 28–4 A commercially prepared disposable clean-catch kit.

- *Quantitative albumin* (24 hours): Determines the daily amount of albumin lost in the urine in such conditions as kidney disease, hypertension, drug toxicity, or severe heart failure involving kidney damage.

- *Amino acid* (24 hours): Determines acquired or congenital disease of the kidneys.

- *Amylase* (2, 12, or 24 hours): Determines the amount of amylase, a pancreatic enzyme that may be excreted in the urine in certain diseases of the pancreas.

- *Quantitative chlorides* (24 hours): Determines the total excretion of chloride; may be performed in the management of cardiac clients who are on low-salt diets.

- *Concentration and dilution:* Determines disorders of the kidney tubules in concentrating and diluting urine. These specimens are collected over varying periods of time. Specimens are commonly collected at hourly intervals for 2 to 4 hours after the client has been given a specified amount of clear fluid to drink.

- *Creatinine* or *creatinine clearance* (24 hours): Reflects the degree of kidney impairment. Creatinine is formed in the muscles from creatine in relatively constant daily amounts and is excreted in the urine. Elevated creatinine content indicates a disturbance in kidney function.

- *Estriol determination* (24 hours): Measures the level of this hormone in the urine of high-risk pregnant women, e.g., those with toxemia or dia-

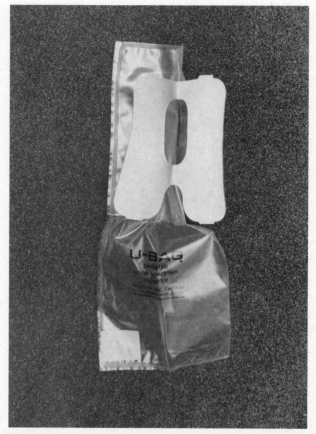

FIGURE 28–5 A plastic disposable infant urine collection bag.

betes. Estriol is the major form in which estrogen is excreted in the urine. Low levels can indicate inadequate function of the placenta and possible fetal distress.

- *Glucose tolerance* (24 hours): Determines disorders of glucose metabolism that may arise from malfunction of the liver or pancreas. Tests are performed on both the blood and the urine after the client is given a large amount of glucose orally or intravenously.

- *17-hydroxycorticosteroid* (24 hours): Assesses the functioning of the adrenal cortex. Corticosteroids are hormones that are produced in the adrenal cortex, altered, and then excreted in the urine.

- *Urobilinogen* (random times or 2 hours): Determines obstruction of the biliary tract, excessive destruction of red blood cells, or liver damage. These specimens need to be protected from light.

Routine urine examination is usually done on the first voided specimen in the morning, because it tends to have a higher, more uniform concentration and a more acidic pH than specimens later in the day. Plastic disposable urine collection bags are available to collect urine specimens from an infant. These are specially designed clear plastic bags with an adhesive backing and an opening that is applied over the infant's urethral meatus or penis (Figure 28–5).

Before collecting the specimen, the nurse determines whether the client can assist with the technique and obtains any special directions for collecting the specimen. Often, the client is able to provide the specimen independently. Male clients generally have little difficulty, but female clients usually need to stand or sit over a toilet bowl and hold the container between their legs during the process of voiding. About 120 ml (4 oz) of urine is generally required. Check agency policy.

For an explanation of how to collect a routine urine specimen from an adult or child who has urinary control, a clean-catch urine specimen for culture and sensitivity, a timed urine specimen, and a urine specimen from an infant, see Techniques 28–1, 28–2, 28–3, and 28–4, respectively.

28-1   Collecting a Routine Urine Specimen from an Adult or Child Who Has Urinary Control

PURPOSE
- To screen the client's urine for abnormal constituents

ASSESSMENT FOCUS
> Client's ability to provide the specimen; medications that may discolor urine or affect the test results.

EQUIPMENT

- Nonsterile gloves as needed
- Clean bedpan, urinal, or commode for clients who are unable to void directly into the specimen container
- Wide-mouthed specimen container
- Completed laboratory requisition
- Completed specimen identification label

INTERVENTION

1. Give ambulatory clients the following information and instructions.

- Explain the purpose of the urine specimen and how the client can assist.

- Explain that all specimens must be free of fecal contamination, so voiding needs to occur at a different time from defecation.

- Instruct female clients to discard the toilet tissue in the toilet or in a waste bag rather than in the bedpan, because tissue in the specimen makes laboratory analysis more difficult.

- Give the client the specimen container, and direct the client to the bathroom to void 120 ml (4 oz) into it.

2. Assist clients who are seriously ill, physically incapacitated, or disoriented.

- Provide required assistance in the bathroom, or help the client to use a bedpan or urinal in bed.

- Wear gloves when assisting the client to void into a bedpan or urinal and transferring the urine from the bedpan, urinal, or commode to the specimen container.

- Empty the bedpan or urinal.

- Remove gloves if worn, and wash your hands.

3. Ensure that the specimen is sealed and the container clean.

- Put the lid tightly on the container. *This prevents spillage of the urine and contamination of other objects.*

- If the outside of the container

▶ **Technique 28–1 Collecting a Routine Urine Specimen** *CONTINUED*

has been contaminated by urine, clean it with soap and water. *This prevents the spread of microorganisms.*

4. Label and transport the specimen to the laboratory.

• Ensure that the specimen label and the laboratory requisition have the correct information on them. Attach them securely to

the specimen container. *Inappropriate identification of the specimen can lead to errors of diagnosis or therapy for the client.*

• Arrange for the specimen to be taken immediately to the laboratory or placed in a refrigerator. *Urine deteriorates relatively rapidly from bacterial contamination when left at room temperature;*

specimens should be analyzed immediately after collection.

5. Document all relevant information.

• Document the collection of the specimen on the client's chart. Include the date and time of collection and the appearance and odor of the urine.

EVALUATION FOCUS

Color, odor, and character of the urine.

SAMPLE RECORDING

Date	Time	Notes
02/27/93	0600	Random urine specimen collected for admission urinalysis. Urine clear, straw colored, and without odor. Specimen sent to lab.———Joyce Daynard, SN

KEY ELEMENTS OF COLLECTING A ROUTINE URINE SPECIMEN FROM AN ADULT OR CHILD WHO HAS URINARY CONTROL

• Provide the client or parent with appropriate instructions to collect the specimen.

• Use aseptic technique.

• Wear gloves if there is a possibility that your hands will touch the client's urine.

• Ensure that the specimen is free of fecal contamination and toilet tissue.

• Ensure that the specimen labels and the labo-

ratory requisition have the correct information on them and are attached securely to the specimen containers.

• Take the specimen immediately to the laboratory, or refrigerate it.

• Assess color, odor, and character of the urine.

• Note medications the client is receiving that may discolor urine or affect the test results.

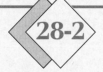
28-2

Collecting a Urine Specimen for Culture and Sensitivity by Clean Catch

PURPOSE

• To determine the presence of microorganisms, the type of organism(s), and the antibiotics to which the organisms are sensitive.

ASSESSMENT FOCUS

Ability of the client to provide the specimen; color, odor, and consistency of the urine; presence of clinical signs of urinary tract infection (e.g., frequency, urgency, dysuria, hematuria, flank pain, cloudy urine with foul odor).

▶ Technique 28–2 Collecting a Urine Specimen for Culture and Sensitivity *CONTINUED*

EQUIPMENT

Equipment used varies from agency to agency. Some agencies use commercially prepared disposable clean-catch kits. Others are agency-prepared sterile trays. Both prepared trays and kits generally contain the following items:

- Disposable gloves
- Antiseptic, such as povidone-iodine
- Sterile cotton balls or 2 × 2 gauze pads
- Sterile specimen container
- Specimen identification label
- Completed laboratory requisition form
- Bath blanket and urine receptacle if the client is not ambulatory

INTERVENTION

1. Instruct and assist the client appropriately.

- Inform the client that a urine specimen is required; give the reason, and explain the method to be used to collect it.

- Ask an *ambulatory* client to wash and dry the genitals and perineum thoroughly with soap and water. *A clean perineum is essential to reduce the number of skin bacteria and to minimize contamination of the specimen.*

- Assist the *ambulatory* client to the bathroom. The preferred method to collect specimens from ambulatory clients is to have them provide the specimen while standing over the toilet in the bathroom.

- Assist *nonambulatory* clients to an upright sitting position on a urine receptacle. Provide appropriate covers for the client: Drape the client in a bath blanket, exposing only the perineal area.

- Assist *female* clients to spread their legs enough to ensure that the urine does not touch the legs.

2. Prepare the equipment and implement body fluid precautions.

- Open the sterile kit or tray, using sterile technique. *Sterile technique is essential to maintain the sterility of the specimen container.*

 • Put on the sterile gloves.

- Pour the antiseptic solution over the cotton balls.

3. Clean the area at the external urinary meatus with the antiseptic. *The antiseptic reduces the number of bacteria near the urethral opening and minimizes contamination of the urine specimens.*

For female clients

- Swab the labia minora from front to back, using one swab for each wipe. *Swabbing from front to back cleans from the area of least contamination to the area of greatest contamination.*

- Spread the labia minora well apart, using the thumb and another finger (e.g., the third finger) of one hand.

- Swab between the labia minora over the urethra from front to back. *The urethra is considered less contaminated than the vagina and anus.*

For male clients

- Hold the penis with one hand, and clean the urinary meatus using a circular motion. First retract the foreskin of an uncircumcised male.

- Wash outward from the meatus in a circular motion, using one swab for each wipe and moving down the shaft of the penis a few inches. *This cleans from the area of least contamination to the area of greatest contamination.*

4. Collect the specimen.

- Ask the client to start voiding. *Initial voiding clears additional external contaminants at the urethral opening.*

- After the client has begun to void, place the specimen container under the stream of urine near to, but not touching, the meatus.

- Collect 30 to 60 ml of midstream urine.

- Handle only the outside of the container. *This protects the sterility of the inside.*

- Put the sterile cap tightly on the specimen container, touching only the outside of the cap. *Capping the container prevents spillage of urine and contamination of other objects. Touching only the outside of the cap retains the sterility of the inside of the cap.*

- If spillage occurs on the outside of the container, clean the outer surface with a disinfectant. *This prevents the transfer of microorganisms to others.*

- Remove your gloves, and wash hands.

5. Label and transport the specimen to the laboratory.

- Ensure that the specimen label and the laboratory requisition carry the correct information. Attach them securely to the specimen. *Inaccurate identification*

▶ **Technique 28–2 Collecting a Urine Specimen for Culture and Sensitivity** *CONTINUED*

and/or information on the specimen container can lead to errors of diagnosis or therapy.

• Arrange for the specimen to be sent to the laboratory immediately. *Bacterial cultures must be started immediately, before any contaminating organisms can grow, multiply, and produce false results.*

6. Document pertinent data.

• Record collection of the specimen, any pertinent observations of the urine in terms of color, odor, or consistency, and any difficulty in voiding that the client experienced.

EVALUATION FOCUS

Appearance and odor of urine.

SAMPLE RECORDING

Date	Time	Notes
02/28/93	0330	Clean-voided midstream urine specimen collected for culture and sensitivity and sent to lab. Urine appears cloudy. No complaints of dysuria. ———————————————————————— Marie Mandola, S.N.

KEY ELEMENTS OF COLLECTING A URINE SPECIMEN FOR CULTURE AND SENSITIVITY BY CLEAN CATCH

• Ask the client to clean the genitals and perineum before the collection.
• Use sterile technique.
• Clean the client's vulvar area or tip of the penis with antiseptic before the collection.

• Collect the urine midstream.
• See also Key Elements for Technique 28–1.

28-3 Collecting a Timed Urine Specimen

For timed urine specimens, appropriate specimen containers with or without preservative in accordance with the specific test are generally obtained from the laboratory and placed in the client's bathroom or in the utility room. Alert signs are placed in the client's unit to remind staff of the test in progress. Specimen identification labels need to indicate the date and time of each voiding in addition to the usual identification information. They may also be numbered sequentially, e.g., 1st specimen, 2nd specimen, 3rd specimen.

PURPOSES

• To assess the ability of the kidney to concentrate and dilute urine
• To determine disorders of glucose metabolism, e.g., diabetes mellitus
• To determine levels of specific constituents, e.g., albumin, amylase, creatinine, urobilinogen, certain hormones (e.g., estriol or corticosteroids) in the urine

▶ **Technique 28–3 Collecting a Timed Urine Specimen** *CONTINUED*

ASSESSMENT FOCUS	Client's ability to understand instructions and to provide urine samples independently; any fluid or dietary requirements associated with the test; any medication restrictions or requirements for the test.

EQUIPMENT

- Appropriate specimen containers with or without preservative in accordance with the specific test
- Completed specimen identification labels
- Completed laboratory requisition
- Bedpan or urinal
- Alert card on or near the bed indicating the specific times for urine collection
- Antiseptic

INTERVENTION

1 Give the client the following information and instructions.

- The purpose of the test and how the client can assist.

- When the specimen collection will begin and end. For example, a 24-hour urine test commonly begins at 0700 hours and ends at the same hour the next day.

- That all urine must be saved and placed in the specimen containers once the test starts.

- That the urine must be free of fecal contamination and toilet tissue.

- That each specimen must be given to the nursing staff immediately so that it can be placed in the appropriate specimen bottle.

2. Start the collection period.

- Ask the client to void in the toilet or bedpan or urinal. Discard this urine (check agency procedure), and document the time the test starts with this discarded specimen. Collect all subsequent urine specimens, including the one at the end of the period.

- Ask the client to ingest the required amount of liquid for certain tests or to restrict fluid intake. Follow the test directions.

- Instruct the client to void all subsequent urine into the bedpan or urinal and to notify the nursing staff when each specimen is provided. Some tests require voiding at specified times.

- Number the specimen containers sequentially, e.g., 1st specimen, 2d specimen, 3d specimen, if separate specimens are required.

- Place alert signs in the client's unit to remind staff of the test in progress.

3. Collect all of the required specimens.

- Place each specimen into the appropriately labeled container. For some tests, each specimen is not kept separately but is poured into a large bottle in the laboratory refrigerator.

- If the outside of the specimen container is contaminated with urine, clean it with soap and water. *Cleaning prevents the transfer of microorganisms to others*.

- Ensure that each specimen is refrigerated throughout the timed collection period. If not refrigerated, specimens are often kept on ice. *Refrigeration or other form of cooling prevents bacterial decomposition of the urine.*

- Measure the amount of each urine specimen as required.

- Ask the client to provide the last specimen 5 to 10 minutes before the end of the collection period.

- Inform the client that the test is completed.

- Remove the alert signs and the specimen equipment from the client's unit and bathroom.

5. Document all relevant information.

- Record the starting time of the test and completion of the specimen collection on the client's chart. Include the date and specific time. In addition, if indicated for the specific test, note the time each urine specimen was collected, the volume of each specimen, the appearance of the urine, and other relevant data such as fluid intake or restrictions.

► **Technique 28–3 Collecting a Timed Urine Specimen** *CONTINUED*

EVALUATION FOCUS | Each urine specimen for color, odor, and clarity; results of laboratory analysis when available.

SAMPLE RECORDING

Date	Time	Notes
03/21/93	0700	24 hour urine collection for quantitative albumin started after client voided. Client informed of need to save all urine and inform nursing staff after each voiding. Specimen collection bottle labeled and placed on ice in bathroom. ————————— Annette Campinola, R.N.
03/22/93	0700	24 hour urine collection for albumin completed. Specimen sent to lab. Urine cloudy. ————————— Thomas Timothy, R.N.

KEY ELEMENTS OF COLLECTING A TIMED URINE SPECIMEN

- On or near the client's bed, place an alert card indicating the specific times for urine collection.
- Provide the client or parent with appropriate instructions to collect the specimen.
- Use aseptic technique.
- Wear gloves if there is a possibility that your hands will touch the client's urine.
- Ensure that the specimen is free of fecal contamination and toilet tissue.
- Ensure that the specimen labels and the laboratory requisition have the correct information on them and are attached securely to the specimen containers.
- Take the specimen immediately to the laboratory, or refrigerate it.
- Document the starting and completion time of the test on the client's record.
- Preserve the specimen appropriately (e.g., by refrigeration).

28-4 Collecting a Urine Specimen from an Infant

PURPOSE | • To screen the infant's urine for abnormal constituents

ASSESSMENT FOCUS | Skin status of infant's perineal area.

EQUIPMENT

- Plastic disposable urine collection bag
- Sterile cotton balls
- Soap and a basin of water

- Antiseptic solution
- Sterile water
- Diaper
- Specimen container

- Disinfectant
- Completed specimen label
- Completed laboratory requisition form

▶ **Technique 28–4 Collecting a Urine Specimen from an Infant** CONTINUED

INTERVENTION

1. Prepare the parents and the infant.

- If parents are present, explain why a urine specimen is being taken and the method of obtaining it.

- Before and throughout the procedure, handle the infant gently, and talk in soothing tones.

- Remove the infant's diaper and clean the perineal-genital area with soap and water and then with an antiseptic. *Cleaning is necessary to remove powder, baby oil, lotions, secretions, and fecal matter from the genitals. It also reduces the number of microorganisms on the skin and subsequent contamination of the voided urine.*

  a. For girls, separate the labia and wash, rinse, and dry the perineal area from the front to the back (clitoris to anus) on each side of the urinary meatus, and then over the meatus (Figure 28–6). Repeat this procedure, using the antiseptic solution to clean, the sterile water to rinse, and some dry cotton balls to dry.

  b. For boys, clean and disinfect both the penis and the scrotum in the manner described above. Wash the penis in a circular motion from the tip toward the scrotum, and wash the scrotum last (Figure 28–7). Retract the foreskin of an uncircumcised boy. *Freeing the skin of all moisture and secretions facilitates proper adhesion of the urine collection bag and prevents leakage of urine.*

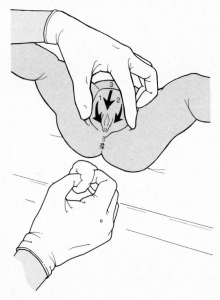

FIGURE 28–6 Cleaning the perineal area of a female infant.

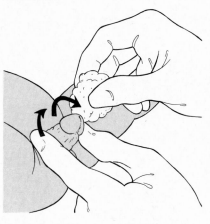

FIGURE 28–7 Cleaning the tip of the penis.

2. Apply the specimen bag.

- Remove the protective paper from the bottom half of the adhesive backing of the collection bag (Figure 28–8).

- Spread the infant's legs apart as much as possible. *Spreading the legs separates and flattens the folds of the skin.*

- Place the opening of the collection bag over the urethra or the penis and scrotum. The base of the opening needs to cover the vagina or to fit well up under the

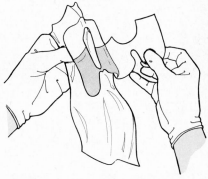

FIGURE 28–8 Removing the bottom half of the adhesive backing.

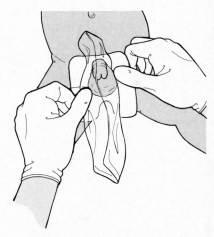

FIGURE 28–9 Placing the opening of the collection bag over the penis and scrotum.

scrotum (Figure 28–9).

- Press the adhesive portion firmly against the infant's skin, starting at the perineum (the area between the anus and the genitals) and working outward. *This method prevents wrinkles, which could cause leakage of urine.*

- Remove the protective paper from the top half of the adhesive backing, and press it firmly in place, working from the top center outward.

- Apply a loose-fitting diaper. *A diaper helps keep the urine bag in place.*

- Elevate the head of the crib mattress to semi-Fowler's position.

► **Technique 28–4 Collecting a Urine Specimen from an Infant** *CONTINUED*

Semi-Fowler's position aids the flow of urine by gravity into the collection portion of the urine bag.

3. Remove the bag, and transfer the specimen.

- After the child has voided a desired amount, gently remove the bag from the skin.

- Empty the urine from the bag through the opening at its base into the specimen container.

- Discard the urine bag.

- Tightly apply the lid to the specimen container. *The lid will pre-* *vent spillage of urine from the container and contamination of other objects.*

- If the outside of the specimen container has been contaminated, clean it with a disinfectant. *Cleaning the outside of the container prevents the spread of microorganisms.*

4. Ensure client comfort.

- Apply the infant's diaper.

- Leave the infant in a comfortable and safe position held by a parent or in a crib.

5. Transport the specimen.

- Ensure that the specimen label and the laboratory requisition have the correct information on them. Attach them securely to the specimen. *Incorrect identification of the specimen can lead to subsequent errors of diagnosis or therapy for the infant.*

- Arrange for the specimen to be sent to the laboratory immediately or refrigerate it.

6. Document all relevant information.

- Record collection of the urine specimen and your assessments.

EVALUATION FOCUS

See Technique 28–1.

KEY ELEMENTS OF COLLECTING A URINE SPECIMEN FROM AN INFANT

- Clean the perineal-genital area with soap and water and then an antiseptic.
- Apply the bottom half of the collection bag before the top half.
- Spread the infant's legs apart as much as possible to flatten skinfolds.
- Secure the bag with a loose-fitting diaper.

- Place the infant in semi-Fowler's position to aid the flow of urine into the bag.
- Ensure client safety after specimen collection.
- Label the specimen accurately, and send it immediately to the laboratory or refrigerate it.

Routine Urine Testing

Several simple urine tests are often done by nurses on the nursing units or are taught to clients, who perform them independently. Tests commonly performed on urine include those for specific gravity, pH, and presence of glucose and occult blood.

Specific Gravity

Specific gravity is the weight or degree of concentration of a substance compared with that of an equal volume of another, such as distilled water, taken as a standard. The specific gravity of distilled water is 1.00 g/ml (in other words, 1 ml of water weighs 1 g).

The specific gravity of urine can be measured by

a urinometer **(hydrometer),** calibrated in units of 0.001. The instrument is placed in a glass cylinder containing the urine (Figure 28–10). The scale on the urinometer progresses from 1.000 at the top to 1.060 at the bottom. The specific gravity of urine is normally about 1.010 to 1.025 g/ml. A low specific gravity is often the result of overhydration or a disease that affects the kidneys' ability to concentrate solutes in the urine. A high specific gravity may indicate dehydration or a disease that increases water reabsorption by the kidneys, causing concentrated urine. False positive results are caused by drugs such as dextran and radiopaque materials used in X-ray examination of the urinary tract.

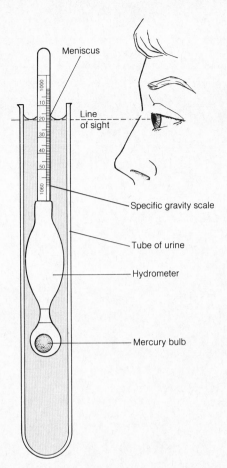

Labels on figure: Meniscus; Line of sight; Specific gravity scale; Tube of urine; Hydrometer; Mercury bulb

FIGURE 28–10 A urinometer measurement of specific gravity is taken at the base of the meniscus.

Urinary pH

Urinary pH is a measurement of the concentration of hydrogen ions in the client's urine, which indicates its acidity or alkalinity. Discrete measurements of pH are made on a scale of 1 to 14, in which the value 7 is neutral, below 7 is acid, and above 7 is alkaline (base). Such quantitative measurements, however, are conducted in the agency laboratory, where specific reactive agents are used. Nurses can make less discrete measurements of urinary pH using litmus paper (i.e., to determine whether the urine is acidic or alkaline).

Urine becomes increasingly acidic when increasing amounts of sodium and excess acid are retained in the body. Ingestion of various foods also affects urinary pH. A diet rich in animal protein and cranberry juice decreases the pH and produces an acid urine. A diet high in citrus fruits, most vegetables, milk, and other dairy products increases the pH and produces an alkaline urine. Urine left at room temperature for several hours gradually becomes alkaline because of bacterial action.

Control of the urine pH is an important factor in certain medical therapies. For example, the formation of renal stones is partially dependent on the urinary pH; therefore, clients being treated for stones are often given diets or medications to alter the pH and prevent stone formation. Certain medications, such as streptomycin, neomycin, and kanamycin, are more effective for treating urinary tract infections if the urine is alkaline.

Glucose

Urine is tested for glucose to screen clients for diabetes mellitus or to follow the progress of a known diabetic. Normally, the amount of glucose in the urine is negligible, although individuals who have ingested large amounts of sugar may show small amounts of glucose in their urine.

Several commercial products are commonly used to test for the presence of glucose, e.g., Clinitest tablets and Clinistix, Diastix, and Tes-Tape reagent strips. Each uses a color scale to measure the quantity of glucose in the urine, but the scales are not interchangeable from one product to the other. The scales grade the results as negative, trace, one plus (1+, or +), two plus (2+, or ++), three plus (3+, or +++), etc. Each grade reflects a specific percentage of glucose, which varies from one testing product to another. For example, a 2+ result from a Clinitest reaction indicates 75% glucose in the urine, whereas a 2+ result from a Tes-Tape strip indicates 25% glucose.

False readings can arise from medications a client is receiving, depending on the type of chemical product used to test the urine for glucose. For example, tetracycline and large doses of ascorbic acid and chloral hydrate can generate false positive results from Clinitest tablets. For this reason, many agencies stock more than one testing product. Nurses need to compare the medications a client is receiving with the literature about each product and choose the appropriate product for the test.

Ketone Bodies

Ketone bodies are products of incomplete fat metabolism and appear in the urine in instances of fasting, very low intake of carbohydrates, and uncontrolled diabetes mellitus. Usually, the urine is tested for ketone bodies at the same time it is tested for glucose. Tablets or reagent strips are used.

Occult Blood

Normal urine is free of blood. When blood is present, it may be clearly visible or not visible (**occult**). Commercial reagent strips are used to test for occult blood in the urine.

Technique 28–5 describes how to test urine for specific gravity, pH, glucose, ketones, and occult blood.

28-5 Testing Urine for Specific Gravity, pH, Glucose, Ketones, and Occult Blood

PURPOSES

- To determine the client's hydration status from a specific gravity measurement
- To determine the acidity or alkalinity of the client's urine
- To determine the presence of glucose and ketone bodies in the urine
- To determine the presence of occult blood in the urine

EQUIPMENT

For All Tests
- Gloves

For Specific Gravity
- Urinometer (hydrometer) and a glass cylinder
  or
- Spectrometer or refractometer

For Urine pH
- Litmus paper (red or blue)

For Glucose
- Reagent tablet or reagent test strip
- Appropriate color scale

- Clean test tube and a dropper, if a tablet is used

For Ketone Bodies
- Reagent tablet or test strip

For Occult Blood
- Reagent strip

INTERVENTION

1. To measure specific gravity:

- If a controlled specimen is ordered, ask the client to withhold fluids for the specified time, e.g., 8 to 12 hours. When routine specific gravity measurements are being taken (e.g., for clients with burns), fluids are not withheld.

- To measure with a *urinometer*:

  a. Don gloves, and pour at least 20 ml of a fresh urine sample in the glass cylinder, or fill the cylinder three-quarters full.

  b. Place the urinometer into the cylinder, and give it a gentle spin to prevent it from adhering to the sides of the cylinder.

  c. Hold the urinometer at eye level, and read the measurement at the base of the meniscus at the surface of the urine (Figure 28–10, earlier). *The concentration of the urine affects the degree to which the urinometer will float. The depth to which it sinks indicates the specific gravity.*

- To measure with a *spectrometer or refractometer*:

  a. Be sure to follow the manufacturer's directions.

  b. Don gloves, and place one or two drops of urine on the slide.

  c. Turn on the instrument light, and look into the instrument. The specific gravity will appear on a scope.

  d. Write down the number, then turn off the instrument.

  e. Remove the urine with a damp towel or gauze.

2. To measure pH:

- Put on a glove, and dip a strip of either red or blue litmus paper into the urine specimen.

- Observe the color of the litmus paper, and compare it to a standardized color chart on the bottle. The blue litmus paper, more commonly used, remains blue if the urine is alkaline and turns red if it is acidic. The red litmus paper remains red in the presence of acidic urine and turns blue if the urine is alkaline. Whichever litmus strip is used, red always indicates acidic urine and blue always indicates alkaline urine.

3. To test for glucose:

- Obtain a freshly voided specimen. Most agencies require a *second-voided specimen*: Ask the client to void, and in 30 minutes to void again, providing a specimen for the test this time. *A second-voided specimen more accurately reflects the present condition of the body. Urine that has accumulated in the bladder, e.g., overnight, reflects the condition of the body at the time the urine was produced, e.g., 0300 hours.*

- Select the appropriate equipment and testing product for the client. If Clinitest tablets are used, obtain a clean test tube and dropper.

- To carry out the test, put on gloves and follow the directions specified by the manufacturer. If Clinitest tablets are used, be careful not to touch the bottom

▶ Technique 28–5 *CONTINUED*

of the test tube because it becomes extremely hot when the tablet boils in the presence of urine and water.

- Compare the results with the appropriate color chart, and record them on the client's chart. (Most agencies now record the findings as a percentage of glucose in the urine rather than as 2+ or 3+.)

4. **To test for ketone bodies:**
   - Put on a glove, and place one or two drops of urine on a reagent tablet (e.g., an Acetest tablet) or dip a reagent test strip (e.g., Ketostix) into the urine.
   - Observe and compare the results with the appropriate color chart to determine the quantity of ketones present.
   - Record the results in accordance with the product used and agency practice. The results may be graded as negative, small, moderate, or large amounts or as negative, positive, or strongly positive amounts.

5. **To test for occult blood:**
   - Don a glove, and dip the reagent strip (e.g., Hemastix) into a sample of urine.
   - Compare the color change with a color chart in the same manner as with other reagent strips.

6. **For all tests:**
   - Discard the urine following the tests. Clean the equipment with soap and water. Remove gloves.
   - Document the results of the test on the client's record.

KEY ELEMENTS OF TESTING URINE FOR SPECIFIC GRAVITY, PH, GLUCOSE, KETONES, AND OCCULT BLOOD

- Use a fresh urine sample.
- Follow the manufacturer's instructions.

Applying External Urinary Devices

The application of a **condom,** also referred to as a *urinary sheath* or *external catheter,* and attachment of its base to a urinary drainage system are commonly prescribed for incontinent males. Use of a condom appliance is preferable to insertion of a retention catheter, because it avoids entrance into the urethra and bladder and minimizes the risk of urethral or bladder infection.

Methods of applying condoms vary according to the length of time the condom is to be worn. Condoms that are to be worn for short periods are generally applied with elastic tape only; if the condom is to be worn for longer periods (e.g., a few days), additional measures are required to protect the foreskin and to ensure secure attachment. The nurse needs to follow manufacturer's instructions when applying a condom. Before applying the condom, the nurse determines when the client experiences incontinence. Some clients may require a condom appliance at night only, others continuously. Technique 28–6 describes how to apply and remove a drainage condom.

28-6 Applying a Drainage Condom

PURPOSES

- To collect urine and control urinary incontinence
- To permit the client physical activity without fear of embarrassment because of leaking urine
- To prevent skin irritation as a result of urine incontinence

ASSESSMENT FOCUS

Times of urinary incontinence; amount of urine passed (e.g., large, dribble); skin irritation, excoriation, swelling, and discoloration of penis.

▶ **Technique 28–6 Applying a Drainage Condom** CONTINUED

EQUIPMENT

- Leg drainage bag with tubing or urinary drainage bag with tubing
- Condom sheath
- Bath blanket
- Disposable gloves
- Basin of warm water and soap
- Washcloth and towel
- Elastic tape or Velcro strap

INTERVENTION

1. Prepare the equipment.

- Assemble the leg drainage bag or urinary drainage bag for attachment to the condom sheath.

- Roll the condom outward onto itself to facilitate easier application. On some models an inner flap will be exposed. *This flap is applied around the urinary meatus to prevent the reflux of urine* (Figure 28–11).

2. Position and drape the client.

- Position the client in either a supine or a bed-sitting position.

- Drape the client appropriately with the bath blanket, exposing only the penis.

3. Inspect and clean the penis.

- Don gloves.

- Inspect the penis for skin irritation (contact dermatitis), excoriation, swelling, or discoloration. *The nurse needs to obtain baseline data.*

- Clean the genital area, and dry it thoroughly. *This minimizes skin irritation and excoriation after the condom is applied.*

4. Apply and secure the condom.

- Roll the condom smoothly over the penis, leaving 2.5 cm. (1 in) between the end of the penis and the rubber or plastic connecting tube (Figure 28–12). *This space prevents irritation of the tip of the penis and provides for full drainage of urine.*

- Secure the condom firmly, but not too tightly, to the penis by wrapping a strip of elastic tape

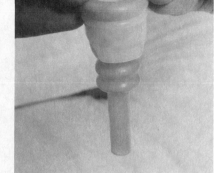

FIGURE 28–11 Before application, roll the condom outward onto itself.

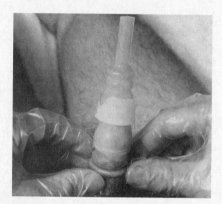

FIGURE 28–12 Rolling the condom over the penis.

or Velcro around the base of the penis over the condom. *Ordinary tape is contraindicated because it is not flexible and can stop blood flow. The elastic or Velcro strip should not come in contact with the skin and should hold the condom in place without impeding blood circulation to the penis.*

5. Securely attach the urinary drainage system.

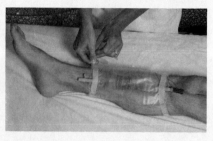

FIGURE 28–13 Attaching the urinary drainage bag to the leg.

- Make sure that the tip of the penis is not touching the condom and that the condom is not twisted. *A twisted condom could obstruct the flow of urine.*

- Attach the urinary drainage system to the condom.

- Remove gloves.

- If the client is to remain in bed, attach the urinary drainage bag to the bed frame.

- If the client is ambulatory, attach the bag to the client's leg (Figure 28–13). *Attaching the drainage bag to the leg helps control the movement of the tubing and prevents twisting of the thin material of the condom appliance at the tip of the penis.*

6. Teach the client about the drainage system.

- Instruct the client to keep the drainage bag below the level of the condom and to avoid loops or kinks in the tubing.

7. Document pertinent data.

- Record the application of the condom, the time, and pertinent observations, such as irritated areas on the penis.

▶ **Technique 28–6** *CONTINUED*

8. Inspect the penis 30 minutes following the condom application, and check urine flow.

⚠ • Assess the penis for swelling and discoloration, which indicates that the condom is too tight.

• Assess urine flow. Normally, some urine is present in the tube if the flow is not obstructed.

9. Change the condom daily, and provide skin care.

• Remove the elastic or Velcro strip, and roll off the condom.

• Wash the penis with soapy water, rinse, and dry it thoroughly.

• Assess the foreskin for signs of irritation, swelling, and discoloration.

EVALUATION FOCUS

Penis swelling and discoloration; urine flow; skin irritation.

KEY ELEMENTS OF APPLYING A DRAINAGE CONDOM

• Inspect the skin integrity of the foreskin before application.

• Clean and dry the penis thoroughly before condom application.

• Secure the condom firmly without impairing blood circulation.

• Allow space between the tip of the penis and the condom.

• Ensure that the drainage system allows free flow of urine.

• Inspect the penis for swelling or discoloration within 30 minutes after application.

• Change the condom, and assess the status of the foreskin daily.

Urinary Catheterization

Urinary catheterization is the introduction of a catheter through the urethra into the urinary bladder. This is usually performed only when absolutely necessary, because the procedure incurs certain hazards. Because the urinary structures are normally sterile except at the end of the urethra, the danger exists of introducing microorganisms into the bladder. This hazard is greatest for clients who have lowered resistance due to disease processes. Once an infection is introduced into the bladder, it can ascend the ureters and eventually involve the kidneys. Even after the catheter has been inserted and left in place for a time, the hazard of infection remains, because microorganisms can be introduced through the catheter lumen. Thus, strict sterile technique is used for catheterization. Guidelines to prevent catheter-associated infections are shown in the box on page 700.

Another hazard is trauma, particularly in the male client, whose urethra is longer and more tortuous. It is important to insert a catheter along the normal contour of the urethra. Damage to the urethra can occur if the catheter is forced through strictures or at an incorrect angle. In females, the urethra lies posteriorly, then takes a slightly anterior direction toward the bladder (Figure 28–2, earlier). In males, the urethra is normally curved (Figure 28–1, earlier), but it can be straightened by elevating the penis to a position perpendicular to the body.

Catheters are tubes commonly made of rubber or plastics, although certain types are made of woven silk or metal. *Urethral catheters* are inserted through the urethra into the urinary bladder. Two categories of urethral catheters are straight catheters and retention catheters. The *straight,* or *Robinson, catheter* is a single-lumen tube with a small eye or opening about 1¼ cm (½ in) from the insertion tip (Figure 28–14, A on page 700).

The *retention,* or *Foley, catheter* contains a second, smaller tube throughout its length on the inside. This tube is connected to a balloon near the insertion tip. After catheter insertion, the balloon is inflated to hold the catheter in place within the bladder. The outside end of the retention catheter is bifurcated, that is, it has two openings, one to drain the urine, the other to inflate the balloon (Figure 28–14, *B*).

Another type of straight catheter is the *coudé*

Preventing Catheter-Associated Urinary Infections

- Have an established infection control program.
- Catheterize clients only when necessary, by using aseptic technique, sterile equipment, and trained personnel.
- Maintain a sterile closed-drainage system.
- Do not disconnect the catheter and drainage tubing unless absolutely necessary.
- Remove the catheter as soon as possible.
- Follow and reinforce good handwashing technique.
- Changing indwelling catheters at arbitrary, fixed intervals and regular bacteriologic monitoring of catheterized clients are not cost-effective practices and should not be performed.
- Avoid other measures until further data are available. New products that appear to be questionable or gimmicky probably should be avoided.
- Although instillation of H_2O_2 into the outlet tube of the drainage set or into the drainage bags has been associated with a reduction in bag contamination, studies indicate no difference in the rate of bag-source infection in clients with the suggested instillation of H_2O_2 into the drainage bag when compared with clients who had conventional closed-drainage systems (Epstein 1985).

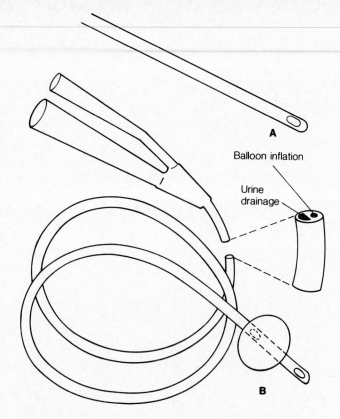

FIGURE 28–14 Two types of commonly used catheters: *A*, a straight (Robinson) catheter; *B*, a retention (Foley) catheter with the balloon inflated.

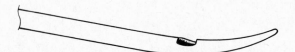

FIGURE 28–15 The coudé catheter, a urethral catheter with a curved tip.

(elbowed) *catheter*, which has a curved tip (Figure 28–15). This is sometimes used for elderly men who have a hypertrophied prostate, because its passage is often less traumatic to the gland than the passage of a straight catheter. It is somewhat stiff and is more readily controlled.

There are several other types of retention catheters. One that is frequently used for a client requiring continual or periodic bladder irrigations is the *three-way Foley catheter* (Figure 28–16, *A*). It is similar to the two-way Foley catheter described earlier, except that it has a third channel through which sterile fluid can flow into the urinary bladder. From the bladder, the fluid then flows through a second channel into a receptacle. Other types are the *de Pezzer*, or *mushroom*, *catheter* (Figure 28–16, *B*), which has a single channel and a noncollapsible mushroom tip, and the *Malecot catheter*, which has a single channel and a tip with two or four wings (Figure 28–16, *C*). The wings collapse when traction is applied, e.g., when the catheter is removed from the urinary bladder.

Catheters are sized by the diameter of the lumen

and are graded on a French scale of numbers; the larger the number, the larger the lumen. Small sizes, such as #8 or #10, are used for children; #14, #16, and #18 are commonly used for adults. Men frequently require a larger size than women. Only even numbers are available.

The balloons of retention catheters are sized by the volume of fluid or air used to inflate them. The two commonly used sizes are 5 ml and 30 ml balloons. The size of the balloon is indicated on the catheter along with the diameter, e.g., "#18 Fr.—5 ml."

Techniques 28–7 and 28–8 describe how to perform female and male urinary catheterization using a straight catheter. For the steps involved in inserting, obtaining a specimen from, and removing a retention catheter, see Techniques 28–9, 28–10, and 28–11.

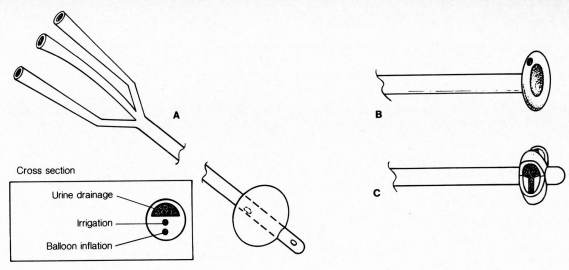

Cross section

Urine drainage

Irrigation

Balloon inflation

FIGURE 28–16 Three types of retention catheters: *A*, a three-way Foley; *B*, a de Pezzer (mushroom); *C*, a Malecot.

28-7 Female Urinary Catheterization Using a Straight Catheter

Before inserting a urinary catheter, determine (a) the order for the catheterization; (b) whether the order specifies a maximum amount of urine to be removed during the catheterization (if the client is retaining urine); usually no more than 750 ml is removed at one time, to avoid redirection of the blood supply to the pelvic blood vessels, leading to hypovolemic shock; and (c) any direction on the client's chart about the type or size of catheter to use.

PURPOSES
- To relieve discomfort due to bladder distention and/or to provide gradual decompression of a distended bladder
- To assess the amount of residual urine if the bladder empties incompletely
- To obtain a urine specimen
- To empty the bladder completely prior to surgery

ASSESSMENT FOCUS

> When the client last voided and amount; presence of urinary retention; symptoms of urinary infection; voiding pattern; ability to maintain position during catheterization.

EQUIPMENT
- ☐ Flashlight or lamp
- ☐ Mask, if required by agency policy
- ☐ Bath blanket
- ☐ Soap, a basin of warm water, a washcloth, and a towel
- ☐ Disposable gloves
- ☐ A sterile catheterization kit containing

Gloves
Drapes
Fenestrated drape (optional) to place over the perineum
Antiseptic solution
Cotton balls or gauze squares
Forceps

Water-soluble lubricant
Catheter of appropriate size (e.g., #14 or #16)
Receptacle for the urine
Specimen container if necessary
- ☐ Bag or receptacle for disposal of the cotton balls

▶

► **Technique 28–7 Female Urinary Catheterization** CONTINUED

INTERVENTION

1. **Percuss and palpate the bladder to assess for urinary retention.**

- To percuss the bladder, place the middle finger of one hand against the skin, and strike it sharply with the middle finger of the other hand. When the bladder is full, the resulting sound will be duller than normal.

- To palpate the bladder, indent the skin more than 1.3 cm (0.5 in) just above the symphysis pubis by pressing the fingers of one hand on the fingers of the other. See Figure 11–90, page 268. *This increases the pressure for palpation.*

2. **Prepare the client.**

- Explain the catheterization to the client, and provide privacy. *Exposure of the genitals is embarrassing to most clients.* Some people fear that the procedure will be painful; explain that normally a catheterization is painless and that there may be a sensation of pressure. *Relieving the client's tension can facilitate insertion of the catheter, because the urinary sphincters are more likely to be relaxed.*

- Assist the client to a supine position, with knees flexed and thighs externally rotated. Pillows can be used to support the knees and to elevate the buttocks. *Raising the client's pelvis gives the nurse a better view of the urinary meatus and reduces the risk of contaminating the catheter.*

- Drape the client. *This maintains comfort and prevents unnecessary exposure.* Cover the client's chest and abdomen with a bath blanket. Pull the client's gown up over her hips. Cover her legs and feet with the bed sheet or another blanket. Place it diagonally on the client with a corner around each foot. See Figure 11–1 on page 201.

- Wash the perineal-genital area with warm water and soap. Wear disposable gloves. *Cleaning reduces the number of microorganisms around the urinary meatus and the possibility of introducing microorganisms with the catheter.*

- Rinse and dry the area well. *Rinsing removes soap that could inhibit the action of the antiseptic later.*

- Obtain assistance if the client requires help in maintaining the required position. *The client must remain still throughout the procedure to maintain a clear view of the urinary meatus and prevent contamination of the sterile field.*

3. **Prepare the equipment.**

- Adjust the light to view the urinary meatus. It may be necessary to use a flashlight or to place a gooseneck lamp at the foot of the bed, so that it focuses on the perineal area.

- Put on a mask, gown, and/or cap if required by agency policy (e.g., for reverse isolation).

4. **Create a sterile field.**

- At the client's bedside, open a sterile kit and the catheter, if it is packaged separately, and put on the sterile gloves (see Technique 9–8, page 153).

- Drape the client with the sterile drapes, being careful to protect the sterility of the drapes and your gloves. Use the first drape as an underpad, and place it under the buttocks. Keep the underpad edges cuffed over your gloves. *This prevents contamination of the gloves against the client's buttocks.* If the other drape is fenestrated, place it over the perineal area, exposing only the labia. If a fenestrated drape is not available, place the two thigh drapes so that they overlap between the client's thighs. Place the thigh drapes from the side farthest to the side nearest you. *This prevents reaching across a sterile field and possible contamination of the new drape.*

- Place the sterile kit on the drape between the client's thighs. *This facilitates access to supplies.*

- Pour the antiseptic solution over the cotton balls, if they are not already prepared.

- Lubricate the insertion tip of the catheter liberally, and place it in the sterile container ready for use. *Water-soluble lubricant facilitates insertion of the catheter by reducing friction. Lubricate at this point because you will subsequently have only one sterile hand available.*

- Open the urine specimen container, and keep the top sterile. *This prepares the container for specimen collection.*

5. **Clean the meatus (if recommended by agency practice).**

- With the nondominant hand, separate the labia majora with the thumb and finger, and clean the labia minor on each side, using forceps and cotton balls soaked in antiseptic. Use a new swab for each stroke. *This prevents the transfer of microorganisms.* Move downward from the pubic area to the anus (Figure 28–17). *Cleaning from anterior to posterior cleans from the area of least contamination to the area of greatest contamination.*

- Then, separate the labia minora with two other fingers, still using the nondominant hand (Figure 28–18).

▶ **Technique 28–7** *CONTINUED*

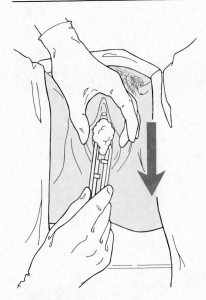

FIGURE 28–17 When cleaning the labia minora, move the swab downward.

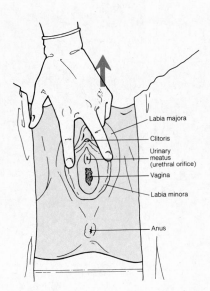

Labia majora

Clitoris

Urinary meatus (urethral orifice)

Vagina

Labia minora

Anus

FIGURE 28–18 To expose the urinary meatus, separate the labia minora and retract the tissue upward.

 • Expose the urinary meatus adequately by retracting the tissue of the labia minora in an upward (anterior) direction (Figure 28–18). Clean first from the meatus downward and then on either side, using a new swab for each stroke. Once the meatus is cleaned, do not allow the labia to close over it. *Keeping the labia apart prevents the risk of contam-*

inating the urinary meatus.
Note: The hand that touches the client becomes unsterile. It remains in position exposing the urinary meatus, while the other hand remains sterile holding the sterile forceps.

6. Inspect the meatus.

• Assess any signs, such as excoriation of the tissues surrounding the urinary meatus, swelling of the urinary meatus, or the presence of discharge around the urinary meatus. *This assessment provides baseline data.* If any discharge is present, refer to the nurse in charge for a culture order.

7. Insert the catheter until urine flows.

Place the drainage end of the catheter in the urine receptacle. Pick up the insertion end of the catheter with your uncontaminated, sterile, gloved hand, holding it about 5 cm (2 in) from the insertion tip. *Because the adult female urethra is approximately 4 cm (1.5 in) long, the catheter is held far enough from the end to allow full insertion into the bladder and to maintain control of the tip of the catheter so it will not accidentally become contaminated.*

• Gently insert the catheter into the urinary meatus until urine flows. Insert the catheter in the direction of the urethra. If the catheter meets resistance during insertion, do not force it. *Forceful pressure exerted against the urethra can produce trauma.* Ask the client to take deep breaths. *This helps relax the external sphincter.* If this does not relieve the resistance, discontinue the procedure, and report the problem to the nurse in charge. Exercise caution to prevent the catheter tip from becoming contaminated. If it becomes contaminated, discard it.

• When the urine flows, transfer your hand from the labia to the catheter to hold it in place 2 cm from the meatus. *This prevents its expulsion by a possible bladder contraction.*

8. Collect a urine specimen.

• Pinch the catheter, and transfer the drainage end of it into the sterile specimen bottle. Usually, 30 ml of urine is sufficient for a specimen. Securely place the top on the specimen container, and set it aside for labeling later.

9. Empty or partially drain the bladder, and then remove the catheter.

• For adults experiencing urinary retention, some orders limit the amount of urine drained to 700 to 1000 ml. Whether to limit the amount of urine drained has been a controversial issue. *Rapid removal of large amounts of urine is thought to induce engorgement of the pelvic blood vessels and hypovolemic shock. However, retained urine may serve as a reservoir for microorganisms to multiply.* Usually, agency policy or the physician indicates the amount to be removed and times at which the remaining urine is to be withdrawn. Bristol, Fadden, Fehring, Rohde, Prue, and Wohlitz (1989, p. 345) concluded from research that *complete drainage of a distended bladder is likely to be more comfortable* and certainly seems as safe as threshold clamping.

• Pinch the catheter. *This prevents leakage of urine.* Remove the catheter slowly.

10. Promote client comfort.

• Dry the client's perineum with a towel or drape. *Excess lubricant and solution in the area can irritate the skin.*

▶

▶ **Technique 28–7 Female Urinary Catheterization** *CONTINUED*

11. Assess the urine.

• Inspect the urine for color, clarity, odor, and the presence of any abnormal constituents, such as blood.

• Measure the amount of urine.

12. Document the catheterization.

• Include assessments before and after the procedure; type and

size of catheter inserted; time; characteristics and amount of urine obtained; whether a specimen was sent to the laboratory; and client response to the procedure.

EVALUATION FOCUS

Signs of urinary infection; discomfort; bladder distention; amount, color, and clarity of urine.

SAMPLE RECORDING

Date	Time	Notes
01/26/93	1900	C/o pubic discomfort. Has not voided since surgery. Intake 2000 ml. Bladder palpable above symphysis pubis. Is restless. Catheterized with #14F catheter for 650 ml clear amber urine. States, "am more comfortable." Less restless. — Sylvia F. Tompkins, RN

KEY ELEMENTS OF FEMALE URINARY CATHETERIZATION USING A STRAIGHT CATHETER

• Determine whether the amount of urine drained is to be limited.

• Obtain assistance for a client who needs help to maintain the required position.

• Clean the perineal area before catheterization.

• Use strict aseptic technique.

• Lubricate the insertion tip of the catheter and do so before swabbing the labia with antiseptic.

• Keep the labia apart once the meatus is cleaned.

• Pick up and insert the catheter with your uncontaminated, sterile, gloved hand.

• Do not force a catheter beyond a major resistance.

• Assess the amount, color, and clarity of the urine.

28-8 Male Urinary Catheterization Using a Straight Catheter

PURPOSES:

See Technique 28–7, page 701.

ASSESSMENT FOCUS

See Techniques 28–7, page 701.

EQUIPMENT

☐ See Technique 28–7. A #16 or #18 catheter is usually used for an adult male

▶ **Technique 28–8 Male Urinary Catheterization** *CONTINUED*

INTERVENTION

1. Percuss and palpate the bladder as in Technique 28–7, step 1.

2. Prepare the client.

- Explain the catheterization, as in Technique 28–7.

- Assist the client to a supine position, with the knees slightly flexed and the thighs slightly apart. *This allows greater relaxation of the abdominal and perineal muscles and permits easier insertion of the catheter.*

- Drape the client by folding the top bedclothes down so that the penis is exposed and the thighs are covered. Use a bath blanket to cover the client's chest and abdomen.

- Wash the perineal area, as in Technique 28–7.

🔺 **3. Create a sterile field.**

- Open the sterile tray, and don the sterile gloves (see Technique 9–8, page 153).

- Place a drape under the penis and a second drape above the penis over the pubic area. If a fenestrated drape is available, place it over the penis and pubic area, exposing only the penis.

- Place the sterile kit on the sterile drape over the client's thighs or next to the thigh.

- Pour the antiseptic solution over the cotton balls, if they are not already prepared.

- Lubricate the insertion tip of the catheter liberally for about 5 to 7 cm (2 to 3 in). Place it in the sterile container ready for insertion. *Water-soluble lubricant facilitates insertion of the catheter by reducing friction. Do this step before cleaning because you will*

subsequently have only one sterile hand available.

4. Clean the urinary meatus.

- Grasp the penis firmly behind the glans with the nondominant hand, and spread the meatus between the thumb and forefinger. Retract the foreskin of an uncircumcised male. The hand holding the penis is now considered contaminated. *Firmly grasp the penis to avoid stimulating an erection.*

🔺 - With the dominant hand, use sterile forceps to pick up a swab. Clean the meatus first, and then wipe the tissue surrounding the meatus in a circular motion. Discard each swab after only one wipe. *Using forceps maintains the sterility of your gloves.*

5. Insert the catheter.

- Place the drainage end of the catheter in the urine receptacle. Then, pick up the insertion end of the catheter with your uncontaminated, sterile, gloved hand, holding it about 8 to 10 cm (3 to 4 in) from the insertion tip for an adult or about 2.5 cm (1 in) for a baby or small boy. In some agencies, the catheter is picked up with forceps. *The male urethra is approximately 20 cm (8 in) long. Holding the catheter far enough from the end to maintain control of the tip of the catheter avoids accidental contamination.*

- Lift the penis to a position perpendicular to the body (90° angle), and exert slight traction (pulling or tension upward). Insert the catheter steadily about 20 cm (8 in) or until urine begins to flow. *Lifting the penis so that it is perpendicular to the body straightens the downward curvature of the urethra.*

- To bypass slight resistance at the sphincters, twist the catheter, or wait until the sphincter relaxes. Ask the client to take deep breaths or try to void. If difficult 🔺 resistance is met, discontinue the procedure, and report the problem to the nurse in charge. *Slight resistance is normally encountered at the external and internal urethral sphincters. Deep breathing can help to relax the external sphincter. Forceful pressure exerted against a major resistance can traumatize the urethra.*

- While the urine flows, lower the penis, and transfer your hand to hold the catheter in place at the meatus.

6. Drain the urine from the bladder.

- Collect a urine specimen (if required) after the urine has flowed for a few seconds. Pinch the catheter, and transfer the drainage end of the catheter into the sterile specimen bottle. Usually, 30 ml of urine is sufficient for a specimen.

- Empty the bladder, or drain the amount of urine specified in the order. See Technique 28–7, step 9.

7. Make the client comfortable.

- Dry the penis with a towel or drape.

🔺 - Replace the foreskin. *This prevents a mechanical phimosis (constriction), which may compromise circulation to the glans.*

8. Assess the client and the urine, as in Technique 28–7, and document the procedure and the assessments.

▶ **Technique 28–8 Male Urinary Catheterization Using a Straight Catheter** CONTINUED

EVALUATION FOCUS	See Technique 28–7, page 701.

KEY ELEMENTS OF MALE URINARY CATHETERIZATION USING A STRAIGHT CATHETER.

See the Key Elements of Technique 28–7.

• Position the client appropriately to relax the abdominal and perineal muscles.

• Retract the foreskin of an uncircumcised client, and keep it back during the catheterization.

• Lift the penis perpendicular to the body before catheterization.

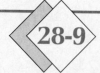

28-9 Inserting a Retention Catheter

PURPOSES	• To manage incontinence when other measures have failed • To provide for intermittent or continuous bladder drainage and irrigation • To prevent urine from contacting an incision after perineal surgery • To facilitate accurate measurement of urinary output for critically ill clients whose output needs to be monitored hourly
ASSESSMENT FOCUS	Distention of urinary bladder; signs of urinary infection; voiding pattern; ability to maintain position during catheterization.

EQUIPMENT

In addition to the equipment used for a straight catheterization, the following equipment is needed:

□ Retention catheter, #14 or #16 for adults, #8 or #10 for children
□ Prefilled syringe (sterile water is often used)
□ Nonallergenic tape
□ Safety pin or clip

INTERVENTION

1. Prepare the client and the equipment.

• Explain to the client why the retention catheter is to be inserted, how long it will be in place, and how the urinary drainage equipment needs to be handled to maintain and facilitate the drainage of urine. Reassure the client that the procedure is painless. Some clients fear spillage of urine when they experience the urge to void during insertion of the catheter and for a short pe-riod of time after the catheter is in place. Reassure these clients that the catheter drains the urine and that the urge to void will disappear.

• Follow procedure as for straight catheterization up to and including draping the client.

2. Test the catheter balloon.

• Attach the prefilled syringe to the balloon valve, and inject the fluid. The balloon should inflate appropriately and not leak. With-draw the fluid, and set aside the catheter with the syringe attached for later use. If the balloon leaks or does not inflate adequately, replace the catheter. In such a case, withdraw the fluid, and detach the syringe for later use. Ask another nurse to obtain a second catheter and open the package for you, then test the new balloon.

or

Remove the equipment, and obtain another catheter. Then be-

▶ **Technique 28–9 Inserting a Retention Catheter** *CONTINUED*

gin again with the new sterile equipment.

3. Follow steps as for straight catheterization.

- Lubricate the insertion tip of the catheter.

- Remove the sterile cap from the specimen container.

- Separate and clean the urinary meatus and surrounding tissues.

- Insert the catheter.

- Collect a urine specimen as required.

4. Move the catheter farther into the bladder, and inflate the balloon.

- Insert the catheter an additional 2.5 to 5 cm (1 to 2 in) beyond the point at which urine began to flow. The balloon of the catheter is located behind the opening at the insertion tip, and sufficient space needs to be provided to inflate the balloon. *This ensures that the balloon is inflated inside the bladder and not in the urethra, where it could produce trauma.*

- Inflate the balloon by injecting the contents of the prefilled syringe into the valve of the catheter (Figure 28–19, *A*). Placement of the catheter and balloon in a male client is shown in Figure 28–19, *B*. If the client complains of discomfort or pain during the balloon inflation, withdraw the fluid, insert the catheter a little farther, and inflate the balloon again. Insert no more fluid than the balloon size indicates (e.g., 5 ml or 30 ml), and remove the syringe. A special valve prevents backflow of the fluid out of the catheter.

- Follow agency policy when using a 30-ml balloon. Some agency policies state that only 15 ml of fluid is injected for inflation.

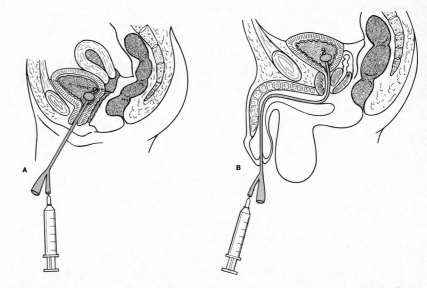

FIGURE 28–19   Placement of catheter and inflated balloon in *A*, female client; and *B*, male client.

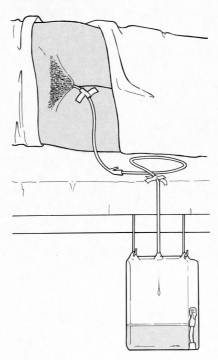

FIGURE 28–20   Tape the catheter to the inside of a female's thigh.

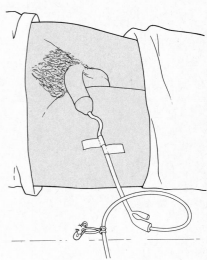

FIGURE 28–21   Tape the catheter to the thigh or abdomen of a male client.

5. Ensure effective balloon inflation.

- When the balloon is safely inflated, apply slight tension on the catheter until you feel resistance. *Resistance indicates that the catheter balloon is inflated appropriately, and that the catheter is well anchored in the bladder.*

- Then, release the resistance on the catheter. This keeps the balloon from exerting undue pressure on the neck of the bladder.

6. Anchor the catheter.

- Tape the catheter with nonallergenic tape to the inside of a female's thigh or to the thigh or abdomen of a male client (Figures 28–20 and 28–21). Some nurses prefer taping the catheter to the abdomen whenever there is increased risk of penile scrotal

▶ **Technique 28–9 Inserting a Retention Catheter** *CONTINUED*

excoriation. *Taping restricts the movement of the catheter, thus reducing friction and irritation in the urethra when the client moves. It also prevents skin excoriation at the penile-scrotal junction in the male.*

7. Establish effective drainage.

• Ensure that the emptying base of the drainage bag is closed.

• Secure the drainage bag to the bed frame, using the hook or strap provided. Suspend the bag off the floor, but keep it below the level of the client's bladder (Fig-

ure 28–20). *Urine flows by gravity from the bladder to the drainage bag. The bag should be off the floor so that the emptying portion does not become grossly contaminated.*

• Coil the drainage tubing loosely beside the client, so that the remaining tubing runs in a straight line down to the drainage bag. Fasten the vertical tubing to the bedclothes with tape, a tubing clamp, or a safety pin and elastic band (Figures 28–20 and 28–21). *The drainage tubing should not loop below its entry into the*

drainage bag, because this impedes the flow of urine by gravity.

8. Document pertinent data.

• Record the time and date of the catheterization; the reason; number of milliliters used to inflate the balloon; assessments before and after the procedure, including amount, color, and consistency of urine obtained; whether a specimen was taken and sent to the laboratory; whether all urine was emptied from the bladder; and the client's response.

EVALUATION FOCUS	Amount, color, and clarity of urine; any discomfort; fluid intake, palpable bladder.

SAMPLE RECORDING

Date	Time	Notes
07/12/93	2000	#18 5-ml Foley catheter inserted and connected to drainage. 600 ml clear amber urine drained. Stated burning pain over pubic area relieved. Instructed about I & O. ——————————————— Ron J. Randall, SN

KEY ELEMENTS OF INSERTING A RETENTION CATHETER

See the key elements of Technique 28–7.

• Test the balloon before insertion to see that it is intact.

• Before inflating the balloon of the catheter, insert the catheter an additional 2.5 to 5 cm (1 to 2 in) beyond the point at which urine began to flow.

• Inflate the balloon with no more fluid than the balloon size indicates.

• After balloon inflation, apply slight tension on the catheter to check that the balloon is well anchored in the bladder, then move the catheter slightly back into the bladder.

• Tape the catheter to the client appropriately.

• Make sure the drainage system allows free flow of urine and is well sealed or closed.

28-10

Obtaining a Urine Specimen from a Retention Catheter

Sterile urine specimens can be acquired from closed drainage systems by inserting a sterile needle attached to a 3-ml syringe through a drainage port in the tubing. Note that aspiration of urine from catheters can be done only with self-sealing rubber catheters, not plastic, silicone, or silastic catheters. When self-sealing rubber catheters are used, the needle is

► **Technique 28–10 Obtaining a Urine Specimen from a Retention Catheter** *CONTINUED*

inserted just above the place where the catheter is attached to the drainage tubing. The area from which to obtain urine may be marked by a patch on the catheter.

PURPOSES
- To analyze the urine for abnormal constituents
- To determine the presence of microorganisms

ASSESSMENT FOCUS

Clinical signs of urinary tract infection, e.g., cloudy urine with sediment, fever, flank pain, hematuria; type of indwelling catheter to determine presence of sampling port.

EQUIPMENT

- Tubing clamp
- Disinfectant swab
- Sterile syringe (3 ml or 30 ml) and sterile 1-inch needle (#21 to #25 gauge)

- Sterile culture tube or unsterile bottle, depending on the purpose of the specimen

- Specimen identification label and laboratory requisition

INTERVENTION

1. Clamp the catheter drainage tubing.

- Clamp the drainage tubing for about 30 minutes. *This allows fresh urine to collect in the catheter.*

2. Clean the entry site of the needle.

- Wipe the area where the needle will be inserted with a disinfectant swab. The site should be remote from the tube leading to the balloon to avoid puncturing this tube. *Disinfecting the needle insertion site removes or destroys any microorganisms on the surface of the catheter, thereby avoiding contamination of the needle and the entrance of microorganisms into the catheter.*

3. Obtain the specimen.

- Unclamp the catheter.

- Insert the needle at a 30° to 45° angle (Figure 28–22). *This angle of entrance facilitates self-sealing of the rubber.*

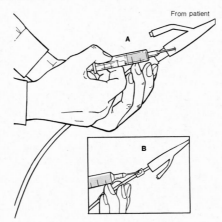

From patient

A

B

FIGURE 28–22 Obtaining a urine specimen from a retention catheter: *A*, from a specific area, sometimes designated by a patch, near the end of the catheter; *B*, from a drainage port in the tubing.

- If urine is not readily available, elevate the tubing slightly to return urine to the area or clamp the tubing about 5 to 7 cm (3 in) from its tip for 15 minutes or until urine appears.

- Withdraw the required amount of urine, e.g., 3 ml for a urine culture or 30 ml for a routine urinalysis.

4. Transfer the specimen and send it to the laboratory.

- Transfer the urine to the specimen container. Make sure the needle does not touch the outside of the container, if a sterile culture tube is used.

- Cap and label the container, and send the urine to the laboratory immediately for analysis or refrigeration.

5. Ensure client comfort.

- If the tubing was clamped, unclamp it. *Failure to unclamp the tubing may result in a distended bladder and cause discomfort for the client.*

6. Document all relevant information.

- Record collection of the specimen and any pertinent observations of the urine on the appropriate records.

EVALUATION FOCUS

Appearance of urine; patency of urinary drainage system; results of laboratory analysis when available.

►

► **Technique 28–10 Obtaining a Urine Specimen from a Retention Catheter** CONTINUED

SAMPLE RECORDING

Date	Time	Notes
04/06/93	1320	Catheter tubing clamped for 30 min. 30 mL urine aspirated from drainage port on catheter tubing. Specimen sent to lab for culture and sensitivity. Urine cloudy and blood tinged. Catheter unclamped. —————————————————— Sheila S. Morrow, R.N.

KEY ELEMENTS OF OBTAINING A URINE SPECIMEN FROM A RETENTION CATHETER

- Clamp the catheter for 30 minutes before collecting the specimen.
- Use a sterile syringe and needle.

- Disinfect the collection port of the catheter beforehand.
- Unclamp the catheter after the specimen is obtained.

28-11 Removing a Retention Catheter

Retention catheters are removed after their purpose has been achieved, usually on the order of the physician. A few days prior to removal the catheter may be clamped for specified periods of time (e.g., 2 to 4 hours) and then released. This causes some distention of the bladder and stimulation of the bladder musculature.

ASSESSMENT FOCUS

Amount, color, and clarity of urine in the drainage bag; size of the catheter balloon.

EQUIPMENT

- Disposable gloves
- Clean, disposable towel

- Sterile syringe and needle to deflate the balloon

- Receptacle for the catheter after its removal, e.g., a disposable basin

---

INTERVENTION

1. Prepare the client.

- Ask the client to assume a back-lying position.

- Obtain a sterile urine specimen if ordered or recommended by agency protocol.

- Remove the tape attaching the catheter to the client.

2. Prepare the equipment.

- Don gloves.

- Place the towel between the legs of the female client and over the thighs of the male client.

3. Remove the catheter.

- Insert the needle of the syringe into the balloon of the inflation

tube of the catheter.

- Withdraw all the fluid from the balloon. *This will permit the balloon to deflate.* If not all the fluid can be removed, report this fact to the nurse in charge before proceeding. *Do not* pull the catheter while the balloon is inflated. *The urethra may be injured.*

▶ **Technique 28–11 Removing a Retention Catheter** CONTINUED

- Gently withdraw the catheter, observe for intactness, and place in the waste receptacle. *If the catheter is not intact, parts may remain in the bladder. Report this immediately to the nurse in charge or physician.*

- Dry the perineal area with the towel.

4. Measure the urine in the drainage bag.

5. Document the procedure and any assessments.

- Record the time the catheter was removed; the intactness of the catheter; and the amount, color, and clarity of the urine.

6. Determine time of first void- ing and the amount voided over the first 8 hours. Compare this with the fluid intake. *When the fluid output is considerably less than the fluid intake the bladder may be retaining urine.*

7. If urine retention is suspected, palpate the bladder for fullness.

EVALUATION FOCUS

Intactness of the catheter; amount, color, and clarity of urine; amount of urine voided after catheter removal.

SAMPLE RECORDING

Date	Time	Notes
08/15/93	1015	Foley catheter removed intact. Oral fluids encouraged. ——— Gail Sim, SN
08/15/93	1100	Taking oral fluids. Voided 200 mL clear yellow urine. Slight burning on voiding. ——— Gail Sim, SN

KEY ELEMENTS OF REMOVING A RETENTION CATHETER

- Wear gloves.
- Deflate the balloon completely before removing it from the urethra.
- Observe the intactness of the catheter.

- Measure the urine in the drainage bag.
- Assess the frequency and amount of urine voided after catheter removal.

Urinary Irrigations

An **irrigation** is a flushing or washing-out with a specified solution. A *bladder irrigation* is carried out on a physician's order, usually to wash out the bladder and/or apply an antiseptic solution to the bladder lining to treat a bladder infection. Sterile technique is used. *Catheter irrigations* are usually carried out to maintain or restore the patency of a catheter, e.g., to remove pus or blood clots that have formed in the bladder and are blocking the catheter. A physician's order may or may not be required, depending on agency protocol.

There are three ways of irrigating a catheter or bladder: (1) maintaining the closed system and injecting the solution through an aspiration port (closed intermittent irrigation), (2) irrigating through a three-way catheter (closed intermittent or continuous irrigation), and (3) irrigating through a catheter after separating the catheter and tubing (open intermittent system). Although the open system may be used in some agencies, closed sterile drainage systems are recommended.

In the usual bladder irrigation, a two-way Foley catheter is usually in place. For a bladder irrigation, the frequency and the type, amount, and strength of solution to be used are ordered by the physician. If the physician has not specified these on the client's

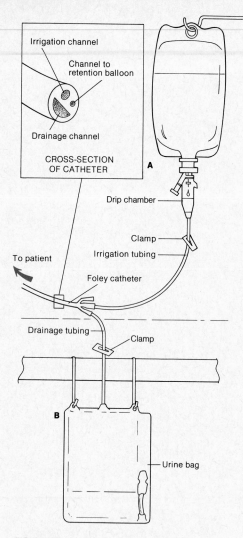

FIGURE 28–23 An intermittent bladder irrigation.

chart, the nurse checks agency policies. Some agencies recommend the use of sterile normal saline at room temperature for both catheter and bladder irrigations. To irrigate an adult bladder, 1000 ml is commonly used for the entire irrigation; for a catheter irrigation, 200 ml is normally required.

Irrigations performed via straight gravity drainage are referred to as *plain irrigations*. A variation of the plain irrigation is the intermittent irrigation, in which one lumen of a three-way catheter is connected by tubing to a drip chamber and then to a container of sterile solution. The second lumen is attached to tubing and then to a urine receptacle (Figure 28–23). There are clamps on both tubes. The clamp from the solution container (*A*) is released while the clamp to the urine bag (*B*) is closed. The fluid enters and remains in the bladder. The nurse then reclamps the container tubing and unclamps the urine receptacle tubing, permitting the solution to flow out of the bladder. This process is carried out regularly. The nurse can use the same system for continuous irrigations by carefully regulating the flow of fluid, leaving the solution container and permitting the solution to flow freely out of the bladder into the urine bag.

There are several variations of this irrigation system. One requires a specific fluid pressure to build up in the urinary bladder before the irrigation system "trips," allowing the solution to flow out of the bladder into a receptacle. These systems are usually set up by a physician and monitored by nurses.

Technique 28–12 outlines the steps in irrigating a catheter or bladder (closed system).

28-12 Irrigating a Catheter or Bladder (Closed System)

Before irrigating a catheter or bladder, determine (a) the order for a bladder irrigation (in most agencies, a physician's order is required); and (b) the type of solution, amount, and strength to be used. If these are not specified on the client's chart, check agency protocol.

PURPOSES

- To maintain the patency of a urinary catheter and tubing (continuous irrigation)
- To free a blockage in a urinary catheter or tubing (intermittent irrigation)

ASSESSMENT FOCUS

Amount, clarity, and color of urine; comparison of fluid intake to output; presence of bladder distention; level of discomfort.

► **Technique 28–12** *CONTINUED*

EQUIPMENT

- Sterile gloves
- Disposable, water-resistant sterile towel
- Sterile 30- or 50-ml syringe with a #19 to #23 needle
- Sterile antiseptic swabs
- Sterile receptacle

INTERVENTION

1. Determine that the catheter and tubing are indeed blocked.

- Palpate the client's bladder to assess for urine retention.
- Compare the amount of urine in the bag with the drainage on the previous shift or with the client's fluid intake.
- If urine does not appear to be running freely, "milk" the catheter and tubing, working from the client toward the drainage bag. *This can dislodge an obstruction, avoiding the necessity of an irrigation to remove it. "Milk" away from the client so that the obstruction, e.g., a blood clot, is forced into the drainage bag and not into the urinary bladder.*

2. Prepare the client.

- Explain the procedure to the client. A bladder or catheter irrigation should not be painful, although solution that is not at body temperature may be uncomfortable to the client.
- Assist the client to a dorsal recumbent position. *This position facilitates the flow of the irrigating fluid into the bladder.*
- Fold back the top bedclothes to expose the retention catheter. Place a bath blanket across the client's chest and abdomen if they are exposed.
- Determine the amount of urine in the drainage bag. *This amount has to be deducted from subsequent measurements of the irrigating fluid returns.*

3. Prepare the equipment.

- Open the sterile set beside or between the client's thighs, using sterile technique.

- Don gloves.
- Place the sterile towel under the end of the catheter.
- For a bladder irrigation, clamp the drainage tubing distal to the irrigation port. *Clamping prevents the urine and solution from draining into the drainage bag.* For a catheter irrigation, leave the tubing unclamped.
- Remove the cap from the needle, and draw the irrigation solution into the syringe, maintaining the sterility of the syringe and the solution.
- Using the antiseptic swab, wipe the place on the catheter lumen or the port on the drainage tubing through which the solution is to be instilled. The correct place on the catheter lumen is usually marked.

4. Instill the fluid into the catheter.

- Insert the needle into the port (Figure 28–22, earlier).
- Infuse the solution gently into the catheter. For each catheter infusion, instill about 30 to 40 ml of fluid for an adult; for each bladder infusion, instill about 100 to 200 ml. Use smaller amounts for children. *Gentle instillation avoids injury to the lining of the bladder and bladder spasms.*
- Remove the needle from the port.

5. Drain the fluid.

- For a catheter irrigation, immediately lower the catheter so that the fluid will run toward the distal end of the catheter into the drainage tubing.

or

For a bladder irrigation, unclamp the drainage tubing so that the solution will run out of the bladder through the catheter and tubing.

- Repeat the process outlined in step 4 until all of the solution has been used or until the purpose of the irrigation has been accomplished.

6. Calculate the amount of urine drained.

- Empty the urine bag and subtract the amount of solution used from the volume of fluid in the bag.

7. Assess both the client and the drainage.

- Note any change in discomfort.
- Assess the drainage for color, clarity, and presence of abnormal constituents.
- Assess the flow of urine in the catheter and tubing.

8. Document the irrigation.

- Include assessments before and after the irrigation.

VARIATION: Continuous Irrigation Using a Three-Way Foley Catheter

1. Assemble the equipment.

- Expell air from the tubing connected to the irrigation bag.
- Connect one port of the three-way catheter to the irrigation tubing which in turn is connected to the irrigation solution in a bag. Connect the second port of the catheter to the drainage tubing and bag, and the third port to the catheter balloon (Figure 28–23, earlier).

▶ **Technique 28–12 Irrigating a Catheter or Bladder** CONTINUED

2. Irrigate the bladder.

- Open the flow clamp on the drainage tubing.

- Adjust the flow rate, using the clamp on the irrigation tubing, as specified by the physician. If the order does not specify, the rate should be 40 to 60 drops per minute or according to agency protocol.

- Inspect the fluid returns for amount, color, and clarity. The amount of returning fluid should correspond to the amount of fluid entering the bladder.

3. Document the assessments as above.

VARIATION: Irrigating a Catheter or Bladder Using the Open System

- After disinfecting the ends, separate the catheter from the drainage tubing, and place the tubing protector over the end of the tubing. Hold the catheter and the tubing at least 2.5 cm (1 in) from their ends. *By maintaining this distance, you avoid contaminating the ends of the catheter and tubing.*

- Draw the fluid into the syringe, then gently inject it into the catheter, maintaining the sterility of the end of the catheter, the syringe, and the solution. Remove the syringe, and allow the fluid to return through the catheter into the drainage receptacle. Repeat until the catheter is running freely or until the purpose of the irrigation has been accomplished.

- Reattach the catheter to the tubing, maintaining the sterility of the ends of the tubing and the catheter.

- Coil the drainage tubing carefully on the bed so that the urine can flow through it freely.

- Make assessments as for irrigating using a closed system.

EVALUATION FOCUS

Catheter patency; amount, color, and clarity of urine; any discomfort.

SAMPLE RECORDING

Date	Time	Notes
04/24/93	1400	Bladder irrigated with 200 ml normal saline at room temperature. Returns slightly blood-tinged with some small blood clots. Catheter running freely. No discomfort. ———————————————— Sandi R. Bailey, NS

KEY ELEMENTS OF IRRIGATING A CATHETER OR BLADDER (CLOSED SYSTEM)

All Irrigations

- Wear gloves.
- Use strict aseptic technique.
- Maintain the integrity of closed systems.
- Instill the correct amount and type of irrigating solution or medication.
- Instill the fluid gently and slowly.
- Determine the amount of urine in the drainage bag beforehand.
- Assess the color and consistency of the urine drainage.

Catheter Irrigation

- Confirm that the catheter or tubing is blocked.
- Leave the catheter unclamped when instilling fluid.

Bladder Irrigation

- Clamp the drainage tubing before instilling the fluid.

- Unclamp the drainage tubing after instilling the fluid.

Irrigations Using a Three-Way Foley Catheter

- Determine whether the irrigation is to be continuous or intermittent.
- Expel air from the tubing before attaching it to the catheter.
- Set the drip rate as ordered.
- Empty the drainage bag as necessary, and measure the amount of fluid inflow and output.

Catheter or Bladder Irrigation Using the Open System

- Disinfect tubing ends before separating the catheter from the tubing.
- After instilling the fluid for a bladder irrigation, remove the syringe to allow fluid to return through the catheter.

Suprapubic Catheter Care

A suprapubic catheter is inserted through the abdominal wall above the symphysis pubis into the urinary bladder (Figure 28–24). The physician inserts the catheter using local anesthesia (in the client's bed unit) or using general anesthesia in conjunction with bladder or vaginal surgery (in the operating room). The catheter may be secured in place with sutures, with a commercial retention body seal, or with both sutures and a body seal. The catheter is then attached to a closed drainage system. When the catheter is removed, the muscle layers of the bladder contract over the insertion site to seal off the opening. Suprapubic catheters have several advantages over urethral catheters:

- They are associated with a lower rate of urinary tract infections.

- They are more comfortable for the client.

- They allow the opportunity to evaluate the client's ability to void normally; the client can void normally when the suprapubic catheter is clamped. The urethral catheter, by contrast, must be removed before the client's ability to void normally can be assessed.

- They facilitate evaluation of the client's residual urine.

Two commonly used suprapubic catheters are the *Cystocath* and the *Bonanno catheter* (Figure 28–25). These are narrow-lumen catheters with a curl at the distal end that prevents the catheter from being expelled by the bladder through the urethra. The Cystocath has a disc that holds the catheter in place on the abdominal wall; the Bonanno catheter has wings for that purpose. Attachments of the catheter to the drainage system tubing also vary: The Cystocath is joined with a stopcock, the Bonanno with a Luer-Lok adapter.

The most common problem with the suprapubic catheter is blockage of drainage by sediment or clots or obstruction of the catheter or catheter tip by the bladder wall itself. Dislodgement of the catheter and hematuria following the use of a large-bore catheter are less common problems. Care of clients with suprapubic catheters includes regular assessments of the client's urine, fluid intake, and comfort; maintenance of a patent drainage system; skin care around the insertion site; periodic clamping of the catheter preparatory to removing it; and measurement of residual urine. Orders generally include leaving the catheter open to drainage for 48 to 72 hours, then clamping the catheter for 3- to 4-hour periods during the day until the client can void satisfactory amounts. Sat-

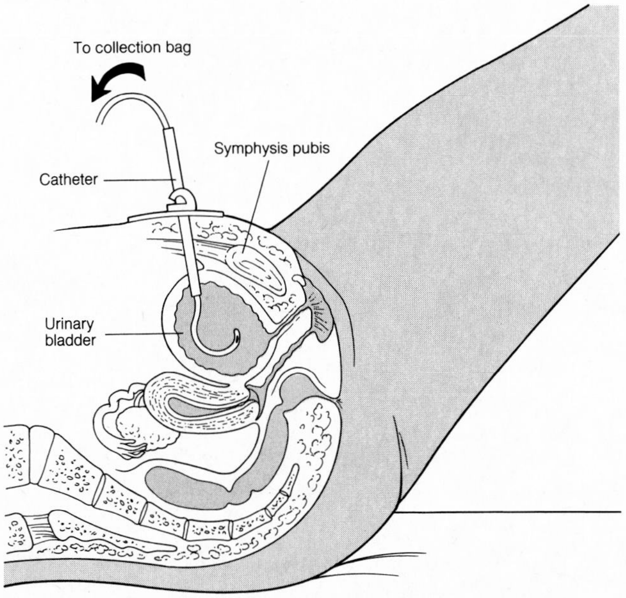

FIGURE 28–24 A suprapubic catheter in place.

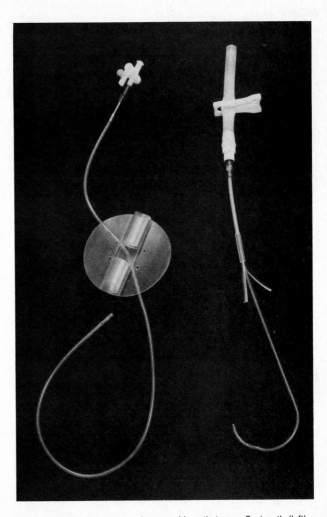

FIGURE 28–25 Two types of suprapubic catheters; a Cystocath (left) and a Bonanno (right).

isfactory voiding is determined by measuring the client's residual urine after voiding. Care of the catheter insertion site involves sterile technique. See Technique 39–2 on page 924 and follow agency protocol.

Kidney Impairment and Peritoneal Dialysis

Normally, the kidneys produce urine continuously at the rate of 60 to 120 ml per hour (720 to 1440 ml per day) in the adult. Newborns need to start micturition within 24 to 36 hours of birth. Anuria, oliguria, and urinary suppression can occur as a result of kidney disease, severe heart failure, burns, and shock. These signs can be fatal if some other means, such as an artificial kidney, is not used to remove the body wastes. Other critical signs of renal failure are the presence of uremic frost (urea crystals) on the skin, an elevated blood urea nitrogen (BUN) level, an aromatic odor to the skin, and signs of fluid and electrolyte imbalances.

Peritoneal dialysis, also referred to as *peritoneal exchange*, is used as a temporary or permanent measure when kidney function is impaired. **Peritoneal dialysis** is the instillation and drainage of a solution (a dialysate) from the peritoneal cavity. Its purpose is to remove impurities, excess fluid, and electrolytes from the blood that would normally be excreted through the kidneys. The peritoneum is used as the dialyzing surface.

The dialysate solution contains water, glucose, and normal serum electrolytes but no body waste products. When the solution is instilled into the peritoneal cavity, the body's waste products, excess electrolytes, and excess fluids pass by diffusion and osmosis across the semipermeable peritoneal membrane to the dialysate. The dialysate containing these waste products is then removed from the peritoneal cavity and replaced with fresh dialysate. This process replaces kidney function and permits the kidneys to rest.

For peritoneal dialysis, the physician inserts a catheter into the peritoneal cavity. This may be done at the bedside or in the operating room. Nurses assist with the insertion of the catheter, change the dressing at the catheter site, perform fluid exchanges, and assist with removal of the catheter. The basic peritoneal dialysis system and its components are shown in Figure 28–26.

There are currently three types of peritoneal dialysis: intermittent peritoneal dialysis (IPD), continuous ambulatory peritoneal dialysis (CAPD), and continuous cycling peritoneal dialysis (CCPD). Intermittent peritoneal dialysis is performed within the acute care setting and is the focus of Technique 28–

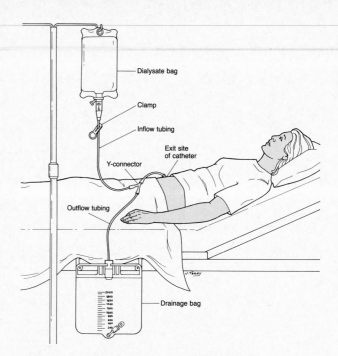

FIGURE 28–26 Basic equipment for peritoneal dialysis.

13. IPD involves the infusion of one bag of dialysate solution at a time. Continuous cycling peritoneal dialysis is performed both in the acute care setting and at home by some clients who are capable of operating the cyclers. CCPD involves the use of as many as eight to twelve bags of dialysate solution, with premeasured amounts of dialysate simultaneously infused through a mechanical fluid regulator and warmer. Continuous ambulatory peritoneal dialysis is also performed by clients and allows the clients to go home with a peritoneal catheter in place and perform the exchange on themselves. Often they need to do this three to six times a day to eliminate waste products from the body. The client is ambulatory and free to resume normal activities between exchanges. With CAPD, the focus of nursing care is on teaching the client and family to perform the dialysis treatments at home.

Most hospital and dialysis unit protocols require persons performing dialysis procedures to wear sterile gloves and masks for even the most basic of dialysis-related procedures. Gowns and goggles should also be worn, as appropriate, when there is a risk of additional contact with contaminated peritoneal fluid through splashing or other means. The client and any family or visitors in the immediate environment should also wear masks. Appropriate handwashing protocols should be followed before, during, and after dialysis procedures.

28-13   Managing Peritoneal Dialysis

Before initiating dialysis, determine the physician's order specifying the amount and type of solution for each peritoneal exchange, the number of exchanges, the length of time the fluid is to remain in the peritoneal cavity, and the amount of fluid to be withdrawn from the peritoneal cavity.

PURPOSE

• To remove impurities, excess fluid, and electrolytes from the blood that would normally be excreted through the kidneys

ASSESSMENT FOCUS

Vital signs, for baseline data; weight, for baseline data and subsequent comparisons; abdominal girth, as an indication of fluid retention; respiratory status (rate, character, and breath sounds) as an indication of fluid retention; presence of edema; status of electrolytes, blood glucose level, and hematology profile studies.

EQUIPMENT

For Inserting a Peritoneal Catheter

□ Sterile gloves, masks, caps, goggles, and gowns for physician, nurse, and anyone assisting; mask for client and family
□ Sterile peritoneal dialysis set containing
   Peritoneal catheter
   Local anesthetic (e.g., lidocaine), #25 gauge ⅝-inch needle, and 3-ml syringe
   Alcohol sponges
   Scalpel with a blade
   Precut gauze to place around the catheter
   Drape
   Tubing and clamp
   Sutures, needles, and needle driver

   Trocar
   Connector
   4 × 4 gauze square
   Specimen container
   Antiseptic ointment, e.g., povidone-iodine
   Protective catheter cap
   10-ml syringe and 1 ½-inch needle
   Scissors
□ Skin preparation set containing
   Povidone-iodine solution
   Razor and blade
   Gauze sponges
   Nonallergenic tape

For Infusing the Dialysate
□ 1000- or 2000-ml container of peritoneal solution at body temperature, of the amount

and kind ordered by the physician
□ IV pole
□ Drainage bag
□ Sterile peritoneal dialysis administration set
□ Dialysis log or flow sheet
□ Gloves, mask, goggles, gown

For Changing the Catheter Site Dressing
□ Sterile gloves and masks (gowns and goggles as needed)
□ Sterile cotton-tipped applicators
□ Hydrogen peroxide
□ Povidone-iodine solution
□ Povidone-iodine ointment
□ Precut sterile 2 × 2 gauze or slit transparent occlusive dressing
□ Nonallergenic tape

INTERVENTION

1. Explain the technique and its purpose to the client and family.

• Explain that since the kidneys are not functioning properly, this procedure will rid the blood and body of excess waste and fluid that are normally excreted by the kidneys.

• Explain that inserting the trocar (which is the physician's responsibility) may be uncomfortable. If the client tenses the abdominal muscles as if for a bowel move-

ment, the discomfort can be reduced.

• Explain that the purpose of the masks, gowns, gloves, and caps is to reduce the possibility of infection (peritonitis). Then explain that the client and any family in the room will also need to wear masks.

2. Prepare the client.

• Ask the client to urinate before the procedure. *Emptying the*

bladder lessens the danger that it will be punctured by the trocar.

• Assist the client to a supine position, and arrange the bedding to expose the area around the umbilicus. *The insertion site is usually in the midline just below the umbilicus.*

• Provide a mask.

3. Prepare the solution and the tubing.

• Check the label on the solution

▶ **Technique 28–13 Managing Peritoneal Dialysis** *CONTINUED*

container and the solution itself. The solution should be clear and the seals unbroken.

- Add any prescribed medication to the dialysate solution. Heparin is sometimes added to prevent the accumulation of fibrin in the catheter; povidone-iodine solution or antibiotics may be added to prevent the growth of microorganisms; potassium is often added to prevent excessive loss of potassium.

- Spike the solution container, close the clamp, and hang the container on the IV pole.

- Prime the tubing (see Technique 25–1, step 5, on page 595). Close the tubing clamp. *This rids the tubing of air that could enter the peritoneal cavity, causing discomfort and preventing free drainage outflow.*

4. Implement surgical aseptic practices and body fluid precautions according to agency protocol.

- Don a mask, and provide masks to the client and anyone else present. *Applying masks prior to breaking the seals on the containers reduces the chance of solution contamination.*

- Don a cap, a gown, and goggles.

- Open the sterile supplies.

- Don sterile gloves.

5. Assist the physician as needed during and after the catheter insertion.

- Connect the end of the tubing from the solution to the catheter.

- Connect the drainage receptacle to the outflow tubing. Close the outflow tubing clamp.

- Cover the catheter site with the precut sterile gauze, and tape the dressing in place.

6. Infuse the peritoneal dialysate.

- Open the clamp on the inflow tubing so that the dialysate can flow into the peritoneal cavity for the time period specified by the order. If no rate is specified, the client can usually tolerate a steady open flow.

- After the fluid has infused, clamp the inflow tubing. *With the tubing clamped, air will not enter the peritoneal cavity.*

- Leave the fluid in the cavity for the designated time period. This "dwell" time may range from 10 minutes to 4 hours.

7. Ensure client comfort and safety.

- Assist the client into a comfortable position.

- Place the call light within the client's reach, lift all bed rails, and lower the bed to its lowest position.

- Monitor the client's vital signs every 15 minutes for the first exchange and hourly on subsequent exchanges.

- Periodically assess the client's respiratory status and the status of comfort or discomfort during the dwell time.

8. Remove the fluid.

- Reapply gloves, gown, goggles, and mask according to agency protocol.

- Unclamp the outflow tubing, and permit the fluid to drain into the drainage bag by gravity for about 30 minutes.

- If the fluid does not drain freely, assist the client to change position, or raise the head of the bed. Drain only the amount specified by the order.

9. Assess the outflow fluid.

- Assess the appearance of the out-

flow fluid. *A cloudy, pink-tinged or blood-tinged return may indicate peritonitis.* During the first two to four exchanges, the return may be blood-tinged but should quickly progress to a straw-color return.

- Measure the amount of outflow fluid, and discard the fluid in an appropriate area.

10. Calculate the fluid balance for each exchange.

- Compare the amount of outflow fluid with the amount of solution infused for each exchange.

- If more fluid was infused than removed, the client's fluid balance is positive (+); if more fluid was removed than infused, the fluid balance is negative (−).

Example:
```
+ 2000 ml 2.5% dialysate
          solution infused
− 1500 ml dialysate fluid
          returned in
          drainage bag
_____
+  500 ml balance for
          this exchange
```

- Repeat steps 6 through 10 for each exchange.

11. Calculate the cumulative fluid balance. The cumulative fluid balance should be negative.

- Add the balance from each exchange (from step 10) to the total exchange balance:

Example:

Previous cumulative exchange balance	− 100 ml
Present exchange balance	+ 500 ml
Cumulative exchange balance	+ 400 ml

12. Check the dressing at the catheter site.

- Wear a mask and sterile gloves when assessing the dryness or wetness of the dressing. *The*

▶ **Technique 28–13** *CONTINUED*

dressing should remain dry during dialysis.

• To change the catheter site dressing, follow Technique 39–2 on page 924.

13. Disconnect the catheter from the tubing, and cover the end of the catheter with a new sterile cap. *This allows the catheter*

to remain in place between each of the exchanges without contamination of the catheter.

14. Document all relevant information.

• Record the date and time of the procedure or the time during which the fluid infused; exchange number; dialysate and additives used; weight of each di-

alysate outflow bag (required by some institutions); amount of time fluid remains in abdomen for each exchange; color of outflow dialysate return from client; client's response; appearance of exit site and dressing; and client's weight before and after the set of exchanges.

EVALUATION FOCUS	Appearance and amount of outflow dialysate; respiratory status (breath sounds, rate, and character); other vital signs; mental status; presence of pain or discomfort; abdominal girth measurement; status of dressing and catheter exit site; client's weight; fluid balance for each exchange; cumulative fluid balance.

SAMPLE RECORDING

Date	Time	Notes
06/09/92	1500	Dialysis #1 2000 ml 2.5 dialysate commenced. BP 100/40; P 102; R 20 shallow. Abd. girth 115 cm. Weight before dialysis 88 kg. Rosie Lam, SN
06/09/92	1600	1500 cloudy pink tinged dialysate returned. Vital signs unchanged. ——————— Rosie Lam, SN

CRITICAL THINKING CHALLENGE

The physician has ordered an indwelling catheter for Anne Jenkins, a 44-year-old female, who is scheduled for an abdominal hysterectomy. When inserting the catheter, you insert it into the vagina instead of the urinary meatus. What action should you take? Why?

RELATED RESEARCH

Brown, J.; Meikle, J.; and Webb, C. March 27–April 2, 1991. Collecting midstream specimens of urine—the research base. *Nursing Times* 87:49–52.

Burgener, S. March 1987. Justification of closed intermittent urinary catheter irrigation/instillation: A review of current research and practice. *Journal of Advanced Nursing* 12:229–34.

Clarey, B., and Malone-Lee, J. February 1991. Reducing the leakage of body-worn incontinence pads. *Journal of Advanced Nursing* 16:187–93.

REFERENCES

Barnett, J. March 6–12, 1991. Preventive procedures . . . catheter care. *Nursing Times* 87:66, 68.

Birdsall, C. May 1986. How do you manage peritoneal dialysis. *American Journal of Nursing* 86:592, 596.

Bristol, S. L.; Fadden, T.; Fehring, R. J.; Rohde, L.; Prue, K. S.; and Wohlitz, B. A. March 1989. The mythical danger of rapid urinary drainage. *American Journal of Nursing* 89:344–45.

Classen, D. C.; Larsen, R. A.; Burke, J. P.; and Stevens, L. E. June 1991. Prevention of catheter-associated bacteriuria: Clinical trial of methods to block three known pathways of infection. *American Journal of Infection Control* 19:136–42.

Epstein, S. E. December 1985. Cost-effective application of the Centers for Disease Control Guidelines for prevention of catheter-associated urinary tract infections. *American Journal of Infection Control* 13:272–75.

Ignataviticus, D., and Bayne, M. 1991. *Medical surgical nursing: A nursing approach.* Philadelphia: W. B. Saunders Co.

Jensen, S. R.; Davidson, M.; Pomeroy, M.; Cox, M.; et al. October 1989. Evaluation of dressing protocols that reduce peritoneal dialysis catheter exit site infections. *American Nephrology Nurses' Association Journal* 16(6):425–31.

Meeusen, M., and Giroux, J. June 1991. What do you think? . . . bladder management. *SCI Nursing* 8:55.

Powers, I., and Williams, D. March/April 1991. Urinary incontinence. *Advancing Clinical Care* 6:10–15.

Richard, C. J. 1986. *Comprehensive Nephrology Nursing.* Boston: Little, Brown & Co.

Roe, B. October 24–30, 1990. Do we need to clamp catheters? *Nursing Times* 86:66–67.

Strangio, L. January 1988. Peritoneal dialysis made easy. *Nursing 88* 18:43–46.

Warren, H. May 1989. Changes in peritoneal dialysis nursing. *American Nephrology Nurses' Association Journal* 16(3):237–38, 240–41.

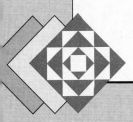

29

Ostomy Care

OBJECTIVES

- Identify various types of bowel and urinary diversion ostomies

- Describe major ways ostomies are constructed

- Discuss selected nursing interventions for clients with bowel diversion ostomies

- Differentiate between distal and proximal stomas of bowel diversion ostomies

- Explain how and why the character of drainage differs among selected "ostomy" sites

- Identify pertinent assessment data related to an ostomy client

- Change bowel diversion ostomy and urinary diversion ostomy appliances

- Irrigate a colostomy

- Give reasons for selected steps underlying the techniques in this chapter

- Document essential information related to ostomy care

CONTENTS

NURSING PROCESS GUIDE
OSTOMY CARE

ASSESSMENT

Determine

- The kind of ostomy and its placement on the abdomen. Surgeons often draw diagrams when there are two stomas. It is important to confirm which is the functioning stoma, if it is a bowel diversion ostomy.

- The type and size of appliance currently used and the special barrier substance applied to the skin, according to the nursing care plan.

- Tape allergy.

- A 24-hour tape-patch test, experimenting with at least three or four different types of tape (silk, paper, and foam) is usually done *before* the client has surgery and on the nonoperative side.

Assess

- Stoma color: The stoma should appear red, similar in color to the mucosal lining of the inner cheek. Very pale or darker-colored stomas with a bluish or purplish hue indicate impaired blood circulation to the area.

- Stoma size and shape: Most stomas protrude slightly from the abdomen. New stomas normally appear swollen, but swelling generally decreases over 2 or 3 weeks or for as long as 6 weeks. Failure of swelling to recede may indicate a problem, e.g., blockage.

- Stomal bleeding: Slight bleeding initially when the stoma is touched is normal, but other bleeding should be reported.

- Status of peristomal skin: Any redness and irritation of the peristomal skin—the 5 to 13 cm (2 to 5 in) of skin surrounding the stoma—should be noted. Transient redness after removal of adhesive is normal.

- Amount and type of feces: For ileal effluent and feces (colostomy effluent), assess the amount, color, odor, and consistency. Inspect for abnormalities, such as pus or blood. For a urinary diversion ostomy, assess the amount, color, clarity, and odor of the urine.

- Complaints. Complaints of burning sensation under the faceplate may indicate skin breakdown. The presence of abdominal discomfort and/or distention also needs to be determined.

- The client's and family members' learning needs regarding the ostomy and self-care.

- The client's emotional status.

RELATED DIAGNOSTIC CATEGORIES

- Body image disturbance
- High risk for Fluid volume deficit
- Knowledge deficit
- Self-esteem disturbance
- High risk for Impaired skin integrity

PLANNING

Client Goals
The client will

- Avoid complications associated with a stoma.
- Manage ostomy care independently.
- Achieve a positive body image and self-esteem.

Outcome Criteria
The client

- Has intact peristomal skin.
- Voices minimal abdominal discomfort.
- Has a fluid output in balance with fluid intake.
- Has a red-colored stoma.
- Experiences a reduction in stomal size over a period of 2 to 3 weeks.
- Evacuates effluent without pus or blood (*or* evacuates urine that is amber colored and clear).
- Identifies foods that may cause obstruction of the stoma.
- Identifies signs and symptoms of fluid and electrolyte imbalance.
- Demonstrates application of the ostomy appliance as taught.
- Demonstrates the correct procedure for irrigating the colostomy.
- Describes changes in thoughts and feelings about self.
- Verbalizes acceptance of physical changes that have occurred.
- Looks at and touches the changed body part.
- Shares feelings about self with significant others.
- Expresses satisfaction with own achievements.

Bowel Diversion Ostomies

An **"ostomy"** is an opening on the abdominal wall for the elimination of feces or urine. There are many types of ostomies. A **gastrostomy** is an opening through the abdominal wall into the stomach. A **jejunostomy** is an opening through the abdominal wall into the jejunum. An **ileostomy** is an opening into the ileum (small bowel). A **colostomy** is an opening into the colon (large bowel). A **ureterostomy** is an opening into the ureter. Gastrostomies and jejunostomies are generally performed to provide an alternate feeding route. The purpose of bowel and urinary ostomies is to divert and drain fecal or urinary material. Urinary diversion ostomies are discussed later in this chapter. Bowel diversion ostomies are often classified according to (a) their status as permanent or temporary, (b) their anatomic location, and (c) the construction of the **stoma**, the opening created in the abdominal wall by the "ostomy."

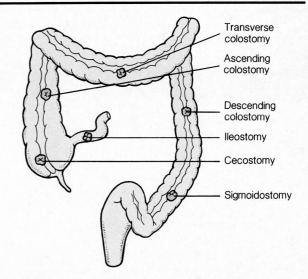

FIGURE 29–1 The locations of bowel diversion ostomies.

Permanence

Colostomies can be either temporary or permanent. Temporary colostomies are generally performed for traumatic injuries or inflammatory conditions of the bowel. They allow the distal diseased portion of the bowel to rest and heal. Permanent colostomies are performed to provide a means of elimination when the rectum or anus is nonfunctional as a result of disease or birth defect. They are commonly performed for diseases such as cancer of the bowel. The diseased portion may or may not be removed.

Anatomic Location

An ileostomy generally empties from the distal end of the small intestine. A cecostomy empties from the cecum (the first part of the ascending colon). An ascending colostomy empties from the ascending colon. A transverse colostomy empties from the transverse colon. A descending colostomy empties from the descending colon. A sigmoidostomy empties from the sigmoid colon (Figure 29–1).

The location of the ostomy influences the character and management of the fecal drainage. The farther along the bowel, the more formed the stool, since the large bowel reabsorbs water from the fecal mass. In addition, more control over the frequency of stomal discharge can be established. For example:

- An ileostomy produces liquid fecal drainage. Drainage is constant and cannot be regulated. Ileostomy drainage contains some digestive

enzymes, which are damaging to the skin. For this reason, ileostomy clients must wear an appliance continuously and take special precautions to prevent skin breakdown. Compared to colostomies, however, odor is minimal because fewer bacteria are present.

- An ascending colostomy is similar to an ileostomy in that the drainage is liquid and cannot be regulated, and digestive enzymes are present. Odor, however, is a problem requiring control (e.g., a deodorant inside the appliance).

- A transverse colostomy produces a malodorous, mushy drainage because some of the liquid has been reabsorbed. There is usually no control.

- A descending colostomy produces increasingly solid fecal drainage. Stools from a sigmoidostomy are of normal or formed consistency, and the frequency of discharge can be regulated. People with a sigmoidostomy may not have to wear an appliance at all times, and odors can usually be controlled.

The length of time that an ostomy is in place also helps to determine the consistency of the stool, particularly with transverse and descending colostomies. Over time, the stool becomes more formed because the remaining functioning portions of the colon tend to compensate by increasing water reabsorption.

Construction

There are three major types of stoma constructions: the loop colostomy, the double-barreled colostomy, and the end colostomy.

• For a loop colostomy (Figure 29–2, A), a loop of bowel is brought out onto the abdomen. To keep the bowel from slipping back, the surgeon may place a plastic rod underneath the bowel loop, opened (unfolded) so that it lies flat against the abdomen, and sutured to the skin. The rod holds the bowel in place until the underlying abdominal incision heals (7 to 10 days). During surgery or 2 to 3 days after surgery, one or two openings are made into the bowel loop by cautery or by inci-

sion. If two openings are made, the proximal (or functioning) opening discharges fecal material. The other opening is the distal or nonfunctioning end. It discharges only mucus unless emergency surgery was performed without the usual bowel preparation. In this instance some fecal matter may be discharged. When only one opening is made, it connects to both proximal and distal parts of the bowel. The loop colostomy is relatively large and cumbersome. It is created generally for an emergency, e.g., an acute bowel obstruction or bowel injury. Complete diversion of fecal matter is not achieved with this procedure because the bowel is not separated.

• In the double-barreled colostomy (Figure 29–2, B), two separate stomas are constructed. One is the proximal, or functioning, stoma, and the other is the distal, or resting, stoma. The stomas are generally adjacent to one another—one above the other or side by side.

• An end colostomy has only one stoma (Figure 29–2, C), which arises from the end of the proximal portion of the bowel. The distal end of the bowel and rectum is either resected (abdominoperineal resection, which is removal through abdominal and perineal incisions) or is closed off by sutures and remains in the abdominal space. The latter is often referred to as an "end colostomy and Hartmann pouch," the pouch referring to the remaining distal portion of the bowel.

Stoma and Skin Care

Care of the stoma (Figure 29–3) and skin is important for all clients who have ostomies. The fecal material from a colostomy or ileostomy is irritating to the peristomal skin. This is particularly true of ileal effluent, which contains digestive enzymes. It is important to assess the peristomal skin for irritation each time the appliance is changed. Any irritations or skin breakdown need to be treated immediately. The skin is kept clean by washing off any excretion and then dried thoroughly. A barrier such as karaya is applied over the skin around the stoma to prevent contact with any excretion. An appliance (bag) is then fitted to the stoma so that there is no leakage around it. It is exceedingly important to dry the skin before attaching the appliance. The pouch will not adhere to moist skin, causing effluent to leak onto the skin. Numerous pouch systems are commercially available. All appliances have three features in common: a pouch to collect the effluent, an outlet at the bottom for easy emptying, and a faceplate. Temporary, disposable pouches are made of transparent plastic and have a

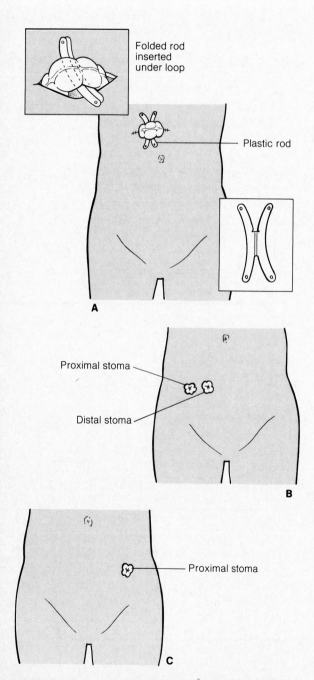

Folded rod inserted under loop

Plastic rod

A

Proximal stoma

Distal stoma

B

Proximal stoma

C

FIGURE 29–2 Three types of colostomies: A, the loop colostomy using a plastic rod; B, the double-barreled colostomy; C, the end colostomy.

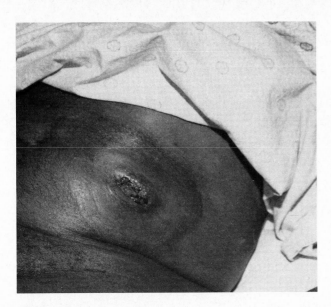

FIGURE 29–3 A colostomy stoma.

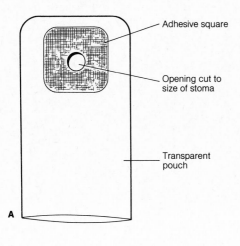

Adhesive square

Opening cut to size of stoma

Transparent pouch

A

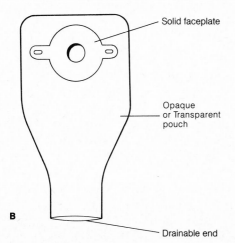

Solid faceplate

Opaque or Transparent pouch

B

Drainable end

FIGURE 29–4 Ostomy appliances: *A*, temporary, disposable; *B*, permanent, reusable.

peel-off adhesive square into which a hole the size of the stoma is cut. Permanent pouches may be clear or opaque, rubber or vinyl and have a solid ring faceplate that fits around the stoma (Figure 29–4).

Odor control is essential to clients' self-esteem. As soon as clients are ambulatory, they can learn to work with the ostomy in the bathroom to avoid odors at the bedside. Selecting the appropriate kind of appliance promotes odor control. An intact appliance contains odors. The appliance should be rinsed thoroughly when it is emptied. Deodorizers can be placed in the pouch of the appliance, or pouches with charcoal filter discs are available. Some recommend oral intake of charcoal or bismuth subcarbonate, which should be taken only with the physician's approval. See the box below for criteria for ostomy appliances. Many agencies employ an enterostomal therapy nurse who can assist in selecting the appliance.

Disposable ostomy appliances can be applied for up to 7 days. They need to be changed whenever the effluent leaks onto the peristomal skin or when it cannot be rinsed completely away. Many people prefer to change them daily or whenever they become soiled, but this practice can be detrimental to the integrity of the peristomal skin and is expensive.

Criteria for Ostomy Appliances

The ostomy appliance should

- Be odor-resistant.
- Protect peristomal skin. The faceplate opening needs to fit closely around the stoma.
- Stay secure for 3 to 5 days.
- Be nonallergenic (bags with adhesive-backed discs).
- Be readily available, affordable, and appealing to the client.
- Be invisible underneath clothing.

Disposable postoperative pouches should be

- Transparent, to allow assessment of the stoma.
- Odorproof, to enhance client acceptability.
- Drainable, so that the pouch need not be removed to be emptied.
- Adjustable, so that the size of the opening can be altered to accommodate changes in stoma shape and size as edema resolves.

Check agency practice in this regard. Erickson (1987, p. 314) recommends removing the pouch and skin barrier twice a week to clean and inspect the peristomal skin. If the peristomal skin is erythematous, Broadwell (1987, p. 331) recommends removing and changing the system every 48 to 72 hours; if the skin is eroded, denuded, or ulcerated, it should be changed every 24 to 48 hours to allow appropriate treatment of the skin. More frequent changes are recommended if the client complains of pain or discomfort. Technique 29–1 explains how to change a bowel diversion ostomy appliance.

Changing a Bowel Diversion Ostomy Appliance

Before changing a bowel diversion ostomy appliance, determine the kind of ostomy and its placement on the abdomen. It is important to confirm which is the functioning stoma and any orders about the care of the stomas.

PURPOSES
- To assess and care for the peristomal skin
- To collect effluent for assessment of the amount and type of output
- To minimize odors for the client's comfort and self-esteem

ASSESSMENT FOCUS

Stoma size and shape; color of stoma; presence of swelling; status of peristomal skin; amount and type of effluent; allergy to tape; type and size of appliance currently used; complaints of discomfort; client and family learning needs; client's emotional status (see Nursing Process Guide on page 722).

EQUIPMENT

- Disposable gloves
- Electric or safety razor
- Bedpan
- Solvent (presaturated sponges or liquid)
- Moistureproof bag (for disposable pouches)
- Cleaning materials, including tissues, warm water, mild soap (optional), washcloth or cotton balls, towel

- Tissue or gauze pad
- Peristomal skin paste or powder
- Skin barrier (liquid protective covering or peristomal skin barrier)
- Measuring guide
- Pen or pencil
- Scissors
- Clean ostomy appliance, with optional belt

- Tail closure or elastic band
- Special adhesive and brush, if needed
- Stoma guidestrip, if needed
- Deodorant (liquid or tablet) for a nonodorproof colostomy bag
- Tape for securing a detachable faceplate as necessary

INTERVENTION

1. Determine the need for appliance change.

- Assess the used appliance for leakage of effluent. *Effluent can irritate the peristomal skin.*

- Ask the client about any discomfort at or around the stoma. *A burning sensation may indicate breakdown beneath the faceplate of the pouch.*

- Assess the fullness of the pouch. Pouches need to be emptied when they are one-third to one-half full. *The weight of an overly full bag may loosen the faceplate and separate it from the skin, causing the effluent to leak and irritate the peristomal skin.*

- If there is pouch leakage or discomfort at or around the stoma,

change the appliance.

2. Select an appropriate time.

- Avoid times close to meal or visiting hours. *Ostomy odor and effluent may reduce appetite or embarrass the client.*

- Avoid times immediately after the administration of any medications that may stimulate bowel

▶ **Technique 29–1** *CONTINUED*

evacuation. *It is best to change the pouch when drainage is least likely to occur.*

3. Prepare the client and support persons.

- Explain the procedure to the client and support persons. Changing an ostomy appliance should not cause discomfort, but it may be distasteful to the client. *Support persons are often more supportive if properly informed.*

- Communicate acceptance and support to the client. It is important to change the appliance competently and quickly and not to convey disgust.

- Provide privacy, preferably in the bathroom, where clients can learn to deal with the ostomy as they would at home.

- Assist the client to a comfortable sitting or lying position in bed or preferably a sitting or standing position in the bathroom. *Lying or standing positions may facilitate smoother pouch application, i.e., avoid wrinkles.*

- Don gloves, and unfasten the belt if the client is wearing one.

4. Shave the peristomal skin of well-established ostomies as needed.

- Use an electric or safety razor on a regular basis to remove excessive hair. *Hair follicles can become irritated or infected by repeated pulling out of hairs during removal of the appliance and skin barrier.*

5. Empty and remove the ostomy appliance.

- Empty the contents of the pouch through the bottom opening into a bedpan. *Emptying before removing the pouch prevents spillage of effluent onto the client's skin.*

- Assess the consistency and the amount of effluent.

- If needed, apply an adhesive solvent to remove the appliance. This is not needed in most cases and should be used only when absolutely necessary.

- Peel the bag off slowly while holding the client's skin taut. *Holding the skin taut minimizes client discomfort and prevents abrasion of the skin.*

- If the appliance is disposable, discard it in a moistureproof bag.

6. Clean and dry the peristomal skin and stoma.

- Use toilet tissue to remove excess stool.

- Use warm water, mild soap (optional), and cotton balls or a washcloth and towel to clean the skin and stoma. Check agency practice on the use of soap. *Soap is sometimes not advised because it can be irritating to the skin.*

- Use a special skin cleanser to remove dried, hard stool. *This emulsifies the stool, making removal less damaging to the skin.*

- Dry the area thoroughly by patting with a towel or cotton swabs. *Excess rubbing can abrade the skin.*

7. Assess the stoma and peristomal skin.

- Inspect the stoma for color, size, shape, and bleeding.

- Inspect the peristomal skin for any redness, ulceration, or irritation. Transient redness *after the removal of adhesive* is normal.

- Place a piece of tissue or gauze pad over the stoma, and change it as needed. *This absorbs any seepage from the stoma.*

8. Apply paste-type skin barrier if needed.

- Fill in abdominal creases or dimples with paste. *This establishes a smooth surface for application of the skin barrier and pouch.*

- Allow the paste to dry for 1 to 2 minutes or as recommended by the manufacturer.

9. Prepare and apply the skin barrier (peristomal seal).

For a Solid Wafer or Disc Skin Barrier

- Use the guide (Figure 29–5) to measure the size of the stoma.

- On the backing of the skin barrier, trace a circle the same size as the stomal opening.

- Make a template (mold) out of cardboard or heavy paper of the stoma pattern. Keep this template for future use. *A template aids other nurses and the client with future appliance changes.* However, the template will need to be adjusted as the stoma size decreases.

- Cut out the traced stoma pattern to make an opening in the skin barrier.

- Remove the backing to expose the sticky adhesive side.

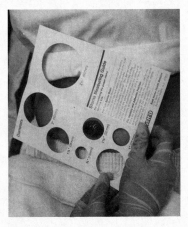

FIGURE 29–5 A guide for measuring the stoma.

▶ **Technique 29–1 Changing an Ostomy Appliance** *CONTINUED*

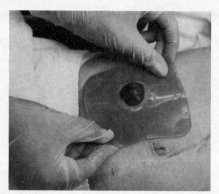

FIGURE 29–6 Centering the skin barrier over the stoma.

• Center the skin barrier over the stoma, and gently press it onto the client's skin, smoothing out any wrinkles or bubbles (Figure 29–6).

For Liquid Skin Sealant

• Cover the stoma with a gauze pad. *This prevents contact with the skin sealant.*

• Either wipe the product evenly around the peristomal skin, or use a brush to apply a thin layer of the liquid plastic coating to the same area.

• Allow the skin barrier to dry until it no longer feels tacky.

10. Fill in any exposed skin around an irregularly shaped stoma.

• Apply paste to any exposed skin areas. Use a nonalcohol-based product if the skin is excoriated. *Alcohol may cause stinging and burning.*
or
Sprinkle peristomal powder on the skin, wipe off the excess, and dab the powder with a slightly moist gauze or an applicator moistened with a liquid skin barrier. *This creates a barrier or seal.*

11. Prepare and apply the clean appliance.

• Remove the tissue over the stoma before applying the pouch.

For a Disposable Pouch with Adhesive Square

• If the appliance does not have a precut opening, trace a circle ⅛ to ⅙ inch larger than the stoma size on the appliance's adhesive square. *The opening is made slightly larger than the stoma to prevent rubbing, cutting, or trauma to the stoma.*

• Cut out a circle in the adhesive. Take care not to cut any portion of the pouch.

• Peel off the backing from the adhesive seal.

• Center the opening of the pouch over the client's stoma, and apply it directly onto the skin barrier (Figure 29–7).

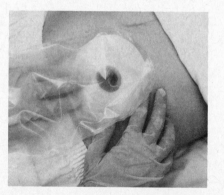

FIGURE 29–7 Applying the disposable pouch.

• Gently press the adhesive backing onto the skin and smooth out any wrinkles, working from the stoma outward. *Wrinkles allow seepage of effluent, which can irritate the skin or soil clothing.*

• Remove the air from the pouch. *Removing the air helps the pouch lie flat against the abdomen.*

• Place a deodorant in the pouch (optional).

• Close the pouch by turning up the bottom a few times, fanfolding its end lengthwise and securing it with a rubber band or tail closure clamp.

For a Reusable Pouch with Faceplate Attached

• Apply either adhesive cement or a double-faced adhesive disc to the faceplate of the appliance, depending on the type of appliance being used. Follow the manufacturer's directions.

• Insert a coiled paper guidestrip (15-cm [6-in] strip of 1.3-cm [½-in] wide paper) into the faceplate opening (Figure 29–8). The strip should protrude slightly from the opening and expand to fit it. *The guidestrip helps you center the appliance over the stoma and prevents pressure or irritation to the stoma due to an ill-fitting appliance.*

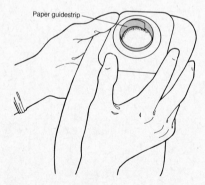

Paper guidestrip

FIGURE 29–8 The coiled paper guidestrip in the faceplate opening.

• Using the guidestrip, center the faceplate over the stoma.

• Firmly press the adhesive seal to the peristomal skin. The guidestrip will fall into the pouch; commercially prepared guidestrips will dissolve in the pouch.

• Place a deodorant in the bag if the bag is not odorproof. Most pouches are odorproof.

▶ **Technique 29–1** *CONTINUED*

- Close the end of the pouch with the designated clamp.

- Attach the pouch belt, and fasten it around the client's waist (optional).

12. Dispose of or clean reusable equipment.

- Discard disposable bags in plastic bags before placing in the waste container.

- If feces is liquid, measure its volume before emptying the feces into a toilet or hopper.

- Wash reusable bags with cool water and mild soap, rinse, and dry.

- Wash a soiled belt with warm water and mild soap, rinse, and dry.

- Remove and discard gloves.

13. Report and record pertinent assessments and interventions.

- Report to the nurse in charge any increase in stoma size, change in color indicative of circulatory impairment, and presence of skin irritation or erosion.

- Record on the client's chart discoloration of the stoma; the appearance of the peristomal skin; the amount and type of drainage; the client's fatigue, discomfort, and significant behavior about the ostomy; and skills learned.

- Adjust the teaching plan and nursing care plan as needed. Include on the teaching plan the equipment and procedure used. *Client learning is facilitated by consistent nursing implementations.*

VARIATION: Applying a Reusable Pouch with Detachable Faceplate

- Note allergies and the results of tape patch test performed before surgery.

- Some nurses recommend applying a skin sealant (e.g., Skin Prep) to the faceplate before attaching the adhesive disc. *This makes it easier to remove the adhesive disc from the faceplate.*

- Remove the protective paper strip from one side of the double-faced adhesive disc.

- Apply the sticky side to the back of the faceplate.

- Remove the remaining protective paper strip from the other side of the adhesive disc.

- Center the faceplate over the stoma and skin barrier, then press and hold the faceplate against the client's skin for a few minutes to secure the seal.

- Press the adhesive around the circumference of the adhesive disc.

- Tape the faceplate to the client's abdomen using four or eight 7.5-cm (3-in) strips of hypoallergenic tape. Place the strips around the faceplate in a "picture-framing" manner, one strip down each side, one across the top, and one across the bottom (Figure 29–9). The additional four strips can be placed diagonally over the other tapes to secure the seal.

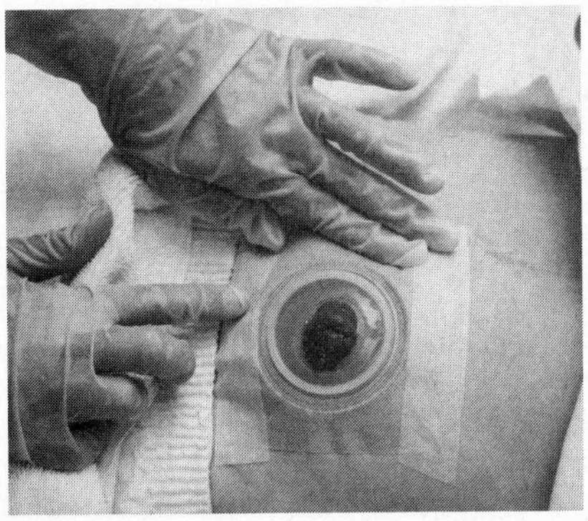

FIGURE 29–9 Taping the faceplate to the client's abdomen.

- Stretch the opening on the back of the pouch, and position it over the base of the faceplate. Ease it over the faceplate flange.

- Place the lock ring between the pouch and the faceplate flange (Figure 29–10) to seal the pouch against the faceplate.

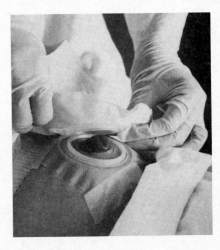

FIGURE 29–10 Sealing the pouch against the faceplate.

- Close the base of the pouch with the appropriate clamp.

- Attach the pouch belt, and fasten it around the client's waist (optional).

VARIATION: Applying the Skin Barrier and Appliance as One Unit

If a disc- or wafer-type skin barrier is used, the skin barrier and appliance can be applied as one unit. Applying the skin barrier and the appliance together not only is quicker but also is thought to reduce the chance of wrinkles. It also is easier for the client to apply without help.

- Prepare the skin barrier by measuring the size of the stoma, tracing a circle on the backing of the skin barrier, and cutting out the traced stoma pattern to make an opening in the skin barrier.

► **Technique 29–1 Changing an Ostomy Appliance** *CONTINUED*

- Prepare the appliance by cutting an opening ⅛ to ⅙ inch larger than the stoma size (if not already present) and peeling off the backing from the adhesive seal.

- Center the opening of the pouch over the skin barrier.

- Remove the skin barrier backing to expose the sticky adhesive side.

- Center the skin barrier and appliance over the stoma, and press it onto the client's skin.

EVALUATION FOCUS

Color and size of stoma; amount, color, and consistency of feces; status of peristomal skin; client responses.

SAMPLE RECORDING

Date	Time	Notes
10/05/93	1400	Colostomy appliance changed. 350 ml dark brown liquid feces. Stoma pink, 8 cm. Peristomal skin intact. States no discomfort. Helped to clean the peristomal skin. ———————— Ramona L. de Santo, NS

KEY ELEMENTS OF CHANGING A BOWEL DIVERSION OSTOMY APPLIANCE

- Communicate acceptance and support.
- Assess the stoma, peristomal skin, and effluent.
- Wear gloves.
- Determine allergies to adhesives.
- Empty the pouch when only one-half to one-third full.
- Hold the skin taut when removing the appliance.
- Keep adhesive solvent off the stoma.
- Thoroughly clean and dry the skin before applying the skin barrier.

- Apply skin barriers appropriately.
- Make sure the appliance is the correct size.
- Use a guidestrip to center the faceplate of a reusable pouch over the stoma.
- Smooth out any wrinkles of a disposable appliance.
- Make sure the appliance is fastened securely to the abdomen.
- Determine the client's readiness to participate in colostomy care.

Colostomy Irrigation

A colostomy irrigation, similar to an enema, is a form of stoma management used only for clients who have a sigmoid or descending colostomy. The purpose of irrigation is to distend the bowel sufficiently to stimulate peristalsis, which promotes evacuation. Clients who achieve a regular evacuation pattern usually need not wear a colostomy pouch.

Whether to perform routine daily irrigations to control the time of elimination is ultimately the client's decision. Some clients prefer to control the time of elimination through rigid dietary regulation, thus avoiding irrigations, which can take up to an hour to complete. Clients who elect to perform irri-

gations should perform them at the same time each day. Control by irrigations also necessitates some control of the diet. For example, clients need to avoid laxative foods that might cause an unexpected evacuation.

For most clients, a relatively small amount of fluid (300 to 500 ml) stimulates evacuation. Others may need up to 1000 ml, since a colostomy has no sphincter and the fluid tends to return as it is instilled. This problem is reduced by the use of a cone on the irrigating catheter. The cone helps to hold the fluid within the bowel during the irrigation.

Before starting an irrigation, assess the client's readiness to select and use the equipment. Because many types of irrigation sets are available, clients

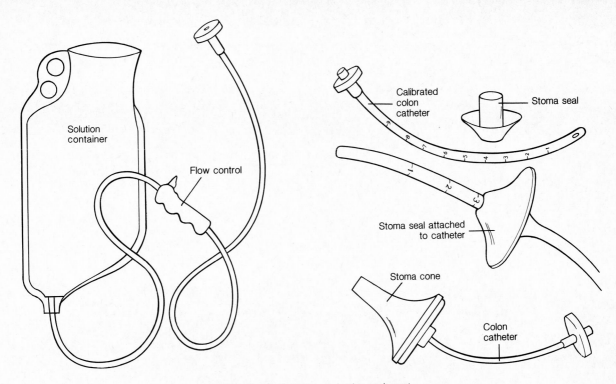

FIGURE 29–11 Colostomy irrigation equipment.

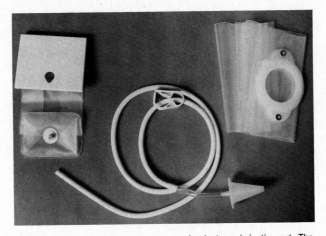

FIGURE 29–12 A commercially prepared colostomy irrigation set. The irrigation solution bag is on the left and the collecting bag (irrigation drainage sleeve) on the right; the stoma cone is fitted to the catheter.

should begin with a "starter set" until they are familiar with the colostomy and the problems of irrigating it. Later, with the help of an enterostomal therapy nurse or a qualified person from a surgical supply house, the client can select the set most appropriate for the client's needs. Both commercially prepared equipment and standard equipment are available (Figures 29–11 and 29–12).

The physician initially is responsible for determining whether a colostomy should be irrigated, what solution should be used, and how much should be used. The last may be preestablished by agency protocol. Technique 29–2 describes how to irrigate a colostomy.

If the client has had a colostomy for a long time, the irrigation needs to be given at the time the client has established, or the pattern of regularity will be disrupted. For a newly established colostomy, select a time based on the client's previous bowel habits and one that will allow the client to participate in usual daily activities. Encourage the client to select the time and to maintain it.

29-2 Irrigating a Colostomy

Before commencing a colostomy irrigation, determine (a) whether the stoma needs to be dilated; (b) which is the distal stoma and which is the proximal stoma, if the colostomy is not an end colostomy; and (c) why the irrigation is being performed and which stoma is to be irrigated (usually the proximal stoma is irrigated, to stimulate evacuation of the bowel; however, it may be necessary to irrigate the distal stoma in preparation for diagnostic procedures (e.g., roentgenography).

PURPOSE
• To distend the bowel and stimulate peristalsis and evacuation of feces

ASSESSMENT FOCUS
Bowel sounds; presence of abdominal distention; type of colostomy and functioning stoma; client readiness to select and use the equipment; client's mobility status to determine where the irrigation will be done.

EQUIPMENT

- Disposable bedpad and a bedpan, if the client is to remain in bed
- Bath blanket
- Irrigation equipment
  A bag to hold the solution
  Tubing attached to the bag
  Tubing clamp or flow regulator

- #28 rubber colon catheter, calibrated in either centimeters or inches, with a stoma cone or seal
  Disposable stoma-irrigation drainage sleeve with belt to direct the fecal contents into the toilet or bedpan
- IV pole

- Moisture-resistant bag
- Clean gloves to protect the nurse's hands from contamination, and one glove to dilate the stoma if ordered by the physician
- Lubricant
- Clean colostomy appliance or dressings

INTERVENTION

1. Prepare the client.

• Assist the client who must remain in bed to a side-lying position. Place a disposable bedpad on the bed in front of the client, and place the bedpan on top of the disposable pad, beneath the stoma.

• Assist an ambulatory client to sit on the toilet or on a commode in the bathroom. Ensure that the client's gown or pajamas are moved out of the way to prevent soiling, and cover the client appropriately with the bath blanket to prevent undue exposure.

• Throughout the technique, provide explanations, and encourage the client to participate.

2. Prepare the equipment.

• Fill the solution bag with 500 ml of warm (body temperature) tap

water, or other solution as ordered.

• Hang the solution bag on an IV pole so that the bottom of the container is at the level of the client's shoulder, or 30 to 45 cm (12 to 18 in) above the stoma. *This height provides a pressure gradient that allows fluid to flow into the colon.*

• Attach the colon catheter securely to the tubing.

• Open the regulator clamp, and run fluid through the tubing to expel all air from it. Close the clamp until ready for the irrigation. *Air should not be introduced into the bowel because it distends the bowel and can cause cramps.*

3. Remove the colostomy bag and then position the irrigation drainage sleeve.

• Remove the soiled colostomy bag, and place it in the moisture-resistant bag. *Placing the colostomy bag in this container prevents the transmission of microorganisms and helps reduce odor.*

• Center the irrigation drainage sleeve over the stoma, and attach it snugly. *This prevents seepage of the fluid onto the skin.*

• Direct the lower, open end of the drainage sleeve into the bedpan or between the client's legs into the toilet.

4. If ordered by the physician, dilate the stoma.

• Put on gloves.

• Lubricate the tip of the little finger.

• Gently insert the finger into the stoma, using a massaging mo-

► **Technique 29–2** *CONTINUED*

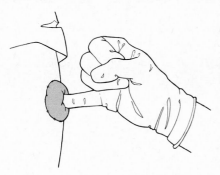

FIGURE 29–13 Dilating a colostomy stoma.

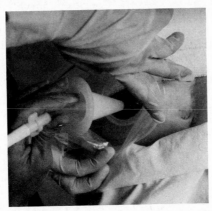

FIGURE 29–14 The client is participating in the colostomy irrigation by directing the cone.

tion (Figure 29–13). *A massaging motion relaxes the intestinal muscles.*

- Repeat the previous two steps, using progressively larger fingers, until maximum dilation is achieved. *Stoma dilation is performed to stretch and relax the stomal sphincter and to assess the direction of the proximal colon prior to an irrigation.*

5. Insert the stoma cone or colon catheter.

- Lubricate the tip of the stoma cone or colon catheter. *Lubricating the tip of the cone or catheter eases insertion and prevents injury to the stoma.*

- Using a rotating motion, insert the catheter or stoma cone through the opening in the top of the irrigation drainage sleeve and gently through the stoma (Figure 29–14). *A rotating motion on insertion helps to open the stoma.*

- Insert a catheter only 7 cm (3 in); insert a stoma cone just until it fits snugly. Many practitioners prefer using a cone to avoid the risk of perforating the bowel.

- If you have difficulty inserting the catheter or cone, do not apply force. *Forcing the cone or catheter may traumatize or perforate the bowel.*

6. Irrigate the colon.

- Open the tubing clamp, and allow the fluid to flow into the bowel. If cramping occurs, stop the flow until the cramps subside and then resume the flow. *Fluid that is too cold or administered too quickly may cause cramps.*

- If the fluid flows out as fast as you put it in, press the stoma cone or seal more firmly against the stoma to occlude it. If a stoma cone or seal is not available, press around the stoma with your fingers to close the stoma against the catheter.

- After all the fluid is instilled, remove the catheter or cone and allow the colon to empty. Although not always indicated, you may ask the client to gently massage the abdomen and sit quietly for 10 to 15 minutes until initial

emptying has occurred. *Massaging the abdomen encourages initial emptying.* In some agencies the stoma cone is left in place for 10 to 15 minutes before it is removed.

7. Seal the drainage sleeve and allow complete emptying of the colon.

- Clean the base of the irrigation drainage sleeve, and seal the bottom with a drainage clamp, following the manufacturer's instructions.

- Encourage an ambulatory client to move around for about 30 minutes. *Complete emptying of the colon often takes up to half an hour. Moving around promotes peristalsis.*

8. Empty and remove the irrigation sleeve.

9. Ensure client comfort.

- Clean the area around the stoma, and dry it thoroughly.

- Put a colostomy appliance on the client as needed. See Technique 29–1.

10. Document and report relevant information.

- Document all assessments and interventions. Include the time of the irrigation, the type and amount of fluid instilled, the returns, any problems experienced, and the client's response.

- Promptly report to the nurse in charge any problems, such as no fluid or stool returns, difficulties inserting the tube, peristomal skin redness or irritation, and stomal discoloration.

EVALUATION FOCUS	Amount and consistency of fluid returns; status of stoma and peristomal skin; any difficulties encountered inserting the tube or dilating the stoma; client's response and participation.

▶ **Technique 29–2 Irrigating a Colostomy** CONTINUED

SAMPLE RECORDING

Date	Time	Notes
12/05/93	0900	Colostomy irrigated with 750 ml warm tap water. Water and large amount soft brown stool expelled. Tube inserted without difficulty. Peristomal skin intact. Stoma is pink. Asked questions about irrigation, looked at stoma for first time. Observed stoma care and pouch application. ———————— — Chung-Hao Jen, NS

KEY ELEMENTS OF IRRIGATING A COLOSTOMY

- If two stomas are present, determine which stoma is to be irrigated.
- Wear gloves.
- Obtain the correct type and amount of irrigating fluid.
- Expel air from the irrigating tube before inserting it.
- Apply the irrigation drainage sleeve appropriately.
- Dilate the stoma only if ordered.
- Lubricate the tip of the stoma cone or catheter.
- Use a rotating motion to insert the stoma cone or catheter.

- Insert a catheter only 3 in (7.5 cm).
- Avoid inserting the stoma cone or catheter against resistance.
- Administer body-temperature fluid slowly.
- Stop the flow of solution temporarily if cramps occur.
- Securely fasten the base of the irrigation drainage sleeve after the irrigation.
- Thoroughly clean and dry the peristomal skin after the irrigation.

Urinary Diversions

A **urinary diversion** is the surgical rerouting of the urine produced in the kidneys to a site other than the bladder. These operations are often necessary when the urine flow is obstructed by, for example, a malignancy of the bladder.

Permanent urinary diversions are indicated for any condition that requires a total cystectomy, e.g., cancer of the bladder. Temporary urinary diversion stomas are indicated for any condition requiring partial cystectomy, trauma to the lower urinary tract, or severe chronic urinary tract infections. One type of urinary diversion is the *continent vesicostomy* in which the anterior wall of the bladder is sutured to the abdominal wall, and a stoma is formed from the bladder wall. Urine drains through this type of vesicostomy only after a catheter is inserted through the stoma into the bladder pouch.

Clients with urinary diversions usually are required to wear an external pouch to collect the urine. An exception is the person with a continent vesicostomy, who needs a small dressing over the stoma to protect the clothing from mucous drainage. Clients with urinary diversions may experience problems with their body image and may require assistance in coping with these changes and managing the stoma. People are usually able to resume their normal activities and life-style.

The nurse's responsibilities include assessment of the amount and character of urine drainage; stoma size, shape, and color; status of the peristomal skin; allergies to tape; and the learning needs of the client and support persons. Essential interventions include peristomal care, application of a clean appliance when required, and teaching the client and support persons self-care.

Generally, a urinary diversion appliance adheres to the client's skin for 2 to 5 days. They are usually changed twice a week. Because urinary diversion ostomies drain constantly, the nurse can expedite application of a clean pouch by attaching the peristomal skin barrier to the faceplate of the ostomy appliance before its application.

Application of a urinary diversion ostomy appliance is similar to application of a bowel diversion ostomy. Like colostomy appliances, urinary diversion appliances include plastic disposable pouches with adhesive squares, soft rubber reusable pouches with faceplates attached, and reusable pouches with detachable faceplates. The enterostomal therapy nurse selects the pouch that best suits the client by considering the type of ostomy, the stoma location and shape, and the peristomal skin surface, as well as the client's body size and contour, physical and mental abilities, skin allergies, financial status, and life-style.

Temporary disposable urinary diversion appliances are often attached to a urinary drainage system, especially during the night, to prevent accumulation and stagnation of urine in the appliance. To avoid separation of the appliance from the skin, pouches that are *not* attached to a drainage system must be emptied several times a day into a graduated receptacle when they are one-third to one-half full.

Peristomal skin barriers such as Skin Prep liquid or wipes or a similar product, or ready-made wafer-type or disc-type barriers are used according to the manufacturer's directions. The Karaya ring seal, although effective in protecting the skin, is less effective with urinary ostomies than with bowel ostomies because urine tends to melt the product.

When teaching the client self-care, the nurse must ensure consistent nursing interventions to promote client learning. Therefore, specific equipment and procedures, as well as the client's achievements, should be included on the teaching plan. The client will also need to learn ways to reduce odor. Use of deodorant tablets in the appliance, soaking a reusable pouch in dilute vinegar solution, a diet that makes the urine more acid, and drinking plenty of fluids all help control odor. A high fluid intake dilutes the urine, making it less odorous. Ascorbic acid and cranberry juice increase the acidity of urine, which in turn inhibits bacterial action and odor. Information about ostomy clubs and other community services available should also be included.

CRITICAL THINKING CHALLENGE

The surgeon has provided a temporary colostomy to rest the bowel for Dorothy Mathers, a 45-year-old female who has Crohn's disease. An important part of Ms Mathers' care is to learn self-care of the colostomy appliance. What behaviors would indicate that Ms Mathers is ready to participate in self-care? What actions can the nurse take to encourage Ms Mathers' participation in self-care?

RELATED RESEARCH

Deeny, P., and McCrea, H. January 1991. Stoma care: The patient's perspective. *Journal of Advanced Nursing* 16:39–46.

Hedrick, J. K. November/December 1987. Effects of nursing interventions on adjustment following ostomy surgery. *Journal of Enterostomal Therapy* 14:229–39.

Wade, B. E. November 1990. Colostomy patients: Psychological adjustment to 10 weeks and 1 year after surgery in districts which employed stoma-care nurses and districts which did not. *Journal of Advanced Nursing* 15:1297–1304.

REFERENCES

Alterescu, K. B. June 1987. Colostomy. *Nursing Clinics of North America.* 22:281–89.

Broadwell, D. C. June 1987. Peristomal skin integrity. *Nursing Clinics of North America* 22:321–32.

Erickson, P. J. June 1987. Ostomies: The art of pouching. *Nursing Clinics of North America* 22:311–20.

McCann, J. A. S. March 1990. A guide to colostomies. *Nursing 90* 20:32.

Rolstad, B. S. June 1987. Innovative surgical procedures and stoma care in the future. *Nursing Clinics of North America* 22:341–56.

Salter, M. May 2–8, 1990. Overcoming the stigma . . . irrigation and continent pouches. *Nursing Times* 86:67–69, 71.

Shipes, E. June 1987. Psychosocial issues: The person with an ostomy. *Nursing Clinics of North America* 22:291–302.

30

Respiratory Assistive Devices and Postural Drainage

CONTENTS

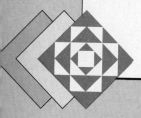

NURSING PROCESS GUIDE

RESPIRATORY ASSISTIVE DEVICES AND POSTURAL DRAINAGE

ASSESSMENT

Determine

- *Current respiratory problems:* What recent changes has the client experienced in breathing pattern (e.g., shortness of breath, difficulty breathing, need to be in upright position to breathe, or rapid and shallow breathing)? See below for cough, sputum, and pain. Which activities might cause the above symptom(s) to occur? What pollutants has the client been exposed to?

- *History of respiratory disease:* Has the client had colds, allergies, croup, asthma, tuberculosis, bronchitis, pneumonia, or emphysema? How frequently have these occurred? How long did they last? And how were they treated?

- *The presence of a cough:* Is it productive or nonproductive? If a cough is productive, when is sputum produced? What is the amount, color, thickness, and odor (e.g., thick, frothy, pink, rusty, or blood-tinged)?

- *Life-style:* Does the client smoke? If so, how much? Does any member of the client's family smoke? Are there any occupational hazards, e.g., inhaling fumes?

- *Pain:* Does the client experience any pain associated with breathing or activity? Where is the pain located? What words does the client use to describe the pain? How long does it last, and how does it affect breathing? What activities precede the pain?

- *Medication history:* Has the client taken or does the client take any over-the-counter or prescription medications for breathing? Which ones? And what are the dosages, times taken, and effects on the client, including side-effects?

Observe*

- Breathing pattern (rate, rhythm, depth, and quality). Note any signs of hyperventilation, hypoventilation, tachypnea, bradypnea.

- Ease or effort of breathing and posture assumed for breathing (e.g., orthopneic).

---

*See the box on page 739 for a definition and description of terms.

- Breath sounds audible without amplification, e.g., stridor, stertor, wheeze, bubbling.

- Chest movements, e.g., retractions, flail chest, or paradoxical breathing. Note the specific location of retractions: intercostal, substernal, suprasternal, supraclavicular, or tracheal tug.

- Clinical signs of hypoxia or anoxia, e.g., increased pulse rate, rapid or deep respirations, cyanosis of the skin and nail beds, restlessness, anxiety, dizziness (vertigo), or faintness (syncope).

- The location of any surgical incision in relation to the muscles needed for breathing. An incision can impede appropriate lung expansion.

Palpate for

- Respiratory excursion (see Chapter 11, page 246).

- Lungs for vocal (tactile) fremitus (see Chapter 11, page 246).

Percuss the chest for

- Diaphragmatic excursion (see Chapter 11, page 247).

- Chest sounds (flatness, dullness, resonance, hyperresonance, tympany). (See Table 11–3, page 204.)

Auscultate the lungs for

- Breath sounds (normal, adventitious, or absent). (See Tables 11–8 and 11–9, on pages 244 and 245.)

Determine the results of

- Sputum analysis.

- Venous blood samples (e.g., complete blood count).

- Arterial blood samples (blood gases).

- Pulmonary function tests.

- Pulse oximetry.

RELATED DIAGNOSTIC CATEGORIES

- Activity intolerance

- Ineffective airway clearance

- Ineffective breathing pattern

- Impaired gas exchange

PLANNING

Client Goals

The client will

- Restore or maintain adequate ventilation and breathing pattern.

- Resume usual activities of daily living.

Nursing Process Guide CONTINUED

Outcome Criteria
The client with **Ineffective airway clearance**

- Has a patent airway.
- Readily expectorates secretions.
- Has clear breath sounds bilaterally.
- Has normal respiratory rate, rhythm, and depth.
- Has skin, nails, lips, and earlobes of natural color.
- Explains medications and treatments for home use and plans for follow-up care.

The client with **Ineffective breathing pattern** or **Impaired gas exchange**

- Establishes a normal effective respiratory pattern of 12 to 20 per minute, effortless breathing (no use of accessory muscles), and symmetric chest expansion on inhalation.
- Is free of cyanosis.
- Has normal arterial blood gases.
- Has adequate O_2 saturation as demonstrated by pulse oximetry.
- Performs activities of daily living without shortness of breath.
- Demonstrates appropriate life-style changes.
- Explains purposes and side-effects of medications (e.g., bronchodilator, expectorant, anti-infective, anti-histamine, corticosteroid).
- Explains treatments for home care and plans for follow-up care.

Lung Inflation Techniques

Lung inflation techniques include diaphragmatic breathing exercises, apical and basal lung expansion exercises, and use of sustained maximal inspiration (SMI) devices or intermittent positive pressure breathing (IPPB) apparatuses. While facilitating the client's lung expansion, these techniques promote the exchange of gases in the lungs and strengthen the muscles used for breathing.

These maneuvers can also clear the respiratory tract of secretions and improve oxygenation. In a healthy, active person, secretions do not normally accumulate in the lungs; rather, air passages are kept clear by the mucous membrane lining, which contains **cilia** (hairlike projections of the respiratory mucous membrane). Mucus entraps organisms or other small foreign material while the cilia move the trapped material. The cilia in the lower respiratory passageways (e.g., the bronchi) beat upward; the cilia in the nose beat downward.

The cough and sneeze reflexes are also clearing mechanisms. The cough reflex helps clear the lower respiratory passage, whereas the sneeze reflex clears the upper nasal passages. The sneeze reflex is not unlike the cough reflex. The initiating stimulus is usually some irritation of the nasal passages.

When a person is immobilized, i.e., confined to bed, not all lung tissue may become aerated, and secretions may accumulate. Other conditions that predispose clients to accumulation of lung secretions are chronic lung disease (e.g., emphysema), unconsciousness, and mechanical ventilation of the lungs.

Adequate hydration is an important aspect of healthy respiratory mucosa. Normally, respiratory tract secretions are thin and readily moved by the cilia. When these secretions are thickened, increased oral fluids and the use of humidifiers can help to thin the secretions. Oral fluid intake should be increased only as the client's health permits.

Terms commonly used in recording physical assessment findings related to respiratory function are shown in the box on page 739.

Sputum, Nose, and Throat Specimens

Sputum is the mucous secretion from the lungs, bronchi, and trachea. It is important to differentiate it from *saliva*, the clear liquid secreted by the salivary glands in the mouth, sometimes referred to as "spit." Healthy individuals do not produce sputum.

Clients need to cough to bring sputum up from the lungs, bronchi, and trachea into the mouth and expectorate it into a collecting container. Sputum specimens are often collected in the morning. On awakening, the client can cough up the secretions that have accumulated during the night. Sometimes specimens are collected during postural drainage, when the client can usually produce sputum. When a client cannot cough, the nurse must sometimes use pharyngeal suctioning (see Chapter 31) to obtain a specimen.

Sputum specimens are ordered for culture and sensitivity to identify a specific microorganism and

Abnormal Breathing Patterns and Sounds

Breathing Patterns

Rate

- *Tachypnea*—rapid respiration marked by quick, shallow breaths
- *Bradypnea*—abnormally slow breathing
- *Apnea*—cessation of breathing

Volume/Depth

- *Hyperventilation*—an increase in the amount of air in the lungs; characterized by prolonged and deep breaths; may be associated with anxiety
- *Hypoventilation*—reduction in the amount of air in the lungs; characterized by shallow respirations

Rhythm

- *Cheyne-Stokes breathing*—rhythmic waxing and waning of respirations, from very deep to very shallow breathing and temporary apnea; often associated with cardiac failure, increased intracranial pressure, or brain damage

Ease or Effort

- *Dyspnea*—difficult and labored breathing during which the individual has a persistent, unsatisfied need for air and feels distressed
- *Orthopnea*—ability to breathe only in upright sitting or standing positions

Breath Sounds

Audible Without Amplification

- *Stridor*—a shrill, harsh sound heard during inspiration with laryngeal obstruction
- *Stertor*—snoring or sonorous respiration, usually due to a partial obstruction of the upper airway
- *Wheeze*—continuous, high-pitched musical squeak or whistling sound occurring on expiration and sometimes on inspiration when air moves through a narrowed or partially obstructed airway
- *Bubbling*—gurgling sounds heard as air passes through moist secretions in the respiratory tract

Audible by Stethoscope

- *Crackles* (formerly called *rales*)—dry or wet crackling sounds simulated by rolling a lock of hair near the ear; generally heard on inspiration as air moves through accumulated moist secretions. *Fine to medium crackles* occur when air passes through moisture in small air passages and alveoli; *medium to coarse crackles* occur when air passes through moisture in the brochioles, bronchi, and trachea.
- *Gurgles* (formerly called *rhonchi*)—coarse, dry, wheezy, or whistling sound more audible during expiration as the air moves through tenacious mucus or narrowed bronchi
- *Pleural friction rub*—coarse, leathery, or grating sound produced by the rubbing together of inflamed pleural

Chest Movements

- *Intercostal retraction*—indrawing between the ribs
- *Substernal retraction*—indrawing beneath the breast bone
- *Suprasternal retraction*—indrawing above the breast bone
- *Supraclavicular retraction*—indrawing above the clavicles
- *Tracheal tug*—indrawing and downward pull of the trachea during inspiration
- *Flail chest*—the ballooning out of the chest wall through injured rib spaces; results in *paradoxical breathing*, during which the chest wall balloons on expiration but is depressed or sucked inward on inspiration

Secretions and Coughing

- *Hemoptysis*—the presence of blood in the sputum
- *Productive cough*—a cough accompanied by expectorated secretions
- *Nonproductive cough*—a dry, harsh, cough without secretions

its drug sensitivities. Cytology studies of the respiratory system often require serial collection of three early morning specimens, which are tested to identify cancer in the lung and its specific cell type. Tests to determine the presence of *acid-fast bacillus* (AFB), also known as the *tubercle bacillus* (TB), also require serial collection of sputum specimens (often taken for 3 consecutive days). Some agencies use a special glass container when the presence of AFB is suspected.

A **throat culture** sample is collected from the mucosa of the oropharynx and tonsillar regions using a culture swab. The sample is then cultured and examined for the presence of disease-producing microorganisms.

A **nose culture** sample is collected from the mucosa of the nasal passages using a culture swab.

Technique 30–1 describes how to collect a sputum specimen; Technique 30–2 describes how to obtain nose and throat specimens.

30-1 Collecting a Sputum Specimen

Before collecting a sputum specimen, identify the purpose for which it is to be obtained. This often determines the number of specimens to obtain and the time of day to obtain them (see pages 738 and 739).

PURPOSES
- To identify a specific microorganism and its drug sensitivities or the presence of cancerous cells
- To assess the effectiveness of therapy

ASSESSMENT FOCUS

Client's ability to cough and expectorate secretions; type of assistance required to produce the specimen (e.g., the need to splint an abdominal incision, the need to be placed in postural drainage position beforehand, or the need to perform deep-breathing exercises beforehand); skin color and rate, depth, and pattern of respiration as baseline data.

EQUIPMENT

- Container with a cover
- Disposable gloves (if assisting the client)
- Disinfectant and swabs, or
- liquid soap and water
- Paper towels
- Completed label
- Completed laboratory requisition
- Mouthwash

INTERVENTION

1. Give the client the following information and instructions:

- The purpose of the test and how to provide the sputum specimen.
- Not to touch the inside of the sputum container.
- To expectorate the sputum directly into the sputum container.
- To keep the outside of the container free of sputum, if possible.
- How to hold a pillow firmly against an abdominal incision if the client finds it painful to cough.
- The amount of sputum required. Usually 1 to 2 tsp (5 to 10 ml) of sputum is sufficient for analysis.

2. Provide necessary assistance to collect the specimen.

- Assist the client to a standing or a sitting position (e.g., high- or semi-Fowler's position or on the edge of a bed or in a chair). *These positions allow maximum lung ventilation and expansion.*

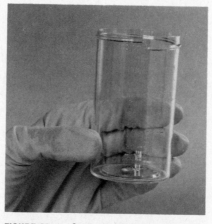

FIGURE 30–1 Sputum specimen container.

- Ask the client to hold the sputum cup on the outside, or, for a client who is not able to do so, don gloves and hold the cup (Figure 30–1).
- Ask the client to breathe deeply and then cough up secretions. *A deep inhalation provides sufficient air to force secretions out of the airways and into the pharynx.*
- Hold the sputum cup so that the client can expectorate into it, making sure that the sputum

does not come in contact with the outside of the container. *Containing the sputum within the cup restricts the spread of microorganisms to others.*

- Assist the client to repeat coughing until a sufficient amount of sputum has been collected.
- Cover the container with the lid immediately after the sputum is in the container. *Covering the container prevents the inadvertent spread of microorganisms to others.*
- If spillage occurs on the outside of the container, clean the outer surface with a disinfectant. Some agencies recommend washing the outside of all containers with liquid soap and water and then drying with a paper towel.
- Remove gloves.

3. Ensure client comfort.

- Assist the client to rinse the mouth with a mouthwash as needed.

► **Technique 30–1** *CONTINUED*

- Assist the client to a position of comfort that allows maximum lung expansion as required.

4. Label and transport the specimen to the laboratory.

- Ensure that the specimen label and the laboratory requisition carry the correct information. Attach them securely to the specimen. *Inaccurate identification*

and/or information on the specimen container can lead to errors of diagnosis or therapy.

- Arrange for the specimen to be sent to the laboratory immediately or refrigerated. *Bacterial cultures must be started immediately, before any contaminating organisms can grow, multiply, and produce false results.*

5. Document all relevant information.

- Document the collection of the sputum specimen on the client's chart. Include the amount, color, consistency, and odor of the sputum, any measures needed to obtain the specimen (e.g., postural drainage), the general amount of sputum produced, and any discomfort experienced by the client.

EVALUATION FOCUS

Amount, color, and consistency (thick, tenacious, watery) of sputum; presence of hemoptysis; respiration rate and any abnormalities or difficulty breathing after the specimen collection; color of the client's skin and mucous membranes, especially any cyanosis, which can indicate impaired blood oxygenation.

SAMPLE RECORDING

Date	Time	Notes
06/21/93	0600	Sputum specimen sent to laboratory. Produced approximately 2 tbsp of green-yellow thick sputum. States has "sharp, knifelike pain" in right anterior lower chest when coughing. ———————— Sheila D. Wry, NS

KEY ELEMENTS OF COLLECTING A SPUTUM SPECIMEN

- Determine the reason for collecting the specimen, and obtain the appropriate container.
- Give the client appropriate instructions to provide the specimen.
- Wear gloves.

- Use aseptic technique.
- Ensure appropriate labeling of the specimen and laboratory requisition.
- Transport a specimen for culture and sensitivity immediately to the laboratory, or refrigerate it.

Obtaining Nose and Throat Specimens

Before collecting a nose or throat specimen, determine (a) whether the client is suspected of having a contagious disease, e.g., diptheria, which requires special precautions; and (b) whether a specimen is required from the nasal cavity as well as from the pharynx and/or the tonsils.

PURPOSE

- To identify the presence of specific organisms and their sensitivities

►

▶ Technique 30–2 Obtaining Nose and Throat Specimens CONTINUED

ASSESSMENT FOCUS	Appearance of nasal mucosa and throat (note in particular areas of inflammation and purulent drainage); complaints of soreness or tenderness; clinical signs of infection (e.g., fever, chills, fatigue).

EQUIPMENT

- ☐ Gloves (optional)
- ☐ Two sterile swabs in sterile culture tubes
- ☐ Penlight
- ☐ Tongue blade (optional)

- ☐ Otoscope with a nasal speculum
- ☐ Container for the used nasal speculum

- ☐ Completed labels for each specimen container
- ☐ Completed requisition

INTERVENTION

1. Prepare the client and the equipment.

- Assist the client to a sitting position. *This is the most comfortable position for many people and the one in which the pharynx is most readily visible.*

- Don gloves if the client's mucosa will be touched.

- Remove the cap from one culture tube. Lay the cap on a firm surface, inner side upward. *This prevents the inside of the cap from coming into contact with microorganisms on the surface.*

- Remove one sterile applicator, and hold it carefully by the stick end, keeping the remainder sterile. *The swab end is kept from touching any objects that could contaminate it.*

2. Collect the specimen.

For a Throat Specimen

- Ask the client to open the mouth, extend the tongue, and say "ah." *When the tongue is extended, the pharynx is exposed. Saying "ah" relaxes the throat muscles and helps minimize contraction of the constriction muscle of the pharynx (the gag reflex).*

- If the posterior pharynx cannot be seen, adjust the light, and depress the tongue with a tongue blade. Depress the tongue firmly

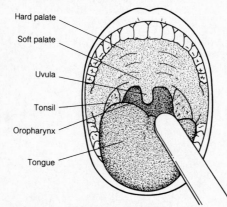

Hard palate
Soft palate
Uvula
Tonsil
Oropharynx
Tongue

FIGURE 30–2 Diagram of the mouth.

without touching the throat (Figure 30–2). *Touching the throat stimulates the gag reflex.*

- Insert a swab into the mouth, taking care not to touch any part of the mouth or tongue. *The swab should not pick up microorganisms in the mouth.*

- Quickly run the swab along the tonsils, making sure to contact any areas on the pharynx that are particularly erythematous (reddened) or that contain exudate. *By moving the swab quickly, you can avoid initiating the gag reflex or causing discomfort. Erythematous areas and areas with exudate will likely have the most microorganisms.*

- Remove the swab without touching the mouth or lips. *This prevents the swab from transmitting microorganisms to the mouth.*

- Insert the swab into the sterile tube containing transport medium without allowing it to touch the outside of the container. Make sure the swab is placed in the correctly labeled tube. *Touching the outside of the tube could transmit microorganisms to it and then to others.*

- Place the top securely on the tube, taking care not to touch the inside of the cap. *Touching the inside of the cap could transmit additional microorganisms into the tube.*

- Repeat the above steps with the second swab.

- Discard the tongue blade in the waste container.

- Discard gloves.

For a Nasal Specimen

- Gently insert the lighted nasal speculum up one nostril.

- Insert the sterile swab carefully through the speculum, without touching the edges. *This prevents the swab from picking up microorganisms from the speculum.*

- Wipe along the reddened areas or the areas with the most exudate.

- Remove the swab without touching the speculum, and place it in a sterile tube.

- Repeat the above steps for the other nostril.

▶ **Technique 30–2** *CONTINUED*

3. Label and transport the specimens to the laboratory.

• See Technique 30–1, step 4.

4. Document all relevant information.

• Record the collection of the nose and/or throat specimens on the client's chart. Include the assessments of the nasal mucosa and pharynx, and any discomfort the client experienced.

EVALUATION FOCUS	Appearance of nasal mucosa and throat; color of any drainage; any complaints of the client.

SAMPLE RECORDING

Date	Time	Notes
06/22/93	0800	Throat specimen for culture and sensitivity sent to lab. Throat is inflamed with patches of yellow discharge on tonsillar pillars. Unable to swallow fluids without soreness. ————————— Glenda Irvine, RN

KEY ELEMENTS OF OBTAINING NOSE AND THROAT SPECIMENS

• Wear gloves.

• Use aseptic technique.

• Obtain specimen from areas that are erythematous or contain exudate.

• Avoid initiating the gag reflex when taking throat specimens.

• While taking the specimen, assess the pharynx and tonsils (nares) for appearance and color and the amount and consistency of any exudate.

• Ensure appropriate labeling of the specimen and laboratory requisition.

• Transport the specimen immediately to the laboratory, or refrigerate it.

Deep-Breathing Exercises

Breathing exercises are frequently indicated for clients with restricted chest expansion, i.e., those with chronic obstructive pulmonary disease (COPD) or recovering from thoracic or upper abdominal surgery. Commonly employed breathing exercises are abdominal (diaphragmatic) and pursed-lip breathing, apical expansion, and basal expansion exercises.

Apical expansion exercises are often required for clients who restrict their upper chest movement because of pain from a severe respiratory disease or surgery, e.g., lobectomy (removal of a lung lobe). Basal expansion exercises are often required for people with restricted bilateral chest movements due to pain from a respiratory disorder, chest surgery, or upper abdominal surgery.

Technique 30–3 explains how to teach clients to perform deep-breathing exercises.

30-3 Teaching Deep-Breathing Exercises

Before starting to teach deep-breathing exercises, determine (a) the location of a surgical incision that could impede lung expansion, and (b) the presence of hypoxemia, respiratory acidosis, or respiratory alkalosis from the laboratory records.

PURPOSES	• To increase pulmonary ventilation and lung expansion • To loosen respiratory secretions • To promote breathing deeply with less effort, thereby conserving energy • To prevent untoward effects of anesthesia and/or hypoventilation

▶

► **Technique 30–3 Teaching Deep Breathing Exercises** CONTINUED

ASSESSMENT FOCUS	Vital signs; breathing pattern (rhythm, ease or effort of breathing, volume); chest movements (retractions, flail chest); amount and character of secretions; type of cough (productive or nonproductive); breath sounds; pallor or cyanosis; clinical signs of hypoxia or anoxia (e.g., restlessness, increased heart rate, anxiety, rapid or deep respirations).

INTERVENTION

Abdominal (Diaphragmatic) and Pursed-Lip Breathing

1. Prepare the client.

- Wash hands.

- Explain to the client that diaphragmatic breathing can help the person breathe more deeply and with less effort.

- Assist the client to assume either a comfortable semi-Fowler's position with knees flexed, back supported, and one head pillow, or a supine position with one head pillow and knees flexed. After learning the exercise, the client can practice first in either semi-Fowler's or supine position and then when sitting upright, standing, and walking. *The semi-Fowler's and supine positions with knees flexed help relax the abdominal muscles.*

- Have the client place one or both hands on the abdomen just below the ribs.

2. Perform abdominal breathing and pursed-lip breathing.

- Instruct the client to breathe in deeply through the nose with the mouth closed, to stay relaxed, not to arch the back, and to concentrate on feeling the abdomen rise as far as possible. *When a person breathes in, the diaphragm contracts (drops), the lungs fill with air, and the abdomen rises or protrudes.*

- If the client has difficulty raising the abdomen, instruct the person to take a quick, forceful inhalation through the nose. *With a quick sniff, the client will feel the abdomen rise.*

- Instruct the client to purse the lips as if about to whistle; to breathe out slowly and gently, making a slow "whooshing" sound; to avoid puffing out the cheeks; to concentrate on feeling the abdomen fall or sink; and to tighten (contract) the abdominal muscles while breathing out. *Pursing the lips creates a resistance to air flowing out of the lungs, increases pressure within the bronchi, and minimizes the collapse of smaller bronchioles, a common problem for clients with COPD. While the client breathes out, the diaphragm relaxes (rises), and the abdomen sinks. Tightening the abdominal muscles helps a person to exhale more effectively.*

- If the client has COPD, teach the "double cough" technique. Have the client

  a. Breath in through the nose and inflate the lungs to the midinspiration point, rather than to the full deep inspiration point.

  b. Simultaneously exhale and cough two or more abrupt, sharp coughs in rapid succession. *A very forceful cough by a client with COPD can cause small airway collapse. With two or more abrupt coughs, the first one*

loosens secretions, while subsequent coughs facilitate movement of secretions toward the upper airways.

- Instruct the client to use this exercise whenever feeling short of breath and to increase it gradually 5 to 10 minutes four times a day. *Regular practice enables a person eventually to do this type of breathing without conscious effort.*

Apical Expansion Exercises

3. Position your hands or the client's hands.

- Place your fingers below the client's clavicles and exert moderate pressure, or have the client place his or her fingers over the same area (Figure 30–3). *This position allows you to evaluate the depth of apical inhalation.*

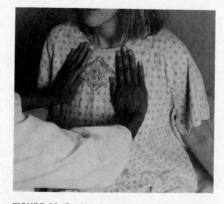

FIGURE 30–3 Hand position to evaluate the depth of apical inhalation.

4. Perform apical expansion exercises. Instruct the client to do the following:

► **Technique 30–3** *CONTINUED*

- Inhale through the nose and concentrate on pushing the upper chest upward and forward against the fingers. *This helps to aerate the apical areas of the upper lung lobes.*

- Hold the inhalation for a few seconds. *This promotes aeration of the alveoli.*

- Exhale through the mouth or nose slowly, quietly, and passively while concentrating on moving the upper chest inward and downward.

- Perform the exercise for at least five respirations four times a day. *Repeating the exercise helps to reexpand lung tissue, eliminate secretions, and minimize flattening of the upper chest wall.*

Basal Expansion Exercises

5. Prepare the client.

- For the postsurgical client, obtain a pillow splint to support the incision, if required. *The splint helps minimize pain.*

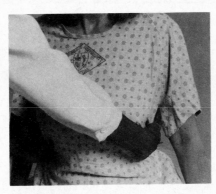

FIGURE 30–4   Hand position to evaluate the depth of bilateral basal expansion.

- Place the palms of your hands in the area of the lower ribs along the midaxillary lines and exert moderate pressure, or have the client place the hands over the same area (Figure 30–4). *This hand position enables you to evaluate and compare the depth of bilateral basal inspiration.*

6. Perform basal expansion exercises. Instruct the client to do the following:

- Inhale through the nose and concentrate on moving the lower chest outward against the hands.

- Hold the inhalation for a few seconds.

- Exhale through the nose or mouth slowly, quietly, and passively. If the person has COPD, observe the rate and character of the exhalation. Normal exhalation is slow, and the upper chest appears relaxed. If the exhalation appears difficult or there is indrawing of the upper chest, encourage pursed-lip exhalation (see step 2).

- Perform this exercise at least five respirations four times a day. *Repetition helps to reexpand lung tissue and eliminate secretions.*

7. Document the teaching and assessments for the exercises performed, and update the teaching plan.

EVALUATION FOCUS Client's ability to perform exercises; compliance to instructions; effectiveness of exercises.

SAMPLE RECORDING

Date	Time	Notes
12/15/93	0930	Crackles present in left lateral and lower lung field. Respirations 18; decreased left basal lung expansion. Deep breathing exercises performed.
	0945	Cough produced moderate amount of thick yellow sputum. Crackles cleared. Encouraged to increase fluid intake by 500 ml. —— Mary Murakami, SN

KEY ELEMENTS OF TEACHING DEEP-BREATHING EXERCISES

- Know the purpose of the exercise.
- Teach the client the exercise appropriate for health status.
- Have the client demonstrate the exercises.
- Assess the client's ability to perform the exercise independently.

- Inform the client about the number and frequency of the exercises.
- Document client teaching and the client's response to it.

Lung Inflation Devices

Sustained Maximal Inspiration (SMI) Devices

Sustained maximal inspiration devices (SMIs), also referred to as **incentive spirometers**, measure the flow of air inhaled through the mouthpiece. They therefore offer an incentive to improve inhalation. Two general types are the flow-oriented spirometer and the volume-oriented spirometer. The *flow-oriented SMI* consists of one or more clear plastic chambers containing freely movable colored balls or discs. The balls or discs are elevated as the client inhales. The client is asked to keep them elevated as long as possible with a maximal sustained inhalation. Figure 30–5 shows a Triflo II SMI. Flow-oriented SMIs are low-cost devices, are often disposable, and can be used independently by clients. They do not measure the specific volume of air inhaled, however.

Volume-oriented SMIs measure the inhalation volume maintained by the client. A plastic *disposable* device is shown in Figure 30–6. When the client inhales, the accordion-pleated cylinder rises from the bottom as the cylinder collapses. Markings on the side indicate the volume of inspiration achieved by the client. The goal is to make the cylinder collapse as much as possible.

More expensive *nondisposable volume-oriented SMIs* measure very precisely the inhalation volume maintained by the client. These devices contain pistons or bellows that are raised by the client's inhalation to a predetermined volume. Some volume-oriented devices feature an achievement counter or light. The light will not turn on until the inspiration is held at the minimum predetermined volume for a specified time period.

When nondisposable devices are used in the hospital setting, the nurse will need to check the physician's or respiratory therapist's order and set the spirometer to the predetermined volume. Volume ranges vary from 0 to 5000 ml, depending on the type of spirometer. Battery-operated SMIs will also need to be checked for proper functioning. In all situations, the nurse should auscultate the client's lungs before and after the procedure and compare the findings. Technique 30–4 describes how to assist a client with an SMI.

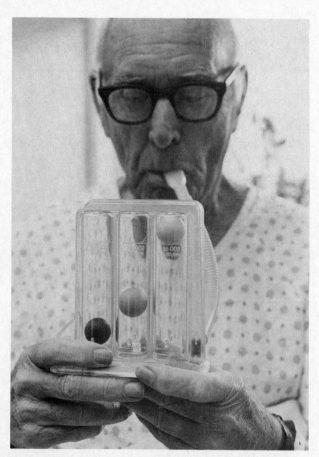

FIGURE 30–5 Sustained maximal inspiration device (SMI).

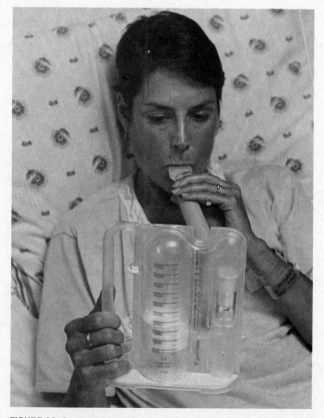

FIGURE 30–6 Plastic disposable volume-oriented SMI.

30-4 Assisting a Client to Use a Sustained Maximal Inspiration (SMI) Device

Before assisting a client to use an SMI device, determine the prescribed inspiratory volume level.

PURPOSES
- To improve pulmonary ventilation
- To counteract the effects of anesthesia and/or hypoventilation
- To loosen respiratory secretions
- To facilitate respiratory gaseous exchange
- To expand collapsed alveoli

ASSESSMENT FOCUS

Vital signs; breathing pattern (rhythm, ease or effort of breathing, volume); chest movements (retractions, flail chest); character of secretions and cough; breath sounds; presence of pallor or cyanosis; presence of clinical signs of hypoxia or anoxia (e.g., restlessness, increased heart rate, anxiety, rapid or deep respirations); location of a surgical incision that could impede lung expansion.

EQUIPMENT

- Flow-oriented or volume-oriented SMI
- Mouthpiece or breathing tube
- Sterile water
- Label for mouthpiece
- Nose clip (optional)

INTERVENTION

1. Prepare the client.
- Explain the procedure.

- Assist the client to an upright sitting position in bed or in a chair. If the person is unable to assume a sitting position for a flow spirometer, have the person assume any position. *A sitting position facilitates maximum ventilation of the lungs.*

For a Flow-Oriented SMI

2. Set the spirometer.
- If the spirometer has an inspiratory volume-level pointer, set the pointer at the prescribed level. The physician's or respiratory therapist's order should indicate the level.

3. Instruct the client to use the spirometer as follows:
- Hold the spirometer in the upright position. *A tilted spirometer requires less effort to raise the balls or discs.*

- Exhale normally.

- Seal the lips tightly around the mouthpiece; take in a slow deep breath to elevate the balls: and then hold the breath for 2 seconds initially, increasing to 6 seconds (optimum), to keep the balls elevated if possible. Instruct the client to avoid brisk low-volume breaths that snap the balls to the top of the chamber. The client may use a noseclip if the person has difficulty breathing only through the mouth. *A slow, deep breath ensures maximal ventilation. Greater lung expansion is achieved with a very slow inspiration than with a brisk shallow breath, even though a slow inspiration may not elevate or keep the balls elevated while the client holds the breath* (Luce, Tyler, and Pierson 1984). *Sustained eleva-*

tion of the balls ensures adequate alveolar ventilation.

- Remove the mouthpiece, and exhale normally.

- Cough productively, if possible, after using the spirometer. *Deep ventilation may loosen secretions, and coughing can facilitate their removal.*

- Relax, and take several normal breaths before using the spirometer again.

- Repeat the procedure several times and then four or five times hourly. *Practice increases inspiratory volume, maintains alveolar ventilation, and prevents atelectasis.*

For a Volume-Oriented SMI

4. Set the spirometer.
- Set the spirometer to the predetermined volume. Check the

▶

► **Technique 30–4 Assisting a Client to Use an SMI Device** *CONTINUED*

physician's or respiratory therapist's order.

- Since some SMIs are battery-operated, ensure that the spirometer is functioning. Place the device on the client's bedside table.

5. Instruct the client to use the spirometer as follows:

- Exhale normally.

- Seal the lips tightly around the mouthpiece, and take in a slow, deep breath until the piston is elevated to the predetermined level. The piston level may be visible to the client, or lights or the word "Hold" may be illuminated to identify the volume obtained.

- Hold the breath for 6 seconds to ensure maximal alveolar ventilation.

- Remove the mouthpiece, and exhale normally.

- Cough productively, if possible, after using the spirometer. *Deep ventilation may loosen secretions, and coughing can facilitate their removal.*

- Relax, and take several normal breaths before using the spirometer again.

- Repeat this procedure several times and then four or five times hourly. *Practice increases inspiratory volume, maintains alveolar ventilation, and prevents atelectasis.*

For All Devices

6. Clean and put away the equipment.

- Clean the mouthpiece with sterile water, and shake it dry. Label the mouthpiece and a disposable SMI with the client's name, and store them in the bedside unit. *Only the mouthpiece of a volume SMI is stored with the client because volume SMIs are used by many clients.* Disposable mouthpieces are changed every 24 hours.

7. Document all relevant information.

- Record the technique, including type of spirometer, number of breaths taken, volume or flow levels achieved, and results of auscultation.

- For a flow SMI, calculate the volume achieved by multiplying the setting by the length of time the client kept the balls elevated. For example, if the setting was 500 ml and the balls were kept suspended for 2 seconds, the volume is 500×2, or 1000 ml.

- For a volume SMI, take the volume directly from the spirometer, e.g., 1500 ml.

EVALUATION FOCUS	Sounds heard on auscultation of the lungs to compare with those heard before technique.

SAMPLE RECORDING

Date	Time	Notes
07/06/93	1100	Instructed in use of Triflo II spirometer. 5 breaths taken at volume of 1,000 ml (500 ml × 2 sec). Bilateral breath sounds normal on auscultation before and after spirometry. ———————————— Nicholas Coscos, SN

KEY ELEMENTS OF ASSISTING A CLIENT TO USE AN SMI DEVICE

- Auscultate the lungs before and after the technique.
- Position the client appropriately.
- Make sure the client seals the lips tightly around the mouthpiece.
- Assess the client's ability to perform the technique as taught.
- Inform the client about the number and frequency of the exercises.

- Set the spirometer at the prescribed level.
- Instruct the client to
  a. Hold the spirometer upright.
  b. Take in a *slow, deep* breath (not brisk low-volume breaths) before holding the breath.
  c. Progressively increase the time for holding the breath.
  d. Cough productively after using the spirometer.

Intermittent Positive Pressure Breathing (IPPB) Devices

Intermittent positive pressure breathing (IPPB) is a lung inflation technique for delivering air or oxygen into the lungs at positive (above atmospheric) pressure during inspiration and releasing the pressure automatically when the predetermined positive pressure level is reached in the air passages. Thus, expiration occurs passively. Some IPPB machines can exert pressure during expiration, and the abbreviations IPPB/I (inspiratory) and IPPB/E (expiratory) are sometimes used to differentiate the two methods. Generally, however, IPPB refers to positive pressure therapy administered during inspiration, a safer and more common practice.

Use of IPPB therapy has decreased since the advent of incentive spirometers. Advocates of IPPB therapy, however, believe that IPPB devices are more effective in expanding the lungs, moving secretions, promoting coughing, and delivering aerosol medications into the deeper, smaller air passages. Because they require less effort by the client, they are prescribed for selected clients.

Various IPPB machines are marketed. Two commonly used types are the Bird respirator and the Bennett respirator. Respiratory therapists usually handle the assembly and maintenance of respirators. The machine is connected to an oxygen supply and is equipped with an in-line humidifier, which must be filled with distilled water. The client breathes through a mouthpiece or a mask attached to the end of the respirator tubing (Figure 30–7).

The Bird Respirator

There are several types of Bird respirators; all are equipped with six basic controls (Figure 30–8):

- The *pressure control setting* establishes the pressure that will be received at the height of an inspiration before the client enters the expiratory phase. It measures the pressure in centimeters of water pressure, from 0 to 60 cm. Usually, the pressure is started low, at 15 or 20 cm H_2O, and gradually increased as the client becomes accustomed to the machine.

- The *flow rate control* adjusts the inspiratory time and switches the ventilator from off to on. It is similar to a water tap: The more it is turned on, the faster the flow of gas. Low numbers on this dial indicate slow rates, and higher numbers indicate faster rates. Since the aim of therapy is usually to achieve deep respirations and transfer of gases deep into the alveoli, the flow rate is generally set at 10 or less to coincide with the client's inspiratory effort. Fast flow rates tend to flood only the upper respiratory tract. The nurse can assess the effectiveness of the flow rate by observing the client's chest expansion during therapy.

- The *air mix plunger* determines the proportion of oxygen and air delivered to the client. It has two positions. When the plunger is pushed in, 100% of oxygen is delivered. When it is pulled out, a mixture of 40% oxygen and 60% air is delivered. These proportions cannot be varied as they can on more sophisticated respirators. Generally, the oxygen/air mixture is used.

- The *sensitivity control* adjusts the inspiratory effort required by the client to trigger or trip the machine (start the flow of gas). Once the machine is triggered, the pressure automatically builds to the peak pressure that was set by the pressure

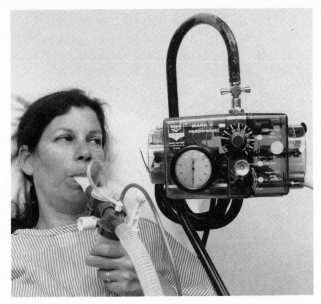

FIGURE 30–7 Intermittent positive pressure breathing (IPPB).

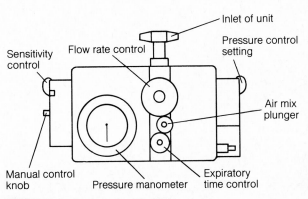

FIGURE 30–8 A schematic of the Bird respirator.

control knob. The smaller the number set on the sensitivity control, the higher the sensitivity (i.e., the less effort required by the client to start the machine). People who are weak often require a high sensitivity control (low number setting) to start the machine, but people who need to be encouraged to breathe deeply should use a low sensitivity control (high number), which offers more resistance and requires more effort. The sensitivity control is usually set at 15 at the start of therapy.

- The *manual control knob*, a pink knob or pin below the sensitivity control, can be pushed in manually to trigger the ventilator. It is mostly used to check respirator function before applying it to the client.

- The *expiratory time control* is turned to "off" for client-cycled IPPB. It is used only for people who are apneic or who require continuous assisted ventilation.

The Bennett Respirator

The Bennett respirator (Figure 30–9) is different in appearance from the Bird respirator, but its operation is similar. The PR-1 model, which is frequently used, has many of the basic controls of the Bird machine:

- The *pressure control knob*, capable of delivering 0 to 45 cm H_2O pressure, is rotated clockwise and generally set at 15 to 20 cm H_2O for adults or 10 to 12 cm H_2O for children. The initial pressure setting may be lower.

- The *control pressure gauge* records the pressure that is reached by turning the pressure control knob.

- The *system pressure gauge* records the pressure that is required by the client and should equal that measured by the control pressure gauge at the end of inspiration.

- The *air dilution control* is usually pushed in to allow for an air/oxygen mixture. When it is pulled out, 100% oxygen is delivered.

- The *sensitivity control* determines the amount of inspiratory effort required to start inspiration and is used only if the client has difficulty triggering the machine. Such difficulty is indicated when the client sucks or draws on the machine to no avail or when the system pressure gauge needle deflects to the negative side. In these instances, the sensitivity control should be set

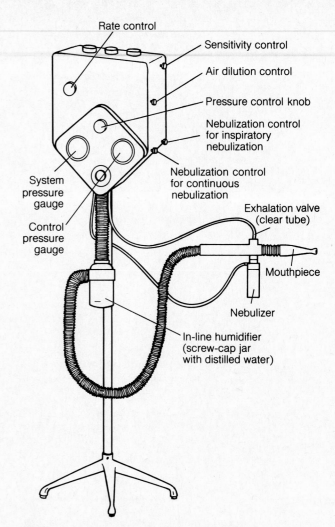

FIGURE 30–9 A schematic of the Bennett respirator.

higher so that less effort is required by the client to trigger the machine.

- The *rate control* regulates the rate of automatic cycling and is turned to the "off" position for client-cycled IPPB.

- The *nebulization controls* provide power to the side steam nebulizer to deliver aerosol medications. One knob sets the nebulizer for continuous therapy, the other for inspiratory nebulization. If a client is receiving a medicated treatment, the inspiration knob is generally turned one revolution to ensure adequate nebulization on inspiration. With the use of the continuous knob, the medication is delivered immediately upon inspiration.

Technique 30–5 describes how to assist a client with IPPB therapy.

30-5

Assisting Clients with Intermittent Positive Pressure Breathing

Before assisting a client with intermittent positive pressure breathing, determine (a) whether aerosol medications are to be administered and (b) when the IPPB treatments are scheduled. They are often prescribed for five to six breaths hourly during waking hours. They should not be scheduled right before or after a meal because they can induce nausea and because a full stomach can prevent maximum lung expansion.

PURPOSES
- To increase lung expansion
- To facilitate the clearing of bronchial secretions
- To provide moisture to the respiratory mucous membranes
- To administer aerosol medications to the lower airways
- To prevent or relieve atelectasis
- To improve oxygenation

ASSESSMENT FOCUS

Chest wall expansion; respiratory rate and depth. See also Assessment Focus in Technique 30–4, page 747.

EQUIPMENT

- Mouthpiece
- Noseclip (optional)
- IPPB machine
- Mask (to be used only if a mouthpiece and a noseclip are not effective)
- Source of pressurized air and oxygen if the machine does not have an internal compression unit
- Sterile normal saline solution or the prescribed aerosol medication, e.g., 1% isoetharine hydrochloride (Bronkosol)
- 3-ml syringe with a needle
- Respirometer (optional) and an exhaled volume collector
- Tissues and a moistureproof receptacle for expectorated secretions

INTERVENTION

1. Confirm the details of the therapy.

- Verify the orders, and check whether aerosol medications are to be administered during therapy. Bronchodilators, mucolytics, or antibiotics may be ordered.

2. Prepare the client.

- Explain that the therapy will assist the client to achieve deep lung expansion and will promote coughing and removal of secretions.

- Assist the client to a Fowler's position in bed or to sit upright in a chair. *These positions facilitate maximal lung expansion.*

- Teach the client to breathe normally through the mouth by using the mouthpiece and to refrain from breathing through the nose. Have the client practice breathing only through the mouthpiece prior to therapy. Ensure that the lips completely seal the mouthpiece. Have the client use a noseclip if breathing only through the mouth is difficult. *Mouth breathing and an airtight seal around the mouthpiece are essential for efficient operation of the IPPB system.*

3. Set up the equipment.

- Adjust the pressure control setting on a Bird respirator (Figure 30–8) or the pressure control knob on a Bennett respirator (Figure 30–9) to 10 to 15 cm H_2O. *This control sets the pressure that will be received at the height of an inspiration.*

- Fill the nebulizer with sterile saline or prescribed medication, reattach it, and set the nebulization control if necessary (Figure 30–10). If a medication is used, prepare it before going to the client. *Nebulization delivers prescribed medications and/or moisture to the respiratory mucous membranes. IPPB therapy must be given with medication or sterile saline in the nebulizer unless a mainstream humidifier is used. Air that is not moisturized dries the airways and impedes the mobilization of secretions.*

- Set the oxygen/air mix control as

▶

▶ **Technique 30–5 Assisting Clients with IPPB** *CONTINUED*

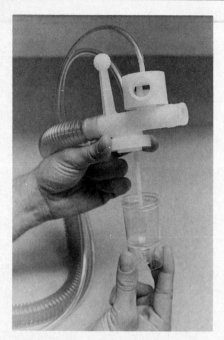

FIGURE 30–10 Reattaching the nebulizer after filling it with saline or the ordered medication.

ordered. For a mixture of air and oxygen, pull the knob of a Bird respirator out,
or
push the knob of a Bennett respirator in.

- Occlude the end of the tubing that will be attached to the mouthpiece, and manually cycle the machine to operate. *This ensures that the system is airtight and that it cycles off at the preset pressure.* If the desired pressure is not reached, check for a leak in the system, e.g., disconnection in the nebulizer.

- Attach the mouthpiece to the machine's tubing.

4. Assist the client with the treatment.

- Have the client place the lips tightly around the mouthpiece, relax, and inhale deeply and slowly through the mouth as the machine cycles on. *The machine will not start until the client breathes in.*

- Encourage the client to breathe in until the lungs are maximally inflated. Explain that the machine will cycle off when the preset pressure is met or when the client breathes out. *Allowing the pressure to reach its peak before exhaling brings about maximal lung expansion when the appropriate pressure is set.*

- *Optional:* After full inspiration, have the client hold the breath for a few seconds. *This provides greater distribution of oxygen, air, and nebulized particles.*

- Instruct the client to exhale normally in a relaxed and passive manner. *Forced exhalation can increase small airway obstructions.*

- Observe the client for adequate chest expansion with each inhalation and for a relaxed, passive exhalation. Observe that the needle gauges reach the preset pressure levels as the client inhales. See the pressure manometer in Figure 30–8 and the system pressure gauge in Figure 30–9. *Although the degree of lung expansion can be observed visually, the gauges on the respirator provide more reliable measures. If the needle gauge on the respirator reaches the preset level during inhalation, the setting is usually satisfactory.*

or

It is preferable to attach a measuring device such as a Wright respirometer to the expiratory port of the IPPB manifold (Figure 30–11). *The Wright respirometer specifically measures the expired tidal volume and indicates whether the client is receiving adequate deep lung inflations.* Tidal volume is the volume of air inspired and expired with a normal breath, about 500 ml (Figure 30–12).

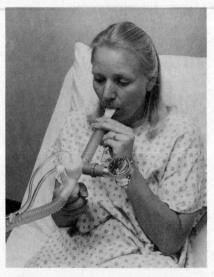

FIGURE 30–11 A respirometer attached to the expiratory port of the IPPB apparatus.

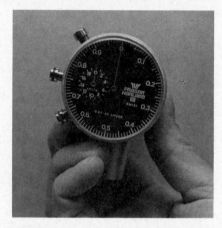

FIGURE 30–12 A respirometer dial showing the scales for measuring expiratory tidal volume.

5. Determine whether the machine is functioning correctly.

- If there is inadequate or no deflection of the needle on the gauges

  a. Determine that the system is airtight. The client may not have sealed the lips around the mouthpiece adequately. If this is the case, decrease the pressure setting until the client feels comfortable, and then grad-

▶ **Technique 30–5** *CONTINUED*

ually increase the pressure. A noseclip may be necessary.

b. Observe whether the client is relaxed. Perhaps the person is not breathing normally or is blowing back into the mouthpiece before the lungs are filled. If this is the case, encourage the client to breathe normally. Some clients have a tendency to force their breathing or to struggle with the apparatus. When advised not to force breaths, to relax, to breathe slowly, and to allow time for expiration (which takes longer than inspiration), people normally adjust to the therapy readily. Remind the client that the client controls the machine: With each inhalation the machine starts; each time the client breathes out, the machine stops at peak inspiration. Extra effort by the client is not required.

c. Determine that the machine is triggering. Perhaps the client does not exert sufficient inspiratory effort to start the machine. In that case, adjust the sensitivity gauge to a lower number. If the needle deflection is neg-

ative, the client may be sucking or using too much inspiratory effort, or the peak flow could be too low.

6. Monitor the client during the treatment.

• Monitor the blood pressure and pulse rate during the therapy, especially at the initial treatment. Stay with the person throughout the treatment. Stop the treatment and notify the charge nurse or physician if there is a sudden significant increase in pulse rate (20 or more beats per minute) or a sudden change in blood pressure (10 mm Hg or more). During subsequent IPPB sessions, blood pressure assessment is necessary only if the client has a history of cardiovascular disease, hypotension, or sensitivity to any medications given during therapy. *Some bronchodilators, e.g., isoproterenol and isoetharine, significantly increase the heart rate. IPPB therapy increases intrathoracic pressure and may cause a temporary decrease in cardiac output and venous return, indicated by hypotension, headache, and tachycardia.*

• If vital signs are stable, continue the IPPB therapy, if indicated, until all the medication in the nebulizer is administered or 15 to 20 minutes.

• Following or during the therapy, encourage the client to expectorate respiratory secretions, as needed. Note the amount of sputum expectorated.

• Auscultate the lung fields, and compare the pretherapy assessment. Note any improvement in aeration and absence of or diminished adventitious breath sounds, e.g., crackles (rales), gurgles (rhonchi), wheezes, or friction. Improvements may not be observable until 10 to 20 minutes after the therapy.

7. Clean and put away the equipment.

• Clean the mouthpiece and nebulizer with sterile water, and dry them thoroughly. Store the mouthpiece in a plastic bag at the bedside or in accordance with agency policy. Generally, the mouthpiece is replaced every 24 hours for aseptic reasons.

8. Document all relevant information.

• Record the IPPB therapy, its duration, the medication administered, the pressure used, the volume achieved, the breath sounds, and other assessments before and after the therapy, e.g., the amount of sputum expectorated by the client.

EVALUATION FOCUS	Pulse rate; respiratory rate; blood pressure; amount and character of expectorated secretions; and breath sounds.

SAMPLE RECORDING

Date	Time	Notes
09/02/93	1500	IPPB administered, 800-ml volume at 15 cm H$_2$O pressure with sterile normal saline nebulization for 15 min. Adventitious breath sounds absent 15 min. after treatment. BP 120/70, P 78, stable, before and after therapy. No secretions expectorated. ——————————————————— Constance S. Boyd, RN

▶ **Technique 30–5 Assisting Clients with IPPB** *CONTINUED*

KEY ELEMENTS OF ASSISTING CLIENTS WITH IPPB

- Verify the orders about aerosol medications to be given with the IPPB.
- Auscultate the client's lungs before and after therapy.
- Measure blood pressure and pulse rate before, during, and after the therapy.
- Observe the client for adequate chest expansion with each inhalation and for a relaxed, passive exhalation.

- Observe that the needle gauges reach the preset pressure levels.
- Discontinue the therapy if the client has an untoward reaction, e.g., hypotension or tachycardia.
- Clean the mouthpiece and nebulizer appropriately following therapy.
- Replace the mouthpiece every 24 hours.

Percussion, Vibration, and Postural Drainage (PVD)

Chest physiotherapy (CPT) includes chest percussion, vibration, postural drainage, deep breathing, and coughing. Deep breathing involves exercises that expand the various segments of the lungs. See Technique 30–3. In this context, coughing means controlled coughing that removes bronchial secretions. It should be learned by all preoperative clients. See Technique 42–1 on page 986.

Percussion, sometimes called *clapping*, is forceful striking of the skin with cupped hands. Mechanical percussion cups and vibrators are also available. When the hands are used, the fingers and thumb are held together and flexed slightly to form a cup, as one would to scoop up water. Percussion over congested lung areas can mechanically dislodge tenacious secretions from the bronchial walls. Cupped hands trap the air against the chest. The trapped air sets up vibrations through the chest wall to the secretions. Before persussion, the nurse ensures that the area to be percussed is covered, e.g., by a gown or towel, because percussing the unprotected skin can cause discomfort. When done correctly, the percussion action should produce a hollow, popping sound. Percussion is avoided over certain easily injured structures, such as the breasts, sternum, spinal column, and kidneys.

Vibration is a series of vigorous quiverings produced by hands that are placed flat against the client's chest wall. Vibration is used after percussion to increase the turbulence of the exhaled air and thus loosen thick secretions. It is often done alternately with percussion.

Postural drainage is the drainage, by gravity, of secretions from various lung segments. Secretions that remain in the lungs or respiratory airways promote bacterial growth and subsequent infection. They also can obstruct the smaller airways and cause atelectasis. Secretions in the major airways, such as the trachea and the right and left main bronchi, are usually coughed into the pharynx, where they can be expectorated, swallowed, or effectively removed by suctioning.

A wide variety of positions is necessary to drain all segments of the lungs, but not all positions are required for every client. Only those positions that drain specific affected areas are used. See Table 30–1. The lower lobes require drainage most frequently, since the upper lobes drain during normal daily activities. Prior to postural drainage, the client may be given a bronchodilator medication or nebulization therapy to loosen secretions. See Chapter 35, page 847. Frequently, postural drainage treatments are scheduled two or three times daily, depending on the degree of lung congestion. The best times include before breakfast, before lunch, in the late afternoon, and before bedtime. It is best to avoid hours shortly after meals because postural drainage at these times can be tiring and can induce vomiting.

The nurse needs to evaluate the client's tolerance of postural drainage by assessing the stability of the client's vital signs, particularly the pulse and respiratory rates, and by noting signs of intolerance, such as pallor, diaphoresis, dyspnea, and fatigue. Some clients do not react well to certain drainage positions, and the nurse must make appropriate adjustments. For example, some clients become dyspneic in Trendelenburg's position and require only a moderate tilt or a shorter time in those positions.

Text continues on p. 755

TABLE 30–1   POSTURAL DRAINAGE FOR ADULTS

Upper Lobes

Lung Segment
Apical segments

Client Position
Lies back at 30° angle

Percussion/Vibration Area
Between the clavicles and above the scapulae

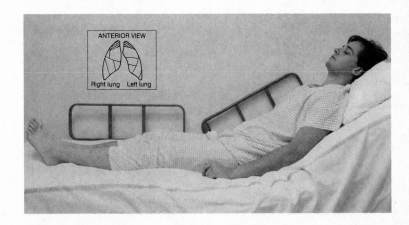

Lung Segment
Posterior segments

Client Position
Sits upright in a chair or in bed with head bent slightly forward

Percussion/Vibration Area
Between the clavicles and the scapulae

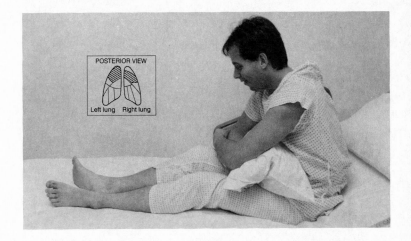

Lung Segment
Anterior segments

Client Position
Lies on a flat bed with pillows under the knees to flex them

Percussion/Vibration Area
Upper chest below the clavicles down to the nipple line, except for women

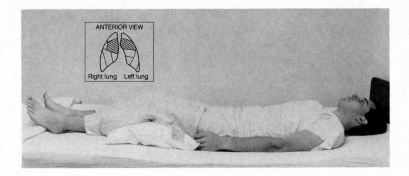

Table continues on pp. 756–757

The sequence for percussion, vibration, and postural drainage (PVD) is usually as follows: positioning, percussion, vibration, and removal of secretions by coughing or suction. Usually, the client assumes each position for 10 to 15 minutes, although beginning treatments may be shorter and gradually increase.

Usually, the entire treatment, including preparatory nebulization and deep breathing as well as all postures, takes 30 minutes. Postural drainage position and percussion areas for specific lung segments are discussed in Technique 30–6.

▶ **Table 30–1** POSTURAL DRAINAGE FOR ADULTS *CONTINUED*

Right Middle Lobe

Lung Segment
Right lateral and medial segments

Client Position
Lies on the left side and leans back slightly (about a quarter turn) against pillows, extending at the back from the shoulder to the hip. Nurse elevates foot of bed about 15° or 40 cm (15 in).

Percussion/Vibration Area
For *male* client: Over the right side of the chest at the level of the nipple between the fourth and sixth ribs

For *female* client: Beneath the breast, with the heel of the nurse's hand positioned toward her axilla, cupped fingers extending forward beneath the breast

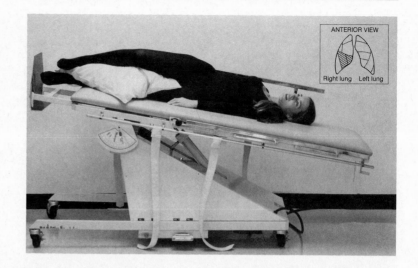

Lower Division of Left Upper Lobe (Lingula)

Lung Segment
Left lingular segments

Client Position
As above for right middle lobe, but on the *right* side

Percussion/Vibration Area
As above for right middle lobe, but on the *left* side

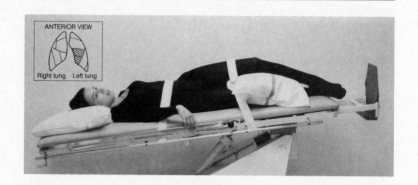

Lower Lobes

Lung Segment
Superior segments

Client Position
Lies on the abdomen on a flat bed, and nurse places two pillows under the hips

Percussion/Vibration Area
The middle area of the back (below the scapulae) on both sides of the spine

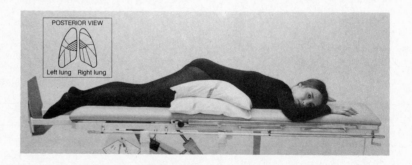

▶ **Table 30–1** *CONTINUED*

Lower Lobes *(continued)*

Lung Segment
Anterior basal segments

Client Position
Lies on unaffected side with the upper arm over the
head and pillow between knees. Nurse elevates the
foot of the bed about 30° or 45 cm (18 in) or to height
tolerated by the client. A pillow under the head is
optional.

Percussion/Vibration Area
Over the lower ribs inferior to the axilla on the affected
side of the chest

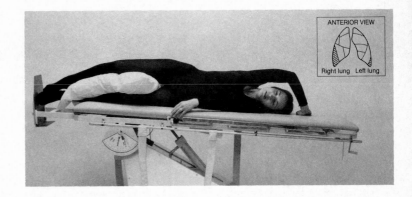

Lung Segment
Lateral basal segments

Client Position
Lies partly on unaffected side and partly on the
abdomen. Nurse elevates the foot of the bed about 30°
or 45 cm (18 in) or to height tolerated, or elevates
client's hips with pillows.

Percussion/Vibration Area
The uppermost side of the lower ribs

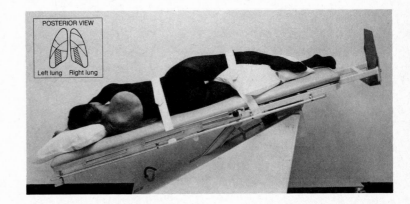

Lung Segment
Posterior basal segments

Client Position
Lies prone. Nurse elevates foot of bed about 45 cm
(18 in), and elevates client's hips on two or three
pillows to produce a jackknife position from the knees
to the shoulders

Percussion/Vibration Area
Over the lower ribs on both sides close to the spine,
but not directly over the spine or kidneys

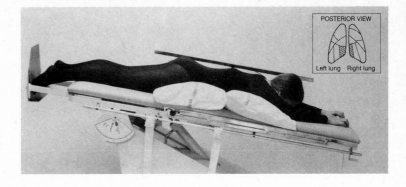

Administering Percussion, Vibration, and Postural Drainage (PVD) to Adults

Before administering PVD to an adult client, determine (a) the lung segments affected; (b) the ordered sequence of percussion, vibration, and postural drainage and the length of time specified; (c) whether the bronchodilator or moisturizing nebulization therapy is ordered prior to the postural drainage (secretions are easier to raise after the bronchi are dilated and secretions are thinned); and (d) preexisting or potential respiratory conditions.

PURPOSES
- To assist the removal of accumulated secretions
- To prevent the accumulation of secretions in clients at risk, e.g., the unconscious and those receiving mechanical ventilation

ASSESSMENT FOCUS

Lung sounds by auscultation; whether the cough is productive or nonproductive; color, amount, and character of expectoration; respiration rate and character; vital signs.

EQUIPMENT

- Bed that can be placed in Trendelenburg's position
- Pillows
- Gown or pajamas
- Towel
- Sputum container
- Tissues
- Mouthwash
- Specimen label and requisition, if a specimen of sputum is required
- Suction, as needed

INTERVENTION

1. Prepare the client.

- Provide visual and auditory privacy. *Coughing and expectorating secretions can embarrass the client and disturb others.*

- Explain which positions the client will need to assume, and explain about percussion and vibration techniques.

2. Assist the client to the appropriate position for the postural drainage.

- See Table 30–1, earlier.

- Use pillows to support the client comfortably in the required positions.

3. Percuss the affected area.

- Ensure that the area to be percussed is covered, e.g., by a gown or towel. *Percussing the skin directly can cause discomfort.*

- Ask the client to breathe slowly and deeply. *Slow deep breathing promotes relaxation.*

- Cup your hands, i.e., hold your fingers and thumb together, and flex them slightly to form a cup, as you would to scoop up water. *Cupped hands trap the air against the chest. The trapped air sets up vibrations through the chest wall to the secretions, helping to loosen them.*

- Relax your wrists, and flex your elbows. *Relaxed wrists and flexed elbows help obtain a rapid, hollow, popping action.*

- With both hands cupped, alternately flex and extend the wrists rapidly to slap the chest (Figure 30–13). *The hands must remain cupped so that the air cushions the impact and injury to the client can be avoided.*

- Percuss each affected lung segment for 1 to 2 minutes. The per-

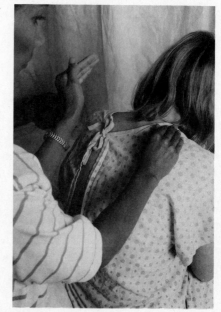

FIGURE 30–13 Percussing the upper posterior chest.

cussing action should produce a hollow, popping sound when done correctly.

▶ **Technique 30–6** *CONTINUED*

4. Vibrate the affected area.

- Place your flattened hands, one over the other (or side by side) against the affected chest area (Figure 30–14).

- Ask the client to inhale deeply through the mouth and exhale slowly through pursed lips or the nose.

- During the exhalation, straighten your elbows, and lean slightly against the client's chest while tensing your arm and shoulder muscles in isometric contractions. *Isometric contractions will transmit fine vibrations through the client's chest wall.*

- Vibrate during five exhalations over one affected lung segment.

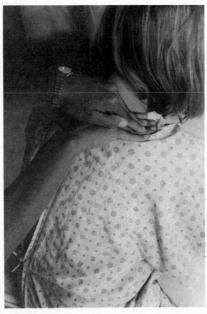

FIGURE 30–14   Vibrating the upper posterior chest.

- Encourage the client to cough and expectorate secretions into the sputum container. Offer the client tissues and mouthwash as required.

- Auscultate the client's lungs, and compare the findings to the baseline data.

5. Label and transport the specimen, if obtained.

- Ensure that the specimen label and requisition carry the correct information.

- Arrange for the specimen to be sent to the laboratory immediately, or refrigerated.

6. Document the percussion, vibration, and postural drainage and assessments.

EVALUATION FOCUS

> Amount, appearance, and character of secretions; tolerance of therapy (note signs of intolerance such as pallor, diaphoresis, dyspnea, or fatigue); change in breath sounds and rate and character of respirations.

SAMPLE RECORDING

Date	Time	Notes
06/06/93	0600	PVD for right anterior basal segment performed for 5 min. Large amount thick grey sputum produced. Specimen sent to lab. No pain or dyspnea. Inspiratory crackles unchanged. ——————— Robert Loo, RN

KEY ELEMENTS OF ADMINISTERING PVD TO ADULTS

- Auscultate the client's breath sounds; observe the rate, depth, and ease of respirations and the amount, character, and color of any expectorated secretions before and after the technique.
- Position the client appropriately.
- Cover the area to be percussed with a gown or towel.

- Position your hands appropriately for percussion.
- Perform vibration during exhalations only.
- Avoid percussing or vibrating over the breasts of a female, the spine, or the kidneys.
- Encourage the client to cough and expectorate secretions after vibrating.

PVD for Infants and Children

Percussion, vibration, and postural drainage for infants and children is similar to that of the adult. It is usually performed three to four times daily and is more effective following bronchodilation and/or nebulization therapy. The length and duration of therapy depend on the child's condition and tolerance. To minimize the chance of vomiting, PVD is performed before meals (or 1 to 1½ hours after meals) and at bedtime. In a hospital setting, an older child can be positioned over the elevated knee rest of the hospital bed. Smaller children and infants can be positioned with pillows or over the nurse's lap. See Table 30–2.

Various methods may be employed to stimulate deep breathing, e.g., blowing feathers, blowing up balloons, using whistle toys, or using blow bottles designed to move colored liquid from one container to another. Because many children have difficulty coughing when in a dependent position, they should be allowed to sit up while they cough. The nurse can also reinforce the child's efforts by encircling the chest with the hands and compressing the sides of the lower chest during the cough.

For an infant whose chest is too small for conventional hand percussion, a small face mask or a bulb syringe cut in half can be used. Cut the syringe, leaving the nozzle with one half, and tape the cut edge to cushion it. Hold the bulb by the nozzle for percussion (Figure 30–15 on page 763). To make a vibrator for an infant, remove the brush from a portable electric toothbrush and tape padding over the vibrating end.

Technique 30–7 on page 763 explains how to provide PVD to infants and children.

TABLE 30-2 POSTURAL DRAINAGE FOR INFANTS AND CHILDREN

Upper Lobes

Lung Segment
Apical segments

Client Position
Seated on nurse's lap leaning back about 30°

Percussion/Vibration Area
Between the clavicles and scapulae

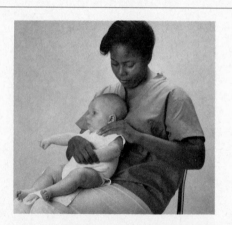

Lung Segment
Posterior segments

Client Position
Seated on nurse's lap leaning forward about 20° over a pillow

Percussion/Vibration Area
Upper back on both sides

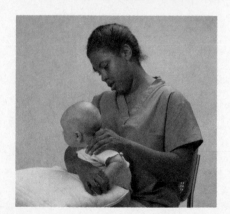
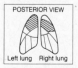

▶ **Table 30–2** *CONTINUED*

Lung Segment
Anterior segments

Client Position
Lies supine on a flat bed or nurse's lap

Percussion/Vibration Area
Upper chest below the clavicles down to the nipple line

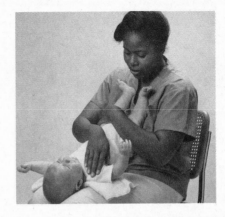

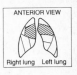

Middle Lobe or Lingular Segments

Lung Segment
Right lateral and medial segments

Client Position
Almost supine on nurse's lap, head slanted down about 15°, turned on the left side about a quarter turn, with the right shoulder slightly elevated and the hips higher than the chest

Percussion/Vibration Area
Over the right nipple

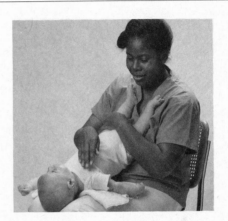

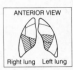

Lung Segment
Left lingular segments

Client Position
As for right lateral and medial segments

Percussion/Vibration Area
Over the left side of the chest at the level of the nipple between the fourth and sixth ribs

Lower Lobes

Lung Segment
Superior segments

Client Position
Prone on a pillow over the nurse's knees, with the hips slightly elevated

Percussion/Vibration Area
Middle area of the back just below each scapula

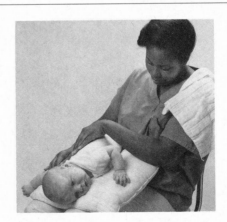

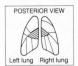

▶ **Table 30–2** POSTURAL DRAINAGE FOR INFANTS AND CHILDREN *CONTINUED*

Lung Segment
Anterior basal segments

Client Position
On unaffected side on a pillow over nurse's knees, with head lowered about 30°

Percussion/Vibration Area
At the side of the chest over the lower ribs beneath the axilla, avoiding the stomach

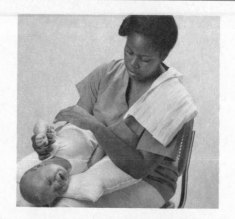
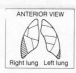

Lung Segment
Lateral basal segments

Client Position
Almost prone on a pillow on nurse's knees, with head lowered about 30°, a pillow placed under the affected side to elevate that side, and the upper body turned a quarter turn

Percussion/Vibration Area
Affected side over lower ribs

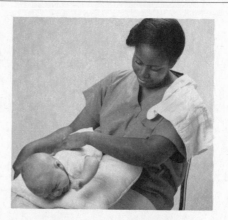
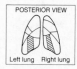

Lung Segment
Posterior basal segments

Client Position
Prone on pillow over nurse's lap, with the head lowered about 30°

Percussion/Vibration Area
Over lower ribes on both sides close to the spine, but not directly over the spine or the kidneys

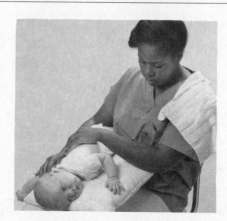
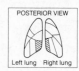

30-7   Administering Percussion, Vibration, and Postural Drainage (PVD) to Infants and Children

Before administering PVD to an infant or child, determine (a) the lung segments affected; (b) the ordered sequence of percussion, vibration, and postural drainage and the length of time specified; (c) whether the bronchodilator or moisturizing nebulization therapy is ordered prior to the postural drainage (secretions are easier to raise after the bronchi are dilated and secretions are thinned); and (d) preexisting or potential respiratory conditions.

PURPOSES
- To assist the removal of accumulated secretions
- To prevent the accumulation of secretions

ASSESSMENT FOCUS

Lung sounds; whether the cough is productive or nonproductive; color, amount, and character of expectorations; respiration rate and character; vital signs.

EQUIPMENT
- Pillows
- Gown or shirt and diapers
- Towel
- Face mask or other percussion device for small infant
- Sputum container
- Tissues
- Mouthwash, if the child is old enough to use it
- Suction apparatus as required
- Specimen label and requisition, if a specimen of sputum is required

INTERVENTION

1. Prepare the infant or child.
- Provide an explanation that is suitable to the child's age.
- Assist the child to the appropriate position for postural drainage. See Table 30–2, earlier.
- Use pillows to support the client comfortably in the required positions.

2. Perform PVD as ordered.
- Percuss the affected area, using a percussion device if appropriate (Figure 30–15) or three fingertips flexed and held together.
- Vibrate the affected area as appropriate, using a vibrator ap-

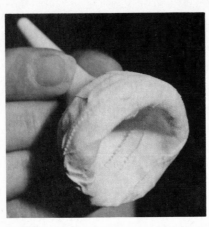

FIGURE 30–15   A bulb syringe modified for chest percussion.

propriate to the child's age. See Technique 30–6, step 4, page 759.

- Instruct the child to sit up, and encourage deep breathing and coughing to remove loosened secretions.

or

Suction airway (see Technique 31–1, page 767).

- Repeat percussion, vibration, deep breathing, and coughing for each lobe requiring drainage.

7. Document the PVD and all assessments.
- See Sample Recording in Technique 30–6, page 759.

EVALUATION FOCUS

Changed breath sounds; cough; amount, color, and character of expectorated secretions; rate and character of respirations; dyspnea; tolerance of treatment.

▶ **Technique 30–7 Administering PVD to Infants and Children** *CONTINUED*

KEY ELEMENTS OF ADMINISTERING PVD TO INFANTS AND CHILDREN

- Auscultate the child's breath sounds; observe the rate, depth, and ease of respirations and the amount, character, and color of any expectorated secretions before and after the technique.
- Position the child appropriately.
- Cover the area to be percussed with clothing or a towel.

- Position your fingers appropriately for percussion.
- Perform vibration during exhalations only.
- Avoid percussing or vibrating over the spine or the kidneys.
- Encourage the child to cough and expectorate, or suction secretions after vibrating.

CRITICAL THINKING CHALLENGE

Marilyn Evans, an obese 44-year-old female, is recovering from abdominal surgery. Her physician has ordered deep-breathing exercises to prevent respiratory complications. Ms Evans is concerned that the exercises will increase the pain related to her surgery. She states she is tired and needs rest. What factors place Ms Evans at risk for respiratory complications? How will you respond to her concerns? What actions will you take to ensure her compliance with the treatment plan?

REFERENCES

Guyton, A. C. 1986. *Textbook of medical physiology*, 7th ed. Philadelphia: W. B. Saunders Co.

Luce, J. M.; Tyler, M. L.; and Pierson, D. J. 1984. *Intensive respiratory care*. Philadelphia: W. B. Saunders Co.

Spearing, C., and Cornell, D. J. September 1987. Incentive spirometry: Inspiring your patient to breathe deeply. *Nursing 87* 17:50–51.

Stevens, S. A., and Becker, K. L. January 1988. How to perform picture-perfect respiratory assessment. *Nursing 88* 18:57–63.

Waterson, M. March 1978. Teaching your patients postural drainage. *Nursing 78* 8:51–53.

31

Oropharyngeal and Nasopharyngeal Suctioning

OBJECTIVES

- Differentiate oropharyngeal, nasopharyngeal, and endotracheal suctioning

- Describe the purposes of suctioning

- Identify indications for suctioning

- Identify two problems associated with suctioning

- Identify essential assessment data required before and after suctioning

- Give rationales underlying selected steps of the techniques in this chapter

- Perform oropharyngeal, nasopharyngeal, and endotracheal suctioning safely and effectively

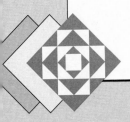

NURSING PROCESS GUIDE
PHARYNGEAL SUCTIONING

ASSESSMENT

See the Nursing Process Guide for Chapter 30. Essential data include the following:

- Rate, depth, rhythm, and character of respirations. Make special note of noisy, wet respirations, which indicate the presence of secretions in the respiratory tract that are impeding the flow of air. Auscultate the chest with a stethoscope, if necessary, to assess the condition of the airways and the lungs.

- The color of the skin and mucous membranes. Be alert to cyanosis and pallor.

- Dyspnea and orthopnea.

- Ability to cough and produce sputum. Note the color, consistency, amount, and odor of the sputum.

- Any drainage from the mouth, if the client is unconscious.

RELATED DIAGNOSTIC CATEGORIES

- Anxiety

- Ineffective airway clearance
- Fear (of suffocation)
- High risk for Infection

PLANNING

Client Goal
The client will restore or maintain airway patency and adequate respiratory ventilation.

Outcome Criteria
The client

- Has clear breath sounds bilaterally.

- Has normal respiratory rate, rhythm, and depth, i.e., an effective respiratory pattern of 12 to 20 per minute, effortless breathing (no use of accessory muscles), and symmetric chest expansion on inhalation.

- Has skin, nails, lips, and earlobes of natural color.

- Has normal arterial blood gases.

- Has normal heart rhythm and rate within 20 beats of normal.

- Has a maximum systolic blood pressure of 140 mm Hg and maximum diastolic blood pressure of 90 mm Hg.

Suctioning Oropharyngeal and Nasopharyngeal Cavities

The nurse must sometimes apply suction to the oropharynx and nasal passages of clients who have difficulty swallowing or expectorating secretions. **Suctioning** is the aspiration of secretions, often through a rubber or polyethylene catheter connected to a suction machine or wall outlet. It is recommended that sterile technique be used for all suctioning, so that microorganisms are not introduced into the pharynx, where they can multiply and move into the trachea and bronchi. This is particularly important for debilitated clients, who are more susceptible to infection.

Several types of catheters are available for suctioning. The open-tipped catheter has an opening at the end and several openings along the sides (Figure 31–1, A). It is effective for thick mucus plugs, but it

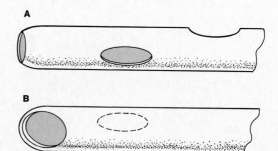

FIGURE 31–1 Types of pharyngeal suction catheters: *A*, open-tipped; *B*, whistle-tipped.

can irritate tissue. The whistle-tipped catheter has a slanted opening at the tip (Figure 31–1, B). Most catheters have a thumb port on the side, which is used to control the suction. The tip of a suction catheter has several openings along the sides to distribute the negative pressure of the suction over a wide area, thus preventing excessive irritation of any one area of the respiratory mucous membrane.

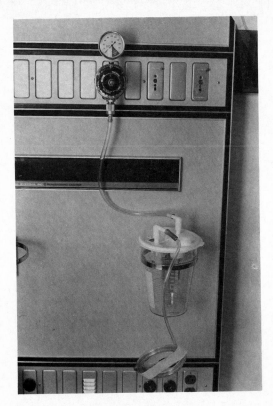

FIGURE 31–2 A wall suction unit.

The suction apparatus includes a collection bottle, a tubing system connected to the suction catheter, and a gauge that registers the degree of suction. These apparatus are either portable or wall mounted (Figure 31–2).

Oropharyngeal or *nasopharyngeal suctioning* remove secretions from the upper respiratory tract. Deeper suctioning, called *endotracheal suctioning*, removes secretions from the trachea and the bronchi. Deep suctioning requires considerably more skill and is usually carried out by a critical-care nursing specialist or an experienced nurse.

Suctioning of the upper respiratory airways is indicated when the client (a) is unable to expectorate coughed secretions, (b) is unable to swallow, and (c) makes light bubbling or rattling breath sounds that signal the accumulation of secretions. The client may also be dyspneic or appear cyanotic. Whether and how often to suction are decisions that require judgment on the part of the nurse. Irritation of the mucous membranes by the suction catheter can increase secretions. Suctioning can also cause some hypoxia. Guidelines for oropharyngeal and nasopharyngeal suctioning are described in Technique 31–1.

31-1 Oropharyngeal and Nasopharyngeal Suctioning

PURPOSES
- To remove secretions that obstruct the airway
- To facilitate respiratory ventilation
- To obtain secretions for diagnostic purposes
- To prevent infection that may result from accumulated secretions

ASSESSMENT FOCUS

Clinical signs indicating the need for suctioning: restlessness; gurgling sounds during respiration; adventitious breath sounds when the chest is auscultated; change in mental status, skin color, rate and pattern of respirations, and pulse rate and rhythm.

EQUIPMENT

- Towel or pad
- Portable or wall suction machine with tubing and collection receptacle
- Sterile disposable container for sterile fluids
- Sterile normal saline or water
- Sterile gloves

- Sterile suction catheter (#12 to #18 Fr. for adults, #8 to #10 Fr. for children, and #5 to #8 Fr. for infants); if both the oropharynx and the nasopharynx are to be suctioned, one sterile catheter is required for each

- Water-soluble lubricant
- Y-connector
- Sterile gauzes
- Moisture-resistant disposal bag
- Sputum trap, if specimen is to be collected

▶ **Technique 31–1 Oropharyngeal and Nasopharyngeal Suctioning** *CONTINUED*

INTERVENTION

1. Prepare the client.

- Explain to the client that suctioning will relieve breathing difficulty and that the procedure is painless but may stimulate the cough, gag, or sneeze reflex. *Knowing that the procedure will relieve breathing problems is often reassuring and enlists cooperation of the client.*

- Position a *conscious* person who has a functional gag reflex in the semi-Fowler's position with the head turned to one side for oral suctioning or with the neck hyperextended for nasal suctioning. *These positions facilitate the insertion of the catheter and help prevent aspiration of secretions.*

- Position an *unconscious* client in the lateral position, facing you. *This position allows the tongue to fall forward, so that it will not obstruct the catheter on insertion. Lateral position also facilitates drainage of secretions from the pharynx and prevents the possibility of aspiration.*

- Place the towel or pad over the pillow or under the chin.

2. Prepare the equipment.

- Set the pressure on the suction gauge, and turn on the suction. Many suction devices are calibrated to three pressure ranges:

Wall unit

Adult: 100 to 120 mm Hg
Child: 95 to 110 mm Hg
Infant: 50 to 95 mm Hg

Portable unit

Adult: 10 to 15 mm Hg
Child: 5 to 10 mm Hg
Infant: 2 to 5 mm Hg

- Open the sterile suction package.

  a. Set up the cup or container, touching only its outside.

b. Pour sterile water or saline into the container.

c. Don the sterile gloves, or don a nonsterile glove on the nondominant hand and then a sterile glove on the dominant hand. *The sterile gloved hand maintains the sterility of the suction catheter, and the unsterile glove prevents the transmission of the microorganisms to the nurse.*

- With your sterile gloved hand, pick up the catheter, and attach it to the suction unit (Figure 31–3).

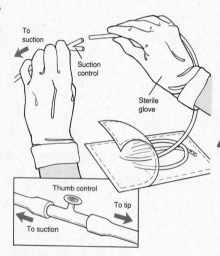

FIGURE 31–3 Attaching the catheter to the suction unit.

- Open the lubricant if performing nasopharyngeal suctioning.

3. Make an approximate measure of the depth for the insertion of the catheter and test the equipment.

- Measure the distance between the tip of the client's nose and the earlobe, or about 13 cm (5 in) for an adult. The appropriate distance for an infant or small child is 4 to 8 cm (1.6 to 3.2 in) or 8 to 12 cm (3.2 to 4.8 in) for an older child.

- Mark the position on the tube with the fingers of the sterile gloved hand.

- Test the pressure of the suction and the patency of the catheter by applying your sterile gloved finger or thumb to the port or open branch of the Y-connector (the suction control) to create suction.

4. Lubricate and introduce the catheter.

- For nasopharyngeal suction, lubricate the catheter tip with water-soluble lubricant; for oropharyngeal suction, moisten the tip with sterile water or saline. *This reduces friction and eases insertion.*

For an Oropharyngeal Suction

- Pull the tongue forward, if necessary, using gauze.

- Do not apply suction during insertion. *Doing so causes trauma to the mucuous membrane.*

- Advance the catheter about 4 to 6 inches along one side of the mouth into the oropharynx. *Directing the catheter along the side prevents gagging.*

For a Nasopharyngeal Suction

- Without applying suction, insert the catheter the premeasured or recommended distance into either naris, and advance it along the floor of the nasal cavity. *This avoids the nasal turbinates.*

- Never force the catheter against an obstruction. If one nostril is obstructed, try the other.

5. Perform suctioning.

- Apply your finger to the suction control port to start suction, and gently rotate the catheter. *Gentle rotation of the catheter ensures that all surfaces are reached and prevents trauma to any one area*

▶ **Technique 31–1** CONTINUED

of the respiratory mucosa due to prolonged suction.

- Apply suction for 5 to 10 seconds; then remove your finger from the control, and remove the catheter.

- A suction attempt should last only 10 to 15 seconds. During this time, the catheter is inserted, the suction applied and discontinued, and the catheter removed.

- It may be necessary during oropharyngeal suctioning to apply suction to secretions that collect in the vestibule of the mouth and beneath the tongue.

6. Clean the catheter, and repeat suctioning as above.

- Wipe off the catheter with sterile gauze if it is thickly coated with secretions. Dispose of the used gauze in a moisture-resistant bag.

- Flush the catheter with sterile water or saline.

- Relubricate the catheter, and repeat suctioning until the air passage is clear.

- Allow 20- to 30-second intervals between each suction, and limit suction to 5 minutes in total. *Applying suction for too long may cause secretions to increase or decrease the client's oxygen supply.*

- Alternate nares for repeat suctionings.

7. Encourage the client to breathe deeply and to cough between suctions. *Coughing and deep breathing help carry secretions from the trachea and bronchi into the pharynx, where they can be reached with the suction catheter.*

8. Obtain a specimen if required. Use a sputum trap (Figure 31–4) as follows:

- Attach the suction catheter to the

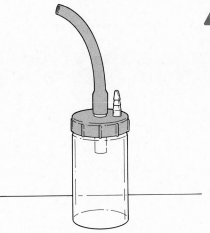

FIGURE 31–4 A sputum collection trap.

rubber tubing of the sputum trap.

- Attach the suction tubing to the sputum trap air vent.

- Suction the client's nasopharynx or oropharynx. The sputum trap will collect the mucus during suctioning.

- Remove the catheter from the client. Disconnect the sputum trap rubber tubing from the suction catheter. Remove the suction tubing from the trap air vent.

- Connect the rubber tubing of the sputum trap to the air vent. *This retains any microorganisms in the sputum trap.*

- Flush the catheter to remove secretions from the tubing.

9. Promote client comfort.

- Offer to assist the client with oral or nasal hygiene.

10. Dispose of equipment and ensure availability for the next suction.

- Dispose of the catheter, gloves, water, and waste container. Wrap the catheter around your sterile glove and roll it inside the glove for disposal.

- To ensure that equipment is

available for the next suctioning, change suction collection bottles and tubing daily or more frequently as necessary.

11. Assess the effectiveness of suctioning.

- Auscultate the client's breathing sounds to ensure they are clear of secretions.

12. Document relevant data.

- Record the procedure: the amount, consistency, color, and odor of sputum (e.g., foamy, white mucus; thick, green-tinged mucus; or blood-flecked mucus) and the client's breathing status before and after the procedure.

- If the technique is carried out frequently, e.g., q1h, it may be appropriate to record only once, at the end of the shift; however, the frequency of the suctioning must be recorded.

VARIATION: Endotracheal Suctioning

Endotracheal suctioning is similar to pharyngeal suctioning; the main difference is that the suction catheter is inserted farther into the client's trachea and/or bronchi. For an adult, it is usually inserted 20 cm, or 8 inches. To ascertain the correct length to insert the catheter for nasal tracheal suctioning, measure the distance from the tip of the nose to the earlobe and then along the side of the neck to the thyroid cartilage (Adam's apple). For oral tracheal suctioning, measure from the mouth to the midsternum. To prevent unnecessary trauma to the tracheal mucosa, always premeasure the correct length for catheter insertion prior to suctioning a child.

Having the client inhale while you insert the catheter facilitates its entry into the trachea because the epiglottis is open during inhalation. Hyperextending the head and ex-

▶ **Technique 31–1 Oropharyngeal and Nasopharyngeal Suctioning** *CONTINUED*

tending the tongue with the mouth open places the glottis in line with the trachea, thereby easing entry into the trachea rather than into the esophagus.

If the catheter needs to be inserted into one or both of the bronchi, turn the client's head to the right to help direct the catheter into the left bronchus. Turn the head to the left to help direct the catheter into the right bronchus. If the catheter meets resistance when it has been inserted the recommended distance, it is probably against the carina. In this instance, pull the catheter back about 1 cm (0.4 in) before applying suction or advancing it farther.

Tracheal and bronchial suctioning should be done intermittently, and the catheter should remain in the client no more than 10 seconds to avoid hypoxemia and cardiopulmonary complications. Once the client coughs, secretions are frequently dislodged to the upper airway, requiring pharyngeal suctioning.

SAMPLE RECORDING

Date	Time	Notes
05/12/93	0200	Oropharyngeal suctioning for 2 min. Thick, greenish sputum. Respirations 20/min, wet. Cyanotic. No response to painful stimuli. Positioned in left Sims'. ———————————————— Rozelle L. Schwartz, RN

SAMPLE RECORDING

Date	Time	Notes
05/12/93	0700	Nasopharyngeal suctioning q.1h. for 3 min × 6. Nares alternated. Thick greenish sputum obtained with 6 suctionings. Respirations remain dyspneic, 30–32/min. No response to painful stimuli. Position changed q.1h. × 6. ———————————————— Rozelle L. Schwartz, RN

EVALUATION FOCUS	Appearance of secretions suctioned; breath sounds; respiratory rate, rhythm, and depth; pulse rate and rhythm; skin color.

KEY ELEMENTS OF OROPHARYNGEAL AND NASOPHARYNGEAL SUCTIONING

- Assess the client's respirations (rate, depth, rhythm, character, and sound); skin and mucous membrane color; difficulty breathing; lung sounds (by auscultation); ability to cough and produce sputum; and level of consciousness before and after the technique.

- Maintain sterility of the suction catheter, flushing solution, and gauzes used to wipe the catheter.

- Position conscious clients appropriately:
  a. For nasal suctioning, hyperextend the neck.
  b. For oral suctioning, turn the head to one side.
  c. For tracheal suctioning, hyperextend the head and have the client extend the tongue.
  d. For the left bronchus, turn the head to the right.
  e. For the right bronchus, turn the head to the left.

- Prevent aspiration of sputum in the unconscious client by positioning the person in the lateral position.

- Measure the correct length for catheter insertion before the procedure.

- Moisten the catheter tip before insertion.

- Insert the catheter *without applying suction* and for tracheal suctioning while the client inhales.

- Never force the catheter against an obstruction.

- Gently rotate the catheter while applying suction.

- Prevent or minimize hypoxia: Apply suction for no more than 15 seconds each time and for no longer than 5 minutes in total.

- Encourage deep breathing and coughing between suctions.

- Flush the catheter between suctions.

- Change suction collection bottles and tubing at least daily.

Infant Bulb Suctioning

A bulb syringe is frequently used to suction the oral and nasal cavities of infants and children, particularly when secretions are not severe enough to require deeper suctioning. This technique may be used for a newborn who has amniotic fluid in the air passages or an infant with increased mucus that is causing labored breathing. The technique requires medical aseptic practice rather than surgical asepsis, since only the mouth or nose is entered, not the pharynx. The bulb syringe should be sterile initially, but it can be rinsed and used for subsequent suctions without resterilizing. The same syringe can be used for the nose and mouth. See Technique 31–2.

31-2 Bulb Suctioning an Infant

PURPOSES
- To establish and maintain a patent airway
- To prevent or relieve labored respirations

ASSESSMENT FOCUS
> Rate and depth of respirations; presence or absence of breath sounds and chest movements: color and pulse rate; color, consistency, and amount of secretions.

EQUIPMENT

- Large towel or blanket
- Clean towel or bib
- Bulb syringe
- Kidney basin or other receptacle
- Disposable gloves as needed

INTERVENTION

1. Position the infant appropriately for the procedure.

- Bundle the infant in a large towel or blanket to restrain the arms, or cradle the child in your arm, tucking the infant's near arm behind your back and holding the other arm securely with your hand (Figure 31–5).

- Put the bib or towel under the infant's chin.

2. Suction the oral and nasal cavities.

- Compress the bulb of the syringe with your thumb before inserting the syringe (Figure 31–6). *Compressing the bulb while the tip is in the mouth or nose can force secretions deeper into the respiratory tract.*

- Keeping the bulb compressed, insert the tip of the syringe into the infant's nose or mouth.

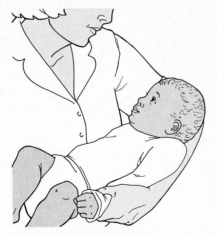

FIGURE 31–5 Restraining the arms of an infant for bulb suctioning. The infant's right arm is tucked behind the nurse's back.

- Release the bulb compression gradually, and slowly move it outward to aspirate the secretions.

- Remove the syringe, hold the tip over the waste receptacle, and compress the bulb again. *Com-*

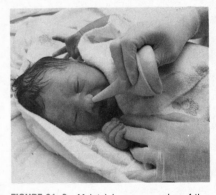

FIGURE 31–6 Maintaining compression of the bulb of the syringe during insertion into the nose. *Source:* S. B. Olds, M. L. London, and P. W. Ladewig, *Maternal-newborn nursing: A family-centered approach,* 4th ed. (Redwood City, Calif.: Addison-Wesley Nursing, 1992), p. 899.

pressing the bulb expels the contents into the waste receptacle.

- Repeat the above until the infant's nares and mouth are clear of secretions and the breathing sounds are clear.

▶ Technique 31–2 Bulb Suctioning an Infant CONTINUED

3. Ensure infant comfort and safety.

🅢 • Cuddle and soothe the infant as necessary, and place the infant in a side-lying or prone position after suctioning. *In a back-lying position, the infant is more likely to aspirate secretions.*

4. Ensure availability of the equipment for the next suction.

• Rinse the syringe and the waste receptacle.

• Place the syringe in a clean folded towel at the cribside for use as needed.

5. Document all relevant information.

• Report to the nurse in charge any problems or untoward responses of the infant.

• Record the procedure and relevant observations in the appropriate records.

VARIATION: The DeLee Suction Device (Mucus Trap)

The DeLee mucus trap is a negative-pressure mouth suction device used for infants (Figure 31–7). To use the device, carefully insert the catheter to 12 cm (3 to 5 in) into the infant's nose or mouth without applying suction, and connect the other end to low suction. Apply suction as the tube is removed. Continue to reinsert the tube and provide suction as long as fluid is aspirated. Avoid excessive suctioning. *This can cause vagal stimulation and subsequent bradycardia.*

🅢 The DeLee device is commonly used in the delivery room to clear the neonate's nose, mouth, and pharynx of mucus and amniotic fluid and to initiate breathing. Suctioning of the mouth is often needed as soon as the neonate's head presents. The mouth is suctioned before the nose. *Nasal stimulation can precipitate the sneezing reflex and cause the infant to inhale and*

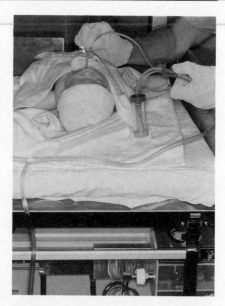

FIGURE 31–7 Suctioning a neonate using the DeLee suction device. *Source:* S. B. Olds, M. L. London, and P. W. Ladewig, *Maternal-newborn nursing: A family-centered approach,* 4th ed. (Redwood City, Calif.: Addison-Wesley Nursing, 1992), p. 678.

aspirate any secretions in the mouth. Suctioning is often repeated after the neonate's first cry.

EVALUATION FOCUS	Response to suctioning in terms of respiratory rate, rhythm, and depth; pulse rate and rhythm; skin color; and appearance of secretions suctioned.

SAMPLE RECORDING

Date	Time	Notes
11/02/93	0730	Admitted to nursery from delivery room. Color pink, heart rate 142, respiratory rate 30. Clear mucous drainage removed from mouth and nose with bulb syringe. Placed in side-lying position. ——————— Kay Kergstra, RN

KEY ELEMENTS OF BULB SUCTIONING AN INFANT

• Restrain the infant's arms.

• Compress the bulb before inserting the syringe.

• Release the bulb compression gradually while aspirating secretions.

• Place the infant in a prone or side-lying position after suctioning to prevent aspiration of the secretions.

• Clean the syringe in readiness for the next suction.

• When suctioning a newborn, suction the mouth before the nose.

CRITICAL THINKING CHALLENGE

When suctioning the client, you note that there are no returns in the bottle. What client assessments should you make? What should you do to determine the problem with the suction? What would you say to the client?

RELATED RESEARCH

Curran, J. F.; Stanek, K. S.; and Kacmarek, R. M. April 1991. Portable airway-suction systems: A comparison of performance. *Respiratory Care* 36:259–66.

Witmer, M. T.; Hess, D.; and Simmons, M. August 1991. An evaluation of the effectiveness of secretion removal with the Ballard closed-circuit suction catheter. *Respiratory Care* 36:844–48.

REFERENCES

Fuchs, P. L. May 1984. Streamlining your suctioning techniques. Part 1. Nasotracheal suctioning. *Nursing 84* 14:55–61.

Reed, J. Jr. November 1987. Orotracheal and nasotracheal intubation. *Emergency Care Quarterly 2* 3:1–6.

Somerson, S. W.; Kozole, A.; Andrea, J.; and Sheehy, S. B. November/December 1990. Suctioning a neonate: Nose or mouth first? *Journal of Emergency Nursing* 16:378.

Oxygen Therapy

32

OBJECTIVES

- Identify essential assessment data required during oxygen therapy

- Describe various methods used to administer oxygen

- Outline safety precautions necessary during oxygen therapy

- Assemble an oxygen cylinder for use

- Assemble wall-outlet oxygen for use

- Give rationales underlying selected steps of the techniques in this chapter

- Administer oxygen by cannula, mask, face tent, and humidity tent safely and effectively

CONTENTS

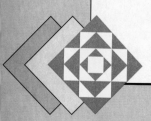

NURSING PROCESS GUIDE

OXYGEN THERAPY

ASSESSMENT

See the Nursing Process Guide for Chapter 30. Observe

- Skin and mucous membrane color. Note whether cyanosis is present.

- Breathing patterns. Note depth of respirations and presence of tachypnea, bradypnea, orthopnea.

- Chest movements. Note whether there are any intercostal, substernal, suprasternal, supraclavicular, or tracheal retractions during inspiration or expiration.

- Chest wall configuration, e.g., kyphosis.

- Lung sounds audible by auscultating the chest and by ear.

- Presence of clinical signs of hypoxemia: tachycardia, tachypnea, restlessness, dyspnea, cyanosis, and confusion. Tachycardia and tachypnea are often early signs. Confusion is a later sign of severe oxygen deprivation.

- Presence of clinical signs of hypercarbia (hypercapnia), restlessness, hypertension, headache, lethargy, tremor.

- Presence of clinical signs of oxygen toxicity: tracheal irritation and cough, dyspnea, and decreased pulmonary ventilation.

Determine

- Vital signs, especially pulse rate and quality, and respiratory rate, rhythm, and depth.

- Whether the client has chronic obstructive pulmonary disease (COPD). Low-flow oxygen systems are essential for these individuals. A high carbon dioxide level in the blood is the normal stimulus to breathe. However, people with COPD may have a high carbon dioxide level, and their stimulus to breathe is hypoxemia. Low flows of oxygen (2 L/min) stimulate breathing for such persons by maintaining slight hypoxemia. This depends on the client's inspiratory flow and normal ventilation. During continuous oxygen administration, levels of oxygen (PO_2) and carbon dioxide (PCO_2) in arterial blood are measured periodically to monitor hypoxemia and adjust the liter flow as needed. PO_2 is normally 80 to 100 mm Hg. PCO_2 is normally 35 to 45 mm Hg.

- Results of diagnostic studies.

- Hemoglobin, hematocrit, complete blood count.

- Arterial blood gases.

- Pulmonary function tests.

RELATED DIAGNOSTIC CATEGORIES

- Activity intolerance
- Ineffective airway clearance
- Anxiety
- Ineffective breathing pattern
- Decreased cardiac output
- Impaired gas exchange
- Ineffective individual coping

PLANNING

Client Goals
The client will

- Restore or maintain adequate ventilation.

- Reduce cardiac workload.

- Increase tissue perfusion and cellular oxygenation.

Outcome Criteria
The client

- Has clear breath sounds bilaterally.

- Has normal respiratory rate, rhythm, and depth, i.e., respiratory pattern of 12 to 20 per minute, effortless breathing (no use of accessory muscles), and symmetric chest expansion on inhalation.

- Has skin, nails, lips, and earlobes of natural color for the individual.

- Has normal arterial blood gases of 80–100 mm Hg (PO_2) and 35–45 mm Hg (PCO_2).

- Performs activities of daily living without shortness of breath or fatigue or alters activities to reduce cardiac workload.

- Has normal heart rhythm and rate within 20 beats of normal.

- Has a maximum systolic blood pressure of 140 mm Hg and a maximum diastolic blood pressure of 90 mm Hg.

- Has warm extremities of a color normal for the individual.

Oxygen Therapy

Additional oxygen is indicated for numerous clients who have **hypoxemia** (low partial pressure of oxygen or low saturation of oxyhemoglobin in the arterial blood), for example, people who have reduced lung diffusion of oxygen through the respiratory membrane, heart failure leading to inadequate transport of oxygen, or substantial loss of lung tissue due to tumors or surgery. See assessment guide for clinical signs of hypoxemia. Oxygen therapy is prescribed by the physician, who specifies the specific concentration, method, and liter flow per minute. The concentration is of more importance than the liter flow per minute. When the administration of oxygen is an emergency measure, the nurse may initiate the therapy.

Oxygen is supplied in hospitals in two ways: by liquid portable systems (cylinders) and from wall outlets. Oxygen cylinders are made of steel. Large ones contain 244 cubic feet of oxygen stored at a pressure of 2200 pounds per square inch (psi). Smaller cylinders are available for emergency and ambulatory use. Piped-in oxygen is stored at much lower pressure, usually 50 to 60 psi.

Oxygen administered from a cylinder or wall-outlet system is dry. Dry gases dehydrate the respiratory mucous membranes. Humidifying devices that add water vapor to inspired air are thus an essential adjunct of oxygen therapy, particularly for liter flows over 2 liters per minute. These devices provide 20% to 40% humidity. The oxygen passes through sterile distilled water and then along a line to the device through which the moistened oxygen is inhaled (e.g., a cannula, nasal catheter, or oxygen mask).

Humidifiers prevent mucous membranes from drying and becoming irritated and loosen secretions for easier expectoration. Oxygen passing through sterile water picks up water vapor before it reaches the client. The more bubbles created during this process, the more water vapor is produced. Very low liter flows (e.g., 1 to 2 liters per minute by nasal cannula) do not require humidification.

Generally, oxygen cylinders are encased in metal carriers equipped with wheels for transport and a broad flat base on which the cylinder stands at the bedside to prevent it from falling. A cap on the top protects the valves and outlets. Accidentally opened outlets can turn a stable tank into a dangerous projectile. A regulator and a humidifier must be attached before the cylinder is used. The purpose of the regulator is to release oxygen at a safe level and at a desirable rate. The regulator has two gauges: the *cylinder contents gauge* nearest the tank indicates the

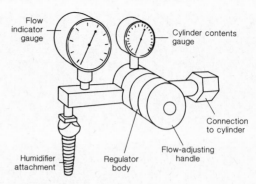

FIGURE 32–1 An oxygen regulator.

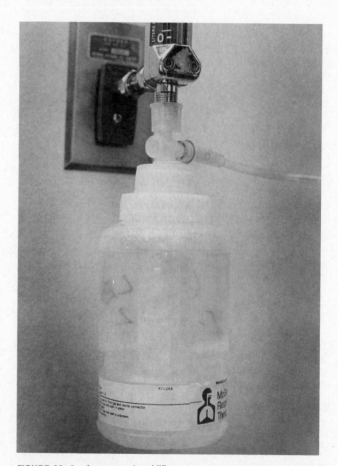

FIGURE 32–2 An oxygen humidifier.

pressure or amount of oxygen in the tank; the *flow meter gauge* or *flow indicator gauge* indicates the gas flow in liters per minute (Figure 32–1). To ensure that the regulator is firmly attached, the inlet nut is tightened with a wrench. A humidifier bottle with distilled water is then attached below the flow meter gauge, and the specific oxygen tubing and equipment prescribed for the client, e.g., nasal cannula or mask, is attached to the bottle (Figure 32–2).

Before the regulator is attached, any dust particles in the outlets must be removed to prevent them from being forced into the regulator. The nurse accomplishes this task by slightly opening the handwheel at the top of the cylinder counterclockwise and then quickly closing it. This procedure, referred to as "cracking the cylinder," releases a small amount of oxygen that flushes out the outlet. The force of this oxygen release causes a loud hissing noise that is startling and frightening to most people. Nurses should therefore forewarn clients and others or prime the tank away from the client. Oxygen cylinders need to be handled and stored with caution and strapped securely in wheeled transport devices or stands to prevent possible falls and outlet breakages. They should be placed away from traffic areas and heaters.

To use an oxygen wall outlet, the nurse carries out these steps:

1. Attach the flow meter to the wall outlet, exerting firm pressure. The flow meter should be in the OFF position (Figure 32–3).

2. Fill the humidifier bottle with distilled water. (This can be done before coming to the bedside.)

3. Attach the humidifier bottle to the base of the flow meter (Figure 32–2, earlier).

4. Attach the prescribed oxygen tubing and delivery device to the humidifier.

5. Regulate the flow meter to the prescribed level.

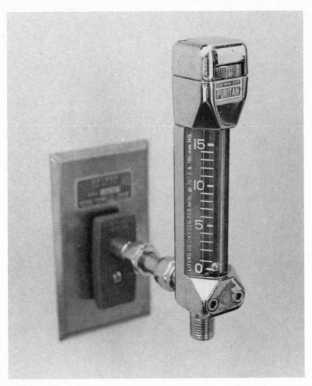

FIGURE 32–3   An oxygen flow meter attached to a wall outlet.

Home Care Equipment

Three major oxygen systems for home care use are available in most communities: cylinders or tanks of compressed gas, liquid (cryogenic) oxygen, and oxygen concentrators.

1. *Cylinders.* These are the system of choice for clients who need oxygen episodically, e.g., on a p.r.n. basis. Advantages are that cylinders deliver all liter flows (1 to 15 L/min), and oxygen evaporation does not occur during storage. Two or more cylinders can be manifolded together and stored in the home. Disadvantages are that the 150-pound cylinders are large and awkward to move (smaller portable cylinders are available, however), the supply company must be notified when a refill is needed, and they are costly for the high-use client.

2. *Liquid oxygen.* Liquid oxygen reservoirs store liquid oxygen at minus 212 C (minus 350 F) in a smaller amount of space than compressed gas. The oxygen is vaporized by adding heat from the surroundings. Advantages are that these reservoirs are lighter in weight and cleaner in appearance than cylinders, they are not as difficult to operate, and they are equipped with a walker accessory resembling a Thermos bottle that can be easily filled from the stationary reservoir. The portable unit is beneficial for the client with COPD who needs continuous oxygen therapy but also needs rehabilitative activities, such as mild exercise, to resume a more normal life-style. Disadvantages of liquid oxygen are that many home care medical supply and service companies are not able to handle it, oxygen evaporation occurs when the unit is not used, only low flows (1 to 4 L/min) can be used or freezing occurs, and the portable unit designed to be carried over the shoulder weighs ten pounds, a burden to the typically weak and emaciated COPD client. Although wheeled carts are available from the oxygen manufacturers, the cost factor is significant; a luggage cart or folding grocery cart is a less expensive alternative.

3. *Oxygen concentrators.* Concentrators are electrically powered systems that manufacture oxygen from room air. At 1 L/min, such a system can deliver a concentration of about 95% oxygen, but the concentration drops when the flow rate increases (e.g., 75% concentration at 4 L/min). Many models of oxygen concentrators are manufactured. Advantages are that they are more attractive in appearance, resembling furniture rather than medical equipment; they eliminate the need for regular delivery of oxygen or refilling of cylinders; because the supply of oxygen is constant, they alleviate the client's anxiety about running out of oxygen; they are the most economical system when continuous use is required; and the client's automobile can be equipped with a special alternator to allow the concentrator to operate from the car battery. The cost of the alternator and its installation is high, however, too expensive for most people. Major disadvantages of a concentrator are that it lacks portability (the smallest unit weighs 45 pounds); it tends to be noisy; it is powered by electricity, and, where the cost of electricity is high, the additional monthly cost can be substantial; an emergency backup unit (e.g., an oxygen tank) must be provided for clients for whom a power failure could be life-threatening; and heat produced by the concentrator motor is a problem for those who live in trailers, small houses, or warm climates, where air conditioners are required. The oxygen concentrator must also be checked periodically with an O_2 analyzer to ensure that it is providing an adequate delivery of oxygen. This service is usually provided by the oxygen supplier on a contractual basis.

Another type of oxygen concentrator is the *oxygen enricher*. It uses a plastic membrane that allows water vapor to pass through with the oxygen, thus eliminating the need for a humidifying device. It is also thought to filter out bacteria present in the air. The enricher provides an O_2 concentration of 40% at all flow rates, it tends to be quieter than the concentrator, there is less chance of combustion (since the gas is only 40% oxygen), it has only two moving parts (thus decreasing the risk of something going wrong), and a nebulizer can be operated off the enricher because of the high flow rate.

The nurse needs to ensure that the client has appropriate help in choosing a reputable home oxygen vendor, since several companies offer home oxygen service. Services furnished should include:

- A 24-hour emergency service.
- Trained personnel to make the initial delivery and instruct the client in safe, appropriate use of the oxygen and maintenance of the equipment.
- At least monthly follow-up visits to check the equipment and reinstruct the client as necessary.
- A regular cost review to assure that the system is the most cost-effective one for that client, with routine notification of the physician or home care professional if it seems that another system is more appropriate.

The nurse needs to also ensure that the client knows about the financial reimbursements available from Medicare and Medicaid or other insurance agencies. In Canada's system of socialized health care, the cost of home oxygen therapy is fully covered.

Oxygen Therapy Safety Precautions

- Place cautionary signs reading "No Smoking: Oxygen in Use" on the client's door, at the foot or head of the bed, and on the oxygen equipment.
- Instruct the client and visitors about the hazard of smoking with oxygen in use.
- Request other clients in the room and visitors to smoke in areas provided elsewhere in the hospital.
- Make sure that electrical equipment, such as razors, hearing aids, radios, televisions, and heating pads, is in good working order to prevent the occurrence of short-circuit sparks.
- Avoid materials that generate static electricity, such as woolen blankets and synthetic fabrics. Cotton blankets are used, and nurses are advised to wear cotton fabrics.
- Avoid the use of volatile, flammable materials, such as oils, greases, alcohol, and ether, near clients receiving oxygen. Avoid alcohol back rubs, and take nail polish removers or the like away from the immediate vicinity.
- Ground electric monitoring equipment, suction machines, and portable diagnostic machines.
- Make known the location of fire extinguishers, and make sure personnel are trained in their use.

Safety Precautions for Oxygen Therapy

Safety precautions are essential during oxygen therapy (see the box above). Although oxygen by itself will not burn or explode, it does facilitate combustion. For example, a bed sheet ordinarily burns slowly when ignited in the atmosphere; however, if saturated with free-flowing oxygen and ignited by a spark, it will burn rapidly and explosively. The greater the concentration of the oxygen, the more rapidly fires start and burn, and such fires are difficult to extinguish. Because oxygen is colorless, odorless, and tasteless, people are often unaware of its presence.

Oxygen Delivery Equipment

Oxygen is administered by either low-flow or high-flow systems. In *low-flow systems*, gas is delivered via small bore tubing at a rate shown on the flowmeter. Because room air is also inhaled along with oxygen, the fraction of inspired oxygen (FiO_2) will vary depending on the respiratory rate, tidal volume, and liter flow. Low-flow systems are generally used for clients who have a respiratory rate below 25 per minute and a regular and consistent respiratory pattern. They are contraindicated for clients who require carefully monitored concentrations of oxygen. Low-flow administration devices include the nasal cannula, simple face mask, partial rebreathing mask, humidity tent, and oxygen tent.

High-flow systems supply all of the gas required during ventilation in precise amounts, regardless of the client's respiratory status. The ratio of room air to oxygen is regulated and does not vary with the client's respirations. Thus it is a precise and consistent method for controlling the client's FiO$_2$. In high-flow systems, gas is delivered via a Venturi device and large-bore tubing placed near the client. The Venturi mask is an example of a high-flow administration device.

Some devices can be used for both low- and high-flow administration, e.g., the face tent and the oxygen hood. Both low-flow and high-flow systems can deliver a variety of oxygen concentrations.

Cannula

The **nasal cannula** (nasal prongs) is the most common inexpensive low-flow device used to administer oxygen. It consists of a rubber or plastic tube that extends around the face, with 0.6- to 1.3-cm (¼- to

½-in) curved prongs that fit into the nostrils. One side of the tube connects to the oxygen tubing and oxygen supply. The cannula is often held in place by an elastic band that fits around the client's head or under the chin (Figure 32–4). For clients who are confused or particularly active, it may be helpful to secure the cannula in place with small pieces of tape on each side of the face.

The nasal cannula is easy to apply and does not interfere with the client's ability to eat or talk. It also is relatively comfortable, permits some freedom of movement, and is well tolerated by the client. It delivers a relatively low concentration of oxygen (24% to 45%) at flow rates of 2 to 6 liters per minute. Higher concentrations and flow rates can be administered; however, above 6 liters per minute there is a tendency for the client to swallow air and for the nasal and pharyngeal mucosa to become irritated. In addition, the FiO$_2$ is *not* increased.

Administering oxygen by cannula is detailed in Technique 32–1 on page 783.

Face Mask

Face masks that cover the client's nose and mouth may be used for oxygen inhalation. Most masks are made of clear, pliable plastic or rubber that can be molded to fit the face. They are held to the client's head with elastic bands. Some have a metal clip that can be bent over the bridge of the nose for a snug fit. There are several holes in the sides of the mask (exhalation ports) to allow the escape of exhaled carbon dioxide.

Some masks have reservoir bags, which provide higher oxygen concentrations to the client. A portion of the client's expired air is directed into the bag. Because this air comes from the upper respiratory passages (e.g., the trachea and bronchi), where it does not take part in gaseous exchange, its oxygen concentration remains the same as that of inspired air.

A variety of oxygen masks are marketed:

- The *simple face mask* (low-flow system) delivers oxygen concentrations from 40% to 60% at liter flows of 5 to 8 liters per minute respectively (Figure 32–5).

- The *partial rebreather mask* (low-flow system) delivers oxygen concentrations of 60% to 90% at liter flows of 6 to 10 liters per minute respectively. The oxygen reservoir bag that is attached allows the client to rebreathe about the first third of the exhaled air in conjunction with oxygen (Figure 32–6). Thus it increases the FiO$_2$ by recycling expired oxygen. The partial rebreather bag must not totally deflate during inspiration to avoid car-

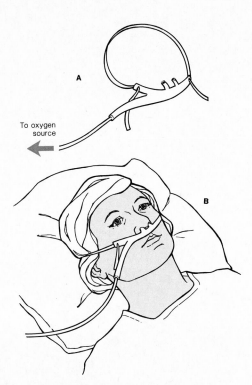

To oxygen source

FIGURE 32–4 *A*, nasal cannula; *B*, the cannula in place.

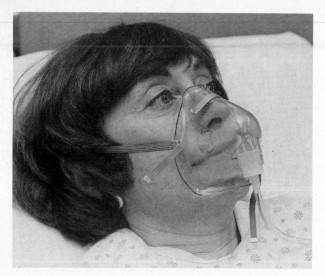

FIGURE 32–5 A simple face mask for a low-flow oxygen system.

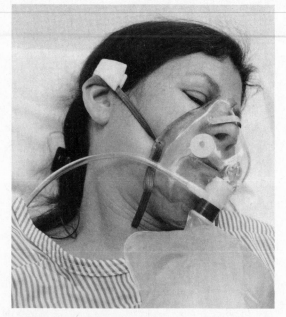

FIGURE 32–7 A nonrebreather mask for a low-flow or a high-flow oxygen system.

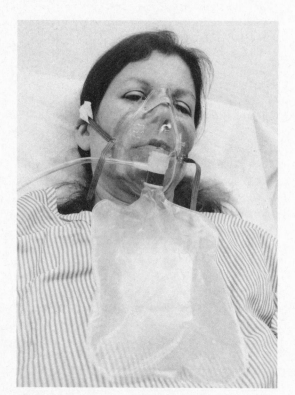

FIGURE 32–6 A partial rebreather mask for a low-flow oxygen system.

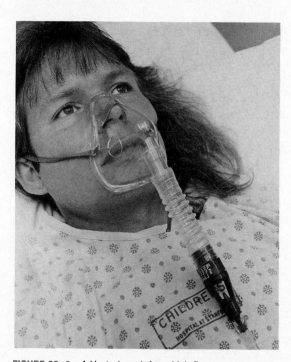

FIGURE 32–8 A Venturi mask for a high-flow oxygen system.

bon dioxide buildup. If this problem occurs, the nurse increases the liter flow of oxygen.

- The *nonrebreather mask* (low-flow system) delivers the highest oxygen concentration possible by means other than intubation or mechanical ventilation, i.e., 95% to 100%, at liter flows of 10 to 15 liters per minute. Using a nonrebreather mask, the client breathes only the source gas from the bag. One-way valves on the mask and between the reservoir bag and the mask prevent the room

air and the client's exhaled air from entering the bag (Figure 32–7). To prevent carbon dioxide buildup, the nonrebreather bag must not totally deflate during inspiration. If it does, the nurse can correct this problem by increasing the liter flow of oxygen.

- The *Venturi mask* (high-flow system) delivers oxygen concentrations precise to within 1% and is often used for clients with COPD (Figure 32–8). Oxygen concentrations vary from 24% to 40% or

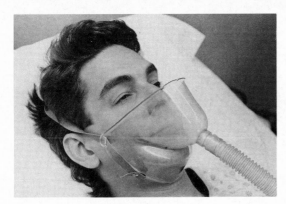

FIGURE 32–9 An oxygen face tent.

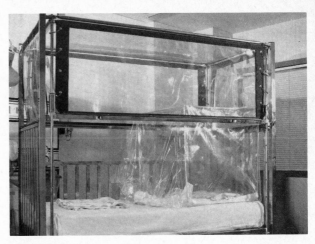

FIGURE 32–10 A humidity tent.

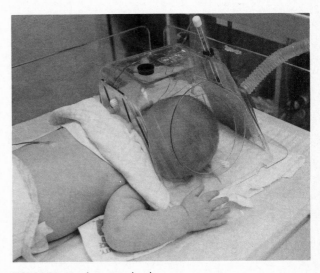

FIGURE 32–11 An oxygen hood.

50%, depending on the brand, at liter flows of 4 to 10 liters per minute. The Venturi mask is designed with wide-bore tubing and various color-coded jet adapters. Each color code corresponds to a precise oxygen concentration and a specific liter flow. For example, a blue adapter delivers a 24% concentration of oxygen at 4 liters per minute, and a green adapter delivers a 35% concentration of oxygen at 8 liters per minute. Optional humidification adapters are also available for clients who require them, e.g., those receiving oxygen concentrations in excess of 30%.

Initiating oxygen by mask is much the same as initiating oxygen by cannula, except that the nurse must find a mask of appropriate size. Smaller sizes are available for children. Administering oxygen by mask is detailed in Technique 32–1 on page 783.

Face Tent

Face tents (Figure 32–9) can replace oxygen masks when masks are poorly tolerated by clients, e.g., children. When a face tent alone is used to supply oxygen, the concentration of oxygen varies; therefore, it is often used in conjunction with a Venturi system. Face tents provide varying concentrations of oxygen, e.g., 30% to 50% concentration of oxygen at 4 to 8 liters per minute. Frequently inspect the client's facial skin for dampness or chafing, and dry and treat as needed. As with face masks, the client's facial skin must be kept dry. Administering oxygen by face tent is detailed in Technique 32–1 on page 783.

Humidity Tent and Incubator

A variety of humidity/oxygen tents are available for children beyond early infancy until they are old enough to cooperate and use a nasal cannula. Each unit generally comes with the manufacturer's instructions for use. However, all have common elements. The tent consists of a rectangular, clear, plastic canopy with outlets that connect to an oxygen or compressed air source and to a humidifier that moisturizes the air or oxygen (Figure 32–10). Because the enclosed tent becomes very warm, some type of cooling mechanism such as an ice chamber or a refrigeration unit is provided to maintain the desired temperature. Administering oxygen by humidity tent is discussed in Technique 32–2.

Oxygen Hood

An oxygen hood (Figure 32–11) is a rigid plastic dome that encloses an infant's head. It is both a low-flow and a high-flow delivery system and provides precise oxygen levels and high humidity. The gas should not be allowed to blow directly into the infant's face, and the hood should not rub against the infant's neck, chin, or shoulder.

Oxygen Analyzer

Oxygen analyzers (Figure 32–12) measure the concentration of oxygen being received by the client. The analyzer is first used to measure the concentration of oxygen in the room. It should register 0.21 (21%).

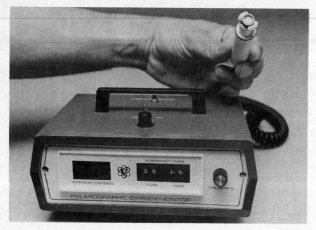

FIGURE 32-12 An oxygen analyzer.

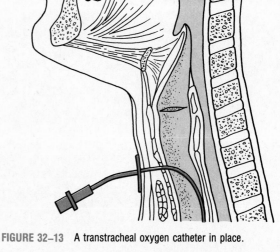

FIGURE 32-13 A transtracheal oxygen catheter in place.

If it does not, the nurse adjusts the dial to this calibration. The nurse then places the sample tube next to the client's nose, monitors the reading on the analyzer, and adjusts the oxygen flow rate to obtain the desired fraction of inspired oxygen (FiO_2).

Home Delivery Devices

Home delivery devices are now available to clients who require continuous oxygen therapy at home. *Transtracheal oxygen delivery* refers to oxygen given through a small, narrow plastic cannula that is inserted through the skin at the base of the neck directly into the trachea (Figure 32–13). A chain around the neck holds the catheter in place. The nurse keeps the catheter patent by injecting 1.5 ml normal saline into it, moving a cleaning rod in and out of it and then injecting another 1.5 ml of saline solution. This is done two or three times a day.

A new device referred to as *Oxy-Frames* delivers oxygen through specially designed eyeglasses that provide the same liter flow as nasal cannulae. The oxygen tubing is camouflaged in grooves on the inside of the frames. It extends down the inside of the frames and around the perimeter of the lens and terminates in a small plastic cannula that enters the nares. The portion of the cannula entering the nares can be detached for maintenance or replacement.

Another option is the *Nocturnal Cannula*, oxygen tubing held in place with a headband. The plastic tubing extends from the headband around the forehead along the sides of the nose into the nares. This device is useful for clients whose nasal cannula tends to become dislodged during sleep. It can also be used during the day to relieve pressure points on the cheeks and ears obtained from the nasal cannula.

Reservoir cannulae, or *Oxymizers*, are nasal cannula devices with plastic reservoirs that store oxygen and deliver a 20-ml bolus of oxygen during the first part of the inspiratory cycle. The plastic reservoirs inflate with 20 ml of oxygen during expiration and deflate at the beginning of inspiration when delivering this 20-ml bolus, which goes directly to the alveoli. After the bolus is delivered, oxygen is received as usual through the nasal cannula.

One type of oxymizer consists of a reservoir worn under the nose in the mustache area. Another, less viisble, type is the oxymizer pendant, which consists of a large storage pendant and tubing larger than standard.

Demand devices (Pulsair, Oxymatic) are battery-operated devices that deliver a bolus of oxygen *only* at the beginning of inhalation. They conserve oxygen, because they do not deliver oxygen during exhalation and late inhalation. These devices are triggered to deliver oxygen when negative pressure at the tip of the nasal cannula is sensed.

Administering Oxygen by Cannula, Face Mask, or Face Tent

Before administering oxygen, determine (a) whether the client has COPD; (b) the levels of oxygen (PO_2) and carbon dioxide (PCO_2) in the client's arterial blood (PO_2 is normally 80 to 100 mm Hg; PCO_2 is normally 35 to 45 mm Hg); and (c) the order for oxygen, including the administering device and the liter flow rate (L/min) or the percentage of oxygen.

PURPOSES

Cannula
- To deliver a relatively low concentration of oxygen when only minimal O_2 support is required
- To allow uninterrupted delivery of oxygen while the client ingests food or fluids

Face Mask
- To provide moderate O_2 support and a higher concentration of oxygen and/or humidity than is provided by cannula

Face Tent
- To provide high humidity
- To provide oxygen when a mask is poorly tolerated
- To provide a high flow of oxygen when attached to a Venturi system

ASSESSMENT FOCUS

Vital signs; arterial blood gas levels; signs of hypoxia (e.g., tachycardia, tachypnea, dyspnea); signs of hypercarbia (e.g., restlessness, hypertension, headache); lung sounds; patency of nares (if nasal cannula is to be used); mental status; signs of oxygen toxicity (e.g., tracheal irritation, cough, decreased pulmonary ventilation).

EQUIPMENT

Cannula
- ☐ Oxygen supply with a flow meter
- ☐ Humidifier with sterile distilled water
- ☐ Nasal cannula and tubing
- ☐ Tape
- ☐ Gauzes

Face Mask
- ☐ Oxygen supply with a flow meter
- ☐ Humidifier with sterile distilled water
- ☐ Prescribed face mask of the appropriate size
- ☐ Padding for the elastic band

Face Tent
- ☐ Oxygen supply with a flow meter
- ☐ Humidifier with sterile distilled water
- ☐ Face tent of the appropriate size

INTERVENTION

1. Determine the need for oxygen therapy, and verify the order for the therapy.

- Perform a respiratory assessment to determine the need for O_2 therapy. See the Assessment in the Nursing Process Guide on page 775.

2. Prepare the client and support persons.

- Assist the client to a semi-Fowler's position if possible. *This position permits easier chest expansion and hence easier breathing.*

- Explain that oxygen is not dangerous when safety precautions are observed and that it will ease the discomfort of dyspnea. Inform the client and support persons about the safety precautions connected with oxygen use.

3. Set up the oxygen equipment and the humidifier. See page 777.

4. Turn on the oxygen at the prescribed rate, and ensure proper functioning.

- Check that the oxygen is flowing freely through the tubing. There should be no kinks in the tubing,

▶

► **Technique 32–1 Administering Oxygen** *CONTINUED*

and the connections should be airtight. There should be bubbles in the humidifier as the oxygen flows through the water. You should feel the oxygen at the outlets of the cannula.

- Set the oxygen at the flow rate ordered, e.g., 2 to 6 liters per minute.

5. Apply the appropriate oxygen delivery device.

Cannula

- Put the cannula over the client's face, with the outlet prongs fitting into the nares and the elastic band around the head. Some models have a strap to adjust under the chin.

- If the cannula will not stay in place, tape it at the sides of the face.

- Slip gauze pads under the tubing over the cheekbones to prevent skin irritation as necessary.

Face Mask

- Guide the mask toward the client's face, and apply it from the nose downward.

- Fit the mask to the contours of the client's face. *The mask should mold to the face, so that very little oxygen escapes into the eyes or around the cheeks and chin.*

- Secure the elastic band around the client's head so that the mask is comfortable but snug.

- Pad the band behind the ears and over bony prominences. *Padding will prevent irritation from the mask.*

Face Tent

- Place the tent over the client's face, and secure the ties around the head.

- Turn on the oxygen at the prescribed flow rate.

6. Assess the client regularly.

- Assess the client's level of anxiety, color, and ease of respirations, and provide support while the client adjusts to the cannula.

- Assess the client in 15 to 30 minutes, depending on the client's condition, and regularly thereafter. Assess vital signs, color, breathing patterns, and chest movements.

- Assess the client regularly for

clinical signs of hypoxia; tachycardia, confusion, dyspnea, restlessness, and cyanosis. Obtain arterial blood gas results, if they are available.

Nasal Cannula

- Assess the client's nares for encrustations and irritation. Apply a water-soluble lubricant as required to soothe the mucous membranes.

Face Mask or Tent

- Inspect the facial skin frequently for dampness or chafing, and dry and treat it as needed.

7. Inspect the equipment on a regular basis.

- Check the liter flow and the level of water in the humidifier in 30 minutes and whenever providing care to the client.

- Maintain the level of water in the humidifier.

- Make sure that safety precautions are being followed.

8. Document relevant data.

- Record the initiation of the therapy and all nursing assessments.

EVALUATION FOCUS

Vital signs; signs of hypoxia, hypercarbia; bilateral lung sounds; blood gas levels; color of skin, nails, lips, and earlobes; activity tolerance; level of anxiety.

SAMPLE RECORDING

Date	Time	Notes
12/5/93	0730	BP 140/90, P 96, R 24. Slightly cyanotic, dyspneic on exertion, and restless, crackles loud at base of left lung. O_2 by cannula at 3 L/min. applied. ———————————————— Susan de Camillis, SN
	0800	No cyanosis apparent. P 84, R 16. States "breathing is easier." Is less restless, crackles loud at base of left lung. ———————— Susan de Camillis, SN

▶ **Technique 32–1** *CONTINUED*

KEY ELEMENTS OF ADMINISTERING OXYGEN

Cannula, Face Mask, Face Tent

- Determine whether the client has COPD.
- Assess the client's vital signs, skin and mucous membrane color, breathing patterns, chest movements, and lung sounds before and regularly during the oxygen administration.
- Establish and maintain oxygen safety precautions.
- Establish and maintain the correct liter flow.
- Establish and maintain the level of water in the humidifier

Face Mask

- Apply and mold the mask from the nose downward.
- Prevent irritation over bony prominences.
- For a Venturi mask, prevent occlusion of the air entrainment ports.
- Maintain the integrity of the facial skin.

Face Tent

- Maintain the integrity of the facial skin.

 32-2 # Administering Oxygen by Humidity Tent

Before administering oxygen by humidity tent, determine (a) whether the damper valve is to be kept open, kept partially open, or intermittently closed and opened; and (b) whether aerosol medications are to be administered. Check the physician's orders.

PURPOSES
- To facilitate breathing by humidifying respiratory membranes and loosening secretions
- To increase blood oxygenation levels if oxygen is required
- To cool the body and reduce body temperature to normal range

ASSESSMENT FOCUS

See Technique 32–1, page 783.

EQUIPMENT

- ☐ Gown or cotton blanket
- ☐ Humidity tent
- ☐ Ice
- ☐ Sterile distilled water
- ☐ Oxygen source or compressed air
- ☐ Additional gowns and bath blankets
- ☐ Small pillow or rolled towel

INTERVENTION

1. Verify the physician's orders.

2. Prepare the child.

- Provide an explanation appropriate to the age of the child, and offer emotional support.

- Cover the child with a gown or a cotton blanket. Some agencies provide gowns with hoods, or a small towel may be wrapped around the head. *The child needs protection from chilling and from* *the dampness and condensation in the tent.*

3. Prepare the humidity tent.

- Close the zippers on each side of the tent.

▶

► **Technique 32–2 Administering Oxygen by Humidity Tent** CONTINUED

- Fanfold the front part of the canopy into the bedclothes or into an overlying drawsheet, and ensure that all sides of the canopy are tucked well under the mattress (Figure 32–10, earlier).

- If cool mist is ordered, fill the trough with ice to the depth indicated by a line on the trough.

- Ensure that the drainage tube for the trough is in place.

- Fill the water jar with sterile distilled water. *The water moisturizes the air or the oxygen.*

- Connect the tent to the wall oxygen or compressed air.

- Flood the tent with oxygen by setting the flow meter at 15 liters per minute for about 5 minutes. Then, adjust the flow meter according to orders, e.g., 10 to 15 liters per minute. *Flooding the tent quickly increases the oxygen to the desired level.*

- Open the damper valve for about 5 minutes to increase humidity. The valve controls mist output and may be left open or partially open.

4. Place the child in the tent, and assess the child's respiratory status.

- Assess vital signs, skin color, breathing, and chest movements.

5. Provide required care for the child.

- Change the bedding and clothing as they become damp.

- Place a small pillow or rolled towel at the head of the tent. *This padding prevents bumping of the child's head and helps absorb excess moisture.*

- When administering care, be sure to maintain the humidity of the air and oxygen therapy. The

canopy can be moved up around the infant's head and neck and secured under a pillow while care is being provided.

6. Monitor the functioning of the humidity tent.

- Monitor air or oxygen flows frequently to maintain required concentrations, and ensure that all connections are airtight.

- Minimize opening of the tent to avoid lowering the prescribed oxygen concentration. Plan care accordingly.

- Monitor the concentration of oxygen inside the tent according to agency protocol.

- Maintain the temperature of the tent at 20 to 21 C (68 to 70 F).

7. Document relevant data.

- Record the initiation of therapy, all assessments, and the data from oxygen analyzer.

EVALUATION FOCUS	Vital signs; cough; skin color; lung sounds; signs of hypoxia, hypercarbia; blood gas levels.

SAMPLE RECORDING

Date	Time	Notes
5/5/93	0600	Placed in humidity tent. T 98.6, P 108, R 32, Slightly cyanotic. O_2 set at 8 L/min., mist continuous. ——————————————— Nina Sims, SN
	0630	P 96, R 24, no cyanosis, Resting ——————————————— Nina Sims, SN

KEY ELEMENTS OF ADMINISTERING OXYGEN BY HUMIDITY TENT

See the Key Elements of Technique 32–1, page 785.

- Maintain oxygen and humidity concentrations while providing care.

- Monitor the concentration of oxygen in the tent according to agency protocol.

- Change clothing and bedding as they become damp.

Pulse Oximetry

A **pulse oximeter** is a noninvasive device that measures a client's arterial blood oxygen saturation (SaO_2) (Figure 32–14) by means of a sensor attached to the client's finger (Figure 32–15), toe, nose, earlobe, or forehead (or around the hand or foot of a neonate). The pulse oximeter can detect hypoxemia before clinical signs and symptoms, such as dusky skin color and dusky nailbeds color develop.

The pulse oximeter's *sensor* has two parts: (a) two light-emitting diodes (LEDs)—one red, the other infrared—that transmit light through nails, tissue, venous blood, and arterial blood; and (b) a photodetector placed directly opposite the LEDs (e.g., the other side of the finger, toe, or nose). The photodetector receives red and infrared light. By a process known as **spectrophotometry**, the photodetector measures the amount of red and infrared light absorbed by oxygenated and deoxygenated hemoglobin in arterial blood: Oxygenated hemoglobin absorbs more infrared light; deoxygenated hemoglobin, more red light. The SaO_2 is computed on the basis of the amount of light (red and infrared) that reaches the photodetector. Normal SaO_2 is 95% to 100%. An SaO_2 below 70% is life-threatening.

Because pulse oximetry measures only the **functional hemoglobin** (the ratio of oxygen bound to hemoglobin compared to the amount of hemoglobin that is available for binding), it can create misleading results if the client's hemoglobin is bound to another substance, such as carbon monoxide. Pulse oximetry doesn't account for hemoglobin bound to carbon monoxide.

Pulse oximeters with various types of sensors are available from several manufacturers. Table 32–1 indicates the types of sensors appropriate for various client weight limits and locations for their use.

The *oximeter unit* consists of an inlet connection for the sensor cable, a faceplate that indicates (a) the oxygen saturation measurement (expressed as a percentage) and (b) the pulse rate. A present alarm system signals high and low SaO_2 measurements and a high and low pulse rate. The high and low SaO_2 levels for adults are generally preset at 100% and 85%, respectively (95% and 80% for neonates). The high and low pulse rates for adults are usually preset at 140 and 50 beats per minute (200 and 100 for neonates). These alarm limits can, however, be changed according to the manufacturer's directions. Technique 32–3 explains how to set up and use a pulse oximeter.

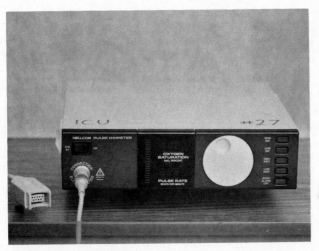

FIGURE 32–14 A pulse oximeter.

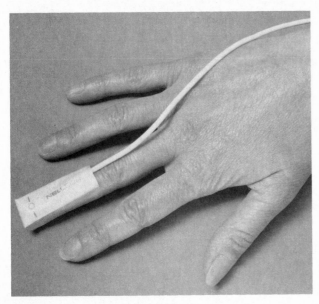

FIGURE 32–15 A finger clip pulse oximeter sensor.

TABLE 32–1   TYPES OF PULSE OXIMETER SENSORS

Type of Sensor	Client's Weight	Location
Adhesive neonatal	Less than 3 kg or more than 40 kg	Around a neonate's hand or foot
Adhesive infant	From 1 kg to 20 kg	Toe or finger
Adhesive pediatric	From 10 kg to 50 kg	Index, middle, or ring finger or toe
Adhesive adult	More than 30 kg	Same as pediatric
Adhesive adult nasal	More than 50 kg	Cartilaginous part of nose below the bridge
Finger clip	More than 40 kg	Finger only

Source: Adapted from G. Sonnesso. Are you ready to use pulse oximetry? *Nursing 91*, August 1991, 21:61.

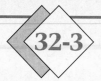

32-3 Using a Pulse Oximeter

PURPOSES
- To measure the arterial blood oxygen saturation (SaO_2)
- To detect the presence of hypoxemia before visible signs develop

ASSESSMENT FOCUS

Risk factors for development of hypoxemia (e.g., respiratory or cardiac disease); vital signs and skin and nailbed color as baseline data; allergy to adhesive; tissue perfusion of extremities; hemoglobin level.

EQUIPMENT

- Pulse oximeter
- Alcohol wipe
- Nail polish remover as needed
- Sheet or towel

INTERVENTION

1. Select an appropriate sensor.

- Choose a sensor appropriate for the client's weight and size. Because weight limits of infant, pediatric, and adult sensors overlap, a neonatal sensor could be used for an infant or a pediatric sensor for a small adult. See the manufacturer's directions for weight limits and Table 32–1.

- If the client is allergic to adhesive, use a clip or reflectance sensor without adhesive.

2. Select an appropriate site.

- Use a location appropriate for the type of sensor. See Table 32–1 on page 787.

- If using an extremity, assess the proximal pulse and capillary refill at the point closest to the site. *Decreased circulation can alter the SaO_2 measurements.*

- If the client has low tissue perfusion due to peripheral vascular disease or therapy using vasoconstrictive medications, use a nasal sensor or a reflectance sensor on the forehead.

- Avoid using lower extremities that have a compromised circulation and extremities that are used for infusions or other invasive monitoring.

3. Prepare the site.

- Clean the site with an alcohol wipe before applying the sensor.

- Remove a female client's nail polish or acrylic nails. *These items can interfere with accurate measurements.*

4. Apply the sensor, and connect it to the pulse oximeter.

- Make sure the LED and photodetector are accurately aligned, i.e., opposite each other on either side of the finger, toe, nose, or earlobe. Many sensors have markings to facilitate correct alignment of the LEDs and photodetector. *Correct alignment is essential for accurate SaO_2 measurement.*

- Attach the sensor cable to the connection outlet on the oximeter. Appropriate connection will be confirmed by an audible beep indicating each arterial pulsation. Turn on the machine according to the manufacturer's directions. Some devices have a wheel that can be turned clockwise to increase the pulse volume and counterclockwise to decrease it.

- Ensure that the bar of light or waveform on the face of the oximeter fluctuates with each pul-

sation and reflects the pulse volume or strength. *A signal that is too weak will not produce an accurate SaO_2 measurement.*

5. Set and turn on the alarm.

- Check the preset alarm limits for high and low oxygen saturation and high and low pulse rates.

- Change these alarm limits according to the manufacturer's directions as indicated.

- Ensure that the audio and visual alarms are on before you leave the client. A tone will be heard and a number will blink on the faceplate.

6. Ensure client safety.

- Inspect and/or move or change the location of an adhesive toe or finger sensor every 4 hours and a spring-tension sensor every 2 hours. *Movement prevents tissue necrosis due to prolonged pressure.*

- Inspect the sensor site tissues for irritation from adhesive sensors.

7. Ensure the accuracy of measurement.

- Minimize motion artifacts by using an adhesive sensor, or immobilize the client's monitoring site. *Movement of the client's fin-*

▶ **Technique 32–3** *CONTINUED*

ger or toe may be misinterpreted by the oximeter as arterial pulsations.

- Cover a sensor with a sheet or towel to block large amounts of light from external sources (e.g., sunlight, procedure lamps, or bilirubin lights in the nursery).

Large amounts of outside light may be sensed by the photodetector and alter the SaO₂ value.

- Verify that the client's hemoglobin level is normal. *An SaO₂ measurement may register normal when the client's hemoglobin is low because the available hemo-*

globin to carry oxygen is fully saturated.

8. Document all relevant information.

- Record the application of the pulse oximeter, its type and size, and all nursing assessments.

EVALUATION FOCUS	Oxygen saturation level; pulse rate and other vital signs; tissue response to the sensor.

SAMPLE RECORDING

Date	Time	Notes
4/12/93	1430	Adult adhesive pulse oximeter sensor applied to L index finger. BP 126/88, R 22 and shallow, P 98. Skin color pink. Continuous oxygen by nasal cannula at 5 L/minute. ——————————————————— Paula Prince, RN

KEY ELEMENTS OF USING A PULSE OXIMETER

- Determine allergies to adhesive and the client's hemoglobin level beforehand.

- Use a sensor appropriate for the client's weight and size, taking into account the client's adequacy of circulation in the extremity selected.

- Before applying the sensor, clean the site selected with an alcohol swab, and remove nail polish or acrylic nails.

- Ensure that the alignment of the LEDs and photodetector is accurate.

- Ensure adequate functioning of the alarm system.

- Inspect an adhesive finger or toe sensor site every 4 hours and a spring-tension sensor every 2 hours.

- Immobilize the sensor site, and protect it from external light sources.

CRITICAL THINKING CHALLENGE

Ralph Ogden, a 66-year-old male, has been admitted to the nursing unit with congestive heart failure. The physician has ordered oxygen via nasal cannula at a flow rate of 6 liters per minute. You note that Mr. Ogden continues to be restless, his pulse rate and respiratory rate are increased, and he continues to breathe through his mouth. He keeps pulling the cannula out, complaining that it's uncomfortable and stating that "no one can breathe with this in their nose." How would you respond? What action would you take? What is your rationale?

RELATED RESEARCH

Winslow, E. H.; Lane, L. D.; and Gaffney, F. A. May/June 1985. Oxygen uptake and cardiovascular responses in control adults and acute myocardial infarction patients during bathing. *Nursing Research* 34:164–69.

REFERENCES

Crocco, J. A.; Francis, P. B.; and Lefrak, S. S. May 15, 1987. When the patient needs oxygen—stat. *Patient Care* 21:83–86, 89.

Hoffman, L. A., and Wesmiller, S. W. April 1988. Home oxygen: Transtracheal and other options. *American Journal of Nursing* 88:464–69.

Mims, B. C. July 1987. The risks of oxygen therapy. Part 2. *RN* 50:20–26.

Riedel, K. July 1989. Pulse oximetry: A new technology to assess patient oxygen needs in the neonatal intensive care unit. *Journal of Perinatal and Neonatal Nursing* 1:49–57.

Scacci, R. December 1990. Air entrainment masks: Jet mixing is how they work; the Bernoulli and Venturi principles are how they don't. *Respiratory Care* 35:1261–64.

Schnapp, L. M., and Cohen, N. H. November 1990. Pulse oximetry: Uses and abuses. *Chest* 98:1244–50.

Siegman, W. L. December 1990. Oxygen tents go streamlined at Johns Hopkins. *Respiratory Care* 35:1241–42.

Sonnesso, G. August 1991. Are you ready for pulse oximetry? *Nursing 91* 21:60–64.

33

Artificial Airways

CONTENTS

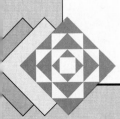

NURSING PROCESS GUIDE
ARTIFICIAL AIRWAYS

ASSESSMENT

See the Nursing Process Guide for Chapter 30, page 737. Essential data include the following:

- The rate, depth, rhythm, and character of respirations.

- The pulse rate, volume, and rhythm.

- Breath sounds that are audible without amplification and those audible by stethoscope.

- Secretions (color, character, amount) from the tracheostomy site.

- Clinical signs of secretions accumulating in the respiratory tract: restlessness or anxiety, pallor, increased heart rate, increased respiratory rate, bubbling or rattling breath sounds, and/or shallow respirations or dyspnea.

- Clinical signs of hypoxia or anoxia: increased pulse rate, rapid or deep respirations, cyanosis of the skin and nail beds, restlessness, anxiety, vertigo, or syncope (faintness).

- Color of skin and nail beds.

RELATED DIAGNOSTIC CATEGORIES

- Ineffective airway clearance

- High risk for Aspiration

PLANNING

Client Goal
The client will restore or maintain a patent airway and adequate ventilation.

Outcome Criteria
The client:

- Has clear breath sounds bilaterally.

- Has normal respiratory rate, rhythm, and depth, i.e., a respiratory pattern of 12 to 20 per minute, effortless breathing (no use of accessory muscles), and symmetric chest expansion on inhalation.

- Has skin, nails, lips, and earlobes of natural color.

- Breathes effectively through the established airway.

- Has secretions that are liquefied and easily mobilized.

- Has intact skin around the artificial airway.

Artificial Airways

Artificial airways are inserted to maintain a patent air passage for clients whose airway has become or may become obstructed. A patent airway is necessary so that air can flow to and from the lungs. The insertion of a tube is known as **intubation**. Four of the more common types of intubation are oropharyngeal, nasopharyngeal, endotracheal, and tracheostomy.

Oropharyngeal intubation is done most frequently for clients who have had general anesthesia and for those who are semiconscious and are likely to obstruct their own airways with their tongues. An **oropharyngeal tube** is inserted in some instances for pharyngeal suctioning. It is not inserted in clients who are conscious, because it stimulates the gag reflex and thus can cause vomiting. Oropharyngeal tubes are somewhat S-shaped and usually made of plastic. Adult, child, and infant sizes are available. The tube is inserted through the mouth and terminates in the posterior pharynx (Figure 33–1). See Technique 33–1 for insertion and maintenance.

Nasopharyngeal intubation is carried out if the oropharyngeal route is contraindicated, e.g., following oral surgery, or to protect the nasal and pharyngeal mucosa during nasopharyngeal or nasotracheal

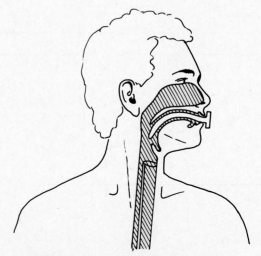

FIGURE 33–1 An oropharyngeal tube in place.

suctioning. The **nasopharyngeal tube** is inserted through a nostril and terminates in the pharynx, below the upper edge of the epiglottis (Figure 33–2). Tubes vary in size for adults, children, and infants. They are usually made of latex rubber. See Technique 33–1 for insertion and maintenance.

Endotracheal tubes are most commonly inserted for clients who have had general anesthetics or for those in emergency situations where mechanical ventilation is required. An **endotracheal tube** is a curved polyvinylchloride tube that is inserted through either the mouth or the nose and into the trachea with the guide of a laryngoscope (Figure 33–3). It terminates just superior to the bifurcation of the trachea into the bronchi. Because an endotracheal tube passes through the epiglottis and splits it open, an inflated cuff is needed to close the system. See the accompanying box for interventions to main-

tain an endotracheal tube. Note: Only nurses with special preparation perform endotracheal intubation.

Tracheostomy tubes are inserted to provide and maintain a patent airway, to remove tracheobronchial secretions from clients unable to cough, to replace endotracheal tubes, to permit the use of positive pressure ventilation, and to prevent unconscious clients from aspirating secretions.

A **tracheostomy tube** is a curved tube that is inserted into a *tracheostomy*, a surgical incision in the trachea just below the first or second tracheal cartilage (Figure 33–4). The tube extends through the tracheostomy stoma into the trachea (Figure 33–5).

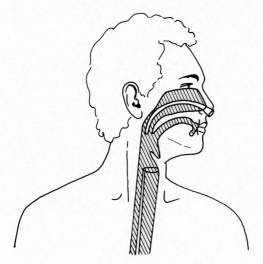

FIGURE 33–2 A nasopharyngeal tube in place.

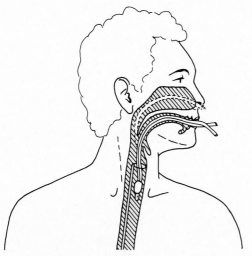

FIGURE 33–3 An endotracheal tube in place.

CLINICAL GUIDELINES

Nursing Interventions for Clients with Endotracheal Tubes

- Maintain the client in a lateral or semiprone position so that blood, vomitus, or secretions can drain from the mouth and are not aspirated.
- Provide oral or nasal hygiene every 3 hours or as needed.
- For an oral insertion, provide a bite block so that the client cannot bite the tube and occlude the airway.
- Assess the condition of the nasal or oral mucosa for irritation, and notify the physician should the need to change a nasal endotracheal tube arise; reposition an oral endotracheal tube from one side of the mouth to the other every 8 hours or as required.
- Closely monitor the air pressure in the endotracheal cuff. If it is greater than 20 mm Hg, necrosis of the tracheal tissues can result.
- Tape the airway in place to prevent accidental slippage or extubation.
- Change the tape daily, and position the tube on the opposite side of the mouth at each change.
- Provide continuous humidification or aerosol therapy to prevent undue drying and irritation of the mucous membranes, if the tube is left in for more than a short time (e.g., for days or weeks).
- Deflate and reinflate the cuff according to the manufacturer's directions.
- Communicate frequently with the client, and provide a notepad or other means for the client to communicate. Most clients cannot speak with an inflated cuff, because no air can pass over the vocal chords.

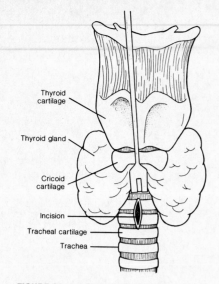

Thyroid cartilage

Thyroid gland

Cricoid cartilage

Incision

Tracheal cartilage

Trachea

FIGURE 33–4   Site of a tracheostomy incision.

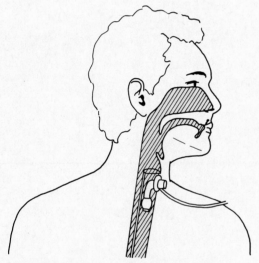

FIGURE 33–5   A tracheostomy tube in place.

Tracheostomy tubes come in different sizes and may be made of metal, plastic, or foam. Plastic tubes are increasingly popular because they are lightweight, their parts are interchangeable, and crusting from the tissues rarely forms on plastic materials.

The main parts of a tracheostomy set are the outer tube, the inner tube or inner cannula, and the obturator (Figure 33–6). The obturator is used only to insert the outer tube. It is removed once the outer tube is in place. The outer tube usually has ties to secure it around the client's neck, although many plastic tubes are cuffed with a soft balloon that can be inflated to hold the tube in place (see below). Fitted inside the outer tube is an inner cannula. (Some plastic sets do not have this, because it is unnecessary to change the tube. They are called *single-cannula tubes.*) In double-cannula sets, the inner cannula is inserted and locked in place after the obturator is removed; it acts as a removable liner for the more permanent, outer cannula. The inner tube is withdrawn for brief periods to be cleaned.

Cuffed tracheostomy tubes are surrounded by an inflatable cuff that produces an airtight seal between the tube and the trachea. This seal prevents aspiration of oropharyngeal secretions and air leakage between the tube and the trachea. Cuffed tubes are often used immediately after a tracheostomy in adults and infants and are essential when ventilating a tracheostomy client with a ventilator. Children do not require cuffed tubes, because their tracheas are resilient enough to seal the air space around the tube.

Some tubes have high-pressure cuffs; others have low-pressure cuffs. Some high-pressure tubes are double-cuffed; these can be inflated alternately to alter the pressure points on the trachea and prevent tracheal irritation and tissue damage. Alternate infla-

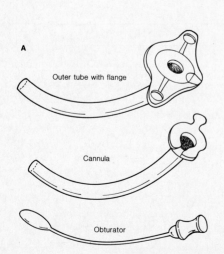

A

Outer tube with flange

Cannula

Obturator

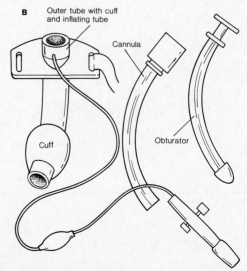

B

Outer tube with cuff and inflating tube

Cannula

Cuff

Obturator

FIGURE 33–6   Two types of tracheostomy sets: *A,* noncuffed; *B,* cuffed.

tion also allows uninterrupted respirator function for people using ventilators. Commercially prepared cuffs are available for use on cuffless tracheostomy tubes.

Different cuffed tubes have different advantages and disadvantages. Cuffs that are bonded to the tracheostomy tube eliminate the risk of accidental detachment inside the trachea. Low-pressure cuffs, which are more costly than others, distribute a low, even pressure against the trachea, thus decreasing the risk of tracheal tissue necrosis. They do not need to be deflated periodically to reduce pressure on the tracheal wall. Double-cuffed high-pressure tubes may reduce the risk of tissue necrosis with alternate inflation of cuffs, but *only* if there is rigid adherence to the alternate inflation schedule. If tracheal damage does occur, a larger area of the trachea is involved with double-cuffed tubes.

A variation of the cuffed tube is the foam cuff. It does not require injected air; instead, when the port is opened, ambient air enters the balloon, which then conforms to the client's trachea (Figure 33–7). The physician removes air from the cuff prior to insertion or removal of the tube.

A **minitracheostomy (MT)** is a technique in which a cannula with an internal diameter of 4 mm is inserted into the trachea, through the cricothyroid membrane. It is not recommended for children under age 12 years. MT is easily performed in the nursing unit under local anesthesia without sedation. Before the development of MT, the treatment of sputum retention depended on nasal/oropharyngeal suction and endotracheal intubation or tracheostomy. Because nasal or oral suction is very unpleasant for conscious clients and intubation interferes with talking and coughing abilities, MT offers distinct advan-

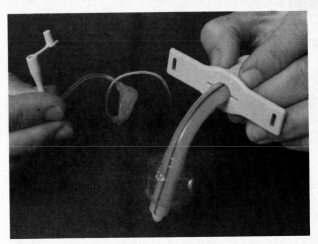

FIGURE 33–7 A tracheostomy tube with a foam cuff.

tages for specific clients (Preston, Matthews, and Ready 1986, p. 496):

- The client still breathes normally through the mouth and nose, thereby filtering and humidifying the air and reducing the risk of superadded infection.
- No respiratory crises occur if the MT becomes blocked.
- The client can talk and cough normally (when otherwise able).
- The client can eat and drink normally.
- The MT can remain in situ long term if necessary.
- The small stab incision heals very quickly after decannulation and is often airtight within one day.

 33-1 ## Inserting and Maintaining a Pharyngeal Airway

PURPOSES
- To prevent obstruction of the airway by the tongue of an unconscious client (oropharyngeal tube)
- To maintain a patent air passage for clients who have or may become obstructed

ASSESSMENT FOCUS

Level of consciousness and presence or absence of gag reflex; clinical signs indicating need for airway (e.g., upper airway "gurgling," labored respiration, increased respiratory and pulse rates).

▶ **Technique 33–1 Inserting and Maintaining a Pharyngeal Airway** CONTINUED

EQUIPMENT

- ☐ Disposable gloves
- ☐ Tongue blade (for oropharyngeal tube)
- ☐ Water-soluble lubricant or cool water
- ☐ Sterile oropharyngeal airway of the appropriate size (length should extend from the teeth to the end of the jawline)

or

- ☐ Nasopharyngeal airway of the appropriate size (diameter should be slightly narrower than the client's naris)
- ☐ Soft tissues or washcloth
- ☐ Topical anesthetic, if ordered (for nasopharyngeal tube)
- ☐ Tape
- ☐ Suction equipment

INTERVENTION

1. Insert the airway.

Oropharyngeal Airway

- Place the client in a supine position with the neck hyperextended or with a pillow placed under the shoulders. *This position prevents the tongue from falling back to block the pharynx.* Note: This position may be contraindicated for clients with head, neck, or back injuries.

- Don disposable gloves, open the client's mouth, and place a tongue depressor on the anterior half of the tongue. *This flattens the tongue and facilitates airway insertion.*

- Remove dentures, if present.

- Lubricate the airway with a water-soluble lubricant or with cool water.

- Turn the airway upside down, with the curved end upward or sideways, and advance it along the roof of the mouth.

- When the airway passes the uvula (or is at the posterior half of the tongue), rotate the airway until the curve of the airway follows the natural curve of the tongue.

- Remove excess lubricant from the client's lips with a soft tissue or washcloth.

Nasopharyngeal Airway

- Assess the patency of each naris. Ask the client, if conscious, to breathe through one naris while occluding the other.

- Ask the client, if conscious, to blow the nose to clear it of excess secretions.

- Lubricate the entire tube with a topical anesthetic (if ordered). *This prevents irritation of the nasopharyngeal mucosa and undue discomfort.*

- Hold the airway by the wide end, and insert the narrow end into the naris, applying gentle inward and downward pressure when advancing the airway. Follow the natural course of the nasal passage.

- Advance the airway until the external horn fits against the outer naris.

- If resistance is felt, try the other naris.

- Remove excess lubricant from the nares, as required.

2. Tape the airway in position, if required. *Stabilizing the airway maintains the airway's position and prevents injury to the oropharyngeal or nasopharyngeal mucosa.* Smith and Johnson (1990) recommend the following method:

- Prepare two long strips of tape—one 35 cm (14 in), and the other 60 cm (24 in). This should be performed before donning the gloves.

- Lay the longer strip down, sticky side up.

- Place the shorter strip, sticky side down, over the center (Figure 33–8).

- Split each end of the longer tape (Figure 33–9).

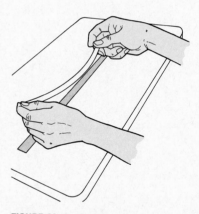

FIGURE 33–8 Attaching the shorter tape over the center of the longer tape.

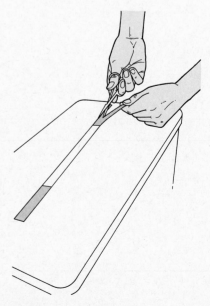

FIGURE 33–9 Splitting one end of the longer tape.

▶ **Technique 33–1** *CONTINUED*

- Place the nonsticky tape under the client's neck.

- For an *oral airway,* press half of the split tape across the upper airway flange and the other across the lower flange (Figure 33–10).
  or
  For a *nasal airway,* press half of the split tape across the upper lip and the other half around the tube without occluding the nares. Repeat for the other side.

3. Ensure the client's comfort and safety.

Oropharyngeal Tube

- Maintain the client in a lateral or semiprone position so that any blood, vomitus, and mucus will

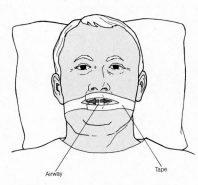

FIGURE 33–10 An oral airway taped in place.

drain out of the mouth and not be aspirated.

- Suction secretions as required.

- Provide mouth care as required to maintain moisture and tissue integrity.

- Remove the airway once the cli-

ent has regained consciousness and has the swallow, gag, and cough reflexes.

Nasopharyngeal Tube

- Remove the tube, clean it in warm, soapy water, and insert it in the other nostril at least every 8 hours, or as ordered by the physician, to prevent irritation of the mucosa.

- Provide nasal hygiene every 4 hours or more often if needed.

4. Document all relevant information.

- Record the time the airway was inserted, type of airway inserted, client response to insertion, and character of any secretions suctioned.

EVALUATION FOCUS

Client response to insertion (e.g., comparison of respiratory rate and depth and pulse rate to baseline data); integrity of oral or nasal mucous membrane and lips; character of secretions suctioned.

SAMPLE RECORDING

Date	Time	Notes
4/6/93	0930	Responding to painful stimuli only. Gurgling during aspiration. R-14, P-88. Oral airway inserted. Clear secretions suctioned from mouth. Turned to L lateral position. Mouth care given. Skin on lips and oral mucous membrane intact. ———————————————— Mary Beth Holly, RN

KEY ELEMENTS OF INSERTING AND MAINTAINING A PHARYNGEAL AIRWAY

- Use tubes of the appropriate size.

Oral Airway

- Wear disposable gloves to insert the airway, if there is time.

- Remove dentures, if present.

- Insert the airway with the curve upward or turned to the side.

- Rotate the airway only after it has advanced to the posterior aspect of the tongue.

- Secure the airway with tape.

- Position the client in lateral or semiprone position.

- Suction secretions and provide required mouth care.

Nasal Airway

- Assess the patency of both nares.

- Lubricate the entire tube before insertion.

- Follow the natural course of the nasal passage during tube insertion.

- Remove the tube and insert it into the other nostril at least every 8 hours.

- Suction secretions, and provide required nasal hygiene.

Endotracheal Suctioning

Following a tracheostomy, the trachea and surrounding respiratory tissues are irritated and react by producing excessive secretions. Suctioning is necessary to remove these secretions and maintain a patent airway. The frequency of suctioning depends on the client's health and how recently the tracheostomy was done.

Suctioning is associated with several complications: hypoxemia, trauma to the airway, nosocomial infection, and cardiac dysrythmia, which is related to the hypoxemia. Suctioning also stimulates the cough reflex and stimulates cells in the bronchi to secrete more mucus (Noll, Hix, and Scott 1990, p. 318). Suctioning should therefore be done only when breath sounds indicate that the need is present, or according to the physician's routine orders.

Several techniques that minimize or decrease these complications have evolved over the past decade:

- *Hyperinflation.* This involves giving the client breaths that are 1 to 1.5 times the tidal volume set on the ventilator through the ventilator circuit or via a manual resuscitation bag. Three to five quick breaths are delivered before and after each pass of the suction catheter.

- *Hyperoxygenation.* This can be done with a manual resuscitation bag or through the ventilator and is performed by increasing the oxygen flow (usually to 100%) before suctioning and between suction attempts.

- *Oxygen insufflation suction catheter.* A double-lumen catheter system has been developed that allows oxygen insufflation during the suctioning procedure *except* during the suctioning phase. This 22-inch, #14 Fr. catheter has a second lumen of oxygen insufflation (Bodai, Watson, Briggs, and Goldstein 1987, p. 39). The suction port is equivalent to a regular #12 Fr. suction catheter. The oxygen port has five side holes to allow oxygen dispersal within the trachea. This

port accommodates a flow rate of 15 liters per minute. The end of the catheter has a fingertip control valve. When the valve tabs are compressed, suction is applied, and the oxygen circuit is occluded. Oxygen is thus administered before suction is applied.

- *Closed tracheal suction systems.* The closed tracheal suction system (CTSS) is the newest technology for facilitating suctioning and reducing such complications as hypoxemia, cardiac dysrhythmias, and infection. Two CTSS systems are currently available: the Ballard Trach Care Suction System (Ballard Medical Products, Midvale, UT) and the Steri-Cath (Concord/Portex, Keene, NH). In both systems, the catheter is enclosed in a plastic sheath that is connected to a specially designed T-piece attached to the airway or to a ventilator circuit. The T-piece contains a washer to prevent gas leakage around the catheter and to remove secretions from the outside of the catheter as it is withdrawn from the airway. A port on the T-piece allows for rinsing of the catheter and instillation of irrigating solutions. A thumb port on the proximal end of the catheter allows for suction control. This port can be locked off to prevent accidental application of suction. The CTSS is used for a 24-hour period. Reported advantages of CTSS include improved oxygenation, decreased clinical signs of hypoxemia, infection control, and reduced client anxiety.

For tracheostomy and endotracheal suctioning, the diameter of the suction catheter should be about half the inside diameter of the tracheostomy tube so that hypoxia can be prevented. The nurse uses sterile technique to prevent infection of the respiratory tract.

If the client's secretions are thick, the nurse performs *tracheal lavage* before suctioning. This is the insertion of sterile normal saline through the tracheostomy tube into the trachea. See Technique 33–2. To clean a double-cannula tracheostomy tube, see Technique 33–3.

 33-2 ## Suctioning a Tracheostomy or Endotracheal Tube

PURPOSES
- To maintain a patent airway and prevent airway obstructions
- To promote respiratory function (optimal exchange of oxygen and carbon dioxide into and out of the lungs)
- To prevent pneumonia that may result from accumulated secretions

▶ **Technique 33–2** *CONTINUED*

ASSESSMENT FOCUS	Presence of congestion on auscultation of the thorax; client's inability to remove the secretions through coughing. See also the Assessment in the Nursing Process Guide, page 792.

EQUIPMENT

- □ Wrist restraints
- □ Resuscitation bag (Ambu bag) connected to 100% oxygen
- □ Sterile towel
- □ Sterile 2- to 10-ml syringe and sterile normal saline
- □ Equipment for suctioning the oropharyngeal cavity (see Technique 31–1, page 767)
- □ Goggles and mask if necessary
- □ Gown (if necessary)
- □ Sterile gloves
- □ Moisture-resistant bag

INTERVENTION

1. Prepare the client.

- Inform the client that suctioning usually causes some intermittent coughing and that this assists in removing the secretions.

- If not contraindicated because of health, place the client in semi-Fowler's position to promote deep breathing, maximum lung expansion, and productive coughing. *Deep breathing oxygenates the lungs, counteracts the hypoxic effects of suctioning, and may induce coughing. Coughing helps to loosen and move secretions.*

- **P** Secure an assistant to stabilize a child's head, and apply wrist restraints. *These actions help prevent accidental dislodgement and contamination of the tracheostomy or endotracheal tube.*

2. Prepare the equipment.

- Attach the resuscitation apparatus to the oxygen source (Figure 33–11). Adjust the oxygen flow to "100% flush."

- Open the sterile supplies in readiness for use.

- Place the sterile towel, if used, across the client's chest, below the tracheostomy.

- Prepare the saline for instillation by opening the ampules and drawing up the saline in a syringe.

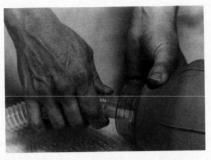

FIGURE 33–11   Attaching the resuscitation apparatus to the oxygen source.

- Turn on the suction, and set the pressure in accordance with agency policy. For a wall unit, pressure of about 100 to 120 mm Hg is normally used for adults, 50 to 95 mm Hg for infants and children.

- Put on goggles and mask (and gown if necessary).

- Put on sterile gloves. Some agencies recommend putting a sterile glove on the dominant hand and an unsterile glove on the nondominant hand to protect the nurse.

- Holding the catheter in the dominant hand and the connector in the nondominant hand, attach the catheter to the Y-connector or straight connector (see Figure 31–3 on page 768).

3. Flush and lubricate the catheter.

- Using the dominant hand, place the catheter tip in the sterile saline solution.

- Using the thumb of the nondominant hand, occlude the thumb control, and suction a small amount of the sterile solution through the catheter. *This determines that the suction equipment is working properly and lubricates the outside and the lumen of the catheter. Lubrication eases insertion and reduces tissue trauma during insertion. Lubricating the lumen also helps prevent secretions from sticking to the inside of the catheter.*

4. If the client does *not* have copious secretions, hyperventilate the lungs with a resuscitation bag before suctioning.

- Summon an assistant, if one is available, for this step.

- Using your nondominant hand, turn on the oxygen to 12 to 15 liters per minute.

- If the client is receiving oxygen, disconnect the oxygen source from the tracheostomy tube using your nondominant hand.

- Attach the resuscitator to the tracheostomy or endotracheal tube (Figure 33–12 on page 800).

- Compress the Ambu bag three to five times as the client *inhales*. This is best done by a second person, who can use both hands to compress the bag, providing a greater inflation volume.

- Observe the rise and fall of the

▶ **Technique 33–2 Suctioning a Tracheostomy Tube** CONTINUED

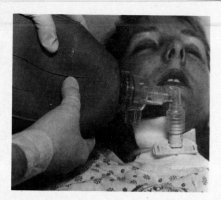

FIGURE 33–12 Attaching the resuscitator to the tracheostomy.

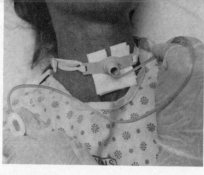

FIGURE 33–13 Inserting the catheter into the trachea through the tracheostomy tube.

client's chest to assess the adequacy of each ventilation.

• Remove the resuscitation device, and place it on the bed or the client's chest with the connector facing up.

5. If the client has copious secretions, do *not* hyperventilate with a resuscitator. Instead:

• Keep the regular oxygen delivery device on, and increase the liter flow for a few minutes before suctioning. *Hyperventilating a client who has copious secretions can force the secretions deeper into the respiratory tract.*

6. Quickly, but gently, insert the catheter without applying any suction.

• With your nondominant thumb off the suction port, quickly but gently insert the catheter into the trachea through the tracheostomy tube (Figure 33–13). *To prevent tissue trauma and oxygen loss, suction is not applied during insertion of the catheter.*

• Insert the catheter about 12.5 cm (6 in) for adults, less for children, or until the client coughs or you feel resistance. Resistance usually means that the catheter tip has reached the bifurcation of the trachea. To prevent damaging the mucous membranes at the bifurcation, withdraw the

catheter about 1 to 2 cm before applying suction.

7. Perform suctioning.

• Apply intermittent suction for 5 to 10 seconds by placing the nondominant thumb over the thumb port. *Suction time is restricted to 10 seconds or less to minimize oxygen loss.*

• Rotate the catheter by rolling it between your thumb and forefinger while slowly withdrawing it. *This prevents tissue trauma by minimizing the suction time against any part of the trachea.*

• Withdraw the catheter completely, and release the suction.

• Hyperventilate the client.

8. If secretions are thick, flush the catheter and perform tracheal lavage according to agency protocol.

• Flush the catheter with sterile water or saline.

• For adults, insert 2 to 5 ml of sterile saline solution through the tracheostomy tube into the trachea. For infants, use 0.5 to 1 ml; for children, use 2 ml. *This liquefies tenacious secretions so that they are more easily suctioned out.*

• Then suction again.

9. Reassess the client's oxygen-

ation status, and repeat suctioning as above.

• Observe the client's respirations and skin color. With your clean hand, check the client's pulse if necessary.

• Encourage the client to breathe deeply and to cough between suctions.

• Allow 2 to 3 minutes between suctions when possible. *This provides an opportunity for reoxygenation of the lungs.*

• Flush the catheter, and repeat suctioning until the air passage is clear and the breathing is relatively effortless and quiet.

• After each suction, pick up the resuscitation bag with your clean hand, and ventilate the client with five breaths.

10. Dispose of equipment and ensure availability for the next suction.

• Flush the catheter and suction tubing.

• Turn off the suction, and disconnect the catheter from the suction tubing.

• Wrap the catheter around your sterile hand, and peel the glove off, so that it turns inside out over the catheter.

• Discard the glove and the catheter in the moisture-resistant bag.

• Replenish the sterile fluid and supplies so that the suction is ready to be used again. *Clients who require suctioning often require it quickly, so it is essential to leave the equipment at the bedside ready for use.*

11. Provide for client comfort and safety.

• Assist the client to a comfortable, safe position that aids breathing. If the person is conscious, a

▶ **Technique 33–2** *CONTINUED*

semi-Fowler's position is frequently indicated. If the person is unconscious, Sims' position can assist the drainage of secretions from the mouth.

• Remove the restraints, and re-

 main until the child is relaxed. Cuddle and stroke the child to facilitate relaxation.

12. Document relevant data.

• Record the suctioning, including

the amount and description of suction returns, the amount of sterile saline instilled, and any other relevant assessments.

EVALUATION FOCUS	Respiratory rate, depth, and character after suctioning; tracheal breath sounds; color of skin and nail beds; character and amount of secretions suctioned; changes in vital signs.

SAMPLE RECORDING

Date	Time	Notes
8/12/93	1030	Coarse rales noted in bilateral upper lobes. Cough weak. Tracheostomy suctioned with #14 catheter for moderate return of thin white mucus. Respirations 16, regular and not labored. Anterior and posterior lung sounds clear bilaterally after suctioning. Skin pink. Nail beds pink. P-78. Teresa McMahon, RN

KEY ELEMENTS OF SUCTIONING A TRACHEOSTOMY TUBE

• Maintain the sterility of the dominant glove, suction catheter, normal saline, and syringe, if used.

• Assess the client's respirations, pulse, color, breath sounds, and behavior before and after the procedure.

• For clients who do *not* have copious secretions, hyperventilate the lungs with a resuscitation bag before suctioning.

• For clients who have copious secretions, increase the oxygen liter flow before suctioning.

• Use appropriate suction pressure.

• Lubricate the suction catheter with saline before insertion.

• Insert the catheter *without* applying suction.

• Rotate the catheter during suctioning and withdrawal.

• Add sterile saline solution to the trachea if secretions are thick.

• Restrict each suction time to 10 seconds.

• Reapply supplementary oxygen as required during and after the procedure.

• Replenish supplies in readiness for the next suction.

33-3   Cleaning a Double-Cannula Tracheostomy Tube

Double-cannula tracheostomy tubes are cleaned whenever necessary, but at least once per shift.

PURPOSES

• To maintain cleanliness and prevent infection at the tracheostomy site
• To maintain airway patency
• To prevent skin breakdown around the tracheostomy stoma

▶ **Technique 33–3 Cleaning a Tracheostomy Tube** CONTINUED

ASSESSMENT FOCUS	Presence of excessive peristomal secretions, excessive tube secretions, or soiled tracheostomy dressing or ties; labored breathing indicating diminished air flow through tracheostomy tube.

EQUIPMENT

- □ Sterile bowls
- □ Hydrogen peroxide and sterile normal saline
- □ Sterile gloves (1 pair and 1 glove or 2 pairs)

- □ Clean (nonsterile) glove
- □ Sterile nylon brush or pipe cleaners

- □ Sterile gauze squares or sterile cotton-tipped applicator sticks

INTERVENTION

1. Don gloves, and suction the tracheostomy tube.

- Put a nonsterile glove on the non-dominant hand and a sterile glove on your dominant hand.

- Suction the entire length of the inner cannula prior to its removal to remove secretions and ensure a patent airway. (See Technique 33–2.)

2. Remove and soak the inner cannula.

- With the nondominant hand, unlock the inner cannula by turning the lock about 90° counterclockwise. *The nondominant hand is used to handle the flange of the cannula, which is not sterile.*

- With the nondominant hand, remove the inner cannula by gently pulling it out toward you in line with its curvature.

- Soak the inner cannula in the hydrogen peroxide solution for several minutes. *This moistens and loosens dried secretions.*

3. Change gloves, and clean the cannula.

- Remove the gloves, and replace them with sterile gloves on both hands. Both hands are needed to clean the tube. *To maintain sterile technique, both hands must be gloved.*

- Remove the cannula from the soaking solution.

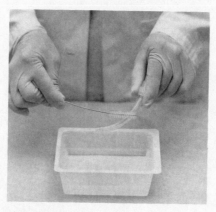

FIGURE 33–14 Cleaning the inner cannula with a brush.

- Clean the lumen and entire inner cannula thoroughly, using the pipe cleaners or brush moistened with sterile saline (Figure 33–14).

- Agitate the cannula for several seconds in the sterile saline. *This thoroughly rinses the cannula and provides a thin film of moisture to lubricate for insertion.*

- Inspect the cannula for cleanliness by holding it at eye level and looking through it into the light. If encrustations are evident, repeat above steps.

- After rinsing the cannula, gently tap it against the inside edge of the sterile solution bowl. *This removes excess liquid from the cannula and prevents possible aspiration of it by the client.*

4. Dry the *inside* of the cannula.

- Use two or three pipe cleaners twisted together to dry the inside of the cannula. Do not dry the outer surface. *A thin film of moisture on the outer surface acts as a lubricant for insertion.*

5. Suction the outer cannula. *Secretions must be removed to prevent adherence of the two tubes when the inner cannula is inserted.*

6. Insert the clean inner cannula, and secure it.

- Grasp the outer flange of the inner cannula, and insert the cannula in the direction of its curvature.

- Lock the inner cannula in place by turning the lock clockwise about 90° to an upright position.

- Gently pull on the inner cannula to ensure that the position is secure.

7. Clean the flange of the outer cannula if necessary.

- Use clean cotton-tipped applicators or gauze squares moistened with sterile saline to clean the flange.

8. Document relevant data.

- On the client's chart record the removal, cleaning, and reinsertion of the cannula and all assessments.

VARIATION: For the Client on a Ventilator

▶ **Technique 33–3** *CONTINUED*

For the client with a double-cannula tracheostomy tube attached to a ventilator, a spare inner cannula is kept on hand in a sterile container because ventilation cannot be discontinued long enough to clean the inner cannula. Additional equipment is required: a clean towel, which is placed across the client's chest (the disconnected ventilator tubing is placed on it); and a handheld resuscitator.

- Prepare the tracheostomy suctioning and cleaning equipment.

- Hyperventilate the client by using the ventilator's sigh mechanism. If the ventilator does not have a built-in sigh mechanism, use a manual resuscitation bag, such as an Ambu bag, connected to an oxygen source; adjust the oxygen flowmeter to deliver 12 to 15 liters per minute.

- Disconnect the ventilator tubing, and place it on the clean towel.

- Don sterile gloves, and suction the tracheostomy tube.

- Quickly remove the inner cannula using the nondominant hand, and replace it with the clean cannula:

  a. Use the nondominant hand to remove the lid of the container holding the spare cannula. *The lid of the container is exposed to the air and is not sterile.*

  b. Use the sterile dominant hand to pick up the cannula and insert it. Lock it in place. *The cannula is sterile and therefore must be handled by a sterile glove.*

  c. Reattach the client to the ventilator.

  d. Change gloves, and clean the soiled cannula as above.

EVALUATION FOCUS

Character and amount of secretions; client's respiration status compared to baseline data; tracheal breath sounds.

SAMPLE RECORDING

Date	Time	Notes
11/17/93	1600	Respirations labored and stertorous. Tracheostomy suctioned for copious thick white secretions. Inner cannula cleaned and replaced. R.16 and eased. ———————————————————————— Antonia Wong, RN

KEY ELEMENTS OF CLEANING A DOUBLE-CANNULA TRACHEOSTOMY TUBE

- Suction the inner cannula before its removal.
- Remove the tracheostomy dressing and inner cannula with your nondominant hand.
- Wear sterile gloves on both hands to clean the tube.

- Inspect the cannula for cleanliness, and remove excess liquid from it before insertion.
- Suction the outer cannula before inserting the inner cannula.
- Lock the inner cannula after insertion.

Changing a Tracheostomy Dressing and Tie Tapes

A tracheostomy dressing and the tie tapes need to be changed whenever they become soiled. Soiled dressings harbor microorganisms and can be a potential source of skin excoriation, breakdown, and infection. Usually, the dressing is changed after the cannula is cleaned, but a more frequent dressing change may be necessary. The dressing technique is described in Chapter 39.

Before applying a new dressing, the nurse needs to check any special orders or agency protocol (e.g., the application of antibiotic ointment to the stoma after cleaning it). Noncotton-filled squares are used to clean the wound because cotton fibers can pull off and remain in the wound, where they encourage bacterial growth and contamination. Technique 33–4 describes how to change a tracheostomy dressing and tie tapes.

Changing a Tracheostomy Dressing and Tie Tapes

PURPOSES
- To prevent skin excoriation and infection of the tracheostomy site
- To provide comfort

ASSESSMENT FOCUS

Character of secretions from the tracheostomy site; clinical signs of infection at the tracheostomy site (e.g, inflammation, purulent discharge, odor); pulse and respiratory rates.

EQUIPMENT

- Disposable gloves
- Moistureproof bag
- Sterile gloves
- Cleaning solutions (e.g., sterile normal saline and hydrogen peroxide)
- Sterile containers
- Sterile noncotton-filled gauze squares and sterile cotton-tipped applicator sticks
- Antibiotic ointment if ordered or recommended by agency policy
- Commercially prepared dressing or sterile 4 × 4 gauze square
- Cotton twill tape
- Gauze square and tape

INTERVENTION

1. Prepare the client and the equipment.

- Assist the client to a semi-Fowler's position to promote lung expansion.

- While wearing a disposable glove, remove the tracheostomy dressing. Discard the dressing and glove in the moistureproof bag.

- Inspect the tracheostomy wound and drainage.

- Open the sterile equipment, and don the sterile gloves.

2. Clean the incision site and tube flange.

- Clean around the incision site with gauze squares or applicator sticks dampened with sterile normal saline (Figure 33–15). If encrustations are difficult to remove, use hydrogen peroxide at the ordered strength, e.g., 50% hydrogen peroxide and 50% sterile saline.

- Wipe only once with each gauze square, and then discard it. *This*

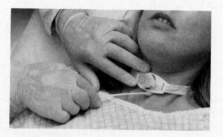

FIGURE 33–15 Using an applicator stick to clean the tracheostomy site.

avoids contaminating a clean area with a soiled gauze square.

- Thoroughly rinse the cleaned area, using gauze squares moistened with sterile normal saline. *Hydrogen peroxide can be irritating to the skin.*

- Clean the flange of the tube in the same manner.

- Thoroughly dry the client's skin and tube flanges with dry gauze squares.

3. Apply a sterile dressing.

- Use an applicator stick to apply antibiotic ointment around the incision site if ordered or recommended by agency policy.

- For the insertion site, use a commercially prepared tracheostomy dressing of nonraveling material, if available.
  or
  Open and refold a 4 × 4 gauze as shown in Figure 33–16, *A* to *D*.

- Place the gauze as shown in Figure 33–16, *E*.

- Avoid using cotton-filled gauze squares, and avoid cutting the 4 × 4 gauze. *The client might aspirate cotton lint or frayed fibers, which could subsequently create a tracheal abscess.*

- While applying the dressing, ensure that the tracheostomy tube is securely supported. *Excessive movement of the tracheostomy tube irritates the trachea.*

4. Change the tie tapes.

Two-Strip Method

- Cut two strips of cotton twill tape, one about 25 cm (10 in) long and the other 50 cm (20 in) long. *When one tape is longer than the other, they can be fastened at*

▶ **Technique 33–4** *CONTINUED*

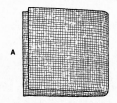
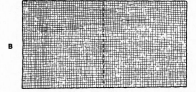
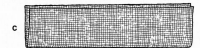
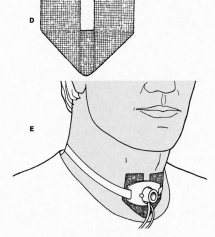

FIGURE 33–16 Folding a 4 × 4 gauze to make a tracheostomy dressing.

the side of the client's neck for easy access. A knot at the back of the neck could create pressure and irritate the skin.

- Cut a 1-cm (0.5-in) slit approximately 2.5 cm (1 in) from one end of each strip. This is best achieved by folding the end of the tape back onto itself about 2.5 cm and then cutting a slit in the middle of the tape from its folded edge.

- Have an assistant don a sterile glove and hold the tracheostomy tube in place while you change the ties. If an assistant is not available, fasten the clean ties before removing the soiled ties. *Holding the tube prevents acci-*

dental expulsion of it if the client coughs or moves.

- Detach and remove the soiled tapes from the client. The ties can be cut or untied.

- Thread the slit end of one clean tape through the eye of the tracheostomy faceplate from the bottom side; then thread the other end of the tie through the slit of the tape, pulling it taut until it is securely fastened to the faceplate. *This method avoids the use of knots, which produce pressure, discomfort, and skin irritation.*

- Repeat the above step for the second tie.

- Ask the client to flex the neck, and have the assistant place one or two fingers under the tapes while you tie the tapes together at the side of the client's neck (Figure 33–17). *Flexion of the neck increases neck circumference the way coughing does. The client's neck flexion and the assistant's finger placement prevent the nurse from making the ties too tight, which could cause choking or pressure on the jugular veins.*

- Tie the tapes using two square knots. Cut off any long ends. *Two square knots will prevent slippage and loosening, allowing the tube to dislodge.*

One-Strip Method

- Determine the length of twill tape required:

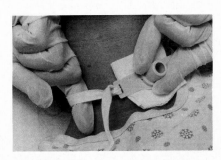

FIGURE 33–17 Placing a finger underneath the tie tape before tying it.

a. Hold one end of the tape at the slot on one side of the tracheostomy faceplate.

b. Pull the tape around the back of the client's neck to the slot on the other side.

c. Multiply this length by 2.5.

- Apply the tie as follows:

a. Thread one end of the tape into the upper half of the slot on one side.

b. Bring both ends of the tape together, and take them around the client's neck, keeping them flat and untwisted.

c. Thread the piece of tape closest to the client's neck from back to front through the other slot.

d. Tie square knots with the loose tape ends as described above.

5. Pad the tie tape knot.

- Place a folded 4 × 4 gauze square under the tie where it is knotted, and apply tape over the knot. *Gauze under the knot prevents skin irritation. Taping over the knot prevents confusing the dressing ties with the client's gown ties.*

6. Check the tautness of the tracheostomy tie.

- Frequently check the tautness of the tracheostomy tie, particularly for clients whose neck diameter may increase from swelling (e.g., those with radical neck surgery, neck trauma, or cardiac failure) or for clients who are restless and may loosen their ties.

7. Document all relevant information.

- Record the dressing change, the application of any ointments, and your assessments.

▶ **Technique 33–4 Changing a Tracheostomy Dressing** *CONTINUED*

EVALUATION FOCUS

Character of secretions from tracheostomy site; appearance of tracheostomy wound; pulse and respiratory rates compared to baseline data; complaints of pain or discomfort at tracheostomy site.

SAMPLE RECORDING

Date	Time	Notes
12/22/93	0945	Tracheostomy dressing and tie tapes changed. Dressing saturated with 2.5 × 3 cm serosanguineous drainage. Incision site slightly reddened. No complaints of discomfort. ——————— Antonia Wong, RN

KEY ELEMENTS OF CHANGING A TRACHEOSTOMY DRESSING AND TIE TAPES

- Wear a disposable glove to remove the dressing.
- Wear sterile gloves to handle sterile gauzes and to clean the incision site and tube flanges.
- Assess the status of the incision and surrounding skin.

- Use noncotton-filled gauze squares for cleaning and for the dressing.
- Thoroughly rinse areas cleaned with hydrogen peroxide.

Deflating and Inflating a Cuffed Tracheostomy Tube

The nurse must check the physician's orders to determine when a cuffed tracheostomy tube should be inflated. Cuffed tracheostomy tubes are generally inflated

- During the first 12 hours after a tracheostomy
- When the client is being ventilated or receiving IPPB therapy, to prevent air leakage
- When the client is eating or receiving oral med-

ications and for a prescribed period of time following meals or medications (e.g., 30 minutes), to prevent aspiration

- When the client is comatose, to prevent aspiration of oropharyngeal secretions

At other times the cuff may be deflated, unless a low-pressure cuff is used. If double-cuffed tubes are used, deflation and inflation must be done at regular intervals according to the manufacturer's directions (e.g., every 1 or 2 hours). Technique 33–5 explains how to deflate and inflate a cuffed tracheostomy tube.

33-5 Deflating and Inflating a Cuffed Tracheostomy Tube

PURPOSES
- To prevent aspiration of oropharyngeal secretions while the client is comatose or is eating or receiving oral medications
- To prevent tracheal edema, ulceration, and necrosis

ASSESSMENT FOCUS

Size of cuff; maximum cuff inflation pressure recommended by the manufacturer; physician's orders and agency policy about the prescribed schedule for deflation and inflation; client respiratory rate and character; breath sounds.

▶ **Technique 33–5 Deflating and Inflating a Cuffed Tracheostomy Tube** *CONTINUED*

EQUIPMENT

- ☐ Equipment needed for suctioning the oropharyngeal cavity
- ☐ 5- or 10-ml syringe
- ☐ Manual resuscitator (Ambu bag)

- ☐ Stethoscope
- ☐ Soft-tipped hemostat
- ☐ Manometer specifically designed to measure cuff

pressure, or blood pressure manometer

- ☐ Sterile three-way stopcock (optional)

INTERVENTION

1. Position the client appropriately.

- Assist the client to a semi-Fowler's position unless contraindicated.

- Place clients receiving positive pressure ventilation in a supine position. *This position enables secretions above the cuff site to move up into the mouth.*

2. Deflate the cuff.

- First suction the oropharyngeal cavity. See Technique 31–1 on page 767. *Suctioning prevents pooled oral secretions from descending into the trachea after the cuff is deflated. The secretions could cause irritation and infection.*

- Discard the catheter. *This catheter is discarded to avoid introducing microorganisms into the lower airway when it is suctioned later.*

- If a soft-tipped hemostat is clamping the cuff inflation tube, unclamp it. Some tubes have one-way valves that replace the hemostat.

- Attach the 5- or 10-ml syringe to the distal end of the inflation tube, making sure the seal is tight.

- While the client inhales, *slowly* withdraw the amount of air from the cuff indicated by the manufacturer (e.g., about 5 ml), or as orders indicate, while providing a positive pressure breath with a manual resuscitator (an Ambu bag). *Removal of air on inhalation*

under positive pressure allows secretions to ascend from the bronchi. Slow deflation allows positive lung pressure to move secretions upward from the bronchi.

- Keep the syringe attached to the tubing. *The syringe is left attached for reinflation of the cuff.*

- If the cough reflex is stimulated during cuff-deflation, suction the lower airway with a sterile catheter. *Cuff deflation can stimulate the cough reflex, which may produce additional secretions.*

- Assess the client's respirations, and suction the client as needed. If the client experiences breathing difficulties, reinflate the cuff immediately.

3. Reinflate the cuff to the minimal occluding volume (MOV) using the minimal air leak technique (MLT).

- Use a stethoscope over the client's neck adjacent to the trachea while inflating the cuff (Figure 33–18). *The stethoscope helps you gauge the proper cuff inflation point.*

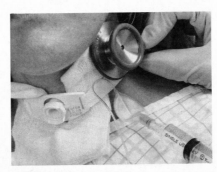

FIGURE 33–18 Inflating a cuff while auscultating breath sounds over the neck beside the trachea.

- Inflate the cuff on inhalation, and inject the least amount of air needed (usually 2 to 5 ml) to achieve a tracheal seal. *This prevents tracheal damage.*

- Continue to inflate the cuff until you cannot hear an air leak, i.e., a harsh, squeaking, or gurgling sound.

- Stop cuff inflation when there is no audible air leak on auscultation. The cuff is sufficiently inflated when

  a. You cannot hear the client's voice.

  b. You cannot feel any air movements from the client's mouth, nose, or tracheostomy site.

  c. You hear no leak from the positive pressure ventilation when auscultating the neck adjacent to the trachea during inspiration.

- Establish a minimum air leak by listening to the client's neck with your stethoscope and aspirating a small amount of air (e.g., 0.1 to 0.3 ml) until a slight leak (i.e., a slight hissing sound) is detected. *This creates a minimal air leak, which indicates that the cuff is inflated at the lowest pressure possible to create an adequate seal. An air leak that is audible without a stethoscope is greater than a minimal leak.*

- Note the exact amount of air used to inflate the cuff to achieve a minimal air leak. *This prevents*

▶

▶ **Technique 33–5 Deflating and Inflating a Cuffed Tracheostomy Tube** *CONTINUED*

overinflation in subsequent cuff inflations and detects tracheal problems if more air is consistently needed.

- If the tube does not have a one-way valve, clamp the inflation tube with a soft-tipped hemostat, or apply a one-way valve.

- Remove the syringe.

4. Measure the cuff pressure.

- Make sure the client is in the same position for each pressure cuff reading. *A change in position can alter the pressure needed to make an adequate seal.*

- Attach the cuff's pilot port to the cuff pressure manometer tubing.

- Read the dial on the manometer. The pressure should not exceed 15 to 20 mm Hg or 25 cm H_2O. Check physician's orders. *Excessive cuff pressure causes tracheal edema, ulceration, and necrosis. Underinflation may cause inadequate ventilation and may allow aspiration of blood, food, or secretions.*

- If the pressure is appropriate, clamp the inflation tube with a soft-tipped hemostat, provided that tube does not have a one-way valve.

- Remove the syringe.

- See also the variation below.

5. Ensure client comfort and safety.

- Check cuff pressure every 8 to 12 hours or as recommended by agency protocol. Note whether

the minimal occlusive volume increases or decreases.

- Suspect an air leak if

    a. Air injection fails to inflate the cuff or increase cuff pressure.

    b. You are not able to inject the amount of air withdrawn.

    c. The client can speak.

    d. You can hear harsh gurgling breath sounds without a stethoscope.

- Make sure the client is comfortable and that the call signal and communication aids are within easy reach.

6. Document all relevant information.

- Document the time of the deflation and/or inflation, the amount of air withdrawn and/or injected, and your assessments.

VARIATION: Using a Stopcock to Measure Cuff Pressure

- Attach the ends of the stopcock to the manometer tubing, the syringe, and the pilot port of the cuff (Figure 33–19).

- Make sure the stopcock dial to the pilot balloon port is in the "off" position when you connect the setup to the pilot balloon port. *This prevents air leakage during equipment attachment.*

- Ensure a tight seal at all connections. *A tight seal prevents an air leak that could alter cuff pressure.*

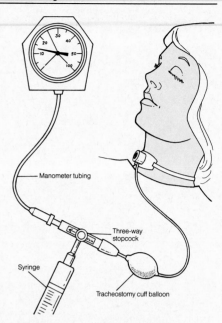

FIGURE 33–19 A stopcock attached to manometer tubing, a syringe, and the pilot port of the cuff.

- Turn the stopcock dial to the "off" position to the syringe. *This establishes the connection between the cuff and the manometer.*

- Note the pressure reading on the manometer as the client exhales.

- If the amount of air needs to be adjusted, inflate or deflate the cuff by first turning the stopcock dial to the "off" position to the manometer. *This establishes a connection between the syringe and the cuff.*

- Turn the stopcock dial to the "off" position to the pilot balloon, and disconnect the apparatus.

EVALUATION FOCUS

Respiratory rate and depth; pulse rate; tracheal breath sounds; skin and nail bed color.

▶ **Technique 33–5** *CONTINUED*

SAMPLE RECORDING

Date	Time	Notes
7/21/93	1700	Oropharyngeal cavity suctioned and tracheal cuff deflated. 3.7 ml air withdrawn from cuff. No coughing after deflation. R 16, regular, and nonlabored, P 84. —————————————————————————— Sally S. Lee, RN
	1800	Tracheal cuff inflated to 15 mm Hg. Respirations 14, regular, and eupneic. Lung sounds clear bilaterally. Skin color and nailbeds pink. ——————————— Sally S. Lee, RN

KEY ELEMENTS OF DEFLATING AND INFLATING A CUFFED TRACHEOSTOMY TUBE

- Assess the client's respirations, pulse, color, breath sounds, and behavior before and after the procedure.
- Verify the physician's orders about cuff deflation and inflation.

For Cuff Deflation

- Maintain asepsis when suctioning.
- Suction the oropharyngeal cavity adequately before cuff deflation.
- Withdraw the correct amount of air while the client inhales and while providing a positive pressure breath if ordered.

- If the cough reflex is stimulated after deflation, suction the lower airway.

For Cuff Inflation

- Inflate the cuff on inhalation.
- Follow the minimal air leak technique.
- Make sure the cuff pressure does not exceed 15 to 20 mm Hg or 25 cm H_2O.
- Clamp the inflation tube if required.
- Document the exact amount of air used to inflate the cuff.

Plugging a Tracheostomy Tube

A tracheostomy plug is usually inserted into a tracheostomy tube for specified lengths of time before the tube is removed. While the tube is plugged, the client is carefully monitored for signs of respiratory distress. Often the length of time the tube is plugged is increased over a number of days if the person tolerates the procedure well. The nurse must check the physician's orders to determine the length of time the tracheostomy tube should remain plugged. Technique 33–6 describes how to plug a tracheostomy tube.

33-6   Plugging a Tracheostomy Tube

PURPOSE
- To establish ventilation through the natural airway

ASSESSMENT FOCUS

Pulse and respirations before plugging the tube; excessive secretions in the respiratory tract (may contraindicate plugging of the tube).

EQUIPMENT

- Suction apparatus
- Sterile suction catheters
- Sterile 10-ml syringe
- Sterile gloves
- Sterile tracheostomy plug

▶

► **Technique 33–6 Plugging a Tracheostomy Tube** *CONTINUED*

INTERVENTION

1. Position the client.

• Assist the client to a semi-Fowler's position if not contraindicated. *This position enhances lung expansion and may decrease fears about not being able to breathe.*

2. Suction the airways.

• Suction the client's nasopharynx if there are any secretions present.

• Change suction catheters, and suction the tracheostomy. If there are excessive secretions, report this finding to the nurse in charge or physician to determine whether to proceed with the procedure.

3. Deflate the tracheal cuff if ordered.

• See Technique 33–5 on page 806.

• Suction the tracheostomy tube again if secretions are present.

4. Insert the tracheostomy plug.

• Using sterile gloves, fit the tracheostomy plug into either the inner or the outer cannula, depending on whether the tracheostomy tube has a double or single cannula.

• Monitor the client closely for 10 minutes for signs of respiratory distress, e.g., noisy and/or rapid respirations and use of accessory muscles for breathing. At the first signs of distress, remove the tracheostomy plug, and suction the tracheostomy if necessary.

• Clean the inner cannula, if it was removed, so that it is ready to be reinserted.

• Observe the client frequently while the tube is plugged.

5. Remove the plug at the designated time.

• After removing the plug, suction the tracheostomy if indicated, and replace the inner cannula if removed.

• Reinflate the cuff if ordered.

6. Document all relevant information.

• Document the amount, color, and consistency of the secretions, the times the plug was inserted and removed, and your assessments.

EVALUATION FOCUS

> Respiratory status while the tube is plugged (i.e., breath sounds, respiratory rate, and the use of accessory muscles for breathing).

SAMPLE RECORDING

Date	Time	Notes
7/11/93	1500	P-82 regular, R-14 and effortless. Tracheostomy tube plugged after suctioning nasopharynx and tracheostomy tube. Cuff deflated—2.5 ml air withdrawn.
	1515	Breathing effortless while plug in place, pulse rate and respiratory rate unchanged. Plug removed. ———————— Briona R. King, SN

KEY ELEMENTS OF PLUGGING A TRACHEOSTOMY TUBE

• Assess the amount of respiratory secretions before plugging the tube.

• Suction the tracheostomy if secretions are excessive.

• Monitor the client closely for signs of respiratory distress while the tube is plugged.

CRITICAL THINKING CHALLENGE

John White, a 54-year-old client with Guillain-Barré syndrome, has had a tracheostomy performed to support his ventilation. He is awake and mentally alert. While the tracheostomy tube is in place, he will be unable to communicate verbally. How can you establish a means of communication with Mr. White?

RELATED RESEARCH

Balazs, I. B.; Walton, C. B.; Briggs, S.; and Goldstein, M. January 1987. A clinical evaluation of an oxygen insufflation/suction catheter. *Heart and Lung* 16:39–46.

Bostick, J., and Wendelgass, S. T. September 1987. Normal saline instillation as part of the suctioning procedure: Effects on PaO$_2$ and amount of secretions. *Heart and Lung* 16:532–37.

Czarnik, R. E.; Stone, K. S.; Everhart, C. C., Jr. March 1991. Differential effects of continuous versus intermittent suction on tracheal tissue. *Heart and Lung* 20:144–51.

Gunderson, L. P.; Stone, K. S.; and Hamlin, K. L. May/June 1991. Endotracheal suctioning—induced heart rate alterations. *Nursing Research* 40:139–43.

Pierce, J. B., and Piazza, D. E. January 1987. Differences in postsuctioning arterial blood oxygen concentration values using two postoxygenation methods. *Heart and Lung* 16:34–38.

REFERENCES

Bodai, B. I.; Walton, C. B.; Briggs, S.; and Goldstein, M. January 1987. A clinical evaluation of an oxygen insufflation/suction catheter. *Heart and Lung* 16:39–46.

Carroll, P. F. May 1988. Lowering the risks of endotracheal suctioning. *Nursing 88* 18:46–50.

Dunleap, E. August 1987. Safe and easy ways to secure breathing tubes. *RN* 50:26–27.

Hoffman, L. A., and Maszkiewicz, R. C. January 1987. Airway management for the critically ill patient. *American Journal of Nursing* 87:39–53.

Lockhart, J. S., and Griffin, C. April 1987. Action STAT! Occluded trach tube. *Nursing 87* 17:33.

Mapp, C. S. July 1988. Trach care: Are you aware of all the dangers? *Nursing 88* 18:34–43.

Noll, M. L.; Hix, C. D.; and Scott, G. August 1990. Closed tracheal suction system: Effectiveness and nursing implications. *AACN Clinical Issues in Critical Care Nursing* 1:318–28.

Preston, I. M.; Matthews, H. R., and Ready, A. R. October 10, 1986. Minitracheostomy: A new technique for tracheal suction. *Physiotherapy* 72:494–97.

Reed, J. Jr. November 1987. Orotracheal and nasotracheal intubation. *Emergency Care Quarterly* 2 3:1–6.

Shekleton, M. E., and Nield, M. March 1987. Ineffective airway clearance related to artificial airway. *Nursing Clinics of North America* 22:167–78.

Smith, A. J., and Johnson, J. Y. 1990. *Nurses' guide to clinical procedures.* Philadelphia: J. B. Lippincott Co.

34

Chest Drainage

CONTENTS

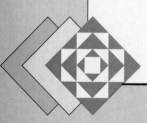

<table>
<tr><td>

NURSING PROCESS GUIDE

CHEST DRAINAGE

ASSESSMENT

See the Nursing Process Guide for Chapter 30. Essential data include the following:

- *Vital signs* for baseline data and then every 4 hours.

- *Breath sounds.* Auscultate bilaterally for baseline data. Diminished or absent breath sounds after chest drainage is established indicate inadequate lung expansion and recurrent pneumothorax.

- *Clinical signs of pneumothorax* before and after chest tube insertion. Leakage or blockage of a chest tube can seriously impair ventilation. Signs include sharp pain on the affected side; weak, rapid pulse; pallor; vertigo; faintness; dyspnea; diaphoresis; excessive coughing; and blood-tinged sputum.

- *Chest expansion* (respiratory excursion). See Chapter 11, pages 246 and 249 and Figures 11–62 and 11–66.

- *Chest movements*, such as retractions, flail chest, or paradoxical breathing. Note the specific location of retractions: intercostal, substernal, suprasternal, supraclavicular, or tracheal tug.

- *Dressing site.* Inspect the dressing for excessive and abnormal drainage, such as bleeding or foul-smelling discharge. Palpate around the dressing site, and listen for a crackling sound indicative of subcutaneous emphysema. Subcutaneous emphysema can result from a poor seal at the chest tube insertion site. It is manifested by a "crackling" sound that is heard when the area around the insertion site is palpated.

- *Level of discomfort* with and without activity. Analgesics often need to be administered before the client

</td><td>

moves or does deep-breathing and coughing exercises.

RELATED DIAGNOSTIC CATEGORIES

- Anxiety
- Fear
- Ineffective breathing pattern
- Impaired gas exchange
- High risk for Infection
- Pain

PLANNING

Client Goal
The client will restore or maintain adequate ventilation and an effective breathing pattern.

Outcome Criteria
The client

- Has stable vital signs.

- Establishes a normal effective respiratory pattern of 12 to 20 per minute, effortless breathing (no use of accessory muscles), and symmetric chest expansion on inhalation.

- Has clear breath sounds bilaterally.

- Has skin, nails, lips, and earlobes of natural color.

- Has minimal clear or slight serosanguineous drainage at tube insertion site.

- Has minimal chest pain.

- Verbalizes awareness of feelings of anxiety.

- Discusses fears.

- Reports an increase in psychologic and physiologic comfort.

</td></tr>
</table>

Chest Tubes

Chest tubes are usually inserted through an intercostal space into the pleural cavity. They are used following chest surgery or trauma and for pneumothorax and/or hemothorax. A **pneumothorax** is a collection of air or other gas in the pleural space that causes the lung to collapse (atelectasis). A **hemothorax** is the accumulation of blood and fluid in the pleural cavity, usually as a result of trauma or surgery. Clinical signs of pneumothorax are provided in the Nursing Process Guide, above.

Chest tubes that are used to remove air are usually inserted superiorly (i.e., through the second intercostal space) and anteriorly because air tends to rise in the pleural cavity. Tubes used to drain fluids are inserted more inferiorly, often in the eighth or ninth intercostal space, and more posteriorly. Sometimes a tube used to drain air is inserted inferiorly and threaded superiorly in the pleural space. When a client requires drainage of both fluid and air, two chest tubes may be inserted. These are sometimes joined externally by a Y-connector.

Drainage Systems

Because the pleural cavity normally has negative pressure which allows lung expansion, any drainage system connected to it must be sealed so that air or liquid cannot enter. Such a drainage system is called a water-sealed (underwater) drainage or a disposable pleural drainage system. In water-sealed drainage, fluid in the bottom of the container prevents air from entering the chest tube and thus entering the pleural cavity. The system must be kept below the level of the client's chest so that the fluid in the container is not drawn into the pleural cavity by gravity. It is also very important to maintain the patency of the tubing.

Drainage systems use three mechanisms to drain fluid and air from the pleural cavity; positive expiratory pressure, gravity, and suction. When the pleural cavity contains some air or fluid, a positive pressure develops during expiration. This positive pressure is abnormal, but it does help expel the air and to some extent fluid from the space. Placing the tubing so that it descends from the insertion site to the drainage receptacle allows gravity to act as an evacuation force. Suction is used in conjunction with the other two forces in some drainage systems.

There are several kinds of water-sealed drainage systems: one- and two-bottle gravity systems, two- and three-bottle suction systems, and disposable unit systems.

Bottle Systems

In a *one-bottle system*, a single receptacle receives both the fluid and/or air from the client and seals the system (Figure 34–1, *A*). The air or fluid enters through the collection inlet, which terminates under sterile water. The air then exits through the water and through the air vent; the fluid remains in the bottle. The fluid in this bottle then is a combination of fluid from the client and sterile water—it forms the water seal. The one-bottle system depends on gravity and positive expiratory pressure for drainage.

A *two-bottle system* uses one bottle to receive the fluid or air from the client and the second bottle to create the water seal (Figure 34–1, *B*). The air or fluid from the pleural cavity is received into bottle 1. The air from bottle 1 is passed into bottle 2. The air then passes through the sterile water and exits from bottle 2 through the air vent. The fluid from the pleural cavity remains in bottle 1. This system uses gravity and positive expiratory pressure for drainage.

The *three-bottle system* has a collection bottle (1), a water-seal bottle (2), and a suction-control bottle (3) (Figure 34–1, *C*). Fluid from the pleural cavity collects in bottle 1, which is connected to a tube in bottle 2 that terminates below the fluid level. Bottle 2 is then connected to bottle 3 by a short tube. Bottle 3 also has a manometer tube submerged in sterile

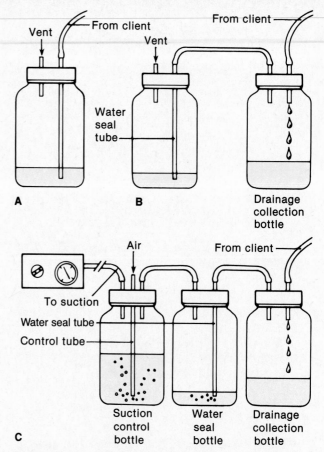

FIGURE 34–1 Drainage systems for chest tubes: *A*, one-bottle system; *B*, two-bottle system; *C*, three-bottle system.

water. The depth to which this tube is submerged determines the amount of suction exerted in the pleural cavity. The suction-control bottle has another inlet, for suction. This system uses positive expiratory pressure, gravity, and suction for drainage.

Disposable Unit Systems

Several types of disposable unit systems are available commercially. Two commonly seen are the Pleur-evac system and the Argyle system. A newer system is the Thora-Drain III system. The *Pleur-evac system* consists of three chambers (Figure 34–2). Chamber A is the collection chamber. It receives fluid and/or air from the pleural cavity and is divided into three subchambers. The client's fluid remains in this chamber, while air from the client passes on to chamber B, the water-seal chamber. This chamber is U-shaped, and air from the pleural cavity passes through the water seal and exits at the suction outlet side of the U. Chamber C, the suction chamber, is also U-shaped. The height of the fluid in chamber C determines the amount of suction pressure exerted upon the client. Atmospheric air enters on the far left of this chamber, passes through the suction-control water, and joins the air from the client. These then pass into the suction outlet.

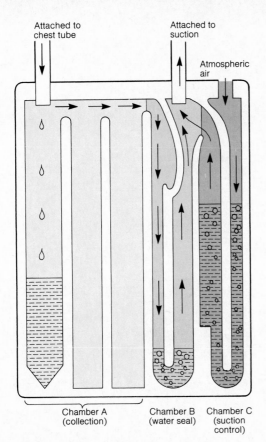

FIGURE 34–2   A Pleur-evac chest drainage system.

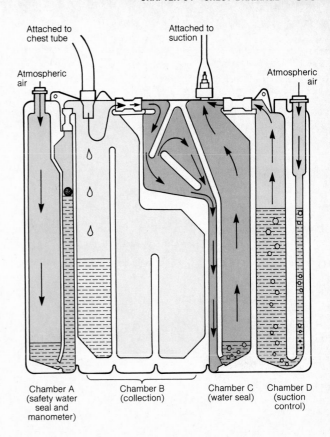

FIGURE 34–3   An Argyle chest drainage system.

The *Argyle double-seal system* consists of four chambers (Figure 34–3). Chamber A is a water-seal chamber with a manometer. Chamber B is the collection chamber. Chamber C is another water seal. Chamber D is for suction control. Normally, the client's pleural air passes from chamber B into chamber C and to the suction source; however, if the suction becomes obstructed, the air can pass to chamber A and to the atmosphere. Chamber A thus serves as a safety vent.

The *Thora-Drain III system* consists of three chambers; a collection chamber, a water-seal chamber, and a suction-control chamber. The unique feature of this system is its replaceable collection chamber. When the collection chamber is filled with drainage, it can be changed or replaced without interrupting the entire system.

Steps for setting up a disposable water-seal drainage system are shown in the box on page 816.

Assisting Clients with Chest Tubes

Chest tubes are inserted and removed by the physician with the nurse assisting. Both procedures require sterile technique and must be done without introducing air or microorganisms into the pleural cavity. After the insertion, an X-ray film is taken to confirm the position of the tube.

The major objective of nursing care of clients with chest tubes is to facilitate drainage of fluid and air, thus promoting lung reexpansion. Essential aspects of care include maintaining the water seal, maintaining patency of the drainage system, and assessing the client's respiratory and cardiovascular status. Policies and procedures vary considerably from agency to agency in regard to chest drainage interventions. Certain interventions, such as milking a chest tube to maintain patency, may be prohibited. The nurse must therefore review agency protocols before intervening. Techique 34–1 provides guidelines for monitoring the client with a chest tube.

Chest tubes are generally removed within 5 to 7 days. Before removal, the tube is clamped with two large, rubber-tipped clamps for 1 to 2 days to assess for signs of respiratory distress and to determine whether air or fluid remains in the pleural space. An X-ray film of the chest is generally taken 2 hours after tube clamping to determine full lung expansion. If the client develops signs of respiratory distress or the film indicates pneumothorax, the tube clamps are removed, and chest drainage is maintained. If neither occurs, the tube is removed. Another X-ray film of the chest is often taken after removal to confirm full lung expansion.

Setting Up a Disposable Water-Seal Drainage System (Pleur-evac or Argyle System)

Nurses must follow strict surgical aseptic technique when setting up chest drainage to prevent microorganisms from entering the system and subsequently entering the client's pleural cavity. To set up the system,

• Open the packaged unit.

• Remove the plastic connector from the tube attached to the water-seal chamber. (The Argyle system has two water-seal chambers; do both.)

• Using a 50-ml Asepto syringe with the bulb removed, fill the water-seal chamber with sterile distilled water up to the 2-cm mark (Figure 34–4). Then reattach the plastic connector.

• If the physician has ordered suction, remove the diaphragm (cap) on the suction-control chamber (Figure 34–5).

• Using the 50-ml syringe, fill the suction-control chamber with distilled water to the ordered level or 20 to 25 cm, and replace the cap.

• Place the system in the rack supplied, or attach it to the bed frame.

• Attach the longer tube from the collection chamber to the client's chest tube.

• If suction is ordered, attach the remaining shorter tube to the suction source, and turn it on. Inspect the suction

chamber for bubbling. Gentle bubbling indicates an appropriate suction level.

• If suction has not been ordered, keep the shorter rubber tube unclamped. This maintains negative or equal pressure in the system.

• Tape all tubing connections, but do not completely cover the tubing connectors with tape (Figure 34–6). Not covering the connectors allows drainage to be seen.

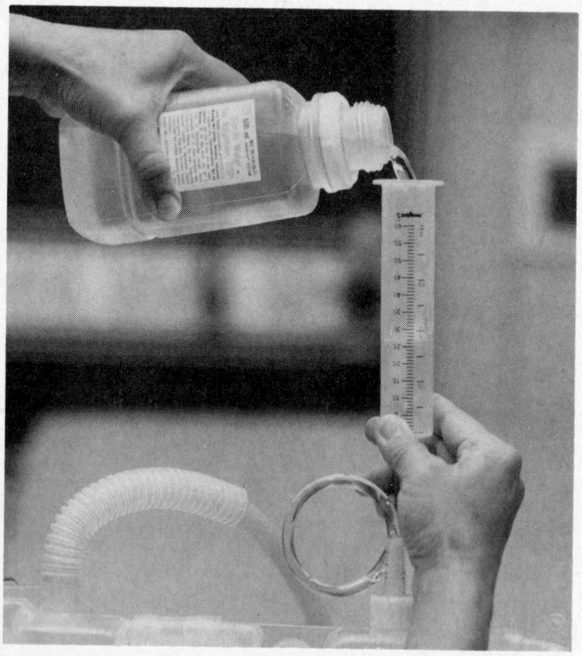

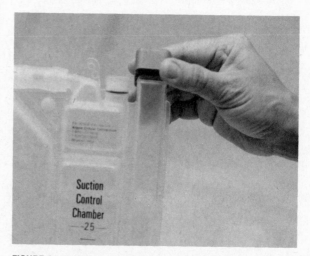

FIGURE 34–5 Removing the cap on the suction-control chamber.

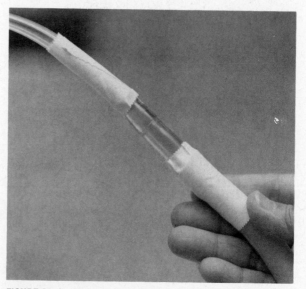

FIGURE 34–4 Filling the water-seal chamber with sterile distilled water

FIGURE 34–6 Taped tubing connection with the connector exposed for observation of drainage.

34-1 Monitoring a Client with Chest Drainage

PURPOSES
- To maintain patency of the chest drainage system and facilitate lung reexpansion
- To prevent complications associated with chest drainage (e.g., infection)

ASSESSMENT FOCUS

See Intervention, step 1.

EQUIPMENT

To Remedy Tube Problems
- Sterile gloves
- Two rubber-tipped Kelly clamps
- Sterile petrolatum gauze
- Sterile drainage system
- Antiseptic swabs
- Sterile 4 × 4 gauzes
- Air-occlusive tape

To Milk Tubing
- Lubricating gel, soap, hand lotion, or alcohol sponge

To Obtain a Specimen
- Povidone-iodine swab
- Sterile #18 or #20 gauge needle
- 3- or 5-ml syringe

- Needle protector
- Label for the syringe
- Laboratory requisition

INTERVENTION

1. Assess the client.

- Assess vital signs every 4 hours, or more often, as indicated.

- Determine ease of respirations, breath sounds, respiratory rate and depth, and chest movements.

- Monitor the client for signs of pneumothorax (see page 813).

- Inspect the dressing for excessive and abnormal drainage, such as bleeding or foul-smelling discharge. Palpate around the dressing site, and listen for a crackling sound indicative of subcutaneous emphysema. *Subcutaneous emphysema can result from a poor seal at the chest tube insertion site. It is manifested by a "crackling" sound that is heard when the area around the insertion site is palpated.*

- Assess level of discomfort. *Analgesics often need to be administered before the client moves or does deep-breathing and coughing exercises.*

🄢 2. Implement all necessary safety precautions.

- Keep two 15- to 18-cm (6- to 7-in) rubber-tipped Kelly clamps within reach at the bedside, to clamp the chest tube in an emergency, e.g., if leakage occurs in the tubing.

- Keep one sterile petrolatum gauze within reach at the bedside to use with an air-occlusive material if the chest tube becomes dislodged.

- Keep an extra drainage system unit available in the client's room. In most agencies, the physician is responsible for changing the drainage system except in emergency situations, such as malfunction or breakage. In these situations:

  a. Clamp the chest tube close to the insertion site with two rubber-tipped clamps placed in opposite directions (Figure 34–7).

  b. Reestablish a water-sealed drainage system.

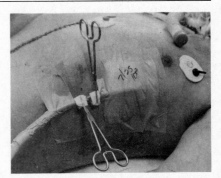

FIGURE 34–7 Clamping a chest tube.

  c. Remove the clamps, and notify the physician.

- Keep the drainage system below chest level and upright at all times, unless the chest tubes are clamped. *Keeping the unit below chest level prevents backflow of fluid from the drainage chamber into the pleural space. Keeping the unit upright maintains the glass tube below the water level, forming the water seal.*

3. Maintain the patency of the drainage system.

- Check that all connections are secured with tape to ensure that the system is airtight.

▶ **Technique 34–1 Monitoring Chest Drainage** *CONTINUED*

- Inspect the drainage tubing for kinks or loops dangling below the entry level of the drainage system.

- Coil the drainage tubing and secure it to the bed linen, ensuring enough slack for the client to turn and move (Figure 34–8). *This prevents kinking of the tubing and impairment of the drainage system.*

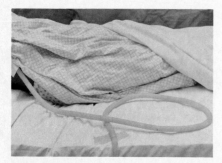

FIGURE 34–8 Coiled drainage tubing secured to the bed linen.

- Inspect the air vent in the system periodically to make sure it is not occluded. A vent must be present to allow air to escape. *Obstruction of the air vent causes an increased pressure in the system that could result in pneumothorax.*

- Milk or strip the chest tubing **as ordered and only in accordance with agency protocol.** *Too vigorous milking can create excessive negative pressure that can harm the pleural membranes and/or surrounding tissues.* Always verify the physician's orders before milking the tube; milking of only short segments of the tube may be specified (e.g., 10 to 20 cm, or 4 to 8 in). To milk a chest tube, follow these steps:

  a. Lubricate about 10 to 20 cm (4 to 8 in) of the drainage tubing with lubricating gel, soap, or hand lotion, or hold an alcohol sponge between your fingers and the tube. *Lubrication reduces friction*

and facilitates the milking process.

  b. With one hand, securely stabilize and pinch the tube at the insertion site.

  c. Compress the tube with the thumb and forefinger of your other hand and milk it by sliding them down the tube, moving away from the insertion site. *Milking the tubing dislodges obstructions, such as blood clots. Milking from the insertion site downward prevents movement of the obstructive material into the pleural space.*

  d. If the entire tube is to be milked, reposition your hands farther along the tubing, and repeat steps **a** through **c** in progressive overlapping steps, until you reach the end of the tubing.

4. Assess any fluid level fluctuations and bubbling in the drainage system.

- In gravity drainage systems, check for fluctuation (tidaling) of the fluid level in the water-seal glass tube of a bottle system or the water-seal chamber of a commercial system as the client breathes. Normally, fluctuations of 5 to 10 cm (2 to 4 in) occur until the lung has reexpanded. In suction drainage systems, the fluid line remains constant. *Fluctuations reflect the pressure changes in the pleural space during inhalation and exhalation. The fluid level rises when the client inhales and falls when the client exhales. The absence of fluctuations may indicate tubing obstruction from a kink, dependent loop, blood clot, or outside pressure (e.g., because the client is lying on the tubing), or may indicate that full lung reexpansion has occurred.*

- To check for fluctuation in suction systems, temporarily turn off the suction. Then observe the fluctuation.

- Check for intermittent bubbling in the water of the water-seal bottle or chamber. *Intermittent bubbling normally occurs when the system removes air from the pleural space, especially when the client takes a deep breath or coughs. Absence of bubbling indicates that the pleural space has healed and is sealed. Continuous bubbling or a sudden change from an established pattern can indicate a break in the system, i.e., an air leak, and should be reported immediately.*

- Check for gentle bubbling in the suction-control bottle or chamber. *Gentle bubbling indicates proper suction pressure.*

5. Assess the drainage.

- Inspect the drainage in the collection container at least every 30 minutes during the first 2 hours after chest tube insertion and every 2 hours thereafter.

- Every 8 hours, mark the time,

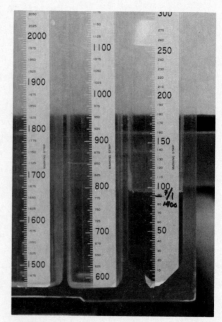

FIGURE 34–9 Marking the date, time, and drainage level.

► **Technique 34–1** CONTINUED

date, and drainage level on a piece of adhesive tape affixed to the container, or mark it directly on a disposable container (Figure 34–9).

• Note any sudden change in the amount or color of the drainage.

Ⓢ • If drainage exceeds 100 ml per hour or if a color change indicates hemorrhage, notify the physician immediately.

6. **Watch for dislodgement of the tubes, and remedy the problem promptly.**

• If the chest tube becomes disconnected from the drainage system,

   a. Have the client exhale fully.

   b. Clamp the chest tube close to the insertion site with two rubber-tipped clamps placed in opposite directions. *Clamping the tube prevents external air from entering the pleural space. Two clamps ensure complete closure of the tube.*

   c. Quickly clean the ends of the tubing with an antiseptic, reconnect them, and tape them securely.

   d. Unclamp the tube as soon as possible. *Having the client exhale and clamping the tube for no longer than necessary prevents an air or fluid build-up in the pleural space, which can cause further lung collapse.*

   e. Assess the client closely for respiratory distress (dyspnea, pallor, diaphoresis, blood-tinged sputum, or chest pain).

   f. Check vital signs every 10 minutes.

• If the chest tube becomes dislodged from the insertion site,

   a. Remove the dressing, and immmediately apply pressure with the petrolatum gauze, your hand, or a towel.

   b. Cover the site with sterile 4 × 4 gauze squares.

   c. Tape the dressings with air-occlusive tape.

   d. Notify the physician immediately.

   e. Assess the client for respiratory distress every 10 to 15 minutes or as client condition indicates.

• If the drainage system is accidentally tipped over,

   a. Immediately return it to the upright position.

   b. Ask the client to take several deep breaths. *Deep breaths help force air out of the pleural cavity that might have entered when the water seal was not intact.*

   c. Notify the nurse in charge and the physician.

   d. Assess the client for respiratory distress.

7. **If continuous bubbling persists in the water-seal collection chamber, indicating an air leak, determine its source.** *Continuous bubbling in the water-seal collection chamber normally occurs for only a few minutes after a chest tube is attached to drainage, because fluid and air initially rush out from the intrapleural space under high pressure.*

• To detect an air leak, follow the next steps sequentially (Quinn 1986 and Palau 1986):

   a. Check the tubing connection sites. Tighten and retape any connection that seems loose. *The tubing connection sites are the most likely places for leaks to occur. Bub-*

bling will stop if these are the sources of the leak.

   b. If bubbling continues, clamp the chest tube near the insertion site, and see whether the bubbling stops while the client takes several deep breaths. *Clamping the chest tube near the insertion site will help determine whether the leak is proximal or distal to the clamp. Chest tube clamping must be done only for a few seconds at a time. Clamping for long periods can aggravate an existing pneumothorax or lead to a recurrent pneumothorax.*

   c. If bubbling stops, proceed with the next step. The source of the air leak is above the clamp, i.e., between the clamp and the client. It may be either at the insertion site or inside the client.

   d. If bubbling continues, the source of the air leak is below the clamp, i.e., in the drainage system below the clamp. See next step below.

• To determine whether the air leak is at the insertion site or inside the client:

   a. Unclamp the tube and palpate gently around the insertion site. If the bubbling stops, the leak is at the insertion site. To remedy this situation, apply a petrolatum gauze and a 4 × 4 gauze around the insertion site, and secure these dressings with adhesive tape.

   b. If the leak is not at the insertion site, it is inside the client and may indicate a dislodged tube or a new pneumothorax, a new disruption of the pleural space.

►

▶ **Technique 34–1 Monitoring Chest Drainage** CONTINUED

In this instance, leave the tube unclamped, notify the physician, and monitor the client for signs of respiratory distress.

• To locate an air leak below the chest tube clamp,

a. Move the clamp a few inches farther down and keep moving it downward a few inches at a time. Each time the clamp is moved, check the water-seal collection chamber for bubbling. The bubbling will stop as soon as the clamp is placed between the air leak and the water-seal drainage.

b. Seal the leak when you locate it by applying tape to that portion of the drainage tube.

c. If bubbling continues after the entire length of the tube is clamped, the air leak is in the drainage device. To remedy this situation, replace the drainage system according to agency protocol.

8. Take a specimen of the chest drainage as required.

• Specimens of chest drainage may be taken from a disposable chest drainage system because these systems are equipped with self-sealing ports. If a specimen is required,

a. Use a povidone-iodine swab to wipe the self-sealing diaphragm on the back of the drainage collection chamber. Allow it to dry.

b. Attach a sterile #18 or #20 gauge needle to a 3- or 5-ml

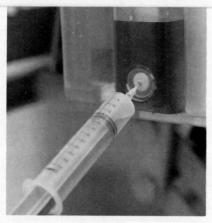

FIGURE 34–10 Obtaining a specimen through a self-sealing port.

syringe, and insert the needle into the diaphragm (Figure 34–10).

c. Aspirate the specimen (discard the needle in the appropriate container), label the syringe, and send it to the laboratory with the appropriate requisition form.

9. Ensure essential client care.

• Encourage deep-breathing and coughing exercises every 2 hours if indicated (this may be contraindicated in clients with a lobectomy). Have the client sit upright to perform the exercises, and splint the tube insertion site with a pillow or with a hand to minimize discomfort. *Deep breathing and coughing help remove accumulations from the pleural space, facilitate drainage, and help the lung to reexpand.*

• While the client takes deep breaths, palpate the chest for thoracic expansion. Place your hands together at the base of the sternum so that your thumbs meet. As the client inhales, your thumbs should separate at least

2.5 to 5 cm (1 to 2 in). Note whether chest expansion is symmetric.

• Reposition the client every 2 hours. When the client is lying on the affected side, place rolled towels beside the tubing. *Frequent position changes promote drainage, prevent complications, and provide comfort. Rolled towels prevent occlusion of the chest tube by the client's weight.*

• Assist the client with range-of-motion exercises of the affected shoulder three times per day to maintain joint mobility.

• When transporting and ambulating the client:

a. Attach rubber-tipped forceps to the client's gown for emergency use.

b. Keep the water-seal unit below chest level and upright.

c. If it is necessary to clamp the tube, remove the clamp as soon as possible or in accordance with the client's condition.

d. Disconnect the drainage system from the suction apparatus before moving the client, and make sure the air vent is open.

10. Document all relevant information.

• Record patency of chest tubes; type, amount, and color of drainage; presence of fluctuations, appearance of insertion site; laboratory specimens, if any were taken; respiratory assessments; client's vital signs and level of comfort; and all other nursing care provided to the client.

▶ **Technique 34–1** *CONTINUED*

| EVALUATION FOCUS | Amount and appearance of drainage; respiratory rate and character; breath sounds, pulse, blood pressure, and body temperature; complaints of discomfort; status of chest tube insertion site; amount and appearance of insertion site drainage. |

SAMPLE RECORDING

Date	Time	Notes
8/6/93	0800	Respirations 12 and effortless. Breath sounds auscultated in all lung lobes. Chest expansion is symmetric. T-37.6, P-78, BP 126/78. 25 ml of serosanguineous chest drainage in last hour. Fluid level in water-seal chamber fluctuating with respiration. Dressing dry and intact. Chest tubes intact. ————— Holly Wilson, RN

KEY ELEMENTS OF MONITORING A CLIENT WITH CHEST DRAINAGE

- Assess the client for signs of pneumothorax.
- Keep two rubber-tipped Kelly clamps, one sterile petrolatum gauze, and an extra drainage system available for emergency situations.
- Always keep the drainage system below chest level.
- Empty drainage systems only if ordered.
- Make sure the system is airtight.

- Make sure there is fluctuation or bubbling in the appropriate bottle or chambers.
- Keep air vents open.
- Prevent tubing obstruction.
- Know what to do if the chest tube becomes disconnected or dislodged or if the drainage system tips over.

CRITICAL THINKING CHALLENGE

Following a lobectomy, Thomas Evans has two chest tubes in place: one in the upper anterior chest, the other in the lower lateral chest. You notice the lower tube is not draining. What is the purpose of each chest tube? What specific assessments should you make for each tube? How can you facilitate drainage from each tube? Why might the lower tube not be draining?

RELATED RESEARCH

Gitt, A. G.; Bolgiano, C. S.; and Cunningham, J. March 1991. Sensations during chest tube removal. *Heart and Lung* 20:131–37.

REFERENCES

Carroll, P. F. December 1986. The ins and outs of chest drainage systems. *Nursing 86* 16:26–34.

Knauss, P. J. December 1985. Chest tube stripping: Is it necessary? *Focus on Critical Care* 12:41–43.

Miller, K. S. February 1987. Chest tubes: Indications, techniques, management and complications. *Chest* 91:258–64.

Palau, D., and Jones, S. October 1986. Test your skill at trouble shooting chest tubes. *RN* 49:43–45.

Quinn, A. September 1986. Thora-Drain III: Closed chest drainage made simpler and safer. *Nursing 86* 16:46–51.

35

Oral and Topical Medications

OBJECTIVES

- Identify essential assessment data before administering oral and topical medications

- Identify various types of drug preparations

- Describe essential legal aspects of medication administration

- Identify clients' rights in relation to medications

- Describe ten common routes of drug administration

- Identify four common medication orders

- Identify essential parts of a drug order

- Compare three systems of drug measurement

- Identify essential guidelines in preparing, administering, and documenting medications and in evaluating the client's response

- Administer oral and topical medications accurately

- Perform eye, ear, nose, vaginal, and rectal instillations safely

- Perform eye, ear, and vaginal irrigations safely

- Assist clients with metered dose nebulizers

CONTENTS

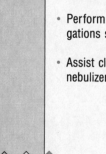

NURSING PROCESS GUIDE

ORAL AND TOPICAL MEDICATIONS

ASSESSMENT

All Medications
Determine

- The client's diagnosis.

- The client's medication history. Include prescription drugs, over-the-counter drugs (e.g., antacids, alcohol, and tobacco), and nonsanctioned drugs (e.g., marijuana). Sometimes one or more of these drugs may affect the choice of another, different medication, because they may be incompatible.

- The client's allergies to medications.

- Specific drug action.

- Signs and symptoms of side-effects or adverse reactions.

- The client's age and developmental stage.

- Any problems in self-administering a medication (e.g., poor eyesight, unsteady hands).

- The client's ability to understand and follow verbal instructions.

- The client's ability to cooperate during administration of instillations and irrigations.

- The client's knowledge of and learning needs about medications.

Oral Medications
Determine

- The client's ability to take oral medications (e.g., pres-

ence of swallow reflex, state of consciousness, presence of nausea or vomiting, uncooperative behavior).

Sublingual Medications

- Assess the status of tissues underneath the tongue. The presence of excoriation or pain contraindicates the use of this route.

Topical Medications

- Inspect skin or mucous membrane areas for lesions, rashes, erythema, and breakdown. Note size, color, distribution, and configuration of lesions (see Chapter 11, pages 209 and 210).

- Determine the presence of symptoms of skin irritation (e.g., pruritus, burning sensation, pain).

- Note the presence of excessive body hair that may require removal before the application of a topical medication.

- For *instillations and irrigations*, observe the condition of the structure receiving the medication and the status of surrounding tissues, and determine the presence of itching, burning, or pain.

- See also the Assessment Focus in each technique.

RELATED DIAGNOSTIC CATEGORIES

Diagnoses relate to the client's health status; e.g., a client receiving aminophylline for difficult breathing may have a nursing diagnosis of **Ineffective breathing pattern**.

PLANNING

Client goals and outcome criteria relate to the stated nursing diagnosis. Using the example above, refer to client goals and outcome criteria for **Ineffective breathing pattern**, pages 737–738.

Types of Medications

A **medication** is a substance administered for the diagnosis, cure, treatment, mitigation (relief), or prevention of disease. In the health care context, the words *medication* and *drug* are generally used interchangeably. The term **drug** also has the connotation of an illicitly obtained substance such as heroin, cocaine, or amphetamines. The written direction for the preparation and administration of a drug is called a **prescription**.

Medications are often available in a variety of

forms. Common types of drug preparations are described in Table 35–1 on page 824.

Legal Aspects of Medication Administration

Dispensing medications is the responsibility of pharmacists. The pharmacist may dispense directly to the client or to a person who will administer the drug. In some agencies, a senior nurse may be delegated the responsibility of dispensing drugs in the absence of

TABLE 35–1 TYPES OF DRUG PREPARATIONS

Type	Description	Type	Description
Aqueous solution	One or more drugs dissolved in water	Ointment	A semisolid preparation of one or more drugs used for application to the skin and mucous membrane
Aerosol spray or foam	A liquid, powder, or foam deposited in a thin layer on the skin by air pressure	Paste	A preparation like an ointment, but thicker and stiffer, that penetrates the skin less than ointment
Aqueous suspension	One or more drugs finely divided in a liquid such as water	Pill	One or more drugs mixed with a cohesive material, in oval, round, or flattened shapes
Capsule	A gelatinous container to hold a drug in powder, liquid, or oil form	Powder	A finely ground drug or drugs; some are used internally, others externally
Cream	A nongreasy, semisolid preparation used on the skin	Spirit	A concentrated alcoholic solution of a volatile substance
Elixir	A sweetened and aromatic solution of alcohol used as a vehicle for medicinal agents	Suppository	One or several drugs mixed with a firm base such as gelatin and shaped for insertion into the body; the base dissolves gradually at body temperature, releasing the drug
Extract	A concentrated form of a drug made from vegetables or animals		
Fluid extract	An alcoholic solution of a drug from a vegetable source; the most concentrated of all fluid preparations	Syrup	An aqueous solution of sugar often used to disguise unpleasant-tasting drugs
Gel or jelly	A clear or translucent semisolid that liquefies when applied to the skin	Tablet	A powdered drug compressed into a hard small disc; some are readily broken along a scored line; others are enteric-coated to prevent them from dissolving in the stomach
Liniment	An oily liquid used on the skin		
Lotion	An emollient liquid that may be a clear solution, suspension, or emulsion used on the skin		
Lozenge (troche)	A flat, round, or oval preparation that dissolves and releases a drug when held in the mouth	Tincture	An alcoholic or water-and-alcohol solution prepared from drugs derived from plants

a pharmacist, e.g., on the night shift or on a holiday. Each state has its own laws governing nursing practice.

In most agencies, graduate nurses are permitted to administer all types of medications (oral, topical, and parenteral), unless the unit-dose system is used and pharmacy personnel are delegated this function. Agency protocol determines who is permitted to administer intravenous medications; agency policies vary. Nurse practice acts also vary from state to state, especially in regard to the scope of practice for licensed practical nurses, specifically in regard to the administration of intravenous medications.

Nurses need to (a) know how nursing practice acts in their areas define and limit their functions and (b) be able to recognize the limits of their own knowledge and skill. To function beyond the limits of nursing practice acts or one's ability is to endanger client's lives and leave oneself open to malpractice suits. Under the law, nurses are responsible for their own actions, regardless of whether there is a written order. If a physician writes an incorrect order (e.g., Demerol 500 mg instead of Demerol 50 mg), a nurse who administers the written incorrect dosage is responsible for the error. Therefore, nurses should question any order that appears unreasonable and

refuse to give the medication until the order is clarified.

Another aspect of nursing practice governed by law is the use of narcotics and barbiturates. In hospitals, narcotics and, often, barbiturates are kept under double lock in a drawer or cupboard. Agencies have special forms for recording narcotics. The information required usually includes the name of the client, date and time of administration, name of the drug, dosage, and signature of the person who prepared and gave the narcotic. The name of the physician who ordered the narcotic may also be part of the record.

Clients' rights relating to medications are shown in the box on page 825.

Routes of Administration

Pharmaceutical preparations are generally designed for one or two specific routes of administration. See Table 35–2 on page 826. The route of administration should be indicated when the drug is ordered. When administering a drug, the nurse should ensure that the pharmaceutical preparation is appropriate for the route specified.

Client's Rights According to the Patient's Bill of Rights

- To be informed of the drug's name, purpose, action, and any possible adverse side-effects
- To refuse any medication
- To have a qualified person, i.e., nurse or physician, assess your medication history, including allergies
- To have complete information about the experimental use of any drug and to refuse or consent to its use
- To receive labeled medications safely
- To receive appropriate therapy adjunctive to the drug therapy
- Not to be given unnecessary medications

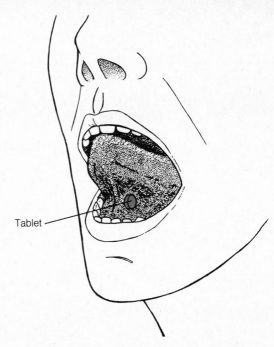

Tablet

FIGURE 35–1 Sublingual administration of a tablet.

Oral Oral administration is the most common, least expensive, and most convenient route for most clients. Because the skin is not broken as it is for an injection, oral administration is also a relatively safe method.

The major disadvantages are possible unpleasant taste of the drugs, possibility of choking or aspiration (especially if the client is confused or unconscious), irritation of the gastric mucosa, irregular absorption from the gastrointestinal tract, slow absorption, and, in some cases, harm to the client's teeth. For example, hydrochloric acid can damage the enamel of teeth. Oral medications are contraindicated for unconscious clients and those whose absorption from the gastrointestinal tract is poor (e.g., those with malabsorption syndrome or diarrhea).

Sublingual A drug may be placed under the tongue (**sublingual** administration), where it dissolves (Figure 35–1). In a relatively short time, the drug is largely absorbed into the blood vessels on the underside of the tongue. The medication should not be swallowed. Drugs such as nitroglycerin may be given in this manner.

Buccal Buccal means "pertaining to the cheek." In buccal administration, a medication (e.g., a tablet) is held in the mouth against the mucous membranes of the cheek until the drug dissolves. The drug may act locally on the mucous membranes of the mouth or systemically when it is swallowed in the saliva.

Parenteral Parenteral administration is administration other than through the alimentary tract, i.e., by needle. Some of the more common routes for parenteral administration are **subcutaneous**, or **hypodermic** (into the subcutaneous tissue, just below the skin); **intramuscular** (into a muscle); **intradermal** (under the epidermis, i.e., into the dermis); and **intravenous** (into a vein).

Some of the less commonly used routes for parenteral administration are **intra-arterial** (into an artery), **intra-cardiac** (into the heart muscle), **intraosseous** (into a bone), and **intrathecal** or **intraspinal** (into the spinal canal). These less common injections are normally administered by physicians. Sterile equipment and sterile drug solution are essential for all parenteral therapy. The main advantage is fast absorption. See Chapter 36.

Topical Topical applications are those applied to a circumscribed surface area of the body. They affect only the area to which they are applied. Topical applications include

- *Dermatologic preparations*—applied to the skin.
- *Instillations and irrigations*—applied into body cavities or orifices such as the urinary bladder, eyes, ears, nose, rectum, or vagina.
- *Inhalations*—administered into the respiratory tract by inhalers, nebulizers, or positive pressure breathing apparatuses. Air, oxygen, and vapor are generally used to carry the drug into the lungs.

Transdermal Transdermal medication systems are being used increasingly to administer sustained-action medications (e.g., nitroglycerine, estrogen, scopalamine, and nicotine). These systems consist of multilayered rectangular or circular films containing the drug. The layers usually include:

TABLE 35–2 ROUTES OF ADMINISTRATION

Route	Advantages	Disadvantages
Oral	Most convenient	Inappropriate for clients nauseated or vomiting
	Usually least expensive	Drug may have unpleasant taste or odor
	Safe, does not break the skin barrier	Inappropriate when gastrointestinal tract has reduced motility
	Administration usually does not cause stress	Inappropriate when client cannot swallow or is unconscious
		Cannot be used before certain diagnostic tests or surgical procedures
		Drug may discolor teeth, harm tooth enamel
		Drug may irritate gastric mucosa
		Drug can be aspirated by seriously ill clients
		Compliance may become a problem if the medication is self-administered
Sublingual	Same as for oral, *plus:*	If swallowed, drug may be inactivated by gastric juice
	Drug can be administered for local effect	Drug must remain under tongue until dissolved and absorbed
	Drug is rapidly absorbed into the bloodstream	
	Ensures greater potency because drug directly enters the blood and bypasses the liver	
Buccal	Same as for sublingual	Same as for sublingual
Rectal	Can be used when drug has objectionable taste or odor or when the client is unconscious or vomiting	Dose absorbed is unpredictable
	Drug released at slow, steady rate	
Skin	Provides a local effect	May be messy and may soil clothes
	Few side-effects	Drug can rapidly enter body through abrasions and cause systemic effects
Transdermal	Convenient application	May cause skin redness, irritation, and hypersensitivity
	Drug released at controlled rate	
Subcutaneous	Onset of drug action faster than oral	Must involve sterile technique because breaks skin barrier
		More expensive than oral
		Can administer only small volume
		Slower than intramuscular administration
		Some drugs can irritate tissues and cause pain
		Can be anxiety-producing
Intramuscular	Pain from irritating drugs is minimized	Breaks skin barrier
	Can administer larger volume than by subcutaneous route	Can be anxiety-producing
	Drug is rapidly absorbed	
Intradermal	Absorption is slow (this is an advantage when testing for allergies)	Amount of drug administered must be small
		Breaks skin barrier
Intravenous	Rapid effect	Limited to highly soluble drugs
		Drug distribution may be inhibited by poor circulation
Inhalation	Introduces drug throughout the respiratory tract	Drug intended for localized effect can have systemic effect
	Rapid localized relief	Only of use for the respiratory system
	Drug can be administered when client is unconscious	

1. A backing layer of polyester film

2. The drug reservoir

3. A microporous membrane that controls the rate of delivery of the drug from the system to the skin surface

4. An adhesive layer

5. A protective peel strip that covers the adhesive layer and which must be removed before application

The rate of delivery of the drug or systemic absorption is controlled and varies with each product. For example, Nitroderm (nitroglycerine), used for the treatment of acute episodes of angina pectoris, is usually applied once daily and left on for 12 to 14 hours and then removed. Transderm-V (scopalamine), an antiemetic, is designed to deliver the drug over a 3-day period. Estraderm (estrogen) is applied twice weekly.

When administering transdermal patches, the nurse and/or client must follow the manufacturer's instructions provided with each product. Generally, the patch is applied to a hairless, clean area of skin that is not subject to excessive movement or wrinkling (i.e., the trunk or lower abdomen). It may also be applied on the side, lower back, or buttocks. Scopalamine, however, is applied to an area of intact skin behind the ear. Patches should not be applied to areas with cuts, burns, or abrasions, or on distal parts of extremities (e.g., the forearms). If hair is likely to interfere with patch adhesion or removal, clipping may be necessary before application.

Just before application, the nurse or client should wash and dry the hands thoroughly. Upon removal, the system should be discarded and the hands and application site washed well to remove residual traces of the drug. Scopalamine, for example, may cause temporary dilation of the pupils if it comes into direct contact with the eyes.

Reddening of the skin with or without mild local itching or burning, as well as allergic contact dermatitis, may occasionally occur. Upon removal of the patch, any slight reddening of the skin usually disappears within a few hours. All applications should be changed regularly to prevent local irritation, and each successive application should be placed on a different site. All clients need to be assessed for allergies to the drug and to materials in the patch before the patch is applied.

Medication Orders

A physician usually determines the clients' medications needs and orders medications, although in some settings nurse practitioners now order some drugs and, in some settings (such as emergency and intensive care units), nurses may follow drug protocols for given medical conditions until the physician is contacted. Usually, the order is written, although telephone and verbal orders are acceptable in a number of agencies. Nursing students need to know the agency policies about medication orders. In some hospitals, for example, only licensed nurses are permitted to accept telephone and verbal orders.

Policies about physicians' orders may vary considerably from agency to agency. For example, a client's orders are frequently automatically canceled after surgery or an examination involving an anesthetic agent. New orders must then be written. Most agencies also have lists of abbreviations officially accepted for use in the agency. Both nurses and physicians may need to refer to these lists if they have been working in a different agency. These abbreviations can be used on legal documents, such as clients' charts. See Table 35–3 on page 828.

Types of Medication Orders

Four common medication orders are the stat order, the single order, the standing order, and the prn order:

1. A **stat order** indicates that the medication is to be given immediately and only once, e.g., Demerol 100 mg IM stat.

2. The **single order** is for a medication to be given once at a specified time, e.g., Seconal 100 mg hs before surgery.

3. The **standing order** may or may not have a termination date. A standing order may be carried out indefinitely (e.g., multiple vitamins daily) until an order is written to cancel it, or it may be carried out for a specified number of days (e.g., Demerol 100 mg IM q4h × 5 days). In some agencies, standing orders are automatically canceled after a specified number of days and must be reordered.

4. A **prn order** permits the nurse to give a medication when, in the nurse's judgment, the client requires it, e.g., Amphojel 15 ml prn. The nurse must use good judgment about when the medication is needed and when it can be safely administered.

Essential Parts of a Drug Order

The drug order has six essential parts, and unless it is a standing order, it should state the number of doses or the number of days the drug is to be administered.

The *client's full name*, that is, the first and last names and middle initials or names, should always be used to avoid confusion between two clients who have the same last names. In some agencies, the

TABLE 35-3 COMMON ABBREVIATIONS USED IN MEDICATION ORDERS

Abbreviation	Explanation	Example of Administration Time	Abbreviation	Explanation	Example of Administration Time
ac	before meals	0700, 1100, and 1700 hrs	qAM (om)	every morning	1000 hours
ad lib	freely, as desired		qh (q1h)	every hour	
agit	shake, stir		q2h	every 2 hours	0800, 1000, 1200 hours, and so on
aq	water		q3h	every 3 hours	0900, 1200, 1500 hours, and so on
aq dest	distilled water		q4h	every 4 hours	1000, 1400, 1800 hours, and so on
bid	twice a day	0900 and 2100 hours	q6h	every 6 hours	0600, 1200, 1800, 2400 hours
c̄	with		qhs	every night at bedtime	
cap	capsule		qid	four times a day	1000, 1400, 1800, 2200 hours
comp	compound				
dil	dissolve, dilute		qod	every other day	0900 hours on odd dates
elix	elixir				
h	an hour		qs	sufficient quantity	
hs	at bedtime		rept	may be repeated	
IM	intramuscular		Rx	take	
IV	intravenous		s̄	without	
M or m	mix		sc	subcutaneous	
no.	number		Sig or S	label	
non rep	do not repeat		sos	if it is needed	
OD	right eye		ss or s̄s̄	one half	
OS or ol	left eye		stat	at once	
OU	both eyes		sup or supp	suppository	
pc	after meals	0900, 1300, and 1900 hours	susp	suspension	
po	by mouth		tid	three times a day	1000, 1400, and 1800 hours
prn	when needed				
q	every		Tr or tinct	tincture	

client's admission number is put on the order as further identification. Some hospitals imprint the client's name and hospital number on all forms. This imprinter is on the nursing unit; it is much like the credit card imprinters used in shops.

In addition to *the day, the month, and the year* the order was written, some agencies also require that the *time of day* be written. Writing the time of day on the order can eliminate errors when nursing shifts change and makes clear when certain orders automatically terminate. For example, in some settings, narcotics can be ordered only for 48 hours after surgery. Therefore, a drug that is ordered at 1600 hours February 1, 1993 is automatically canceled at 1600 hours February 3, 1993. Many health agencies use the 24-hour clock, which eliminates confusion between morning and afternoon times. Time with the 24-hour clock starts at midnight, which is 0000 hours. See Figure 3–10, page 57.

The *name of the drug* to be administered must be clearly written. In some settings, only generic names are permitted; however, trade names are widely used in hospitals and health agencies.

The *dosage of the drug* includes the amount, the times or frequency of administration, and in many instances the strength; for example, tetracycline *250 mg* (the amount) *four times a day* (frequency); *sodium sulfacetamide 10%* (strength) *1 or 2 drops* into lower conjunctival sac (amount) *every two or three hours during the day and less frequently at night* (time and frequency). Dosages can be written in apothecaries' or metric systems.

Also included in the order is the *method of administering* the drug. This part of the order, like other parts, is frequently abbreviated. See Table 35–3 for abbreviations of routes of administration. Nurses must familiarize themselves with the list of accepted abbreviations approved by the agency in which they are employed.

It is not unusual for a drug to have several possible routes of administration; therefore, it is important that the *route* be included in the order.

The *signature* of the ordering physician or nurse makes the drug order a legal request. An unsigned order has no validity, and the ordering physician or nurse needs to be notified if the order is unsigned.

In agencies where telephone orders are taken, the nurse usually indicates the name of the person who phoned in the order. The nurse signs the order, but usually the person who ordered the drug must also sign at a later date. Some hospitals have policies that those who give orders by telephone must sign those orders within a certain time, for example, 48 hours after they have communicated the order.

When a physician writes a prescription for a client, the prescription also includes information for the pharmacist. Therefore, a prescription's content differs from that of a medication order in a hospital.

Systems of Measurement

Three systems of measurement are used in North America: the metric system, the apothecaries' system, and the household system, which is similar to the apothecaries' system.

Metric System

The metric system, devised by the French in the latter part of the 18th century, is the system prescribed by law in most European countries and in Canada. The metric system is logically organized into units of ten; it is a decimal system. Basic units can be multiplied or divided by ten to form secondary units. Multiples are calculated by moving the decimal point to the right, and divisions by moving the decimal point to the left.

Basic units of measurement are the meter, the liter, and the gram. Prefixes derived from Latin designate subdivisions of the basic unit: deci (1/10 or 0.1), centi (1/100 or 0.01), and milli (1/1000 or 0.001). Multiples of the basic unit are designated by prefixes derived from Greek: deka (10), hecto (100), and kilo (1000). Only the measurements of volume (the liter) and of weight (the gram) are discussed in this chap-

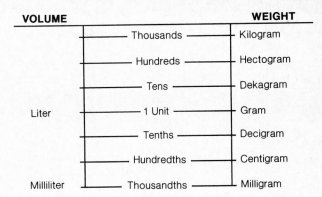

FIGURE 35–2 Basic metric measurements of volume and weight.

ter. These are the measures used in medication administration. See Figure 35–2. In nursing practice, the kilogram (kg) is the only multiple of the gram used, and the milligram (mg) and microgram (mcg or μg) are subdivisions. Fractional parts of the liter are usually expressed in milliliters (ml), for example, 600 ml; multiples of the liter are usually expressed as liters or milliliters, for example, 2.5 liters or 2500 ml. Another volume measurement frequently used in practice is the cubic centimeter (cc). It is equivalent to one milliliter.

Apothecaries' System

The apothecaries' system, older than the metric system, was brought to the United States from England during the colonial period. The basic unit of weight in the apothecaries' system is the *grain*, likened to a grain of wheat, and the basic unit of volume is the **minim**, a volume of water equal in weight to a grain of wheat. The word *minim* means "the least." In ascending order, the other units of weight are the *scruple*, the *dram*, the *ounce*, and the *pound*. Today, the scruple (scr) is seldom used. The units of volume are, in ascending order, the *fluid dram*, the *fluid ounce*, the *pint*, the *quart*, and the *gallon*.

Quantities in the apothecaries' system are often expressed by lowercase Roman numerals, particularly when the unit of measure is abbreviated. The Roman numeral follows rather than precedes the unit of measure. For example, a fluid ounce is abbreviated as f℥. Two fluid ounces are written as f℥ii, and 4 fluid ounces are written as f℥iv. One half fluid ounce is written as f℥ss, and 1½ fluid ounces as f℥iss. See Table 3–2, page 59.

Household System

Household measures may be used when more accurate systems of measure are not required. Included in household measures are drops, teaspoons, tablespoons, cups, and glasses. Although pints and quarts are often found in the home, they are defined as apothecaries' measures. Equivalent units of the household system are in Appendix B.

Converting Units of Weight and Measure

Sometimes drugs are dispensed from the pharmacy in grams when the order specifies milligrams, or they are dispensed in milligrams though ordered in grains. The nurse preparing a medicated irrigation may find that the order calls for quarts and that the solution is dispensed in liter containers. In all situations, it is the nurse's responsibility to convert units of measure or weight; and nurses must therefore be aware of approximate equivalents within each system of measurement and among systems. See Tables 35–4 and 35–5. The nurse may also consult with the agency pharmacist, a valuable source of information regarding appropriate conversions.

Administering Medications Safely

The nurse should always assess a client's physical status prior to giving any medication. The extent of the assessment depends on the client's illness or current condition and the intended drug action and route of administration. For example, the nurse assesses a dyspneic client's respirations carefully before administering any medications that might affect breathing. In general, the nurse assesses the client *prior* to administering any medication to obtain baseline data by which to evaluate the effectiveness of the medication. Clinical guidelines for administering medications are given in the accompanying box.

CLINICAL GUIDELINES

Administering Medications

- Nurses who administer medications are responsible for their own actions. Question any order that you consider incorrect.
- Be knowledgeable about the medications you administer.
- Federal laws govern the uses of narcotics and barbiturates. Keep these medications in a locked place.
- Use only medications that are in a clearly labeled container.
- Return to the pharmacy liquid medications that are cloudy or have changed color.
- Before administering a medication, identify the client correctly using the appropriate means of identification, e.g., identification bracelet and/or asking clients to state their names.
- Do not leave a medication at the bedside, with certain exceptions, e.g., nitroglycerin, cough syrup. Determine agency policy.
- If a client vomits after taking an oral medication, report this to the nurse in charge.
- Take special precautions when administering certain medications; for example, have another nurse check the dosages of anticoagulants, insulin, and certain IV preparations.
- Most hospitals require new orders from the physician for the client's postsurgery care.
- When a medication is omitted for any reason, record the fact together with the reason.
- When a medication error is made, report it immediately to the nurse in charge.

TABLE 35–4 APPROXIMATE VOLUME EQUIVALENTS: METRIC, APOTHECARIES', AND HOUSEHOLD SYSTEMS

Metric	Apothecaries'	Household
1 ml	= 15 minims (min or m)	= 15 drops (gtt)
15 ml	= 4 fluid drams (f3)	= 1 tablespoon (Tbsp)
30 ml	= 1 fluid ounce (f3)	= same
500 ml	= 1 pint (pt)	= same
1000 ml	= 1 quart (qt)	= same
4000 ml	= 1 gallon (gal)	= same

TABLE 35–5 APPROXIMATE WEIGHT EQUIVALENTS: METRIC AND APOTHECARIES' SYSTEMS

Metric		Apothecaries'
1 mg	=	1/60 grain
60 mg	=	1 grain
1 g	=	15 grains
4 g	=	1 dram
30 g	=	1 ounce
500 g	=	1.1 pound (lb)
1000 g (1 kg)	=	2.2 lb

When administering any drug, regardless of the route of administration, the nurse must do the following.

1. *Identify the client.* Errors can and do occur, usually because one client gets a drug intended for another. In hospitals, most clients wear some sort of identification, such as a wristband with name and hospital identification number. Before giving the client any drug, the nurse should check the identification band with the medication card or medication administration record (MAR). As a double check, nurses also ask the client's name or ask another nurse to identify the client before administering any medication.

2. *Administer the drug.* Medication orders and cards or lists need to be read carefully and checked against the name on the medication envelope or, if a medication cart is used, on the drawer in which the client's medications are kept. The medication is then administered in the prescribed dosage, by the route ordered, at the correct time.

3. *Provide adjunctive interventions as indicated.* Clients may need help when receiving medications. They may require physical assistance, for instance, in assuming positions for intramuscular injections, or they may need explanations about the medications and guidance about measures to enhance drug effectiveness and prevent complications, e.g., drinking fluids. Some clients convey fear about their medications. The nurse can allay fears by listening carefully to clients' concerns and giving correct information.

4. *Record the drug administered.* The facts recorded in the chart—in ink or by computer printout—are the name of the drug, dosage, method of administration, specific relevant data such as pulse rate (taken in most settings prior to the administration of digitalis), and any other pertinent information. The record should also include the exact time of administration and the signature of the nurse providing the medication. Many medication records are designed so that the nurse signs once on the page and initials each medication administered. Often, medications that are given regularly are recorded on a special flow record, and prn or stat medications are recorded separately.

5. *Evaluate the client's response to the drug.* The kinds of behavior that reflect the action or lack of action of a drug and its untoward effects (both minor and major) are as variable as the purposes of the drugs themselves. The anxious client may show the desired effects of a tranquilizer by behavior that reflects a lowered stress level (e.g., slower speech or fewer random movements). The effectiveness of a

---

Drug Administration: Five "Rights"

- Right drug
- Right dose
- Right time
- Right route
- Right client

---

sedative can often be measured by how well a client slept; the effectiveness of an antispasmodic, by how much pain the client feels. In all nursing activities, nurses need to be aware of the medications that a client is taking and record their effectivness as assessed by the client and the nurse on the client's chart. The nurse may also report the client's response directly to the senior nurse and physician.

See the box above for the five "rights" to accurate drug administration. In addition to adhering to these five "rights," the nurse should also be aware of clients' rights regarding medications. These are shown on page 825.

Developmental Considerations Related to Medications

Knowledge of growth and development is essential for the nurse administering medications to children. Oral medications for children are usually prepared in sweetened liquid form to make them more palatable. The parents may provide suggestions about what method is best for their child. Necessary foods, such as milk or orange juice, should not be used to mask the taste of medications, because the child may develop unpleasant associations and refuse that food in the future.

Children are often apprehensive about medication administration. Allowing the child to participate, as much as possible, in decision making, e.g., type of fluid to drink with the medication, may increase cooperation. Never refer to medication as "candy." The child may be tempted at home to surreptitiously take the medication and overdose.

Children tend to fear any procedure in which a needle is used because they anticipate pain or because the procedure is unfamiliar and threatening. The nurse needs to acknowledge that the child will feel some pain; denying this fact only deepens the child's distrust. After the injection, the nurse (or the

Physiologic Changes Associated with Aging that Influence Medications

- Altered memory
- Less acute vision
- Decrease in renal function resulting in slower elimination of drugs and higher drug concentrations in the bloodstream for longer periods
- Less complete and slower absorption from the gastrointestinal tract
- Increased proportion of fat to lean body mass, which facilitates retention of fat-soluble drugs and increases potential for toxicity
- Decreased liver function, which hinders biotransformation of drugs
- Decreased organ sensitivity, which means that the response to the same drug concentration in the vicinity of the target organ is less in older people than in the young
- Altered quality of organ responsiveness, resulting in adverse effects becoming pronounced before therapeutic effects are achieved

parent) can cuddle and speak softly to the infant and give the child a toy to dispel the child's association of the nurse only with pain. Holding and cuddling the child after medication administration helps reestablish a sense of security, calm, and trust.

The older person can present special problems, most of which are related to physiologic changes, to past experiences, and to established attitudes toward medications. The physiologic changes in elderly persons that may affect the administration and effectiveness of medications are included in the box above.

Many of these changes enhance the possibility of cumulative effects and toxicity. For example, impaired circulation delays the action of medications given intramuscularly or subcutaneously. Digitalis, which is frequently taken by elderly people, can accumulate to toxic levels and be lethal. It is not uncommon for elderly clients to take several different medications daily. The possibility of error increases with the number of medications taken, whether self-administered at home or administered by nurses in a hospital. The greater number of medications also compounds the problem of drug interactions, because much is yet to be learned about the effects of drugs given in combinations. A general rule to follow is that elderly clients should take as few med- ications as possible.

Elderly persons usually require smaller dosages of drugs, especially sedatives and other central nervous system depressants. Reactions of the elderly to medications, particularly sedatives, are unpredictable and often bizarre. It is not uncommon to see irritability, confusion, disorientation, restlessness, and incontinence as a result of sedatives. Nurses therefore need to observe clients carefully for untoward reactions. The use of alcohol (e.g., brandy) as a bedtime relaxant and as an appetizer before meals is becoming more common. The moderate use of alcohol by people who are accustomed to it can contribute to a sense of well-being. Some medications, however, may have adverse effects when administered with alcohol (e.g., central nervous system depressants and some cephalosporins).

Attitudes of elderly people toward medical care and medications vary. Elderly people tend to believe in the wisdom of the physician more readily than younger people. Some older people are bewildered by the prescription of several medications and may passively accept their medications from nurses but not swallow them, spitting out tablets or capsules after the nurse leaves the room. For this reason, the nurse is advised to stay with clients until they have taken the medications. Others may be suspicious of medications and actively refuse them.

Elderly people are mature adults capable of reasoning. Therefore, the nurse needs to explain the reasons for and effects of medications. This education can prevent clients from taking a medication long after there is a need for it or discontinuing a drug too quickly. For example, clients should know that diuretics will cause them to urinate more frequently and may reduce ankle edema. Instructions about medications need to be given to all clients prior to discharge from a hospital. These instructions should include when to take the drugs, what effects to expect, and when to consult a physician.

Because some clients are required to take several medications daily and because visual acuity and memory may be impaired, the nurse needs to develop simple, realistic plans for clients to follow at home. For example, remembering to take drugs can be difficult for most persons, including the elderly. If medications are scheduled to be taken with meals or at bedtime, clients are not as likely to forget. Some clients may take their medications and then an hour later not remember whether they took them. One solution to forgetfulness is to use a special container or glass strictly for medications. An empty glass or container indicates that the person took the pills. Loss of visual acuity presents problems that can be overcome by writing out the plan in block letters large enough to be read. In some situations, the nurse can enlist the help of a spouse, son, daughter, or home health care nurse.

Oral Medications

The oral route is the most common route by which medications are given. As long as a client can swallow and retain the drug in the stomach, this is the route of choice if the medication is dispensed in tablet or capsular form and if a local effect on the gastrointestinal tract or a systemic effect is desired. See Technique 35–1. Oral medications are contraindicated when a client is vomiting, has gastric or intestinal suction, or is unconscious and unable to swallow. Such clients in a hospital usually are on orders "nothing by mouth" (NPO).

Whenever possible, the oral route is preferred for administering medications to infants and children because of the ease of administration and because most are dissolved or suspended in liquid preparations. Solid preparations are not recommended for children under 5 years of age because of the danger of aspiration, especially if their administration causes marked resistance or crying. Many pediatric medications are supplied in palatable, colorful preparations that most children will swallow with little or no resistance. To accurately describe the taste of a medication to children, nurses are advised to first taste the medication themselves. Drugs that are not available in pediatric preparations need to be crushed with a pill crusher or between two spoons and then mixed with a palatable substance for the child to swallow.

Vehicles to accurately measure and administer medications to children differ from those used for the adult because of the small amounts required. Often many liquid preparations are prescribed in teaspoon measurements but because household teaspoons vary considerably in capacity, the milliliter is a more accurate measurement. One teaspoon is considered by most to be equivalent to 5 ml. The most accurate means for measuring small amounts of medication required for pediatric clients is the syringe, and for volumes less than 1 ml, a tuberculin syringe.

Some facilities use less expensive nonsterile oral syringes for this purpose. Because the medication is administered directly from the syringe, only *plastic* syringes that cannot be broken and cause injury are used. A short length of flexible tubing may be placed on the tip of the syringe for added safety. Measuring spoons specifically made for accurate medication measurement and administration are commercially available, and many parents find these useful for home use. The standard measuring spoon may also be used.

Another convenient method for giving liquid medications to infants is to allow the infant to suck the medication from an empty nipple attached to a needleless syringe. Other methods should be used, however, for unpleasant tasting medicine so that the infant will not associate the unpleasant taste with the nipple. Medication should never be added to the infant's formula feeding for the same reason. Older children who can drink from a cup may use a medicine cup.

35-1 Administering Oral Medications

PURPOSE
- To provide a medication that has systemic effects and/or local effects on the gastrointestinal tract (see specific drug action)

ASSESSMENT FOCUS

Allergies to medication(s); client's ability to swallow the medication; presence of vomiting or diarrhea that would interfere with the ability to absorb the medication; specific drug action; side-effects and adverse reactions; client's knowledge of and learning needs about the medication.

EQUIPMENT
- Medication tray or cart
- Disposable medication cups: small paper or plastic cups for tablets and capsules, waxed or plastic calibrated medication cups for liquids
- Medication cards, medication administration record (MAR), or computer printout
- Pill crusher
  or
  Syringe of appropriate size for child's mouth and medication amount
- Straws to administer medications that may discolor the teeth or to facilitate the ingestion of liquid medication for certain clients

▶ **Technique 35–1 Administering Oral Medications** CONTINUED

INTERVENTION

1. Organize the supplies.

- Assemble the medication tray and cups in the medicine room, or place the medication cart outside the client's room.

- Plan to give medications first to clients who do not require assistance and last to those who do. Arrange the medication cards or records in this order.

- Assemble the medication cards or records for each client together so that medications can be prepared for one client at a time. *Organization of supplies saves time and reduces the chance of error.*

2. Verify the client's ability to take medication orally.

- Determine whether the client can swallow, is on NPO, is nauseated or vomiting, or has gastric suction.

3. Verify the order for accuracy.

- Check the accuracy of the medication card, MAR, or printout with the physician's written order. It should contain the following: (a) client's name, (b) drug name and dosage, (c) time for administration, and (d) route of administration.

- Check the expiration date.

- Report any discrepancies in the order to the nurse in charge or the physician, as agency policy dictates.

4. Obtain the appropriate medication.

- Read the medication card or MAR, and take the appropriate medication from the shelf, drawer, or refrigerator. The medication may be dispensed in the bottle, box, or unit dose package.

- Compare the label of the medication container or unit dose package against the order on the medication card or MAR. If these are not identical, recheck the client's chart. If there is still a discrepancy, check with the nurse in charge and/or the pharmacist.

5. Prepare the medication.

- Prepare the correct amount of medication for the required dose, without contaminating the medication. *Aseptic technique maintains drug cleanliness.*

- While preparing the medication, recheck each medication card or MAR with the prepared drug and container. *This second check reduces the chance of error.*

Tablets or Capsules from a Bottle

- Pour the required number into the bottle cap, and then transfer the medication to the disposable cup without touching the tablets (Figure 35–3). Usually, all tablets or capsules to be given to the client are placed in the same cup.

- Keep medications that require specific assessments, e.g., pulse measurements, respiratory rate or depth, or blood pressure, separate from the others. *This enables the nurse to withhold the medication if indicated.*

- If the client has difficulty swallowing, crush the tablets to a fine powder with a pill crusher or between two medication cups or spoons. Then, mix the powder with a small amount of soft food (e.g., custard, apple sauce).

Liquid Medication

- Remove the cap, and place it upside down on the countertop to avoid contaminating it.

- Hold the bottle with the label next to your palm, and pour the medication away from the label (Figure 35–4). *This prevents the label from becoming soiled and illegible as a result of spilled liquids.*

- Hold the medication cup at eye level, and fill it to the desired level, using the bottom of the **meniscus** (crescent-shaped upper surface of a column of liquid) as the measurement guide (Figure 35–5). *This method ensures accuracy of measurement.*

- Before capping the bottle, wipe the lip with a paper towel. *This prevents the cap from sticking.*

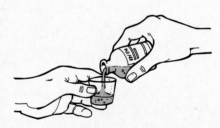

FIGURE 35–4 Pouring a liquid medication from a bottle.

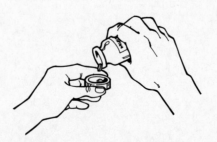

FIGURE 35–3 Pouring a tablet into the container lid.

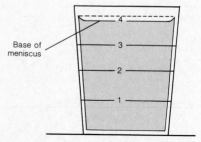

Base of meniscus

FIGURE 35–5 The bottom of the meniscus is the measuring guide.

▶ **Technique 35–1** CONTINUED

Oral Narcotics

- Check the narcotic record for the previous drug count, and compare it with the supply available. Some narcotics are kept in specially designed plastic containers that are sectioned and numbered (Figure 35–6).

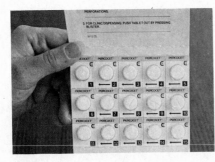

FIGURE 35–6 Commercially packaged narcotics.

- Remove the next available tablet, and drop it in the medicine cup.
- After removing a tablet, record the necessary information on the appropriate narcotic control record, and sign it.

Unit-dose Medication

- Place the *unwrapped* unit-dose medications directly into the medicine cup. *The wrapper keeps the medication clean and facilitates identification.*

All Medications

- Place the prepared medication and medication card together on the tray or cart.
- Return the bottle, box, or envelope to its storage place, and recheck the label on the container. *This third check further reduces the risk of error.*
- Avoid leaving prepared medications unattended. *Accidental disarrangement of the medication could occur.*

6. Administer the medication at the correct time.

- Identify the client by comparing the name on the medication card or list with the name on the client's identification bracelet and by asking the client to tell you his or her name. *Accurate identification is essential to prevent error.*
- Explain the purpose of the medication and how it will help, using language that the client can understand. Include relevant information about effects, e.g., tell the client receiving a diuretic to expect an increase in urine. *Information facilitates acceptance of and compliance with the therapy.*
- Assist the client to a sitting position or, if not possible, to a lateral position. *These positions facilitate swallowing and prevent aspiration.*
- Take the required assessment measures, e.g., pulse and respiratory rates or blood pressure. Take the pulse rate before administering digitalis preparations. Take blood pressure before giving hypotensive drugs. Take the respiratory rate prior to administering narcotics. *Narcotics depress the respiratory center.* If any of the findings are above or below the predetermined parameters, consult the physician before administering the medication.
- Give the client sufficient water or preferred juice to swallow the medication. *Fluids ease swallowing and facilitate absorption from the gastrointestinal tract.* Liquid medications other than antacids or cough preparations are generally diluted with 15 ml (½ oz) of water to facilitate absorption.

- If the client is unable to hold the pill cup, use the pill cup to introduce the medication into the client's mouth, and give only one tablet or capsule at a time. *Putting the cup to the client's mouth maintains the cleanliness of the nurse's hands. Giving one medication at a time eases swallowing.*
- If an older child or adult has difficulty swallowing, ask the client to place the medication on the back of the tongue before taking the water. *Stimulation of the back of the tongue produces the swallowing reflex.*
- If the medication has an objectionable taste, ask the client to suck a few ice chips beforehand, or give the medication with juice, apple sauce, or bread. *The cold will desensitize the taste buds, and juices or bread can mask the taste of the medication.*
- If the client says that the medication you are about to give is different from what the client has been receiving, do not give the medication without checking the original order. Most clients are familiar with the appearance of medications taken previously. *Unfamiliar drugs may signal a possible error.*
- Stay with the client until all medications have been swallowed. *The nurse must see the client swallow the medication before the drug administration can be recorded.* A physician's order or agency policy is required for medications left at the bedside.

7. Document each medication given.

- Record the medication given, dosage, time, any complaints or assessments of the client, and your signature.

▶ **Technique 35–1 Administering Oral Medications** CONTINUED

- If medication was refused or omitted, record this fact on the appropriate record, and document the reason when possible.

8. **Dispose of all supplies appropriately.**

- Return the medication cards or records to the appropriate file for the next administration time.

- Replenish stock, e.g., medication cups, and return cart to medicine room.

- Discard used disposable supplies.

9. **Evaluate the effects of the medication.**

- Return to the client when the medication is expected to take effect (usually 30 minutes) to evaluate the effects of the medication on the client.

▶ VARIATION: Giving Oral Medications to Infants and Children

- Select an appropriate vehicle to measure and administer the medication, i.e., plastic disposable cup, plastic syringe without needle, or tuberculin syringe (see page 833). For young infants, a plastic syringe is usually used. For older infants who can drink from a cup, a medicine cup can be used.

- Dilute the oral medication, if indicated, with a *small* amount of water. *Many oral medications are readily swallowed if they are diluted with a small amount of water. If large quantities of water are used, the child may refuse to drink the entire amount and receive only a portion of the medication.*

- Crush medications not supplied in liquid form and mix them with substances available on most pediatric units, e.g., honey, flavored syrup, jam, or a fruit puree. Note: When selecting a substance to mix with a medication, *avoid essential food items* such as milk, cereal, and orange juice. *If essential food items are used, the child may become intolerant of them and refuse these foods in their diet.*

- Disguise disagreeable tasting medications with sweet-tasting substances mentioned above. However, present any altered medication to the child honestly and not as a food or treat.

- To prevent nausea, pour a carbonated beverage over finely crushed ice and give it before or immediately after the medication is administered.

- To prevent aspiration and choking, position infants in a semi-reclining position and administer the medication slowly in divided doses by spoon or a plastic syringe.

- If using a spoon, retrieve and refeed medication that is thrust outward by the infant's tongue.

- If using a syringe, place it along the side of the infant's tongue. *This position prevents gagging and expulsion of the medication.*

- Partially restrain a child who refuses to cooperate or consistently resists despite explanation, encouragement, and attempt to determine the reason for the behavior.

  a. Place the child in your lap with the right arm behind you.

  b. Grasp the child's left hand firmly by your left hand.

  c. Secure the head between your arm and body.

- Follow all medication with a drink of water, juice, a soft drink, or a Popsicle or frozen juice bar. *This removes any unpleasant aftertaste.*

- For children who take sweetened medications on a long term basis, follow the medication administration with oral hygiene. *These children are at high risk for dental caries.*

EVALUATION FOCUS

Desired effect (e.g., relief of pain or decrease in body temperature); any adverse effects or side-effects (e.g., nausea, vomiting, skin rash, change in vital signs).

SAMPLE RECORDING

Date	Time	Notes
07/09/93	2200	Complaining of insomnia. Seconal sodium 50 mg given. ———————— Mary Markoski, SN
	2330	Client asleep with even, nonlabored respirations; rate 16. ———————— Mary Markoski, SN

▶ **Technique 35–1** *CONTINUED*

KEY ELEMENTS OF ADMINISTERING ORAL MEDICATIONS

- Know the expected action of the medication, undesirable side-effects, and signs of toxicity.
- Check the physician's order against other sources, e.g., the Kardex, medication record, or medication label.
- Confirm the correct route of administration.
- Maintain medical asepsis.
- Take required assessment measures, e.g., pulse and respiratory rates or blood pressure before administering the drug.
- Prepare and administer the correct drug and dosage to the correct client by the right route and at the right time.
- Document the administered medication according to agency protocol.

Topical Medications

Topical medications include dermatologic medications and irrigations and instillations. Irrigations may or may not be medicated.

Dermatologic preparations include lotions, liniments, ointments, pastes, and powders. See Table 35–1, earlier. Unless contraindicated by a specific order, the nurse washes and carefully dries the area, using a patting motion, before applying a dermatologic preparation. Skin encrustations and discharges harbor microorganisms and cause local infections. They can also prevent the medication from coming in contact with the area to be treated. Nurses should always use surgical asepsis when an open wound is present. If a client has lesions, the nurse must wear gloves or use tongue depressors. In this way, the nurse's hand will not come in direct contact with microorganisms in and around the lesions. See Table 35–6 for general guidelines for applying topical medications. Technique 35–2 details the steps in administering topical medications.

TABLE 35–6   TOPICAL APPLICATIONS

Medication	Application
Lotion	Shake before use to distribute suspended particles.
	Pour onto sterile gauze, and pat onto affected area.
	To avoid aggravating affected area, do not rub.
Liniment	Pour onto hands, and rub into client's skin with long, smooth strokes.
Ointment and paste	Usually applied with a tongue blade or with gloves. Some must be applied thinly over the area, e.g., cortisone. Sterile dressing may be applied over ointment. If a corticosteroid is applied, avoid using an occlusive dressing or plastic-covered diaper. Occlusive materials increase the percutaneous absorption of corticosteroids thus increasing the possibility of systemic absorption and effects.
Powder	Sprinkle over the surface and cover with a dressing.

 35-2   **Administering Dermatologic Medications**

PURPOSES
- To decrease itching (pruritus)
- To lubricate and soften the skin
- To cause local vasoconstriction or vasodilation
- To increase or decrease secretions from the skin
- To provide a protective coating to the skin
- To apply an antibiotic or antiseptic to treat or prevent infection
- To reduce inflammation
- To administer sustained-action transdermal medications (see page 827.)

ASSESSMENT FOCUS

Discomfort; pruritus; color of affected and surrounding area (e.g., redness, rash); swelling; discharge; amount of hair on affected area (excessive hair may need to be removed before the medication is applied).

▶

▶ **Technique 35–2 Administering Dermatologic Medications** *CONTINUED*

EQUIPMENT

Use sterile supplies and techniques for all open skin lesions.
- □ Gloves (disposable and sterile if required)
- □ Ordered solution to wash area as ordered
- □ 2 × 2 gauze pads for cleaning
- □ Medication container
- □ Application tube (if required)
- □ Tongue blades
- □ Gauze to cover area (if required)

INTERVENTION

1. Verify the order.

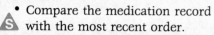

- Compare the medication record with the most recent order.

- Compare the label on the medication tube or jar with the medication record.

- Determine whether area is to be washed before applying medication.

2. Prepare the client.

- Provide privacy.

- Expose the area of the skin to be treated.

3. Prepare the area for the medication.

- Wash hands and don gloves.

- Determine that the body part to be treated is clean; if not, wash it gently as directed, and pat it dry with gauze pads.

4. Apply the medication and dressing as ordered.

- Place a small amount of cream (e.g., emollient) on the tongue blade, and spread it evenly on the skin.
  or
  Pour some lotion on the gauze, and pat the skin area with it.
  or
  If a liniment is used, rub it into the skin with the hands using long, smooth strokes.

- Repeat the application until the area is completely covered. *For complete coverage, no skin should show through cream or ointment.*

- Apply a sterile dressing as necessary.
  or
- Apply a prepackaged transdermal patch as directed.

5. Provide the client comfort.

- Provide a clean gown or pajamas after the application if the medication will come in contact with the clothing. *Agency clothes can be washed more easily than the client's own clothes.*

- Remove gloves.

6. Document all assessments and interventions.

- Record the type of preparation used; the site to which it was applied; the time; and the response of the client, including data about the appearance of the site, discomfort, itching, and so on.

- Return at a time by which the preparation should have acted to assess the reaction, e.g., redness (for a rubefacient, i.e., an agent that reddens the skin), and/or relief of itching, burning, swelling, or discomfort.

EVALUATION FOCUS	Presence of redness or discharge; increased or decreased comfort.

SAMPLE RECORDING

Date	Time	Notes
8/7/93	2100	Thin film of 0.5% Topicort cream applied to affected areas as ordered. Area is dry and has flaky patches (2.5 cm in diameter) scattered on chest, back, and abdomen. States no itching or pain. ———— Lawrence Campbell, RN

KEY ELEMENTS OF ADMINISTERING DERMATOLOGIC MEDICATIONS

See the Key Elements of Technique 35–1.
- Clean and shave the affected area before administering the medication, if required, and assess the condition of the skin.
- Use sterile technique for open skin lesions.
- Apply the correct topical preparation to the appropriate area.

Ophthalmic Irrigations and Instillations

An eye irrigation is administered to wash out the conjunctival sac of the eye. In a hospital, sterile equipment is usually used. Medications for the eyes are instilled in the form of liquids or ointments. Eye drops are packaged in monodrip plastic containers

 that are used to administer the preparation. Ointments are usually supplied in small tubes. All containers must state that the medication is for ophthalmic use. Usually, sterile preparations are used, but sterile technique is not always indicated. Prescribed liquids are usually dilute, e.g., less than 1% strength. Technique 35–3 illustrates how to administer irrigations and instillations.

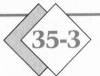 **35-3**

Administering Ophthalmic Irrigations and Instillations

PURPOSES

Instillation
- To provide an eye medication the client requires (e.g., an antibiotic) to treat an infection or for other reasons (see specific drug action)

Irrigation
- To clear the eye of noxious or other foreign material or excessive secretions or in preparation for surgery

ASSESSMENT FOCUS

Allergy to medication; appearance of eye and surrounding structures for lesions, exudate, erythema, or swelling; the location and nature of any discharge; lacrimation, and swelling of the eyelids or of the lacrimal gland; client complaints (e.g., itching, burning, pain, blurred vision, and photophobia); client behavior (e.g., squinting, blinking excessively, frowning, or rubbing the eyes); client's level of consciousness and ability or willingness to cooperate (e.g., restlessness, disorientation); specific drug action and side-effects; client's knowledge about the medication.

EQUIPMENT

Instillation
- ☐ Sterile gloves
- ☐ Sterile absorbent sponges soaked in sterile normal saline
- ☐ Medication
- ☐ Dry sterile absorbent sponges
- ☐ Sterile eye dressing (pad) as needed and paper eye tape to secure it

Irrigation
- ☐ Moistureproof drape
- ☐ Sterile kidney basin
- ☐ Sterile gloves
- ☐ Sterile cotton balls
- ☐ Sterile normal saline (optional)
- ☐ Sterile container for the irrigating solution

- ☐ Irrigating solution (usually 60 to 240 ml (2 to 8 oz) of solution at 37 C (98.6 F) is appropriate)
- ☐ Sterile eye syringe or eye irrigator (eyedropper can be used if only small amounts of solution are required)

INTERVENTION

1. Verify the medication or irrigation order.

Instillation
- Check the physician's order for the preparation, strength, and number of drops. Also confirm

the prescribed frequency of the instillation and which eye is to be treated. Abbreviations are frequently used to identify the eye: OD (right eye), OS (left eye), OU (both eyes).

- Check the expiration date and ensure that the medication is clearly labeled.

Irrigation
- Check the type, amount, temperature, and strength of the so-

▶ **Technique 35–3 Administering Ophthalmic Medications** CONTINUED

lution and the frequency of the irrigation.

2. Prepare the client.

- Explain the technique to the client or to the parents of an infant or child. The administration of an ophthalmic irrigating solution or medication is not usually painful. Ointments are often soothing to the eye, but some liquid preparations may sting initially.

- **P** For a young child, use a doll to demonstrate the procedure. *This facilitates cooperation and decreases anxiety.*

- Assist the client to a comfortable position, either sitting or lying. For an irrigation, tilt the client's head toward the affected eye, and ensure that the light source does not shine into the person's eyes. *The head is tilted so that the irrigating or cleaning solution will run from the eye to the basin at the side, not to the other eye. The light source is directed slightly away from the eye, particularly if the person is photophobic.*

- **P** For a confused or uncooperative client or for a young child or infant, enlist assistance to restrain the arms and head. Use wrist restraints or a mummy restraint. *This prevents interference from the client during medication administration.*

- For an irrigation, place the drape to protect the client and the bedclothes, and position the basin against the cheek below the eye on the affected side.

3. Clean the eyelid and the eyelashes.

- **◊** Don sterile gloves.

- Use sterile cotton balls moistened with sterile irrigating solution or sterile normal saline, and wipe from the inner canthus to the outer canthus: *If not re-*

moved, material on the eyelid and lashes can be washed into the eye. Cleaning toward the outer canthus
S *prevents contamination of the other eye and the lacrimal duct.*

4. Administer the eye medication or irrigation.

Instillation

- Check the ophthalmic preparation for the name, strength, and number of drops if a liquid is used. Draw the correct number of drops into the shaft of the dropper if a dropper is used. If ointment is used, discard the first bead. *Checking medication*
S *data is essential to prevent a medication error. The first bead of ointment from a tube is considered to be contaminated.*

- Instruct the client to look up to the ceiling. Give the client a dry sterile absorbent sponge. *The person is less likely to blink if looking up. While the client looks up, the cornea is partially protected by the top eyelid. A sponge is needed to press on the nasolacrimal duct after a liquid instillation or to wipe excess ointment from the eyelashes after an ointment is instilled.*

- Expose the lower conjunctival sac by placing the thumb or fingers of your nondominant hand on the client's cheekbone just below the eye and gently drawing down the skin on the cheek. If the tissues are edematous, han-
S dle the tissues carefully to avoid damaging them. *Placing the fingers on the cheekbone minimizes the possibility of touching the cornea, avoids putting any pressure on the eyeball, and prevents the person from blinking or squinting.*

- Using a side approach, instill the correct number of drops onto the outer third of the lower conjunctival sac. Hold the dropper 1 to

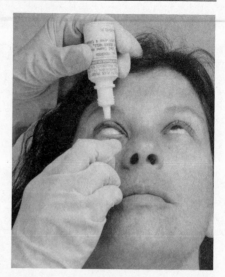

FIGURE 35–7 Instilling an eye drop into the lower conjuctival sac.

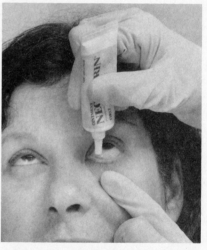

FIGURE 35–8 Instilling an eye ointment into the lower conjunctival sac.

2 cm (0.4 to 0.8 in) above the sac (Figure 35–7). *The client is less likely to blink if a side approach is used. When instilled into the conjunctival sac, drops will not harm the cornea as they might if dropped directly on it. The drop-*
S *per must not touch the sac or the cornea.*
or
Holding the tube above the lower conjunctival sac, squeeze 3 cm (0.8 in) of ointment from the tube into the lower conjunctival sac from the inner canthus outward (Figure 35–8).

▶ **Technique 35–3** *CONTINUED*

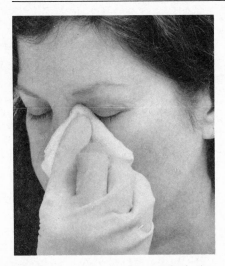

FIGURE 35–9 Pressing on the nasolacrimal duct.

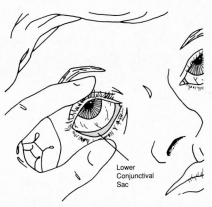

FIGURE 35–10 Exposing the lower conjunctival sac.

• Instruct the client to close the eyelids but not to squeeze them shut. *Closing the eye spreads the medication over the eyeball. Squeezing can injure the eye and push out the medication.*

• For liquid medications, press firmly or have the client press firmly on the nasolacrimal duct for at least 30 seconds (Figure 35–9). Check agency practice. *Pressing on the nasolacrimal duct prevents the medication from running out of the eye and down the duct.*

Irrigation

• Expose the lower conjunctival sac by separating the lids with the thumb and forefinger (Figure 35–10). Or, to irrigate in stages, Ⓢ

first hold the lower lid down, then hold the upper lid up. Exert pressure on the bony prominences of the cheekbone and beneath the eyebrow when holding the eyelids. *Separating the lids prevents reflex blinking. Exerting pressure on the bony prominences minimizes the possibility of pressing the eyeball and causing discomfort.*

• Fill and hold the eye irrigator about 2.5 cm (1 in) above the eye. *At this height the pressure of the solution will not damage the eye tissue, and the irrigator will not touch the eye.*

• Irrigate the eye, directing the solution onto the lower conjunctival sac and from the inner canthus to the outer canthus. *Directing the solution in this way prevents possible injury to the cor-*

nea and prevents fluid and contaminants from flowing down the nasolacrimal duct.

• Irrigate until the solution leaving the eye is clear (no discharge is present) or until all the solution has been used.

• Instruct the client to close and move the eye periodically. *Eye closure and movement help to move secretions from the upper to the lower conjunctival sac.*

• Dry around the eye with cotton balls.

5. Clean the eyelids as needed.

• Wipe the eyelids gently from the inner to the outer canthus to collect excess medication.

6. Apply an eye pad if needed, and secure it with paper eye tape.

7. Assess the client's response.

• Assess responses immediately after the instillation or irrigation and again after the medication should have acted.

8. Document all relevant information.

• Record nursing assessments and interventions relative to the instillation or irrigation. Include the name of the drug, the strength, the number of drops if a liquid, the time, and the response of the client.

EVALUATION FOCUS	Relief of complaints; change in appearance of eye in accordance with drug action; amount and character of exudate; character of irrigation returns; adverse reactions or side-effects of medication.

SAMPLE RECORDING

Date	Time	Notes
12/05/93	0900	C/o burning sensation OD. Moderate amount yellow purulent discharge at inner canthus and on eyelashes. Conjunctiva red. OD irrigated with 90 ml normal saline at 38C. Returns cloudy. Stated "eye feels better" following irrigation. —————— Deborah M. Mondeau, NS

▶ **Technique 35–3 Administering Ophthalmic Medications** *CONTINUED*

KEY ELEMENTS OF ADMINISTERING OPHTHALMIC IRRIGATIONS AND INSTILLATIONS

- Know the expected action of the medication instilled and the purpose of an irrigation.
- Verify the physician's order and confirm which eye is to be treated.
- Assess the eye and associated symptoms and behavior of the client before and after the technique.
- Use sterile technique unless indicated otherwise.
- Wear gloves.
- Clean the eye as needed before administration, wiping from the inner to the outer canthus.
- For a confused client or young child, obtain assistance or use restraints.
- For an irrigation, tilt the client's head toward the affected eye.
- Administer the correct drug and dosage (or irri-gating solution) to the correct client in the correct eye and at the right time.
- Instruct the client to look upward.
- Exert pressure on the bony prominences of the cheekbone and beneath the eyebrow when holding the eyelids open.
- Direct the irrigating solution or eye ointment from the inner to the outer canthus onto the lower conjunctival sac.
- Instill drops onto the outer third of the lower conjunctival sac.
- Avoid touching the conjunctival sac or cornea with the irrigator, eye dropper, or tube.
- Document the administered irrigation or medication according to agency protocol.

Otic Irrigations and Instillations

Irrigations of the external auditory canal are generally carried out for cleaning purposes, although applications of heat and of antiseptic solutions are sometimes prescribed. Irrigations performed in a hospital require sterile supplies and equipment so that microorganisms will not be introduced into the ear. Normal saline at body temperature (37.0 C, or 98.6 F) is frequently used to irrigate the ear. The nurse uses a thermometer to ensure that the temperature of the solution is appropriate. Medical aseptic technique is used to instill medications to the ear unless the tympanic membrane is damaged, in which case sterile technique is used. The position of the external auditory canal varies with age. In the child under 3 years of age, it is directed upward. In the adult, the external auditory canal is an S-shaped structure about 2.5 cm (1 in) long. Technique 35–4 explains how to administer otic irrigations and instillations.

Administering Otic Irrigations and Instillations

PURPOSES

Instillation
- To soften earwax so that it can be readily removed at a later time
- To provide local therapy to reduce inflammation and/or destroy infective organisms in the external ear canal
- To relieve pain

Irrigation
- To clean the canal, e.g., to remove cerumen or pus
- To apply heat
- To remove a foreign object, e.g., an insect

▶ **Technique 35–4 Administering Otic Medications** *CONTINUED*

ASSESSMENT FOCUS	Allergy to medication; the pinna of the ear and meatus for signs of redness and abrasions; the type and amount of any discharge; complaints of discomfort; intactness and appearance of the tympanic membrane and presence of foreign bodies in the ear canal (an irrigation is contraindicated if the membrane is not intact or a foreign body is present); ability to cooperate during the procedure; specific drug action and side-effects; client's knowledge about the medication to be used.

EQUIPMENT

Instillation

- □ Gloves (optional)
- □ Cotton-tipped applicator
- □ Correct medication bottle with a dropper
- □ Flexible rubber tip (optional) for the end of the dropper, which prevents injury from sudden motion, e.g., by a child or disoriented client
- □ Cotton fluff

Irrigation

- □ Moisture-resistant towel
- □ Basin, e.g., kidney basin
- □ Gloves (optional)
- □ Applicator swabs
- □ Irrigating solution at the appropriate temperature, about 500 ml (16 oz) or as ordered
- □ Container for the irrigating solution
- □ Syringe (rubber bulb or Asepto syringe is frequently used)
- □ Absorbent cotton balls

INTERVENTION

Ⓢ 1. Verify the medication or irrigation order.

- Check the physician's order for the kind of medication or irrigation; the time, amount, and dosage (if it is an instillation) or strength (if it is an irrigation); the temperature (if it is an irrigation); and which ear is to be treated.

2. Prepare the client.

- Obtain assistance to restrain an uncooperative child or confused adult. *This prevents injury due to sudden movement during the procedure or medication administration.* Ⓢ

Instillation

- Assist the client to a side-lying position with the ear being treated uppermost (Figure 35–11).

Irrigation

- Explain that the client may experience a feeling of fullness, warmth, and, occasionally, discomfort when the fluid comes in contact with the tympanic membrane.

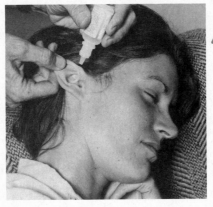

FIGURE 35–11 Instilling ear drops.

- Assist the client to a sitting or lying position with head turned toward the affected ear. *The solution can then flow from the ear canal to a basin.*

- Place the moisture-resistant towel around the client's shoulder under the ear to be irrigated, and place the basin under the ear to be irrigated.

3. Clean the pinna of the ear and the meatus of the ear canal.

- 💧 Don gloves if infection is suspected.

- Use cotton-tipped applicators and solution to wipe the pinna and auditory meatus. *Any discharge is removed so that it will not be washed into the ear canal during an irrigation. It is cleaned before an instillation to remove any drainage.* Ⓢ

4. If doing an irrigation, prepare the equipment. (Omit this step for an instillation.)

- Fill the syringe with solution.
  or
  Hang up the irrigating container, and run solution through the tubing and the nozzle. *Solution is run through to remove air from the tubing and nozzle.*

5. Administer the ear medication or irrigation.

Instillation

- Warm the medication container in your hand, or place it in warm water for a short time. *This promotes client comfort.*

- Partially fill the ear dropper with medication.

▶

► **Technique 35–4 Administering Otic Medications** CONTINUED

- Straighten the auditory canal. For an infant, gently pull the pinna downward. For an adult or a child older than 3 years of age, pull the pinna upward and backward. See Figures 12–7 and 11–33, pages 309 and 226. *The auditory canal is straightened so that the solution can flow the entire length of the canal.*

- Instill the correct number of drops along the side of the ear canal.

- Press gently but firmly a few times on the tragus of the ear. *Pressing on the tragus assists the flow of medication into the ear canal.*

- Ask the client to remain in the side-lying position for about 5 minutes. *This prevents the drops from escaping and allows the medication to reach all sides of the canal cavity.*

- Insert a small piece of cotton fluff loosely at the meatus of the auditory canal for 15 to 20 minutes. Do not press it into the canal. *The cotton helps retain the medication when the client is up. If pressed tightly into the canal, the cotton would interfere with the ac-* tion of the drug and the outward movement of normal secretions.

Irrigation

- Straighten the ear canal.

- Insert the tip of the syringe into the auditory meatus, and direct the solution gently upward against the top of the canal. *The solution will flow around the entire canal and out at the bottom. The solution is instilled gently because strong pressure from the fluid can cause discomfort and damage the tympanic membrane.*

- Continue instilling the fluid until all the solution is used or until the canal is cleaned, depending on the purpose of the irrigation. Take care not to block the outward flow of the solution with the syringe.

- Dry the outside of the ear with absorbent cotton balls. Place a cotton fluff in the auditory meatus to absorb the excess fluid.

- Assist the client to a side-lying position on the affected side. *Lying with the affected side down helps drain the excess fluid by gravity.*

6. Assess the client's response.

Instillation

- Assess the character and amount of discharge, appearance of the canal, discomfort, and so on, immediately after the instillation and again when the medication is expected to act. Inspect the cotton ball for any drainage.

Irrigation

- Assess the client for any discomfort and the appearance and odor of the fluid returns.

7. Document all relevant information.

- Document all nursing assessments and interventions relative to the procedure.

Instillation

- Include the time, the dose, and any complaints of pain. Many agencies use flowsheets; others may require that a notation be made on the nurse's notes.

Irrigation

- Include the type, concentration, amount, and temperature of the solution used; the appearance of the returns; and the presence of any discomfort.

EVALUATION FOCUS | Relief of complaints; change in appearance of ear in accordance with drug action; amount and character of discharge; appearance of tympanic membrane; character of irrigation returns; presence of adverse reactions or side-effects of medication.

SAMPLE RECORDINGS

Date	Time	Notes
12/05/93	1100	Irrigated left ear with 60 ml normal saline at 40 C. Returns clear with several dark brown flecks. No complaints of discomfort. — Josephine A. deSanto, NS

Date	Time	Notes
12/05/93	0900	Auralgan instilled into left ear. States ear less painful. No discharge present. — Margaret N. Kerr, NS

▶ **Technique 35–4** *CONTINUED*

KEY ELEMENTS OF ADMINISTERING OTIC IRRIGATIONS AND INSTILLATIONS

- Know the expected action of the medication instilled and the purpose of an irrigation.
- Verify the physician's order and confirm which ear is to be treated.
- Assess the pinna of the ear, and the external meatus and canal before and after the techniques.
- Use sterile technique unless indicated otherwise.
- Don gloves if the ear is infected.
- Obtain assistance or restrain the uncooperative client or the young child and infant.
- Clean the pinna and external ear meatus before the administration.

- Straighten the ear canal correctly and administer the correct drug and dosage (or irrigating fluid) to the correct client in the correct ear, at the right time.
- Make sure the typanic membrane is intact and the external ear canal is free of foreign bodies before irrigating the ear.
- Instill the irrigating fluid gently, directing it against the top of the ear canal.
- Drain excess irrigating fluid by gravity.
- Have the client remain in the side-lying position for about 5 minutes following an ear instillation.

Nasal Instillations

Nasal instillations (nose drops) usually are instilled for their astringent effect (to shrink swollen mucous membranes), to loosen secretions and facilitate drainage, or to treat infections of the nasal cavity or sinuses. Nasal instillations are sometimes intended for the nasal sinuses, which are hollow cavities in the facial bones. There are four groups of sinuses: sphenoid, ethmoid, frontal, and maxillary. See Figure 11–39, page 231. The sinuses are lined with mucous membrane, which is continuous with the mucous membrane of the nasal passage. Technique 35–5 describes how to administer nasal instillations.

 **35-5** # Administering Nasal Instillations

PURPOSES
- To decrease nasal congestion and improve nasal breathing
- To treat infections, inflammations, or allergies of the nasal cavity or facial sinuses

ASSESSMENT FOCUS

Appearance of nasal cavities; congestion of the mucous membranes and any obstruction to breathing; facial discomfort with or without palpation (see Intervention, step 3).

EQUIPMENT

- Disposable tissues
- Correct medication
- Dropper

▶

▶ Technique 35–5 Administering Nasal Instillations *CONTINUED*

INTERVENTION

1. Verify the medication or irrigation order.

- Carefully check the physician's order for the solution to be used, its strength, the number of drops, the frequency of the instillation, and the area to receive the instillation (e.g., the eustachian (auditory) tube or specific sinuses).

2. Prepare the client.

- If secretions are excessive, ask the client to blow the nose to clear the nasal passages.

- Inspect the discharge on the tissues for color, odor, and thickness.

3. Assess the client.

- Assess congestion of the mucous membranes and any obstruction to breathing. Ask the client to hold one nostril closed and blow out gently through the other nostril. Listen for the sound of any obstruction to the air. Repeat for the other nostril.

- Assess signs of distress when nares are occluded. Block each naris of an infant or young child and observe for signs of greater distress when the naris is obstructed.

- Assess facial discomfort. An infected or congested sinus can cause an aching, full feeling over the area of the sinus and facial tenderness on palpation.

- Assess any crusting, redness, bleeding, or discharge of the mucous membranes of the nostrils. Use a nasal speculum. The membrane normally appears moist, pink, and shiny.

4. Position the client appropriately.

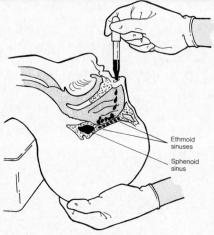
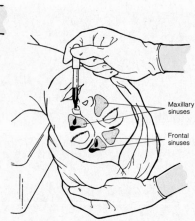

FIGURE 35–12 The Proetz position.

FIGURE 35–13 The Parkinson position.

- To treat the opening of the eustachian tube, have the client assume a back-lying position. *The drops will flow into the nasopharynx, where the eustachian tube opens.*

- To treat the ethmoid and sphenoid sinuses, have the client take a back-lying position with the head over the edge of the bed or a pillow under the shoulders so that the head is tipped backward. This is called the *Proetz position* (Figure 35–12).

- To treat the maxillary and frontal sinuses, have the client assume the same back-lying position, with the head turned toward the side to be treated. This is called the *Parkinson position.* (Figure 35–13). If only one side is to be treated, be sure the person is positioned so that the correct side is accessible. If the client's head is over the edge of the bed, support it with your hand so that the neck muscles are not strained.

5. Administer the medication.

- Draw up the required amount of solution into the dropper.

- Hold the tip of the dropper just above the nostril, and direct the solution laterally toward the midline of the superior concha of the ethmoid bone as the client breathes through the mouth. Do not touch the mucous membrane of the nares. *If the solution is directed toward the base of the nasal cavity, it will run down the eustachian tube. Touching the mucous membrane with the dropper could damage the membrane and cause the client to sneeze.*

- Repeat for the other nostril if indicated.

- Ask the client to remain in the position for 5 minutes. *The client remains in the same position to help the solution come in contact with all of the nasal surface or flow into the desired area.*

- Discard any remaining solution in the dropper, and dispose of soiled supplies appropriately.

6. Document all relevant information.

- Document nursing assessments and interventions.

▶ **Technique 35–5** *CONTINUED*

EVALUATION FOCUS	Relief of complaints (e.g., nasal congestion, difficulty breathing, and discomfort); amount and character of secretions; appearance of nasal mucosa; adverse reactions or side-effects of medication.

SAMPLE RECORDING

Date	Time	Notes
12/6/93	2250	Moderate amount clear secretions cleared from nose by blowing. Neosynephrine 2 gtts administered in both nares. No nasal or facial discomfort. Mucosa is pink. ——————————— Sharona Von Stachenberg, RN

KEY ELEMENTS OF ADMINISTERING NASAL INSTILLATIONS

- Know the expected action of the medication instilled.
- Verify the physician's order, and confirm whether both nostrils or specific sinuses are to be treated.
- Assess the nares and any discharge appropriately before and after the instillation.
- Maintain asepsis.

- Obtain assistance or restrain the pediatric client during the procedure as indicated.
- Administer the correct drug and dosage to the correct client in the correct area at the right time.
- Prevent nasal discomfort and injury; e.g., keep the tip of the dropper off the mucous membrane.
- Document the instillation according to agency protocol.

Nebulizers

A **nebulizer** is used to deliver a fine spray of medication or moisture to a client. **Nebulization** is the production of a fog or mist.

There are two kinds of nebulization: atomization and aerosolization. In *atomization*, a device called an *atomizer* produces rather large droplets for inhalation. In *aerosolization*, or **inhalation therapy**, the droplets are suspended in a gas, such as oxygen. The smaller the droplets, the further they can be inhaled into the respiratory tract. When a medication is intended for the nasal mucosa, it is inhaled through the nose; when it is intended for the trachea, bronchi, and/or lungs, it is inhaled through the mouth.

A *large-volume nebulizer* can provide a heated or cool mist. It is used for long-term therapy, such as that following a tracheostomy. These nebulizers have a 250-ml capacity and deliver oxygen or room air. The *ultrasonic nebulizer* (Figure 35–14) provides 100% humidity and can provide particles small enough to be inhaled deeply into the respiratory tract. There are two types of ultrasonic nebulizers: one has a cup filled with sterile distilled water; the other requires a continuous supply of sterile distilled water from a bag connected by tubing to the nebulizer bottle.

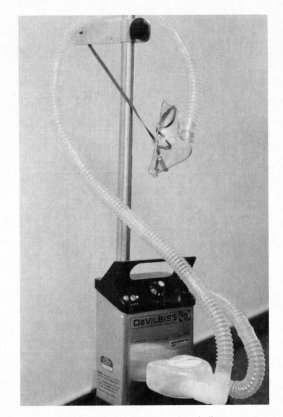

FIGURE 35–14   An ultrasonic nebulizer.

The *hand (metered dose) nebulizer* (Figure 35–15) is a container of medication that can be compressed by hand to release the medication through a nose-piece or mouthpiece. The force with which the air moves through the nebulizer causes the large particles of medicated solution to break up into finer particles, forming a mist or fine spray. Aerosol inhalers must be used properly to ensure correct delivery of the prescribed medication. The *mininebulizer* is used with oxygen or a pressurized gas source, e.g., air. With this device, the client inhales and exhales independently. Medication is administered during inhalation. A *side-stream nebulizer* provides a medication to a client on a ventilator or receiving intermittent positive pressure breathing (IPPB) therapy (Figure 30–7 on page 749). The gas, e.g., oxygen, passes through a device containing the medicated solution and then into the ventilator and to the client.

Technique 35–6 describes how to administer a medication by metered dose nebulizer.

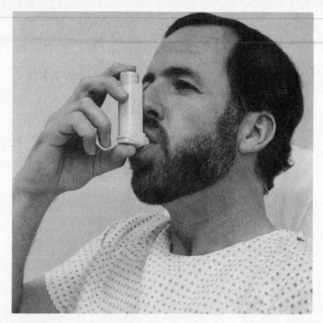

FIGURE 35–15 A hand nebulizer.

 35-6

Administering Medications by Metered Dose Nebulizer

Before administering a medication by metered dose nebulizer, determine the type, strength, and amount of medication to administer.

PURPOSES
- To assist the removal of accumulated lung secretions
- To prevent the accumulation of secretions in clients at risk, e.g., those on mechanical ventilators
- To relieve dyspnea

ASSESSMENT FOCUS

Lung sounds (e.g., crackles (rales) or gurgles (rhonchi)); respiratory rate and depth; cough (productive or nonproductive); amount, color, and character of expectorations; presence of dyspnea; vital signs for baseline data.

EQUIPMENT

☐ Metered dose nebulizer with medication cannister

INTERVENTION

1. Prepare the client.

- Explain that this nebulizer delivers a measured dose of drug with each push of the medication cannister, which fits into the top of the nebulizer (Figure 35–15).

2. Instruct the client to use the metered dose nebulizer as follows:

- Exhale through the nose as deeply as possible.

- Place the mouthpiece of the nebulizer into the mouth with its opening toward the throat or, with some models, hold the mouthpiece 1 to 2 inches from the open mouth. For a nasal instillation, hold a naris closed and place the nosepiece at the opening of the naris.

- Then inhale slowly and deeply

▶ **Technique 35–6** *CONTINUED*

through the mouth while releasing the dose. The dose is released by pressing down on the medication cannister.

- Hold the breath for several seconds. *This allows the aerosol to reach deeper branches of the airways.*

- Exhale slowly through pursed lips. *Controlled exhalation keeps the small airways open during exhalation.*

- Repeat for other naris if administering a nasal instillation.

3. **Caution the client about overuse of the nebulizer.**

- Tolerance to the medication and

serious side-effects (e.g., bronchospasm or adverse cardiac effects) may result.

4. **Document all relevant information.**

- Record the administration of the medication and assessments according to agency protocol.

EVALUATION FOCUS	Relief of dyspnea, crackles (rales) or gurgles (rhonchi); ability to expectorate secretions; stability of vital signs.

SAMPLE RECORDING

Date	Time	Notes
7/11/93	0930	Instructed client on use of metered dose nebulizer. Client returned demonstration correctly. ————————————— Sheila Springfield, RN

KEY ELEMENTS OF ADMINISTERING MEDICATIONS BY METERED DOSE NEBULIZER

- Have the client place the opening of the inhaler in the mouth or at the entrance of one naris, and direct it toward the throat.

- Instruct the client to (a) exhale through the nose as deeply as possible, (b) inhale slowly while

releasing the medication, (c) hold the breath after administering the medication, and (d) exhale slowly through pursed lips.

- Block one naris while inhaling the medication through the other.

Vaginal Irrigations and Instillations

A vaginal irrigation (douche) is the washing of the vagina by a liquid at a low pressure. It is similar to the irrigation of the external auditory canal in that the fluid returns immediately after being inserted. Vaginal irrigations are not necessary for ordinary female hygiene but are used to prevent infection by applying an antimicrobial solution that discourages the growth of microorganisms, to remove an offensive or irritating discharge, and to reduce inflammation or prevent hemorrhage by the application of heat or cold. Commonly a povidone-iodine solution is prescribed.

In hospitals, sterile supplies and equipment are used; in a home, sterility is not usually necessary because people are accustomed to the microorganisms in their environments. Sterile technique is indicated if there is an open wound. Usually, 1000 to 2000

ml of irrigating solution at 40.5 C (105 F) is required. Check agency protocol. Normal saline, tap water, sodium bicarbonate solution (8 ml of sodium bicarbonate to 1000 ml of water), and vinegar solution (8 ml of vinegar to 1000 ml of water) are commonly used. Before taking the equipment to the client, the nurse uses a thermometer to check the temperature of the solution.

Vaginal medications, or instillations, are inserted as creams, jellies, foams, or suppositories to relieve infection or to relieve vaginal discomfort, e.g., itching or pain. Medical aseptic technique is usually used. Vaginal creams, jellies, and foams are applied by using a tubular applicator with a plunger. Suppositories are inserted with the index finger of a gloved hand. Suppositories are designed to melt at body temperature, so they are generally stored in the refrigerator to keep them firm for insertion. See Technique 35–7 for administering vaginal irrigations and instillations.

35-7 | Administering Vaginal Irrigations and Instillations

PURPOSES
- To treat or prevent infection
- To remove an offensive or irritating discharge
- To reduce inflammation
- To relieve vaginal discomfort

ASSESSMENT FOCUS

Allergy to medications or irrigating fluid; vaginal orifice for inflammation; amount, character, and odor of vaginal discharge; complaints of vaginal discomfort (e.g., burning or itching).

EQUIPMENT

Vaginal Instillation
- Drape
- Correct vaginal suppository or cream
- Applicator for vaginal cream
- Disposable gloves
- Lubricant for a suppository
- Disposable towel

- Clean perineal pad and T-binder or sanitary belt

Vaginal Irrigation
- Bedpan
- Roll or pillow
- Moistureproof pad
- Moisture-resistant drape
- Vaginal irrigation set (these are often disposable) containing a

nozzle, tubing and a clamp, and a container for the solution
- IV pole
- Irrigating solution
- Gloves
- Tissues
- Clean perineal pad and T-binder or sanitary belt

INTERVENTION

 1. Verify the medication or irrigation order.

- Carefully check the physician's order for the specific medication or solution ordered, its dosage, and the time of administration.

2. Prepare the client.

- Explain to the client that a vaginal irrigation or instillation is normally a painless procedure and, in fact, may bring relief from itching and burning if an infection is present. It usually takes about 10 minutes. Many people feel embarassed about these procedures, and some may prefer to perform the procedure themselves if instruction is provided.

- Provide privacy, and ask the client to void. *If the bladder is empty, the client will have less discomfort during the treatment, and the*

possibility of injuring the vaginal lining is decreased.

3. Position and drape the client appropriately.

Installation

- Assist the client to a back-lying position with the knees flexed and the hips rotated laterally.

- Drape the client appropriately so that only the perineal area is exposed.

Irrigation

- Assist the client to a back-lying position with the hips higher than the shoulders so that the solution will flow into the posterior fornix of the vagina. Position the client on a bedpan, and provide comfortable support for the lumbar region of the back with a roll or pillow.

- Place the waterproof pad under

the bedpan to protect the bedding.

- Provide a drape for the legs so that only the perineal area is exposed.

4. Prepare the equipment.

Installation

- Unwrap the suppository, and put it on the opened wrapper.
 or
 Fill the applicator with the prescribed cream, jelly, or foam. Directions are provided with the manufacturer's applicator.

Irrigation

- Clamp the tubing. Hang the irrigating container on the IV pole so that the base is about 30 cm (12 in) above the vagina. *At this height, the pressure of the solution should not be great enough to injure the vaginal lining.*

▶ **Technique 35–7** *CONTINUED*

- Run fluid through the tubing and nozzle into the bedpan. *Fluid is run through the tubing to remove air and to moisten the nozzle.*

5. Assess and clean the perineal area.

- Don gloves. *Gloves prevent contamination of the nurse's hands from vaginal and perineal microorganisms.*

- Inspect the vaginal orifice, note any odor or discharge from the vagina, and ask about any vaginal discomfort. (See Assessment Focus, earlier.)

- Provide perineal care to remove microorganisms. *This decreases the chance of moving microorganisms into the vagina.*

6. Administer the vaginal suppository, cream, foam, jelly, or irrigation.

Suppository

- Ⓢ Lubricate the rounded (smooth) end of the suppository, which is inserted first. *Lubrication facilitates insertion.*

- Lubricate your gloved index finger.

- Expose the vaginal orifice by separating the labia with your nondominant hand.

- Insert the suppository about 8 to 10 cm (3 to 4 in) along the posterior wall of the vagina, or as far as it will go (Figure 35–16). The posterior wall of the vagina is about 2.5 cm (1 in) longer than the anterior wall because the cervix protrudes into the uppermost portion of the anterior wall. The anterior wall is usually about 6 to 7.5 cm (2½ to 3 in).

- Ⓢ Withdraw the finger, and remove the gloves, turning them inside out and placing them on the towel. *Turning the gloves inside out*

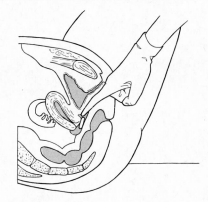

FIGURE 35–16 Instilling a vaginal suppository.

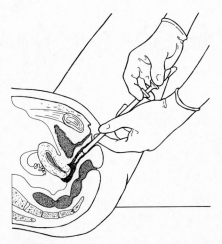

FIGURE 35–17 Using an applicator to instill a vaginal cream.

prevents the spread of microorganisms.

- Ask the client to remain lying in the supine position for 5 to 10 minutes following insertion. The hips may also be elevated on a pillow. *This position allows the medication to flow into the posterior fornix after it has melted.*

Vaginal Cream, Jelly, or Foam

- Gently insert the applicator about 5 cm (2 in).

- Slowly push the plunger until the applicator is empty (Figure 35–17).

- Remove the applicator, and place it on the towel. *The applicator is*

put on the towel to prevent the spread of microorganisms.

- Discard the applicator if disposable or clean it according to the manufacturer's directions.

- Ⓢ Remove the gloves, turning them inside out, and place them on the towel.

- Ask the client to remain in bed in the supine position for 5 to 10 minutes following the instillation.

Irrigation

- Run some fluid over the perineal area, then insert the nozzle carefully into the vagina. Direct the nozzle toward the sacrum, following the direction of the vagina.

- Insert the nozzle about 7 to 10 cm (3 to 4 in), start the flow, and rotate the nozzle several times. *Rotating the nozzle irrigates all parts of the vagina.*

- Ⓢ Use all the irrigating solution, permitting it to flow out freely into the bedpan. *Obstructing the flow of the returns could result in injury to the tissues from pressure.*

- Remove the nozzle from the vagina.

- Assist the client to a sitting position on the bedpan. *Sitting on the bedpan will help drain the remaining fluid by gravity.*

7. Ensure client comfort.

- Dry the perineum with tissues as required.

- Remove the bedpan, if used.

- Remove the moisture-resistant pad and the drape.

- Apply a clean perineal pad and a T-binder if there is excessive drainage.

▶

▶ **Technique 35–7 Administering Vaginal Medications** *CONTINUED*

8. Document all relevant information.

• Record the instillation and assessments as you would other

medications and instillations. See sample below.

• To record the administration of the irrigation, note when it was administered; the amount, type,

strength, and temperature of the irrigating solution; and all nursing assessments.

9. Assess the client's response.

EVALUATION FOCUS	Relief of complaints; amount, character, and odor of discharge; appearance of vaginal orifice to compare to baseline data; character of irrigation returns; adverse reactions or side-effects of medication.

SAMPLE RECORDING

Date	Time	Notes
3/15/93	1000	C/o pruritus around vaginal orifice. Thick, white, foul-smelling discharge apparent. Perineal care provided. Mycostatin cream 4 gm inserted into vagina. —————— Gloria Seng, NS

KEY ELEMENTS OF ADMINISTERING VAGINAL IRRIGATIONS AND INSTILLATIONS

• Know the expected action of the medication instilled and the purpose of an irrigation.
• Verify the physician's order.
• Make sure the client voids before the administration.
• Assess the vaginal orifice and any discharge before and after the techniques.
• Wear gloves.
• Provide perineal care before the administration.
• Administer the correct drug and dosage to the correct client at the right time.

• Hang an irrigating container at the appropriate height.
• Moisten an irrigation nozzle, or lubricate a suppository and your gloved finger before insertion.
• Rotate an irrigation nozzle during the procedure.
• Insert a suppository along the posterior wall of the vagina.
• Have the client remain in supine position for at least 5 minutes following an instillation.
• Document the administered irrigation or medication according to agency protocol.

Rectal Instillations

Insertion of medications into the rectum in the form of suppositories is a frequent practice. Rectal administration is a convenient and safe method of giving certain medications. Advantages include the following:

• It avoids irritation of the upper gastrointestinal tract in clients who encounter this problem.

• It is advantageous when the medication has an objectionable taste or odor.

• The drug is released at a slow but steady rate.

• Rectal suppositories are thought to provide higher bloodstream levels (titers) of medication, because the venous blood from the lower rectum is not transported through the liver.

Technique 35–8 describes how to insert a rectal suppository.

35-8   Inserting a Rectal Suppository

PURPOSES
- To provide a local medicinal effect (e.g., a laxative suppository to soften feces and stimulate defecation)
- To provide a systemic medicinal effect (e.g., an aminophylline suppository to dilate the client's bronchi and enhance breathing)
- To provide an alternate route when the oral route is contraindicated or the client is vomiting

ASSESSMENT FOCUS

Client's need for the medication (e.g., abdominal distention and/or discomfort if the suppository is intended to stimulate defecation); whether the client desires to defecate or time of last defecation (suppositories that are given for a systemic effect should be given when the rectum is free of feces to enhance absorption of the drug); the action of the medication and any side-effects; any contraindications to the rectal route (e.g., recent rectal surgery or rectal pathology, such as bleeding).

EQUIPMENT
- Correct suppository
- Glove
- Lubricant, placed on the disposable towel, in an amount

   sufficient to cover the suppository tip

   and the nurse's index finger
- Disposable towel

INTERVENTION

1. Identify and prepare the client for the procedure.

- Check the client's identification band, and ask the client's name. *This ensures that the right client receives the medication.*

- Assist the client to a left lateral position with the upper leg acutely flexed.

- Fold back the top bedclothes to expose only the buttocks.

2. Prepare the equipment.

- Unwrap the suppository, and leave it on the opened wrapper.

- Don the glove on the hand to be used to insert the suppository. *The glove prevents contamination of the nurse's hand by rectal microorganisms and feces.*

- Lubricate the smooth rounded end of the suppository, or see the manufacturer's instructions. *The smooth rounded end is inserted first. Lubrication prevents anal friction and tissue damage on insertion.*

- Lubricate the gloved index finger.

3. Insert the suppository.

- Ask the client to breathe through the mouth. *This usually relaxes the external anal sphincter.*

- Insert the suppository gently into the anus, rounded end first (or according to the manufacturer's instructions) and along the wall of the rectum with the gloved index finger. For an adult, insert the suppository 10 cm (4

in); for a child or infant, insert it 5 cm (2 in) or less (Figure 35–18). *The rounded end facilitates insertion. The suppository needs to be placed along the wall of the rectum, rather than amid feces, in order to be absorbed effectively.*

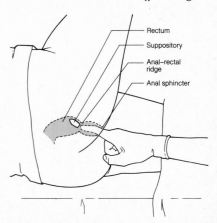

FIGURE 35–18   Inserting a rectal suppository.

▶ **Technique 35–8 Inserting a Rectal Suppository** *CONTINUED*

- Withdraw the finger. Remove the glove by turning it inside out and placing it on the towel. *Turning the glove inside out contains the rectal microorganisms and prevents their spread.*

- Press the client's buttocks together for a few seconds. *This* *helps minimize any urge to expel the suppository.*

- Ask the client to remain flat or in the left lateral position for at least 5 minutes. *This helps prevent expulsion of the suppository.*

- If the client has been given a laxative suppository, place the call light within easy reach to summon assistance for the bedpan or toilet.

4. Document all relevant information.

- Record on the client's record the type of suppository given, the time it was given, the amount of time it was retained if it was expelled, and the results or effects.

EVALUATION FOCUS

The effect of the suppository at the time it is expected to be effective; any signs of side-effects.

SAMPLE RECORDINGS

Date	Time	Notes
2/28/93	0900	Dulcolax suppository 10 mg inserted. ——————— Eric P. Jones, NS
	0935	Large amount soft brown stool and much flatus expelled. ——————— Eric P. Jones, NS

Date	Time	Notes
2/28/93	1025	Marked dyspnea, R 32, P 120. Aminophylline suppository 500 mg inserted. ——————— Margery Smith, NS
	1055	Breathing easier. R 20, P 96. ——————— Margery Smith, NS

KEY ELEMENTS OF INSERTING A RECTAL SUPPOSITORY

- Know the expected action of the medication.
- Verify the physician's order.
- Perform required assessment measures based on the client's health problem and medication administered.
- Wear a glove.
- Lubricate the tip of the suppository and your gloved index finger before administration.

- Administer the correct drug and dosage to the correct client at the right time.
- Insert the suppository along the wall of the rectum.
- Press the client's buttocks together following the insertion.
- Document the administered irrigation or medication according to agency protocol.

CRITICAL THINKING CHALLENGE

Bette Wilson, a 68-year-old client on the medical unit, refuses to take her medication. She tells you that it upsets her stomach and makes her feel sick. How do you feel when a client refuses treatment? What action would you take?

RELATED RESEARCH

Worrell, P. J., and Hodson, E. March/April 1989. Posology: The battle against dosage calculation errors. *Nursing Educators Microworld* 14:27–31.

REFERENCES

Byington, K. C. 1991. Your guide to pediatric drug administration. *Nursing 91*, 21:82, 84, 86–89.

Canadian Pharmaceutical Association. 1992. Compendium of Pharmaceuticals and Specialties, 27th ed. Canadian Pharmaceutical Association Ottawa, Ontario: Canada.

Clayton, M. June 1987. The right way to prevent medication errors. *RN* 50:30–31.

Hahn, K. September 1989. Administering eye medications. *Nursing 89* 19:80.

Hussar, D. A. August 1986. Drug interactions: Another good reason for checking and rechecking before you administer medications. *Nursing 86* 16:34–40.

McConnell, E. A. March 1991. How to irrigate the eye. *Nursing 91* 21:28.

McGovern, K. March 1992. 10 golden rules for administering drugs safely. *Nursing 92* 22:49–56.

Smith, A. J., and Johnson, J. Y. 1990. *Nurse's guide to clinical procedures*. Philadelphia: J. B. Lippincott Co.

36

Parenteral Medications

CONTENTS

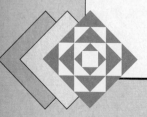

NURSING PROCESS GUIDE
PARENTERAL MEDICATIONS

ASSESSMENT

Determine

- Medication history.

- History of allergies.

- Client's age. Medications are not administered subcutaneously to infants and young children *except* for insulin; intramuscular sites for infants and young children differ from those of adults. Some elderly clients may have muscle atrophy.

- Previous injection sites used, especially those used for insulin and heparin administration. Note planned body rotation sites on the client's nursing care plan or record.

- The expected skin reaction for intradermal skin tests.

- Specific drug action desired.

- Signs and symptoms of side-effects or adverse reactions.

- Client's knowledge of and learning needs about the medication.

Assess

- The injection site for the presence of factors contraindicating the prescribed injection (e.g., decreased local tissue perfusion, presence of lesions, inflammation, ecchymosis, and tissue damage from previous injections).

- Client's level of awareness and response (verbal and nonverbal) toward receiving an injection.

- Client's ability to cooperate during the injection.

RELATED DIAGNOSTIC CATEGORIES

Diagnoses relate to the client's health status; for a client receiving meperidine (Demerol) for pain, for example, the nursing diagnosis is **Pain**.

PLANNING

Client goals and *outcome criteria* relate to the stated nursing diagnosis. Using the example above, refer to client goals and outcome criteria for **Pain** on page 903.

Parenteral Medications

Parenteral medications are given subcutaneously, intramuscularly, intradermally, or intravenously. Because parenteral medications are absorbed more quickly than oral medications and are irretrievable once injected, the nurse must prepare and administer them carefully and accurately. Administering parenteral drugs requires the same nursing knowledge as administering oral and topical drugs, plus considerable manual dexterity and the *use of sterile technique.*

Equipment

Syringes

To administer parenteral medications, nurses use syringes, needles, vials, and ampules. Syringes have three parts: the *tip*, which connects with the needle; the *barrel*, or outside part, on which the scales are printed; and the *plunger*, which fits inside the barrel (Figure 36–1). Most syringes used today are made of plastic and are individually packaged for sterility in

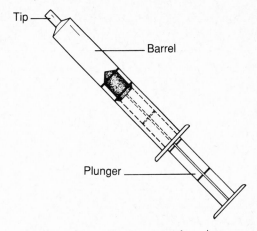

FIGURE 36–1 The three parts of a syringe.

a paper wrapper or a rigid plastic container. Glass syringes are used when the medication is incompatible with plastic.

There are several kinds of syringes, differing in size, shape, and material. The three most commonly

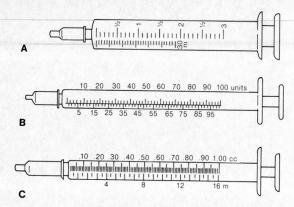

FIGURE 36–2 Three kinds of syringes: *A*, hypodermic; *B*, insulin; *C*, tuberculin.

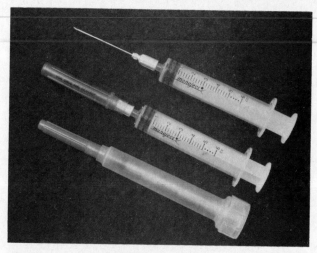

FIGURE 36–3 Disposable plastic syringes and needles: *top*, with syringe and needle exposed; *middle*, with the plastic cup over the needle; *bottom*, with the plastic case over the needle and syringe.

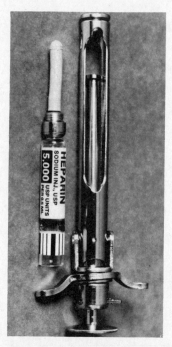

FIGURE 36–4 Metal cartridge holder and prefilled medication cartridge with needle.

used types are the standard hypodermic syringe, the insulin syringe, and the tuberculin syringe (Figure 36–2). *Hypodermic syringes* come in sizes of 2, 2.5, and 3 milliliters. They usually have two scales marked on them: the minim and the milliliter. The milliliter scale is the one normally used; the minim scale is used for very small dosages.

Insulin syringes are similar to hypodermic syringes, but they usually have a nonremovable needle and a scale specially designed for insulin: a 100-unit calibrated scale intended for use with U-100 insulin. Low-dose insulin syringes can hold a maximum of 50 units (½ ml). The *tuberculin syringe* was designed to administer tuberculin. It is a narrow syringe, calibrated in tenths and hundredths of a milliliter (up to 1 ml) on one scale and in sixteenths of a minim (up to 1 minim) on the other scale. This type of syringe can also be useful in administering other drugs, particularly when small or precise measurement is indicated (e.g., pediatric dosages or intravenous push medications). Syringes are made in other sizes as well, for example, 5, 10, 20, and 50 milliliters. These are not generally used to administer drugs directly but can be useful for adding medications to intravenous solutions or for irrigating wounds.

The *disposable plastic syringe* is most frequently used today. The syringe is supplied with a needle, which may have a plastic cap over it. The syringe and needle may be packaged together or separately (Figure 36–3).

Injectable medications are frequently supplied in *prefilled unit-dose syringes* with needles or cartridge-needle units (Figure 36–4). These prefilled syringes and cartridge-needle units are disposable. The cartridge-needle units, however, require special metal or plastic cartridge holders or syringes for administration. These syringes and cartridges come with the manufacturer's directions for use.

Needles

Needles are made of stainless steel, and most are disposable. Reusable needles (e.g., for special procedures) need to be sharpened periodically before resterilization, because the points become dull with use and are occasionally damaged or acquire burrs on the tips. A dull or damaged needle should *never* be used.

A needle has three discernible parts: the *hub*, which fits onto the syringe; the *cannula*, or shaft,

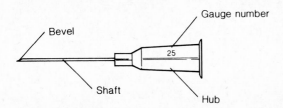

FIGURE 36–5 The parts of a needle.

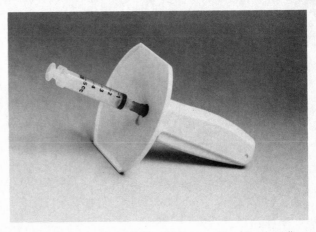

FIGURE 36–6 A needle cap holder to help prevent accidental needle sticks.

which is attached to the hub; and the *bevel*, which is the slanted part at the tip of the needle (Figure 36–5). A disposable needle has a plastic hub. Needles used for injections have three variables:

1. *Slant or length of the bevel.* The bevel of the needle may be short or long. Longer bevels provide the sharpest needles and cause less discomfort and are commonly used for subcutaneous and intramuscular injections. Short bevels are used for intradermal and intravenous injections, because a long bevel can become occluded if it rests against the side of a blood vessel.

2. *Length of the shaft.* The shaft length of commonly used needles varies from ¼ to 5 in.

3. *Gauge (or diameter) of the shaft.* The gauge varies from #14 to #28. The larger the gauge number, the smaller the diameter of the shaft. Smaller gauges produce less tissue trauma, but larger gauges are necessary for viscous medications, such as penicillin.

For subcutaneous injections, it is usual to use a needle of #24 to #26 gauge and ⅜ to ⅝ inches long. Obese clients may require a 1-inch needle. For intramuscular injections, a longer needle, e.g., 1 to 1½ inches, with a larger gauge, e.g., #20 to #22, is used.

Needle Recappers
New devices, such as the On ● Gard Recapper™ (Figure 36–6), allow the nurse to uncap and recap any needle safely and effectively without changing current technique or needle brand. To use the On ● Gard Recapper, the nurse inserts the entire syringe in the center hole of the shield. The Recapper firmly grips the needle cap and holds it in place for recapping.

Pin Cushion Container
The Sharps Pin Cushion™ container for "sharps" disposal consists of a three-piece container: a wide-based holder, a sponge pin cushion insert, and an empty covering top that snaps over the pin cushion insert. It is designed to contain no more than five needles or blades (sharps) that are a maximum of

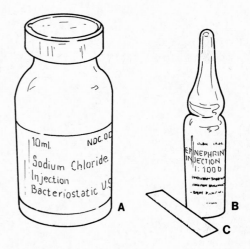

FIGURE 36–7 *A,* vial; *B,* ampule; *C,* ampule file.

7 in long. It will not accommodate butterfly-type needles.

These containers can be placed at each client's bedside. To reduce the risk of injury from sharp instruments, the device should be used in accordance with the manufacturer's instructions.

Ampules and Vials
Ampules and *vials* are frequently used to package sterile parenteral medications (Figure 36–7). Most ampule necks have colored lines around them, indicating where they are prescored for easy opening. If the neck is not scored, the nurse files it with a small file and then breaks it off. Vials come in different sizes, from single to multidose vials. They usually have a metal or plastic cap that protects the rubber seal.

Technique 36–1 explains how to prepare medications from ampules and vials.

36-1 Preparing Medications from Ampules and Vials

EQUIPMENT

- ☐ Medication card, MAR, or computer printout
- ☐ Vial or ampule of sterile medication
- ☐ File and small gauze square

- ☐ Antiseptic wipe
- ☐ Needle and syringe
- ☐ Special filter needle (optional) for withdrawing premixed liquid medications from

multidose vials or for filtering out glass slivers from ampules
- ☐ Sterile water or normal saline, if drug is in powdered form

INTERVENTION

1. Ensure the accuracy of the order and drug administration.

- Check the label on the ampule or vial carefully against the medi-Ⓢ cation card, MAR, or client's chart to make sure that the correct medication is being prepared.

- Follow the three checks for administering medications. Read the label on the medication (a) before it is taken off the shelf, (b) before withdrawing the medication, and (c) after placing it back on the shelf.

2. Prepare the medication ampule or vial for drug withdrawal.

Ampules

- Flick the upper stem of the ampule several times with a fingernail or, holding the upper stem of the ampule, make a large circle with the arm extended. *This will bring all the medication down to the main portion of the ampule.*

- Partially file the neck of the ampule, if necessary, to start a clean break.

- Place a piece of sterile gauze between your thumb and the am-Ⓢ pule neck or around the ampule neck, and break off the top by bending it toward the gauze, i.e., away from you (Figure 36–8). *The sterile gauze protects the fingers from the broken glass.* or

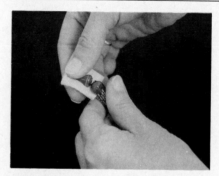

FIGURE 36–8 Breaking the neck of an ampule.

Place the antiseptic wipe packet over the top of the ampule before breaking off the top. *This method ensures that all the glass fragments fall into the packet and reduces the risk of cuts.*

- Dispose of the top of the ampule in the sharps container.

Vials

- Mix the solution, if necessary, by rotating the vial between the palms of the hands, not by shaking. *Some vials contain aqueous suspensions, which settle when they stand. In some instances shaking is contraindicated because it may cause the mixture to foam.*

- Remove the protective metal cap, and clean the rubber cap with an antiseptic wipe, by rubbing in a circular motion. *The antiseptic cleans the cap so that the needle will remain sterile when it is inserted.*

3. Withdraw the medication.

Ampules

- Some nurses recommend using a needle with a filter to withdraw the medication in case there is any broken glass from the ampule in the medication. In this case, disconnect the regular needle, leaving its cap on, and attach the filter needle to the syringe.

- Remove the cap from the needle, insert the needle into the ampule, and withdraw the amount of drug required for the dosage (Figure 36–9).

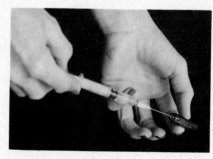

FIGURE 36–9 Withdrawing a medication from an ampule.

- With a single-dose ampule, hold the ampule slightly on its side, if necessary, to obtain all the medication.

- If a filter needle was used to withdraw the medication, replace it with a regular needle before injecting the client.

- If a filter needle was not used, recap the needle and tighten the cap at the hub of the needle.

► **Technique 36-1** *CONTINUED*

Vials

- Attach a special filter needle as agency practice dictates to draw up premixed liquid medications from multidose vials. *The filter prevents any solid material from being drawn up through the needle.*

- Remove the cap from the needle; then draw up into the syringe the amount of air equal to the volume of the medication to be withdrawn.

- Carefully insert the needle into the upright vial through the center of the rubber cap, maintaining the sterility of the needle.

- Inject the air into the vial, keeping the bevel of the needle above the surface of the medication (Figure 36-10). *The air will allow the medication to be drawn out easily, because negative pressure is not created inside the vial. The bevel is kept above the medication to avoid creating bubbles in the medication.*

- Invert the vial to withdraw medication and hold it vertically at eye level to determine the correct dosage of the drug into the syringe (Figure 36-11). *Holding the vial in a vertical position at eye level ensures correct measurement.*

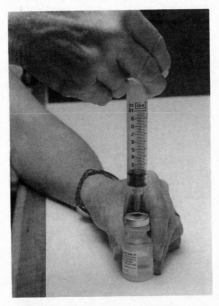
FIGURE 36-10 Injecting air into a vial.

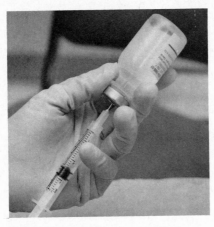
FIGURE 36-11 Withdrawing a medication from a vial.

- Withdraw the needle from the vial, and replace the cap over the needle, thus maintaining its sterility.
  or
  Replace the filter needle with the regular needle.

VARIATION: Preparing Powdered Drugs

- Read the manufacturer's directions.

- Withdraw an equivalent amount of air from the vial before adding the solvent, unless otherwise indicated by the directions.

- Add the amount of sterile water or saline indicated in the directions.

- If a multidose vial is reconstituted, label the vial with the date, time it was prepared, the amount of drug contained in each milliliter of solution, and your initials. *Time is an important factor to consider in the expiration of these medications.*

- Once reconstituted, store the medication in the vial in a refrigerator or as recommended by the manufacturer.

KEY ELEMENTS OF PREPARING MEDICATIONS FROM AMPULES AND VIALS

See the Key Elements of Technique 35-1 on page 837. In addition:
- Maintain sterility of the medication, the syringe, and the needle.
- Open ampules correctly.
- Use a filter needle as agency protocol indicates.

When Using Vials
- Mix solution by rotating rather than shaking the vial.

- Clean the rubber top of a vial with antiseptic before withdrawing the medication.
- Keep the bevel of the needle above the surface of the medication when injecting air into the vial.

When Reconstituting Powdered Drugs
- Carefully follow the manufacturer's directions.
- Label the vial appropriately (with date, time, amount of drug per milliliter, and your initials).
- Store the reconstituted vial appropriately.

Mixing Medications in One Syringe

Frequently, clients need more than one drug injected at the same time. To spare the client the experience of being injected twice, two drugs (if compatible) are often mixed together in one syringe and given as one injection. It is common, for instance, to combine two types of insulin in this manner or to combine injectable preoperative medications such as morphine or meperidine (Demerol) with atropine or scopolamine. Drugs can also be mixed in intravenous solutions. When uncertain about drug compatibilities, the nurse should consult a pharmacist or check a compatibility chart before mixing the drugs.

The nurse must also exercise caution when mixing short- and long-acting insulins, because they vary in content. Chemically, insulin is a protein that, when hydrolyzed in the body, yields a number of amino acids. Some insulin preparations contain an additional modifying protein, such as globulin or protamine, that slows absorption. This fact is particularly relevant to mixing two insulin preparations for injection because many insulin syringes have needles that cannot be changed. A vial of insulin that does *not* have the added protein should never be contaminated with insulin that does have the added protein. For example, a vial of regular insulin (crystalline zinc insulin, CZ) should never be entered with a needle that had been previously used to withdraw Lente, or isophane (NPH) insulins, all of which have added protein (see Figure 36–12, later in this chapter).

Technique 36–2 describes how to mix medications in one syringe.

36-2 — Mixing Medications Using One Syringe

EQUIPMENT

- Medication cards, computer printout, or chart
- Two vials of medication, or one vial and one ampule, or two ampules, or one vial and one cartridge
- Sterile antiseptic-soaked swabs
- Sterile hypodermic or insulin syringe and needle (if insulin is being given, use a small-gauge hypodermic needle, e.g., #26 gauge).
- Additional sterile subcutaneous or intramuscular needle (optional)

INTERVENTION

1. Verify the order for accuracy.

- Check the label on the ampule or vial carefully against the medication card, MAR, or client's chart to make sure that the correct medication is being prepared.

- Follow the three checks for administering medications. Read the label on the medication (a) before it is taken off the shelf, (b) before withdrawing the medication, and (c) after placing it back on the shelf.

- Before preparing and combining the medications, ensure that the total volume of the injection is appropriate for the injection site.

2. Prepare the medication ampule or vial for drug withdrawal.

- See Technique 36–1, step 2.

- Inspect the appearance of the medication for clarity. Some medications are always cloudy. *Preparations that have changed in appearance should be discarded.*

- If using insulin, thoroughly mix the solution in each vial prior to administration. Rotate the vials between the palms of the hands and invert the vials. *Mixing ensures an adequate concentration and thus an accurate dose. Shaking insulin vials can make the medication frothy, making precise measurement difficult.*

- Clean the tops of the vials with disinfectant swabs.

3. Withdraw the medications.

Mixing Medications from Two Vials

- Withdraw a volume of air equal to the volume of medications to be withdrawn from vials A and B.

- Inject a volume of air equal to the volume of medication to be withdrawn into vial A.

- Withdraw the needle from vial A, and inject the remaining air into vial B.

- Withdraw the required amount of medication from vial B. *The same needle is used to inject air into and withdraw medication from the second vial. It must not be contaminated with the medication in vial A.*

- Using a newly attached sterile needle, withdraw the required amount of medication from vial A. If using a syringe with a fused needle, withdraw the medication

Technique 36–2 *CONTINUED*

from vial A. The syringe now contains a mixture of medications from vials A and B. *With this method, neither vial is contaminated by microorganisms or by medication from the other vial.*

- See also the Variation below.

Mixing Medications from One Vial and One Ampule

- First prepare and withdraw the medication from the vial. *Ampules do not require the addition of air prior to withdrawal of the drug.*

- Then withdraw the required amount of medication from the ampule.

Mixing Medications from One Cartridge and One Vial or Ampule

- First ensure that the correct dose of the medication is in the cartridge. Discard any excess medication and air.

- Draw up the required medication from a vial or ampule into the cartridge. Note that when withdrawing medication from a vial, an equal amount of air must first be injected into the vial.

- If the total volume to be injected exceeds the capacity of the cartridge, use a syringe with sufficient capacity to withdraw the desired amount of medication

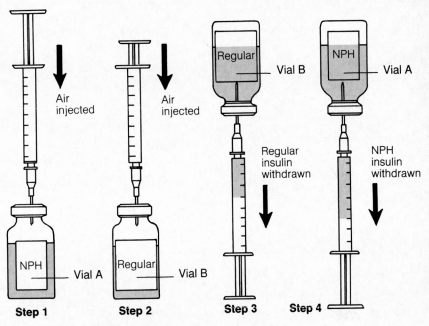

FIGURE 36–12 Mixing together two types of insulin.

from the vial/ampule, and transfer the required amount from the cartridge to the syringe.

VARIATION: Mixing Insulins

The following is an example of mixing 10 units of regular and 30 units of NPH insulin, which contains protamine.

- Inject 30 units of air into the NPH vial, and withdraw the needle. (There should be no insulin in the needle.) The needle should

not touch the insulin (Figure 36–12, step 1).

- Inject 10 units of air into the Regular insulin vial, and immediately withdraw 10 units of Regular insulin (Figure 36–12, steps 2 and 3).

- Reinsert the needle into the NPH insulin vial, and withdraw 30 units of NPH insulin (Figure 36–12, step 4). (The air was previously injected into the vial.)

By using this method, you avoid adding NPH insulin to the Regular insulin.

KEY ELEMENTS OF MIXING MEDICATIONS USING ONE SYRINGE

See the Key Elements of Technique 35–1 on page 837. In addition:

- Make sure the drugs to be mixed are compatible.
- Maintain the sterility of each drug, syringe, and the needle.
- Prevent contaminating the medication in multidose vials with medication from another vial (or ampule).

- When two vials are used, first add air to the vial from which the medication will be withdrawn last.
- Withdraw shorter-acting insulins into the syringe first.
- When one vial and an ampule are used, withdraw medication first from the vial and then from the ampule.

Subcutaneous Injections

Among the many kinds of drugs administered subcutaneously are vaccines, preoperative medications, narcotics, insulin, and heparin. Common sites for subcutaneous injections are the outer aspect of the upper arms and the anterior aspect of the thighs. These areas are convenient and normally have good blood circulation. Other areas that can be used are the abdomen, the scapular areas of the upper back, and the upper ventrogluteal and dorsogluteal areas (Figure 36–13). Clients who administer their own injections, such as diabetics requiring insulin, usually use the abdomen and anterior thigh sites. Heparin, however, is given only in the abdomen (see Technique 36–3).

Subcutaneous injection sites need to be rotated in an orderly fashion to minimize tissue damage, aid absorption, and avoid discomfort. This is especially important for clients who must receive repeated injections, e.g., diabetics. The nurse or client can prepare a diagram indicating the sites to be used and after each injection mark its location on the diagram (Figure 36–14).

Generally, a 2-ml syringe and a #25 gauge needle are used for subcutaneous injections. The length of the needle depends on the amount of adipose tissue at the site and the angle used to administer the injection. Generally, a ⅝-inch needle is used for adults when the injection is administered at a 45° angle; a

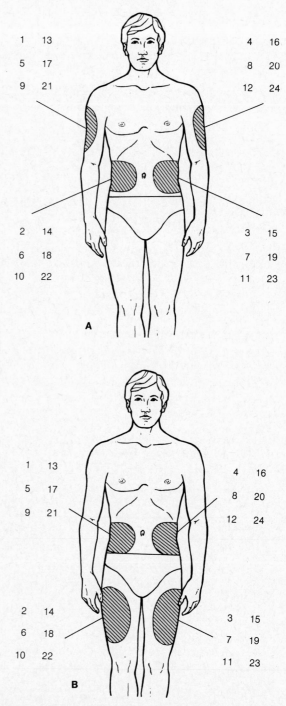

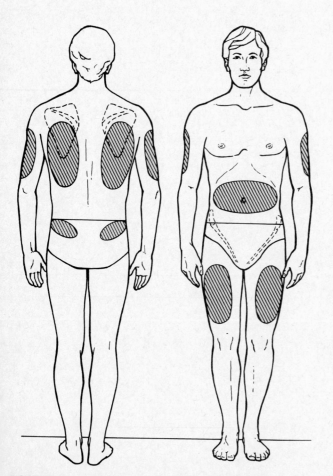

FIGURE 36–13 Body sites commonly used for subcutaneous injections.

FIGURE 36–14 A commonly used system of rotating body injection sites for injecting insulin: *A,* sites used by the nurse; *B,* sites used by the client.

½-inch needle is used at a 90° angle. Shorter needles, e.g., ⅜ inch, may be used for children, and longer ones, e.g., 1 inch, may be necessary for very obese adults. To determine the appropriate length of the needle for a 90° angle injection, the nurse pinches a fold of skin between the thumb and forefinger at the injection site, then measures the width of the skinfold

by placing a needle that will not be used for the injection against the skin surface. The appropriate needle length is one-half the width of the skinfold (Pitel 1971, p. 78). When this method of measuring is used, the needle is inserted without pinching the skin.

The steps for administering a subcutaneous injection are described in Technique 36–3.

 36-3

Administering a Subcutaneous Injection

PURPOSES
- To provide a medication the client requires (see specific drug action)
- To allow slower absorption of a medication compared with either the intramuscular or intravenous route

ASSESSMENT FOCUS

Allergies to medication; specific drug action; side-effects and adverse reactions; client's knowledge and learning needs about the medication; status and appearance of subcutaneous site for lesions, erythema, swelling, ecchymosis, inflammation, and tissue damage from previous injections; ability to cooperate during the injection; and previous injection sites used.

EQUIPMENT
- Client's medication card, MAR, or computer printout
- Vial or ampule of the correct sterile medication
- Sterile syringe and needle (e.g., 2-ml syringe, #25 gauge ⅝- or ½-in needle)
- Sterile antiseptic-soaked swabs
- Dry sterile gauze for opening an ampule (optional)
- Gloves (according to agency protocol)

INTERVENTION

1. Verify the medication order for accuracy.
- See Technique 36–1, step 1.

2. Prepare the medication from the vial or ampule.
- See Technique 36–1, step 2.

3. Identify the client, and assist the client to a comfortable position.
- Check the client's arm band, and ask the client to tell you his or her name.
- Assist the client to a position in which the arm, leg, or abdomen can be relaxed, depending on the site to be used. *A relaxed muscle at the site minimizes discomfort.*
- Obtain assistance in holding an

uncooperative client or small child. *This prevents injury due to sudden movement after needle insertion.*

4. Select and clean the site.
- Select a site free of tenderness, hardness, swelling, scarring, itching, burning, or localized inflammation. Select a site that has not been used frequently. *These conditions could hinder the absorption of the medication and also increase the likelihood of an infection at the injection site.*
- Don gloves if required.
- As agency protocol indicates, clean the site with an antiseptic swab. Start at the center of the site and clean in a widening cir-

cle to about 2 inches. Allow the area to dry thoroughly. *The mechanical action of swabbing removes skin secretions, which contain microorganisms.*
- Place and hold the swab between the third and fourth fingers of the nondominant hand. *Doing so keeps the swab readily accessible when the needle is withdrawn.*

5. Prepare the syringe for injection.
- Remove the needle cap while waiting for the antiseptic to dry. Pull the cap straight off to avoid contaminating the needle by the outside edge of the cap. *The needle will become contaminated if it touches anything but the inside of the cap, which is sterile.*

▶ Technique 36–3 Administering a Subcutaneous Injection *CONTINUED*

• Expel any air bubbles from the syringe by inverting the syringe and gently pushing on the plunger until a drop of solution can be seen in the needle bevel. If air bubbles still remain, flick the side of the syringe barrel.

6. Inject the medication.

• Grasp the syringe in your dominant hand by holding it between your thumb and fingers with palm facing to the side or upward for a 45° angle insertion or with the palm downward for a 90° angle insertion (Figure 36–15).

• Using the nondominant hand, pinch or spread the skin at the site, and insert the needle, using the dominant hand and a firm steady push (Figure 36–16). The nondominant hand can be used to immobilize the extremity of an infant or a young child as the needle is inserted. Recommendations vary about whether to pinch or spread the skin. *Pinching the skin is thought to desensitize the area somewhat and thus lessen the sensation of needle insertion. Spreading the skin can make it firmer and facilitate needle insertion.* Some recommend neither pinching nor spreading the skin (Pitel 1971, p. 79). The nurse needs to judge which method to use depending on the client's tissue firmness.

• When the needle is inserted, move your nondominant hand to the end of the plunger. Some nurses find it easier to move the nondominant hand to the barrel of the syringe and the dominant hand to the end of the plunger. If the nondominant hand is holding the extremity of an infant or small child, use the dominant hand to aspirate and inject the medication.

• Aspirate by pulling back on the

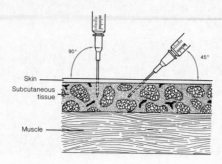

FIGURE 36–15 Inserting a needle into the subcutaneous tissue at 90° and 45° angles.

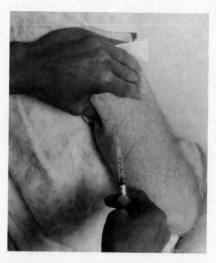

FIGURE 36–16 Administering a subcutaneous injection.

plunger. If blood appears in the syringe, withdraw the needle, discard the syringe, and prepare a new injection. If blood does not appear, continue to administer the medication. *Aspiration determines whether the needle has entered a blood vessel. Subcutaneous medications may be dangerous if placed directly into the bloodstream; they are intended for the subcutaneous tissues, where the absorption time is greater.* See below about heparin variation.

• Inject the medication by holding the syringe steady and depressing the plunger with a slow, even pressure. *Holding the syringe steady and injecting the medication at an even pressure minimizes discomfort for the client.*

7. Remove the needle, and massage the site.

• Remove the needle quickly, pulling along the line of insertion while depressing the skin with your nondominant hand. *Depressing the skin places countertraction on it and minimizes the client's discomfort when the needle is withdrawn.*

• Massage the site lightly with a sterile antiseptic-soaked swab, or apply slight pressure. *Massage is thought to disperse the medication in the tissues and facilitate its absorption. Massaging is omitted with heparin and insulin injections or when contraindicated by the drug manufacturer.*

• If bleeding occurs, apply pressure to the site with a dry sterile gauze until it stops. Bleeding rarely occurs after subcutaneous injection.

8. Dispose of supplies appropriately.

• Discard the uncapped needle and attached syringe into designated receptacles. *Proper disposal protects the nurse and others from injury and contamination. The CDC does not recommend capping before disposal to reduce the risk of needle-prick injuries.*

• Remove gloves, if worn.

9. Document all relevant information.

• Document the medication given, dosage, time, route, any assessments, and add your signature.

• Many agencies prefer that medication administration be recorded on the medication record (see Figure 36–17 for one type of record). The nurse's notes are used when prn medications are given or when there is a special problem.

▶ **Technique 36–3** *CONTINUED*

Injection Record							
SITE	1	2	3	4	5	6	7
right arm							
right abdomen							
right thigh							
left thigh							
left abdomen							
left arm							
left buttock							
right buttock							

FIGURE 36–17   A record for indicating injection sites used.

10. Assess the effectiveness of the medication when it is expected to act.

VARIATION: Administering a Heparin Injection

The subcutaneous administration of heparin requires special precautions because of the drug's anticoagulant properties.

• Select a site on the abdomen away from the umbilicus and above the level of the iliac crests. *These areas are away from major muscles and are not involved in muscular activity, as the arms and legs are; thus, the possibility of hematoma is reduced. In addition, muscular activity increases the absorption of the drug.*

• Use a ½-inch #25 or #26 gauge needle, and insert it at a 90° angle. Draw 0.1 ml of air into the syringe when preparing the heparin, and inject it after the heparin. *This step fills the needle with air and prevents any leakage of heparin into the intradermal layers when the needle is inserted and when the needle is withdrawn.*

• Check agency practices regarding aspiration. *Some nurses recommend not to aspirate to determine needle placement because this can cause the needle to move, possibly damaging tissue and rupturing small blood vessels and causing bleeding as well as severe bruising.*

• Do *not* massage the site after the injection. *Massaging could cause bleeding and ecchymoses and hasten drug absorption.*

• Alternate sites of subsequent injections.

EVALUATION FOCUS

Desired effect (e.g., relief of pain, sedation, lowered blood sugar or decreased urine glucose, a prothrombin time within preestablished limits); any adverse effects (e.g., nausea, vomiting, skin rash); clinical signs of side-effects.

SAMPLE RECORDING

Date	Time	Notes
08/09/93	0700	C/o severe pain in R upper quadrant. Restless and tense. 60 mg. Codeine given. S.C. in left upper arm. ——————————— Ann Tanazaki, RN
	0800	Pain relieved. Facial muscles less tense. Resting quietly. ——————— Ann Tanazaki, RN

KEY ELEMENTS OF ADMINISTERING A SUBCUTANEOUS INJECTION

See the Key Elements of Technique 36–1 on page 861. In addition:

• Select a needle size appropriate for the client.

• Select an appropriate site, one that has not been used frequently and has healthy intact skin.

• Don gloves as required by agency protocol.

• Minimize discomfort:

  a. Hold the syringe steady.

  b. Inject the medication at an even pressure.

  c. Remove the needle quickly while depressing the skin.

• Prevent hematoma formation when administering heparin:

  a. Draw 0.1 ml air into the syringe to inject after the heparin:

  b. Check agency policies about aspiration.

  c. Do not massage the site after the injection.

• Apply pressure to sites that bleed.

• Dispose of the syringe and needle safely.

Insulin Pump

The insulin pump enables the person who has diabetes mellitus to achieve long-term control in preventing *hypoglycemia* (low blood sugar, as evidenced by jitteriness, nervousness, and lightheadedness) and *hyperglycemia* (high blood sugar, as evidenced by headache, hunger, thirst, blurred vision, and frequent urination). The insulin pump consists of five basic parts: the battery, the motor (a computerized "brain"), the drive mechanism, the insulin syringe or reservoir, and the plastic catheter with tubing. The pump can be worn discreetly in a pocket or with a belt (Figure 36–18). An alarm device is built into the pump to alert the wearer to any problem with the pump (e.g., kinks in the tubing, a low battery, or an empty syringe).

The pump delivers a constant dosage (known as the *basal dosage*) of Regular insulin around the clock, but it also allows the person using the pump to deliver various doses (known as *bolus dosages*) as needed when the blood sugar increases. A bolus dosage is calculated according to the client's individual status,

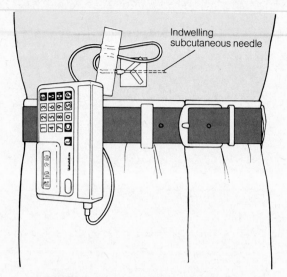

FIGURE 36–18 Schematic of an insulin pump.

prescribed physician's recommendations, anticipated food intake, and glucose levels. The box below describes the use of an insulin pump.

CLINICAL GUIDELINES

Using an Insulin Pump

• Set the pump for operation.

a. Follow the manufacturer's directions for assembling the unit, and always use the tubing and syringe designed for the pump being used.

b. Insert the battery.

c. Insert the insulin reservoir into the drive mechanism.

d. Attach the tubing to the syringe and needle.

e. Program the pump, and prime the tubing.

• Select and prepare the needle site.

a. Select an area of the abdomen that has adequate subcutaneous tissue and has not been used in the last few days.

b. Rotate sites every 3 days to prevent infection. The front part of the upper thighs, the hips, and the fatty tissue on the back and sides of the upper arms may be used.

c. Clean the area with alcohol by making a large circle starting inside and moving outward.

• Insert and secure the needle.

a. Insert the needle at a 45° angle.

b. Secure the needle with hypoallergenic tape.

• Prevent and monitor for infection at the needle site.

a. Wash hands well before handling the needle.

b. Inspect the site for redness, swelling, discoloration, pain, or drainage.

• Monitor the client for hypoglycemia and hyperglycemia.

a. Check the blood glucose at least four times a day to detect any problem.

b. If the blood glucose is above 200 to 250 mg/dl, test the urine for the presence of ketone bodies.

c. Follow recommendations for correcting the low blood glucose (e.g., have the client drink juice or eat hard candy).

d. Check that the pump was programmed correctly.

e. Check for kinks in the tubing, and ensure that all connection points for the device are intact.

f. Check the status of the needle insertion site.

Intramuscular Injections

The intramuscular (IM) injection route is ordered for the following reasons:

- The speed of absorption by the intramuscular route is faster than by the subcutaneous route because the blood supply to the body muscles is greater.

- Muscles can usually take a larger volume of fluid without discomfort than subcutaneous tissues, although the amount varies among individuals, chiefly with muscle size and condition.

- Medications that irritate subcutaneous tissue may safely be given by intramuscular injection.

Usually, a 2- to 5-ml syringe is needed. Some medications, such as paraldehyde, require a glass syringe because the medication interacts with plastic. The standard prepackaged intramuscular needle is 1½ inches and #21 or #22 gauge. However, several factors dictate the size and length of the needle to be used: the muscle, the type of solution, the amount of adipose tissue covering the muscle, and the age of the client. A large muscle, such as the gluteus medius, usually requires a #20 to #23 gauge needle, 1½ to 3 inches long, whereas the deltoid muscle requires a smaller, #23 to #25 gauge needle, ⅝ to 1 inch long. Oily solutions such as paraldehyde require a thicker needle, e.g., #21 gauge instead of #23 gauge. Also, the greater the amount of adipose tissue over the muscle, the longer the needle must be to reach the muscle. Therefore, 3-inch needles may be needed for obese clients, whereas ½-inch needles are used for thinner people. Infants and young children usually require smaller, shorter needles (#22 to #25 gauge, ⅝ to 1 inch long).

A number of body sites are used for intramuscular injections. Frequently used sites are the ventrogluteal, dorsogluteal, vastus lateralis, rectus femoris, and deltoid muscles. Only healthy muscles should be used for injections.

Ventrogluteal Site

The ventrogluteal site, also known as von Hochsteter's site, is in the gluteus medius muscle, which lies over the gluteus minimus (Figure 36–19). The ventrogluteal site is the preferred site for intramuscular injections because the area contains no large nerves or blood vessels and less fat than the buttock area. It is also farther from the rectal area and tends to be less contaminated. These considerations are important when giving injections to incontinent adults.

This site is suitable for infants, children, and adults. It is particularly suitable for immobilized clients whose dorsogluteal muscles may be atrophying.

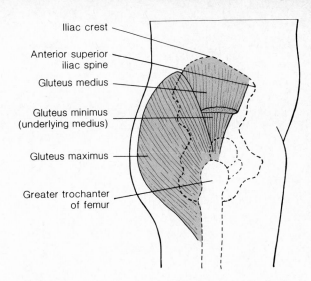

FIGURE 36–19 Lateral view of the right buttock showing the three gluteal muscles used for intramuscular injections.

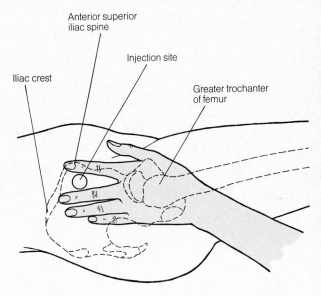

FIGURE 36–20 The ventrogluteal site for an intramuscular injection.

The client position for the injection can be a back- or side-lying position with the knee and hip flexed to relax the gluteal muscles. To establish the exact site, the nurse places the heel of the hand on the client's greater trochanter, with the fingers pointing toward the client's head. The right hand is used for the left hip, and the left hand for the right hip. With the index finger on the client's anterior superior iliac spine, the nurse stretches the middle finger dorsally, palpating the crest of the ilium and then pressing below it. The triangle formed by the index finger, the third finger, and the crest of the ilium is the injection site (Figure 36–20).

Dorsogluteal Site

The dorsogluteal site is composed of the thick gluteal muscles of the buttocks (Figure 36–19). The dorsogluteal site can be used for adults and for children with well-developed gluteal muscles. Because these muscles are developed by walking, this site should not be used for children under 3 years unless the child has been walking for at least 1 year. The nurse must choose the injection site carefully to avoid striking the sciatic nerve, major blood vessels, or bone.

The nurse palpates the posterior superior iliac spine, then draws an imaginary line to the greater trochanter of the femur. This line is lateral to and parallel to the sciatic nerve. The injection site is, then, lateral and superior to this line (Figure 36–21). Palpating the ilium and the trochanter is important; visual calculations alone can result in an injection that is placed too low and injures other structures.

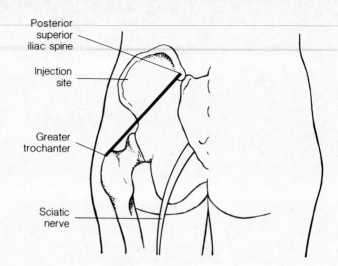

FIGURE 36–21 The dorsogluteal site for an intramuscular injection.

Vastus Lateralis Site

The vastus lateralis muscle is usually thick and well developed in both adults and children. It is increasingly recommended as the site of choice for intramuscular injections for infants because there are no major blood vessels or nerves in the area. It is situated on the anterior lateral aspect of the thigh (Figure 36–22). The middle third of the muscle is suggested as the site. It is established by dividing the area between the greater trochanter of the femur and the lateral femoral condyle into thirds and selecting the middle third (Figure 36–23). The client can assume a back-lying or a sitting position for an injection into this site.

Rectus Femoris Site

The rectus femoris muscle, which belongs to the quadriceps muscle group, can also be used for intra-

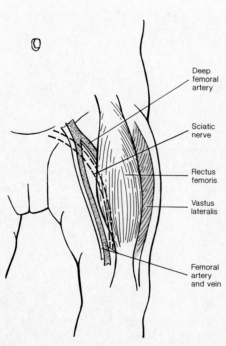

FIGURE 36–22 The vastus lateralis muscle of the upper thigh, used for intramuscular injections.

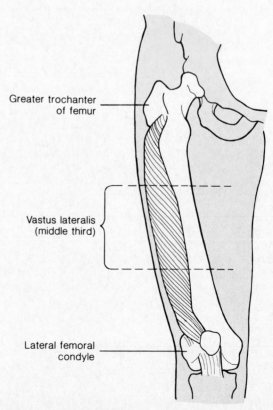

FIGURE 36–23 The vastus lateralis site for an intramuscular injection.

muscular injections. It is situated on the anterior aspect of the thigh (Figure 36–24). This site can be used for occasional injections for infants and children and for adults when other sites are contraindicated.

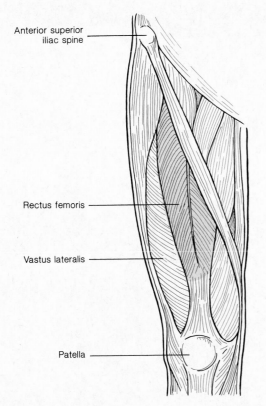

FIGURE 36–24 The rectus femoris muscle of the upper right thigh, used for intramuscular injections.

Its chief advantage is that clients who administer their own injections can reach this site easily. Its main disadvantage is that an injection here may cause considerable discomfort for some people. The client assumes a sitting or back-lying position for an injection at this site.

Deltoid Site

The deltoid muscle is found on the lateral aspect of the upper arm. It is not used often for intramuscular injections because it is a relatively small muscle and is very close to the radial nerve and radial artery. It is sometimes considered for use in adults and children over 18 months of age because of rapid absorption from the deltoid area.

To locate the densest part of the muscle, the nurse palpates the lower edge of the acromion and the midpoint on the lateral aspect of the arm that is in line with the axilla. A triangle within these boundaries indicates the deltoid muscle about 5 cm (2 in) below the acromion process (Figure 36–25). Another method of establishing the deltoid site is to place four fingers across the deltoid muscle, with the first finger on the acromion process; i.e., the site is three finger breadths below the acromion process (Figure 36–26).

Technique 36–4 describes how to administer an intramuscular injection.

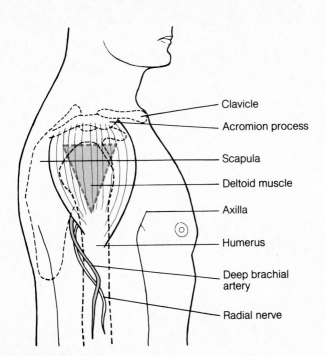

FIGURE 36–25 The deltoid muscle of the upper arm, used for intramuscular injections.

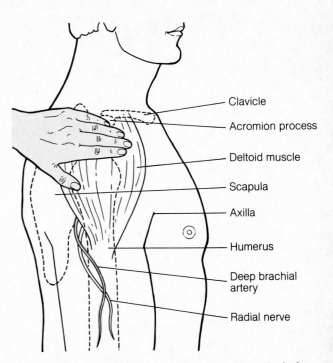

FIGURE 36–26 A method of establishing the deltoid muscle site for an intramuscular injection.

36-4 Administering an Intramuscular Injection

PURPOSE	• To provide a medication the client requires (see specific drug action)
ASSESSMENT FOCUS	Allergies to medication(s); specific drug action, side-effects, and adverse reactions; client's knowledge of and learning needs about the medication; tissue integrity of the selected site; client's age and weight to determine site and needle size; client's ability or willingness to cooperate.

EQUIPMENT

- Medication card, MAR, or computer printout
- Sterile medication (usually provided in an ampule or vial)
- Sterile syringe and needle of a size appropriate for the amount of solution to be administered
- Swab saturated in an antiseptic solution
- Gloves, if required by agency protocol

INTERVENTION

1. Verify the medication order for accuracy.

- See Technique 36–1, step 1.

2. Prepare the medication from the vial or ampule.

- See Technique 36–1, step 2.

- If the medication is particularly irritating to subcutaneous tissue, change the needle on the syringe before the injection. *Because the outside of the new needle is free of medication, it does not irritate subcutaneous tissues as it passes into the muscle.*

3. Identify the client, and assist the client to a comfortable position.

- Check the client's arm band, and ask the client to tell you his or her name.

- Assist the client to a supine, lateral, prone, or sitting position, depending on the chosen site.

- Obtain assistance to immobilize an uncooperative client or an infant or young child. The parent may hold the infant or young child (Figure 36–27). *This prevents accidental injury during the procedure.*

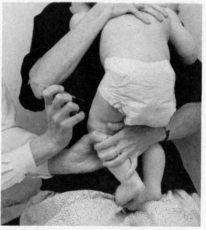

FIGURE 36–27 A parent restraining an infant during an intramuscular injection.

4. Select, locate, and clean the site.

- Select a site free of skin lesions, tenderness, swelling, hardness, or localized inflammation and one that has not been used frequently.

- If injections are to be frequent, alternate sites. If necessary, discuss with the prescribing physician an alternative method of providing the medication.

- Determine whether the size of the muscle is appropriate to the amount of medication to be in-

jected. An average adult's deltoid muscle can usually absorb 0.5 ml of medication, although some authorities believe 2 ml can be absorbed by a well-developed deltoid muscle. The gluteus medius muscle can absorb 1 to 5 ml (Newton and Newton 1979, p. 19), although 5 ml may be very painful.

- Locate the exact site for the injection. See the discussion of sites earlier in this chapter.

- Don gloves, if required.

- Clean the site with an antiseptic swab. Using a circular motion, start at the center and move outward about 5 cm (2 in).

- Transfer and hold the swab between the third and fourth fingers of your nondominant hand in readiness for needle withdrawal.

5. Prepare the syringe for injection.

- Remove the needle cover without contaminating the needle.

- Invert the syringe, and expel excess air, leaving only 0.2 ml of air. *This technique, referred to as*

▶ **Technique 36–4** *CONTINUED*

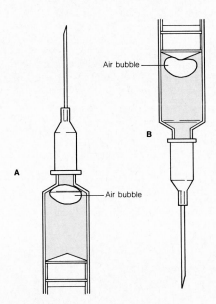

FIGURE 36–28 An air bubble in the medication in the syringe: *A*, needle pointed up; *B*, needle pointed down.

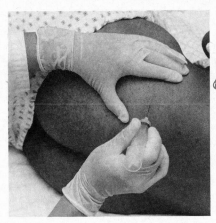

FIGURE 36–29 Administering an intramuscular injection.

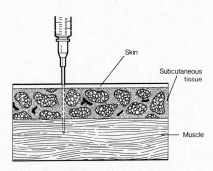

FIGURE 36–30 An intramuscular needle inserted into the muscle layer.

the air-lock or air-bubble technique, prevents tracking of the medication through sensitive subcutaneous tissues in two ways: (a) it keeps the needle clean of medication on insertion, and (b) because the air bubble moves to the end of the plunger when the needle is pointed downward, the air bubble is injected behind the medication into the tissues (Figure 36–28). This provides a seal at the point of insertion, and prevents tracking of the medication. It is particularly helpful when injecting a medication that is irritating to the skin and subcutaneous tissue.

6. Inject the medication.

• Use the nondominant hand to spread the skin at the site. Under some circumstances, e.g., for an emaciated client or an infant, the muscle may be pinched. *Spreading the skin or pinching the muscle makes it firmer and facilitates needle insertion.*

• Holding the syringe between the thumb and forefinger, pierce the skin quickly at a 90° angle (Figure 36–29), and insert the needle

into the muscle (Figure 36–30). *Using a quick motion lessens the client's discomfort.*

• Aspirate by holding the barrel of the syringe steady with your nondominant hand and by pulling back on the plunger with your dominant hand. If blood appears in the syringe, withdraw the needle, discard the syringe, and prepare a new injection. *This step determines whether the needle has been inserted into a blood vessel.*

• If blood does not appear, inject the medication steadily and slowly, holding the syringe steady. *Injecting medication slowly permits it to disperse into the muscle tissue, thus decreasing the client's discomfort. Holding the syringe steady minimizes discomfort.*

7. Withdraw the needle quickly, and massage the site.

• See Technique 36–3, step 7.

8. Discard the uncapped needle and attached syringe into the proper receptacle.

• Remove gloves if worn.

9. Document all relevant information.

• Include the time of administration, drug name, dose, route, and the client's reactions.

VARIATION: Administering a Z-Track Injection

This variation of the standard intramuscular technique is used to administer intramuscular medications that are highly irritating to subcutaneous and skin tissues.

• Follow steps 1 through 4 above.

• Attach a new sterile needle to the syringe. *A new needle will not have any medication adhering to the outside that could be irritating to tissues.*

• Prepare an air lock (see step 5, above).

• With the nondominant hand, pull the skin and subcutaneous tissue about 2.5 to 3.5 cm (1 to 1¼ in) to one side at the injection site (Figure 36–31 on page 874).

• Insert the syringe and medication as in step 6. Withdraw the plunger with the dominant hand while holding the syringe to ascertain placement of the needle.

• Maintain the traction for 10 seconds before withdrawing the needle, and then permit the skin to return to its normal position. *This provides a seal over the injected medication, thus preventing tracking to subcutaneous tissues.*

• Do not massage the site. *This can lead to tissue irritation.*

► **Technique 36–4 Administering an Intramuscular Injection** *CONTINUED*

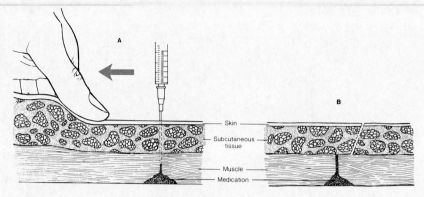

FIGURE 36–31 Inserting the needle using the Z-track method: *A*, skin pulled to the side; *B*, skin released.

EVALUATION FOCUS

Desired effect (e.g., relief of pain or vomiting, reduction in body temperature); any adverse reactions or side-effects.

SAMPLE RECORDING

Date	Time	Notes
08/07/93	1500	C/o general malaise and headache. T-39.9, P-92, R-22 and shallow. States pain in L lower posterior chest when breathing. Has dry hacking nonproductive cough. Cloxacillin 60 mg given I.M. in L ventrogluteal site. ————————— Molly McIntyre, RN

KEY ELEMENTS OF ADMINISTERING AN INTRAMUSCULAR INJECTION

See the Key Elements of Technique 36–1 on page 861. In addition:

- Select a needle size appropriate for the client.
- Select an appropriate muscle, one that has not been used frequently, has healthy intact skin, and adequate muscle mass.
- Locate the correct site for the injection.
- Position the client appropriately.
- Immobilize the injection site of a confused client or infant or young child prior to needle insertion.
- Don gloves as agency protocol indicates.
- Expel air from the syringe before administration unless the air-bubble technique is used.
- Aspirate for blood before injecting the medication.
- Minimize discomfort:

  a. Spread the skin at the site before inserting the needle.

  b. Insert the needle quickly.

  c. Hold the syringe steady.

  d. Inject the medication slowly and steadily.

  e. Remove the needle quickly while depressing the skin.

- Use the Z-track technique for medications that irritate subcutaneous tissues:

  a. Attach a new sterile needle before injection.

  b. Pull the skin to one side before the needle is inserted.

  c. Maintain the skin traction for 10 seconds before withdrawing the needle.

  d. Do not massage the site after the injection.

Intradermal Injections

An intradermal injection is the administration of a drug into the dermal layer of the skin just beneath the epidermis. Usually only a small amount of liquid is used, for example, 0.01 to 0.1 ml. This method of administration is frequently indicated for allergy and tuberculin tests and for vaccinations. Common sites for intradermal injections are the inner lower arm, the upper chest, and the back beneath the scapulae (Figure 36–32). For children, the medial thigh is sometimes used. Commonly the left arm is used for tuberculin tests, and the right arm is used for all other tests. Technique 36–5 details the steps involved in administering an intradermal injection.

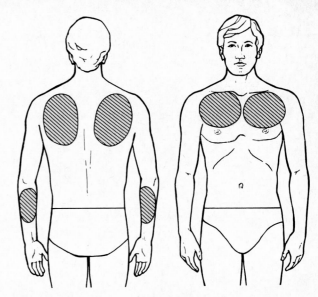

FIGURE 36–32 Body sites commonly used for intradermal injections.

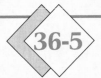 **Administering an Intradermal Injection**

| PURPOSES | • To administer a medication for sensitivity and allergy testing |
| | • To administer some types of immunizations |

| ASSESSMENT FOCUS | Appearance of injection site; specific drug action and expected response; client's knowledge of drug action and response; agency protocol about sites to use for skin tests. |

EQUIPMENT

- Medication card or computer printout
- Vial or ampule of the correct sterile medication
- Sterile 1-ml syringe calibrated into hundredths of a milliliter and a needle ¼ to ⅝ inch

long with #25, #26, or #27 gauge
- Acetone and 2 × 2 sterile gauze square (optional)
- Swab moistened with alcohol or other colorless antiseptic

- Gloves (according to agency protocol)
- Band-Aid (optional)
- Epinephrine, a bronchodilator, and antihistamine on hand

INTERVENTION

1. Verify the order.

- Check the physician's orders carefully for the medication, dosage, and route. ⓢ

2. Prepare the medication from the vial or ampule.

- See Technique 36–1.

3. Identify and prepare the client for the injection.

- Check the client's arm band, and ask the client to tell you his or ⓢ her name.

- Explain that the medication will produce a small bleb like a blister. The client will feel a slight prick as the needle enters the skin. Some medications are absorbed slowly through the capillaries into the general circula-

tion, and the bleb gradually disappears. Other drugs remain in the area and interact with the body tissues to produce redness and induration (hardening), which will need to be interpreted at a particular time, e.g., in 24 or 48 hours. This reaction will also gradually disappear.

- Restrain a confused client or an

▶

▶ **Technique 36–5 Administering an Intradermal Injection** *CONTINUED*

infant or small child. *This prevents accidental injury from sudden movement.*

4. Select and clean the site.

- Select a site (e.g., the forearm about a hand's breadth above the wrist and three or four finger-widths below the antecubital space).

- Avoid using sites that are tender, inflamed, or swollen and those that have lesions.

- Don gloves as agency protocol indicates.

- Defat the skin if agency protocol dictates, using a gauze square or swab moistened with acetone. Start at the center and widen the circle outward.

- Using the same method, clean the site with a swab moistened with alcohol or other colorless antiseptic, according to agency protocol. Allow the area to dry thoroughly. *A colorless antiseptic does not hinder the reading of the test.*

5. Prepare the syringe for injection.

- Remove the needle cap while waiting for the antiseptic to dry.

- Expel any air bubbles from the syringe. Small bubbles that adhere to the plunger are of no consequence. *A small amount of air will not harm the tissues.*

- Grasp the syringe in your dominant hand, holding it between thumb and four fingers, with

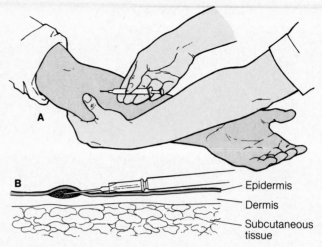

FIGURE 36–33 For an intradermal injection: *A*, the needle enters the skin at a 15° angle; and *B*, the medication forms a bleb under the epidermis.

your palm upward. Hold the needle at a 15° angle to the skin surface, with the bevel of the needle up.

6. Inject the fluid.

- With the nondominant hand, pull the skin at the site until it is taut, and thrust the tip of the needle firmly through the epidermis into the dermis (Figure 36–33, *A*). Do *not* aspirate.

- Inject the medication carefully so that it produces a small bleb on the skin (Figure 36–33, *B*).

- Withdraw the needle quickly while providing countertraction on the skin, and apply a Band-Aid if indicated.

- Do *not* massage the area. *Massage can disperse the medication into the tissue or out through the needle insertion site.*

- Dispose of the syringe and needle safely.

- Remove gloves, if worn.

7. Document all relevant information.

- Record the testing subtance given, the time, dosage, route, site, and nursing assessments.

8. Assess the client.

- Evaluate the client's response to the testing substance. *Some medications used in testing may cause allergic reactions.* An antidotal drug (e.g., epinephrine hydrochloride), may need to be given.

- Evaluate the condition of the site in 24 or 48 hours, depending on the test. Measure and record the area of redness and induration in millimeters at the largest diameter.

EVALUATION FOCUS	Client's response; size of induration and redness at the injection site. See step 8.

▶ **Technique 36-5** *CONTINUED*

SAMPLE RECORDING

Date	Time	Notes
02/26/93	1500	Tuberculin skin test (0.1 ml) administered intradermally in inner aspect of L forearm. No adverse systemic or local response. ————————————————————— Maureen Kirkpatrick, RN
02/28/93	1500	Small wheal (4 mm in diameter) formed. ——— Maureen Kirkpatrick, RN

KEY ELEMENTS OF ADMINISTERING AN INTRADERMAL INJECTION

See the Key Elements of Technique 36-1 on page 861. In addition:

- Explain the reactions that may occur and when the reaction is to be assessed.
- Select the correct site that has healthy, intact skin.
- Restrain the confused client or infant or small child prior to needle insertion.
- Don gloves as agency protocol indicates.
- Use alcohol or other *colorless* antiseptic to disinfect the site.

- Remove excess air from the syringe before the injection.
- Pull the skin taut before the injection.
- Thrust the needle in firmly with the bevel up.
- Inject the medication carefully.
- Withdraw the needle quickly while pressing down on the adjacent skin.
- Do not massage the area.
- Safely dispose of the syringe and needle.

Intravenous Medications

Because intravenous (IV) medications enter the client's bloodstream directly, they are appropriate when a rapid effect is required (e.g., in a life-threatening situation such as cardiac arrest). This route is also appropriate when medications are too irritating to tissues to be given by other routes. When an intravenous line is already established, this route is desirable because it avoids the discomfort of other parenteral routes. Medications are administered intravenously via the following:

- Bottle or bag (continuous infusion)
- Additional container (intermittent infusion by piggyback [IVPB] or partial fill [IVPF])
- Volume-control administration set (often used for children)
- Intravenous push (IVP or bolus)

Other IV drug delivery systems are shown in Table 36-1 on page 878.

There are potential hazards in giving intravenous medications: infection, rapid severe reactions to the medication, and fluid volume overload. The nurse must dilute medication in the smallest possible volume, particularly when administering medication and fluid to infants, small children, elderly clients, or clients with renal failure or heart disease.

To prevent infection, the nurse uses sterile technique during all aspects of administering intravenous medication. To safeguard the client against severe reactions, the nurse must administer the drug slowly, following the manufacturer's recommendations. The nurse assesses the client closely during the administration and discontinues the medication immediately if an untoward reaction occurs.

Technique 36-6 on page 879 describes how to add medications to intravenous fluid containers. To administer intravenous medications using additive sets, see Technique 36-7 on page 882.

TABLE 36–1   IV DRUG DELIVERY SYSTEMS*

System	Description	
Minibag	A reconstituted drug is added to a small plastic bag containing diluent.	
ADD-Vantage	A vital containing the medication is attached to a partially filled IV bag. The nurse must break at the bedside an internal seal that separates the drug from the fluid and then mix the drug and diluent before administration.	
Ready-to-use (RTU) premix	The drug and diluent are premixed in a plastic bag. Less stable drugs may be frozen and must be thawed before use.	
Drug manufacturer's piggyback (DMPB)	The container is prefilled with a single dose of medication to which diluent must be added.	
CRIS adapter	A two-position valve is placed in the primary IV line below the IV container. To this a vial of reconstituted drug is directly attached.	
Minisyringe pump	The reconstituted drug is withdrawn into a syringe. Medication is delivered by mechanical pressure on the syringe plunger.	

*All systems are attached to a check valve Y-site on the primary IV line, *except* the CRIS adapter, which is attached between the IV container and drip chamber.

36-6 Adding Medications to Intravenous Fluid Containers

PURPOSES
- To provide and maintain a constant level of a medication in the blood
- To administer well-diluted medications at a continuous and slow rate

ASSESSMENT FOCUS

Signs of infiltration, infection, or a dislodged needle at the infusion site; redness, pallor, swelling, coldness or edema of the surrounding tissues; vital signs for baseline data; allergies to medications; compatibility of medication(s) and IV fluid.

EQUIPMENT

- Medication card, MAR, or computer printout
- Correct sterile medication
- Diluent for medication in powdered form (see manufacturer's instructions)
- Correct solution container, if a new one is to be attached
- Antiseptic swabs
- Sterile syringe of appropriate size (e.g., 5 or 10 ml) and a 1-
- to 1½-inch, #20 or #21 gauge sterile needle
- Medication label

INTERVENTION

1. Verify the medication order for accuracy, and confirm the compatibility of the drugs and solutions being mixed.

- Check the physician's orders carefully for the medication, dosage, and route. Verify which infusions are to be used with the medication. For example, the order may say to infuse the medication with 1000 ml of 5% dextrose and water rather than with normal saline.

- Consult a pharmacist, if required, to confirm compatibility of the drugs and solutions being mixed.

2. Prepare the medication from a vial or ampule.

- See Technique 36–1, step 2.

- Check the agency's practice for using a special filter needle to withdraw premixed liquid medications from multidose vials or ampules.

3. Confirm the sterility of the solution container (if a new one is to be attached), and locate and clean the injection port.

- Be sure that the solution container has no cracks or leaks, that the fluid is not discolored or has visible particles, that the seal is undamaged, and that the date on the container has not expired.

- For a vented glass container, remove the metal cap and the rubber disc to locate the injection port. An injection port may be designated in several ways, e.g., by a triangle, cross, or circle. Do *not* inject medication through the port for the administration spike or through an air vent port if there is an injection port.

or

For a plastic container, locate the separate, self-sealing, soft rubber injection port.

- Clean the injection port with an antiseptic swab. *This reduces the risk of introducing microorganisms into the container when the needle is inserted.*

4. Inject the medication into the container.

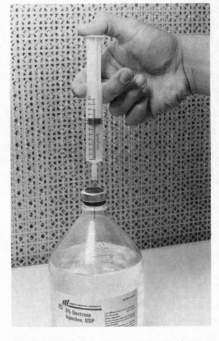

FIGURE 36–34 Inserting a medication into an intravenous bottle.

- Remove the needle cover from the medication syringe, and inject the medication into the port (Figure 36–34).

- Withdraw the needle.

- For a glass container, cover the

▶ **Technique 36–6 Adding Medications to IV Fluid Containers** *CONTINUED*

top immediately either with (a) an antiseptic swab with the metal IV cap taped over it or (b) the special sterile cap provided by the manufacturer. *An open tubing port increases the risk of fluid contamination by microorganisms. Plastic containers have self-sealing ports.*

5. Attach a medication label.

- Apply the medication label to the fluid container so it can be easily read when the container is hanging up.

- See Figure 36–35 for the information to be included on the medication label.

MEDICATION ADDED
PATIENT *Mendoza, Paula S.* RM. *207-A*
DRUG *K-Cl*
AMOUNT *40 mEq*
ADDED BY *N.W. Armstrong, R.N.*
DATE *12/5/93*   TIME *0900*
START TIME *0900* DATE *12/5/93* FLOW RATE *40*
EXP. DATE ———
THIS LABEL MUST BE AFFIXED TO ALL INFUSION FLUIDS CONTAINING ADDITIONAL MEDICATION

FIGURE 36–35 A medication label for an intravenous infusion.

6. Establish the infusion.

- Spike and hang the container.

- Regulate the flow rate according to the dosage required. *This prevents rapid infusion of the medication and fluid and subsequent complications.*

7. Document all relevant information.

- Record the type and amount of solution, medication and dose added, and times of starting and completing the infusion. Some agencies have a special parenteral fluid form for this purpose.

- Record fluid volume on the intake and output record.

8. Monitor the client and the infusion.

- During the administration, observe the client for signs of an adverse reaction, such as noisy respirations, changes in pulse rate, chills, nausea, or headache. If any adverse sign occurs, follow agency policy (i.e., slow rate or stop flow), and notify the physician or nurse in charge. Also monitor the client for signs of the intended action of the medication.

- Carefully monitor the infusion to maintain delivery of the medication and fluid at the specified rate.

VARIATION: Adding Medications to an Infusing Container

IV Container with a Vented Administration Set (Nonvented Container)

- Make sure there is sufficient solution in the bottle to ensure proper dilution of the drug.

- Close the IV flow clamp. *Closing the clamp is essential to prevent the medication from infusing to the client before it is properly diluted with the solution. Undiluted medication can produce a severe reaction.*

- Detach the air vent cap, taking care not to contaminate the end.

- Insert the tip of the medication syringe, *without the needle,* into the air vent port (Figure 36–36).

- Instill the medication.

- Reattach the air vent.

Vented IV bottle

- After ensuring that there is sufficient solution in the bottle, close the IV flow clamp.

- Clean the medication port with an antiseptic swab and allow it

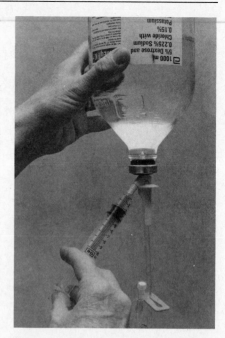

FIGURE 36–36 Instilling a medication into a hanging intravenous bottle.

to dry completely.

- Insert the needle through the port and instill the medication. The medication port is usually marked (e.g., by a triangular imprint).

Plastic IV Bag

- After ensuring that there is sufficient solution in the bag, close the IV flow clamp.

- Clean the medication port with an antiseptic swab and allow it to dry completely.

- While supporting and stabilizing the bag with your thumb and forefinger, carefully insert the syringe needle through the port, and inject the medication (Figure 36–37). *The bag is supported during the injection of the medication to avoid punctures.*

VARIATION: Using a Transfer Needle

A special transfer needle (Figure 36–38) can be used to put medications in vials into a *plastic* IV container, provided the entire amount

▶ **Technique 36–6** *CONTINUED*

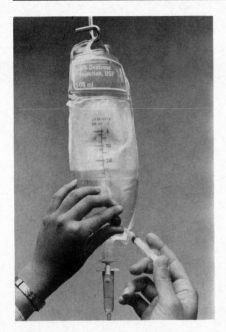

FIGURE 36–37   Instilling a medication into a hanging intravenous bag.

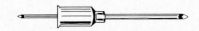

FIGURE 36–38   A transfer needle.

of medication is to be transferred to the IV container. After cleaning the top of the medication vial and the medication port on the IV bag with an antiseptic sponge, insert the small end of the transfer needle into the medication vial and the large end into the port of the IV container. To mix the medication and solution:

• Invert the bag, so that the medication bottle is on top.

• Gently squeeze the bag to transmit some air from the bag into the medication vial.

• Release the pressure on the bag

to allow medication to drain into the bag.

• Repeat squeezing and releasing pressure until all the medication is transferred into the IV solution. The transfer needle may need to be pulled down so that all the medication is obtained from the vial.

• Remove the needle, and gently rotate the bag to disperse the medication.

For All Infusing Methods

• Attach a medication label to the IV container.

• Gently lift and rotate the container to mix the solution and medication.

• Follow steps 6 through 8.

EVALUATION FOCUS

Desired effect of the medication; any adverse reactions or side-effects; change in vital signs; status of the IV site; patency of the IV infusion.

SAMPLE RECORDING

Date	Time	Notes
11/02/93	1045	1000 ml IV D_5 W started with 40 mEq of potassium chloride added. IV regulated at 40 gtts/min. —————————————— Martin Gregory, RN

KEY ELEMENTS OF ADDING MEDICATIONS TO INTRAVENOUS FLUID CONTAINERS

See the Key Elements of Technique 36–1 on page 861. In addition:

• Verify which infusions are to receive medications.

• Confirm the compatibility of the medication and IV solution and equipment.

• Maintain sterility of the IV and medication equipment.

• Attach appropriate medication labels to the IV container.

• When adding medications to infusing containers:

   a. Make sure there is sufficient solution to dilute the drug.

   b. Clamp the IV tubing before adding medications.

   c. Insert medications only through designated medication ports.

   d. If using an air vent port, insert the medication syringe *without the needle.*

36-7 Administering Intravenous Medications Using Additive Sets

Additive sets, i.e., the piggyback alignment and tandem setup, are discussed in Chapter 25, pages 592–593.

PURPOSES

- To intermittently administer IV drugs that cannot be mixed with the primary solution for reasons of incompatibility
- To administer different IV drugs at different times
- To maintain peak levels of a medication in the client's bloodstream by simultaneous infusion

ASSESSMENT FOCUS

See Assessment Focus for Technique 36–6 on page 879.

EQUIPMENT

- Physician's order, medication card, or MAR
- Medication label
- Antiseptic swab
- Sterile needle, syringe, and saline, if medication is incompatible with the primary infusion
- Adhesive tape

Piggyback
- 50- to 100-ml infusion bag with medication (most piggybacks are prepared by the pharmacist)
- Microdrip or macrodrip infusion set
- Needle (1-in, #21 or #23 gauge)
- Extension hook

Tandem Setup
- Solution container with medication added
- Long secondary tubing set

INTERVENTION

 1. Verify the medication order for accuracy, and confirm the compatibility of the medication.

- See Technique 36–1, step 1.

2. Add the medication to the additive set, if required.

- Prepare the medication from an ampule or vial. See Technique 36–1, step 2.

- Add the medication to the additional container. See Technique 36–6, step 4.

- Apply the medication label.

3. Assemble the secondary infusion.

- Spike the secondary infusion container.

- Hang the secondary container at or above the level of the primary infusion. Use the extension hook

to lower the primary infusion if a piggyback setup is required.

- Attach the 1-inch needle to the tubing, prime the tubing, and close the clamp.

4. Attach the secondary infusion to the primary infusion.

- Clean the Y-port on the primary IV line with an antiseptic swab. Clean the *primary port* (that furthest from the client) for a piggyback alignment and the *secondary port* (that closest to the client) for a tandem setup.

- If the medication is *not* compatible with the primary infusion, flush the primary line with a sterile saline solution before attaching the secondary set. To flush the line, wipe the port with an antiseptic swab, clamp the pri-

mary line, and, using a sterile needle and syringe, instill a few milliliters of sterile saline solution through the port to wash any primary infusion fluid out of the infusion tubing.

- Insert the needle of the secondary line through the injection port of the primary line.

- Secure the needle with adhesive tape. *Tape prevents needle dislodgment.* Some agencies recommend that a needle guard be taped alongside the needle to support the needle placement and keep the needle guard handy for use when discontinuing the secondary attachment.

- Attach appropriate label to the tubing.

5. Administer the medication.

► **Technique 36–7** *CONTINUED*

Piggyback

- Ensure that the primary line is unclamped if the port has a back-check valve. *The valve automatically stops the flow of the primary infusion while the additive set infuses and automatically starts it running after the piggyback solution has been administered.*

- Open the clamp on the piggyback line, and regulate it in accordance with the recommended rate for that medication. Usually, medications are administered in 30 to 60 minutes.

Tandem Infusion

- Open the clamp on the secondary line, and regulate its flow.

- For *continuous* infusion, set the secondary solution to the appropriate drip rate for the medication, and then adjust the primary solution to achieve the desired total infusion flow.

- For *intermittent* infusion, clamp the primary line and adjust the primary drip rate after the secondary solution is completed.

6. Document relevant data.

- Record the date, time, medication, dose, route, and solution; assessments of IV site, if appropriate; and client response.

- Enter fluid intake according to agency protocol.

EVALUATION FOCUS

See Evaluation Focus for Technique 36–6 on page 881.

SAMPLE RECORDING

Date	Time	Notes
06/07/93	1530	Aminophylline 500 mg. started as ordered via piggyback set up. ———— ———— Roberta Ness, RN

KEY ELEMENTS OF ADMINISTERING INTRAVENOUS MEDICATIONS USING ADDITIVE SETS

See the Key Elements of Technique 36–1 on page 861. In addition:

- Confirm the compatibility of the medication with the primary IV solution.

- Maintain the sterility of the IV medication and equipment.

- Attach an appropriate medication label to the additive set and an appropriate label to the tubing.

- Flush the primary IV line with saline if the medication is incompatible.

- Secure the additive line to the primary line with adhesive tape.

- Monitor the infusion to ensure the correct delivery rate of the medication and IV fluid(s).

Volume-Control Sets

Intermittent medications may also be administered by **volume-control sets** (e.g., Buretrol, Soluset, Volutrol, Pediatrol). They are small fluid containers (100 to 150 ml in size) attached below the primary infusion container. Volume-control sets are equipped with either a stationary membrane filter or a floating valve filter at the base of the container and are designed for fine control of the amount of infusing fluid. See Figure 25–23 on page 609. Technique 36–8 describes how to administer intravenous medications using volume-control sets.

36-8 Administering Intravenous Medications Using Volume-Control Administration Sets

PURPOSES

- To administer intravenous medications (such as some antibiotics) that do not remain stable for the length of time it takes an entire solution container to infuse
- To administer medications intermittently
- To avoid mixing medications that are incompatible
- To dilute a drug so that it is less irritating to the veins than if given by direct intravenous push
- To deliver medications diluted in precise amounts of fluid

ASSESSMENT FOCUS

See Technique 36–6 on page 879.

EQUIPMENT

- Physician's order, medication card, or MAR
- Correct sterile medication
- Antiseptic swabs
- Sterile syringe of appropriate size (e.g., 5 or 10 ml)
- 1- to 1½-inch, #20 or #21 gauge, sterile needle
- Sterile filter needle if needed to withdraw the medication
- Volume-control administration set
- Correct solution container
- Medication label for the volume-control set

INTERVENTION

1. Verify the medication order, and confirm the compatibility of the medication.

- See Technique 36–1, step 1.

2. Prepare the medication from an ampule or vial.

- See Technique 36–1, step 2.

3. Attach the volume-control set to the infusion container.

- Insert the spike of the volume-control set into the solution container, and hang the container on the pole.
- Open the air vent clamp on the volume-control set.
- Position the lower clamp on the tubing below the drip chamber, and clamp it.

4. Fill the volume-control device, and prime the tubing.

Set with a Stationary Membrane Filter

- Open the upper clamp, and allow the fluid chamber to fill with about 30 ml of solution, then close this clamp.
- Open the lower clamp, and flatten the drip chamber with two fingers and the thumb of your opposite hand. *The membrane filter can be damaged if the drip chamber is squeezed while the lower clamp is closed.*
- While keeping the drip chamber flattened, close the lower clamp. *These actions create a vacuum, so that solution from the fluid chamber will then flow into the drip chamber.*
- Release your pressure on the drip chamber, and reshape it until it becomes about half full.

- Repeat the above steps as necessary.
- Open the lower clamp, prime the tubing, and close the clamp.

Set with a Floating Valve Filter

- Open the upper clamp, and squeeze the fluid chamber until it is filled with about 30 ml of solution.
- Close the clamp, and again gently squeeze the drip chamber until it is about half full.
- Open the lower clamp, prime the tubing, and close the clamp.

5. Administer the medication.

- Ensure that there is sufficient fluid in the volume-control fluid chamber to dilute the medication. Generally, 50 to 100 ml of fluid is used. Check the direc-

► **Technique 36–8** *CONTINUED*

tions from the drug manufacturer or consult the pharmacist.

- Close the inflow to the fluid chamber by adjusting the upper roller or slide clamp above the fluid chamber; also ensure that the clamp on the air vent of the chamber is open.

- Clean the medication port on the volume-control fluid chamber with an antiseptic swab.

- Insert the needle of the medication syringe into the port (Figure 36–39).

- Inject the medication.

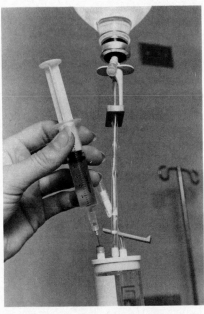

FIGURE 36–39 Adding medication to the port of a volume-control administration set.

- Gently rotate the fluid chamber until the fluid is well mixed.

- Open the line's upper clamp, and regulate the flow by adjusting the lower roller or slide clamp below the fluid chamber.

6. Attach a medication label to the volume-control fluid chamber.

7. Document relevant data, and monitor the client and the infusion.

- See Technique 36–6, steps 7 and 8 on page 880.

EVALUATION FOCUS	See Technique 36–6 on page 881.

SAMPLE RECORDING

Date	Time	Notes
08/07/93	1000	Vibramycin 4.4. mg added to volume control set containing 100 ml Lactated Ringer's solution from primary container. Infusion rate set at 60 gtts/min. IV running well. IV site free of signs of infiltration. —— Robyn Napp, RN

KEY ELEMENTS OF ADMINISTERING INTRAVENOUS MEDICATIONS USING VOLUME-CONTROL ADMINISTRATION SETS

See the Key Elements of Technique 36–1 on page 861. In addition:

- Confirm the compatibility of the medication and IV solution.
- Maintain the sterility of the IV and medication equipment.
- Prime the volume-control set according to its type of filter.
- Attach an appropriate medication label to the volume-control set and appropriate tubing label.

- Before inserting the medication:
  a. Make sure there is sufficient solution in the volume-control set to dilute the medication.
  b. Close the inflow clamp.
  c. Clean the medication port with an antiseptic swab.
- Insert the medication through the appropriate port.
- Regulate the flow appropriately.

Intravenous Push

An **intravenous push (IVP** or **bolus)** is the intravenous administration of a medication that cannot be diluted or that is needed in an emergency. Also, certain drugs are administered this way to achieve maximum effect. It is important to remember that the rapid administration of an IVP could be dangerous for the client. An IVP can be administered directly into a vein through venipuncture, into an existing intravenous apparatus through an injection port (Figure 36–40 in Technique 36–9), or through an intermittent infusion set (heparin lock) when the client does not have an IV running but does have a heparin lock in place. The heparin lock (Figure 36–41 in Technique 36–9), also called a male adapter plug (MAP), is used primarily for clients who require regular intermittent intravenous medications but not the fluid volume of an intravenous infusion. The set usually consists of an indwelling catheter attached to a plastic tube with a sealed injection tip. It is called a **heparin lock** because small amounts of heparin are injected into the catheter to maintain its patency. Some agencies now recommend that saline, rather than heparin, be used. After administering an IVP, the nurse discards the used syringe and needle in a designated container without recapping the needle, as for any other type of injection. See Technique 36–9.

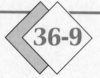

36-9 Administering Intravenous Medications Using IV Push

PURPOSE
- To achieve immediate and maximum effects of a medication

ASSESSMENT FOCUS

Signs of infiltration or infection at the infusion site or heparin lock insertion site; redness, pallor, or swelling of the surrounding skin; coldness and edema of the surrounding tissues; vital signs for baseline data; allergies to medications; compatibility of medication(s) and IV fluid; specific drug action; side-effects; normal dosage; recommended administration time; time of peak of action.

EQUIPMENT

- Physician's order, medication card, or MAR
- Correct sterile medication
- Sterile syringe of the appropriate size for the volume of medication
- Gloves, if required by agency protocol

- Antiseptic swabs
- Sterile 2.5-cm (1-in) #25 gauge needle to prevent large puncture holes in the injection port

In Addition, for a Heparin Lock:
- Sterile syringe and needle with a heparin flush solution (optional)
- One or two syringes and needles, each with 2 ml (or amount prescribed by the agency) of normal saline

---

INTERVENTION

1. Verify the medication order.

- Check the physician's order carefully for the medication, dosage, route, and rate of administration. Medication rate may also come from the agency, pharmacy, or manufacturer's insert. *A medication that is injected too rapidly can create toxic concentrations in the blood plasma.*

2. Prepare the medication and heparin and/or saline as required.

- Prepare the medication according to Technique 36–1. Label the syringe with the name of the medication and the dosage if other syringes for the heparin lock are needed.

- In a separate syringe, prepare the heparin solution according to agency practice, if needed. Many hospital protocols include the use of 100 units/ml of solu-

▶ **Technique 36–9** *CONTINUED*

tion, and 0.5 ml or 1.0 ml is injected. Label this syringe. A prepackaged heparin syringe may be used.

- In other syringes, prepare the saline solution if needed. Label these syringes.

3. Administer the medication.

To Administer Medication into an Existing Line

💧 • Don gloves, if required by agency protocol.

- Inspect the injection site for any signs of infiltration, then identify an injection port nearest the client. Some ports have a circle indicating the site for the needle insertion. *An injection port must be used because it is self-sealing. Any puncture to the plastic tubing will leak.*

- Clean the port with an antiseptic swab.

- Stop the IV flow by closing the clamp or pinching the tubing above the injection port (Figure 36–40).

- While holding the port steady, insert the needle into the port.

- Draw back on the plunger to withdraw some blood into the IV tubing (not into the syringe) *This shows that the needle or catheter is in the vein.*

- Inject the medication at the ordered rate, withdraw the needle, reopen the clamp, and reestablish the intravenous infusion at the correct rate. If the medication is particularly irritating to the veins, run the IV rapidly for about a minute to dilute the medication, and then adjust the rate.

To Administer Medication into an Intermittent Infusion Set

- Swab the injection port with an antiseptic swab and permit it to dry.

- Insert the needle attached to the normal saline syringe into the port, and aspirate for blood return (Figure 36–41). *This ensures that the heparin lock catheter is in the vein. In some situations, blood will not return*

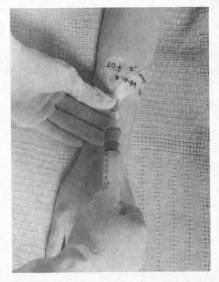

FIGURE 36–41 Administering medication through an intermittent infusion set.

even though the heparin lock is patent.

- Inject ½ to 2 ml of normal saline. This step is *optional.* Check agency practice. *This is done to flush the heparin from the catheter and to verify patency of the vein.* If the client experiences a burning or stinging sensation, this may be normal, or it may indicate that the needle or catheter is not in the vein and the fluid is infiltrating the tissue. In this case, withhold the medication until the heparin lock is replaced.

- Remove the saline syringe.

- Insert the needle attached to the medication syringe into the injection port.

- Inject the medication slowly at the recommended rate of infusion. Observe the client closely for adverse reactions. Remove the needle and syringe when all medication is administered.

- Attach the second saline syringe, and inject the recommended amount of saline. *The saline injection flushes the medication through the catheter and prepares*

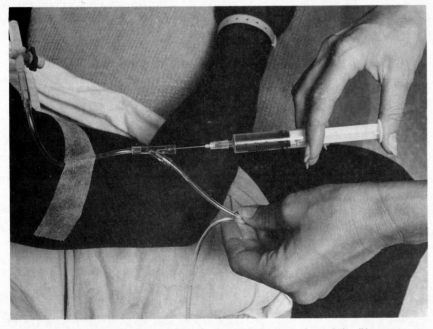

FIGURE 36–40 Administering medication through an injection port of an existing IV apparatus.

▶

▶ **Technique 36–9 Administering IV Medications Using IV Push** *CONTINUED*

the lock for the heparin. Heparin is incompatible with many medications.

- If heparin is to be used, insert the heparin syringe, and inject the heparin slowly into the set (Figure 36–42).

- Check the patency of the heparin lock at least every 8 hours or according to agency practice.

  a. Aspirate for return blood flow.

  b. Flush the catheter with ½ to 2 ml of normal saline.

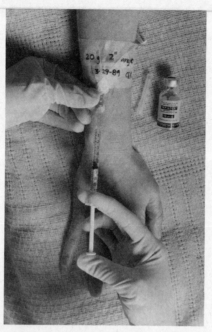

FIGURE 36–42 Injecting heparin into an intermittent infusion set.

  c. Refill the heparin lock with new heparin solution (optional).

- Check agency practice about recommended times for changing the heparin lock. Some agencies advocate a change every 48 to 72 hours.

4. Document all relevant information.

- Record the date, time, drug, dose, and route; client response; and assessments of infusion or heparin lock site if appropriate.

EVALUATION FOCUS

Desired effect of medication; any adverse reactions or side-effects; change in vital signs; status of IV or heparin lock site; patency of IV infusion, if running.

SAMPLE RECORDING

Date	Time	Notes
10/06/93	1930	Fluorouracil 400 mg administered by IV push as ordered. – Meg Tully, RN

KEY ELEMENTS OF ADMINISTERING INTRAVENOUS MEDICATIONS USING IV PUSH

See the Key Elements of Technique 36–1 on page 861. In addition:

- Determine the correct dosage and rate of administration.
- Maintain the sterility of the IV and medication equipment.
- Inspect the infusion site for signs of infiltration.

IV Push into an Existing IV

- Use the injection port nearest the client.
- Stop the IV flow before the injection.
- Aspirate for blood before the injection.

IV Push into an Intermittent Infusion Set

- Label all syringes accurately, i.e., the specific medication and dose, the saline solution, and the heparin solution.
- Aspirate for blood return before the injection.
- Inject solutions in the proper sequence: saline (optional), the medication, the saline solution, and lastly the heparin solution.
- Maintain the patency of the heparin lock.

All Methods

- Inject the medication at the proper rate.

CRITICAL THINKING CHALLENGE

Jeremy Gregor, a 68-year-old client on the surgical unit, has been receiving intramuscular medication for several days. He complains to you that it always hurts when he receives his medication. What can you say? What are the possible reasons for his pain? What can you do to minimize his discomfort?

RELATED RESEARCH

Beecroft, P. C., and Redick, S. July/August 1989. Possible complications of intramuscular injections on the pediatric unit. *Pediatric Nursing* 15:333–36, 376.

Keen, M. F. July/August 1986. Comparison of intramuscular injection techniques to reduce site discomfort and lesions. *Nursing Research* 35:207–10.

Keen, M. F., Bomber, D., and Baer, C. 1989. *Using nursing research: Comparison of intramuscular injection techniques to reduce site discomfort and lesions . . .* The Z track technique. NLN Publication No. 15–2232. pp. 63–69, 70–73, 73–77. New York: National League for Nursing.

REFERENCES

American Diabetic Association. April 1992. Clinical practice recommendations (1991–92): Continuous subcutaneous insulin infusion. *Diabetes Care* 15 (suppl 2): 34–35.

Byington, K. C. 1991. Your guide to pediatric drug administration. *Nursing 1991* 21(8): 82, 84, 86–89.

Cohen, M. R. March 1990. Taking this test will help you avoid errors. *Nursing 90* 20:23–24.

McCrea, D., and McCrea, C. August 1991. Emergency department care of the patient with an insulin pump. *Journal of Emergency Nursing* 17(4): 220–24.

Newton, D. W., and Newton, M. July 1979. Route, site, and technique: Three key decisions in giving parenteral medication. *Nursing 79* 9:18–21, 23, 25.

Pitel, M. January 1971. The subcutaneous injection. *American Journal of Nursing* 71:76–79.

Tomkey, D. June 1989. Tapping the full power of insulin pumps. *RN* 52:46–48.

Wiggins, M. S., and Sesin, P. April 1990. Guidelines for administering I.V. drugs. *Nursing 90* 20:145–52.

Stress Management

37

OBJECTIVES

- Differentiate the concepts of stress as a stimulus, as a response, and as a transaction

- Identify Selye's definition of stress

- Describe the three stages of Selye's general adaptation syndrome

- Describe essential aspects of the Lazarus stress model

- Identify developmental stressors throughout life

- Identify relevant data to assess stress and coping

- Identify clinical indicators of anxiety or stress

- Identify general guidelines to minimize a client's anxiety

- Describe interventions to help clients cope with stress

CONTENTS

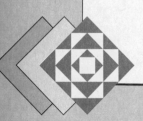

NURSING PROCESS GUIDE
STRESS AND COPING

ASSESSMENT

Determine

- How, on a scale of 1 to 10, the client rates the stress the client is experiencing in the following areas:

  a. Home
  b. Work or school
  c. Finance
  d. Recent illness or loss of loved one
  e. Health
  f. Family responsibilities
  g. Ethnic or cultural group
  h. Religion
  i. Relationships with friends
  j. Relationship with parents or children
  k. Relationship with partner
  l. Recent hospitalization
  m. Other (specify)

- How long the client has been dealing with the above stressor(s).

- How the client usually handles stressful situations:

  a. Cry?
  b. Get angry?
  c. Become verbally abusive?
  d. Talk to someone? Who?
  e. Withdraw from the situation?
  f. Structure and control others or the situation?
  g. Go for a walk or physical exercise?
  h. Try to arrive at a solution?
  i. Pray for wisdom and courage?
  j. Other (specify)?

- How the client's usual coping strategy works.

Assess clinical indicators of anxiety/stress:

- *Physiologic manifestations*: restlessness, pacing, tremors, muscle tension, rigid posture, purposeless activity, rapid pulse, increased respiratory rate, hyperventilation, heart palpitations, diaphoresis, pallor, clammy hands, dry mouth.

- *Perceptual changes*: increased awareness and attending or narrowed focus of attention, inability to focus on what is really happening.

- *Verbalization changes*: increased questioning or information seeking; expressions of concern; feelings of tension, apprehension, nervousness, severe dread; inappropriate verbalization; voice tremors and pitch changes; increased rate and quantity of speech; anger.

RELATED DIAGNOSTIC CATEGORIES

- Anxiety
- Fear
- Decisional conflict
- Defensive coping
- Ineffective individual coping
- Ineffective family coping: Compromised
- Ineffective family coping: Disabling

PLANNING

Client Goals
The client will

- Experience a reduction in the level of anxiety.
- Cope with multiple life changes.
- Receive adequate support for coping.

Outcome Criteria
The client

- Verbalizes awareness of feelings of anxiety.
- Discusses fears.
- Verbalizes fears and concerns regarding choices and responses of others.
- Keeps a log of incidents that arouse anxiety, frustration, or time urgency.
- Reports an increase in psychologic and physiologic comfort.
- Experiences a reduction in the manifestations of anxiety (specify) or in manifestations indicative of fear (e.g., tension, apprehension, panic).
- Has blood pressure and heart rate within normal range, relaxed muscles, and normal pupil size.
- Describes effective and ineffective coping behaviors and consequences.
- Identifies own coping resources.
- Uses adaptive coping methods to reduce anxiety (e.g., relaxation techniques; time management strategies; direct, open discussion; problem-solving skills).
- Identifies personal strengths (skills, knowledge, abilities) to cope with threats.
- Seeks new knowledge and skills to resolve stressful event(s).
- Demonstrates increased objectivity, ability to solve problems, and assertiveness.
- Seeks support as needed for decision making.
- Identifies and assesses available alternatives.

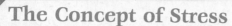

The Concept of Stress

Stress is a universal phenomenon. All people experience it. Stress can have physical, emotional, intellectual, social, and spiritual consequences. Usually, the effects are mixed, because stress affects the whole person.

Although stress is highly individual, certain stressors are common to many people at specific periods in life. See Table 37–1. In addition, pain may be considered a stressor that can occur at any time in a person's life.

Stress is defined in a number of ways: as a stimulus, as a response, and as a transaction.

Stress as a Stimulus

Stress may be defined as a **stimulus**, a life event (sometimes called a "life change") or set of circumstances causing a disrupted response (Lyon and Werner 1987) that increases the individual's vulnerability to illness. Scales have been developed to rate the stress associated with a person's relatively recent experiences, such as divorce, pregnancy, and retirement. A numerical value is assigned to each event.

TABLE 37–1   SELECTED STRESSORS ASSOCIATED WITH DEVELOPMENTAL STAGES

Developmental Stage	Stressors
Child	Resolving conflict between independence and dependence Beginning school Establishing peer relationships and adjustments Coping with peer competition
Adolescent	Accepting changing body physique Developing heterosexual or other relationships Achieving independence Choosing a career
Young adult	Getting married Leaving home Managing a home Getting started in an occupation Continuing one's education Rearing children
Middle adult	Accepting physical changes of aging Maintaining social status and standard of living Helping teenage children to become independent Adjusting to aging parents
Older adult	Accepting decreasing physical abilities and health Accepting changes in residence Adjusting to retirement and reduced income Adjusting to death of spouse and friends

On this view, both positive and negative events are considered stressful.

It is important to caution people about the use of these scales, because the degree of stress the event presents can be highly individual. For example, a divorce may be highly traumatic to one person and cause relatively little anxiety to another. What is important is that research has shown that people who have a high level of stress are often more prone to illness and have a lowered ability to cope with illness and subsequent stress.

Stress as a Response

Stress may also be defined as a **response**, the disruption caused by a noxious stimulus or stressor (Lyon and Werner 1987). In this definition of stress, reactions rather than events are the focus. The response view was developed by Hans Selye (1956, 1976). He defined stress as "the nonspecific response of the body to any kind of demand made upon it" (1976, p.1). Regardless of the cause, situation, or psychological interpretation of a demanding situation, Selye's stress response is characterized by the same chain or pattern of physiologic events. This nonspecific response was called the **general adaptation syndrome (GAS)**, or **stress syndrome**.

To differentiate the cause of stress from the response to stress, Selye created the term **stressor** (1976, p. 51) to denote any factor that produces stress and disturbs the body's equilibrium. Because stress is a state of the body, it can be observed only by the changes it produces in the body. This response of the body, the stress syndrome or general adaptation syndrome, occurs with the release of certain adaptive hormones and subsequent changes in the structure and chemical composition of the body. Body organs affected by stress are the gastrointestinal tract, the adrenals, and the lymphatic structures. With prolonged stress, the adrenals enlarge considerably; the lymphatic structures, such as the thymus, spleen, and lymph nodes atrophy (shrink) and deep ulcers appear in the lining of the stomach. In addition to adapting globally, the body can also react locally; i.e., one organ or a part of the body reacts alone. This is referred to as the **local adaptation syndrome**, or **LAS**. One example of the LAS is inflammation.

Stress as a Transaction

Transactional theories of stress are based on the work of Lazarus (1966). The Lazarus **transactional stress theory** encompasses a set of cognitive, affective, and adaptive (coping) responses that arise out of person-environment transactions. The person and the environment are inseparable; each affects and is affected by the other. **Stress**, in this context, is defined as a particular relationship between the person and the environment that is appraised by the person as taxing or exceeding the person's resources and endangering well-being (Lazarus and Folkman 1984, p. 19). The individual responds to perceived environmental changes by adaptive or coping responses. **Cognitive appraisal** is an evaluative process that determines why and to what extent a particular transaction or series of transactions between the person and the environment is stressful. **Coping** is the process through which the individual manages the demands of the person-environment relationship that are appraised as stressful and the emotions they generate (Lazarus and Folkman 1984, p. 19).

Strategies for Stress Management

Minimizing Anxiety

One way to reduce or perhaps eliminate anxiety is for the nurse and client to establish goals that are attainable. Clients must first recognize that they are anxious. This recognition is best brought about in an atmosphere of warmth and trust. Sometimes anxious clients react negatively to nurses because of personal frustration. In such cases, the nurse needs to understand this response and react to the behavior in a calm, accepting, and confident manner.

After clients realize that they are anxious, it is important that they discuss all the possible reasons for their anxiety. When clients can identify the cause of their anxiety, they may find it helpful to explore the cause with the objective of learning better coping strategies. The following are general nursing guidelines to minimize the client's anxiety and stress:

- *Support the client and family at a time of illness.* By conveying caring and understanding, the nurse can help clients reduce their stress. Feeling that someone else cares is a source of support to stressed people. Often families require time to talk about their worries and anxieties before they can feel assured and less stressed.

- *Orient the client to the hospital or agency.* The nurse helps the client adjust to the role change from, for example, independent wage earner to relatively dependent client. The nurse can help family members by giving information, for instance, about visiting hours and specific unit policies.

- *Give the client in a hospital some way of maintaining identity.* A person's name and clothes are important parts of the person's uniqueness as an individual. Nurses can help clients maintain identity by addressing them by the name they prefer and by assisting them to wear their own clothes in a hospital setting, when this is possible.

- *Provide information when the client has insufficient information.* Fear of the unknown and incorrect information can frequently cause stress. Stressed clients often misunderstand facts related by health personnel. Additional information or clarification can allay stress.

- *Repeat information when the client has difficulty remembering.* Nurses can assist clients by repeating information when it is requested and assisting people to apply it when they so desire. This problem is particularly prevalent among elderly people who are stressed by a change of setting as well as by their illness.

- *Encourage the client to participate in the plan of care.* Loss of the right to determine their own destiny can be very stressful to some people, particularly adults who function independently or who assume responsibility for others in their daily lives.

- *Give the client time to express feelings and thoughts.* Allow time for clients to describe their feelings and worries if they wish. Nurses should be sensitive to clients' needs and neither probe with prying questions nor be too busy to listen.

- *Ensure that expectations are within the client's capabilities.* Whatever the activity, whether an exercise or recreation, the nurse should make sure that it is possible for the client to accomplish it. If an activity is beyond the client's ability, the client is likely to be more stressed by not achieving the goal.

- *Be sensitive to specific situations and experiences that increase anxiety and stress for clients.* For example, a man might appear highly stressed each time he receives an intramuscular injection. A careful remark by the nurse about the stress may elicit information that the nurse can use to assist the client.

- *Assist a client to make a correct appraisal of a situation.* Sometimes, through a lack of knowledge or misinterpretation of a sequence of events, people draw incorrect conclusions. Having valid information might relieve the client's stress.

- *Provide an environment in which a person can function independently to some degree without assistance.* It may be difficult and stressful for an adult to assume the dependent client role even for a short time. By restoring some degree of independent functioning, such as by adapting eating utensils so that clients can feed themselves, nurses can lower clients' stress levels.

- *Reinforce positive environmental factors and recognize negative ones to help reduce stress.* Dwelling on problems and difficulties increases stress, but focusing on what can be accomplished positively usually decreases stress.

- *Arrange for other clients with similar experiences to visit.* Clients with colostomies or similar conditions may be highly stressed and feel that they will never be able to live a normal life again. Meeting another person who has successfully adjusted to a colostomy can lower the stress greatly.

- *Bring clients and their support persons into contact with people in community agencies who can help them make valid plans.* Social workers are familiar with discharge planning and arrangements that a client may need to make. Often people are stressed needlessly because they do not know what help is available to them in the community.

- *Communicate competence, understanding, and empathy rather than stress and anxiety.* When a nurse conveys stress or anxiety, the client and support persons may be concerned about the nurse's ability to function where the client's health and life are involved. To reduce a client's stress, nurses need to know themselves well and be able to function in a nondefensive manner that conveys competence and empathy.

Mediating Anger

Often nurses find clients' anger difficult to handle. Caring for the client who is angry is difficult for two reasons (Gluck 1981, p. 9):

- Clients rarely state, "I feel angry or frustrated," and rarely indicate the reason for their anger. Instead, they may refuse treatment, become verbally abusive or demanding, may threaten violence, or become overly critical. Their complaints rarely reflect the cause of their anger.

- Anger from clients can elicit fear and anger in the nurse, who may respond in a manner that intensifies the client's anger, even to the point of violence. The majority of nurses respond in a way that reduces their own stress rather than the client's stress (Gluck 1981, p. 11).

Responses whose major purpose is to reduce the nurse's stress include defending, providing reassurance, offering advice or persuading, and retaliating aggressively.

Responses that reduce the client's anger and stress include offering help, apologizing, asking relevant questions, and conveying understanding. For example, the nurse might respond by saying, "I guess it's pretty frustrating being alone and having to wait for others to do things for you." Gluck (1981, p. 10) suggests that nurses wishing to provide understanding responses to clients follow these guidelines:

- Focus on the feeling words of the client.

- Note the general content of the message.

- Restate the feeling and content of what the client has communicated.

- Observe the client's body language.

- Ask yourself, "If I were in the client's shoes, what would I be feeling?"

In addition to these general guidelines for minimizing stress, several health promotion strategies are often appropriate as interventions for clients with stress-related nursing diagnoses. Among these are physical exercise and recreation, optimal nutrition, adequate rest and sleep, time management, and relaxation techniques.

Massage

A variety of massage strokes or movements may be used singly or in combination, depending on the outcome desired. These include **effleurage** (stroking), friction, pressure, **petrissage** (kneading or large, quick pinches of the skin, subcutaneous tissue, and muscle), vibration, and percussion.

Historically, the back massage has been used by nurses to enhance or induce relaxation before sleep or to stimulate skin circulation in association with hygienic measures. Support persons, too, can provide the technique to loved ones. See Technique 37–1 for a back massage technique that includes a combination of massage strokes.

The duration of a massage ranges from 5 to 20 minutes, in accordance with the client's tolerance. Before offering a massage, the nurse must ensure that the environment is free of distractions and interruptions and that the room temperature is comfortable for the client with the back uncovered. The nurse must also feel relaxed and convey an attitude that the massage will alleviate pain, stress, and physical and mental tension. Because cultural and religious beliefs regarding personal touch may cause the client emotional discomfort during massage therapy, the nurse must, in addition, ensure that the client is receptive to the therapy.

37-1 Providing Massage

PURPOSES

- To relieve muscle tension
- To promote physical and mental relaxation
- To improve muscle and skin functioning
- To relieve insomnia
- To provide relief from pain

ASSESSMENT FOCUS

Vital signs; signs of stress (e.g., muscle tension); receptability of the client to therapy.

EQUIPMENT

□ Lotion or oil

INTERVENTION

1. Select an appropriate time free of interruptions and distractions.

- Provide massage following the morning bath, before sleeping, and at other times as necessary to achieve relaxation and comfort for the client.
- Assist the client to a prone position in bed. Remove the client's gown, or open the back of the hospital gown.

2. Warm the massage lotion or oil before use.

- Warm the lotion or oil by pouring it into your hands before applying it to the client's back. *Cold lotion may startle the client and increase discomfort.*

3. Effleurage the entire back.

- Place your hands next to the lower spine. Using your palms and fingers, slowly massage upwards to the neck, gradually decreasing pressure as you get close to the neck. Circle your hands over the shoulder blades, and then slowly move them gently down the lateral surface of the back. *Effleurage has a relaxing, sedative effect if slow movement and light pressure are used.*

4. Apply friction strokes next to the spine.

- Use your thumbs to apply friction strokes (strong circular motions).
- Massage the back, moving from side to side in smooth, tiny circles, starting at the neck and ending at the waist.

5. Petrissage the back and shoulders of the client.

- Petrissage first up the vertebral column and then over the entire back. *Petrissage is stimulating, especially if done quickly and with firm pressure.*
- Observe the client carefully to ensure that petrissage does not cause pain or discomfort. If the client grimaces or withdraws from the touch, ease the kneading pressure.

6. Apply hand pressure movements up the back.

- Using moderate pressure, walk your hands up the outer edges of the back from the hips to the neck.

7. Effleurage and petrissage the upper back and shoulders, using long soothing strokes. *This area often experiences the most tension.*

8. Apply pressure strokes along the spinal column.

- Place one hand on top of the other, and move slowly from the lower spine to the top of the spine, using light to moderate pressure.
- Observe the client carefully to ensure that the pressure strokes are not causing the client pain or discomfort.

9. Using gentle pressure, apply large circular movements to the back.

- Start at the outer side of the back at the waistline. Move from the waistline to the lower hip, then across the hip and up the spine.

10. Complete the massage by using light effleurage to the entire back.

- With each massage stroke, lessen the pressure.

11. Assist the client to a position of comfort.

12. Document the massage and the client's response.

▶ **Technique 37–1 Providing Massage** *CONTINUED*

EVALUATION FOCUS	Signs of relaxation and/or decreased pain (e.g., relaxed breathing, decreased muscle tension, drowsiness, and peaceful affect); verbalizations of freedom from pain and tension; areas of redness, broken skin, bruises, or other signs of skin breakdown.

SAMPLE RECORDING

Date	Time	Notes
7/12/93	2200	Stated "I can't get to sleep. I feel so tense and nervous and can't seem to unwind." Respiration 28. Hyperventilating. Pupils dilated. Facial muscles tense. Voice quivering. Back massage provided for 10 minutes. Stated "feels more relaxed now" ———————————————— Bruce Machiavelli, SN
	2300	Sleeping. R 16 and regular. ———————————————— Bruce Machiavelli, SN

KEY ELEMENTS OF PROVIDING MASSAGE

- Ensure that the client is receptive to massage.
- Provide an environment conducive to relaxation.
- Convey a calm and positive attitude.

- Warm the lotion or oil in your hands before application.
- Use a combination of massage strokes to reduce muscle tension.

Shiatsu Massage

Shaitsu massage is a highly specialized form of massage designed to relieve muscle tension and fatigue. It is the application of firm, gentle pressure to the acupuncture points of the body and therefore is sometimes referred to as acupressure. Shiatsu aims to restore the balance of true Qi (pronounced "chee"), a balance of the constantly flowing life energy forces of *yang* and *yin*. True Qi circulates around the body through 12 main channels called meridians, which correspond to 12 organs, including the lungs, heart, and stomach. Clients can use shiatsu on themselves to relieve minor ailments. For example, a frontal headache may be relieved by applying firm pressure behind the head at the base of the skull.

Progressive Relaxation

Relaxation techniques have been used extensively to reduce high levels of stress and chronic pain. Using relaxation techniques enables the client to exert control over the body's responses to tension and anxiety.

For many years, nurses on maternity units have encouraged women in labor to relax and breathe rhythmically.

Progressive relaxation requires that the client (a) tense and then relax successive muscle groups, and (b) focus attention on discriminating the feelings experienced when the muscle group is relaxed in contrast to when it was tense. Jacobsen (1938), the originator of the progressive relaxation technique, found that tension of a muscle group before its relaxation actually achieved a greater degree of relaxation than simply commanding oneself to relax. This technique can result in decreased body oxygen consumption, metabolism, respiratory rate, cardiac rate, muscle tension, and systolic and diastolic blood pressures.

Procedures for teaching progressive relaxation vary. The method for relaxing muscle groups, the specific muscle groups to be relaxed, the number of sessions involved, and the role of the instructor (taped versus live instructions) may differ. Technique 37–2 explains the steps involved in teaching progressive relaxation.

Teaching Progressive Relaxation

PURPOSES
- To reduce stress
- To control chronic pain
- To ease tension
- To obtain maximum benefits from rest and sleep periods
- To enable the client to gain control over body responses to stress and pain

ASSESSMENT FOCUS

Willingness to participate in the relaxation exercises; the nature and location of any pain; vital signs; signs of stress.

INTERVENTION

1. Ensure that the environment is quiet, peaceful, and at a temperature that promotes comfort to the client. *Interruptions or distractions and a room that is too cool interfere with the client's ability to achieve full relaxation.*

2. Tell the client how progressive relaxation works.

- Provide a rationale for the procedure. *This enables the client to understand how stress affects the body.*

- Ask the client to identify the stressors operating in the client's life and the reactions to these stressors.

- Demonstrate the method of tensing and relaxing the muscles. *Demonstration enables the client to understand the complete relaxation procedure clearly.*

3. Assist the client to a comfortable position.

- Ensure that all body parts are supported and the joints slightly flexed, with no strain or pull on the muscles (e.g., arms and legs should not be crossed). *Assuming a position of comfort facilitates relaxation.*

4. Encourage the client to rest the mind.

- Ask the client to gaze slowly around the room, e.g., across the ceiling, down the wall, along a window curtain, around the fabric pattern, and back up the wall. *This exercise focuses the mind outside the body, and creates a second center of concentration, facilitating relaxation.*

5. Instruct the client to tense and then relax each muscle group.

- Progress through each muscle group in the following order, starting with the dominant side:

  a. Hand and forearm
  b. Upper arm
  c. Forehead
  d. Central face
  e. Lower face and jaw
  f. Neck
  g. Chest, shoulders, and upper back
  h. Abdomen
  i. Thigh
  j. Calf muscles
  k. Foot

- Encourage the client to breathe slowly and deeply during the en-

tire procedure. *Slow, deep breathing facilitates relaxation.*

- Encourage the client to focus on each muscle group being tensed and relaxed.

- Speak in a soothing voice that encourages relaxation, and coach the client to focus on each muscle group: e.g., "Make a tight fist," "Clench your fist tightly," "Hold the tension for 5 to 7 seconds," "Let all the tension go," and "Enjoy the feelings as your muscles become relaxed and loose."

6. Ask the client to state whether any tension remains after all muscle groups have been tensed and relaxed.

- Repeat the procedure for muscle groups that are not relaxed.

7. Terminate the relaxation exercise slowly by counting backward from 4 to 1.

- Ask the client to move the body slowly: first the hands and feet; then arms and legs; and finally the head and neck.

8. Document the client's response to the exercise.

EVALUATION FOCUS

Signs of relaxation (e.g., decreased muscle tension, slowed breathing); the client's feelings regarding success or problems with the technique.

▶ **Technique 37–2 Teaching Progressive Relaxation** *CONTINUED*

SAMPLE RECORDING

Date	Time	Notes
9/10/93	1300	Instruction provided for progressive relaxation technique. States has difficulty relaxing and resting because of worries about recent diagnosis of cancer, work pressures, and financial concerns. During the technique respirations slowed to 14 and facial body tension not evident. Stated felt "more peaceful" following the technique.————————————— Sharon Stookey, RN

KEY ELEMENTS OF TEACHING PROGRESSIVE RELAXATION

- Provide an environment conducive to relaxation.
- Ensure that the client assumes a position of comfort.
- Speak in a soothing voice.
- Encourage the client to breathe deeply and slowly throughout the procedure.
- Instruct the client to focus on each muscle group that is being tensed and relaxed.

Guided Imagery

Guided imagery involves the use of self-chosen or instructor-suggested positive images to achieve specific health-related goals. Imagery is "the formation of a mental representation of an object that is usually only perceived through the senses" (Sodergren 1985, p. 104). Images can have visual, auditory, olfactory, gustatory, or tactile-proprioceptive qualities. For examples of the different types of images used to assist in acute and chronic pain control and to augment relaxation techniques, see Table 37–2. Images often evoke more than one sense. For example, the image of waves breaking upon a shore may combine the visual picture with the sound of the waves and the smell of the salt air. Such images focus the mind *away from* the body.

Imagery can be used to enhance other forms of medical and nursing therapies to improve the body's response to therapy (e.g., chemotherapy and radiation therapy). In these instances, an image of power, such as a crocodile, a knight on a white horse, or an intergalactic battleship may be selected to control or eradicate the problem (e.g., a tumor). Such images

TABLE 37–2 TYPES OF IMAGES

Type	Example
Visual	A valley scene with its many shades of greenery
Auditory	Ocean waves breaking rhythmically upon a beach
Olfactory	Freshly baked bread
Gustatory	A juicy hamburger
Tactile-proprioceptive	Stroking a soft, furry cat

focus the mind internally, or *toward* the body.

The nurse and client may explore together what images will be effective in achieving the desired goal. The client's religious and/or spiritual beliefs should be considered when determining helpful images. Images of religious or spiritual bliss can produce physical relaxation and mental peace. Images that are meaningful to the client need to be used.

Technique 37–3 explains the steps involved in assisting a client with guided imagery.

37-3 Assisting with Guided Imagery

PURPOSES
- To improve the body's response to therapy
- To control acute and chronic pain
- To reduce muscle tension
- To augment other relaxation techniques

▶ **Technique 37–3 Assisting with Guided Imagery** *CONTINUED*

ASSESSMENT FOCUS	Willingness to participate in imagery exercises.

INTERVENTION

1. Provide a comfortable, quiet environment free of distractions. *An environment free of distractions is necessary for the client to focus on the selected image.*

2. Explain the rationale and benefits of imagery. *The client is an active participant in an imagery exercise and must understand completely what to do and what the expected outcomes are.*

3. Assist the client to a comfortable position.

- Assist the client to a reclining position, and ask the client to close the eyes. *A position of comfort can enhance the client's focus during the imagery exercise.*

- Use touch only if this does not threaten the client. For some clients, physical touch may be disturbing because of cultural or religious beliefs.

4. Implement actions to induce relaxation.

- Use the client's preferred name. *During imagery exercises, the client is more likely to respond to the preferred name.*

- Speak clearly in a calming and neutral tone of voice. *Positive voice coaching can enhance the effect of imagery. A shrill or loud voice can distract the client from the image.*

- Ask the client to take slow, deep breaths and to relax all muscles.

- Use progressive relaxation exercises as needed to assist the client to achieve total relaxation (see Technique 37–2).

- For pain or stress management, encourage the client to "go to a place where you have previously felt very peaceful."
  or
  For internal imagery, encourage the client to focus on a meaningful image of power and to use it to control the specific problem.

5. Assist the client to elaborate on the description of the image.

- Ask the client to use all the senses in describing the image and the environment of the image. Sometimes clients will think only of visual images. *Using all the senses enhances the client's benefit from imagery.*

6. Ask the client to describe the physical and emotional feelings elicited by the image.

- Direct the client to explore the response to the image. *This enables the client to modify the image. Negative responses can be redirected by the nurse to provide a more positive outcome. Positive responses can be enhanced by describing them in detail.*

7. Provide the client with continuous feedback.

- Comment on signs of relaxation and peacefulness.

8. Take the client out of the image.

- Slowly count backward from 5 to 1. Tell the client that the client will feel rested when the eyes are opened.

- Remain until the client is alert.

9. Following the experience, discuss the client's feelings about the experience.

- Identify anything that could enhance the experience.

10. Encourage the client to practice the imagery technique.

- Imagery is a technique that can be done independently by the client once he knows how.

EVALUATION FOCUS	Signs of relaxation and/or decreased pain (e.g., decreased muscle tension; slow, restful breathing; and peaceful affect); the effectiveness of the image selected.

SAMPLE RECORDING

Date	Time	Notes
8/4/93	1000	States inability to get enough rest because of chronic back pain ("I wake up in the middle of the night and can't get back to sleep. During the day I can't sit in a chair for very long either so I have to walk and move to relieve the pain.") Assisted with guided imagery. Needed encouragement to use her senses of smell and hearing as well as the visual image. States would like to try imagery again this afternoon with assistance. —— Marilyn Morrison, RN

▶ **Technique 37–3 Assisting with Guided Imagery** *CONTINUED*

KEY ELEMENTS OF ASSISTING WITH GUIDED IMAGERY

- Provide a comfortable, nondistracting environment.
- Ensure that the client is comfortable and relaxed.
- Use a calm and neutral tone of voice.

- Encourage the client to use all senses when imaging.
- Help the client explore physical and emotional responses associated with the image.

Biofeedback

Biofeedback is a technique that brings under conscious control bodily processes normally thought to be beyond voluntary command. In the past, most physiologic processes were considered involuntary. However, it has been discovered that many of these processes are partially subject to voluntary control. Studies show that muscle tension, heartbeat, blood flow, peristalsis, and skin temperature, for example, can be controlled voluntarily. The feedback is usually provided through temperature meters that indicate skin temperature changes or an electromyogram (EMG) that shows the electric potential created by the contraction of muscles. Reduced EMG activity reflects muscle relaxation. Biofeedback teaches clients to achieve a generalized state of relaxation characterized by parasympathetic dominance and antagonistic to the pattern of physiologic arousal manifested in stress-related disorders.

Therapeutic Touch

Therapeutic touch (TT) is a process by which energy is transmitted or transferred from one person to another with the intent of potentiating the healing process of one who is ill or injured. It is derived from, but not the same as, the "laying on of hands" associated with Eastern, European, and religious philosophies. Delores Krieger (1979), who coined the term *therapeutic touch,* refers to TT as a healing meditation, since the primary act of the nurse (healer) is to "center" the self and to maintain that center (mental concentration and focusing) throughout the process.

Basic to therapeutic touch are the concepts that the human being has an energy field—or, more properly, *is* an energy field (human field)—and that energy can be intentionally channeled from one person to another. The human field extends beyond the level of the skin and is perceptible to the trained sense (primarily touch) of a healer. This energy field can be most clearly "felt" within several feet of the body. An everyday experience that may demonstrate this field

phenomenon is the feeling of having one's space invaded when someone stands too close in a crowded elevator, even though there is no physical contact.

The body and the environment are considered open systems and constantly exchange energy and matter. The pattern and organization of the human field are constantly affected by the flow of energy from the environment. In situations of disease, illness, or pain, the pattern and organization of the field are disrupted; there may be a loss of energy, a disruption in the flow, an accumulation, or a blockage (Wright 1987, p. 708).

The therapeutic touch process consists of the following four steps (Snyder 1985, p. 203):

1. *Centering* is a meditative step in which the person directs attention inward to achieve a sense of detachment, sensitivity, and balance.

2. *Assessing* is a head-to-toe scanning process in which the nurse holds the palms of both hands 2 to 3 inches over the client's skin surface. This process can be performed by one nurse or two. One nurse scans the client's front while the second nurse simultaneously scans the client's back. The purpose of the assessment is to detect asymmetric differences in the client's energy flow, such as heat, cold, tingling, congestion, pressure, emptiness, or other sensations.

3. *Unruffling* is a process in which an identified congestive energy field is "unruffled," or mobilized, to make the client's energy field more receptive and to enhance the transfer of energy from the nurse to the client. The nurse accomplishes this step by moving the hands (palms facing the client) in a sweeping motion from the area where pressure was perceived down along the long bones of the body.

4. *Transferring energy* is the process in which the actual transference of energy from the nurse to the client occurs . The nurse must know which form of energy to use, how to modulate energy, and where to apply energy. The form of energy has different effects and is related to colors: Blue energy is sedating; yellow energy is stimulating and energizing; and green

energy is harmonizing. The nurse modulates these energy forms by mentally visualizing the color, e.g., visualizing light through a blue stained-glass window. The nurse may apply energy directly over an identified area of congestion or to one of the *chakras* (special channels that serve as entry areas for energy from the environment). These are located in the thoracic or solar plexus. Energy transference helps restore the balance of the energy field and provides additional energy to promote self-healing.

CRITICAL THINKING CHALLENGE

Both nursing students and practicing nurses are faced with many stressors. Identify stressors that cause you tension or stress now. Which of the several relaxation techniques described would you consider using to alleviate your own tension and stress? Consider images that evoke pleasant feelings for you, that might be effective in guided imagery. Try using the progressive relaxation technique.

RELATED RESEARCH

Dewe, P. J. April 1989. Stressor frequency, tension, tiredness and coping: Some measurement issues and a comparison across nursing groups. *Journal of Advanced Nursing* 14:308–20.

McGrath, A.; Reid, N.; and Boore, J. 1989. Occupational stress in nursing. *International Journal of Nursing Studies* 26(4):343–58.

Martin, D. March 1, 1990. Effects of ethical dilemmas on stress felt by nurses providing care to AIDS patients. *Critical Care Nursing Quarterly*, 12:53–57.

REFERENCES

Breakwell, G. M. August 1990. Are you stressed out? *American Journal of Nursing* 90:31–33.

Dugan, D. O. 1987–1988. Essays on the art of caring in nursing: The human spirit in stress management. *Nursing Forum* 23(3):108–17.

Egan, E. C. 1985. Therapeutic touch. In Snyder, M., editor. pp. 199–210. *Independent nursing interventions*. New York: John Wiley and Sons.

Gluck, M. March 1981. Learning a therapeutic verbal response to anger. *Journal of Psychiatric Nursing and Mental Health Services* 19:9–12.

Jacobsen, E. 1938. *Progressive relaxation*. Chicago: University of Chicago Press.

Kaseman, D. F., and Young, S. H. September/October 1988. Stress: An added incapacitator. *Geriatric Nursing* 9:274–77.

Krieger, D. 1979. *The therapeutic touch: How to use your hands to help or heal*. Englewood Cliffs, N.J.: Prentice-Hall.

Lazarus, R. S. 1966. *Psychological stress and the coping process*. New York: McGraw-Hill.

Lazarus, R. S., and Folkman, S. 1984. *Stress, appraisal, and coping*. New York: Springer Publishing Co.

Lyon, B. I., and Werner, J. 1987. Stress. In Fitzpatrick, J. J. and Taunton, R. L., editors. vol. 5, pp. 3–22. *Annual review of nursing research*. New York: Springer Publishing Co.

Roberts, S. L. 1987–1988. A framework for coping with stress and its application in patient care. *Nursing Forum* 23(3): 101–7.

Selye, H. 1956. *The stress of life*. New York: McGraw-Hill.
———. 1976. *The stress of life*. Rev. ed. New York: McGraw-Hill.

Snyder, M. 1985. *Independent nursing interventions*. New York: John Wiley and Sons.

Sodergren, K. M. 1985. Guided imagery. In Snyder, M. pp. 103–24. *Independent nursing interventions*. New York: John Wiley and Sons.

Wilson, L. K. December 1989. Professional Growth Section: High-gear nursing: How it can run you down and what you can do about it. *Nursing 89* 19:81–82, 84, 86, 88.

Wright, S. M. September 1987. The use of therapeutic touch in the management of pain. *Nursing Clinics of North America* 22:705–13.

Zahourek, R. 1988. *Relaxation and imagery: Tools for therapeutic communication and intervention*. Philadelphia: W. B. Saunders Co.

Pain Management

OBJECTIVES

- Describe the three stages of the pain experience

- Compare the gate-control theory and the parallel processing model of pain

- Describe subjective and objective data to be collected and analyzed when assessing pain

- Describe interventions that help prevent or decrease a client's pain

- Assist clients with effective pain management

CONTENTS

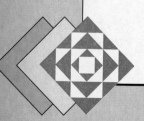

NURSING PROCESS GUIDE
PAIN

ASSESSMENT

Determine

- *Location* of the pain.

- *Intensity* of the pain on a scale of 1 to 10 (with 1 representing the lowest pain level).

- *Quality* of the pain, or how it feels (e.g., aching, burning, constant, cramping, diffuse, dull, excruciating, knifelike, pounding, stabbing, throbbing).

- *Pattern* of the pain in terms of time of onset, duration, and constancy (pain-free periods).

- *Precipitating factors* that trigger the pain or make it worse.

- *Alleviating factors* or methods the client finds helpful in lessening or relieving the pain (including medications).

- *Associated pain symptoms* (e.g., nausea, dizziness, blurred vision, shortness of breath) before, during, or after the pain.

- *Effects of pain on daily life* (e.g., appetite, sleep, concentration, work or school, family and interpersonal relationships).

- *Past pain experiences* and effectiveness of pain relief measures.

- *Meaning of the pain*, i.e., interpretation, outcomes anticipated, and worries.

- *Coping resources* used to deal with the pain.

- *Feelings* associated with the pain (e.g., anxiety, depression, fright, fatigue, irritability).

Assess

- Physiologic responses to pain. Sympathetic stimulation associated with acute pain increases blood pressure, pulse rate, and respiratory rate and causes pallor and diaphoresis. Parasympathetic stimulation associated with chronic pain decreases blood pressure and pulse rate, causes pupil constriction, and makes the skin warm and dry.

- Facial grimaces (e.g., clenched teeth, tightly shut eyes, open somber eyes, and biting of the lower lip).

- Self-induced immobilization of a body part or purposeless movements (e.g., pacing or tossing and turning in bed).

- Rubbing or massaging of the body part.

RELATED DIAGNOSTIC CATEGORIES

- Pain
- Chronic pain
- Anxiety
- Fear
- Hopelessness
- Knowledge deficit (pain control measures)
- Impaired physical mobility
- Sleep pattern disturbance
- Altered health maintenance

PLANNING

Client goals

The client will

- Experience minimal pain that will allow partial or complete resumption of usual daily activities.

- Cope more effectively with the pain experience.

Outcome Criteria

The client

- Reports increased control over pain or increased feelings of comfort.

- Reports a reduction in fatigue.

- Identifies effective and ineffective pain strategies.

- Is free of nonverbal signs of pain (e.g., guarding, protective behavior).

- Resumes prepain activities.

- Modifies activities according to limitations inflicted by the pain experience.

- Resumes normal sleep pattern.

- Uses noninvasive pain control strategy to reduce anxiety (or depression) or to manage the pain.

The Nature of Pain

Pain is a highly unpleasant and very personal sensation that cannot be shared with others. It can occupy all of one's thinking, direct one's activities, and change one's life. Pain often is an important sign that something is physiologically wrong, e.g., that tissues are damaged. McCaffery (1979, p. 11) defines pain as "whatever the experiencing person says it is, existing whenever he says it does." Basic to this definition is the caregiver's willingness to believe the client's pain.

The pain experience can be divided into three stages: reception, transmission/perception, and modulation.

Pain Reception

The skin and certain internal tissues, such as the periosteum, the joint surfaces, and the arterial walls, have many receptors, whereas most other deep tissues have few pain receptors. The alveoli of the lungs and the brain have no pain receptors.

A pain receptor, called a **nociceptor,** is stimulated either directly by damage to the receptor cell or secondarily by the release of chemicals such as bradykinin. Basically, there are three types of stimuli that excite corresponding types of nociceptors: mechanical, thermal, and chemical.

Pain does not necessarily result, however, when the nociceptors are stimulated. Pain occurs only when the pain message is relayed via the spinal cord to the brain, which then interprets the stimuli.

Transmission/Perception

An individual's **pain threshold** is the amount of pain stimulation a person requires before feeling pain. People's pain threshold is generally fairly uniform, although it can be dramatically altered by each person's state of consciousness. For instance, an anesthetized client feels no pain. **Pain tolerance** is the maximum amount and duration of pain that an individual is willing to endure. Some clients are unable to tolerate even the slightest pain, whereas others are willing to endure severe pain rather than be treated for it. Thus, pain tolerance varies greatly among people and is widely influenced by psychologic and sociocultural factors. Pain tolerance appears to increase with age.

Although the precise mechanism of pain transmission and perception is unknown, the following sequence of events is a widely accepted explanation. Pain fibers enter the spinal cord through the dorsal horn (Figure 38–1). Transmission of pain impulses along neurons in the dorsal horn causes the release

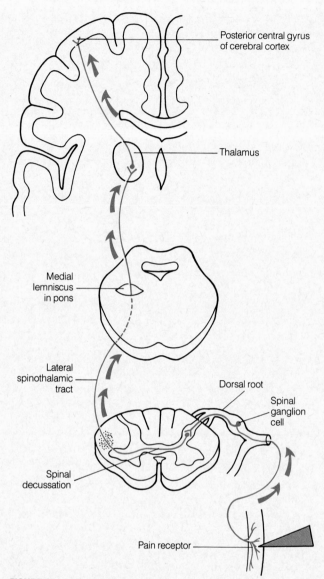

FIGURE 38–1 Acute pain pathway.

of **substance P,** a neurotransmitter that acts to enhance transmission of pain impulses across a synapse to other neurons that cross the spinal cord and enter the lateral spinothalmic tract. This tract ascends in the lateral area of the spinal cord's white matter to the thalamus in the brain. After reaching the thalamus, pain impulses travel to the somatic sensory area in the cerebral cortex for interpretation (Figure 38–2).

Modulation

It appears that there are natural mechanisms within the body that modulate pain transmission and pain perception. **Endogenous opioids** are chemical regulators that may modify pain. Certain pain relief ther-

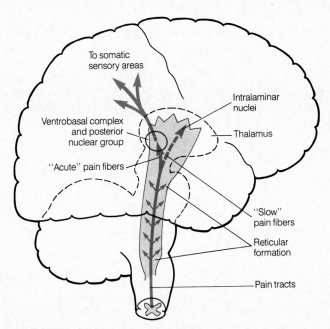

FIGURE 38–2 Transmission of pain signals to the higher brain centers.

apies, such as acupuncture, are thought to work by stimulating the release of endogenous opioids. Three groups of opioids have so far been identified: enkephalins, endorphins, and dynorphins.

Enkephalins (meaning "in the head") combine with opiate receptors in the dorsal horn of the spinal cord and apparently inhibit the release of substance P. Enkephalins are also found outside the spinal cord—in the brain stem, limbic system, hypothalamus, adrenal glands, and gastrointestinal tract.

Endorphins (meaning "morphine within") are synthesized and stored by the pituitary gland. They are also found in the hypothalamus, midbrain, and limbic system of the central nervous system. Some endorphins have been found to be more potent than the enkephalins. It is suggested that they increase with exercise (Whitaker and Warfield 1988, p. 160).

Dynorphins, only recently discovered, are compounds found in the pituitary gland, hypothalamus, and spinal cord. They seem to have an analgesic effect, one that is 50 times greater than that of the most potent endorphins.

Strategies for Pain

Nursing management of pain consists of both independent and collaborative nursing actions. In general, noninvasive measures such as massage, progressive relaxation, and guided imagery (see Chapter 37) may be performed as an independent nursing function, whereas administration of analgesic medications requires a physician's order. However, the decision to administer the prescribed medication is frequently the nurse's, often requiring judgment as to the dose to be given and the time of administration.

Generally speaking, a combination of strategies is best for the client in pain. Sometimes strategies need to be tried and changed until the client obtains effective pain relief.

Acknowledging the Client's Pain

Basic to all strategies for reducing pain is that nurses convey to clients that they believe the client is having pain. The nurse can communicate this belief in several ways:

- Verbally acknowledging the presence of the pain: "I understand your leg is very painful. How do you feel about the pain?"

- Listening attentively to what the client says about the pain.

- Conveying that the nurse is assessing the client's pain to understand it better, *not* to determine if the pain is real. The nurse can do so by asking, for example, "How does your pain feel now?" or "Tell me how it feels compared to an hour ago."

- Attending to the client's needs promptly.

Assisting Support Persons

Support persons often need assistance to respond positively to the client experiencing pain. Nurses can help by giving them accurate information about the pain and providing opportunities for them to discuss their emotional reactions, which may include anger, fear, frustration, and feelings of inadequacy. Enlisting the aid of support persons in the provision of pain relief to the client, such as massaging the client's back, may diminish their feelings of helplessness and foster a more positive attitude toward the client's pain experience. Support persons also may need the nurse's verbal recognition of their concern and participation in the client's care.

Reducing Misconceptions About Pain

Reducing a client's misconceptions about the pain and its treatment may modify pain perception. The nurse should explain to the client that pain is a highly individual experience and that it is only the client who really experiences the pain, although others can understand and empathize. The nurse can also deal with misconceptions by discussing with the client the reasons why pain increases or decreases at certain times. For example, a client whose pain increases in the evening may mistakenly think this is the result of eating dinner rather than fatigue.

Reducing Fear and Anxiety

It is important to help relieve the emotional component, i.e., anxiety or fear, associated with the pain. When clients have no opportunity to talk about their pain and associated fears, their reactions to the pain can intensify. The client may become angry or complain about the nurse's care when the problem really is a belief that the pain is not being attended to. If the nurse is honest and sincere and promptly attends to the client's needs, the client is much more likely to know that the nurse does believe the client is in pain.

By providing accurate information, the nurse can also reduce many of the client's fears, such as fear of addiction or a fear that the pain will always be present. It also helps many clients to have privacy when they are experiencing pain. It is always wise to encourage clients to share their fears and concerns about how they are handling the pain.

Using Distraction Techniques

Distraction draws the person's attention away from the pain and lessens the perception of pain. In some instances, distraction can make a client completely unaware of pain. For example, a client recovering from surgery may feel no pain while watching a football game on television yet feel pain again when the game is over.

The effectiveness of distraction to decrease pain can be explained by the *gate-control theory*. In the spinal cord, the receptor cells receiving the peripheral pain stimuli are inhibited by stimuli from other peripheral nerve fibers carrying different stimuli. Because pain messages are slower then diversional messages, the spinal cord gate, which controls the amount of input to the brain, closes, and the client feels less pain (Cummings 1981, p. 62).

Distraction is most effective at relieving mild or moderate pain, but intense concentration on other subjects can also relieve acute pain. An example of the latter is an adolescent who feels pain from a fractured foot bone only after she finishes playing a basketball game. Certain distractions (e.g., disturbing stimuli such as loud noises, bright lights, unpleasant odors, or an argumentative visitor), however, can increase pain perception. Therefore, the nurse needs to reduce disturbing stimuli. Guidelines for using selected distraction techniques are included in the accompanying box.

Providing Cutaneous Stimulation

Cutaneous stimulation of the skin can reduce pain intensity. Again, this is another refinement of distraction, using tactile stimulation to "distract" the client from the pain experience. Guidelines for using specific techniques for cutaneous stimulation are summarized in the box on page 907.

Applying Heat or Cold

The nurse may need a physician's order before applying heat or cold. Heat is known to stimulate the pro-

Distraction Techniques

- *Slow, rhythmic breathing.* Instruct the client to stare at an object and inhale slowly through the nose while counting from 1 to 4 and then exhale slowly through the mouth while counting to 4 again. Encourage the client to concentrate on the sensation of breathing and to picture a restful scene. Continue until a rhythmic pattern is established.
- *Massage and slow, rhythmic breathing.* Instruct the client to breath rhythmically and at the same time massage a painful body part with stroking or circular movements.
- *Rhythmic singing and tapping.* Ask the client to select a well-liked song and concentrate attention on its words and rhythm. Encourage the client to mouth or sing the words and tap a finger or foot. Loud, fast songs are best for intense pain.
- *Active listening.* Have the client listen to music and concentrate on the rhythm by tapping a finger or foot.
- *Guided imagery.* Ask the client to close the eyes and imagine and describe something pleasurable. As the client describes the image, ask about the sights, sounds, and smells imagined, encouraging the client to provide details. See also Chapter 37, page 898.

duction of serotonin, which in turn helps an individual feel secure, serene, and safe. Heat can be applied as warm soaks, compresses, or pads (see Chapter 41 for more information). Cold stimulates the production of norepinephrine. The secretion of excessive norepinephrine causes the individual to feel powerful, in control, confident, and excited (see also the discussion of cutaneous stimulation earlier).

Administering Analgesics

Analgesics alter perception and interpretation of pain by depressing the central nervous sytem at the thalamus and cerebral cortex. Analgesics are more effective when given *before* the client feels severe pain than *after* the pain becomes severe. For this reason, analgesics are often given at regular intervals, such as every 4 hours (q4h) after surgery.

When administering analgesics, it is essential that the nurse review the side-effects. For example, narcotic analgesics depress respiration and must be used cautiously in clients with respiratory problems. If the client experiences significant respiratory depression (e.g., a drop from 18 to 12) or is overly

---

CLINICAL GUIDELINES

Cutaneous Stimulation

- *Cold packs* slow the conduction of pain impulses to the brain and motor impulses to muscles in the painful area. They provide quicker and longer-lasting pain relief than hot packs (McCaffery 1980, p. 57). Use cold packs to help relieve headaches, muscle strains, joint pain, muscle spasm, and back pain during childbirth.

- *Analgesic ointments* containing menthol relieve pain, but the analgesic mechanism is unknown. These ointments produce immediate sensations of warmth that last for several hours, and even longer if the body part is wrapped in plastic. They can be used to relieve joint or muscle pain. Moreover, menthol ointment rubbed into the neck, scalp, or forehead sometimes relieves tension headaches, and some cultures (e.g., Filipino) use it on the abdomen to relieve gas pains or on the abdomen or lower back to relieve the pain of labor or delivery (McCaffery 1980, p. 57).

- *Counterirritants,* such as mustard plasters, flaxseed poultices, and liniments, may be used to relieve the aching joint pain of rheumatoid arthritis and osteoarthritis. Counterirritants are thought to relieve pain by increasing circulation to the painful area.

- *Contralateral stimulation* can be accomplished by stimulating the skin in an area opposite to the painful area (e.g., stimulating the left knee if the pain is in the right knee). The contralateral area may be scratched for itching, massaged for cramps, or treated with cold packs or analgesic ointments. This method is particularly useful when the painful area cannot be touched because it is hypersensitive, inaccessible by a cast or bandages, or when the pain is felt in a missing part, i.e., phantom pain (McCaffery 1980, p. 57).

ment technique that allows the client to take an active role in managing pain. Clients vary widely in the type and dosage of analgesic they need for adequate pain control. With PCA, the client administers a predetermined dose of a narcotic agent (usually morphine, meperidine, or hydromorphone) by an electronic infusion pump. This allows the person to maintain a more constant level of relief than traditional methods of analgesia therapy can provide. The PCA mode of therapy minimizes the rollercoaster effect of peaks of sedation and valleys of pain that occur with traditional methods of administering analgesics on demand.

Patient-controlled analgesia pumps are designed with built-in safety mechanisms to prevent client overdosage, abusive use, and narcotic theft. The most significant adverse effects are respiratory depression and hypotension; however, they occur rarely. Although electronic PCA pumps vary in design, they all have the same protective features. The line of the PCA pump, a syringe-type pump, is usually introduced into the injection port of a primary IV fluid line (Figure 38–3). Most PCA pumps allow the client to receive continuous narcotic infusion plus self-administered boluses at intervals. Some pumps are key operated; that is, the drug can be accessed only with the key. In addition, parameters for safety limits on dose volume, lockout time, and 4-hour dose limits are programmed into the machine. The client may

sedated, the dosage is excessive. *Before* administering narcotics, the nurse needs to assess a client's respiratory rate and level of alertness for baseline data. The nurse also needs to note other side-effects, such as nausea and vomiting. Nonnarcotics such as aspirin may aggravate gastrointestinal bleeding and therefore are contraindicated in clients with peptic ulcers. *After* medicating the client, the nurse records the response. Some nurses use pain medication flowsheets for this purpose.

Patient-Controlled Analgesia (PCA) Therapy

Patient-controlled analgesia (PCA) is a pain manage-

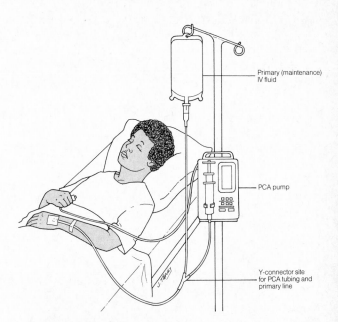

FIGURE 38–3 PCA line introduced into the injection port of a primary line.

attempt to activate the pump to receive a dose as many times as desired, but the machine will deliver only within the preset parameters. Another type of PCA device on the market is a mechanically operated device that the client wears. Although it does not have as many built-in safety features, it permits client mobility and allows the client to deliver a preset dosage of medication within a certain time frame (Figure 38–4). Client teaching about the purpose, benefits, and use of this mode of therapy is essential to its success. Technique 38–1 describes the use of a PCA pump.

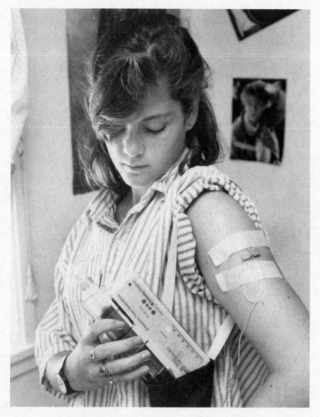

FIGURE 38–4 PCA device worn by a client.

38-1 Managing Pain with a Patient-Controlled Analgesia Pump

Before initiating PCA therapy, determine factors that may contraindicate use (e.g., impaired mental staus, impaired respiratory status), the amount of narcotic specified by the order, bolus and continuous infusion dosage parameters, and type of primary fluid. Calculate the following: (a) the initial bolus dose based on the number of milligrams of drug per milliliter of fluid, (b) the dose per intermittent bolus delivery, and (c) the 4-hour lockout drug limit. Confirm that the drug is premixed with the required amount of dilutent.

PURPOSES
- To enhance pain control
- To decrease opioid requirements
- To facilitate client involvement in controlling pain

▶ **Technique 38–1** *CONTINUED*

ASSESSMENT FOCUS	Pain (intensity, location, presence of radiation, associated factors, precipitating factors, and alleviating factors); client's allergies; baseline vital signs; client's understanding of the pump.

EQUIPMENT

- Gloves
- IV start kit
- IV catheter
- Primary line IV tubing
- Primary IV fluid (per orders)
- PCA pump and appropriate tubing
- Operational manual for specific pump to be used
- Premixed drug to be infused
- PCA flowsheet

INTERVENTION

1. Prepare the client.

- Explain the purpose and operation of the PCA.

2. Set up the primary IV line and fluid.

- Don gloves.

- Start the IV line. *This will secure venous access.*

3. Set up the PCA infusion line according to the manfacturer's instructions.

- Remove the protective caps from the injector (plunger) and premixed drug vial.

- Connect (screw or twist) the injector into the drug vial.

- Remove excessive air from the vial by pushing the injector into the vial.

- Connect the PCA tubing to the injector (Figure 38–3).

- Prime the PCA tubing up to the point of the Y-connector.

- Clamp the tubing above the Y-connector. *This prevents accidental bolusing and flushing of the primary line with the narcotic.*

- Place the injector with attached vial in the PCA machine according to the operational instructions.

4. Connect the PCA infusion line to the primary fluid line.

- Connect the PCA tubing to the primary fluid line at the Y-connector site. (The clamps should still be closed on the primary IV line and the PCA line.)

5. Deliver the loading dose.

- Set the pump for a lockout time of zero minutes.

- Set the volume to be delivered based on calculated dosage volume for the loading dose.

- Inject the loading dose by pressing the loading dose control button.

6. Set the safety parameters for the infusion on the PCA pump according to the manufacturer's instructions. For example:

- Dose volume limits. *This will limit the amount of drug that the client can receive when the client pushes the control button.*

- Lockout interval between each dose. The lockout interval is generally between 5 and 12 minutes. *This sets the minimum time that must elapse before the client can receive another dose of the drug. Lockout time is based on the usual onset of the IV narcotic and the assessment of the client.*

- 4-hour limit. Set the 4-hour dosage limit as specified on the orders. *This is an additional safety feature to limit the amount of medication delivered over 4 hours.*

7. Lock the machine.

- Close the door on the pump.

- Look for any digital cues or alarms that may indicate the machine is not set, and make corrections as needed.

- Lock the machine with the key.

8. Begin the infusion.

- Release the clamp on the Y-connector, and press the start button to begin the infusion.

- Place the client control button within reach.

9. Monitor the client.

- Monitor the status of the client every 2 hours during the first 24 to 36 hours of infusion and regularly thereafter, depending on the client's health and agency protocol.

10. Monitor the infusion.

- Observe the IV site for signs of infiltration and phlebitis.

- Inspect the tubing for kinks that may occlude the line.

- Ascertain the total number of doses received and the total number of attempts by the client to activate a dose delivery.

11. Document all relevant information.

- Record the initiation of PCA, the dose setting, the doses received, pain intensity, and all assessments.

▶

▶ **Technique 38–1 Managing Pain with a PCA Pump** *CONTINUED*

EVALUATION FOCUS

Pain status; respiratory rate and character; amount of medication used and frequency of use.

SAMPLE RECORDING

Date	Time	Notes
4/23/93	1300	PCA therapy initiated with loading dose of MSO_4 5 mg. delivered. Dose volume setting 1 ml (1 mg) MSO_4, lock-out interval setting 15 minutes, 4-hour limit setting 16 mg. States pain intensity 6-7 prior to receiving MSO_4 and beginning PCA infusion. Return demonstrated correct technique for delivering drug. Respirations even and regular, alert and oriented. Reports no nausea or dizziness. IV site clean s̄ redness or edema. ——— Susanna Marshall, SN

KEY ELEMENTS OF MANAGING PAIN WITH A PCA PUMP

- Assess the client at appropriate time frames during PCA infusion.
- Administer the correct medication and dosage.
- Set up the PCA line and primary line correctly.
- Program the parameters for the pump.

- Keep the pump locked at all times.
- Evaluate the client's level of understanding of the purpose and use of the pump.
- Maintain the narcotic records according to agency policy.

Transcutaneous Electric Nerve Stimulation (TENS)

Transcutaneous electric nerve stimulation (TENS) is a noninvasive, nonanalgesic pain control technique that allows the client to assist in the management of acute and chronic pain. It provides an alternative or adjunct to some of the traditional therapies.

The TENS unit consists of a portable battery-operated unit, lead wires, and electrodes (Figure 38–5). It may be applied intermittently or worn discretely by the client throughout the day. The placement of the electrodes depends on the location, nature, and origin of the pain. They may be placed along both sides of an incision, directly over identified pain areas, at an acupressure point, along peripheral nerve areas that innervate the pain area, or along the spinal column.

Many clients receive significant relief with TENS therapy. TENS units used near incision areas have been shown to provide partial relief of postoperative pain, thereby decreasing the amount of analgesia needed. One of the theories behind the development of the TENS unit is the gate-control theory. Cutaneous stimulation from the electronic signals of the TENS unit activate large-diameter fibers to trigger central nervous centers to "close the gate" to signals given to small diameter fibers. Another theory postulates that the electronic signals emitted by the TENS unit cause the release of endorphins from central nervous system centers. Adverse effects of TENS therapy are minimal.

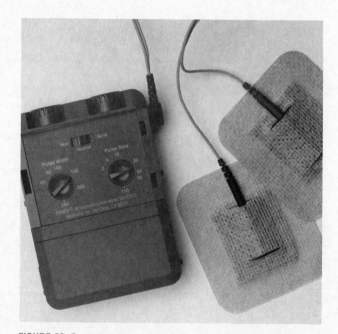

FIGURE 38–5 A transcutaneous electric nerve stimulator (TENS).

Although TENS therapy may help decrease pain, the client may need adjunctive analgesic administration during more intense pain periods. The nurse should monitor the client closely to determine the level of pain relief and the need for adjunctive drug therapy. Technique 38–2 describes the use of a TENS unit.

38-2 Managing Pain with a Transcutaneous Electric Nerve Stimulation Unit

Before applying a TENS unit, determine the presence of factors contra-indicating usage (presence of a cardiac pacemaker; history of dysrhythmias, myocardial ischemia, or myocardial infarction; first-trimester pregnancy; confusion; history of peripheral vascular problems altering neurosensory perception).

PURPOSES

- To reduce chronic and acute pain (especially postoperative pain)
- To decrease opioid requirements and reduce the chances of depressed respiratory function from narcotic usage
- To facilitate client involvement in managing pain control

ASSESSMENT FOCUS

Client's mental status and ability to follow instructions in using the TENS unit; intactness of skin and absence of signs of infection and irritation; appearance of incisional area of postoperative client; characteristics of pain (intensity, location, associated factors, precipitating factors, and alleviating factors); amount of pain medication required before and during treatment.

EQUIPMENT

- TENS Unit
- Bath basin with warm water
- Soap
- Washcloth
- Towel
- Conduction cream, gel, or
- water (see manufacturer's instructions)
- Hypoallergenic tape

INTERVENTION

1. Explain the purpose and application technique to the client and family.

- Explain that the TENS unit may not completely eliminate pain but should reduce pain to a level that allows the client to rest more comfortably and/or carry out everyday activities.

2. Prepare the equipment.

- Insert the battery into the TENS unit to test the status of functioning.
- With the TENS unit off, plug the lead wires into the battery-operated unit at one end, leaving the electrodes at the other end.

3. Clean the application area.

- Wash, rinse, and dry the designated area with soap and water. *This reduces skin irritation and facilitates adhesion of the electrodes to the skin for a longer period of time.*

4. Apply the electrodes to the client.

- If the electrodes are not prejelled, moisten them with a small amount of water or apply conducting gel. (Consult the manufacturer's instructions). *This facilitates electrical conduction.*
- Place the electrodes on a clean, unbroken skin area. Choose the area according to the location, nature, and origin of the pain.
- Ensure that the electrodes make full surface contact with the skin. *This prevents an inadvertent burn.*
- Secure the electrodes with hypoallergenic tape.

5. Turn the unit on.

- Ascertain that the amplitude control is set at level 0.
- Slowly increase the intensity of the stimulus (amplitude) until

the client notes a slight increase in discomfort.

- When the client notes discomfort, slowly decrease the amplitude until the client notes a pleasant sensation. Once this has been achieved, keep the TENS unit set at this level to maintain blockage of the pain sensation.

6. Monitor the client.

- If the client complains of itching, pricking, or burning, explore the following options:

  a. Turn the pulse-width dial down.

  b. Check that the entire electrode surface is in contact with the skin.

  c. Increase the distance between the electrodes.

  d. Select another type of electrode suitable for the model

> ▸ **Technique 38–2 Managing Pain with a TENS Unit** *CONTINUED*

of TENS unit in use.

e. Discontinue the TENS, and consider the possibility of another brand of TENS.

- If the sensation of the stimulus is unpleasant, too intense, or distracting, turn down both the amplitude and the pulse-width dial.

- If the client complains of headache or nausea during application or use, turn down both the amplitude and the pulse-width dial. Repositioning of the electrodes may also be helpful.

- If further troubleshooting is not

effective, discontinue the use of the TENS unit, and notify the physician.

7. Provide client teaching.

- Review with the client instructions for use, and verify that the client understands.

- Have the client demonstrate the use of the TENS unit and verbalize ways to troubleshoot if headache, nausea, or unpleasant sensations occur.

- Instruct the client not to submerge the unit in water but in-

stead to remove and reapply it after bathing.

- Check the manufacturer's instructions for removing electrode gel from the electrodes.

8. Document all relevant information.

- Record the date and time TENS therapy was initiated, the location of electrode placement and status of skin in that area, the character and quality of the pain, settings of TENS unit used, any side-effects experienced, and the client's response.

EVALUATION FOCUS | Response of the client in terms of pain relief or side-effects experienced; self-care abilities.

SAMPLE RECORDING

Date	Time	Notes
4/23/93	1000	TENS unit applied near midline abdominal incision for postoperative pain at intensity level given by client of 6–7. Lead 1 and lead 2 settings on 6.0 Verbalized minimum relief of discomfort upon initiation of treatment.———— ———————————————————————————————— Mark McCormick, SN

KEY ELEMENTS OF MANAGING PAIN WITH A TRANSCUTANEOUS ELECTRIC NERVE STIMULATION UNIT

- Assess skin integrity before application.
- Assess the character and quality of pain before and after therapy.
- Follow the manufacturer's instructions about use.
- Ensure that the unit is turned off before applying the electrodes.

- Ensure that the entire electrode surface is in contact with the skin.
- Secure the electrode with tape.
- Increase the amplitude of the unit slowly to the desired level.

CRITICAL THINKING CHALLENGE

Janet Alexander is a 38-year-old female who has been admitted to the oncology unit with ovarian cancer. Ms Alexander has an order for narcotic analgesic for pain control. Because she dislikes the feeling of being drowsy and drugged, she asks to try guided imagery to increase her control of her pain. After her first imagery session, she becomes discouraged and depressed because she feels no relief. What would you say to her? What else would you do?

RELATED RESEARCH

Camp, L. D. August 1988. A comparison of nurses' recorded assessments of pain with perceptions of pain as described by cancer patients. *Cancer Nursing* 11:237–43.

Giuffre, M.; Keane, A.; Hatfield, S. M.; and Korevaar, W. July/August 1988. Patient-controlled analgesia in clinical pain research measurement. *Nursing Research* 37:254–55.

Holm, K.; Cohen, F.; Dudas, S.; Medema, P. G.; and Allen, B. L. Summer 1989. Effect of personal pain experience on pain assessment. *Image: Journal of Nursing Scholarship.* 21:72–75.

REFERENCES

Collier, M. March/April 1990. Controlling postoperative pain with patient-controlled analgesia. *Journal of Professional Nursing* 6(6):121–26.

Cummings, D. January 1981. Stopping chronic pain before it starts. *Nursing 81* 11:60–62.

Dunwoody, C. J. September/October 1987. Patient-controlled analgesia: Rationale, attributes, and essential factors. *Orthopaedic Nursing* 6:31–36.

Ferrell, B. R., and Ferrell, B. A. July/August 1990. Easing the pain. *Geriatric Nursing* 11:175–78.

Fitzgerald, J. J., and Shammy, P. G. July 1987. Let your patient control his analgesia. *Nursing 87* 17:48–51.

Gedaly-Duff, V. October 1988. Pain theories and their relevance to nursing practices. *Nurse Practitioner* 13:66–68.

Jones, L., and Brooks, J. May 1990. The ABC's of PCA . . . patient-controlled analgesia. *RN* 53:54–60.

Kresl, J. S. September 1988. Patient-controlled analgesia: A new system for pain management. *AORN Journal* 48:481–82, 484, 486–87.

McCaffery, M. 1979. *Nursing management of the patient with pain.* 2d ed. Philadelphia: J. B. Lippincott Co.

———. December 1980. Relieving pain with noninvasive techniques. *Nursing 80* 10:55–57.

———. November 1987. Patient-controlled analgesia: More than a machine. *Nursing 87* 17:63–64.

McCaffery, M., and Beebe, A. 1989. *Pain: Clinical manual for nursing practice.* St. Louis: C. V. Mosby.

Nolan, M. F. January/February 1990. Pain: The experience and its expression. *Clinical Management* 10:22–25.

Paice, J. A. September 1987. New delivery systems in pain management. *Nursing Clinics of North America* 22:715–26.

Whitaker, O. C., and Warfield, C. A. February 15, 1988. The measurement of pain. *Hospital Practice* 23:155–56, 159–62.

39

Wound Care

OBJECTIVES

• Identify assessment data pertinent to wounds

• Describe commonly used dressing materials

• Identify essential aspects of securing a dressing

• Compare primary and secondary intention wound healing

• Identify purposes and essential aspects of dry dressings versus wet-to-dry dressings

• Identify purposes and essential aspects of wound drains and suctions

• Describe various methods of suturing

• Give reasons underlying selected steps of the techniques

• Perform the wound care techniques in this chapter safely

CONTENTS

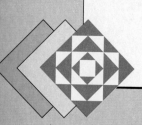

NURSING PROCESS GUIDE
WOUND CARE

ASSESSMENT

Determine the client's allergies to wound-cleaning agents and tape.

Assess the wound for:

- *Appearance.* Inspect the wound itself for signs of healing and approximation of the wound edges. Taylor (1983, p. 44) and Bruno (1979, p. 670) outline the following *sequential* signs of primary intention wound healing:

  a. Absence of bleeding and a clot binding the wound edges together within the first few hours after surgical closure.

  b. Inflammation (redness and swelling) at the wound edges for 1 to 3 days.

  c. Reduction in inflammation when the clot diminishes and as granulation tissue starts to close the wound within 7 to 10 days. (Increased inflammation associated with fever and drainage is indicative of wound infection; the wound edges then appear brightly inflamed and swollen.)

  d. Scar formation. Collagen, which forms scar tissue, is produced 4 days after injury and continues for 6 months or longer.

  e. Diminished scar size over a period of months or years.

- *Size.* To determine the width and length of the wound's surface area or its circumference, use a disposable measuring guide calibrated in centimeters. For irregularly shaped wounds, use a transparent wound dressing, and trace and date the margins of the wounds (Krasner 1992, p. 89).

- *Depth.* To determine wound depth, probe the deepest part of the wound with a sterile swab. Place your forefinger on the swab at surface level, and then measure the distance with a paper measuring guide (Krasner 1992, p. 89).

- *Drainage.* Observe the location, color, consistency, odor, and degree of saturation of dressings. Note the number of gauzes saturated or the diameter of drainage on gauze.

- *Swelling.* Wearing sterile gloves, palpate wound edges for tension and tautness of tissues; minimal to moderate swelling is normal in early stages of wound healing.

- *Pain.* Expect severe to moderate postoperative pain for 3 to 5 days; persistent severe pain or sudden onset of severe pain may indicate internal hemorrhaging or infection.

- *Drains or tubes.* Inspect drain security and placement, amount of character of drainage, and functioning of collecting apparatus, if present.

Assess the client for factors that hinder wound healing:

- *Malnutrition.* A poorly nourished person often has insufficient amounts of the vitamins and trace substances needed to synthesize wound-healing elements. In addition, resistance to infection depends on a well-balanced diet that includes protein, carbohydrates, lipids, vitamins, and minerals.

- *Obesity.* Adipose tissue has a limited blood supply; thus, an obese client is more likely to acquire an infection. In addition, adipose tissue is difficult to suture, increasing the likelihood of wound dehiscence.

- *Medications.* Some medications may retard healing. Immunosuppressive agents, for example, can affect collagen synthesis, and anti-inflammatory drugs such as the corticosteroids can suppress the inflammatory reaction. In addition, the prolonged use of antibiotics can increase the likelihood of infection because of their effect on glucose metabolism and electrolyte balance, for example.

- *Smoking.* People who smoke have a reduced amount of functional hemoglobin, with a resultant reduced level of oxygen in the circulating blood. Oxygen is required for cellular metabolism.

- *Compromised host.* A compromised host is a person at risk for some other reason. For example, clients who have diabetes mellitus or acid-base imbalances may be more likely to get an infection. Some cancer therapies may also delay healing and increase susceptibility to infection.

Determine results of laboratory data pertinent to healing:

- *Leukocyte count.* A deficient leukocyte count can delay healing and increase the possibility of infection.

- *Blood coagulation studies.* Prolonged coagulation times can result in excessive blood loss and prolonged clot absorption. Hypercoagulability can lead to intravascular clotting. Intraarterial clotting can result in ischemia to the wound area.

RELATED DIAGNOSTIC CATEGORIES

- High risk for Infection

- Pain

Continued on page 916

Nursing Process Guide *CONTINUED*

- High risk for Impaired skin integrity (if the wound is draining)
- Knowledge deficit

PLANNING

Client Goals
The client will

- Avoid the complications of wound healing.
- Experience minimal pain.
- Regain skin integrity.

Outcome Criteria
The client

- Maintains normal or baseline vital signs.

- Achieves timely wound healing, as manifested by decreasing inflammation and wound drainage and absence of purulent drainage.
- Accomplishes activities of daily living with minimal or no pain.
- Maintains adequate dietary intake for healing.
- Maintains intact skin around drainage site.
- Resumes normal activities within specified period.
- Demonstrates wound care as instructed.
- Verbalizes understanding of discharge instructions.
- States signs of complications that require notification of the nurse or physician.

Types of Wounds

The skin encloses the body structures and the body fluids, thereby protecting them from external assault. When this protective barrier is penetrated, the inflammatory process of the individual's immune response acts to eliminate the foreign material, if possible, and prepare the injured body area for healing. This injured body area, whether internal or external, is called a **wound**.

Body wounds are either intentional or unintentional. *Intentional* traumas occur during therapy. Examples are operations, venipunctures, or radiation burns. Although removing a tumor is therapeutic, the surgeon must cut into body tissues, thus traumatizing them. *Unintentional* wounds are accidental; e.g., a person may fracture an arm in an automobile collision. If the tissues are traumatized without a break in the skin, the wound is *closed*. The wound is *open* when the skin or mucous membrane surface is broken.

Wounds can also be described according to the likelihood and degree of wound contamination (Garner 1986, p. 73).

- *Clean wounds* are uninfected wounds that are free of inflammation and do not enter the respiratory, alimentary, genital, or urinary tracts. Clean wounds are primarily closed wounds; or, if necessary, they are drained with closed drainage.
- *Clean-contaminated wounds* are surgical wounds in which the respiratory, alimentary, genital, or

urinary tract has been entered. Such wounds show no evidence of infection.

- *Contaminated wounds* include open, fresh, accidental wounds and surgical wounds involving a major break in sterile technique or a large amount of spillage from the gastrointestinal tract. Contaminated wounds show evidence of inflammation.
- *Dirty or infected wounds* include old, accidental wounds containing dead tissue and wounds with evidence of a clinical infection, e.g., purulent drainage.

Wound Healing

Following injury, the process of healing takes place. Only certain tissues of the body are capable of **regeneration** (renewal); those that are not form scars. Healing takes place by primary or secondary intention. **Primary intention healing** occurs where the tissue surfaces have been **approximated** (closed) and there is minimal or no tissue loss; it is characterized by the formation of minimal granulation tissue and scarring. It is also called *primary union* or *first intention healing*. Signs of primary intention healing are described in the Nursing Process Guide on page 915.

A wound heals by secondary intention when it is extensive and there is considerable tissue loss. **Secondary intention healing** differs from primary intention healing in three ways: (a) the repair time is longer; (b) the scarring is greater; and (c) the susceptibility to infection is greater. The complications of wound healing are shown in the accompanying box.

Kinds of Wound Drainage

There are three major types of **exudate** (material, such as fluid and cells, that has escaped from blood vessels during the inflammatory process and is deposited in tissue or on tissue surfaces): **serous** (consisting of serum), **purulent** (containing pus), and **sanguineous** (containing blood). A **serosanguineous** exudate is commonly seen in surgical incisions; it consists of serous and sanguineous drainage. Descriptions of these exudates are given in Table 39–1.

Specimens for culture and sensitivity may be taken from a draining wound to identify microorganisms that are causing an infection. The specimen is often taken when the dressing is changed. Determine agency protocol about cleaning the wound before

Complications of Wound Healing
Clinical Signs of Hemorrhage
Increased pulse rate
Increased respiratory rate
Lowered blood pressure
Restlessness
Thirst
Cold, clammy skin
Clinical Signs of Infection
Redness
Swelling
Pain
Induration (hardening of the tissues)
Fever
Increased leukocyte count
Clinical Signs of Dehiscence
Unexplained fever
Unexplained tachycardia
Unusual wound pain
Prolonged paralytic ileus

TABLE 39–1   KINDS OF WOUND DRAINAGE*

Type	Description	Constitutents
Serous	Watery, clear	Serum, few cells
Purulent	Viscous fluid; varies in color (e.g., blue, white, green)	Leukocytes, liquefied dead tissue debris, dead and living bacteria
Sanguineous (hemorrhagic)	Dark or bright red; liquid	Red blood cells

*Some kinds of drainage are combinations of the above, e.g., serosanguineous and purosanguineous.

obtaining the specimen. In some agencies, the wound is cleaned with sterile water or normal saline to remove excessive exudate before the specimen is obtained. In other agencies, only the area around the wound is cleaned with an alcohol or povidone-iodine sponge to minimize the risk of contaminating the specimen with skin bacteria. Technique 39–1 describes how to obtain a specimen of wound drainage.

39-1 Obtaining a Specimen of Wound Drainage

Before obtaining a specimen of wound drainage determine (a) whether the wound should be cleaned before taking the specimen and (b) whether the site from which to take the specimen has been specified.

PURPOSES

- To identify the microorganisms causing an infection and the antibiotics to which they are sensitive
- To evaluate the effectiveness of antibiotic therapy

▶ Technique 39–1 Obtaining a Specimen of Wound Drainage CONTINUED

ASSESSMENT FOCUS	Pain at the wound site; clinical signs of infection (e.g., fever, chills); appearances of the wound and the character and amount of wound drainage.

EQUIPMENT

- Disposable gloves
- Moisture-resistant (plastic or waxed paper) disposal bag
- Sterile dressing set, including dressings, cleaning solution, scissors, swabs, medications
- Sterile gloves
- Sterile culture tube or sterile syringe and needle (for an *aerobic culture,* use the standard culture tube with transport medium; for an *anaerobic culture,* use either a special culture tube containing carbon dioxide or nitrogen *or* a sterile 10-ml syringe and #21 gauge needle)
- Completed labels for each container
- Completed requisition to accompany the specimens to the laboratory

INTERVENTION

1. Remove any moist outer dressings that cover the wound.

- Put on disposable gloves.

- Remove the outer dressing, and observe any drainage on it. Hold the dressing so that the client does not see the drainage. *The appearance of the drainage could upset the client.*

- Discard the dressing in the moisture-resistant bag. Handle it carefully so that the dressing does not touch the outside of the bag. *Touching the outside of the bag will contaminate it.*

- Remove your gloves and dispose of them properly.

2. Open the sterile dressing set using sterile technique.

- See Technique 9–7, page 149.

3. Assess the wound.

- Put on sterile gloves.

- Assess the appearance of the tissues in and around the wound and the drainage. Infection can cause reddened tissues with a thick discharge, which may be foul-smelling, whitish, or colored.

- Determine the amount of the drainage, e.g., one 2 × 2 gauze saturated with pale yellow drainage.

4. Obtain the culture.

For an aerobic culture

- Open a specimen tube, and place the cap upside down on a firm, dry surface so that the inside will not become contaminated. Hold the tube in one hand, and pick up a swab in the other.

- Using the sterile swab, wipe the drainage at the designated point, i.e., at deep or active drainage areas of the wound. Absorb as much drainage as possible onto the swab. Wipe only once with one swab. *Only one wipe is taken with each swab to prevent contamination of other wound areas.*

- Insert the swab into the sterile container, taking care not to touch the top or the outside of the tube. *The outside of the container must remain free of pathogenic microorganisms to prevent their spread to others.*

- Close the container securely.

- If a specimen is required from another site, repeat the above steps. Specify the exact site (e.g., inferior drain site or lower aspect of incision) on the label of each container, if not labeled previously. Be sure to put each swab in the appropriately labeled tube.

For an anaerobic culture, using a special culture tube containing a swab

- Remove the swab from the inner tube of the anaerobic culture tube without removing the rubber stopper of the larger tube (Figure 39–1, *A*).

- Insert the sterile swab deeply into the draining body cavity.

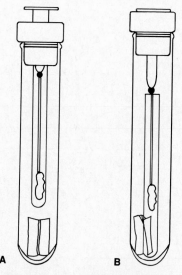

FIGURE 39–1 An anaerobic specimen culture tube with swab: *A,* before specimen collection; *B,* after specimen collection.

► **Technique 39–1** *CONTINUED*

- Rotate the swab gently.

- Remove the swab, and quickly replace it into the inner tube.

- Depress the plunger of the inner tube to force it down into the larger tube. *Pushing the inner tube down into the larger tube exposes the specimen to the carbon dioxide or nitrogen environment* (Figure 39–1, *B*).

- Label the tube appropriately.

For an anaerobic culture, using a sterile syringe and needle

- Insert a sterile 10-ml syringe (without needle) into the wound and aspirate 1 to 5 ml of drainage into the syringe.

- Attach the #21 gauge needle to the syringe, and expel all air from the syringe.

- Immediately inject the drainage into the anaerobic culture tube.
  or
  If a rubber stopper is available, insert the needle into the rubber stopper, and send the syringe of drainage to the laboratory immediately.

- Label the tube or syringe appropriately.

5. Clean and dress the wound.

- Clean the wound, if this step was not done previously.

- Apply any ordered medication to the wound. Cover the wound with sterile dressings. See Technique 39–2.

- Remove gloves, if worn, and dispose of them appropriately.

6. Arrange for the specimen to be transported to the laboratory immediately. Be sure to include the completed requisition.

7. Document all relevant information.

- Record on the client's chart the taking of the specimen.

- Include the date and time; the appearance of the wound; the color, consistency, amount, and odor of any drainage; and any discomfort experienced by the client.

EVALUATION FOCUS

The character of the drainage (amount, color, consistency, and odor); discomfort; appearance of the wound.

SAMPLE RECORDING

Date	Time	Notes
12/05/93	1500	Perineal dressing changed. Incision cleaned with Tr. Hibitane. Two 4 × 4 gauzes saturated with serous drainage at base of incision. Wound clean, edges closely approximated. Specimen taken from inferior part of incision. No redness on incision line or surrounding tissue. 3–4 × 4 gauze and 2 surgipads secured with T-binder. No discomfort. ———— Evangeline R. Puritos, RN

KEY ELEMENTS OF OBTAINING A SPECIMEN OF WOUND DRAINAGE

- Obtain appropriate culture tube or equipment (aerobic or anaerobic).

- Use aseptic technique. Wear clean gloves to remove soiled dressings and sterile gloves or sterile forceps to handle sterile dressings.

- Assess the appearance of tissues in and around the wound and the drainage.

- Take only one wipe of drainage with each swab used.

- Send the specimen immediately to the laboratory.

Preventing Wound Infection

The Centers for Disease Control recommend the following wound care practices for preventing wound infection (Garner 1986, pp. 78–79).

- Wash hands before and after caring for surgical wounds.

- Touch an open or fresh surgical wound only when wearing sterile gloves or using sterile forceps. After the wound is sealed, sterile gloves are no longer required.

- Remove or change dressings over open and closed wounds when they become wet.

- Take a specimen of any drainage from the wound that is suspected of being infected. Send the specimen to the laboratory for culture and Gram stain.

To prevent transmission of human immunodeficiency virus (HIV), the causative agent of acquired immunodeficiency syndrome (AIDS), the CDC (1987) makes the following recommendations specific to wound care:

- Wear gloves when touching blood and body fluids, mucous membranes, or nonintact skin of all clients, and when handling items or surfaces soiled with blood or body fluids.

- Wash hands thoroughly after removing gloves, and if contaminated with blood or body fluids.

- Take precautions to prevent injuries by needles, sharp instruments, or sharp devices.

- Avoid direct client care if you have open or weeping lesions or dermatitis.

- Wear gloves, surgical masks, and protective eyewear as appropriate if procedures commonly cause droplets or splashing of blood or body fluids.

Caring for Open and Closed Wounds

In the *open method* of wound care, no dressings are used. The *closed method* involves applying a dressing.

Prior to the 1960s, open wounds were treated by exposure to the air to encourage scab formation. Studies since then have revealed that superficial wounds heal faster when kept moist than when a scab forms. Studies have also shown that a moist environment speeds up collagen synthesis (Cuzzell and Stotts 1990, p. 54). As a result of these discoveries, a variety of occlusive and semiocclusive wound dressings have been developed, including thin films, hydrocolloids,

and foams. These dressings all hydrate the wound. See Table 39–2.

Cleaning Wounds

Caring for wounds involves cleaning (both open and closed wounds) and covering the wound. Cleaning agents vary considerably. Examples include povidone-iodine (Betadine), 70% isopropyl alcohol, and sterile normal saline. The choice depends on agency protocol and physician preference. Some nurses prefer cotton balls to clean wounds because of their absorbent qualities; others prefer gauze squares, claiming that threads of cotton balls can stick to sutures.

The RYB Color Code

To guide wound care, the nurse can use the RYB color code of wounds developed by Marion Laboratories, Inc. (Cuzzell 1988, p. 1342). This concept is based on the color of an open wound—red, yellow, or black (RYB)—rather than the depth or size of a wound. On this scheme, the goals of wound care are to *protect* red, *cleanse* yellow, and *debride* black. The RYB code can be applied to any wound allowed to heal by secondary intention.

Wounds that are *red* are usually in the late regeneration phase of tissue repair (i.e., developing granulation tissue) and are clean and uniformly pink in appearance. They need to be protected to avoid disturbance to regenerating tissue. Examples are superficial wounds, skin donor sites, and partial-thickness or second-degree burns. The nurse protects red wounds by (a) gentle cleansing, (b) avoiding the use of dry gauze or wet-to-dry saline dressings, (c) applying a topical antimicrobial agent, and/or (d) changing the dressing as infrequently as possible.

Yellow wounds are characterized primarily by liquid to semiliquid "slough" that is often accompanied by purulent drainage. The nurse *cleanses* yellow wounds to absorb drainage and remove nonviable tissue. Methods used may include applying wet-to-dry dressings, irrigating the wound, using absorbent dressing materials, and consulting with the physician about the need for a topical antimicrobial to minimize bacterial growth.

Black wounds are covered with thick necrotic tissue, or **eschar**. Examples are full-thickness or third-degree burns and gangrenous ulcers. Black wounds require **debridement** (removal of the infected and necrotic material) usually by a physician. When the eschar is removed, the wound is treated as yellow, then red. When more than one color is present, the nurse treats the most serious color first, i.e., black, then yellow, then red.

TABLE 39–2   TYPES OF DRESSINGS

Dressing	Description	Purpose
Dry-to-dry	A layer of wide-mesh cotton gauze lies next to the wound surface. A second layer of dry absorbent cotton or Dacron is on top.	Necrotic debris and exudate are trapped in the interstices of the contact (gauze) layer. These are removed when the dressing is removed.
Wet-to-dry	Next to the wound surface is a layer of wide-mesh cotton gauze saturated with saline or an antimicrobial solution. This layer is covered by a moist absorbent material, i.e., moistened with the same solution.	Necrotic debris is softened by the solution and then adheres to the mesh gauze as it dries. It is removed when the dressing is removed. Also, moisture helps dilute viscous exudate.
Wet-to-damp	A variation of the wet-to-dry dressing, this dressing is removed before it has completely dried.	The wound is debrided when the gauze is removed.
Wet-to-wet	A layer of wide-mesh gauze saturated with antibacterial or physiologic solution lies next to the wound surface. Above is a second layer of absorbent material saturated with the same solution. The entire dressing is kept moist with wetting agent.	The wound surface is continually bathed. Moisture dilutes viscous exudate.
Topical enzymes (e.g., Elase ointment)	The preparation is applied according to the manufacturer's instructions.	The preparation hastens separation of necrotic tissue.
Synthetic Dressings Thin film (e.g., Op-site)	Wound fluid is contained beneath a transparent, adhesive, plastic, nonabsorbent film (i.e., the dressing forms an "artificial" blister).	This dressing facilitates wound assessment, retains serous exudate, and keeps the wound moist, thereby hastening healing and reducing the risk of infection.
Hydrocolloid (e.g. DuoDERM)	A moderately absorbent occlusive wafer made of a gumlike material such as karaya and pectin is covered with a water-resistant outer film or foam layer. These dressings vary in translucence, absorbency, and thickness.	The dressing hydrates the wound surface. Wound fluid interacts with the wafer and melts it, forming a moist, jellylike substance that keeps the wound moist and promotes healing.
Hydrogel	A nonadhesive sheet of gelatinous dressing material composed of 95% water and 5% gel-form polymers is placed next to the wound surface.	The dressing keeps the wound moist, but because the dressing absorbs exudate slowly, it can cause maceration of wounds that have excessive exudate.
Foam	A nonadherent sheet of inert material that varies in thickness and degree of absorbency is placed against the wound surface. The sheet requires a cover dressing to seal the edges and obtain an occlusive environment.	The foam prevents cell dessication (drying) of superficial cavities and flat granulating wounds; it also absorbs moderate amounts of exudate.
Liquid gel	A clear, nonabsorbent, hydrating gel coats the wound surface.	The preparation prevents cell dessication.
Absorption powders, flakes, granules, gels, and pastes	Substances of cellulose, gelatin, hydrophilic particles or copolymer starches are applied to the wound surface.	These preparations provide absorptive dressings but also keep the wound surface moist.

Sources: J. Z. Cuzzell, Wound care forum: Artful solutions to chronic problems, *American Journal of Nursing,* February 1985, 85:162–66; J. Z. Cuzzell and N. A. Stotts, Wound care: Trial and error yields to knowledge, *American Journal of Nursing,* October 1990, 90:59; E. Fowler, J. Z. Cuzzell, and J. C. Papen, Healing with hydrocolloid. *American Journal of Nursing,* February 1991, 91:63–64; and S. Bale and K. G. Harding, Foams still find favor: Wound management using foam dressings, *Professional Nurse,* June 1991, 6:510, 512–14, 516.

Dressing Materials

Several sizes of gauze are available to cover wounds (Figure 39–2). The standard sizes are 10 × 10 cm (4 × 4 in) and 10× 20 cm (4 × 8 in). The size and number of pads used depend on the nature of the wound, the amount of exudate, and the location of the wound. These decisions are left to the nurse's judgment. Sometimes the gauze is precut halfway through one side to make it fit around a drain, or it is folded in a special way.

Telfa gauze is a special type. It has a shiny, non-adherent surface on one or both sides and is applied

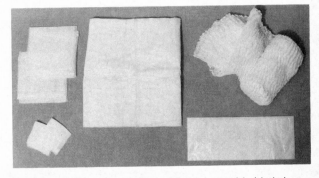

FIGURE 39–2   Some frequently used dressing materials (clockwise from bottom left): 2 × 2 gauze; 4 × 4 gauze; surgipad, or abdominal pad; roller gauze; and nonadherent absorbent dressing.

with the shiny surface on the wound. Exudate seeps through this surface and collects on the absorbent material on the other side or is sandwiched between the two nonadherent surfaces. Since the dressing does not adhere, it does not cause injury to the wound when removed. *Petrolatum* gauze, another nonadherent type, is impregnated with petroleum jelly. It is placed against the wound and usually covered with 4 × 4 gauze. Nonadherent dressings should not be used when wound debridement is desired.

Larger and thicker gauze dressings, called *surgipads* or *abdominal pads*, are used to cover small gauzes. They not only hold the other gauzes in place but also absorb and collect excess drainage. Surgipads are more absorbent on one side, and this side is placed toward the wound; the less absorbent, more protective side is placed outward to protect the wound from external contamination. The outer side is often indicated with a blue stripe.

See also the discussions of moist transparent wound barriers and hydrocolloid dressings on pages 928 and 930.

Securing Dressings

The nurse tapes the dressing over the wound, ensuring that the dressing covers the entire wound and does not become dislodged. The correct type of tape must be selected for the purpose. Elastic tape can provide pressure; nonallergenic tape is used when a client is allergic to other tape. The nurse follows these steps:

1. Place the tape so that the dressing cannot be folded back to expose the wound. Place strips at the ends of the dressing, and space tapes evenly in the middle (Figure 39–3).

2. Ensure that the tape is long and wide enough to adhere to the skin but not so long or wide that it loosens with activity (Figure 39–3).

3. Place the tape in the opposite direction from the body action, e.g., across a body joint or crease, not lengthwise (Figure 39–4).

After surgery, an elastic adhesive tape may be applied over wounds because of its ability to compress, thereby controlling hemorrhage. The original tape is removed during the initial dressing change, and a lighter dressing is applied. The nurse secures the dressing at both ends and across the middle and uses tape of a sufficient width for the dressing and the wound.

Montgomery straps (tie tapes) are commonly used for wounds requiring frequent dressing changes (Figure 39–5). These straps prevent skin irritation and discomfort caused by removing the adhesive each time the dressing is changed. Nonallergenic tie tapes

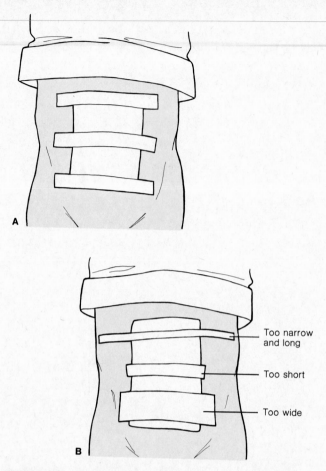

FIGURE 39–3 The strips of tape should be placed at the ends of the dressing and must be sufficiently long and wide to secure the dressing: *A,* correct taping; *B,* incorrect taping.

are available for people with sensitive skin. If these are not available, the nurse can protect the skin by applying tincture of benzoin to the site where the adhesive is to be placed.

Dry Dressings

Sterile dry dressings are used for wounds that have minimal drainage and no tissue loss and heal by *primary intention* (e.g., surgical incisions). Most dressings have three layers:

1. A *nonadhering contact dressing* that covers the incision and part of the surrounding skin and that collects fibrin, blood products, and debris from the wound

2. An *absorbent gauze dressing* that acts as a reservoir for excess secretions

3. A *thicker outer dressing* that protects the wound from external contamination

Not all surgical dressings require changing. Sometimes surgeons in the operating room apply a dressing that remains in place until the sutures are removed, and no further dressings are required. In

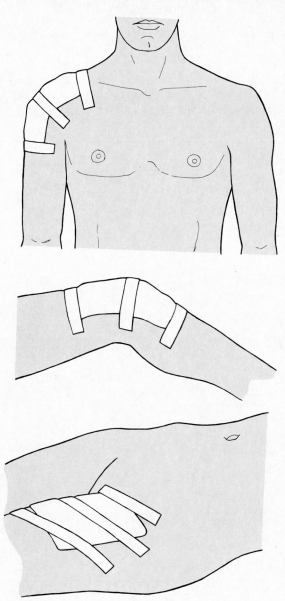

FIGURE 39–4 Dressings over moving parts must remain secure in spite of the movement.

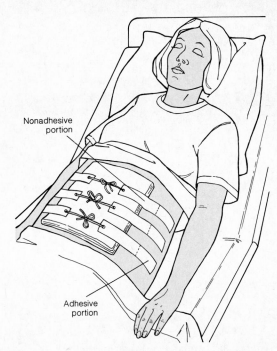

FIGURE 39–5 Montgomery straps, or tie tapes, are used to secure large dressings that require frequent changing.

most situations, however, surgical dressings are changed regularly to prevent the growth of microorganisms.

In some instances, a client may have a Penrose drain inserted. The main surgical incision is considered cleaner than the surgical stab wound made for the drain insertion, because there usually is considerable drainage. The main incision is therefore cleaned first, and under no circumstances are materials used to clean the stab wound used subsequently to clean the main incision. In this way, the main incision is kept free of the microorganisms around the stab wound. Changing a dry sterile dressing is detailed in Technique 39–2.

39-2 Changing a Dry Sterile Dressing

Before changing a dressing, determine any specific orders about the wound or dressing. Also see Nursing Process Guide on page 915.

PURPOSES
- To promote wound healing by primary intention
- To prevent infection
- To assess the healing process
- To protect the wound from mechanical trauma

ASSESSMENT FOCUS

Allergies to wound cleaning agents; the appearance and size of the wound; the amount and character of exudate; complaints of discomfort; the time of the last pain medication; signs of systemic infection (e.g., elevated body temperature, diaphoresis, malaise; leukocytosis).

▶ Technique 39–2 Changing a Dry Sterile Dressing CONTINUED

EQUIPMENT

- ☐ Bath blanket (if necessary)
- ☐ Moistureproof bag
- ☐ Mask (optional)
- ☐ Acetone or another solution (if necessary to loosen adhesive)
- ☐ Disposable gloves
- ☐ Sterile gloves
- ☐ Sterile dressing set; if none is available, gather the following

  sterile items from a central supply cart
  - Drape or towel
  - Gauze squares
  - Container for the cleaning solution
  - Antimicrobial solution
  - Two pairs of forceps (thumb or artery)

  - Gauze dressings and surgipads
  - Applicators or tongue blades to apply ointments
- ☐ Additional supplies required for the particular dressing, e.g., extra gauze dressings and ointment or powder, if ordered
- ☐ Tape, tie tapes, or binder

INTERVENTION

1. Prepare the client, and assemble the equipment.

- Ⓢ Acquire assistance for changing a dressing on a restless or confused adult. *The person might move and contaminate the sterile field or the wound.*

- Assist the client to a comfortable position in which the wound can be readily exposed. Expose only the wound area, using a bath blanket to cover the client, if necessary. *Undue exposure is physically and psychologically distressing to most people.*

- Make a cuff on the moistureproof bag for disposal of the soiled dressings, and place the bag within reach. It can be taped to the bedclothes or bedside table. *Making a cuff keeps the outside of the bag free from contamination by the soiled dressings and prevents subsequent contamination of the nurse's hands or of sterile instrument tips when discarding dressings or sponges. Placement of the bag within reach prevents the nurse from reaching across the sterile field and the wound and potentially contaminating these areas.*

- Don a face mask, if required. *Some agencies require that a mask be worn for surgical dressing changes to prevent contamination of the wound by droplet spray* Ⓢ *from the nurse's respiratory tract.*

2. Remove outer dressings.

- Remove binders, if used, and place them aside. Untie tie tapes, if used.

- Ⓢ If adhesive tape was used, remove it by holding down the skin and pulling the tape gently but firmly toward the wound. *Pressing down on the skin provides countertraction against the pulling motion. Tape is pulled toward the incision to prevent strain on the sutures or wound.*

- Use a solvent to loosen tape, if required. *Moistening the tape with acetone or a similar solvent lessens the discomfort of removal, particularly from hairy surfaces.*

- Don disposable gloves, and remove the outer abdominal dressing or surgipad. *The outer surgipad is considered contaminated by the client's clothing and linen.*

- Lift the dressing so that the underside is away from the client's face. *The appearance and odor of the drainage may be upsetting to the client.*

3. Dispose of soiled dressings appropriately.

- Place the soiled dressing in the moisture-resistant bag without touching the outside of the bag. *Contamination of the outside of the bag is avoided to prevent the spread of microorganisms to the nurse and subsequently to others.*

- Remove gloves, dispose of them in the moisture-resistant bag, and wash your hands.

4. Remove inner dressings.

- Open the sterile dressing set, using surgical aseptic technique.

- Place the sterile drape beside the wound, and don sterile gloves (optional).

- Remove the under dressings with tissue forceps or sterile gloves, taking care not to dislodge any drains. If the gauze sticks to the drain, use two pairs of forceps, one to remove the gauze and one to hold the drain, or secure the drain with one hand. *Forceps or gloves are used to prevent contamination of the wound by the nurse's hands and contamination of the nurse's hands by wound drainage.*

- Assess the location, type (color, consistency), and odor of wound drainage, and the number of gauzes saturated or the diameter of drainage collected on the dressings.

- Discard the soiled dressings in the bag. To avoid contaminating the forceps tips on the edge of the paper bag, hold the dressings 10 to 15 cm (4 to 6 in) above the bag, and drop the dressings into it.

- After the dressings are removed, discard the forceps, or set them

▶ **Technique 39–2** *CONTINUED*

aside from the sterile field. *These forceps are now contaminated by the wound drainage.*

5. Clean the wound.

- Clean the wound, using the second pair of artery or tissue forceps and gauze swabs moistened with antiseptic solution.

- Keep the forceps tips lower than the handles at all times. *This prevents their contamination by fluid traveling up to the handle and nurse's wrist and back to the tips.*

- Clean with strokes from the top to the bottom, starting at the center and continuing to the outside (Figure 39–6).

or

Clean with strokes outward from the incision on one side and then outward on the other side (Figure 39–7). *The wound is cleaned from the least to the most contaminated area, e.g., from the top of the incision, which is drier, to the bottom of the incision, where any drainage will collect and which is considered more contaminated, or from the incision outward.*

- Use a separate swab for each stroke, and discard each swab after use. *This prevents the introduction of microorganisms to other wound areas.*

- If a drain is present, clean it after

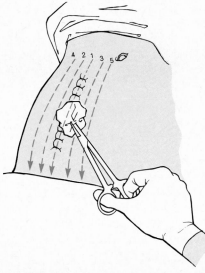

FIGURE 39–6   Cleaning a wound from top to bottom, starting at the center.

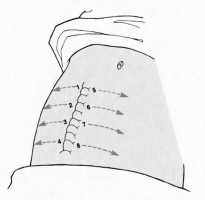

FIGURE 39–7   Cleaning a wound outward from the incision.

the incision.

- For irregular wounds, such as a decubitus ulcer, clean from the center of the wound outward, using circular strokes.

- Repeat the cleaning process until

all drainage is removed.

- Dry the wound with dry gauze swabs as required, using the strokes described above.

6. Assess the overall appearance of the wound.

- See the Nursing Process Guide on page 915.

7. Apply the ordered powder or ointment.

- Shake powders directly onto the wound. Antibiotic powders may be ordered by the physician.

- Use sterile applicators or tongue blades to apply ointments. *Ointments can protect the skin from irritation if drainage is profuse.*

8. Apply sterile dressings.

- Apply sterile dressings one at a time over the wound, using sterile forceps or sterile gloves. Start at the center of the wound and move progressively outward. The final surgipad can be picked up by hand, touching only the outside, which is often marked by a blue line down the center.

- Remove and discard gloves, if worn.

- Secure the dressing with tape, tie tapes, or a binder.

9. Document the change of dressing and all nursing assessments.

EVALUATION FOCUS	Amount of granulation tissue or degree of healing; amount of discharge and its color and odor; presence of inflammation; degree of discomfort associated with wound care.

SAMPLE RECORDING

Date	Time	Notes
12/05/93	1500	Abdominal dressing changed. Incision cleaned with isopropyl alcohol 70%. Two 4 × 4 gauzes saturated with serous drainage at base of incision. Wound clean, edges closely approximated. Slight redness on incision line, no redness on surrounding tissue. 4 × 4 gauze and surgipads secured with tie tapes. No discomfort voiced. ——— Evangeline R. Puritos, RN

▶ **Technique 39–2 Changing a Dry Sterile Dressing** CONTINUED

KEY ELEMENTS OF CHANGING A DRY STERILE DRESSING

- Support the adjacent skin when removing adhesive tape.
- Pull tape toward the wound rather than away from it.
- Wear disposable gloves when removing moist outer dressings.
- Use sterile forceps or gloves to remove under dressings.
- Support a drain appropriately when removing dressings.
- Use separate sterile forceps to clean and dress the wound.

- Use a separate swab for each cleaning stroke.
- Clean the wound from the least to the most contaminated area.
- Clean a drain site after the incision.
- Dry the wound appropriately.
- Apply sufficient dressings to cover the wound and absorb drainage.
- Secure the dressing securely.
- Assess the wound appearance and drainage accurately.

Wet-to-Dry Dressings

Sterile wet-to-dry dressings may be prescribed for debridement of wounds with extensive tissue loss that heal by secondary intention. Examples of such wounds are burns, varicose ulcers, or decubitus ulcers. These wounds are not amenable to suturing.

Wet-to-dry dressings consist of a moistened contact dressing layer that touches the wound surface. This layer is allowed to dry between dressing changes every 4 to 6 hours. The wet gauze traps necrotic material in its spaces as it dries. Dry dressings do not trap the debris as effectively. Wet dressings that do not dry out enough to trap debris promote bacterial growth in the damp environment and can cause tissue breakdown. Generally, 4 × 4 non-cotton-filled gauze dressings are used. Cotton fibers are contraindicated because they can pull loose and remain in the wound, encouraging bacterial growth and contamination. See Table 39–2 on page 921 for types of dressings. Technique 39–3 explains how to apply wet-to-dry dressings.

39-3 Applying Wet-to-Dry Dressings

PURPOSE
- To debride a wound and promote secondary intention healing

ASSESSMENT FOCUS

See Assessment Focus, Technique 39–2, page 923.

EQUIPMENT

- Moistureproof bag
- Mask (optional)
- Disposable gloves
- Sterile gloves

- Sterile dressing equipment (see Technique 39–2).
- Sterile thin, fine-mesh gauze

- Ordered solution
- Tape, tie tapes, bandage, or binder

▶ **Technique 39–3 Applying Wet-to-Dry Dressings** *CONTINUED*

INTERVENTION

1. Ensure that the client's medication has been given before the procedure is begun.

- Check the physician's orders and the nursing progress notes. Clients are usually medicated before this procedure.

2. Assemble all equipment, prepare the client, and remove the outer dressings.

- See steps 1 to 3 in Technique 39–2.

3. Gradually free the wet-to-dry dressing as quickly as possible.

- Do not moisten the dressing. *Wet-to-dry dressings are intended to clean wounds by debridement of the exudate or necrotic tissue.*

- Dispose of soiled dressings appropriately in the moistureproof bag.

- Remove the disposable gloves, and discard them in the bag.

- Wash your hands.

4. Assess the wound.

- Assess the character and amount of drainage on the dressings and the appearance of the wound, i.e., the progress of healing by secondary intention.

- Observe the development and amount of granulation tissue.

5. Apply the wet-to-dry dressing.

- Open the packages of the sterile dressing set, fine-mesh gauze, and sterile solution container.

- Pour the ordered solution into the solution container.

- Don the sterile gloves.

- Place the fine-mesh gauze dressings into the solution container, and thoroughly saturate them with solution. *The entire gauze must be moistened to enhance its absorptive abilities.*

- If agency protocol indicates, clean the wound gently, using a circular motion. Work outward from the center of the wound to its edge and beyond. Use a separate gauze swab for each cleaning stroke.

- Wring out excess moisture from the saturated fine mesh gauze dressings. *Dressings that are too wet will not dry out in 4 to 6 hours.*

- Pack the moistened dressings into all depressions and grooves of the wound, ensuring that all exposed surfaces are covered. If necessary, use forceps to feed the gauze gradually into deep depressed areas. *Necrotic tissue is usually more prevalent in depressed wound areas and needs to be covered with the wet-to-dry gauze.*

6. Cover the wet-to-dry dressing with dry dressings.

- Apply a dry 4 × 4 gauze over the wet dressings. *The dry gauze absorbs excess drainage.*

- Cover the dressings with a surgipad or abdominal pad. *The pad protects the wound from external contaminants.*

- Remove your gloves, and discard them.

- Secure the dressing at the edges only, with tape, tie tapes, bandage, or binder. Do *not* apply an airtight occlusive covering. *Occlusive dressings prevent air circulation and hinder drying of the fine-mesh gauze.*

7. Document the change of dressing and nursing assessments.

EVALUATION FOCUS	Amount of granulation tissue or degree of healing; character and amount of exudate on dressing; level of discomfort associated with wound care.

SAMPLE RECORDING

Date	Time	Notes
06/04/93	1015	Wet-to-dry dressing using sterile normal saline applied to ulcer on L lateral ankle. Ulcer is 3 cm in diameter with 0.5 cm granulation tissue at edges. Inner aspect filled with dark yellow drainage. Dry nonocclusive dressing applied and secured with tape. —————— Robert Tetley-Jones, RN
	1415	Tylenol #3 given for discomfort. —————— Robert Tetley-Jones, RN
	1445	Wet-to-dry dressing removed. Two 4 × 4 gauzes saturated with brownish drainage. No complaints. —————— Robert Tetley-Jones, RN

▶ **Technique 39–3 Applying Wet-to-Dry Dressings** CONTINUED

KEY ELEMENTS OF APPLYING WET-TO-DRY DRESSINGS

- Before applying the dressing, medicate the client as ordered.
- Maintain asepsis.
- Verify the ordered solution, and check agency policy about cleaning the wound.
- Remove the wet-to-dry dressing as quickly as possible, without moistening it.
- Assess the wound appearance and drainage accurately.

- Thoroughly saturate the mesh gauze with solution, and then wring out excess moisture.
- Make sure all depressions and grooves of the wound are packed with the gauze.
- Cover the wet dressings appropriately. Do not apply an airtight occlusive covering.

Moist Transparent Wound Barriers

Transparent wound barriers such as Op-Site, Tegaderm, and Bio-occlusive are often applied to wounds including ulcerated or burned skin areas. These dressings offer several advantages:

- They act as temporary skin.
- They are nonporous, self-adhesive dressings that do not require changing as other dressings do. They are often left in place until healing has occurred or as long as they remain intact.
- Because they are transparent, the wound can be assessed through them.
- Because they are occlusive, the wound remains moist and retains the serous exudate, which pro-

motes epithelial growth, hastens healing, and reduces the risk of infection.

- Because they are elastic, they can be placed over a joint without disrupting the client's mobility.
- They adhere only to the skin area around the wound and not to the wound itself, because the wound is kept moist.
- They allow the client to shower or bathe without removing the dressing.
- They can be removed without damaging wound tissues.

Technique 39–4 describes how to apply a moist transparent wound barrier.

Applying a Moist Transparent Wound Barrier

Before applying or changing a moist transparent wound barrier, (a) verify the physician's orders regarding frequency and type of dressing change, and (b) determine agency protocol about solutions used to clean the wound.

PURPOSES
- To contain exudate and prevent wound infection
- To provide a moist wound environment and promote wound healing
- To protect the wound from trauma
- To facilitate assessment of wound healing

▶ **Technique 39–4 Applying a Moist Transparent Wound Barrier** *CONTINUED*

ASSESSMENT FOCUS	See Technique 39–2 on page 923.

EQUIPMENT

- □ Disposable gloves
- □ Soap and water
- □ Razor (optional) or clippers
- □ Alcohol or acetone
- □ Moistureproof bag
- □ Sterile gloves

- □ Sterile gauze and the wound-cleaning agents specified by the physician or agency (e.g., sterile saline, hydrogen peroxide, or povidone-iodine)

- □ Wound barrier
- □ Scissors
- □ Paper tape
- □ Sterile #26 gauze needle and syringe

INTERVENTION

1. **Obtain assistance as needed.**

- If the size of the wound necessitates it, acquire the assistance of a coworker to help apply the dressing.

2. **Thoroughly clean the skin area around the wound.**

- Don disposable gloves.

- Clean the skin well with soap and water.

- Clip the hair about 5 cm (2 in) around the wound area if indicated.

- Rub the area with alcohol or acetone, and allow it to dry. *Alcohol or acetone defats the skin. Defatted, clean, dry skin ensures better adhesion of the dressing.*

- Remove gloves, and dispose of them in the moistureproof bag.

3. **Clean the wound if indicated.**

- Don sterile gloves.

- Clean the wound with the prescribed solution.

4. **Assess the wound.**
- See the Nursing Process Guide on page 915.

5. **Apply the wound barrier.**

- Remove part of the paper backing on the dressing. If you have an assistant, remove all of the paper backing; the two of you should hold the colored tabs attached to the dressing.

- Apply the dressing at one edge of the wound site, allowing at least 2.5-cm (1-in) coverage of the skin surrounding the wound.

- Gently lay or press the barrier over the wound. Keep it free of wrinkles, but avoid stretching it too tightly. *A stretched dressing restricts mobility.*

- Cut off the colored tabs after the wound is completely covered.

- Remove and discard gloves.

6. **Reinforce the dressing as needed.**

- Apply paper or other porous tape to the edges of the dressing.

7. **Assess the wound at least daily.**

- Determine the extent of serous fluid accumulation under the dressing, wound healing, and the need to repair the dressing.

- If excessive serum has accumulated, use a sterile #26 gauge needle to aspirate the fluid. Then patch the needle hole.

- If the dressing is leaking, remove it, and apply another dressing.

8. **Document the technique and all nursing assessments.**

EVALUATION FOCUS	Amount of granulation tissue or degree of healing; amount of serous fluid under dressing (see step 7); degree of discomfort associated with wound care.

SAMPLE RECORDING

Date	Time	Notes
04/08/93	1030	Moist transparent dressing applied over R ankle ulcer. (2.2 cm in diameter). Wound clean with minimal serous drainage. Edges inflamed. Wound tender when touched. ——————— Jackie Lombardi, RN
04/08/93	1100	Transparent dressing over ulcer inspected. Minimal serous drainage. Dressing borders intact. ——————— Jackie Lombardi, RN

▶ **Technique 39–4 Applying a Moist Transparent Wound Barrier** *CONTINUED*

KEY ELEMENTS OF APPLYING A MOIST TRANSPARENT WOUND BARRIER

- Maintain asepsis.
- Wear appropriate gloves when preparing the surrounding skin and cleaning the wound.
- Clean, thoroughly dry, and defat the surrounding skin before applying a wound barrier.
- Assess the wound accurately before the application and then at least daily.

- Cover the surrounding skin area sufficiently with the dressing.
- Keep the wound barrier free of wrinkles.
- Secure the dressing appropriately.
- Aspirate excessive fluid by using a small sterile needle and syringe as required and then patch the needle hole.

Hydrocolloid Dressings

Hydrocolloid dressings (see Table 39–2), such as DuoDERM, are used to (a) protect granulation tissue from excessive drying and trauma, (b) absorb slight to moderate amounts of wound drainage, and (c) liquefy necrotic tissue by autolysis (Fowler, Cuzzell, and Papen 1991, p. 63). They are frequently used over venous stasis ulcers and pressure ulcers. These dressings offer several advantages:

- They last a long time.
- They do not need a "cover" dressing and are water resistant, so the client can shower or bathe.
- They can be molded to uneven body surfaces.
- They act as temporary skin and provide an effective bacterial barrier.
- They decrease pain and thus reduce the need for analgesics.

- They absorb some drainage and therefore can be used on draining wounds.
- They contain wound odor.

These dressings have certain limitations, however (Fowler, Cuzzell, and Papen 1991, p. 63):

- They are opaque and obscure wound visibility.
- They have a limited absorption capacity.
- They can facilitate anaerobic bacterial growth.
- They can soften and wrinkle at the edges with wear and movement.
- They can be difficult to remove and may leave a residue on the skin.

 Because of these limitations, hydrocolloid dressings should not be used for infected wounds or those with deep tracts or fistulas.

Technique 39–5 describes how to apply colloid dressings.

 39-5 **Applying a Hydrocolloid Dressing**

A hydrocolloid dressing should be changed whenever it becomes dislodged, leaks, or develops an odor. If the wound has substantial drainage or yellow slough, it may need to be changed every 24 to 72 hours. If it is applied to liquefy necrotic material, the change may need to be done more frequently. When drainage subsides, the dressing may be left in place for 3 to 7 days.

PURPOSES
- To maintain a moist wound surface and promote healing
- To prevent the entrance of microorganisms into the wound
- To minimize wound discomfort
- To promote autolysis of necrotic material by white blood cells
- To decrease the frequency of dressing changes

ASSESSMENT FOCUS

See Technique 39–2 on page 923.

▶ **Technique 39–5 Applying a Hydrocolloid Dressing** CONTINUED

EQUIPMENT

- Disposable gloves
- Moistureproof bag
- Soap and water
- Dressing set
- Sterile normal saline or other cleaning agent used by the agency
- Sterile gloves
- Hydrocolloid dressing of appropriate size
- Tape

INTERVENTION

1. Remove the old dressing.

- Put on disposable gloves.

- Pull the dressing off gradually in the direction of hair growth. *This minimizes skin irritation.*

- Dispose of the soiled dressing into the moistureproof bag.

2. Clean the skin area around the wound.

- Gently wash the skin surrounding the wound with soap and water, and dry it thoroughly with gauze squares.

- Leave the residue that is difficult to remove on the skin. It will wear off in time. *Attempts to remove residue can irritate the surrounding skin.*

3. Clean the wound if indicated.

- Open the sterile dressing supplies.

- Pour saline or other cleaning agent into the sterile container.

- Don sterile gloves.

- Clean the wound with the prescribed solution.

4. Assess the wound.

- See the Nursing Process Guide on page 915.

5. Apply the dressing.

- Follow the manufacturer's instructions.

- Remove the sterile gloves by pulling them inside out. *This de-creases the risk of microorganism transmission.*

- Optional: Tape all four sides of the dressing as required or according to agency protocol. *Taping prevents the dressing from sticking to bed linens and the edges from lifting.*

6. Assess and change the dressing as indicated.

- Inspect the dressing at least daily for leakage, dislodgement, odor, and wrinkling.

- Change the dressing if the above signs are present.

7. Document the technique and all nursing assessments.

EVALUATION FOCUS

Amount of granulation tissue or degree of healing; amount and character of any drainage; level of discomfort associated with wound care.

SAMPLE RECORDING

Date	Time	Notes
08/04/93	1330	Sacral ulcer (3.5 cm in diameter) cleaned with normal saline Wound filled with yellow slough and pale yellow drainage. Edges inflammed. No granulation tissue. DuoDERM dressing applied. ———— Malika Marriot, RN

KEY ELEMENTS OF APPLYING A HYDROCOLLOID DRESSING

- Maintain asepsis.
- Wear appropriate gloves when preparing the surrounding skin and cleaning the wound.
- Clean and thoroughly dry the surrounding skin before applying the dressing.
- Assess the wound accurately before the application and then whenever the dressing is changed.

- Cover the surrounding skin area sufficiently with the dressing.
- Secure the dressing with tape over all four edges, if indicated.
- Inspect the dressing at least daily for leaks, dislodgment, or odor.

Wound Drains and Suction

Surgical **drains** are inserted to permit the drainage of excessive serosanguineous fluid and purulent material and to promote healing of underlying tissues. These drains may be inserted and sutured through the incision line, but they are most commonly inserted through stab wounds a few centimeters away from the incision line so that the incision itself may be kept dry. Without a drain, some wounds would heal on the surface and trap the discharge inside. Then the tissues under the skin could not heal because of the discharge, and an abscess might form. These drains, e.g., the **Penrose drain**, have an open end that drains onto a dressing.

Drains vary in length and width. The length can be 25 to 35 cm (10 to 14 in), and the width 2.5 to 4 cm (0.5 to 1.5 in). To facilitate drainage and healing of tissues from the inside to the outside, or from the bottom to the top, the physician may order that the drain be pulled out or shortened 2 to 5 cm (1 to 2 in) each day. When a drain is completely removed, the remaining stab wound usually heals within a day or two. In some agencies, this shortening procedure is performed only by physicians; in others, it is ordered by the physician and performed by nurses. When changing a dressing of a draining wound, the nurse should be careful not to dislodge the drain. Shortening the drain is usually done when the dressing is changed. Technique 39–6 describes cleaning a drain site and shortening a Penrose drain.

A *closed wound drainage system* consists of a drain connected to either an electric suction or a portable

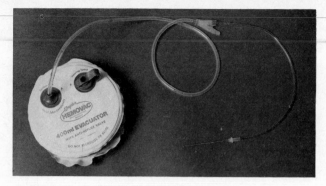

FIGURE 39–8 Closed wound drainage system (Hemovac).

drainage suction, such as a Hemovac (Figure 39–8) or Jackson-Pratt. The closed system eliminates the possible entry of microorganisms into the wound through the drain. The drainage tubes are sutured (stitched) in place and connected to a reservoir. For example, the Jackson-Pratt drainage tube is connected to a reservoir that maintains constant low suction. These portable wound suctions also provide for accurate measurement of the drainage.

The surgeon inserts the wound drainage tube during surgery. Generally, the suction is discontinued from 3 to 7 days postoperatively or when the wound is free from drainage. Nurses are responsible for maintaining the patency of the tube used for wound suction, which hastens the healing process by draining excess exudate that might otherwise interfere with the formation of granulation tissue. Technique 39–7 describes how to establish and maintain a closed wound drainage system.

39-6

Cleaning a Drain Site and Shortening a Penrose Drain

Before cleaning a drain site and shortening a Penrose drain, determine (a) agency protocol about who may shorten drains; (b) that the drain is to be shortened and the length it is to be shortened, e.g., 2.5 cm (1 in); (c) whether the drain has been shortened previously (drains that have not been shortened previously are often attached to the skin by a suture, which must be removed before shortening the drain); (d) the location of the drain; and (e) the type and amount of discharge previously recorded and previous assessments of the appearance of the wound, for baseline data.

PURPOSES

Cleaning a Drain Site
- To remove any discharge from the skin, thereby reducing the danger of skin irritation
- To reduce the number of microorganisms present and therefore decrease the possibility of infection

▶ **Technique 39–6** CONTINUED
───

Shortening a Drain
- To decrease the length of the drain a designated amount, thereby encouraging healing of the wound from the inside toward the outside

ASSESSMENT FOCUS	See Technique 39–2 on page 923.

───

EQUIPMENT

- ☐ Moistureproof bag
- ☐ Mask for the nurse and one for the client, if necessary
- ☐ Disposable gloves
- ☐ Sterile gloves
- ☐ Sterile dressing equipment, including
  - Two pairs of forceps, including at least one hemostat

- Sterile cotton-tipped applicators
- Sterile dressing materials sufficient to cover the surgical incision and the drain site (at least two 4 × 4 gauzes are usually needed to dress the drain site, more if drainage is copious; a sterile precut gauze is needed to apply first

around the drain site)
- Sterile suture scissors (if the drain has *not* been shortened previously)
- Sterile scissors
- Sterile safety pin (add this to the sterile dressing set)
- ☐ Tape, tie tapes, or other binding supplies

───

INTERVENTION

1. Verify the physician's order.

S • Confirm that the drain is to be shortened by the nurse and the length it is to be shortened, e.g., 2.5 cm (1 in).

2. Prepare the client.

- Inform the client that the drain is to be shortened and that this procedure should not be painful.

- Explain that there may be a pulling sensation for a few seconds when the drain is being drawn out before it is shortened.

- Position the client as for a dressing change.

3. Remove dressings, and clean the incision.

- See Technique 39–2, steps 2 to 5, pages 924–925. *The incision is cleaned first because it is considered cleaner than the drain site. Moist drainage facilitates the growth of resident skin bacteria around the drain.*

4. Clean and assess the drain site.

- Clean the skin around the drain site by swabbing in half or full circles from around the drain

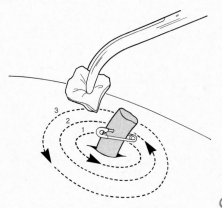
FIGURE 39–9 Cleaning the skin around a drain site.

site outward, using separate swabs for each wipe (Figure 39–9). You may hold forceps in the nondominant hand to hold the drain erect while cleaning around it. Clean as many times as necessary to remove the drainage.

- Assess the amount and character of drainage, including odor, thickness, and color.

5. Shorten the drain.

- If the drain has *not* been shortened before, cut and remove the suture. See Technique 39–9. *The drain is sutured to the skin during*

surgery to keep it from slipping into the body cavity.

- With a hemostat, firmly grasp the drain by its full width at the level of the skin, and pull the drain out the required length. *Grasping the full width of the drain ensures even traction.*

- Wearing sterile gloves, insert the sterile safety pin through the base of the drain as close to the skin as possible by holding the drain tightly against the skin edge and inserting the pin above your fingers (Figure 39–10). *The pin keeps the drain from falling back into the incision. Holding the drain securely in place at the skin level and inserting the pin above the fingers prevents the nurse from*

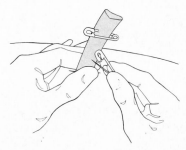
FIGURE 39–10 Pinning a drain.

▶ **Technique 39–6 Shortening a Penrose Drain** *CONTINUED*

pulling the drain further out or pricking the client during this step.

• With the sterile scissors, cut off the excess drain so that about 2.5 cm (1 in) remains above the skin (Figure 39–11). Discard the excess in the waste bag.

6. Apply dressings to the drain site and the incision.

• Place a precut 4 × 4 gauze snugly around the drain (Figure 39–12), or open a 4 × 4 gauze to 4 × 8, fold it lengthwise to 2 × 8, and place the 2 × 8 around the drain so that the ends overlap. *This dressing absorbs the drainage and helps prevent it from excoriating the skin. Using precut gauze or folding it as described, instead of cutting the gauze, prevents any threads from coming loose and get-*

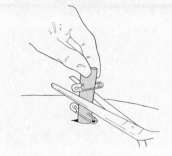

FIGURE 39–11 Shortening a drain.

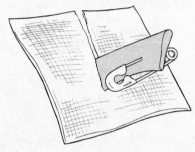

FIGURE 39–12 Precut gauze in place around a drain.

ting into the wound, where they could cause inflammation and provide a site for infection.

• Apply the sterile dressings one at a time, using sterile gloved hands or sterile forceps. Take care that the dressings do not slide off and become contaminated. Place the bulk of the dressings over the drain area and below the drain, depending on the client's usual position. *Layers of dressings are placed for best absorption of drainage, which flows by gravity.*

• Apply the final surgipad by hand; remove gloves, and dispose of them; and secure the dressing with tape or ties.

7. Document the technique and nursing assessments.

EVALUATION FOCUS

Amount of drainage and its color, clarity, thickness, and odor; degree of inflammation; pain at the incision or drain site.

SAMPLE RECORDING

Date	Time	Notes
12/05/93	1025	Penrose drain shortened 2.5 cm. Three 4 × 4 gauzes saturated with brownish yellow drainage. Dry dressings × 4 applied. Skin intact; no redness or irritation. ———————————————————— Maria L. Antonio, RN

KEY ELEMENTS OF CLEANING A DRAIN SITE AND SHORTENING A PENROSE DRAIN

• Verify the physician's order and agency policy about shortening drains.

• Maintain asepsis.

• Clean the incision before cleaning the drain site.

• Assess the appearance of the incision and the amount and character of drainage from the incision and drain site accurately.

• Remove the suture if the drain has not been shortened previously.

• Grasp the drain its full width at the level of the skin.

• Pull the drain out the specified length.

• Hold the drain tightly against the skin edge, and insert the safety pin above your fingers (or forceps).

• Layer sufficient dressings around the drain site, and secure all dressings appropriately.

39-7 Establishing and Maintaining a Closed Wound Drainage System

PURPOSES
- To hasten the healing process by draining excess exudate, which interferes with the formation of granulation tissue in a wound
- To maintain the patency of the wound suction

ASSESSMENT FOCUS

The amount, color, consistency, clarity, and odor of the drainage; discomfort around the area of the drain; clinical signs of infection (e.g., elevated body temperature).

EQUIPMENT

- Disposable gloves
- Drainage receptacle, e.g., solution basin
- Calibrated pitcher

INTERVENTION

1. Establish suction if it has not been already initiated.

- Place the evacuator bag on a solid, flat surface and don disposable gloves.

- Open the drainage plug on top of the bag, without contaminating the bag.

- Compress the bag; while it is compressed, close the drainage plug to retain the vacuum (Figure 39–13).

2. Empty the evacuator bag.

- When the drainage fluid reaches

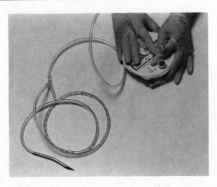

FIGURE 39–13 Compressing the Hemovac.

the line marked "Full," don disposable gloves, and open the drainage plug.

- Invert the bag, and empty it into

the collecting receptacle.

- Reestablish suction as in step 1.

- Using the calibrated pitcher, measure the amount of drainage, and note its characteristics.

3. Document all relevant information.

- Record the emptying of the evacuator bag and nursing assessments on the nursing progress notes.

- Record the amount and type of drainage on the intake and output record.

EVALUATION FOCUS

Amount of drainage and its color, clarity, consistency, and odor; increased or decreased discomfort; clinical signs of infection.

SAMPLE RECORDING

Date	Time	Notes
09/09/93	1030	Hemovac emptied 20 ml dark thick red drainage. Vacuum re-established. Tubing patent and suction functioning. Drain site red, small amount of thick, white discharge. Specimen to lab for culture. No odor. No discomfort. Dry dressing applied. ——————————— Sarah J. Woo, RN

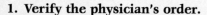

▶ **Technique 39–7 Maintaining a Closed Wound Drainage System** *CONTINUED*

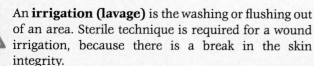

KEY ELEMENTS OF ESTABLISHING AND MAINTAINING A CLOSED WOUND DRAINAGE SYSTEM

- Maintain asepsis.
- Maintain appropriate compression of the evacuator bag.
- Wear gloves when emptying the bag or whenever there is risk of contact with the drainage.

- Empty the evacuator bag when indicated.
- Measure the drainage.

Wound Irrigation

An **irrigation (lavage)** is the washing or flushing out of an area. Sterile technique is required for a wound irrigation, because there is a break in the skin integrity.

Using piston syringes instead of Asepto syringes to irrigate a wound reduces the risk of aspirating drainage. For deep wounds with small openings, a sterile straight catheter may also be necessary. Frequently used irrigation solutions are sterile normal saline, lactated Ringer's solution, and antibiotic solutions. Dakin's solution, hydrogen peroxide, and some antimicrobial solutions, such as the iodophors, are reported to have adverse effects (Rodeaver 1989). See Technique 39–8.

39-8 Irrigating a Wound

Before irrigating a wound, determine (a) the type of irrigating solution to be used, (b) the frequency of irrigations, and (c) the temperature of the solution.

PURPOSES
- To clean the area
- To apply heat and hasten the healing process
- To apply an antimicrobial solution

ASSESSMENT FOCUS

Appearance and size of the wound; the character of the exudate; the time of the last pain medication; clinical signs of systemic infection; allergies to the wound irrigation agent or tape.

EQUIPMENT
- Sterile dressing equipment and dressing materials (see Technique 39–2)
- Sterile irrigating syringes, (e.g., a 50-ml piston syringe)
- Sterile basin for the irrigating solution
- Sterile basin to receive the irrigation returns
- Irrigating solution, usually 200 ml (6.5 oz) of solution at 32 to 35 C (90 to 95 F), according to the agency's or physician's choice
- Sterile gloves
- Moistureproof sterile drape
- Sterile straight catheter, if needed
- Disposable gloves

INTERVENTION
1. Verify the physician's order.
- Confirm the type and strength of the solution.

2. Prepare the client.

- Assist the client to a position in which the irrigating solution will flow by gravity from the upper end of the wound to the lower end and then into the basin.

- Place the waterproof drape over the client and the bed, and position the sterile basin on it below the wound, to catch the irrigating solution.

▶ Technique 39–8 Irrigating a Wound *CONTINUED*

 • Remove the old dressing, and clean the wound. See Technique 39–2.

3. Irrigate the wound.

• Using the syringe, gently instill a steady stream of irrigating solution into the wound. Make sure all areas of the wound are irrigated.

• If you are using a catheter, insert the catheter into the wound until resistance is met. Do not force the catheter. *Forcing the catheter can cause tissue damage*.

• Continue irrigating until the so-lution becomes clear (no exudate is present) or until all the solution has been used. *The irrigation washes away tissue debris and drainage so that later returns are clearer*.

• Using dressing forceps or sterile gloves and sterile gauze, dry the area around the wound. *Moisture left on the skin promotes the growth of microorganisms and can cause skin irritation*.

4. Assess and dress the wound.

• Assess the appearance of the wound, noting in particular the type and amount of exudate and the presence and extent of granulation tissue. See the Nursing Process Guide at the beginning of this chapter.

• Apply a sterile dressing to the wound as described in Technique 39–2.

5. Document all relevant information.

• Document the irrigation, the solution used, the appearance of the irrigation returns, and nursing assessments. Note the presence of any exudate and sloughing tissue.

EVALUATION FOCUS	Character of irrigation returns; the extent of wound healing (i.e., the amount of granulation tissue); the degree of discomfort associated with wound irrigation.

SAMPLE RECORDING

Date	Time	Notes
09/11/93	1000	Gaping incisional abdominal wound irrigated with sterile normal saline using piston syringe. Irrigation returns clear. Gaping area is 5 cm × 2.5 cm and pink in color. No purulent discharge. Sterile petrolatum gauze dressing applied. ——————————————— Toni T. Maximillian, SN

KEY ELEMENTS OF IRRIGATING A WOUND

• Verify the order for type of irrrigating solution and frequency of irrigations.

• Maintain asepsis.

• Assess and clean the wound appropriately before irrigating the wound.

• Instill irrigating fluid gently to all areas of the wound until the returns become clear or until the ordered volume is used.

• Dry the surrounding skin after the irrigation.

• Apply an appropriate sterile dressing to the wound after the procedure.

Sutures

Sutures are stitches used to sew body tissues together. *Suture* can also refer to the material used to sew the stitch. In some agencies, only physicians remove sutures; in others, registered nurses, licensed vocational nurses, and nursing students with appropriate supervision may do so. Various suture materials, e.g., silk, cotton, linen, wire, nylon, and Dacron (polyester fiber) threads are used. Silver wire clips are also available. The physician orders the removal of sutures. Usually, skin sutures are removed 7 to 10 days after surgery. Sterile technique and special suture scissors are used. The scissors have a short, curved cutting tip that readily slides under the suture (Figure 39–14). Wire clips or staples are removed with a special instrument that squeezes the center of the clip to remove it from the skin (Figure 39–15).

Retention sutures (stay sutures) are very large sutures used in addition to skin sutures for some

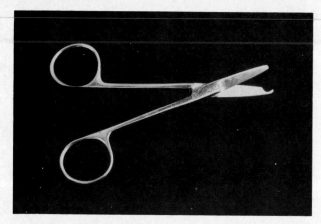

FIGURE 39-14   Suture scissors.

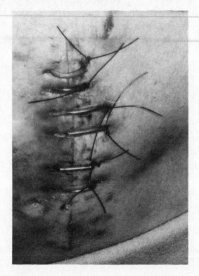

FIGURE 39-16   A surgical incision with retention sutures.

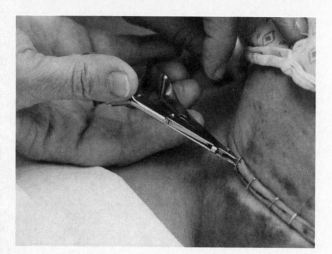

FIGURE 39-15   Removing surgical clips.

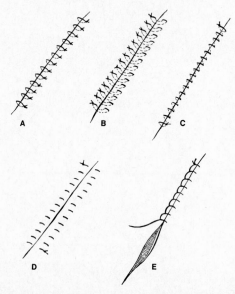

FIGURE 39-17   Common sutures: *A*, plain interrupted; *B*, mattress interrupted; *C*, plain continuous; *D*, mattress continuous; *E*, blanket continuous.

incisions (Figure 39-16). They attach underlying tissues of fat and muscle as well as skin and are used to support incisions in obese individuals or when healing may be prolonged. They are frequently left in place longer than skin sutures (14 to 21 days) but in some instances are removed at the same time as the skin sutures. To prevent these large sutures from irritating the incision, the surgeon may place rubber tubing over them or a roll of gauze under them extending down the incision line. Several forms of retention sutures are used, and agency policies about them may vary. The nurse should verify whether they are to be removed and who may remove them.

There are various methods of suturing. Skin

sutures can be broadly categorized as either *interrupted* (each stitch is tied and knotted separately) or *continuous* (one thread runs in a series of stitches and is tied only at the beginning and at the end of the run). Common sutures are illustrated in Figure 39-17. Removing skin sutures is described in Technique 39-9.

39-9 Removing Skin Sutures

Before removing skin sutures, verify (a) the orders for suture removal (many times only *alternate* interrupted sutures are removed one day, and the remaining sutures are removed a day or two later); and (b) whether a dressing is to be applied following the suture removal. Some physicians prefer no dressing; others prefer a small, light gauze dressing to prevent friction by clothing.

ASSESSMENT FOCUS

> Appearance of suture line; factors contraindicating suture removal (e.g., nonuniformity of closure, inflammation, presence of drainage).

EQUIPMENT

- ☐ Moistureproof bag
- ☐ Sterile gloves
- ☐ Disposable gloves
- ☐ Sterile dressing equipment (see Technique 39–2), including:
  - • Sterile suture scissors
  - • Sterile butterfly tape (optional)
- • Light sterile gauze pad
- ☐ Tape (if a dressing is to be applied)

INTERVENTION

1. Prepare the client.

- Inform the client that suture removal may produce slight discomfort, such as a pulling or stinging sensation, but should not be painful.

2. Remove dressings, and clean the incision.

- See Technique 39–2, steps 2 through 5, pages 924–925.

💧 • Don sterile gloves.

- Clean the suture line with an antimicrobial solution before and after suture removal. *This is generally done as a prophylactic measure to prevent infection.*

3. Remove the sutures.

Plain Interrupted Sutures

- Grasp the suture at the knot with a pair of forceps.

- Place the curved tip of the suture scissors under the suture as close to the skin as possible, either on the side opposite the knot (Figure 39–18) or directly under the knot. Cut the suture. *Sutures are cut as close to the skin as possible on one side of the visible part because the suture ma-*

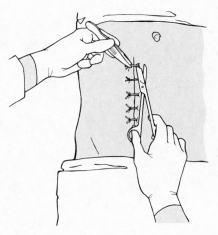

FIGURE 39–18 Removing a plain interrupted skin suture.

terial that is visible to the eye is in contact with resident bacteria of the skin and must not be pulled beneath the skin during removal. Suture material that is beneath the skin is considered free from bacteria.

- With the forceps, pull the suture out in one piece. Inspect the suture carefully to make sure that all suture material is removed. *Suture material left beneath the skin acts as a foreign body and causes inflammation.*

- Discard the suture onto a piece of sterile gauze or into the moistureproof bag, being careful not to contaminate the forceps tips. Sometimes the suture sticks to the forceps and needs to be removed by wiping the tips on a sterile gauze.

- Continue to remove *alternate* sutures, i.e., the third, fifth, seventh, and so forth. *Alternate sutures are removed first so that remaining sutures keep the skin edges in close approximation and prevent any dehiscence from becoming large.*

- If no dehiscence occurs, remove the remaining sutures. If dehiscence does occur, do not remove the remaining sutures, and report the dehiscence to the nurse in charge.

- If a little wound dehiscence occurs, apply a sterile butterfly tape over the gap:

  a. Attach the tape to one side of the incision.

  b. Press the wound edges together.

▶ **Technique 39–9 Removing Skin Sutures** CONTINUED

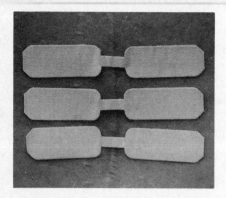

FIGURE 39–19 Butterfly tapes.

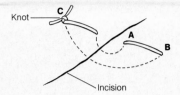

FIGURE 39–20 Mattress interrupted sutures.

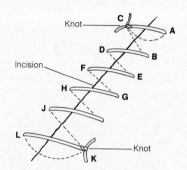

FIGURE 39–21 Plain continuous sutures.

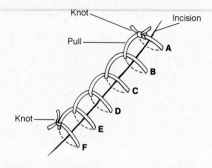

FIGURE 39–22 Blanket continuous sutures.

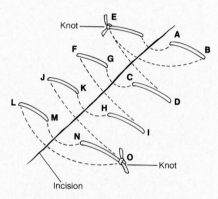

FIGURE 39–23 Mattress continuous sutures.

c. Attach the tape to the other side of the incision (Figure 39–19). *The butterfly tape holds the wound edges as close together as possible and promotes healing.*

- If a large dehiscence occurs, cover the wound with sterile gauze, and report the problem immediately to the nurse in charge or physician.

Mattress Interrupted Sutures

- When possible, cut the visible part of the suture close to the skin at A and B in Figure 39–20, opposite the knot, and remove this small visible piece. Discard it as described above. In some sutures, the visible part opposite the knot may be so small that it can be cut only once.

- Grasp the knot (C) with forceps. Remove the remainder of the suture beneath the skin by pulling out in the direction of the knot.

Plain Continuous Sutures

- Cut the thread of the first suture opposite the knot at A in Figure 39–21. Then cut the thread of the second suture on the same side at B.

- Grasp the knot (C) with the forceps, and pull. This removes the first stitch and the piece of thread beneath the skin, which is attached to the second stitch. Discard the suture.

- Cut off the visible part of the second suture at D, and discard it.

- Grasp the suture at E, and pull out the underlying loop between D and E.

- Cut the visible part at F, and remove it.

- Repeat the above two steps at G through J, until the last knot is reached. Note that after the first stitch is removed, each thread is cut down the same side, below the original knot.

- Cut the last suture at L, and pull out the last suture at K.

Blanket Continuous Sutures

- Cut the threads that are opposite the looped blanket edge; i.e., cut at A through F in Figure 39–22.

- Pull each stitch out at the looped edge.

Mattress Continuous Sutures

- Cut the visible suture at both skin edges opposite the knot (at A and B in Figure 39–23) and the next suture opposite the knot (at C and D). Remove and discard the visible portions as described above.

- Pull the first suture out by the knot at E.

- Lift the second suture between F and G to pull out the underlying suture between G and C. Cut off the visible part at F as close to the skin edge as possible.

- Go to the opposite side between H and I. Lift out the suture between F and I, and cut off all the visible part close to the skin at H.

- Lift the suture between J and K to pull out the suture between H and K, and cut the suture close to the skin at J.

- Repeat the above 2 steps, working from side to side of the incision, until the last suture is reached.

- Cut the visible suture opposite the knot at L and M. Pull out all remaining pieces of suture at O.

5. Clean and cover the incision.

► **Technique 39–9** *CONTINUED*

- Clean the incision again with antimicrobial solution.

- Apply a small, light, sterile gauze dressing if any small dehiscence has occurred or if this is agency practice.

6. Instruct the client about follow-up wound care.

- Generally, if a wound is dry and healing well, the person can take showers in a day or two.

- Instruct the client to contact the physician if wound discharge appears.

7. Document the suture removal and assessment data on the appropriate records.

EVALUATION FOCUS

Status of suture line; any wound separation or discharge.

SAMPLE RECORDING

Date	Time	Notes
12/05/93	1105	All abdominal sutures removed. Wound dry, edges approximated closely. No signs of inflammation or dehiscence. Gauze dressing applied. —————— Gwen E. Owens, NS

KEY ELEMENTS OF REMOVING SKIN SUTURES

- Verify the physician's order and agency policy about removing sutures.
- Maintain asepsis.
- Clean the incision with antiseptic before and after suture removal.
- Identify the method of suturing used, and remove sutures appropriately.
- Remove alternate sutures first if the sutures are interrupted.
- Apply sterile butterfly tapes over a wound dehiscence and then a dry sterile dressing.

CRITICAL THINKING CHALLENGE

Denise Travers, a 54-year-old obese client, has been admitted to the nursing unit from the postanesthesia recovery room following abdominal surgery. When changing her incisional dressing 2 days postoperatively, you note that some of the sutures have broken and the edges of her longitudinal midline abdominal incision have split open, causing wound dehiscence. What actions will you take? In what order will you take them? Provide the rationale for your answer.

RELATED RESEARCH

Frey, K. A.; Briggs, J.; and Broadhead, W. E. December 1990. Postdischarge, postoperative nosocomial infection surveillance using random sampling. *American Journal of Infection Control* 18:383–85.

Zoutman, D.; Pearce, P.; McKenzie, M.; and Taylor, G. August 1990. Surgical wound infections occurring in day surgery patients. *American Journal of Infection Control* 18:277–82.

REFERENCES

Bale, S., and Harding, K. G. February 1990. Using modern dressings to effect debridement. *Professional Nurse* 5:244, 246, 248.

————. June 1991. Foams still find favour: Wound management using foam dressings. *Professional Nurse* 6:510, 512–14, 516.

Bruno, P. December 1979. The nature of wound healing: Implications for nursing practice. *Nursing Clinics of North America* 14:667–82.

Centers for Disease Control: Recommendations for prevention of HIV transmission in health care settings. MMWR 1987:36:55.

Cerrato, P. L. June 1988. Nutritionist on call. What diet does for wound healing. *RN* 51:73–74, 76.

Changing the dressing: Proceed with care. June 1988. *Nursing 88* 18:34–37.

Cooper, D. M. March 1990. Wound healing. *Nursing Clinics of North America* 25:163–64.

————. March 1990. Optimizing wound healing: A practice within nursing's domain. *Nursing Clinics of North America* 25:165–80.

Cuzzell, J. Z. February 1985. Wound care forum: Artful solutions to chronic problems. *American Journal of Nursing* 85:162–66.

———. October 1988. The new RYB color code: Next time you assess an open wound, remember to protect red, cleanse yellow, and debride black. *American Journal of Nursing* 88:1342–46.

Cuzzell, J. Z., and Stotts, N. A. October 1990. Wound care: Trial and error yields to knowledge. *American Journal of Nursing* 90:53–60.

Fowler, E.; Cuzzell, J. Z., and Papen, J. C. February 1991. Healing with hydrocolloid. *American Journal of Nursing* 91:63–64.

Garner, J. S. April 1986. CDC guidelines for the prevention and control of nosocomial infections: Guideline for prevention of surgical wound infections, 1985. *American Journal of Infection Control* 14:71–80.

Krasner, D. May 1992. Wound measurements: Some tools of the trade. *American Journal of Nursing* 92:89–90.

McConnell, E. A. June 1990. How to tape a dressing. *Nursing 90* 20:23.

McDowell, S. July 1991. Are we using too much Betadine? *RN* 54:43–45.

Meehan, P. A., and Mayz, E. J. June 1988. Nursing management of an open abdominal wound. *Critical Care Nurse* 8:29–30, 32–34.

Modic, B. M. December 1990. Myths and facts about chronic wound care. *Nursing 90* 20:68.

Morison, M. J. February 1989. Wound cleansing—which solution? *Professional Nurse* 4:220–22, 224–25.

Piper, S. M. May 1989. Effective use of occlusive wound dressings. *Professional Nurse* 4:402–4.

Rodeaver, G. 1989. Controversies in topical wound management. *Wounds* 1:19–27.

Taylor, D. L. May 1983. Wound healing: Physiology, signs and symptoms. *Nursing 83* 13:44–45.

Thomason, S. S. September/October 1989. Front-line antiseptics. *Geriatric Nursing* 10:235–36.

Van Rijswijk, L., and Cuzzell, J. Z. June 1991. Managing full-thickness wounds. *American Journal of Nursing* 91:18, 22.

Bandages and Binders

CONTENTS

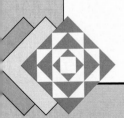

NURSING PROCESS GUIDE
BANDAGES AND BINDERS

ASSESSMENT

Assess the area to be bandaged or to which a binder is to be applied for

- Swelling.

- Presence of and status of wounds (open wounds will require a dressing before a bandage or binder is applied).

- Presence of drainage (amount, color, odor, and viscosity).

- Adequacy of circulation (skin temperature, color, and sensation). Pale or cyanotic skin, cool temperature, tingling, and numbness can indicate impaired circulation.

- Presence of pain (location, intensity, onset, and quality).

Determine

- The client's ability to reapply the bandage or binder when needed.

- The client's ability to carry out activities of daily living (e.g., to eat, dress, write, comb hair, bathe, and drive).

- The amount of assistance the client will require during the convalescence period.

RELATED DIAGNOSTIC CATEGORIES

- High risk for Infection (open wound)
- Altered tissue perfusion: Peripheral
- High risk for Impaired skin integrity
- High risk for Injury
- Impaired physical mobility
- Pain
- Knowledge deficit
- Self-care deficit
- Impaired tissue integrity

PLANNING

Client Goals
The client will

- Maintain support to the injured extremity.
- Maintain immobilization of injured part.
- Avoid edema and altered tissue perfusion to the injured extremity or body part.

Outcome Criteria
The client:

- Maintains normal or baseline vital signs.
- Achieves timely wound healing, as manifested by decreasing inflammation and wound drainage and absence of purulent drainage.
- Accomplishes activities of daily living with minimal or no pain.
- Maintains adequate dietary intake for healing.
- Resumes normal activities within the specified period.
- Demonstrates binder or bandage application as instructed.
- Reports understanding of discharge instructions.
- Identifies signs of complications that require notification of the nurse or physician.

Supporting and Immobilizing Wounds

Bandages and binders serve various purposes:

- Supporting a wound, e.g., a fractured bone

- Immobilizing a wound, e.g., a strained shoulder

- Applying pressure; e.g., elastic bandages apply pressure to the lower extremities to improve venous blood flow

- Securing a dressing, e.g., for an extensive abdominal surgical wound

- Retaining splints (this applies chiefly to bandages)

- Retaining warmth, e.g., a flannel bandage on a rheumatoid joint

There are several types of bandages and binders and several ways in which they are applied. When correctly applied, they promote healing, provide comfort, and can prevent injury.

Bandages

A **bandage** is a strip of cloth used to wrap some part of the body. Bandages are available in various widths, most commonly 1.5 to 7.5 cm (0.5 to 3 in), and are usually supplied in rolls for easy application to a body part.

Many types of materials are used for bandages. Gauze is one of the most commonly used; it is light and porous and readily molds to the body. It is also relatively inexpensive, so it is generally discarded when soiled. Gauze is frequently used to retain dressings on wounds and to bandage the fingers, hands, toes, and feet. It supports dressings and at the same time permits air to circulate; it can also be impregnated with petroleum jelly or other medications for application to wounds.

Many kinds of elasticized bandages are applied to provide pressure to an area. They are commonly used as tensor bandages or as partial stockings to provide support and improve the venous circulation in the legs. Some elasticized bandages have an adhesive backing and can be secured to the skin; these are most frequently used to retain dressings and at the same time provide some support to a wound.

Plastic adhesive bandages are also used to retain dressings. They are waterproof and thus retain wound drainage or keep the area dry. They have some elastic properties and therefore provide some pressure.

The width of the bandage used depends on the size of the body part to be bandaged. For example, a 2.5-cm (1-in) bandage is used for a finger, a 5-cm (2-in) bandage for an arm, and a 7.5-cm or 10-cm (3-in or 4-in) bandage for a leg. The larger the circumference of the part, the wider the bandage. Padding (e.g., abdominal pads and gauze squares) is frequently used to cover bony prominences, such as the elbow, or to separate skin surfaces, such as the fingers.

Before applying a bandage, the nurse needs to know its purpose and to assess the area requiring support. See the assessment guidelines in the Nursing Progress Guide on page 944.

Applying bandages to various parts of the body involves one or more of five basic bandaging turns: circular, spiral, spiral reverse, recurrent, and figure-eight. *Circular* turns are used to anchor bandages and to terminate them. They are also used to bandage certain areas, such as the proximal aspect of a finger

CLINICAL GUIDELINES

Bandaging

- Whenever possible, bandage the part in its normal position, with the joint slightly flexed to avoid putting strain on the ligaments and the muscles of the joint.

- Pad between skin surfaces and over bony prominences to prevent friction from the bandage and consequent abrasion of the skin.

- Always bandage body parts by working from the distal to the proximal end to aid the return flow of venous blood.

- Bandage with even pressure to prevent interference with blood circulation.

- Whenever possible, leave the end of the body part (e.g., the toe) exposed so that you will be able to determine the adequacy of the blood circulation to the extremity.

- Cover dressings with bandages at least 5 cm (2 in) beyond the edges of the dressing to prevent the dressing and wound from becoming contaminated.

- Face the client when applying a bandage to maintain uniform tension and the appropriate direction of the bandage.

or a wrist. Circular turns usually are not applied directly over a wound because of the discomfort the bandage would cause.

Spiral turns are used to bandage parts of the body that are fairly uniform in circumference, e.g., the upper arm or upper leg. *Spiral reverse* turns are used to bandage cylindrical parts of the body that are not uniform in circumference, e.g., the lower leg or forearm. *Recurrent* turns are used to cover distal parts of the body, e.g., the end of a finger, the skull, or the stump of an amputation. *Figure-eight* turns are used to bandage an elbow, knee, or ankle, because they permit some movement after application. The *spica* bandage is a variation of the figure-eight bandage. It is commonly used to bandage the hip, groin, shoulder, breast, or thumb. A 2.5-cm (1-in) bandage is frequently used for a thumb spica, and a 7.5-cm (3-in) bandage for a hip or shoulder spica.

Some basic guidelines for bandaging are listed in the box above. Technique 40–1 illustrates how to apply basic bandages using the turns described above.

40-1 Basic Bandaging

PURPOSES

- To provide comfort
- To prevent further injury
- To promote healing

ASSESSMENT FOCUS

Status of the skin area to which the bandage is to be applied; presence of an open wound; adequacy of circulation to the part; degree of pain.

EQUIPMENT

- ☐ Clean bandage of the appropriate material and width
- ☐ Padding, such as ABD pads or gauze squares
- ☐ Tape, special metal clips, or a safety pin

INTERVENTION

1. Position and prepare the client appropriately.

- Provide the client with a chair or bed, and arrange support for the area to be bandaged. For example, if a hand needs to be bandaged, ask the client to place the elbow on a table, so that the hand does not have to be held up unsupported. *Because bandaging takes a little time, holding up a body part without support can fatigue the client.*

- Make sure that the area to be bandaged is clean and dry. Wash and dry the area if necessary. *Washing and drying remove microorganisms, which flourish in dark, warm, moist areas.*

- Align the part to be bandaged with slight flexion of the joints, ⚠ unless this is contraindicated. *Slight flexion places less strain on the ligaments and muscles of the joint.*

2. Apply the bandage.

Circular Turns

- Hold the bandage in your dominant hand, keeping the roll uppermost, and unroll the bandage about 8 cm (3 in). *This length of unrolled bandage allows good control for placement and tension.*

- Apply the end of the bandage to the part of the body to be bandaged. Hold the end down with the thumb of the other hand (Figure 40–1).

- Encircle the body part a few times or as often as needed, making sure that each turn directly covers the previous turn. *This provides even support to the area.*

- Secure the end of the bandage with tape, metal clips, or a safety pin over an uninjured area. *Clips and pins can cause discomfort when situated over an injured area.*

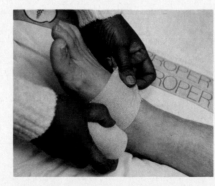

FIGURE 40–1 Starting a bandage with two circular turns.

Spiral Turns

- Make two circular turns. *Two circular turns anchor the bandage.*

- Continue spiral turns at about a 30° angle, each turn overlapping the preceding one by two-thirds the width of the bandage (Figure 40–2).

- Terminate the bandage with two circular turns, and secure the end as described for circular turns.

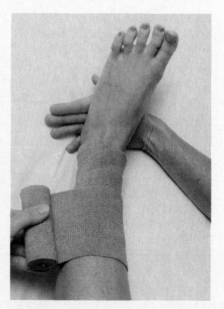

FIGURE 40–2 Applying spiral turns.

► **Technique 40–1** *CONTINUED*

Spiral Reverse Turns

- Anchor the bandage with two circular turns, and bring the bandage upward at about a 30° angle.

- Place the thumb of your free hand on the upper edge of the bandage (Figure 40–3, *A*). *The thumb will hold the bandage while it is folded on itself.*

- Unroll the bandage about 15 cm (6 in), then turn your hand so that the bandage falls over itself (Figure 40–3, *B*).

- Continue the bandage around the limb, overlapping each previous turn by two-thirds the width of the bandage. Make each bandage turn at the same position on the limb so that the turns

of the bandage will be aligned (Figure 40–3, *C*).

- Terminate the bandage with two circular turns, and secure the end as described for circular turns.

Recurrent Turns

- Anchor the bandage with two circular turns.

- Fold the bandage back on itself, and bring it centrally over the distal end to be bandaged (Figure 40–4).

- Holding it with the other hand, bring the bandage back over the end to the right of the center bandage but overlapping it by two-thirds the width of the bandage.

- Bring the bandage back on the left side, also overlapping the first turn by two-thirds the width of the bandage.

- Continue this pattern of alternating right and left until the area is covered. Overlap the preceding turn by two-thirds the bandage width each time.

- Terminate the bandage with two circular turns (Figure 40–5). Secure the end appropriately.

Figure-Eight Turns

- Anchor the bandage with two circular turns.

- Carry the bandage above the joint, around it, and then below it, making a figure eight (Figure 40–6).

- Continue above and below the joint, overlapping the previous turn by two-thirds the width of the bandage.

- Terminate the bandage above the joint with two circular turns, and then secure the end appropriately.

Thumb Spica

- Anchor the bandage with two circular turns around the wrist.

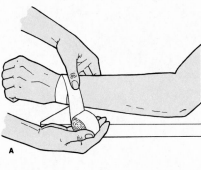

Circular turns

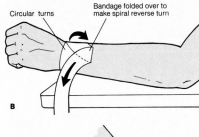

Bandage folded over to make spiral reverse turn

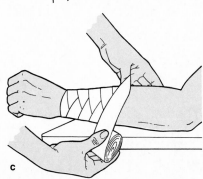

FIGURE 40–3   Applying spiral reverse turns.

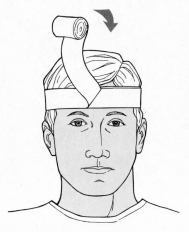

FIGURE 40–4   Starting a recurrent bandage with two circular turns.

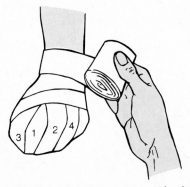

FIGURE 40–5   Completing a recurrent bandage with two circular turns.

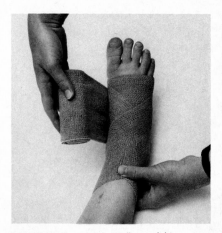

FIGURE 40–6   Applying a figure-eight bandage.

► **Technique 40–1 Basic Bandaging** *CONTINUED*

• Bring the bandage down to the distal aspect of the thumb, and encircle the thumb. Leave the tip Ⓢ of the thumb exposed if possible. *This allows you to check blood circulation to the thumb.*

• Bring the bandage back up and around the wrist, then back down and around the thumb, overlapping the previous turn by two-thirds the width of the bandage.

• Repeat the above two steps, working up the thumb and hand until the thumb is covered (Figure 40–7).

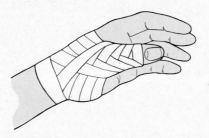

FIGURE 40–7   A thumb spica bandage.

• Anchor the bandage with two circular turns around the wrist, and secure the end appropriately.

3. Document all relevant information.

• Record the type of bandage applied, the area to which it is applied, and nursing assessments, Ⓢ including skin problems or neurovascular problems.

EVALUATION FOCUS

Adequacy of distal circulation to bandaged part (e.g., skin color for pallor or cyanosis, skin temperature, strength of pulse, presence of numbness or tingling); client's ability to reapply the bandage when needed; client's ability to perform ADLs and assistance required.

SAMPLE RECORDING

Date	Time	Notes
04/07/93	0700	Elastic spiral bandage applied to right leg. Toes warm and pink. No numbness. Rt pedal pulse 60 beats per min strong. Laura R. Stenhouse, NS

KEY ELEMENTS OF BASIC BANDAGING

See Clinical Guidelines for Bandaging, earlier in this chapter.

• Assess for baseline data the status of the skin to which the bandage is to be applied.

• If needed, clean the skin before applying the bandage.

• Anchor and terminate all bandages with circular turns.

• Use the bandage size appropriate for the body part to be bandaged.

• Hold the bandage with the roll uppermost.

• Use the appropriate bandaging turn for the body part to be bandaged.

• Overlap preceding turns by two-thirds the bandage width each time.

Stump Bandages

When a limb is amputated, the distal portion of the limb that remains is called the *stump*. A stump bandage is usually applied to retain a dressing after a dressing change. It is also applied to apply pressure, support venous return flow, prevent swelling, and to help shape the stump. Some agencies provide elasticized stump shrinkers to shape the stump in preparation for a prosthesis (Figure 40–8).

If a stump shrinker is not available, the nurse needs to determine the surgeon's preference regarding the type of material and the kind of bandage to apply. Agency protocol may indicate that the stump be wrapped with a figure-eight bandage or a recurrent or a spiral bandage. Commonly, the figure-eight or modified figure-eight bandages are used. An elastic bandage is often used to apply pressure. An 8-cm or 10-cm (3-in or 4-in) bandage is recommended for an

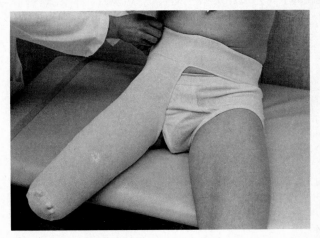

FIGURE 40–8   A stump shrinker.

adult's stump. Technique 40–2 describes how to bandage a leg amputation; the bandaging of arm amputations is similar.

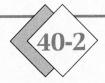

40-2   Applying a Stump Bandage

PURPOSES
- To support the return flow of venous blood
- To apply pressure and minimize bleeding and/or swelling
- To retain a surgical dressing
- To help shape a stump in preparation for a prosthesis

ASSESSMENT FOCUS

The amount of any drainage on the dressing; the color, temperature, and swelling of the skin near the dressing to provide baseline data for evaluating the blood circulation to and from the area after the bandage has been applied; any discomfort, e.g., "phantom" pain (pain or irritation perceived to be in the removed part of the limb).

EQUIPMENT
- Clean bandage
- Tape, safety pins, or metal clips

INTERVENTION

1. Position the client appropriately.
- Assist the client to a semi-Fowler's position in bed or to a sitting position on the edge of the bed.
- Clean the skin or stump wound, and apply a sterile dressing as needed.

2. Apply the bandage.

Figure-Eight Bandage
- Anchor the bandage with two circular turns around the hips.
- Bring the bandage down over the stump and then back up and around the hips (Figure 40–9).
- Bring the bandage down again,

overlapping the previous turn, and make a figure eight around the stump and back up around the hips.
- Repeat, working the bandage up the stump (Figure 40–10).
- Anchor the bandage around the hips with two circular turns.

▶ **Technique 40–2 Applying a Stump Bandage** *CONTINUED*

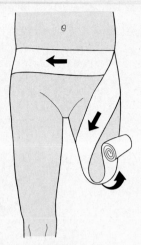

FIGURE 40–9 One way of beginning a figure-eight stump bandage.

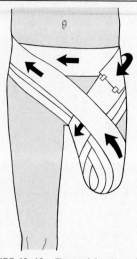

FIGURE 40–10 Figure-eight stump bandage applied around stump and waist.

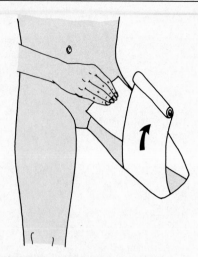

FIGURE 40–11 A second way to begin a figure-eight stump bandage.

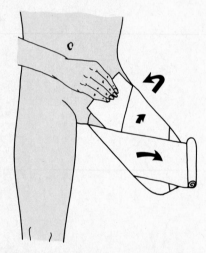

FIGURE 40–12 Figure-eight stump bandage applied around stump only.

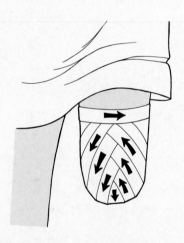

FIGURE 40–13 A recurrent stump bandage.

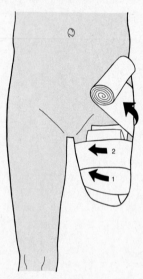

FIGURE 40–14 A spiral stump bandage.

- Secure the bandage with adhesive tape, safety pins, or clips. *or*

- Place the end of the elastic bandage at the top of the anterior surface of the leg, and have the client hold it in place. Bring the bandage diagonally down toward the end of the stump.

- Then, applying even pressure, bring the bandage diagonally upward toward the groin area (Figure 40–11).

- Make a figure-eight turn behind the top of the leg, downward again over and under the stump, and back up to the groin area (Figure 40–12).

- Repeat these figure-eight turns at least twice.

- Anchor the bandage around the hips with two circular turns.

- Secure the bandage with tape, safety pins, or clips.

Recurrent Bandage

- Anchor the bandage with two circular turns around the stump.

- Cover the stump with recurrent turns.

- Anchor the recurrent bandage with two circular turns (Figure 40–13).

- Secure the bandage with tape, safety pins, or clips.

Spiral Bandage

- Make recurrent turns to cover the end of the stump.

- Apply spiral turns from the distal aspect of the stump toward the body (Figure 40–14).

- Anchor the bandage with two circular turns around the hips.

- Secure the bandage with tape, safety pins, or clips.

3. Document all relevant information.

- Record the application of the bandage, all nursing assessments, and the client's response.

▶ **Technique 40–2** *CONTINUED*

EVALUATION FOCUS	Adequacy of circulation to the stump (e.g., skin color for pallor or cyanosis; skin temperature; strength of pulses; presence of numbness or tingling).

SAMPLE RECORDING

Date	Time	Notes
07/11/93	0930	Figure-eight stump bandage removed as ordered. Slight serosanguineous drainage on one 4 × 4 gauze. Sterile dressing applied and figure-eight stump bandage reapplied. Wound is clean with minimal inflammation; stump skin color pink, feels warm to touch. No complaints of numbness or tingling. – ————————————————————— Sam Fields, RN

KEY ELEMENTS OF APPLYING A STUMP BANDAGE

- Before applying the bandage, assess the status of the skin and any wound to which the bandage is to be applied. Note swelling, adequacy of circulation, and the amount and color of wound drainage.

- Clean the skin or stump wound, and apply a sterile dressing as needed before applying bandage.

- Determine the surgeon's preference regarding the type and kind of bandage to apply.

- Apply a figure-eight, recurrent, or spiral bandage correctly.

Binders

A **binder** bandage is designed for a specific body part; for example, the triangular binder (sling) fits the arm. Binders are used to support large areas of the body, such as the abdomen, arm, or chest. Most binders are made of muslin (plain-woven cotton fabric), flannel, or synthetic material that may or may not be elasticized. Some abdominal binders are made of an elasticized netlike material that fits the body contours and allows air to circulate around the body part.

Four types of binders are commonly used:

1. *Triangular arm binder (sling):* Usually applied as a full triangle to support the arm, elbow, and forearm of the client or to reduce or prevent swelling of a hand.

2. *Breast binder:* To provide pressure on the breasts (e.g., when drying up the milk flow after childbirth) or to support the breasts (e.g., after surgery). Breast binders are pinned in the front and usually have shoulder straps to prevent the binder from slipping down.

3. *T-binder (single or double T):* To retain pads, dressings, or packs in the perineal area. Single T-binders are often used for females, and double T-binders for males to prevent undue pressure on the penis. The double T-binder can also provide greater support for large dressings on both males and females.

4. *Straight abdominal binder:* To provide support to the abdomen. This binder is a rectangular piece of material long enough to encircle the client's abdomen with some overlap. It can be made from any material, e.g., a towel.

Abdominal (ABD) pads are used to protect bony prominences (e.g., the iliac crests for an abdominal binder) or to prevent skin surfaces from rubbing together and becoming excoriated (e.g., the skin beneath the breasts for a breast binder).

Technique 40–3 describes how to apply the various binders.

40-3 Applying Binders

PURPOSES

- To support or immobilize a body part
- To provide pressure on a body part
- To prevent or reduce swelling
- To retain pads, dressings, or packs

ASSESSMENT FOCUS

Status of the body area to which the binder is applied (presence of swelling, discoloration, skin abrasions, or discomfort); status of underlying dressing (type and amount of drainage); need for adjunctive measures (e.g., a cold pack); degree of chest expansion and breathing rate for baseline data if an abdominal or chest binder is to be applied; learning needs for self-application of binder or sling.

EQUIPMENT

- Appropriate binder
- Abdominal (ABD) pads as required for padding
- Safety pins or tape

INTERVENTION

1. Prepare the client.

- If the binder is being placed directly against the skin and the area is soiled, wash and dry the area.

- Assist the client to a comfortable lying or sitting position, supporting the area as appropriate.

2. Apply the binder.

Triangular Arm Sling

- Ask the client to flex the elbow to an 80° angle or less, depending on the purpose. The thumb should be facing upward or inward toward the body. *An 80° angle is sufficient to support the forearm, to prevent swelling of the hand, and to relieve pressure on the shoulder joint (e.g., to support the paralyzed arm of a stroke client whose shoulder might otherwise become dislocated).* A more acute angle is preferred if there is swelling of the hand (see how to apply a sling for maximum hand elevation, below).

- Place one end of the unfolded triangular binder over the shoulder of the uninjured side so that the binder falls down the front of the chest of the client with the point of the triangle (apex) under the elbow of the injured side.

- Take the upper corner, and carry it around the neck until it hangs over the shoulder on the injured side.

- Bring the lower corner of the binder up over the arm to the shoulder of the injured side. Using a square knot, secure this corner to the upper corner at the side of the neck on the involved side (Figure 40–15). *A square knot will not slip. Tying the knot at the side of the neck prevents pressure on the bony prominences of the vertebral column at the back of the neck.*

- Make sure the wrist is supported, to maintain alignment.

- Fold the sling neatly at the elbow, and secure it with safety pins or tape. It may be folded and fastened at the front.

- Remove the sling periodically to inspect the skin for indications

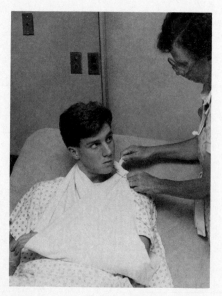

FIGURE 40–15 A large arm sling.

of irritation, especially around the site of the knot.

Small Arm Sling (Cravat Binder)

- Make a cravat binder by folding the triangular binder in on itself, starting at the apex (Figure 40–16, *A*).

- Apply the sling as in Figure 40–16, *B*, with the knot on the affected side.

▶ **Technique 40–3** *CONTINUED*

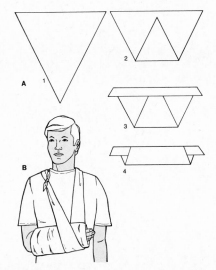

FIGURE 40–16 *A*, Making a cravat: (1) lay the triangular bandage on a flat surface; (2) fold the point up toward the base of the bandage; (3) fold the base over on itself to make a smooth edge; (4) fold the cravat from the other side to the desired width. *B*, The cravat applied as a small arm sling.

Triangular Arm Sling for Maximum Hand Elevation

- Flex the client's arm so that the hand rests on the clavicle of the uninjured side. *This position provides maximum elevation of the hand.*

- Place the binder over the shoulder of the uninjured side and *over the arm* (i.e., in front of the arm) so that the apex of the binder extends beyond the elbow of the injured side (Figure 40–17, *A*).

- Tuck the base of the binder under the arm, bring the free end across the client's back, and—using a square knot—tie it to the other free end at the shoulder on the *uninjured* side. The knot should rest in the hollow of the clavicle to prevent pressure on the clavicle (Figure 40–17, *B*).

- Bring the apex of the sling toward the back, tuck it in, and secure it with a safety pin or pins (Figure 40–17, *C*).

FIGURE 40–17 A triangular arm sling applied to provide hand elevation.

Hand or Foot Mitt

- Apply the triangular bandage as a mitt to cover hand or foot dressings (Figure 40–18).

Breast Binder

- Spread the binder on the bed, and ask the client to lie in a supine position on top of it. Center the binder, place the lower edge at the waistline, and allow adequate armhole space. *Adequate armhole space is needed to prevent the material from chafing the axillae.*

- If the breasts are large, place padding under each breast. *This prevents skin excoriation caused by pressing the two skin surfaces tightly together.*

- Pull the binder tightly across the breast tissue at the nipple line, and fasten it at the midline with a safety pin placed vertically. Ask

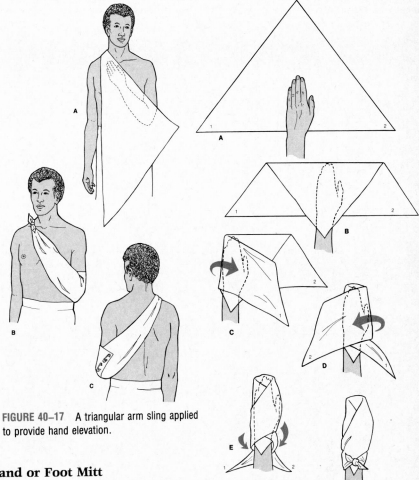

FIGURE 40–18 Wrapping a hand with a triangular bandage: *A*, lay the hand in the center of the triangular bandage; *B*, fold the apex over the wrist; *C*, *D*, wrap the corners (1 and 2) around the hand; *E*, bring the corners around the wrist; *F*, tie a square knot on the dorsum of the wrist.

the client to help by pressing the palms of her hands against the sides of the breasts.

- While continuing to compress the breasts, pin the binder alternately above and below the first fastening. Place the pins vertically except for the lowest one, which is placed horizontally (Figure 40–19 on page 954). *Fastening the pins alternately above and below distributes pressure equally, thereby providing maximum support. Placing the lowest pin hori-*

▶ **Technique 40–3 Applying Binders** CONTINUED

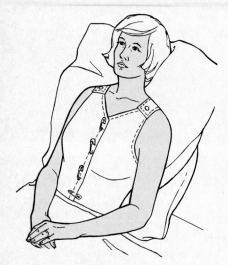

FIGURE 40–19   A breast binder.

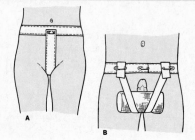

FIGURE 40–20   T-binders: *A*, single tail; *B*, two tails.

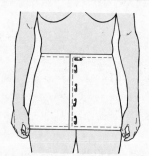

FIGURE 40–21   A straight abdominal binder.

zontally allows for more comfort
when moving.

- Fasten the shoulder straps, if required, with pins.

T-Binder

- Select the appropriate binder for the client, and place it smoothly under the person with the waistband at waist level and the tails running down the midline at the back. Double T-binders may be used for females if a dressing is large (e.g., after extensive surgery).

- Bring the waist tails around the client, overlap them, and secure them with a pin placed horizontally. *The pins placed horizontally*

allow comfort when bending at the waist and moving.

- Bring the center tail up between the legs (Figure 40–20, *A*). The two tails of the double T-binder are brought up on either side of the penis (Figure 40–20, *B*). When dressings are in place, take care to touch only the outside of the dressings to prevent contamination of the wound or yourself.

- Fasten the ties at the waist with a safety pin placed horizontally.

Straight Abdominal Binder

- With the client in a supine position, place the binder smoothly under the body, with the upper border of the binder at the waist and the lower border at the level of the gluteal fold. *A binder placed over the waist interferes with respiration; one placed too low interferes with elimination and walking.*

- Apply padding over the iliac

crests if the client is thin.

- Bring the ends around the client, overlap them, and secure them with pins (Figure 40–21). Place the top pin horizontally at the waist to allow for comfort when moving.

3. Ensure client comfort.

- Ensure that there are no wrinkles or creases against the body. *Wrinkles and creases cause pressure on the skin and subsequent excoriation.*

4. Document all relevant information.

- Determine the agency's policies about recording application of a binder. Binders are generally not recorded when applied to hold a dressing in place. However, an arm sling, breast binder, or abdominal binder may be recorded, together with the assessment data.

EVALUATION FOCUS	Relief of discomfort in affected limb or part; reduced swelling; decreased breast engorgement (breast binder); ability to ventilate during deep breathing (abdominal binder); assistance required for ADLs.

SAMPLE RECORDING

Date	Time	Notes
08/17/93	1000	Breast binder applied. Breasts are enlarged, hard, engorged, and painful. ─────── Page O. Mills, NS

▶ **Technique 40–3** *CONTINUED*

KEY ELEMENTS OF APPLYING BINDERS

All Binders

- Assess the status of the skin to which the binder is to be applied for baseline data.
- If needed, clean the skin before applying the binder.
- Ensure that there are no wrinkles or creases against the body.

Arm Sling

- Position the forearm and hand to prevent swelling of the hand and to maintain wrist alignment.
- Secure the sling with a square knot at the side of the neck.
- Periodically inspect the skin for irritation at the site of the knot.

Breast Binder

- Prevent skin excoriation by ensuring adequate armhole space and padding skin surfaces beneath large breasts.
- Ask the client to compress the breasts while you fasten the binder.
- Fasten the binder by placing pins alternately above and below the first fastening.
- Place all pins, except the lowest waist-level pin, vertically.

T-Binder

- Place the waist pin horizontally.

Abdominal Binder

- Position the binder so that respiratory, elimination, and ambulatory functions are maintained.
- Pad bony prominences.
- Place pins at the waist horizontally.

CRITICAL THINKING CHALLENGE

Kevin Matthews, a 24-year-old male, has a below-the-knee (BK) amputation of his left leg following a traumatic injury. The surgeon has applied an occlusive dressing following surgery. The dressing is not to be changed until the physician orders. When assessing the client's dressing, you note bloody drainage on it. How would you determine the extent of the bleeding problem? What actions will you take?

41

Heat and Cold Therapy

OBJECTIVES

- Identify reasons for administering hot and cold applications

- Identify essential guidelines for applying heat and cold

- Explain the rebound phenomenon

- Identify recommended temperatures for hot and cold applications

- Identify essential assessment data required before administering hot and cold applications

- Identify conditions that contraindicate the use of heat and the use of cold

- Identify conditions that indicate the need for precautions during heat and cold therapy

- Describe methods of applying dry and moist heat

- Describe methods of applying dry and moist cold

- Administer hot and cold applications included in this chapter safely and effectively

CONTENTS

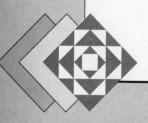

NURSING PROCESS GUIDE
HEAT AND COLD THERAPY

ASSESSMENT

Assess

- *The capacity of the client to recognize when the heat is injurious.* Establish whether the client is aware of heat and cold and can discern a temperature that is too hot or too cold for the tissues.

- *The client's degree of consciousness and general physical condition.* Very young, very old, unconscious, or debilitated clients do not tolerate heat well.

- *The area to be treated* for

  a. *Alterations in skin integrity,* such as the presence of edema, bruises, redness, open lesions, discharge, and bleeding.

  b. *Circulatory status* (color, temperature, and sensation). Tissues that feel cold, have a pale or bluish hue, and lack sensation or feel numb indicate circulatory impairment.

  c. *Level of discomfort* and range of motion if muscle spasm or pain is being treated.

- *Pulse, respirations, and blood pressure.* Assessing these factors is particularly important before hot or cold is applied to large body areas.

Determine the presence of any conditions contraindicating the use of heat:

- *The first 24 hours after traumatic injury.* Heat increases bleeding and swelling.

- *Active hemorrhage.* Heat causes vasodilation and increases bleeding.

- *Noninflammatory edema.* Heat increases capillary permeability and edema.

- *Acute inflammation.* Heat on such areas can increase edema; e.g., it can rupture an appendix.

- *Localized malignant tumor.* Because heat accelerates cell metabolism and cell growth and increases circulation, it may accelerate metastases (secondary tumors).

- *Developing fetus.* Heat to the abdomen of a pregnant woman can cause mutation in the fetal germinal cells and affect fetal growth.

- *Skin disorder that causes redness or blisters.* Heat can burn or cause further damage to the skin.

- *Metallic implants,* such as a pacemaker or knee or hip replacements. Because metal is a good conductor of heat, medical diathermy—which uses electric current to heat deep tissues—can burn deep tissues.

Determine the presence of any conditions contraindicating the use of cold:

- *Open wounds.* Cold can increase tissue damage by decreasing blood flow to an open wound.

- *Impaired circulation.* Cold can further impair nourishment of the tissues and cause tissue damage. In clients with Raynaud's disease, cold increases arterial spasm.

- *Allergy or hypersensitivity to cold.* Some clients have an allergy to cold that may be manifested by an inflammatory response, e.g., erythema, hives, swelling, joint pain, and occasional muscle spasm. Some react with a sudden increase in blood pressure, which can be hazardous if the person is hypersensitive.

Determine the presence of any conditions indicating the need for precautions during heat and cold therapy:

- *Neurosensory impairment.* Persons with sensory impairments are unable to perceive that heat is damaging the tissues and are at risk for burns, or they are unable to perceive discomfort from cold and are unable to prevent tissue injury.

- *Impaired mental status.* Persons who are confused or have an altered level of consciousness need monitoring and supervision during applications to ensure safe therapy.

- *Impaired circulation.* Persons with peripheral vascular disease, diabetes, or congestive heart failure lack the normal ability to dissipate heat via the blood circulation, which puts them at risk for tissue damage with heat applications. Note that cold applications are contraindicated for these people.

- *Open wounds.* Tissues around an open wound are more sensitive to heat and cold.

RELATED DIAGNOSTIC CATEGORIES

- Impaired skin integrity
- High risk for Impaired skin integrity
- High risk for Injury (burn)
- High risk for Infection (open wound)
- Pain
- Knowledge deficit

Nursing Process Guide *CONTINUED*

PLANNING

Client Goals
The client will

• Experience increased comfort.

• Demonstrate wound healing.

Outcome Criteria
The client

• Maintains normal or baseline vital signs.

• Achieves timely wound healing, as manifested by decreasing inflammation and wound drainage and the absence of purulent drainage.

• Accomplishes ADLs with minimal or no pain.

• Maintains a dietary intake adequate for healing.

• Resumes normal activities within a specified period.

Applying Heat and Cold

Heat and cold are applied to the body to promote the repair and healing of tissues. The form of thermal applications generally depends on their purpose. Cold applied to a body part draws heat from the area; heat, of course, warms the area. The application of heat or cold produces physiologic changes in the temperature of the tissues, size of the blood vessels, capillary blood pressure, capillary surface area for exchange of fluids and electrolytes, and tissue metabolism. The duration of the application also affects the response. See Table 41–1 for a summary of the physiologic effects of heat and cold.

Heat Therapy

Heat is an old remedy for aches and pains; people often equate heat with comfort and relief. Heat is often used for clients with musculoskeletal problems, such as joint stiffness from arthritis, contractures, and low back pain, and for those with open wounds needing debridement. See Table 41–2.

TABLE 41–1 PHYSIOLOGIC EFFECTS OF HEAT AND COLD

Body Part or Process	Effect of Heat	Effect of Cold
Local circulatory response	Vasodilation (reddened skin)	Vasoconstriction (pale, bluish skin)
Capillary permeability	Increased	Decreased
Cellular metabolism	Increased	Decreased
Inflammatory process	Increased	Decreased
Muscles	Relaxation	Decreased contractility
Nerves	Increased conduction rate	Decreased conduction rate
Synovial fluid	Increased viscosity	Decreased viscosity
Pain	Promotes comfort	Initial discomfort; later, numbness and paresthesia

TABLE 41–2 SELECTED INDICATIONS FOR HEAT

Indication	Effect of Heat
Muscle spasm	Relaxes muscles and increases their contractility
Inflammation	Increases blood flow, bringing more phagocytes (to facilitate exudate formation) and essential nutrients for healing; also enhances removal of wastes and debris formed in the inflammatory process. Moist heat softens exudates
Contracture	Reduces contractures and increases joint range of motion by allowing greater distention of muscles and connective tissue
Joint stiffness	Reduces joint stiffness by decreasing the viscosity of synovial fluid and increasing tissue distensibility
Pain	Relieves pain, possibly by promoting muscle relaxation, increasing circulation to ischemic areas, promoting psychologic relaxation and a feeling of comfort, and acting as a counterirritant

Source: P. S. Tepperman and M. Devlin, Therapeutic heat and cold: A practitioner's guide, *Postgraduate Medicine*, January 1983, 73:69.

Heat can be applied to the body in both dry and moist forms. Dry heat is applied locally, for heat conduction, by means of a hot water bottle, electric pad, aquathermia pad, or disposable heat pack. The heat lamp and bed cradle provide dry heat by radiation. Moist heat can be provided, through conduction, by compress, hot pack, soak, or sitz bath.

Cold Therapy

Cold therapy is more recent than heat therapy. It is most often used for active young people with sports injuries (e.g., sprains, strains, fractures) to limit postinjury swelling and bleeding. See Table 41–3.

Applications of cold may also be dry or moist. Dry cold is administered for local effect by the use of ice bags, ice collars, ice gloves, and disposable cold packs. Moist cold is applied for either local or systemic effects. Cold moist compresses are administered to body parts for a local effect; tepid sponge baths are given for a systemic cooling effect. Cold is often applied to the body to decrease bleeding by constricting blood vessels; to decrease inflammation by causing vasoconstriction; and to decrease pain by slowing nerve conduction rate, producing numbness, and acting as a counterirritant.

Guidelines for Applying Heat and Cold

An understanding of the adaptive response of thermal receptors, the rebound phenomenon, systemic effects, tolerance to heat and cold, and contraindications are essential when administering hot and cold applications.

Adaptation of Thermal Receptors
Thermal receptors adapt to temperature changes. When a cold receptor is subjected to an abrupt fall in temperature or when a warmth receptor is sub-

jected to an abrupt rise in temperature, the receptor is strongly stimulated initially. This strong stimulation declines rapidly during the first few seconds and then more slowly during the next half hour or more as the receptor adapts to the new temperature (Guyton 1986, p. 604). This adaptive mechanism explains why people feel very cold at first when they go outdoors from a heated room on a cold day or feel very warm when they go from a cold environment to a heated room or from a warm room to a hot tub.

Nurses need to understand this adaptive response when applying heat and cold. Clients may be tempted to change the temperature of a thermal application because of the change in thermal sensation following adaptation. Increasing the temperature of a hot application after adaptation has occurred can result in serious burns. Decreasing the temperature of a cold application can result in pain and serious impairment of circulation to the body part. See Table 41–4 on page 960 for recommended temperatures of hot and cold applications.

Rebound Phenomenon
The **rebound phenomenon** occurs at the time the maximum therapeutic effect of the hot or cold application is achieved and the opposite effect begins. For example, heat produces maximum vasodilation in 20 to 30 minutes; continuation of the application beyond 30 to 45 minutes brings tissue congestion, and the blood vessels then *constrict* for reasons unknown. If the heat application is continued further, the client is at risk for burns, since the constricted blood vessels are unable to dissipate the heat adequately via the blood circulation.

With cold applications, maximum vasoconstriction occurs when the involved skin reaches a temperature of 15 C (60 F). Below 15 C, vasodilation begins. This mechanism is protective: It helps to prevent freezing of body tissues normally exposed to cold, such as the nose and ears. It also explains the ruddiness of the skin of a person who has been walking in cold weather.

TABLE 41–3   SELECTED INDICATIONS FOR COLD

Indication	Effect of Cold
Traumatic injury	Decreases bleeding by constricting blood vessels; decreases edema by reducing capillary permeability
Inflammation	Decreases inflammation by causing vasoconstriction, decreasing capillary permeability, decreasing blood flow, decreasing cellular metabolism, and slowing phagocytosis
Muscle spasm	Increases muscle relaxation by decreasing muscle contractility
Pain	Decreases pain by slowing nerve conduction rate and blocking nerve impulses, by producing numbness, by acting as a counterirritant, and by increasing the pain threshold

Source: P. S. Tepperman and M. Devlin, Therapeutic heat and cold: A practitioner's guide, *Postgraduate Medicine*, January 1983, 73:69.

TABLE 41–4 RECOMMENDED TEMPERATURES FOR HOT AND COLD APPLICATIONS

Description	Centigrade	Fahrenheit	Application
Very cold	Below 15	Below 59	Ice bags
Cold	15 to 18	59 to 65	Cold pack
Cool	18 to 27	65 to 80	Cold compress
Tepid	27 to 37	80 to 98	Alcohol and tepid sponges
Warm	37 to 40	98 to 105	Warm bath
Hot	40 to 46	105 to 115	Aquathermia, soaks, sitz baths, irrigations, moist sterile compresses, hot water bags for debilitated or young clients
Very hot	Above 46	Above 115	Hot water bags for adults, heat cradles

An understanding of the rebound phenomenon is essential for the nurse. Thermal applications must be halted *before* the rebound phenomenon begins.

Systemic Effects

Heat applied to a localized body area, particularly a large body area, may increase cardiac output and pulmonary ventilation. These increases are a result of excessive peripheral vasodilation, which diverts large supplies of blood from the internal organs and produces a drop in blood pressure. A significant drop in blood pressure can cause fainting. Clients who have heart or pulmonary disease and who have circulatory disturbances such as arteriosclerosis are more prone to this effect than healthy persons.

With extensive cold applications and vasoconstriction, a client's blood pressure can increase, because blood is shunted from the cutaneous circulation to the internal blood vessels. This shunting of blood, a normal protective response to prolonged cold, is the body's attempt to maintain its core temperature. Shivering, another generalized effect of prolonged cold, is a normal response as the body attempts to warm itself.

Tolerance and Contraindications

Various parts of the body differ in tolerance to heat and cold. The physiologic tolerance of individuals also varies. See the accompanying box.

Before applying heat or cold, the nurse assesses the area to be treated and the client's history and current health status to (a) determine the client's ability to tolerate the therapy and (b) identify conditions that contraindicate the therapy. The area to which the heat and cold will be applied also needs to be assessed. See the Assessment in the Nursing Process Guide on page 957.

Specific conditions contraindicate the use of hot or cold applications. For example, heat increases bleeding and therefore is not used during the first 24

hours after traumatic injuries. In addition, certain conditions call for precautions in administering heat and cold therapy. See page 957.

Dry Heat

A *hot water bottle or bag* is a common source of dry heat used in the home. It is convenient and relatively inexpensive. However, because of the danger of burning from improper use, many agencies use other means. *Electric pads* provide a constant, even heat, are lightweight, and can be molded to a body part. Electric pads, however, can burn if the setting is too

Variables Affecting Physiologic Tolerance to Heat and Cold

- *Body part.* The back of the hand and foot are not very temperature-sensitive. In contrast, the inner aspect of the wrist and forearm, the neck, and the perineal area are temperature-sensitive.
- *Size of the exposed body part.* The larger the area exposed to heat and cold, the lower the tolerance.
- *Individual tolerance.* Tolerance to heat and cold is to some degree affected by age and condition of the skin, nervous system, and circulatory system. The very young and the very old generally have the lowest tolerance. Persons who have neurosensory impairments may have a high tolerance, but the risk of injury is greater.
- *Length of exposure.* People feel hot and cold applications most while the skin temperature is changing. After a period of time, tolerance increases.
- *Intactness of skin.* Injured skin areas are more sensitive to temperature variations.

high. In some agencies, the controls on the pads are set to a specific temperature to prevent burning.

The *aquathermia* or *aquamatic pad* (also referred to as a *K-pad*) is a device commonly used in hospitals to provide heat to a body part. The pad is attached by tubing to an electrically powered control unit that has an opening for water and a temperature gauge (Figure 41–1). Some aquathermia pads have an absorbent surface through which moist heat can be applied. The other surface of the pad is waterproof. These pads are disposable.

Dry heat can also be supplied by *commercially prepared disposable hot packs* (Figure 41–2). Directions on the package tell how to initiate the heating process, e.g., by striking, squeezing, or kneading the pack. Hot packs provide a specified amount of heat for a specified time.

Lamps also provide dry heat to localized areas. A *heat lamp* is often a gooseneck lamp. Heat lamps containing a 60 or 40 watt light bulb are often applied three times a day as needed to relieve perineal discomfort after delivery.

Technique 41–1 shows how to apply various kinds of dry heat.

An *infant radiant warmer* or similar device is an open heating unit. A row of long lights is positioned at a stationary height from a bedding pad below. The radiant warmer is used to prevent the loss of body heat from the newborn infant. This warming process is crucial to the immature infant who has difficulty maintaining body temperature because of insufficient subcutaneous body fat and inadequate temperature self-regulation mechanisms. If the environmental temperature is not maintained with a radiant warmer or some similar thermal device, the infant will expend significant metabolic energy, with a resultant increase in oxygen and caloric needs. Technique 41–2 describes how to apply an infant radiant warmer.

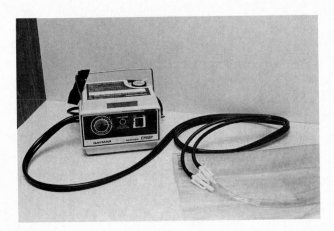

FIGURE 41–1 An aquathermia heating unit.

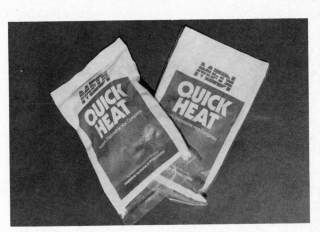

FIGURE 41–2 Commercially prepared disposable hot packs.

41-1 Applying a Hot Water Bottle, Electric Heating Pad, Aquathermia Pad, Commercial Hot Pack, or Perineal Heat Lamp

Before applying dry heat, determine (a) whether the client is required to sign a release for the application of dry heat (if a release is required, check the client's chart for the signed release); (b) the type of heat to be used, the temperature, and the duration and frequency of the application (check the physician's or nursing order); (c) agency protocol about the type of equipment used, the temperature recommended, and the length of heat applications; (d) at what time the heat should be applied, e.g., 1000 and 1900 hours or after a wound dressing is changed (check the nursing care plan); (e) if a heat lamp, if used, is in proper working order.

▶ **Technique 41–1 Applying Dry Heat** CONTINUED

PURPOSES
- To warm a body part and promote comfort, relaxation, and sleep
- To increase blood circulation and promote healing and comfort
- To reduce muscle pain
- To dry the perineal tissues (heat lamp)

ASSESSMENT FOCUS

Any traumatic injury, signs of redness, abraded skin, swelling, or hemorrhage at the area to which the heat is to be applied; other factors contraindicating heat therapy (see Nursing Process Guide, page 957); any discomfort experienced by the client; the client's capacity to recognize when the heat is injurious; the client's general physical condition and mental capability to cooperate with the treatment; the blood circulation to the area.

EQUIPMENT

Hot Water Bottle (Bag)
- ☐ Hot water bottle with a stopper
- ☐ Cover
- ☐ Hot water and a thermometer

Electric Heating Pad
- ☐ Electric pad and control
- ☐ Cover, waterproof if there will be moisture under the pad

when it is applied
- ☐ Gauze ties (optional)

Aquathermia Pad
- ☐ Pad
- ☐ Distilled water
- ☐ Control unit
- ☐ Cover

- ☐ Gauze ties or tape (optional)

Disposable Hot Packs
- ☐ One or two commercially prepared disposable packs

Heat Lamp
- ☐ Perineal heat lamp with 60-watt bulb

INTERVENTION

1. Prepare and assess the client.

- Inspect the area to receive heat. See the Nursing Process Guide for this chapter.

- Fold down the bedclothes to expose the area to which the heat will be applied.

Hot Water Bottle

2. Fill and cover the bottle.

- Fill the hot water bottle about two-thirds full.

- Measure the temperature of the water if this was not done before the bag was filled. Follow agency practice for the appropriate temperature. Temperatures commonly used are

a. 52 C (125 F) for a normal adult.

b. 40.5 to 46 C (105 to 115 F) for a debilitated or unconscious adult.

c. 40.5 to 46 C (105 to 115 F) for a child under 2 years of age.

- Expel the air from the bottle. *Air remaining in the bottle prevents it from molding to the body part being treated.*

- Secure the stopper tightly.

- Hold the bottle upside down, and check for leaks.

- Dry the bottle.

- Wrap the bottle in a towel or hot water bottle cover.

3. Apply the bottle.

- Support the bottle against the body part with pillows as necessary.

- Go to step 14.

Electric Heating Pad

4. Prepare the client and pad for application.

- Ensure that the body area is dry. *Electricity in the presence of moisture can conduct a shock.*

- Check that the electric pad is functioning and in good repair. The cord should be free from cracks, wires should be intact, heating components should not be exposed, and temperature distribution over the pad should be even.

- Place the cover on the pad. Some models have waterproof covers to be used when the pad is placed over a moist dressing. *Moisture could cause the pad to short circuit and burn or shock the client.*

- Plug the pad into the electric socket.

- Set the control dial for the correct temperature.

5. Apply the pad.

- After the pad has heated, place

▶ **Technique 41–1** *CONTINUED*

the pad *over* the body part to which heat is being applied.

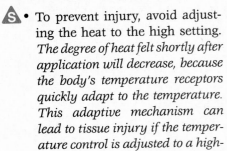• Use gauze ties instead of safety pins to hold the pad in place, if needed. *A pin might strike a wire, damaging the pad and giving an electric shock to the client.*

6. Give the client the following instructions:

• Do not insert any sharp, pointed object, e.g., a pin, into the pad.

• Do not lie directly on the pad. *The surface below the pad promotes heat absorption instead of normal heat dissipation.*

• To prevent injury, avoid adjusting the heat to the high setting. *The degree of heat felt shortly after application will decrease, because the body's temperature receptors quickly adapt to the temperature. This adaptive mechanism can lead to tissue injury if the temperature control is adjusted to a higher setting.*

• Call the nurse if any discomfort is felt.

Aquathermia Pad

7. Assemble the unit.

• Fill the unit with distilled water until it is two-thirds full. The unit will warm the water, which circulates through the pad.

• Remove air bubbles, and secure the top.

• Regulate the temperature with the key if it has not been preset. Normal temperature is 40.5 C (105 F). Check the manufacturer's instructions.

• Cover the pad with a towel or pillowcase.

• Plug in the unit.

8. Apply the pad to the body part.

• Check for any leak or malfunctions of the pad before use.

• Use tape or gauze ties to hold the pad in place. Never use safety pins. *They can cause leakage.*

• If unusual redness or pain occurs, discontinue the treatment, and report the client's reaction.

9. Give the client the following instructions:

• Do not lie directly on the pad.

• Avoid adjusting temperature settings during the application.

• Call the nurse if any discomfort is felt.

Disposable Hot Pack

10. Initiate the heating process.

• Strike, squeeze, or knead the pack according to the manufacturer's directions.

• Note the manufacturer's instructions about the length of time that heat is produced.

Perineal Heat Lamp

11. Prepare the client.

• Expose the area to be treated, and drape the client so that the body is exposed minimally.

• Clean and dry the perineum to remove all secretions, ointments, or perineal sprays. *Cleaning prevents drying of secretions, ointments, or sprays on the perineum.*

• Clean from the front (area of the symphysis pubis) to the back (area around the anus) of the perineum. *This avoids contamination between the anal area and the urethral/vaginal area, thereby preventing infection.*

12. Position the lamp appropriately.

• Plug in the lamp, and, with the lamp turned off, place it approximately 30 cm (12 in) from the

perineum. (Check agency protocol.)

• Do not drape or cover the lamp. *A cover on the lamp may catch fire.*

13. Give the client the following instructions.

• Remain in position.

• Warn the client not to touch the bulb of the heat lamp.

• Call the nurse if any discomfort is felt.

For All Applications

14. Monitor the client during the application.

• Every 5 to 10 minutes, assess the client for any complaints of discomfort, e.g., pain, burning, and skin reaction. Frequency of assessment depends on such factors as the client's previous responses to applications and ability to report problems.

• At the first sign of pain, swelling, or excessive redness, remove the heat and report any sign to the nurse in charge.

15. Remove the heat application.

• Remove the heat before the rebound phenomenon begins, i.e., 20 to 30 minutes. A hot water bottle will usually stay hot for the duration of the treatment. It needs to be replaced for the next application. *Prolonged heat, e.g., 1 hour, decreases the blood flow to the area and can damage skin tissue.*

16. Document all relevant information.

• When the heat is applied, record the application, its purpose, the time, the method used, the site, and any nursing assessments.

• After removal, record the time and all nursing assessments.

▶

▶ **Technique 41–1 Applying Dry Heat** *CONTINUED*

EVALUATION FOCUS	Relief of pain or muscle tension; skin color and temperature (e.g., excessive redness); complaints of excessive heat.

SAMPLE RECORDING

Date	Time	Notes
04/02/93	2000	Aquathermia pad at medium setting applied to lower back for nonradiating pain aggravated by movement. Skin intact. ——— Marilyn March, SN
	2020	Aquathermia pad removed. States pain relieved. Skin warm and pink. ——— Marilyn March, SN

KEY ELEMENTS OF APPLYING A HOT WATER BOTTLE, ELECTRIC HEATING PAD, AQUATHERMIA PAD, COMMERCIAL HOT PACK, OR PERINEAL HEAT LAMP

All Methods of Dry Heat

- Know the purpose of the application.
- Before the application, assess the appearance of the area to be treated, factors that may affect the client's tolerance to heat, conditions that contraindicate the therapy, and conditions that indicate the need for precautions during therapy.
- Apply a protective covering to the device.
- Throughout the application assess the condition of the skin every 5 to 10 minutes and any complaints of the client.
- Remove the heat before the rebound phenomenon occurs (i.e., 20 to 30 minutes) or whenever adverse reactions occur (excessive redness, swelling, discomfort).

For a Hot Water Bottle

- Use the correct water temperature.
- Partially fill the bottle, and expel excess air.
- Secure the stopper tightly, and check for leaks.

Heating Pad

- Make sure the body area is dry before applying the pad.
- Warn the client to protect the pad from sharp pointed objects.
- Correctly set the temperature dial.

Aquathermia Pad

- Fill the unit appropriately, remove air bubbles, and secure the top.

Disposable Hot Pack

- Follow manufacturer's instructions to initiate the heating process.

Perineal Heat Lamp

- Use a 60-watt bulb.
- Position the lamp approximately 30 cm (12 in) from the client.
- Do not cover the lamp.

  Applying an Infant Radiant Warmer

Before applying the radiant warmer, determine (a) that the equipment is in proper working order and (b) the manufacturer's operating instructions and institutional policy regarding the temperature control process and alarm setting protocols.

PURPOSE

- To assist the newborn or immature infant in establishing and maintaining a stable body temperature

▶ **Technique 41–2 Applying an Infant Radiant Warmer** CONTINUED

ASSESSMENT FOCUS	The infant's initial body temperature; parental knowledge of the warmer function.

EQUIPMENT

- Radiant warmer with appropriate skin temperature sensors and reflective sensor covers (according to institutional policy)
- Prewarmed towels and infant blankets
- Infant head cover and diaper (according to institutional policy)
- Appropriate bedding for infant warmer

INTERVENTION

1. Prepare the warmer.

- Using the manual control setting, turn on the radiant warmer. *This prewarms the unit and eases the infant's transition from intrauterine to extrauterine life; it also prevents stressing of the immature infant.*

2. Assess and prepare the infant for the treatment.

- Wipe the blood and vernix from the newborn's head and body using the prewarmed towels. *Prewarmed towels prevent loss of the infant's body heat through evaporation.*

- Wrap the infant in the preheated blankets, transfer the infant to the mother (parents), and then return him or her to the warmer.

- Remove the blankets, and apply a diaper and a head cover (if agency protocol indicates). *This allows maximal infant exposure to the heating element.* The value of a head covering in maintaining infant body heat remains debatable.

- Apply the temperature sensor to the infant's abdomen between the umbilicus and the xiphoid process. *Thin subcutaneous tissue found over the ribcage may prevent recording of an accurate temperature.*

- Cover the temperature sensor with a reflective covering (if indicated in unit manual or institutional policy). *A reflective covering decreases functional interference of the sensor by overhead lights.*

- Turn the warmer control device to the automatic setting. *This permits the infant's body temperature to control the level of heating and prevents accidental overheating or erratic warming.*

3. Initiate the warming process.

- Adjust the temperature setting control to the desired goal temperature. This ranges from 35.1 C (97.0 F) to 37.0 C (98.6 F). *This prevents overheating.*

- Turn the warmer on.

- Set the temperature sensor alarm at the upper limit of the desired temperature range. *The alarm alerts the nurse if the infant's temperature exceeds upper limits of normal.*

4. Monitor the warming process.

- Check the infant's temperature sensor reading every 15 to 30 minutes (or as agency protocol dictates) until the infant's temperature reaches the desired level.

- Check the infant's axillary temperature every 2 to 4 hours (or according to agency protocol). *This verifies the accuracy of the sensor probe and the effectiveness of the treatment.*

- Monitor the sensor probe site and surrounding skin for irritation or breakdown. *Early detection of skin damage facilitates early intervention.*

5. Terminate the warming process.

- When the infant's temperature reaches the desired level, dress the infant in a T-shirt, diaper, and head cover. Wrap the infant in two blankets, and transfer the infant from the warmer to an open crib.

- Check the infant's axillary temperature every 2 to 4 hours (or according to agency protocol). *This allows the nurse to determine the infant's ability to maintain body temperature without assistance.*

- If the infant's temperature drops below 36.1 C (97.0 F), return the infant to the warmer, remove clothing, and reinitiate the warming procedure by performing the steps above.

▶ **Technique 41–2 Applying an Infant Radiant Warmer** *CONTINUED*

EVALUATION FOCUS

Temperature within acceptable range; infant's ability to maintain temperature after therapy is discontinued; vital signs other than temperature within baseline data (indicates absence of environmental stress).

SAMPLE RECORDING

Date	Time	Notes
05/04/93	1032	Baby Jones born by vaginal delivery. Initial temperature 96.2 F. Placed in preheated infant radiant warmer after cleaning and brief visit with parents. Temperature sensor applied to abdomen; equipment operating properly with increase noted in infant's temperature to 96.6 F after 15 minutes. No signs of distress. ——————————————— Pearl Gunther, RN

KEY ELEMENTS OF APPLYING AN INFANT RADIANT WARMER

- Ensure that the warmer is operating properly.
- Prewarm the unit prior to use.
- Remove blood and excess vernix from the infant's head and body.
- Remove all infant clothing except a diaper and (optional) a head covering.
- Apply the temperature sensor to the infant's abdomen.

- Set the temperature control element to the desired goal temperature.
- Place the temperature control unit to the automatic setting.
- Set the unit alarm.
- Monitor the infant's temperature during and after therapy.
- Reinitiate therapy if the infant's temperature drops below 36.1 C (97.0 F).

Hyperthermia and Hypothermia Blankets

Hyperthermia and *hypothermia blankets* are used to increase or decrease a client's body temperature. The blanket has an associated control panel on which the desired temperature is set and the client's core temperature registers (Figure 41–3). Technique 41–3 describes how to manage clients with hyperthermia and hypothermia blankets.

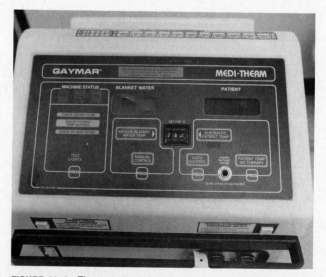

FIGURE 41–3 The control unit for a hyperthermia/hypothermia blanket.

Managing Clients with Hyperthermia and Hypothermia Blankets

PURPOSE	• To increase or decrease the client's body temperature and prevent complications or extremes of temperatures
ASSESSMENT FOCUS	Vital signs as baseline data; skin condition and temperature; presence of shivering; neurologic status.

EQUIPMENT

- ☐ Two pairs of gloves
- ☐ Basin of warm water, soap, washcloths, and towels (for client bath if needed)
- ☐ Hyperthermia/hypothermia control module (should come with rectal probe and blanket)
- ☐ Distilled water
- ☐ Plastic cover or thin sheet
- ☐ Lubricating jelly
- ☐ Tape
- ☐ Linen blanket (optional)

INTERVENTION

1. Prepare the client.

- Don gloves.
- Bathe the client if necessary.
- Remove gloves.
- Apply towels to the extremities according to agency protocol.

2. Prepare the equipment.

- Connect the blanket pad to the modular unit, and inspect for adequate functioning.
- Inspect the pad and cords for frays or exposed wires.
- Screw (twist) the male tubing connectors of the coil blanket tubing into the inlet and outlet opening connectors on the modular unit.
- Check the solution level in the module, and fill with distilled water if necessary. *(The solution should be up to the fill line in order for the blanket temperature to be correct.)*
- Turn the modular unit on *to circulate the solution through the blanket.*

- Check for adequate filling of the coils throughout the blanket as the solution circulates throughout it. If you note leakage, obtain another blanket.
- Turn the client temperature control knob to the desired temperature, and determine whether the temperature gauge is functioning.
- Set the modular control knob or master switch to either the manual or automatic mode, and note the accuracy of the temperature settings.

If using the automatic mode:

- Insert the thermistor probe plug into the thermistor probe jack on modular unit.
- Check the automatic mode light to be sure it comes on.
- Set the machine to the desired temperature.
- Set the limits for the pad temperature.

If using the manual mode:

- Set the master temperature control knob to the desired temperature.

- Check the manual mode light to be sure it is operational.
- If the blanket is nondisposable, cover it with a plastic cover or thin sheet. If the blanket is disposable, cover it with a plastic covering to avoid excess soiling.

3. Apply the blanket to the client.

- Don clean gloves.
- Place the client on the blanket.
- Apply lubricating jelly to the rectal probe, insert the rectal probe 7 to 10 cm (3 to 4 in).
- Secure probe with tape. *The tape should prevent the probe from falling out.*
- Remove gloves.

4. Monitor the client closely.

- Take vital signs every 15 minutes for at least the first hour, every half-hour for the second hour, and every hour thereafter.
- Determine the client's neurologic status regularly as needed.
- Observe the skin for indications of burns, intactness, and color. *Heat and cold can cause burning.*

▶ **Technique 41–3 Managing Hyperthermia and Hypothermia Blankets** CONTINUED

- Determine any intolerance to the blanket. *Shivering may result from increased metabolic activity.*

5. Maintain the therapy as required.

- Remove and clean the rectal probe every 3 to 4 hours or when

the client has a bowel movement. *When the probe is impacted with feces, the temperature reading can be distorted.*

| EVALUATION FOCUS | Vital signs; skin condition; presence of shivering. |

SAMPLE RECORDING

Date	Time	Notes
06/06/93	1035	Hypothermia blanket applied. T 40 C, P 128, R 32, BP 90/40. Blanket set at 28 C. Rectal probe inserted. Skin intact, no abrasions. Hands and feet covered with towels. —————————— Nancy Sun, SN

KEY ELEMENTS OF MANAGING CLIENTS WITH HYPERTHERMIA AND HYPOTHERMIA BLANKETS

- Know the purpose of applying the blanket.
- Before applying the blanket, assess vital signs, neurologic status, and intactness of the skin.

- Monitor the client closely during therapy.

Moist Heat

Moist heat is applied by the use of soaks or sitz baths. A **soak** refers to immersing a body part, e.g., an arm, in a solution or to wrapping a part in gauze dressings and then saturating the dressing with a solution. Sterile technique is generally indicated for open wounds, e.g., a burn or an unhealed surgical incision. Dry dressings are usually applied between the soaks.

A **sitz bath**, or hip bath, is used to soak a client's pelvic area. The client sits in a special tub or chair and is usually immersed from the midthighs to the iliac crests or umbilicus. Special tubs or chairs are preferred (Figure 41–4); when the legs are also immersed, as in a regular bathtub, blood circulation to the perineum or pelvic area is decreased. Disposable sitz baths are also available; they are commonly used in homes but may be used in hospitals as well.

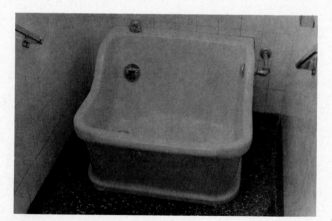

FIGURE 41–4 A sitz bath used in hospitals.

Technique 41–4 describes how to administer hot soaks and sitz baths.

41-4 Administering Hot Soaks and Sitz Baths

Before administering a hot soak or a sitz bath, determine (a) the type and temperature of the solution to be used; (b) the duration, frequency, and purpose of the soak, as indicated on the chart; and (c) agency protocol regarding the temperature and the length of time for soaks. Generally, a temperature of 40 to 43 C (105 to 110 F), as tolerated by the client, is indicated. For a hot soak, determine whether sterile technique is required.

PURPOSES
- To hasten suppuration, soften exudates, and enhance healing
- To apply medications to a designated area
- To clean a wound in which there is sloughing tissue or an exudate
- To promote circulation and enhance healing

ASSESSMENT FOCUS

Appearance of the affected area, e.g., redness, drainage (amount, color, consistency, odor), and swelling; any break in the skin; any discomfort experienced by the client; the client's mental status and ability to cooperate during the procedure; factors contradindicating heat therapy (see the Nursing Process Guide, page 957).

EQUIPMENT

(Use sterile equipment and supplies for an open wound)
- Small basin, special arm or foot bath, or sitz tub or chair
- Specified solution at the correct temperature
- Thermometer
- Disposable and sterile gloves (if the client has any open areas on the skin)
- Moisture-resistant bag
- Towels
- Bath blanket
- Required dressing materials (e.g., gauze squares and roller gauze for an extremity soak, perineal pads and a T-binder for a perineal soak)

INTERVENTION

Hand or Foot Soak

1. Prepare the soak.

- Fill the container at least one-half full and test the temperature of the solution with a thermometer. *A temperature that is too high can cause burning and one that is too low will not produce the desired effect.*

- Pad the edge of the container with a towel. *Padding is necessary to prevent pressure on the body part that rests on the edge of the container.*

- Use sterile solution and a sterile thermometer if the client has an open wound.

2. Prepare and assess the client.

- Assist the client to a well-aligned, comfortable position; the position adopted will be maintained for 15 to 20 minutes. *This position helps prevent muscle strain.*

- Don disposable gloves as required, remove the dressings, and discard them in the bag. Assess the amount, color, odor, and consistency of the drainage on removed dressings.

- Inspect the appearance of the area to be soaked.

3. Commence the soak.

- Immerse the body part com-

pletely in the solution. *The entire affected area must be in contact with the solution.*

- If the soak is sterile, cover the open container with a sterile drape or the container wrapper. *Covering the open container helps prevent accidental contamination.*

- Place a large sheet or blanket over the soak. *This will help maintain the temperature of the solution.*

- Go to step 7.

Sitz Bath

4. Prepare the bath.

- Fill the sitz bath with water at

▶ **Technique 41–4 Administering Hot Soaks and Sitz Baths** CONTINUED

about 40 C (105 F). (The water level in a tub should be at the umbilicus.) The temperature of the water should feel comfortable to the inner aspect of the wrist.

- Pad the tub or chair with towels as required. *Padding prevents pressure on the sacrum or posterior aspects of the thighs.* When a disposable sitz bath on the toilet is used, provide a footstool. *This can prevent pressure on the back of the thighs.*

5. Prepare the client.

- Remove the gown, or fasten it above the waist.

- Don gloves if an open area or drainage is present.

- Remove the T-binder and perineal dressings, if present, and note the amount, color, odor, and consistency of any drainage.

- Assess the appearance of the area to be soaked for redness, swelling, odor, breaks in the skin, and drainage.

- Wrap the bath blanket around the client's shoulders and over the legs as needed. *Draping the client provides warmth and prevents chilling.*

6. Begin the sitz bath.

- Assist the client into the bath, and provide support for the client as needed.

- Leave a signal light within reach. Stay with the client if warranted, and terminate the bath as necessary. *Some clients may become faint or dizzy and need to be able to call a nurse or have the nurse remain with them.*

7. Give the client the following instructions:

- Remain in position, and call the nurse if any discomfort is felt or an untoward reaction occurs.

8. Monitor the client.

Soak

- Assess the client and test the temperature of the solution at least once during the soak. Assess for discomfort, need for additional support, and any reactions to the soak.

- If the solution has cooled, remove the body part, empty the solution, add newly heated solution, and reimmerse the body part.

Sitz Bath

- Assess the client during the bath in terms of discomfort, color, and pulse rate. *An accelerated pulse or extreme pallor may precede fainting.*

- Immediately report any unexpected or adverse responses to the nurse in charge.

- Test the temperature of the solution at least once during the bath. Adjust the temperature as needed.

9. Discontinue the soak or bath.

- At completion of a *soak*, remove the body part from the basin, and dry it thoroughly and carefully. If the soak was sterile, use a sterile towel for drying, and wear sterile gloves. *Drying prevents skin maceration.*

- Assess the appearance of the affected area carefully, and reapply a dressing if required.
  or
- At the completion of a *sitz bath*, assist the client out of the sitz bath, and dry the area with a towel.

- Assess the perineal area, and reapply dressings and garments as required.

10. Document all relevant information.

- Record the soak or sitz bath, including the duration, temperature, and type of solution. Include all assessments.

EVALUATION FOCUS

Redness, drainage, swelling of the affected area; any discomfort; extent of healing.

SAMPLE RECORDING

Date	Time	Notes
12/05/93	0900	43 C saline soak to (L) index finger × 20 min. 2 × 2 gauze saturated with purulent exudate. Finger measures 7 cm (down 1 cm from previous measurement) but continues to be red in color. ——— Toby N. Zacharias, NS

Technique 41–4 *CONTINUED*

KEY ELEMENTS OF ADMINISTERING HOT SOAKS AND SITZ BATHS

Soaks and Sitz Baths

- Know the purpose of the application.
- Before the application, assess the amount, color, odor, and consistency of drainage on dressings; the appearance of the area to be treated; and conditions that indicate the need for precautions during the therapy.
- Maintain asepsis. Use sterile technique as required for a hand or foot soak.
- Wear gloves when removing dressings.
- Before the therapy, pad the edge of the soak container or the edge and base of a sitz bath.
- Prepare the specified solution at the correct temperature.
- Adjust the temperature of the solution as

required halfway through the soak.

- Assess the status of the client at least once during the soak.
- Dry the treated area thoroughly after the treatment, and apply appropriate dressings as required.

Sitz Bath

- Assess the pulse rate for baseline data before the therapy, at least once throughout the soak, and again after the soak.
- Prevent chilling.
- Assist the client as needed to transfer into and out of the bath.
- Leave a signal light within reach, or stay with the client.

Compresses and Moist Packs

Compresses and moist packs can be either hot or cold. A **compress** is a moist gauze dressing applied frequently to an open wound. When hot compresses are ordered, the solution is heated to the temperature indicated by the physician, e.g., 40.5 C (105 F). When there is a break in the skin or when the body part (e.g., an eye) is vulnerable to microbial invasion, sterile technique is necessary; therefore, sterile gloves or sterile forceps are needed to apply the compress, and all materials (solution, container, thermometer, towels, gauze squares, and petroleum jelly) must be sterile. If a sterile thermometer is not available, the nurse pours a small amount of the solution into a clean basin, measures the temperature, and then discards the solution, since it is no longer sterile. The nurse

adjusts the temperature of the solution according to the findings.

A hot or cold **pack** is a hot or cold moist cloth applied to an area of the body. Packs are usually unsterile; after application, they are covered with a water-resistant material (e.g., plastic wrap) to contain the moisture and prevent the transfer of airborne microorganisms to the area. For a sterile moist pack, the container, solution, thermometer, and all materials must be sterile. In addition, sterile gloves or forceps are required to maintain the sterility of the pack when it is wrung out and applied.

After a compress or a pack has been applied, it is advisable to apply external heat or cold, such as a hot water bottle, heating pad, or ice bag, to help maintain the temperature of the application. The application of compresses and moist packs is described in Technique 41–5.

41-5 Applying Compresses and Moist Packs

Before applying compresses or moist packs, determine
- The type of solution, the strength, and the temperature ordered for the compress. Check agency protocol if these are not specified in the order. Some orders require that the pack or compress be applied at the hottest or coldest temperature the client is able to tolerate.
- Whether sterile applications are required. Sterile compresses are needed for an open wound or a vulnerable part of the body, e.g., an eye, so that microorganisms are not transmitted to the wound or body part.

▶ **Technique 41–5 Applying Compresses and Moist Packs** CONTINUED

* Whether the sterile compress is to be replaced with a sterile dressing after the treatment.

PURPOSES

Hot Compress
* To hasten the suppurative process and healing

Hot Pack
* To relieve muscle spasm or pain
* To reduce the pressure of accumulated fluid in a tissue or joint
* To reduce congestion in an underlying organ

Cold Compress
* To decrease or prevent bleeding
* To reduce inflammation

Cold Pack
* To prevent swelling due to tissue trauma and inflammation
* To anesthetize tissues and reduce pain temporarily

ASSESSMENT FOCUS

> Redness, abrasions, or discharge at the area of application (for an open wound, assess the size, appearance, and type and amount of discharge); discomfort, swelling, bleeding; whether blood circulation to the area is impaired (i.e., tingling, cyanosis, coolness to touch); presence of any neurosensory impairment or reduced capacity to discern changes in skin temperature (i.e., very young, very elderly, unconscious, or debilitated clients); pulse, respirations, and blood pressure.

EQUIPMENT

(Use sterile equipment and supplies for an open wound)

Compress
☐ Disposable gloves or sterile gloves (for an open wound)
☐ Container for the solution
☐ Solution at the strength and temperature specified by the physician or the agency
☐ Thermometer
☐ Gauze squares
☐ Sterile gloves, forceps, and cotton applicator sticks (if compress must be sterile)
☐ Petroleum jelly
☐ Insulating towel
☐ Plastic

☐ Ties, e.g., roller gauze or masking tape
☐ Hot water bottle or aquathermia pad (optional)
  or
  Ice bag (optional)
☐ Sterile dressing, if required

Moist Pack
☐ Disposable gloves
☐ Flannel pieces or towel packs
☐ Hot-pack machine for heating the packs
  or
  Basin of water with some ice chips

☐ Thermometer if a specific temperature is ordered for the pack
☐ Sterile gloves, forceps, and cotton applicator sticks (if sterility must be maintained)
☐ Petroleum jelly
☐ Insulating material, e.g., flannel or towels
☐ Plastic
☐ Hot water bottle (optional)
  or
  Ice bag (optional)
☐ Sterile dressing, if required

INTERVENTION

1. Prepare the client.
* Assist the client to a comfortable position.
* Expose the area for the compress or pack.

* Provide support for the body part requiring the compress or pack.
* Don disposable gloves, and remove the wound dressing, if

present. A dry, sterile dressing is often placed over open wounds between applications of moist heat or cold.

2. Moisten the compress or the pack.

▶ **Technique 41–5** *CONTINUED*

• Place the gauze in the solution.
or
Heat the flannel or towel in a steamer, or chill it in the basin of water and ice chips.

3. Protect the surrounding skin as indicated.

• With a cotton swab or an applicator stick, apply petroleum jelly to the skin surrounding the wound, not on the wound or open areas of the skin. *Jelly protects the skin from possible burns, maceration, and the irritating effects of some solutions.*

4. Apply the moist compress or pack.

• Wring out the gauze compress so that the solution does not drip from it. For a sterile compress, use sterile forceps or sterile gloves to wring out the gauze (Figure 41–5).

• Apply the gauze lightly and gradually to the designated area (Fig-

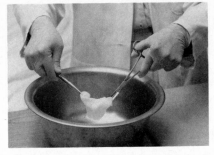

FIGURE 41–5   Using sterile forceps to wring out the gauze.

ure 41–6), and, if tolerated by the client, mold the compress close to the body. Pack the gauze snugly against all wound surfaces. *Air is a poor conductor of cold or heat, and molding excludes air.*
or

• Wring out the flannel (for a sterile pack, use sterile gloves).

• Apply the flannel to the body area, molding it closely to the body part.

5. Immediately insulate and secure the application.

• Cover the gauze or flannel quickly with a dry towel and a piece of plastic. *This step helps maintain the temperature of the application and thus its effectiveness.*

• Secure the compress or pack in place with gauze ties or tape.

• Optional: Apply a hot water bottle or aquathermia pad or ice bag

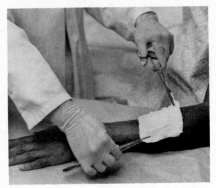

FIGURE 41–6   Applying a sterile compress.

over the plastic to maintain the heat or cold.

6. Monitor the client.

• Assess the client for discomfort at 5- to 10-minute intervals. If the client feels any discomfort, assess the area for erythema, numbness, maceration, or blistering.

• For applications to large areas of the body, note any change in the pulse, respirations, and blood pressure.

• In the event of unexpected reactions, terminate the treatment and report to the nurse in charge.

7. Remove the compress or pack at the specified time.

• Compresses and packs with external heat or cold usually retain their temperature anywhere from 15 to 30 minutes. Without external heat or cold, they need to be changed every 5 minutes.

• Apply a sterile dressing if one is required.

8. Document all relevant information.

• Document the technique, the time, and the type and strength of the solution.

• Record assessments, including the appearance of the wound and surrounding skin area.

EVALUATION FOCUS	Increased or decreased discomfort, inflammation, swelling, discharge and/or bleeding; extent of healing if applicable; vital signs.

SAMPLE RECORDING

Date	Time	Notes
05/12/93	0910	Sterile normal saline compress with K-Matic 37.7 C applied to 2.5 cm sacral ulcer. Pink tissue surrounding ulcer. 1 cm diameter serosanguineous discharge on dressing. No discomfort voiced. ——— Olga R. Resnicoff, NS
	0940	Compress removed. No further discharge. Ulcer packed with petrolatum gauze and sterile dry dressing applied. ——— Olga R. Resnicoff, NS

▶ **Technique 41–5 Applying Compresses and Moist Packs** *CONTINUED*

KEY ELEMENTS OF APPLYING COMPRESSES AND MOIST PACKS

- Know the purpose of the application.
- Before the application, assess the appearance of the area to be treated; factors that may affect the client's tolerance to the application; and conditions that indicate the need for precautions during the therapy.
- Use sterile technique for open wounds.
- Protect the surrounding skin of open wounds from injury.

- Apply the compress or pack lightly and gradually until tolerance is determined.
- Make sure all wound surfaces are covered appropriately by the gauze or pack.
- Prevent heat or cold loss by insulating the compress or pack appropriately.
- After the treatment, assess the appearance of the area, and apply a sterile dressing as required.

Dry Cold

The *ice bag*, commonly used in many homes and hospitals, is a moderate-sized rubber or plastic bag with a removable cap. Ice is placed inside the bag. Commercially prepared ice bags are available in some agencies. Such bags are filled with an alcohol-based solution and sealed; they are kept in freezing units in a central supply area. An *ice collar* is similar to an ice bag but is long and narrow. It is designed for use around the neck, although it can be used on other body parts. An *ice glove* is simply a plastic glove filled with ice chips or a solution of alcohol and water and tied at the open end. It is applied to a small body area, such as the eye. Ice gloves can be stored in the freezer when not in use.

Disposable cold packs (Figure 41–7) are similar to disposable hot packs. They come in a variety of sizes and shapes and provide a specific degree of coldness for a specified period of time, as indicated on the package. By striking, squeezing, or kneading the package, the nurse activates chemical reactions that release the cold. The manufacturer's instructions

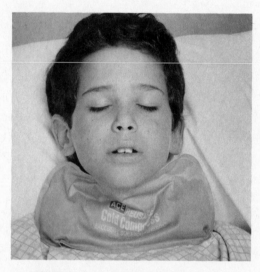

FIGURE 41–7 A disposable ice pack in place.

must be followed. Most commercially prepared cold packs have soft outer coverings so that they can be applied directly to the body part.

Technique 41–6 describes how to apply an ice bag, collar, or glove or disposable cold pack.

41-6

Applying an Ice Bag, Ice Collar, Ice Glove, or Disposable Cold Pack

Before applying dry cold, verify the order for the cold application, including when, where, why, and for how long the cold is to be applied.

PURPOSES

- To relieve headaches caused by vasodilation
- To prevent swelling of tissues immediately following an injury or surgery
- To prevent, decrease, or terminate bleeding following an injury or surgery
- To reduce joint pain from the pressure of accumulated fluid

▶ **Technique 41–6** Applying Dry Cold *CONTINUED*

ASSESSMENT FOCUS	Evidence of circulatory deficiencies at the area of application (e.g., bluish purplish color, feeling of cold, decreased sensation or numbness); other factors contraindicating cold therapy (see Nursing Process Guide, page 957); any discomfort experienced by the client; swelling; client's ability to cooperate during the procedure.

EQUIPMENT

- ☐ Ice bag, collar, glove, or cold pack
- ☐ Ice chips
- ☐ Protective covering
- ☐ Roller gauze, a binder or a towel, and tape

INTERVENTION

1. Prepare and assess the client.

- Assist the client to a comfortable position, and support the body part requiring the application.

- Expose only the area to be treated, and provide warmth to avoid chilling. Privacy may or may not be necessary, depending on the location of the application and the client's wishes.

- Assess the area to which the cold will be applied. See the Assessment Focus above and the Nursing Process Guide on page 957.

Ice Bag, Collar, or Glove

2. Fill and cover the device.

- Fill the device one-half to two-thirds full of crushed ice. *Partial filling makes the device more pliable so that it can be molded to a body part.*

- Remove excess air by bending or twisting the device. *Air inflates the device so that it cannot be molded to the body part.*

- Insert the stopper securely into an ice bag or collar, or tie a knot at the open end of a glove. *This prevents leakage of fluid when the ice melts.*

- Hold the device upside down, and check it for leaks.

- Cover the device with a soft cloth cover, if it is not already equipped with one. *The cover absorbs moisture that condenses on the outside of the device. It is also more comfortable for the client.*

3. Apply the cold device.

- Apply the device for the time specified. The device is usually applied for no longer than 30 minutes because of the rebound phenomenon.

- Hold it in place with roller gauze, a binder, or a towel. Secure with tape as necessary.

Disposable Cold Pack

4. Initiate the cooling process.

- Strike, squeeze, or knead the cold pack according to the manufacturer's instructions. *The action activates the chemical reaction that produces the cold.*

- Cover with a soft cloth cover, if the pack does not have a cover. Most commercially prepared cold packs have soft outer coverings to permit application directly to the body part.

All Applications

5. Instruct the client as follows:

- Remain in position for the duration of the treatment.

- Call the nurse if discomfort is felt.

6. Monitor the client during the application.

- Assess the client in terms of comfort and skin reaction (e.g., pallor, mottled appearance) as frequently as necessary for the client's safety, e.g., every 5 to 10 minutes. Factors such as previous responses to applications and the client's ability to report any problems need to be considered.

- Report untoward reactions to the nurse in charge, and remove the application.

7. Remove the application.

- Remove the cold application at the designated time. *This avoids the harmful effects of prolonged cold.*

8. Document all relevant information.

- At the time of application, document the cold application, its purpose, the method used, the site, and nursing assessments.

- After removal, record the time and all nursing assessments.

EVALUATION FOCUS	Presence or absence of signs of impaired blood circulation to the area; appearance of affected tissues (e.g., any swelling); any discomfort experienced by the client.

► **Technique 41–6 Applying Dry Cold** *CONTINUED*

SAMPLE RECORDING

Date	Time	Notes
08/10/93	1145	Disposable ice pack applied to left ankle as ordered. Ankle very swollen and painful especially with weight-bearing. Skin pink. Popliteal and pedal pulses strong. ———————————————————— Roberta Victor, RN
	1205	Ice pack removed. Skin pale and slightly mottled. Ankle remains swollen. ———————————————————— Roberta Victor, RN

KEY ELEMENTS OF APPLYING AN ICE BAG, ICE COLLAR, ICE GLOVE, OR DISPOSABLE COLD PACK

- Know the purpose of the application.
- Before the application, assess the appearance of the area to be treated, in particular, the circulatory status of the area; factors that may affect the client's tolerance to cold; conditions that contraindicate the therapy; and conditions that indicate the need for precautions.
- Partially fill ice bags (collars, gloves), and expel excess air.

- Ensure that the appliance is leakproof and has a protective covering.
- Prevent chilling of the client.
- Throughout the application assess the condition of the skin at least every 10 minutes.
- Remove the application before the rebound phenomenon occurs or whenever adverse reactions occur (e.g., pain, pallor, skin insensitivity).

Cooling Sponge Bath

The cooling sponge bath consists of water or a combination of alcohol and water that is below body temperature. Alcohol evaporates at a low temperature and therefore removes body heat rapidly. However, alcohol-and-water sponge baths are less frequently used than in the past because alcohol has a drying effect on the skin. The temperatures for cooling sponge baths range from 18 to 32 C (65 to 90 F). A *tepid* sponge bath generally refers to one in which the water temperature is 32 C (90 F) throughout the bath. For a *cool* sponge bath, the water temperature is 32 C (90 F) at the beginning of the bath and is gradually lowered to 18 C (65 F) by adding ice chips during the bath. A fan is sometimes used to increase air movement around the client, which lowers the body temperature through convection. In this case, drafts are not usually eliminated during the sponge bath. Cool sponge baths are used with extreme caution because of potential deleterious effects, such as shock.

The decision to give a tepid sponge bath is generally made only after a marked fever is noted or a temperature increase of 1 to 2 C (2 to 3 F). Some agencies require a physician's order; others permit a decision by the nurse in charge. Technique 41–7 describes how to administer a cooling sponge bath.

41-7 Administering a Cooling Sponge Bath

Before administering a cooling sponge bath, determine agency protocol. Some agencies recommend sponging the entire body. To avoid chilling, others recommend sponging only the face, arms, legs, back, and buttocks (*not* the chest and abdomen).

PURPOSE

- To reduce a client's fever by promoting body heat loss through conduction and vaporization

▶ **Technique 41–7 Administering a Cooling Sponge Bath** *CONTINUED*

ASSESSMENT FOCUS	Body temperature, pulse, respirations for baseline data; other signs of fever (e.g., skin warmth, flushing, complaints of feeling hot or chilly, diaphoresis, irritability, restlessness, general malaise, or delirium).

EQUIPMENT

- Thermometer to measure the client's temperature
- Bath blanket
- Several washcloths and bath towels (fewer are needed if ice
- bags or cold packs are used)
- Basin for the solution
- Bath thermometer
- Solution at the correct temperature (water or equal
- portions of 70% alcohol and water)
- Ice bag or cold pack (optional)
- Fan (optional)

INTERVENTION

1. Obtain all relevant baseline data.

- If not already recorded prior to the sponge bath, measure the client's body temperature, pulse, and respirations to provide comparative baseline data.
- Assess the client for other signs of fever (see the Assessment Focus above).

2. Prepare the client.

- Remove the gown, and assist the client to a comfortable supine position.
- Place a bath blanket over the client.
- If ice bags or cold packs are not used, place bath towels under each axilla and shoulder. *Bath towels protect the lower bed sheet from getting wet.*

3. Sponge the face.

- Sponge the client's face with plain water only, and dry it.
- Apply an ice bag or cold pack to the head for comfort.

4. Place cold applications in the axillae and groins.

- Wet four washcloths; wring them out so that they are very damp but not dripping. *Washcloths need to be as moist as possible to be effective.*

- Place washcloths in the axillae and groins.
or
Place ice bags or cold packs in these areas. *The axillae and groins contain large superficial blood vessels, which aid the transfer of heat.*

- Leave washcloths in place for about 5 minutes, or until they feel warm. Rewet and replace them as required during the bath. *Washcloths warm up relatively quickly in such vascular areas.*

5. Sponge the arms and legs.

- Place a bath towel under one arm and sponge the arm *slowly* and *gently* for about 5 minutes or as tolerated by the client. *Slow, gentle motions are indicated because firm rubbing motions increase tissue metabolism and heat production. Cool sponges given rapidly or for a short period of time tend to increase the body's heat production mechanisms by causing shivering.*

or

Place a saturated towel over the extremity, and rewet it as necessary. Give the client enough time to adjust to the initial reaction of chilliness and for the body to cool.

- Dry the arm, using a patting motion rather than a rubbing motion.
- Repeat the above steps for the other arm and the legs.
- When sponging the extremities, hold the washcloth briefly over the wrists and ankles. *The blood circulation is close to the skin surface in the wrists and ankles.*

6. Reassess the client's vital signs after 15 minutes.

- Compare findings with data taken before the bath. *The vital signs are checked to evaluate the effectiveness of the sponge bath.* Proceed with the bath if the temperature is above 37.7 C (100 F); discontinue if the temperature is below 37.7 C (100 F), or if the pulse rate is significantly increased and remains so after 5 minutes.

7. (Optional) Sponge the chest and abdomen.

- Sponge these areas for 3 to 5 minutes and pat them dry.

8. Sponge the back and buttocks.

- Sponge the back and buttocks for 3 to 5 minutes.
- Pat these areas dry.

9. Remove the cold applications from the axillae and groins.

▶ **Technique 41–7 Administering a Cooling Sponge Bath** *CONTINUED*

10. Reassess vital signs.

11. Document assessments, including the vital signs, as well as the type of sponge bath given.

VARIATION: Pediatric Bathing

Cooling baths for children can be given in the tub, or the bed or crib. Immersion of a child in a tepid tub bath for 20 to 30 minutes is a simple and effective method to reduce an elevated temperature.

Tub

• While the child is in the tub, firmly support the child's head and shoulders and gently squeeze water over the back and chest or gently spray water from a sprayer over the body.

• To make a tub bath more effective, lay a small infant or older child down in the water and support the head on your arm or a

padded support. Small children, however, may resist any effort to place them in a horizontal position.

• For conscious children, use a floating toy or other distraction during the bath.

• Always stay with the child in a tub for safety reasons.

• Discontinue the cooling bath if there is evidence of chilling. The process of shivering generates additional heat and defeats the purpose of the bath and chilling causes vasoconstriction so that minimal blood is carried to the skin surface.

• Dry and dress the child in lightweight clothing or only a diaper and cover the child with a light cotton blanket.

• Retake the temperature 30 min-

utes after removal from the tub and repeat measurement as often as indicated.

Bed or Crib Sponge

• Place the undressed child on an absorbent towel.

• Follow the steps above for a sponge bath, or use the following towel method:

   a. Apply a cool cloth or icebag to the forehead.

   b. Wrap each extremity in a towel moistened with tepid water.

   c. Place one towel under the back and another over the neck and torso.

   d. Change the towels as they warm.

   e. Continue the procedure for about 30 minutes.

EVALUATION FOCUS | Vital signs and changes in baseline assessments.

SAMPLE RECORDING

Date	Time	Notes
09/18/93	1645	T40.2, P94, R18 and shallow. C/o "burning up," face flushed, diaphoretic, and states feels "miserable and muscles aching." Dr. Kirkpatrick notified. Cooling sponge bath given. ———————— Jennifer Newton, RN
	1700	T39.4, P90, R16. Face less flushed. States "feels cooler." ———— Jennifer Newton, RN
	1715	T38.8, P90, R14. ———————— Jennifer Newton, RN

KEY ELEMENTS OF ADMINISTERING A COOLING SPONGE BATH

• Determine agency policies about administering cooling sponge baths in regard to need for physician's order, and type and temperature of solution used.

• Obtain temperature, pulse, and respiration measurements before the bath for baseline data, after 15 minutes, and then at the end of the procedure.

• Place damp washcloths or ice bags or cold packs on the forehead, axillae, and groins. If using damp washcloths, rewet and replace them every 5 minutes.

• Use slow gentle motions when using damp washcloths.

• Hold the washcloth briefly over the wrists and ankles.

• Use a patting motion to dry each area.

• Remove washcloths or cold packs from the axillae and groins following the procedure, and dry these areas.

CRITICAL THINKING CHALLENGE

Grant Williams was admitted to the neurosurgical unit with a closed head injury. He is unresponsive to command and minimally responsive to pain. His physician has ordered a hypothermia blanket to maintain his body temperature at 36.1 C (97 F) to decrease oxygen demand by the brain. When assessing Mr. Williams, you observe that he is shivering. What effect will shivering have on the planned goal of hypothermia therapy? What action would you take?

REFERENCES

Guyton, A. C. 1986. *Textbook of medical physiology.* 7th ed. Philadelphia: W. B. Saunders Co.

James, S. R., and Mott, S. R. 1988. *Child health nursing. Essential care of children and families.* Redwood City, Calif.: Addison-Wesley Nursing.

Kozier, B.; Erb, G.; and Olivieri, R. 1991. *Fundamentals of nursing: Concepts, process and practice.* 4th ed. Redwood City, Calif.: Addison-Wesley Nursing.

Lehmann, J. F., and DeLateur, B. J. 1982a. *Therapeutic heat and cold.* 3d ed. Baltimore: Williams and Wilkins Co.

————. 1982b. Diathermy and superficial heat and cold therapy. In Kottke, F. J.; Stillwell, G. K.; and Lehmann, J. F. *Krusen's handbook of physical medicine and rehabilitation.* 3d ed. Philadelphia: W. B. Saunders Co.

Olds, S. B., London, M. L.; and Ladewig, P. W. 1992. *Maternal-newborn nursing.* 4th ed. Redwood City, Calif.: Addison-Wesley Nursing.

Tepperman, P. S., and Devlin, M. January 1983. Therapeutic heat and cold: A practitioner's guide. *Postgraduate Medicine* 73:69.

Perioperative Nursing

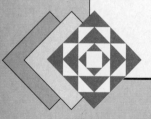

NURSING PROCESS GUIDE
PERIOPERATIVE NURSING

PERIOPERATIVE PERIOD

ASSESSMENT

Determine the client's

- *Age and developmental stage.* The nurse often needs to adapt preoperative teaching to the special needs of children and the elderly.

- *Mental attitude.* Mild anxiety is a normal response to surgery; severe anxiety can increase surgical risk.

- *Understanding of surgical procedure.* A well-informed client knows what to expect and in general accepts and copes more effectively with surgery and convalescence.

- *Previous experience.* This may influence the physical and psychologic responses to the planned surgery.

- *Expected outcomes.* The results of the surgery may alter a client's body image and life-style to varying degrees.

- *Current medications.* Certain medications, such as anticonvulsants and insulin, must be continued throughout the operative period to prevent adverse effects. A physician's order to this effect is required, however. The regular use of certain medications can increase surgical risk:

  a. *Anticoagulants* increase blood coagulation time.

  b. *Tranquilizers* may cause hypotension and thus contribute to shock.

  c. *Heroin and other depressants* decrease central nervous system responses.

  d. *Antibiotics* may be incompatible with anesthetic agents, resulting in untoward reactions.

  e. *Diuretics* may precipitate electrolyte (especially potassium) imbalances.

- *Smoking habits.* Smokers' lung tissue may be chronically irritated, and a general anesthetic agent irritates it further.

- *Use of alcohol.* Heavy, consistent use can lead to problems during anesthesia, surgery, and recovery.

- *Readiness to learn.* See Chapter 5.

- *Coping resources.* Employing previously effective coping mechanisms or developing new strategies (e.g., diversional activities such as reading and relaxation exercises) may be helpful.

- *Self-concept.* A healthy, positive self-concept predisposes clients to approach a surgical experience with confidence that they can handle it successfully.

- *Body image.* Possible disfigurement or change in physical identity may be a concern prior to surgery. Providing accurate information often allays fears based on misconceptions.

Determine the presence of any health problems that increase surgical risk:

- *Cardiac conditions,* such as angina pectoris, recent myocardial infarction, severe hypertension, and severe congestive heart failure. Well-controlled cardiac problems generally pose minimal operative risk.

- *Blood coagulation disorders* that may lead to severe bleeding, hemorrhage, and subsequent shock.

- *Upper respiratory tract infections or chronic obstructive lung diseases,* such as emphysema. These conditions, especially when exacerbated by the effects of general anesthesia, adversely affect pulmonary function. They also predispose the client to postoperative lung infections.

- *Renal disease* that impairs the regulation of the body's fluids and electrolytes, e.g., renal insufficiency.

- *Diabetes mellitus,* which predisposes the client to wound infection and delayed healing.

- *Liver disease,* e.g., cirrhosis, which impairs the liver's abilities to detoxify medications used during surgery, produce the prothrombin necessary for blood clotting, and metabolize nutrients essential for healing.

- *Uncontrolled neurologic disease,* such as epilepsy.

Determine the results of preoperative screening tests:

- Urinalysis.

- Chest roentgenography.

- Electrocardiography.

- Complete blood count (CBC).

- Blood grouping and cross matching.

- Serum electrolytes (Na^+, K^+, Mg^{2+}, Ca^{2+}, H^+).

- Fasting blood sugar.

- Blood urea nitrogen (BUN) or creatinine.

Assess the client's

- *General appearance,* e.g., color and energy level. Note pallor, cyanosis, or marked fatigue.

- *Vital signs.* Measure blood pressure in supine and upright positions.

Nursing Process Guide *CONTINUED*

- *Nutrition status.* Observe any signs of malnutrition (see Chapter 22), and measure weight and height.

- *Hydration status.* Measure fluid intake and output, and test tissue turgor.

- *Cardiopulmonary status.* Auscultate breath and heart sounds, and observe the presence of dyspnea, cough, or edema.

- *Peripheral vascular status.* Inspect and palpate the extremities for

  a. Signs of inadequate arterial blood circulation, such as cool skin temperature in a warm environment; pallor; shiny, taut skin; mild edema.

  b. Signs of insufficient venous return, such as thickening of the skin, increased pigmentation around the ankles, pitting edema, peripheral cyanosis, and the appearance or presence of distended superficial veins in the legs. (Normally, veins may appear distended in a dependent position but collapse when the limb is elevated.)

  c. Posterior tibial and dorsalis pedis pulse rates, volumes, and rhythms.

  d. Pain in the calf of the leg. Dorsiflex the foot abruptly and firmly while the knee is straight or slightly flexed (Homans' sign). The presence of pain is a positive Homans' sign.

- *Mobility status.* Determine gait, balance, range of motion, and motor coordination; muscle strength in upper and lower extremities; and the need for ambulation aids.

RELATED DIAGNOSTIC CATEGORIES

- Anxiety

- Fear (about the effects or outcome of surgery)

- Knowledge deficit

- Anticipatory grieving (for possible loss of body part)

PLANNING

Client Goals

The client will

- Experience minimal anxiety preoperatively.

- Understand the preoperative regimen and rationales and the surgical procedure to be performed.

- Be physically and psychologically prepared for surgery.

Outcome Criteria

The client

- Describes in general terms the proposed surgical procedure, reason for it, subsequent therapy, and expected length of stay in hospital.

- Verbalizes understanding of events (e.g., transfers to postanesthesia room or intensive care unit) and therapeutic devices (e.g., monitoring equipment, infusions) in all perioperative phases.

- States reasons for preoperative and postoperative procedures (e.g., skin prep, bowel prep) and practices (e.g., deep breathing, coughing, turning, leg exercises).

- Demonstrates deep breathing, coughing, splinting, leg exercises, and moving techniques as taught.

- Verbalizes expectations and understanding of usual postoperative pain control and activity.

- Expresses feelings about the surgery and its expected outcomes.

- Expresses feelings of achieving adequate rest and sleep.

- Demonstrates balanced fluid intake and output.

- Remains free from infection, as manifested by baseline temperature and pulse rate.

POSTOPERATIVE PERIOD

ASSESSMENT

Assess

- *Vital signs: pulse, respirations, and blood pressure.* Compare them with data from the recovery room. Many hospitals have postoperative routines for regular assessment of clients. In some agencies, assessments are made every 15 minutes until vital signs stabilize, every hour thereafter the same day, and every 4 hours for the next 2 days. Body temperature is usually assessed every 4 hours for the first few days. *It is very important that the assessments be made as frequently as the person's condition requires.* An elevated temperature along with other signs can indicate infection of the respiratory tract, urinary tract, or incision. A rapid, weak pulse and increased respiratory rate along with other signs can indicate infection, hemorrhage, or shock. A lowered blood pressure along with other signs can indicate hemorrhage, shock, or pulmonary embolism.

- *Skin color and temperature.* The color of the lips and nail beds are indicators of **tissue perfusion** (passage of blood through the vessels). Pale, cyanotic, cool, and moist skin may be a sign of circulatory problems.

- *Level of consciousness.* At this point, most clients are conscious but drowsy.

- *Bleeding.* Inspect the dressings for bleeding and the bedclothes underneath the client for pooled blood.

Later, when dressings are changed, inspect the wound for signs of localized infection.

- *Intravenous infusion.* Observe the type of solution, amount in the bottle, the drip rate, and the venipuncture site. Determine additional solutions ordered.

- *Patency of drainage tubes.* Note also the amount, color, consistency, and character of the drainage.

- *Fluid balance.* Measure the client's fluid intake and output for at least 2 days or until fluid balance is stable without an IV.

- *Pain or discomfort and when the client last had an analgesic.* Note the location, note the type of pain, and determine the cause. Pain is usually greatest 12 to 36 hours after surgery, decreasing on the second or third day. Analgesics are usually administered every 3 or 4 hours the first day, and by the third day most clients require only oral analgesics. Signs of acute pain include pallor, perspiration, tension, and reluctance to perform deep-breathing and coughing exercises or to move or ambulate.

- *Any difficulties with voiding and/or bladder distention.*

- *Return of peristalsis.* Auscultate the client's abdomen to confirm the return of peristalsis. Note the passage of flatus and stool.

- *Tolerance of food and fluids ingested.*

Determine any clinical signs of postoperative complications:

- *Pneumonia:* Elevated temperature, cough, expectoration of blood-tinged or purulent sputum, dyspnea, chest pain.

- *Atelectasis:* Marked dyspnea, cyanosis, pleural pain, prostration, tachycardia, increased respiratory rate, fever, productive cough, auscultatory crackling sounds.

- *Pulmonary embolism:* Sudden chest pain, shortness of breath, cyanosis, shock (tachycardia, low blood pressure).

- *Thrombophlebitis:* Aching, cramping pain; affected area is swollen, red, and hot to touch; vein feels hard; discomfort in calf when foot is dorsiflexed or when client walks (Homans' sign).

- *Thrombus or embolus:* Same as for pulmonary embolism; if lodged in heart or brain, assess cardiac or neurologic signs.

- *Urinary retention:* Fluid intake larger than output; inability to void or frequent voiding of small amounts, bladder distention, suprapubic discomfort, restlessness, bladder palpable above the symphysis pubis.

- *Urinary infection:* Burning sensation when voiding, urgency, cloudy urine, lower abdominal pain.

- *Constipation:* Absence of stool elimination, abdominal distention and discomfort.

- *Tympanites:* Obvious abdominal distention, abdominal discomfort (gas pains), absence of bowel sounds.

- *Wound infection:* Purulent exudate, redness, tenderness, elevated body temperature, wound odor.

- *Wound dehiscence:* Increased incision drainage, tissues underlying skin become visible along parts of the incision.

- *Wound evisceration:* Opening of incision and visible protrusion of organs.

RELATED DIAGNOSTIC CATEGORIES

Because surgery can involve many body systems—both directly and indirectly—and is a complex experience for the client, the nursing diagnoses focus on a wide variety of actual and potential problems. Certain diagnoses, however, are more likely to apply.

- Ineffective airway clearance

- Ineffective breathing pattern

- High risk for Injury

- High risk for Infection

- Pain

- High risk for Fluid volume deficit

- Urinary retention

- Knowledge deficit (wound care and activity restrictions after discharge)

- Self-care deficit: Bathing/hygiene, dressing/grooming, toileting

PLANNING

Client Goals

The client will

- Be free of surgical complications.

- Experience minimal discomfort.

- Achieve adequate rest.

- Be free of injury.

- Maintain a healthy attitude toward self.

- Resume the highest possible level of wellness.

Outcome Criteria

The client

- Maintains normal baseline vital signs.

- Performs deep-breathing exercises and voluntary coughing every 2 hours when awake, as instructed.

- Has adequate respiratory excursion (depth).

Nursing Process Guide *CONTINUED*

- Has clear lung sounds on auscultation.

- Performs specified leg exercises at least every 4 hours when awake, as instructed.

- Has negative Homans' sign.

- Has balanced fluid intake and output.

- Has good tissue turgor of the skin.

- Has clear amber urine.

- Experiences no burning sensation or urgency when voiding.

- Has active bowel sounds within 48 hours.

- Resumes normal defecation within 3 days.

- Is free of purulent wound drainage.

- Ambulates, performs self-care activities, and rests with minimal or no pain.

- Reports satisfactory sleep pattern each night.

- Reports feelings of increasing wellness each day.

The Perioperative Period

Operations are traumatic for both clients and their support persons. Although increasing numbers of elective and minor surgical procedures are being performed in day-surgery centers, most operations still take place in hospitals.

The **perioperative period** is the time before, during, and after an operation; it encompasses three phases: preoperative, intraoperative, and postoperative. The **preoperative phase** begins when the decision for surgical intervention is made, and it ends when the client is transferred to the operating room bed. The preoperative client is prepared psychologically and physically for surgery. An important aspect of preoperative nursing is teaching clients what they need to know. The **intraoperative phase** begins when the client is transferred to the operating room bed, and it terminates when the client is admitted to the postanesthesia area. The main intraoperative nursing function is to maintain the client's safety.

The **postoperative phase** is the time following surgery. It begins with admission to the postanesthetic care unit (PACU), also referred to as the recovery room (RR), and ends when the client has completely recovered from the surgery.

Prior to any surgical procedure, clients must sign a surgical consent form. This requirement protects clients from having any surgical procedure they do not want or do not know about. It also protects the hospital and the health personnel from a claim by client or family that permission was not granted. The consent form becomes a part of the client's record and goes to the operating room with the client.

Obtaining legal, informed consent to perform surgery is the responsibility of the surgeon. Informed consent is possible only when the client is told in advance of the character and importance of the surgery, its probable consequences, the chances for success, and alternative measures. Often a nurse is responsible for witnessing a consent. Nurses must be aware of their responsibilities regarding consents and of the particular hospital's policies.

Preoperative Teaching

An explanation of perioperative care informs the client and the support persons about the perioperative period. Usually, people are anxious at this time, and many have misconceptions about surgery and surgical care. Clients often ask nurses about the operation after the surgeon has gained informed consent and left the client's room. The surgeon should be notified if the client is anxious about the procedure or has questions about the surgery that the nurse cannot answer.

Clients and their support persons need to know the time and type of surgery. The surgeon usually arranges the date and may specify it in the orders. The exact time may not be known until the surgical schedule for the hospital is distributed.

The nurse needs to listen attentively and carefully to help the client identify specific concerns or fears and talk them through. This is also the time to clarify any misconceptions the client may have. Providing accurate information and acting supportively will help the client deal with identified concerns. The nurse should not dismiss the client's concerns by saying, "Everything will be all right." Unknowns or misconceptions can produce unrealistic fears and anxiety.

The client also may have specific learning needs regarding postoperative care. For example, learning to attend to a colostomy requires preparation *before* surgery. Pain is common postoperatively; learning *beforehand* how to minimize it (e.g., by holding a pillow against the abdomen when moving after abdominal surgery) reassures the client. It also is important that clients know they will receive analgesics postoperatively to minimize discomfort.

Whenever possible, preadmission of pediatric clients should be carried out (see page 106 and Technique 7–2, page 113). The role of the parent or support person in the interactive process with children is extremely important. Often, the parent must be approached and prepared first, and then the parent may prepare the child. Nursing interventions requiring communication with the pediatric client—such as interviewing and client teaching—require that the nurse consider the age and developmental stage of the child and adapt the interaction appropriately.

The nurse needs to consult the parent and child to determine priorities and the best timing for teaching of the pediatric client. The client who participates in the formulation of the teaching plan is generally more motivated to work toward the achievement of desired outcomes. Preoperative teaching objectives must be achievable within a short period of time for young children with short attention spans. Children may require more time to digest small amounts of material.

The nurse may use a doll or puppet to demonstrate procedures to young preschool and school-age children. For older children and adolescents, pictures, booklets, and audiovisual aids may also be used to explain important preoperative preparation, key aspects of the operative process, and postoperative care measures. The nurse should encourage the child to handle the equipment and to perform the procedure on the doll or puppet. The child who is old enough may draw pictures or write to express feelings and reactions related to the impending surgery. A group learning approach may be utilized when appropriate, but brief follow-up individualized teaching sessions with the child and parents may provide greater understanding.

When choosing content for the preoperative instruction of a child, the nurse should consult the parent or guardian of a minor child regarding appropriate content and approach. Preoperative teaching should address topics about which the child or parent has expressed concern, and then proceed to other unknown aspects.

The nurse should provide explanations in a language they can understand and at a rate that keeps their attention and does not overwhelm them. It will also help to show the child the anesthetic equipment and the postanesthesia room ("wake-up room") before surgery, explaining all postoperative care and discomfort clearly and simply, for example, "You will have a sore tummy." Confirm when the parents will visit, because this is the most essential piece of information the nurse can give the child.

Elderly clients, too, often have special needs regarding surgical preparation. See Table 42–1.

TABLE 42–1 RISK FACTORS FOR THE ELDERLY SURGICAL CLIENT

Physiologic Change	Preoperative Nursing Interventions
Integumentary System Vulnerable skin due to venous stasis and poor venous return	Teach passive and active exercises. Determine the need for antiemboli stockings (see box on page 990).
Cardiovascular System Reduced cardiac reserve due to changes in the myocardium	Determine usual pattern of ADLs and how quickly the client tires.
Tachycardia from anxiety, which is tolerated poorly in the elderly heart	Teach about and support anxiety reduction.
Decreased compliance of blood vessels due to atherosclerosis	Teach leg exercises and turning. Obtain baseline data re vital signs. Monitor blood pressure closely for hypertension.
Respiratory System Reduced vital capacity due to lowered expansibility of the rib cage	Teach deep breathing and coughing. Obtain baseline data re respirations.
Urinary System Reduced blood flow to the kidneys	Obtain baseline urine output for 24 hours.
Reduced ability to excrete toxins due to reduced glomerular filtration	Initiate fluid intake and output recordings.
Fluids and Electrolytes Dehydration from repeated enemas	Assess hydration status for baseline data.
Hypokalemia due to diarrhea	Monitor fluid intake and output.
Neurologic System Reduced sensory acuity	Orient client to surroundings.
Decreased reaction time	Allow time for client to proceed at own pace.

All clients need to be informed about what activities to expect, when to expect them, and why they are being done. Technique 42–1 provides guidelines for teaching moving, leg exercises, deep-breathing exercises, and coughing.

42-1 Teaching Moving, Leg Exercises, Deep-Breathing Exercises, and Coughing

Before commencing to teach moving, leg exercises, deep-breathing exercises, and coughing, determine (a) the type of surgery, (b) the time of the surgery, (c) the name of the surgeon, (d) the preoperative orders, (e) the agency's practices for preoperative care, and (f) the learning needs of the client. Also, verify that the physician has completed the medical history and physical examination and that the consent form has been signed by the client or the family.

PURPOSES

Moving
- To maintain blood circulation
- To stimulate respiratory function
- To decrease stasis of gas in the intestine
- To facilitate early ambulation

Leg Exercises
- To stimulate blood circulation, thereby preventing thrombophlebitis and thrombus formation

Deep Breathing and Coughing
- To facilitate lung aeration, thereby preventing atelectasis and pneumonia
- To promote blood circulation to and from the lungs, thereby preventing pulmonary embolism

ASSESSMENT FOCUS

Vital signs; discomfort; temperature and color of feet and legs; breath sounds; presence of dyspnea or cough.

INTERVENTION

1. Show the client ways to turn in bed and to get out of bed.

- Instruct a client who will have a right abdominal incision or a right-sided chest incision to turn to the left side of the bed and sit up as follows:

a. Flex the knees.

b. Hold the left arm and hand or a small pillow against the incision to splint the wound.

c. Turn to the left while pushing with the right foot and grasping a partial side rail on the left side of the bed with the right hand.

d. Come to a sitting position on the side of the bed by using the right arm and hand to push down against the mattress.

- Ask a client with a left abdominal or left-sided chest incision to perform the same procedure but splint with the right arm and turn to the right.

- For clients with orthopedic surgery (e.g., hip surgery), use special aids, such as a trapeze, to assist with movement.

2. Teach the client the following three leg exercises.

- Alternate dorsiflexion and plantar flexion of the feet. *This exercise is sometimes referred to as calf pumping, since it alternately contracts and relaxes the calf muscles, including the gastrocnemius muscles.*

- Flex and extend the knees, and press the backs of the knees into the bed while dorsiflexing the feet (Figure 42–1). Instruct clients who cannot raise their legs to do isometric exercises that contract and relax the muscles.

- Raise and lower the legs alternately from the surface of the bed. Extend the knee of the mov-

▶ **Technique 42–1** *CONTINUED*

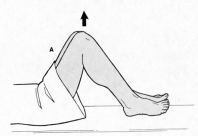

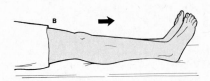

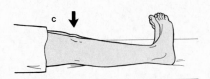

FIGURE 42–1 Flexing and extending the knees.

FIGURE 42–2 Raising and lowering the legs.

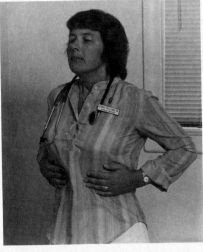

FIGURE 42–3 Demonstrating deep breathing.

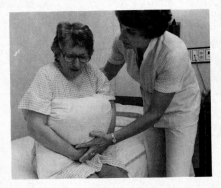

FIGURE 42–4 Splinting an incision with a pillow.

ing leg (Figure 42–2). *This exercise contracts and relaxes the quadriceps muscles.*

3. Demonstrate deep-breathing (diaphragmatic) exercises as follows.

- Place your hands palms down on the border of your rib cage, and inhale slowly and evenly through the nose until the greatest chest expansion is achieved (Figure 42–3).

- Hold your breath for 2 to 3 seconds.

- Then exhale slowly through the mouth.

- Continue exhalation until maxi-

mum chest contraction has been achieved.

4. Help the client perform deep-breathing exercises.

- Ask the client to assume a sitting position.

- Place the palms of your hands on the border of the client's rib cage to assess respiratory depth.

- Ask the client to perform deep breathing, as described in step 3.

5. Instruct the client to cough voluntarily after a few deep inhalations.

- Ask the client to inhale deeply, hold the breath for a few seconds, and then cough once or twice.

- Ensure that the client coughs deeply and does not just clear the throat.

6. Demonstrate ways to splint the abdomen when coughing, if the incision will be painful when the client coughs.

- Show the client how to support the incision by placing the palms of the hands on either side of the incision site or directly over the incision site, holding the palm of one hand over the other. *Cough-*

ing uses the abdominal and other accessory respiratory muscles. Splinting the incision may reduce pain while coughing if the incision is near any of these muscles.

- Show the client how to splint the abdomen with clasped hands and a firmly rolled pillow held against the client's abdomen (Figure 42–4).

7. Inform the client about the expected frequency of these exercises.

- Instruct the client to start the exercises as soon after surgery as possible.

- Encourage clients with abdominal or chest surgery to carry out deep breathing and coughing at least three or four times daily and at each session to take a minimum of five breaths. Note, however, that the number of breaths and frequency of deep breathing varies with the client's condition. People who are susceptible to pulmonary problems may need deep-breathing exercises every hour. People with chronic respiratory disease may need special breathing exercises, e.g., pursed-lip breathing, abdominal breathing, exercises using various kinds of incentive spirometers. See Chapter 30.

8. Document the teaching and all assessments.

▶ **Technique 42–1 Teaching Exercises** *CONTINUED*

EVALUATION FOCUS	Client's demonstrated ability to perform moving, leg exercises, deep-breathing and coughing exercises.

SAMPLE RECORDING

Date	Time	Notes
09/06/93	1030	Taught turning in bed, leg exercises, coughing and deep breathing. Returned demonstrations. No difficulty with turning or exercises. Simone Lentley, SN

KEY ELEMENTS OF TEACHING MOVING, LEG EXERCISES, AND COUGHING AND DEEP-BREATHING EXERCISES

- Assess the client's ability to perform each exercise

- Have the client demonstrate the exercises.

Surgical Skin Preparation

The surgeon usually indicates the type of surgery in the preoperative orders on the client's chart. From this information, the nurse determines the kind and extent of skin preparation required (if not already specified on the order). Agencies often have protocols to follow regarding skin preparation areas; for example, the area should be larger than the incision area. In many hospitals skin preparation is done by operating room personnel.

The Association of Operating Room Nurses states that cleansing can be accomplished before surgery by having the client shower, by washing the operative site in the client unit, and/or by washing the operative site immediately before applying the antimicrobial agent in the operating room. (AORN 1988, p. 950).

Hair removal of an operative site is not recommended unless the hair interferes with the surgical procedure, e.g., craniotomy. If hair removal at the operative site is required, the nurse should perform it in a client care area that provides privacy and good lighting. There are three methods.

1. Applying a **depilatory** (cream hair remover), which can be used before the client's arrival in the surgical suite (a skin sensitivity test should be done before application)

2. Using an electric clipper with a disposable or removable head that can be sterilized between clients

3. Shaving with a sharp, well-designed disposable or terminally sterilized razor.

Hair should be shaved only when other methods of hair removal are not available or when time does not permit their use. Shaving should be done as close to the time of the operative procedure as possible. The wet method of shaving is preferred. Persons performing the shave prep should wear protective gloves (AORN 1988, p. 951). Preparing the operative site is detailed in Technique 42–2.

42-2

Preparing the Operative Site

Before commencing the surgical skin preparation, determine the surgeon's order, relevant protocols, and recorded allergies to any solutions used in the skin preparation.

PURPOSE

- To reduce the risks of postoperative wound infection by removing soil and transient microbes from the skin, reducing the resident microbial count to subpathogenic levels in a short time and with the least amount of tissue irritation, inhibiting rapid rebound growth of microbes

▶ **Technique 42–2 Preparing the Operative Site** CONTINUED

ASSESSMENT FOCUS	Presence of growths, moles, rashes, pustules, irritations, exudate, abrasions, bruises, or broken or ischemic areas.

EQUIPMENT

□ Adequate lighting for clear visibility of the hair on the skin
□ Bath blanket

Depilatory

□ Cream hair remover with or without applicator
□ Washcloth
□ Gauze squares

□ Lukewarm water

Clipping

□ Electric clippers with sharp heads and unbroken teeth
□ Scissors for long hair, if needed
□ Antimicrobial solution and applicators, if needed

Wet Shave

□ Disposable gloves
□ Skin preparation set containing a disposable razor, compartmentalized basin for solutions, moistureproof drape, soap solution, sponges, and cotton-tipped applicators
□ Warm water

INTERVENTION

1. Drape the client appropriately.

• Expose only the area to be prepared. If using clippers or a razor, expose only small areas at a time. You will clip or shave about 15 cm (6 in) at a time.

2. If a depilatory is to be used, test the client's reaction to it. *Some people may experience irritation or an allergic reaction, even after prior use without an adverse effect.*

• Apply a small amount of the depilatory on a small part of the area where hair is to be removed. Use an area at the periphery of the skin prep area or area advised by the agency policy.

• Apply the cream to the test area smoothly and thickly. Do not rub it in.

• Leave the cream on for the specified time.

• Remove the depilatory by rinsing the area thoroughly with lukewarm water and a washcloth. Do not use soap.

• Pat, rather than rub, the area dry with gauze squares.

• Wait for 24 hours, and assess the client's skin for redness or other responses.

3. Remove hair.

Depilatory

• If the client's skin appears normal after the skin test, apply the depilatory.

  a. Apply the depilatory as described above, and leave it in place for the *minimum* time specified by the manufacturer.

  b. Check a small area. If hair does not wipe off easily, wait a few minutes and check again, but do not leave the cream on longer than the *maximum* time recommended by the manufacturer.

  c. Remove all the depilatory as described in step 2, and pat the area dry.

Clipping

• Make sure the area is dry.

• Remove hair with clippers; do not apply pressure. *Pressure can cause abrasions, particularly over bony prominences.*

• Move the drape, and repeat the above steps until the entire area to be prepared is clipped.

• If applying antimicrobial solution, follow step 4.

Wet Shave

• Don disposable gloves.

• Place the moistureproof towel under the area to be prepared.

• Lather the skin well with the soap solution. *Lathering makes the hair softer and easier to remove.*

• Stretch the skin taut, and hold the razor at about a 45° angle to the skin.

• Shave in the direction in which the hair grows. Use short strokes, and rinse the razor frequently. *Rinsing removes hairs and lather that can obstruct the blade.*

• Wipe excess hair off the skin with the sponges.

• Move the drape, and repeat the above steps until the entire area to be prepared is shaved.

4. Clean and disinfect the surgical area according to agency practice.

• This may be done in the operating room.

• Clean any body crevices, such as the umbilicus, nails, and ear canals, with applicators and solutions. Dry with swabs.

► **Technique 42–2 Preparing the Operative Site** *CONTINUED*

- If an antimicrobial solution is used, apply to the area immediately after it is clipped. Leave it for the designated time, then dry the area with clean swabs. Agency policy will guide you on whether to use an antimicrobial solution and, if so, which to use and how long to leave it on.

5. Inspect the skin after hair removal.

- Closely observe the skin for reddened or broken areas.
- Report to the nurse in charge any skin lesions.

6. Dispose of used equipment appropriately.

- Dispose of razor blade, if used,

according to agency policy to prevent injury to others.

- Discard disposable supplies.

7. Document all relevant information.

- Record the technique, area prepared, and status of skin in the skin preparation area.

EVALUATION FOCUS

Presence of hairs on operative area; see also Assessment Focus.

SAMPLE RECORDING

Date	Time	Notes
12/05/93	0830	Area clipped on left lower extremity. Skin intact. Appeared tense. Stated: "I hope the scar won't show much."———————— Eunice L. Lentz, NS

KEY ELEMENTS OF PREPARING THE OPERATIVE SITE

- Assess the skin preparation area for lesions or broken areas.
- Determine allergies to any skin preparation solution or cream.
- If using clippers, avoid applying pressure.
- If wet shaving, first lather the skin well with soap, hold the skin taut, and shave in the direction of hair growth while holding the razor at a 45° angle.
- Thoroughly clean any body crevices.

Antiemboli Stockings

Antiemboli (elastic) stockings are indicated for clients who have or may have problems with circulation to their feet and legs. The elastic material compresses the veins of the legs and thereby facilitates the return of venous blood to the heart. These stockings are frequently applied preoperatively as well as postoperatively.

There are several types of stockings. One type extends from the foot to the knee and another from the foot to midthigh. These stockings usually have a partial foot that exposes either the heel or toes so that extremity circulation can be assessed. Elastic stockings usually come in small, medium, and large sizes. The accompanying box summarizes the assessments the nurse should make before applying antiemboli stockings.

Technique 42–3 describes how to apply antiemboli stockings. Many agencies use a measuring guide supplied by the stocking manufacturer.

Criteria for the Use of Antiemboli Stockings

- *Inadequate arterial blood circulation:* cool skin temperature in a warm environment; pallor; shiny, taut skin; mild edema.
- *Insufficient venous blood return:* thickening of the skin; increased pigmentation around the ankles; pitting edema (edema in which firm finger pressure on the skin produces an indentation, or pit, that remains for several seconds); peripheral cyanosis.
- *Altered posterior tibial* and *dorsalis pedis pulses:* rates, volumes, and rhythms.
- *Pain in the calf of the leg:* The nurse dorsiflexes the client's foot abruptly and firmly while the client's knee is straight or slightly flexed to assess pain in the calf (Homans' sign). The presence of pain is a positive Homans' sign.
- *Distended superficial veins in the legs:* Normally veins may appear distended in a dependent position but collapse when the limb is elevated.

42-3 Applying Antiemboli Stockings

Before applying antiemboli stockings, determine any potential or present circulatory problems and the surgeon's orders involving the lower extremities.

PURPOSES
- To improve arterial blood circulation to the legs and feet
- To improve venous blood circulation from the legs and feet
- To reduce or prevent edema of the legs or feet

ASSESSMENT FOCUS
Blood circulation to and from the feet and legs. See the box on page 990.

EQUIPMENT

- ☐ Size chart
- ☐ Correct size of elastic stockings

INTERVENTION

1. Select an appropriate time to apply the stockings.

- Apply stockings in the morning, if possible, before the client arises. *In sitting and standing positions, the veins can become distended, and edema occurs; the stockings should be applied before this happens.*

- Wash the legs and feet daily.

- Assist the client who has been ambulating to lie down and elevate the legs for 15 to 30 minutes before applying the stockings. *This facilitates venous return and reduces swelling.*

2. Apply the elastic stocking to the foot.

- Assist the client to a lying position in bed.

- Dust the ankle with talcum powder, and ask the client to point the toes. *These measures ease application.*

- Turn the stocking inside out by inserting your hand into the stocking from the top and grabbing the heel pocket from the inside. The foot portion should now be inside the stocking leg.

- Remove your hand, and, with the

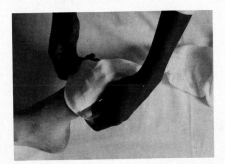

FIGURE 42-5 Applying the inverted stocking over the client's toes.

heel pocket downward, hook your index and middle fingers of both hands into the foot section.

- Face the client, and slip the foot portion of the stocking over the client's foot, toes, and heel (Figure 42-5). As you move up the foot, stretch the stocking sideways.

- Support the client's ankle with one hand while using the other hand to pull the heel pocket under the heel.

- Center the heel in the pocket.

3. Apply the remaining inverted portion of the stocking.

- Gather the remaining portion of the stocking up to the toes, and

pull only this part over the heel. With the foot already covered, the remainder of the stocking should slide easily over it.

- At the ankle, grasp the gathered portion between your index and middle fingers, and pull the stocking up the leg to the knee. You may need to support the ankle with one hand and use the other hand to stretch the stocking and distribute it evenly.

- For *thigh-* or *waist-length stockings,* ask the client to straighten the leg while stretching the rest of the stocking over the knee.

- Ask the client to flex the knee while pulling the stocking over the thigh. Stretch the stocking from the top (front and back) to distribute it evenly over the thigh. The top should rest 2.5 to 7.5 cm (1 to 3 in) below the gluteal fold.

- For a *waist-length stocking,* ask the client to stand and continue extending the stocking up to the top of the gluteal fold.

- Apply the adjustable belt that accompanies thigh- and waist-length stockings, making sure that it does not interefere with

▶ **Technique 42–3 Applying Antiemboli Stockings** *CONTINUED*

any incision or external device (e.g., drainage tube or catheter).

• Adjust the foot section by tug-ging on the toe section to ensure toe comfort and smoothness of the stocking. Make sure a toe window is properly positioned.

4. Document the application of the antiemboli stockings.

EVALUATION FOCUS	Skin temperature and color; presence of edema; posterior tibial and dorsalis pedis pulses; pain in the calf; appearance of leg veins.

SAMPLE RECORDING

Date	Time	Notes
05/05/93	1800	Both feet warm, pink color. No edema. Tibial and pedis pulses 60/bm, equal. No pain, leg veins not visible. Applied antiemboli stockings to both legs. — ————————— Rosie Blakefield, SN

KEY ELEMENTS OF APPLYING ANTIEMBOLI STOCKINGS

• Apply stockings before the client gets out of bed in the morning.

• Clean the skin of the legs and feet daily.

• Assess the adequacy of arterial and venous circulation to the legs and feet.

Preparing for the Postoperative Client

While the client is in the operating room, the client's bed and room are prepared for the postoperative phase. In some agencies, the client is brought back to the unit on a stretcher and transferred to the bed in the room. In other agencies, the client's bed is brought to the recovery room (RR), and the client is transferred there. In the latter situation, the surgical bed needs to be made as soon as the client goes to the operating room so that it can be taken to the RR at any time. In addition, the nurse must obtain and set up special equipment as needed, such as an intravenous pole, suction, oxygen equipment, and orthopedic appliances (e.g., traction). If these are not requested on the client's record, the nurse should consult with the nurse in charge.

The surgical bed is also referred to as the *recovery bed, anesthetic bed,* or *postoperative bed*. It may be used not only for clients who have undergone surgical procedures but also for clients who have been given anesthetics for certain examinations. Technique 42–4 provides instructions for making a surgical bed.

42-4 Making a Surgical Bed

PURPOSES

• To arrange the top bed linen so that the client can be readily transferred to the bed
• To provide as clean an environment as possible for the client
• To provide a bed foundation that can be changed quickly and easily if it becomes soiled
• In some instances, to provide extra warmth through the use of flannelette sheets

▶ **Technique 42–4 Making a Surgical Bed** *CONTINUED*

EQUIPMENT

- ☐ Two clean sheets
- ☐ Clean cotton drawsheet
- ☐ Clean flannelette sheet
- ☐ Clean bedspread
- ☐ Disposable incontinence or drainage pad (optional)

INTERVENTION

1. Strip the bed.

- See Technique 18–1, step 3, on page 447.

- Place and leave the pillows on the bedside chair. *Pillows are left on a chair to facilitate transferring the client into the bed.*

2. Make the foundation of the bed.

- See Technique 18–1, steps 4 and 5.

- Place the flannelette sheet on the foundation of the bed, if this is agency practice. *A flannelette sheet provides additional warmth.*

- Place a disposable pad for the client's head (optional)

3. Apply and fanfold the top bedding.

- Spread the top covers on the bed. Do not tuck them in, miter the corners, or make a toe pleat.

- Fold the hanging edges of the top covers up over the top of the bed so that the folds are at the mattress edge (fold the sides first, then the top and bottom). Then fanfold the covers in either of the following ways:

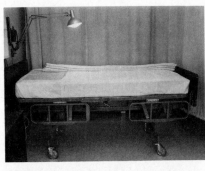

FIGURE 42–6 Surgical bed with top covers folded to the side.

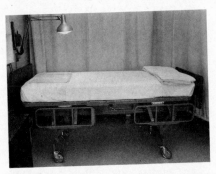

FIGURE 42–7 Surgical bed with top covers folded to the bottom.

a. Fanfold them lengthwise at one side of the bed (Figure 42–6).

b. Fanfold them crosswise at the bottom of the bed (Figure 42–7). *The covers are fanfolded for ease in transferring the client into bed.*

4. Arrange the furniture and equipment appropriately.

- Arrange the furniture and equipment so that there is room near the bed for a stretcher or room to move the bed out of the room if the bed is to be transported to the operating room.

- Make sure any additional equipment, e.g., suction, is in readiness for use when the client returns from surgery.

5. Stabilize and raise the bed.

- Lock the wheels of the bed if the bed is not to be moved. *Locking the wheels keeps the bed from rolling when the client is transferred from the stretcher to the bed.*

- Leave the bed in the high position to meet the level of the stretcher. *The high position facilitates the transfer of the client.*

6. Notify the appropriate people that the surgical bed is ready.

- In some hospitals, a porter service or the like takes the bed to the recovery room.

KEY ELEMENTS FOR MAKING A SURGICAL BED

- Use clean bed linen.
- Fold the top bed clothes for the client's easy access to the bed.

- Leave the bed in high position.

The Postoperative Phase

Immediate postanesthetic care is usually provided in a postanesthetic room (PAR) or recovery room (RR). Recovery room nurses have specialized skills to care for clients recovering from anesthesia and surgery. Once the health status has stabilized, the client is returned to the nursing unit or, in the case of a day-surgery client, to the day-surgery area, for *continuing postoperative care*.

As soon as the client returns to the nursing unit, the nurse conducts an initial assessment. See Figure 42–8 for a postoperative checklist. The sequence of these activities varies with the situation. For example, the nurse may need to check the physician's stat orders before conducting the initial assessment; in such a case, nursing interventions to implement the orders can be carried out at the same time as assessment. The nurse records the client's condition, including the assessment, on the chart.

At this point, most postoperative clients are conscious but often drowsy. A fully conscious person responds verbally, is alert, and is aware of time, place, and person. The nurse notifies the support persons that the client has returned from surgery. It may be necessary to caution them about the client's drowsiness and about not staying too long. Special assessments should be made with older adults. See Table 42–1, earlier.

Assessment continues throughout the postoperative period. See the postoperative assessment guidelines in the Nursing Process Guide on page 982 regarding potential postoperative problems. Nursing interventions designed to prevent these problems include early ambulation, deep breathing and coughing exercises, adequate hydration, leg exercises, monitoring fluid intake and output, and early recognition of signs of complications.

Nursing interventions for postoperative clients include the so-called stir-up regime, in which the client is mobilized as much as possible, i.e., turned, ambulated early, and encouraged frequently to do deep-breathing, coughing, and leg exercises without creating undue fatigue. See the box below for additional guidelines for ongoing postoperative care.

Techniques commonly implemented in the postoperative period are discussed elsewhere in this book. For example, intravenous therapy techniques are discussed in Chapter 25; parenteral medications in Chapter 36; assisting clients to move and ambulate in Chapter 21; and wound care in Chapter 39. This chapter includes the technique of managing gastrointestinal suction.

POSTOPERATIVE INITIAL ASSESSMENT CHECKLIST

1. **Time of arrival** _____
2. **Vital signs**
   Pulse _____ Respirations _____ Blood pressure _____
3. **Skin**
   Color _____
   Condition _____
4. **Level of consciousness**
   Conscious ____ Semiconscious ____ Unconscious ____
5. **Dressing**
   Dry _____ Drainage present _____
   Blood _____ Intact _____
6. **Intravenous**
   Type of solution _____
   Amount in bottle _____ Drip rate _____
   Venipuncture site _____
7. **Drainage tubes**
   Type _____
   Attached to suction or drainage container _____
   Appearance and amount of drainage _____
   _____
8. **Patient position** _____
9. **Side rails** _____
10. **Pain**
    Type of analgesic _____
    Time last given _____
11. **Other discomforts** _____
    _____
    _____

FIGURE 42–8 A sample postoperative checklist.

CLINICAL GUIDELINES

Ongoing Postoperative Care

- Watch for signs indicating acute pain: pallor, perspiration, tension, and reluctance to perform deep-breathing and coughing exercises or to move or ambulate.

- Give analgesics *before* activities (e.g., ambulation or meals) or rest periods (e.g., at bedtime) and assess the effectiveness of the analgesics.

- Do not assume that the pain is caused by the incision (other causes include tight dressings, irritation from drainage tubes, or muscle strains resulting from positioning on the operating table).

- Assess the abdominal area. Note and report the passage of flatus or abdominal distention.

- Inspect dressings regularly to ensure that they are clean, dry, and intact. Excessive drainage can indicate hemorrhage, infection, or dehiscence. See the box on page 983. Change dressings, using sterile technique as required, when they are soiled with drainage or in accordance with the surgeon's or nursing orders. (See Chapter 39).

- Report wound separations promptly to the nurse in charge and the surgeon. If a large dehiscence or evisceration occurs, cover the wound with sterile, moist saline towels or dressings.

Suction

The manner in which suction is applied to drainage tubes depends on the type of equipment available in the agency and the amount of suction required. The following are most commonly used:

• *Portable electric motor suction.* Portable electric units are plugged into electric wall outlets. The units have an on-off switch, a motor that generates the negative pressure, and a drainage bottle. The bottle needs to be monitored regularly to prevent overflow of drainage into the motor, which can cause irreparable damage to the apparatus.

• *Gomco thermotic pump.* The Gomco pump (Figure 42–9) is electrically operated but consists of a pump rather than a motor. It provides intermittent suction by alternating the air pressure, i.e., expanding and contracting the air. As the pressure alternates, red and green lights flash on and off. The amount of suction is regulated by a "high" or "low" pressure button. The pump is commonly used to suction gastrointestinal tubes.

• *Wall suction.* In some agencies, wall suction units with piped-in negative pressure are available. These units consist of a suction pressure regulator and a drainage receptacle, which needs to be checked regularly to prevent overflow. See Figure 31–2, page 767.

• *Closed wound suction.* Closed wound drainage, e.g., the *Hemovac,* is used to apply suction to wounds. See Chapter 39. The nurse creates suction by manually compressing and releasing the sides of the apparatus.

Some clients return from surgery with a gastric or intestinal tube in place and orders to connect the tube to suction. For more information about gastrointestinal tubes, see Chapter 23, page 560. The suction ordered can be continuous or intermittent. Intermittent suctioning is less likely to harm the

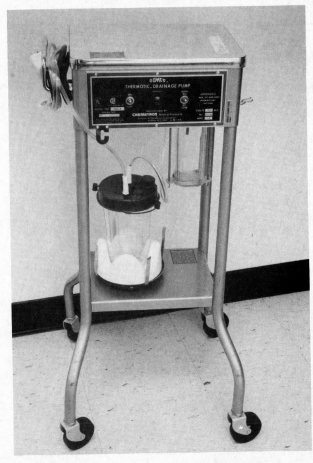

FIGURE 42–9 A Gomco thermotic drainage pump.

mucous membrane lining near the tip of the suction tube.

Nasogastric tubes are generally irrigated (a) before and after the installation of medications, (b) before and after tube feedings, and (c) as ordered to prevent clogging. Check agency policies and practices. Nasogastric irrigation may require a physician's order. Excessive irrigation can lead to metabolic alkalosis.

Technique 42–5 describes the management of gastrointestinal suction.

42-5 Managing Gastrointestinal Suction

Before initiating gastric suction, determine (a) whether the suction is continuous or intermittent; (b) the ordered suction pressure (a low suction pressure is between 80 and 100 mm Hg, and a high pressure is between 100 and 120 mm Hg); and (c) whether there is an order to irrigate the gastrointestinal tube and, if so, the type of solution to use.

PURPOSES

• To relieve abdominal distention
• To maintain gastric decompression after surgery
• To remove blood and secretions from the gastrointestinal tract

▶ **Technique 42–5 Managing Gastrointestinal Suction** CONTINUED

- To relieve discomfort, i.e., when a client has a bowel obstruction
- To maintain the patency of the nasogastric tube

ASSESSMENT FOCUS	Presence of abdominal distention on palpation; auscultated bowel sounds; abdominal discomfort; vital signs for baseline data.

EQUIPMENT

Initiating Suction

- ☐ Gastrointestinal tube in place in the client
- ☐ Basin
- ☐ 50-ml syringe with an adapter
- ☐ Stethoscope
- ☐ Suction device for either continuous or intermittent suction

- ☐ Connector and connecting tubing
- ☐ Disposable gloves

Maintaining Suction

- ☐ Graduated container as required to measure gastric drainage
- ☐ Basin of water
- ☐ Cotton-tipped applicators
- ☐ Ointment or lubricant

- ☐ Disposable gloves

Irrigation

- ☐ Disposable gloves
- ☐ Stethoscope
- ☐ Disposable irrigating set containing a sterile 50-ml syringe, moisture-resistant pad, basin, and graduated container
- ☐ Sterile normal saline (500 ml) or the ordered solution

INTERVENTION

Initiating Suction

1. Position the client appropriately.

- Assist the client to semi-Fowler's position if it is not contraindicated because of health. *In semi-Fowler's position the tube is not as likely to lie against the wall of the stomach and will therefore suction most efficiently. Semi-Fowler's position also prevents reflux of gastric contents, which could lead to aspiration.*

2. Confirm that the tube is in the stomach.

- Don gloves.

- Aspirate stomach contents, and check their acidity.

- Insert air into the tube with the syringe and listen with a stethoscope over the stomach (just below the xiphoid process) for a swish of air.

- Use other methods in accordance with agency protocol. See Chapter 23, pages 560 to 561.

3. Set and check the suction.

- Adjust the suction machine for the recommended suction pressure, in accordance with agency policy or the physician's order. Some suctions are preset and cannot be adjusted. If using a Gomco thermotic pump, the suction is usually set on intermittent "low" suction for a single-lumen nasogastric tube or on "high" suction for a double-lumen nasogastric tube (e.g., Salem sump tube).

- Turn on the suction machine, and check that the suction is working. The Gomco thermotic drainage pump has a red indicator light in the middle of the front panel; it blinks continuously when the machine is functioning. When using other suction machines, test for proper suctioning by holding the open end of the suction tube to the nurse's ear. Suctioning is confirmed by a sucking noise.

4. Establish gastric suction.

- Connect the gastrointestinal tube

to the tubing from the suction by using the connector.

- If a Salem sump tube is in place, connect the larger lumen to the suction equipment. This double-lumen tube has a smaller tube running inside the primary suction tube. *The smaller tube provides a continuous flow of atmospheric air through the drainage tube at its distal end and prevents excessive suction force on the gastric mucosa at the drainage outlets. Damage to the gastric mucosa is thus avoided.*

- Always keep the air vent tube of a Salem sump tube open when suction is applied. *Closing the vent would stop the sump action and cause mucosal damage.*

- After suction is applied, watch the tubing for a few minutes until the gastric contents appear to be running through the tubing into the receptacle. A Salem sump tube makes a soft, hissing sound when it is functioning correctly.

- If the suction is not working properly, check that the rubber

▶ **Technique 42–5** *CONTINUED*

stopper in the collection bottle and all tubing connections are tightly sealed and that the tubing is not kinked.

- Coil and pin the tubing on the bed so that it does not loop below the suction bottle. *If the tubing falls below the suction bottle, the suction may be obstructed because of the pressure required to push the fluid against gravity.*

5. Assess the drainage.

- Observe the amount, color, odor, and consistency of the drainage. Normal gastric drainage has a mucoid consistency and is either colorless or yellow-green because of the presence of bile. A coffee-grounds color and consistency may indicate bleeding.

- Test the gastric drainage for pH and blood (by using Hematest) when indicated. A person who has had gastrointestinal surgery can be expected to have some blood in the drainage.

Maintaining Suction

6. Assess the client and the suction system regularly.

- Assess the client regularly, e.g., every 30 minutes until the system is running effectively and then every 2 hours, or as the client's health indicates, to ensure that the suction is functioning properly. If the client complains of fullness, nausea, or epigastric pain or if the flow of gastric secretions is absent in the tubing or the collection bottle, ineffective suctioning or blockage of the nasogastric tube is likely.

- Inspect the suction system for patency of the system, e.g., kinks or blockages in the tubing, and tightness of the connections. *Loose connections can permit air to enter and thus decrease the ef-*

fectiveness of the suction by decreasing the negative pressure.

7. Relieve blockages if present.

- Don gloves.

- Milk the suction tubing.

- Check the suction equipment. To do this, disconnect the nasogastric tube from the suction over a collecting basin (to collect gastric drainage), and then, with the suction on, place the end of the suction tubing in a basin of water. If water is drawn into the drainage bottle, the suction equipment is functioning properly, but the nasogastric tube is either blocked or positioned incorrectly.

- Reposition the client, e.g., to the other side, if permitted. *This may facilitate drainage.*

- Rotate the nasogastric tube, and reposition it. This step is contraindicated for clients with gastric surgery. *Moving the tube may interfere with gastric sutures.*

- Irrigate the nasogastric tube as agency protocol states or on the order of the physician. See steps 11 to 13.

8. Prevent reflux into the vent lumen of a Salem sump tube. Reflux of gastric contents into the vent lumen may occur when stomach pressure exceeds atmospheric pressure. In this situation gastric contents follow the path of least resistance and flow out the vent lumen rather than the drainage lumen. To prevent reflux:

- Place the vent tubing above the client's midline. *A vent lumen placed below the midline acts as a siphon and allows gastric contents to flow through the air vent lumen.*

- Always keep the drainage receptacle below the client's midline.

A drainage receptacle placed above midline and the fluid level in the client's stomach will cause reflux of gastric contents through the air vent lumen. To avoid reflux when wall suction units are used, place the drainage container on the side of the bed or on the floor, and attach a connecting tube from the drainage container to the wall outlet.

- Keep the drainage lumen free of particulate matter that may obstruct the lumen. See irrigating a nasogastric tube in steps 11 to 13.

9. Ensure client comfort.

- Clean the client's nostrils every 3 hours or as needed, using the cotton-tipped applicators and water. Apply a water-soluble lubricant or ointment.

- Provide mouth care every 3 hours or as needed. Some postoperative clients are permitted to suck ice chips or a moist cloth to maintain the moisture of the oral mucous membranes.

10. Empty the drainage receptacle every 8 hours, or whenever it becomes three-quarters full.

- Clamp the nasogastric tube, and turn off the suction.

- Don gloves.

- If the receptacle is graduated, determine the amount of drainage.

- Disconnect the receptacle.

- If not already measured, empty the contents into a graduated container and measure.

- Inspect the drainage carefully for color, consistency, and presence of substances, e.g., blood clots.

- Rinse the receptacle with warm water.

- Reattach the receptacle to the suction.

▶ **Technique 42–5 Managing Gastrointestinal Suction** *CONTINUED*

- Turn on the suction and unclamp the nasogastric tube.

- Observe the system for several minutes to make sure function is reestablished.

- Go to step 14.

Irrigating a Gastrointestinal Tube

11. Prepare the client and the equipment.

- Place the moisture-resistant pad under the end of the gastrointestinal tube.

- Turn off the suction.

 - Don gloves.

- Disconnect the gastrointestinal tube from the connector.

- Determine that the tube is in the stomach. See step 2 above and Technique 23–1, step 5, page 563. *This ensures that the irrigating solution enters the client's stomach.*

12. Irrigate the tube.

- Draw up the ordered volume of irrigating solution in the syringe; 30 ml of solution per instillation is usual, but up to 60 ml may be given per instillation if ordered.

- Attach the syringe to the nasogastric tube, and slowly inject the solution.

- Gently aspirate the solution. *Forceful withdrawal could damage the gastric mucosa.*

- If you encounter difficulty in withdrawing the solution, inject 20 ml of air and aspirate again, and/or reposition the client or the nasogastric tube. *Air and repositioning may move the end of the tube away from the stomach wall.* If aspirating difficulty continues, reattach the tube to intermittent low suction, and notify the nurse in charge or physician.

- Repeat the above steps until the ordered amount of solution is used.

- Note: A Salem sump tube can also be irrigated through the vent lumen without interrupting suction. However, only small quantities of irrigant can be injected via this lumen compared to the drainage lumen.

- After irrigating a Salem sump tube, inject 10 to 20 ml of air into the vent lumen while applying suction to the drainage lumen.

This tests the patency of the vent and ensures sump functioning.

13. Reestablish suction.

- Reconnect the nasogastric tube to suction.

- If a Salem sump tube is used, inject the air vent lumen with 10 ml of air after reconnecting the tube to suction.

- Observe the system for several minutes to make sure it is functioning.

14. Document all relevant information.

- Record the time suction was started. Also record the pressure established, the color and consistency of the drainage, and nursing assessments.

- During maintenance, record assessments, supportive nursing measures, and data about the suction system.

- When irrigating the tube, record verification of tube placement; the time of the irrigation; the amount and type of irrigating solution used; the amount, color, and consistency of the returns; the patency of the system following the irrigation; and nursing assessments.

EVALUATION FOCUS	Relief of abdominal distention or discomfort; bowel sounds; character and amount of gastric drainage; integrity of nares; hydration of oral mucous membranes; patency of tube; system functioning.

SAMPLE RECORDINGS

Date	Time	Notes
09/10/93	1400	Suction initiated 100 mm Hg. Returns watery, bright red. Abdomen firm and slightly distended. Bowel sounds irregular and high pitched. ———— Molly Jones, RN
	1600	250 ml light brown thick drainage. No complaints of pain. Bowel sounds hyperactive, increased pitch. Abdomen soft upon palpation. No irritation in nostrils. Nostrils cleaned with water and lubricant applied. Vital signs q2h. BP 140/80, P 90, R 18 and stable. ———— Roberta Loo, SN
09/11/93	0600	Tube placement confirmed by injecting 10 ml air. Tube irrigated with 30 ml normal saline × 2. 30 ml × 2 returns cloudy, pink with small clots. Suction running with drainage noted. Abdomen soft, no discomfort, vital signs stable. ———— Roberta Loo, SN

► **Technique 42–5** *CONTINUED*

KEY ELEMENTS OF MANAGING GASTROINTESTINAL SUCTION

- Confirm the placement of the nasogastric tube before establishing suction.
- Place an air vent appropriately and maintain its patency by injecting air.
- Test the functioning of the suction system before connecting it.
- Prevent kinks or blockages in the tubing.
- Keep all connections well sealed.
- Inspect the flow of gastric secretions into the drainage bottle.

- Clean the nares at least every 3 hours.
- Provide mouth care.

Irrigations
- Obtain the physician's order if needed.
- Confirm the placement of the tube before irrigation.
- Reconnect the tube and attach it to suction following the procedure.
- Assess the amount and character of the drainage and client comfort and distention.

CRITICAL THINKING CHALLENGE

Maria Elena Rodriguez is a 54-year-old client who is scheduled to have surgery. During her admission assessment, you noted that she has difficulty communicating in English, as she has only recently immigrated to the United States from Cuba. You are concerned about whether she fully understands the proposed surgery. What action would you take? How can you reassure Mrs. Rodriguez?

RELATED RESEARCH

Raleigh, E. H.; Lepcyzyk, M.; and Rowley, C. August 1990. Significant others benefit from preoperative information. *Journal of Advanced Nursing* 15:841–45.

Schepp, K. G. January/February 1991. Factors influencing the coping effort of mothers of hospitalized children. *Nursing Research* 40(1):42–46.

Yount, S. T.; Edgell, Sr. J.; and Jakovec, V. February 1990. Preoperative teaching: A study of nurses' perceptions. *AORN Journal* 51:572, 574–75, 577–79.

REFERENCES

Association of Operating Room Nurses. 1986. *AORN standards and recommended practices for perioperative nursing.* Denver: Association of Operating Room Nurses, Inc.

———. November 1988. Recommended practices: Preoperative skin preparation. *AORN Journal* 48:950–51, 953–55, 958.

Erickson, R. July 1982. Tube talk principles of fluid flow in tubes. *Nursing 82* 12:54–61.

Garner, J. S. April 1986. CDC guidelines for the prevention and control of nosocomial infections: Guideline for prevention of surgical wound infections, 1985. *American Journal of Infection Control* 14:71–80.

Kozier, B.; Erb, G.; and Olivieri, R. 1991. *Fundamentals of nursing: Concepts, Process, and Practice.* 4th ed. Redwood City, Calif.: Addison-Wesley Nursing.

Leckrone, L. July 1991. Preparing your patient for surgery. *Nursing* 21: 46–49.

McConnell, E. A. September, 1975. All about gastrointestinal intubation. *Nursing 75* 5:30–37.

———. March 1977. After surgery. *Nursing 77* 7:32–39.

———. September 1977. Ensuring safer stomach suctioning with a Salem sump tube. *Nursing 77* 7:54–57.

———. April 1979. Ten problems with nasogastric tubes . . . and how to solve them. *Nursing 79* 9:78–81.

Mott, S. R.; James, S. R.; and Sperhac, A. M. 1990. *Nursing care of children and families.* 2d ed. Redwood City, Calif.: Addison-Wesley Nursing.

Smith, A. P., editor. 1991. *Comprehensive child and family nursing skills.* St. Louis: Mosby-Year Book, Inc.

Whaley, L. F., and Wong, D. L. 1991. *Nursing care of infants and children.* 4th ed. St. Louis: Mosby-Year Book, Inc.

43

Cast Care

CONTENTS

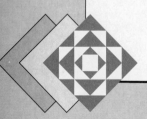

NURSING PROCESS GUIDE

CAST CARE

ASSESSMENT

Assess the neurovascular status of the affected limbs. The first three items below are often referred to as CMS (color, movement, and sensation) checks.

- *Color of the skin:* Compare it to the color of the unaffected extremity. Pallor or cyanosis can indicate circulatory impairment.

- *Motor ability or movement:* Have the client move the fingers and wrist or toes and ankle as indicated in Table 43–1. The inability to do so suggests compression of a nerve and potential paralysis. Commonly affected nerves are the peroneal, tibial, radial, median, and ulnar nerves (Figure 43–1). If the peroneal nerve is compressed, the client is unable to dorsiflex the foot. With compression of the tibial nerve, the client is unable to plantar flex the foot. With compression of the radial nerve, the client is unable to hyperextend the thumb or wrist. With compression of the ulnar nerve, the client is unable to abduct all the fingers in unison. With compression of the median nerve, the client is unable to flex the wrist and oppose the thumb and little finger.

- *Sensation:* Ask the client about the presence or absence of sensation, e.g., numbness, tingling, or the inability to feel pain. These symptoms can indicate increasing pressure within the cast. Pinch all toes or fingers, and ask the client to identify which one you are pinching. All toes and fingers must be checked, because they are innervated by different nerves. If the client does not feel sensation in one or more digits, conduct the necessary sensory function tests outlined in Table 43–1. Have the client close the eyes, use the pointed end of a safety pin to prick the specific areas, and ask whether the client feels the stimulus. A lack of sensation in any of the areas noted can indicated impaired function of the associated nerves.

- *Temperature of the skin:* Feel both extremities (affected and unaffected), and compare the temperatures. Excessive coldness can indicate circulatory impairment.

- *Degree of swelling:* Some swelling can be expected, and swelling does not always indicate circulatory impairment.

- *Blanching sign (capillary refill):* Compress the nail of the thumb or large toe for a few seconds until it blanches, and note the return flow of blood. Blood should return instantly on release of pressure. If it

returns too slowly, there may be venous congestion or arterial insufficiency.

- *Distal pulse,* when obtainable, of the extremity in the cast: Palpate the pulse for presence and strength, and compare it with the pulse in the opposite extremity. A weak or absent pulse may indicate decreased circulation to the area.

Inspect the cast for

- Rough edges, cracking, and moisture.

- Signs of bleeding or drainage from under the cast.

- Odor emanating through the cast.

Assess the client for

- Skin irritation at the edge of the cast.

- Complaints of a burning sensation or pain beneath the cast.

- Edema distal and proximal to the cast

- Signs of fat emboli (see page 1003).

- Signs of venous thromboembolism (see page 1003).

RELATED DIAGNOSTIC CATEGORIES

- Body image disturbance

- High risk for Disuse syndrome

- Fear (of falling)

- Impaired home maintenance management

- High risk for Infection (open reductions)

- High risk for Injury

- Knowledge deficit (e.g., cast care)

- Impaired physical mobility

- Pain

- Self-care deficit: Bathing/hygiene, dressing/grooming, toileting

- Impaired skin integrity

- Altered tissue perfusion: Peripheral

PLANNING

Client Goals
The client will

- Maintain adequate neurovascular status and tissue perfusion of the affected limb.

- Maintain skin integrity at the cast edges.

- Experience minimal physical and psychologic discomfort.

Nursing Process Guide *CONTINUED*

- Demonstrate understanding of essential facts and procedures required to restore or maintain self-care.

Outcome Criteria
The client

- Maintains baseline vital signs.

- Has normal skin color of toes and fingers in affected extremity.

- Is able to move all fingers or toes in casted extremity.

- Feels normal sensation in all fingers or toes in casted extremity.

- Has skin temperature in affected extremity equal to that of the opposite limb.

- Has normal capillary refill in the nail of the large thumb or toe of the affected limb.

- Has a peripheral pulse in the affected limb equal in rate and volume to that of the opposite limb.

- Has minimal swelling in the affected limb.

- Has intact clean skin around the cast edges.

- Has cast edges that are intact.

- Voices minimal discomfort.

- Experiences minimal or no bleeding through the cast.

- Demonstrates the correct and safe use of required walking aids.

- Verbalizes signs and symptoms that require notification of the physician.

- Verbalizes understanding of self-care required to maintain cast integrity and muscle tone.

Fractures

Fractures are breaks in the continuity of bones. They are described in terms of type, location, and special features. All fractures are designated either simple (closed) or compound (open). *Simple*, or *closed*, fractures are the most common. The bone is broken in one place only, and there is no skin wound. Hence, the bone is protected from contamination.

In a *compound*, or *open*, fracture, there is a skin wound, and the bone is therefore vulnerable to infection through the opening in the skin. The skin wound may be caused from the outside (e.g., a gunshot, which breaks the skin before it fractures the bone) or from the inside (the fracture occurs first, and it lacerates the tissues and skin).

Fracture Repair

Bleeding at the fracture site produces a hematoma (blood clot), which is the basis for repair. This clot becomes an interlacing mesh composed of fibrin from the clotted blood, lymph, and inflammatory exudate. It forms a bridge across the fracture site, and—eventually—granulation tissue is formed. Calcium is deposited into this tissue, and when this occurs the tissue is called **callus** (early bone). The callus is usually more abundant than appears necessary. Callus will not stand much muscle stress, strain, or weight bearing. The process of calcium depositing goes on until the callus becomes hard bone. The larger the bone, the longer the healing process. A radius or ulna

heals in about 2 months, a humerus in about 3 months, and a femur in about 6 months. Age and blood circulation are also significant. Children heal much more rapidly than adults, and a good blood supply promotes timely healing. With normal use, the bone eventually assumes a shape that resembles the original bone. This takes place over a period of months, and frequently a year is needed to complete the process.

Complications of Fractures

Three major complications of fractures are compartment syndrome, fat embolism, and venous thromboembolism. Prevention or early detection of symptoms related to these complications is an essential nursing responsibility.

Compartment syndrome is the condition in which increased pressure in a limited space, such as a splint or cast, compromises or reduces the circulation and function of the tissues within the space. The outcome is hypoxia, ischemia, and neurovascular impairment. Signs and symptoms of compartment syndrome include **hypesthesia** (abnormally decreased sensitivity to stimulation), weakness, muscle pain evoked when the muscle is passively stretched; and complaints of pain out of proportion to that expected for the type of injury. Peripheral pulses are not typically affected by compartment syndrome but should be assessed to rule out arterial injury (Slye 1991, p. 115). Because peripheral nerves may be the

TABLE 43–1   NERVE FUNCTION ASSESSMENTS

Nerve	Motor Function Tests	Sensory Function Tests
Radial	Instruct client to hyperextend thumb or wrist and straighten all four fingers.	Prick web space between thumb and index finger.
Median	Instruct client to oppose thumb and little finger and flex wrist.	Prick distal fat pad of index finger.
Ulnar	Instruct client to abduct all fingers.	Prick fat pad at distal end of small finger.
Peroneal	Instruct client to dorsiflex ankle and extend toes.	Prick web between great toe and second toe or lateral surface of great toe and medial surface of second toe.
Tibial	Instruct client to plantar flex ankle and flex toes.	Prick medial and lateral surfaces of sole of foot.

first to be affected, assessment of the client's sensory status is essential. See Table 43–1 and Figure 43–1.

Fat embolism may occur following fractures when fat globules are released from the bone marrow and from local tissue trauma into the blood circulation. When the emboli pass through the pulmonary circulation, the globules lodge in the lung, occlude capillaries and small arterioles, and cause pulmonary insufficiency. Fat embolism is commonly associated with multiple fractures and those involving the pelvis, femur, tibia, or ribs. Clients who experience hypovolemic shock after traumatic injury are at a greater risk of developing fat emboli. Signs and symptoms are dyspnea, restlessness, agitation, confusion, tachypnea (i.e., more than 30 breaths per minute), tachycardia (i.e., more than 140 beats per minute), fever, diffuse lung crackles, and hypoxemia (i.e., a PO_2 of less than 80 mm Hg arterial blood). A petechial skin rash indicative of capillary fragility occurs in about 50% of clients.

Venous thromboembolism is commonly associated with clients who have hip fractures and those undergoing total hip or knee replacements or reconstructions. *Deep vein thrombosis (DVT)* resulting from immobility and venous stasis is manifested by pain, swelling, and redness in the involved extremity, usually the calf. A positive Homans' sign may or may not be present. Key signs and symptoms of *pulmonary embolism* are dyspnea, pleuritic chest pain, anxiety, cough, hemoptysis, tachypnea, tachycardia, and localized lung crackles. Hypoxemia, the end product

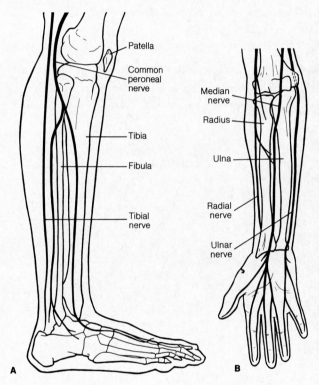

FIGURE 43–1   *A*, the peroneal and tibial nerves; *B*, the radial, median, and ulnar nerves. These nerves can be injured by prolonged compression in a cylindrical cast.

of pulmonary embolism, is indicated by a PO_2 of less than 80 mm Hg (arterial blood).

Technique 43–1 on page 1004 explains the steps involved in applying a splint.

43-1 Applying a Splint at the Scene of an Accident

PURPOSES
- To immobilize a fractured limb and maintain good alignment
- To minimize pain and further injury to surrounding tissues

ASSESSMENT FOCUS

Location of the fracture; appearance of the fracture site (i.e., whether the fracture is open or closed and whether bleeding is present); complaints of discomfort.

EQUIPMENT

- Pressure dressing, if necessary
- Padding material (e.g., a piece of cloth, towel, or blanket)
- Splint (e.g., pieces of wood or rolled pillows, magazines, or blankets)

or
- Air splint, if available
- Strips of cloth, rope, or tape

INTERVENTION

1. Control hemorrhage, and prevent further injury.

- Move the person to a safe place if life is in danger.

- Apply direct pressure and a pressure dressing.

- Move the affected limb as little as possible. *This helps prevent further injury to the surrounding tissues.*

2. Apply padding.

- Pad joints, bony prominences, and exposed skin areas as much as possible. *This helps prevent skin damage from the splint.*

- Avoid padding areas such as the axilla or groin that may affect circulation to the area.

3. Apply the splint.

- Splint a leg in the extended position.

- Splint an arm in a flexed or extended position.

- If splint material is not available, use parts of the person's body for support. For example, splint an arm to the trunk; a leg to the other leg; or toes or fingers together.

- If pillows or blankets are used for splinting, reinforce them with a rolled magazine or other material. *This helps make the splint more firm.*

- Include joints proximal and distal to the fracture in the splint to ensure maximum immobilization of the body part.

- Strap the splint firmly to the limb to immobilize the limb.

4. Assess the circulatory status of the involved extremity.

- Assess the pulse distal to the fracture, capillary refill, and the color and temperature of the involved limb.

5. Transport the person to a medical facility.

VARIATION: Applying an Air Splint

Air splints are most commonly used to splint a forearm or lower leg. Before applying this splint, cover a compound fracture with absorbent material. To apply the splint:

- Place the splint over the fractured limb.

- Inflate the splint by blowing into the mouthpiece.

- Assess the tension of the splint by pressing your finger into the splint. It should dimple to a depth of 1.25 cm (½ in).

- Follow steps 4 and 5 above.

EVALUATION FOCUS

Circulatory status of the involved limb (see step 4); movement and sensation of digits (toes and fingers); complaints of numbness, tingling, or other discomfort.

Reduction and Immobilization of Fractures

Reduction is the realignment of fractured bone fragments to their normal position. Reduction can be accomplished by three methods.

1. *Closed reduction* is manual **traction** (exertion of a pulling force) and manipulation of the bone fragments. The client may be given a general anesthetic. After reduction, a cast is applied to immobilize the part. See Technique 43–2.

2. *Open reduction* includes surgical exposure of the fracture. The bone may be immobilized by pins, nails, screws, plates, or rods.

3. *Traction* for a period of days or weeks may be necessary to reduce some fractures, e.g., of the femur or humerus where the large muscles make manual traction and manipulation impossible. See Chapter 44 for further discussion.

Casts

Casts are generally applied to immobilize a body part so that healing can take place without further injury. The degree of immobilization of the person varies with the type of cast. Some people are confined to bed for weeks or even months, whereas others are able to resume most daily activities with only slight inconvenience from the cast. Although casts are applied for reasons other than fractures, this chapter focuses on clients who have fractures.

Cast Materials

In addition to the traditional plaster of paris (POP) cast material, several synthetic materials are now available: polyester and cotton, fiberglass, and thermoplastics. See Table 43–2.

Padding Materials

Before the plaster of paris or synthetic casts are applied, the affected area must be padded. *Stockinette*, a soft, flexible, tubular, cloth material, is commonly placed over the body part before the cast material is applied. The most common sizes are 5 to 25 cm (2 to 12 in) in flattened width. Usually, one thickness of stockinette is used for extremity casts and two thicknesses for casts covering the trunk of the body. Two thicknesses may also be used beneath thermoplastic casts to protect the skin from this hot application (Figure 43–2 on page 1006). If the client's fracture is severe and the limb very painful, stockinette may not be used, because its application is difficult and may enhance pain.

Cotton sheet wadding or padding is often applied directly over the skin or stockinette or to pad bony prominences or between skin surfaces. Sheet wadding clings and molds to the contours of the limb. It is available in 2-, 3-, and 4-inch rolls. *Felt padding* may be needed over bony prominences or joints that are vulnerable to skin breakdown. Padding (available

---

TABLE 43–2 CAST MATERIALS

Type of Material	Description	Application	Setting Time and Weight-Bearing Restrictions
Plaster of Paris (POP)	Open-weave cotton rolls or strips saturated with powdered calcium sulfate crystals (gypsum)	Applied after being soaked in tepid water for a few seconds until bubbling stops	Dries in 48 hours, no weight-bearing allowed until dry
Synthetics			
Polyester and Cotton (e.g., Cutter Cast)	Open-weave polyester and cotton tape permeated with water-activated polyurethane resin	Applied after being soaked in cool water, 26 C (80 F); used within 2 to 3 minutes of soaking	Sets in 7 minutes, weight-bearing allowed in 15 minutes
Fiberglass; water-activated (e.g., Scotchcast, Delta-lite) or light-cured (e.g., Lightcast II)	Open-weave fiberglass tape impregnated with water-activated polyurethane resin (Scotchcast) or photosensitive polyurethane resin (Lightcast II)	Applied after being immersed in tepid water for 10 to 15 seconds (Scotchcast); applied with silicone type hand cream to keep it from sticking (Lightcast II)	Sets in 15 minutes, weight-bearing allowed in 30 minutes (Scotchcast); sets after being exposed for 3 minutes to a special ultraviolet lamp, weight-bearing allowed immediately (Lightcast II)
Thermoplastic (e.g., Hexcelite)	Knitted thermoplastic polyester fabric in rigid rolls	Applied after being heated in water at 76 to 82 C (170 to 180 F) for 3 to 4 minutes to make the rolls soft and pliable. Remove excess water by squeezing between towels before applying	Sets in 5 minutes, weight-bearing allowed in 20 minutes

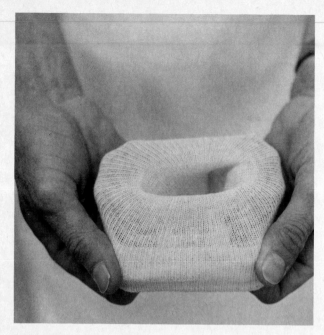

FIGURE 43–2 Rolling stockinette to facilitate its application.

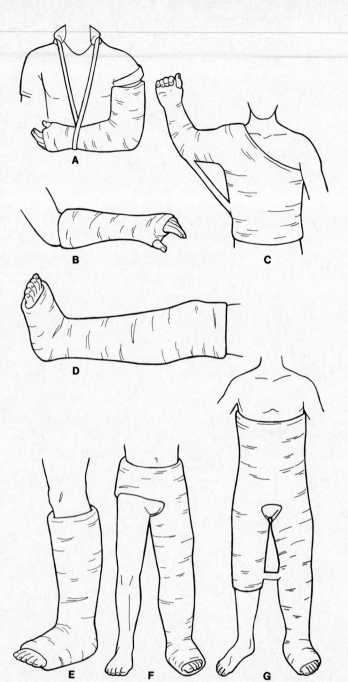

FIGURE 43–3 Types of cylindrical casts: *A,* hanging arm cast; *B,* short arm cast; *C,* shoulder spica cast; *D,* long, or full, leg cast; *E,* short leg cast; *F,* single hip spica cast; *G,* one-and-one-half hip spica.

in 4- or 2-inch thicknesses) is cut to fit the desired area and is incorporated within the folds of cotton sheet wadding. *Plaster splints* may be used to add strength over areas susceptible to breakage, e.g., over a knee joint or the heel. Splints are flat strips of cast material 3 × 15, 4 × 15, or 4 × 30 inches in length. These are prepared like the POP cast rolls and may be applied in four to eight layers.

Types of Casts

The *hanging arm cast* (Figure 43–3, *A*) extends from the axilla to the fingers of the hand, usually allowing for elbow flexion. It immobilizes the wrist, the humerus, the radius, and the ulna. The *short arm cast* (Figure 43–3, *B*) extends from below the elbow to the fingers. It immobilizes the wrist, the radius, and the ulna. The *shoulder spica cast* (Figure 43–3, *C*) extends around the chest and the entire arm to the fingers. The arm is usually abducted to immobilize the shoulder bones, e.g., the clavicle.

The *long,* or *full, leg cast* (Figure 43–3, *D*) extends from above the knee to the toes. The *short leg cast* (Figure 43–3, *E*) begins just below the knee and extends to the toes. The *hip spica cast* (Figure 43–3, *F*) begins at waist level or above. It immobilizes the hip joint and the femur, extends down one entire leg, and may cover all or part of the second leg. A single spica covers one leg only. A *one-and-one-half hip spica* (Figure 43–3, *G*) covers the second leg to the knee. A double hip spica covers both legs to the toes. The *body* cast extends from the axillae to encompass the entire trunk. It is often used to immobilize the spine.

Casts are usually applied, adjusted, split, and removed only by physicians. The major role of the nurse during cast application is to hold and support the fractured extremity.

Care for Clients with Casts

Essential nursing for clients who have casts includes continual assessment and implementations to prevent pressure on underlying blood vessels, nerves, and the skin; to maintain the integrity of the cast itself; and to prevent problems associated with immobility. Common cast pressure areas are shown in Table 43–3.

TABLE 43–3 COMMON CAST PRESSURE AREAS

Type of Cast	Common Pressure Areas
Short arm cast	Radial styloid Ulnar styloid Joint at base of thumb
Hanging arm cast	Radial styloid Ulnar styloid Olecranon Lateral epicondyle
Short leg cast	Heel Achilles tendon Malleolus
Long leg cast	Heel Achilles tendon Malleolus Popliteal artery behind knee Peroneal nerve at side of knee
Hip spica	As above for long leg cast Sacrum Iliac crests

Because a POP cast is porous and will absorb water or urine, every effort is made to keep the cast dry. Casts that become wet soften, and their function is impaired; thus, tub baths and showers are contraindicated. Casts that become soiled with feces develop an unremovable odor. Elimination presents a particular problem for people with long leg, body, and hip spica casts. There is no effective way to keep a POP cast clean other than wiping it with a damp cloth. Before a client is discharged, a cast may be cleaned by applying more wet plaster over the soiled area. The best approach is to prevent soils and stains, especially those from food spills, urine, and feces.

Synthetic casts can be cleaned readily and may, with the physician's agreement, be immersed in water if polypropylene stockinette and padding were applied.

Techniques 43–2 and 43–3 explain the client care required immediately after cast application, and continuing care, respectively.

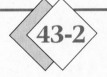

43-2 Client Care Immediately After Cast Application

PURPOSES
- To maintain the integrity of the cast
- To reduce swelling
- To assess problems associated with the cast

ASSESSMENT FOCUS

Neurovascular status of affected limb; the degree of swelling distal to the cast; the amount and character of drainage through the cast; complaints of discomfort (e.g., a burning sensation or pain beneath the cast); any odor emanating through the cast.

EQUIPMENT
- Soft, pliable pillows

INTERVENTION

1. Assess the neurovascular status of the affected limbs.

- Assess the toes and fingers for nerve or circulatory impairments every 30 minutes for four hours following cast application, and then every 3 hours for the first 24 to 48 hours or until all signs and symptoms of impairment are negative. See the Nursing Process Guide on page 1001. *Rapid swelling under a cast can cause neurovascular problems necessitating frequent neurovascular assessments by the nurse.* Increase the frequency of neurovascular assessments in accordance with the client's condition, e.g., presence of circulatory impairment.

2. Support and handle the cast appropriately.

- Immediately after the cast is applied, place it on pillows. Avoid using plastic or rubber pillows. *The pillows provide even pressure and support the curves of the cast and promote venous blood return, thereby decreasing the possibility of swelling. Plastic or rubber pil-*

▶

▶ **Technique 43–2 Client Care After Cast Application** *CONTINUED*

lows do not allow the heat of a drying cast to dissipate and so cause discomfort.

- Until a cast has set or hardened (10 to 20 minutes), support the cast in the palms of your hands rather than with the fingertips, and extend your fingers so that your fingertips do not touch the plaster (Figure 43–4). *Fingertip pressure can cause dents in unset plaster and subsequent skin pressure areas.*

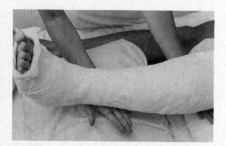

FIGURE 43–4 Handling an unset plaster cast with the palms of the hands and fingers extended.

- When the cast is set, continue to handle the cast in your palms, but you may then wrap your fingers around the contour of the cast.

3. Implement measures to reduce swelling.

- Controll swelling by elevating arms or legs on pillows or, for a leg fracture, by elevating the foot of the bed. Immediately after injury and surgery, elevate the limb well above the level of the client's heart. Generally, three pillows are needed to achieve high elevation of a leg. As circulation improves and healing progresses, the elevation can be gradually reduced to two pillows (moderate elevation) and then to one pillow (low elevation). *Swelling can cause neurovascular impairment.*

- Apply ice packs to control perineal edema associated with a hip spica cast. Although ice packs are a less effective method of control, elevation of the area is obviously difficult.

- Report excessive swelling and indications of neurovascular impairment to the physician or nurse in charge. The physician may bivalve a cast if it appears to be too tight. Bivalving a cast is cutting the cast and the underlying padding on each side, thus making two separate shells (Figure 43–5, *A*). *This relieves the pressure of the cast but still provides support.* Bivalved casts are usually fastened in place with Velcro straps, buckled webbing straps, or elastic bandages (Figure 43–5, *B*).

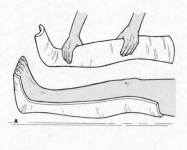

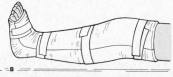

FIGURE 43–5 *A*, A bivalved cast; *B*, A bivalved cast strapped in place.

4. Use appropriate means to dry the cast thoroughly.

- Extremity POP casts usually take 24 to 48 hours to dry completely; spica or body casts require 48 to 72 hours. Drying time depends on the temperature, humidity, size of the cast, and method used for drying. The cast is dry when it no longer feels damp. A dry cast feels dry and looks white and shiny and is odorless, hard, and resonant when tapped.

- Expose the cast to the circulating air. Place sheets and blankets only over areas that do not have the cast.

- Check agency policy about the recommended turning frequency for clients with different kinds of casts. *Frequent turning promotes even drying of the cast.*

- Turn the client with an extremity cast or body spica every 2 to 4 hours. See Technique 43–3, step 5.

- Use regular pillows. *Plastic or rubber pillows hinder drying and do not allow the heat of a drying cast to dissipate.*

- Avoid the use of artificial means to facilitate drying. These means include fans, hair driers, infrared lamps, and electric heaters. *Artificial methods dry the outer surface of the cast while the inner portion remains soft and spongy. Such a cast cracks readily at points of strain. Natural methods dry the cast evenly.*

5. Monitor bleeding if an open reduction was done or if the injury was a compound fracture.

- Monitor blood stains or other drainage on the cast for 24 to 72 hours after surgery or injury or longer if necessary.

- Outline the stained area with a pen every 8 hours or at the change of shift, and note the time and date, so that any further bleeding can be determined (Figure 43–6).

6. Assess pain and pressure areas.

- Never ignore any complaints of pain, burning, or pressure. If a client is unable to communicate,

▶ **Technique 43–2** *CONTINUED*

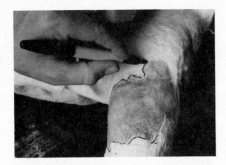

FIGURE 43–6 Outlining drainage on a cast.

be alert to changes in temperament, restlessness, or fussiness.

- Determine particularly whether the pain is persistent and if it occurs over a bony prominence or joint. See Table 43–3 for common pressure points associated with various casts.

- Give pain medication selectively. *Pain medication can mask symptoms.*

- Do not disregard the cessation of persistent pain or discomfort complaints. *Cessation of complaints can indicate a skin slough. When a skin slough occurs, superficial skin sensation is lost and the client no longer feels pain.*

- When a pressure area under the cast is suspected, the physician may either bivalve the cast so that all of the skin beneath the cast can be inspected or cut a window in the cast over only the area of concern. When a cast is windowed

  a. Retain the piece (cast and padding) that was cut out. Some physicians order that it be taped back if there is no skin problem present but that it be left out if there is a pressure area present. *Putting back the piece prevents window edema, which*

  occurs when skin pressure at the window is not equal to that from the remainder of the cast.

  b. Inspect the skin under the window at scheduled time intervals.

7. Document all relevant information.

- Record each assessment (whether or not there are problems) and implementation. Examples of documentation include: "Toes warm to touch, color pink," "Blanching sign satisfactory," "Moves toes readily; states no numbness or tingling; states leg painful." Record specific nerve function assessments such as "Able to hyperextend R thumb," "Sensation felt at web space between R thumb and index finger."

EVALUATION FOCUS	Skin color, temperature, and sensation of toes or fingers; blanching sign; ability to move toes or fingers; complaints of numbness, tingling, and/or pain.

SAMPLE RECORDING

Date	Time	Notes
04/06/93	1500	Toes cold, pale, and edematous. Slow return of blood from blanching sign. C/o numbness and tingling in toes. Unable to extend toes but sensation felt between great toe and second toe. —————— Marlin M. Mysak, RN

KEY ELEMENTS OF CLIENT CARE IMMEDIATELY AFTER CAST APPLICATION

- Assess and document the neurovascular status of the affected limb regularly.

- Use regular rather than plastic or rubber pillows to support the cast and to elevate the involved extremity.

- Support a wet cast in the palms of your hands rather than with the fingertips.

- Promptly report indications of neurovascular impairment.

- Allow the cast to dry naturally rather than by artificial methods.

- Monitor drainage for at least 24 to 72 hours after surgery or injury.

- Assess, document, and attend to complaints of pain, burning, or pressure.

43-3 Continuing Care for Clients with Casts

PURPOSES

- To prevent skin irritation at the edges of a cast
- To keep the cast dry
- To prevent the formation of pressure areas
- To prevent joint stiffness and muscle atrophy

ASSESSMENT FOCUS

Status of skin at the cast edges and over bony prominences; neurovascular status of the affected limb; degree of swelling distal to the cast; odor emanating through the cast; integrity of the cast; learning needs.

EQUIPMENT

Skin Care

- Duckbilled cast bender
- Rubbing alcohol
- Mineral, olive, or baby oil

Covering Rough Cast Edges

- Adhesive tape 2.5 cm (1 in) wide

- Scissors

Keeping the Cast Clean and Dry

- Bib or towel
- Damp washcloth, slipper (fracture) pan, and plastic or

other waterproof material (for POP casts)

- Warm water and a mild soap (for synthetic casts)

Comfort

- Pillows

INTERVENTION

1. Continue to assess the client for problems.

- Assess the neurovascular status of the affected limb (see the Nursing Process Guide, page 1001) at regular intervals in accordance with agency protocol.

- Inspect the skin near and under the cast edges whenever neurovascular assessments are made and/or whenever the client is turned.

- Check the cast daily for a foul odor. *This kind of odor may indicate skin excoriation from pressure or an infected area beneath the cast.*

2. Implement measures to prevent skin irritation at the edges of the cast.

- Wash crumbs of plaster from the skin with a damp cloth and feel along the cast edges to check for rough edges or areas that press into the client's skin. *As a POP cast dries, small bits of plaster frequently break off from its rough*

edges. If they fall inside the cast, they can cause discomfort and irritation.

- Remove the resin of synthetic casting materials with a swab moistened with alcohol, acetone, or nail polish remover. Check the manufacturer's directions.

- It may be necessary to use a duckbilled cast bender to bend cast edges that may irritate the skin (Figure 43–7). Excessive bending or trimming of the cast should not be done without a physician's order.

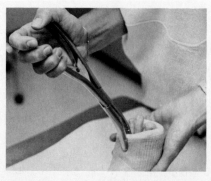

FIGURE 43–7 Using a duckbilled cast bender.

- Cover any rough edges of the cast when it is dry. If stockinette has not been used to line the cast, "petal" the edges with small strips of adhesive tape as follows (Figure 43–8):

  a. Cut several strips of 2.5 cm (1 in) *nonwaterproof* adhesive, 5 to 7.5 cm (2 to 3 in)

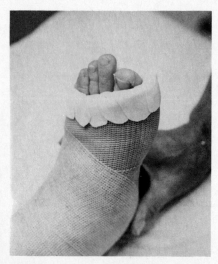

FIGURE 43–8 "Petals" applied to the edges of the cast.

▶ **Technique 43–3** *CONTINUED*

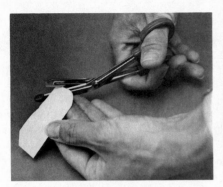

FIGURE 43–9 Making a "petal" for the cast edge.

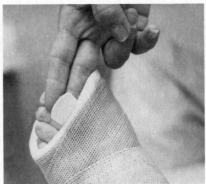

FIGURE 43–10 Applying a "petal" to the inside of the cast.

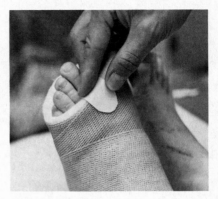

FIGURE 43–11 Applying the "petal" to the outside edge of the cast.

long. Then curve all corners of each strip (Figure 43–9). *Square or pointed ends tend to curl. Nonwaterproof adhesive is more adherent.*

b. Insert one end of each strip as far as possible inside the cast, and bring the other end out over the cast edge (Figure 43–10).

c. Press the petals firmly against the plaster (Figure 43–11).

d. Overlap successive petals slightly.

3. Provide skin care to all areas vulnerable to pressure.

• Apply alcohol to all areas vulnerable to pressure and breakdown at least every 4 hours. For clients with sensitive skin or potential skin problems, provide care every 2 hours during the day and every 3 hours at night. *Alcohol cleans and toughens the skin and evaporates without making the cast soggy.*

a. Reach under the cast edges as far as possible and massage the area.

b. Also provide skin care over all bony prominences not under the cast, e.g., the sacrum, heels, ankles, wrists, elbows, and feet. *These are*

potential pressure areas while the client is confined to bed.

4. Keep the cast clean and dry.

POP Cast

• Place a bib or towel over a body cast to catch spills. If a spill does wet the cast, allow the area to air dry.

• Use a slipper (fracture) bedpan for people with long leg, hip spica, or body casts. *The flat end placed correctly under the client's buttocks lessens the chance of spillage and minimizes the amount of lifting required by the client and/or nurse.*

• Before placing the client on the bedpan, tuck plastic or other waterproof material around the top of a long leg cast or in around the perineal cutout. For a perineal cutout, funnel one end of the plastic into the bedpan.

• Remove the plastic when elimination is completed. *If left in place, waterproof material makes the cast edge airtight and prevents evaporation of perspiration, which is irritating to the skin.*

• For people with long leg casts, keep the cast supported on pillows while the client is on the bedpan. *If the cast dangles, urine may run down the cast.*

• For clients with hip spica casts, support both extremities and the back on pillows so that they are as high as the buttocks. *This prevents urine from running back into the cast.*

• When removing the bedpan, hold it securely while the client is turning or lifting the buttocks. *This prevents dripping and spilling.*

• After removing the bedpan, thoroughly clean and dry the perineal area.

Synthetic Cast

• Wash the soiled area with warm water and a mild soap.

• Thoroughly rinse the soap from the cast.

• Dry thoroughly to prevent skin maceration and ulceration under the cast.

• If the cast is immersed in water, dry the cast and underlying padding and stockinette thoroughly. First, blot excess water from the cast with a towel. Then use a hand-held blow drier on the cool or warm setting, directing the air stream in a sweeping motion over the exterior of the cast for about 1 hour or until the client no longer feels a cold clammy sensation like that produced by a wet bathing suit. *This drying*

▶ Technique 43–3 Continuing Care for Clients with Casts CONTINUED

procedure is essential to prevent skin maceration and ulceration.

5. Turn and position the client in correct alignment to prevent the formation of pressure areas.

- Place pillows in such a way that

  a. Body parts press against the edges of the cast as little as possible.

  b. Toes, heels, elbows, and so on, are protected from pressure against the bed surface.

  c. Body alignment is maintained.

- Plan and implement a turning schedule that will incorporate all the possible positions. *Repositioning prevents pressure areas.* Generally, clients can be placed in lateral, prone, and supine positions unless surgical procedures or any other factors contraindicate them. Attach a trapeze to the Balkan frame to enable the client to assist with moving.

- Turn people with large casts or those unable to turn themselves at least once every 4 hours. If the person is at risk for skin breakdown, turn every 1 to 3 hours as needed.

- When turning the client in a long leg cast to the unaffected side, place a pillow between the legs to support the cast.

- Use at least three persons to turn a person in a *damp* hip spica cast. When the cast is dry, the individual can usually turn with the assistance of one nurse. To turn a client from the supine to prone position, follow these steps:

  a. Remove the support pillows only when an assistant is supporting the cast.

  b. Move the client to one side of the bed.

  c. Ask the client to place the arms above the head or along the sides.

  d. Have two assistants go to the other side of the bed while you remain to provide security for the person who is at the edge of the bed.

  e. Place pillows along the bed surface to receive the cast when the client turns.

  f. Roll the client toward the two assistants onto the pillows.

  g. Adjust the pillows as needed so that they provide proper support and comfort, and prevent pressure areas.

6. Encourage range-of-motion (ROM) and isometric exercises.

- Unless contraindicated, encourage active ROM exercises for all joints on the unaffected extremities, as well as on the joints proximal and distal to the cast. If active exercises are contraindicated, implement active-assistive or passive exercises, depending on the client's abilities and disabilities. *Exercise helps prevent joint stiffness and muscle atrophy.*

- Encourage the client to move toes and/or fingers of the casted extremity as frequently as possible. *Moving these extremities enhances peripheral circulation and decreases swelling and pain.*

- Teach isometric (muscle-setting) exercises for extremities in a cast. *Isometric exercise will minimize muscle atrophy in the affected limb.*

  a. Teach the isometric exercises on the client's unaffected

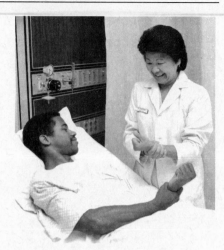

FIGURE 43–12 Teaching muscle-setting exercises.

limb before the person applies it to the affected limb.

  b. Demonstrate muscle palpation while the client is carrying out the exercise (Figure 43–12). *Palpation enables the person to feel the changes that occur with muscle contraction and relaxation.*

7. Provide client teaching to promote self-care, comfort, and safety.

- Teach parents of young children ways to prevent the child from placing small items under the cast. One approach is to avoid giving the child small play items such as marbles, pencils, or crayons. Parents also need to ensure that the top of a body cast is covered during meals so that food does not fall inside the cast.

- Teach people immobilized in bed with large body casts ways to turn and to move safely by using a trapeze, the side rails, and other such devices.

- Instruct clients with leg casts about ways to walk effectively with crutches. See Technique 21–5, page 529.

► **Technique 43–3** *CONTINUED*

- Instruct people with arm casts how to apply slings. See Technique 40–3, page 952.

- Teach clients how to resolve itching under the cast safely.

  a. Discourage the person from using long sharp objects to scratch under the cast. *These objects can break the skin and cause an infection, because bacteria flourish in the warm, dark, moist environment under the cast.*

  b. Suggest that the client tap the cast or, at home, to use a hair drier on cool, a vacuum cleaner on reverse, or an ice bag over the outside of the itching area. *These are safer ways to resolve itching and less irritating to the skin.*

- Before discharge from the hospital, instruct the client to

  a. Observe for indications of nerve or circulatory impairment, such as extreme coldness or blueness of toes or fingers; extreme continuous swelling of casted toes or fingers; numbness or tingling ("pins and needles" sensation) in casted toes or fingers; continuous complaints of pain; or inability to move the toes or fingers.

  b. Keep the cast dry.

  c. Avoid strenuous activity and follow medical advice about exercises.

  d. Elevate the arm or leg frequently to prevent dependent edema.

  e. Move the toes or fingers frequently.

  f. Observe the skin around the cast edges frequently, and keep it clean and dry.

  g. Report any increase in pain; unexplained fever; foul odor from within the cast; decreased circulation; numbness; inability to move the fingers or toes; or a weakened, cracked, loose, or tight cast.

- When healing is complete and the cast is removed, the underlying skin is usually dry, flaky, and encrusted, since layers of dead skin have accumulated. Instruct clients to remove this debris gently and gradually.

  a. Apply oil (e.g., mineral, olive, or baby oil).

  b. Soak the skin in warm water and dry it.

  c. Caution the client not to rub the area too vigorously. *Vigorous rubbing can cause bleeding or excoriation.*

  d. Repeat steps a and b for several days. *Gradual removal of skin exudate avoids skin irritation.*

8. Document assessments and nursing implementations on the appropriate records.

EVALUATION FOCUS	Ability to perform self-care; ability to perform exercises; understanding of all instructions provided. See also the Assessment Focus on page 1010.

KEY ELEMENTS OF CONTINUING CARE FOR CLIENTS WITH CASTS

- Remove crumbs of plaster from the skin, "petal" rough cast edges, and clean and massage skin areas under cast edges with alcohol.
- For bed-confined clients, provide skin care over all bony prominences, and turn the clients at least every 4 hours.
- Keep the cast clean and dry.
- Encourage clients to move the toes or fingers of the casted extremity frequently.
- Provide necessary instructions about cast care, ways to move safely, activity allowed, exercises, elevating the involved extremity, signs of neurovascular problems, and ways to handle itching.
- Assess and document assessments and interventions.

CRITICAL THINKING CHALLENGE

Jenny Allen, a 23-year-old college student, suffered an open fracture of the left leg in a motorcycle accident. Following reduction of the fracture and suturing of the laceration, the physician applied a long leg cast and admitted Ms Allen to the nursing unit. During a routine assessment of her cast, Ms Allen complains that her foot is cold and numb. What would you do? What should you say?

REFERENCES

Hansell, M. J. January/February 1988. Fractures and the healing process. *Orthopaedic Nursing* 7:43–50.

Hoyt, N. J. September/October 1986. Infections following orthopaedic injury. *Orthopaedic Nursing* 5:15–24.

Mather, M. L. S. January 1987. The secret to life in a spica. *American Journal of Nursing* 87:56–58.

Ryan, B. March 1986. Assessing for neurovascular deficiency following orthopaedic peripheral surgery. *CONA Journal* 8:13–15.

Slye, D. B. March 1991. Orthopedic complications: Compartment syndrome, fat embolism syndrome, and venous thromboembolism. *Nursing Clinics of North America* 26:113–32.

Wienke, V. K. July/August 1987. Pressure sores: Prevention is the challenge. *Orthopaedic Nursing* 6:26–30.

Traction Care

OBJECTIVES

- State the purposes of selected tractions

- Differentiate four types of traction

- Identify six types of skin traction

- Identify three types of skeletal traction

- Outline essential assessment data for clients with traction

- Identify potential problems associated with specific tractions

- List nursing measures to prevent problems for clients with selected tractions

- Apply nonadhesive skin traction

- Provide essential nursing interventions to clients in traction

CONTENTS

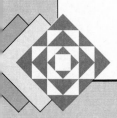

NURSING PROCESS GUIDE
TRACTION CARE

ASSESSMENT

Assess

- *The neurovascular status of the affected extremity,* i.e., the status of peripheral pulses, color, amount of movement, temperature, capillary filling, edema, numbness, sensation. See the Nursing Process Guide for Chapter 43.

- *The presence of pain in the area:* exact location, degree, duration, and description of the pain (e.g., sharp, needlelike) and identification of any movement or activity that would initiate the pain.

- *Clinical signs of thrombi and emboli:* Regularly assess the client's pulse, blood pressure, respirations, mental status, and breath sounds for evidence of emboli. Inspect the client's involved extremity for redness, swelling, and pain. See page 1003 in Chapter 43 for further information.

- *Pressure areas* for signs of skin irritation or breakdown. Note in particular (a) bony prominences (e.g., the heels, ankles, sacrum, elbows, chin, and shoulders) and (b) areas susceptible to pressure from the traction (e.g., the iliac crests for a pelvic girdle, or the legs for Buck's extension).

- *Inflammation and drainage at the pin sites* for skeletal traction.

Inspect the traction apparatus:

- Is the appropriate countertraction provided?

- Are the correct weights applied?

- Is there free play of the ropes on the pulleys; i.e., does the groove of the pulley support the rope? Are the knots positioned no closer than 12 inches to the nearest pulley?

- Do all weights hang freely and not rest against or on the bed or floor?

- Are the ropes intact, i.e., not frayed, knotted, or kinked between their points of attachment?

- Are the ropes securely attached with slip knots and the short ends of ropes attached with tape?

- Is the line of the traction straight and in the same plane as the long axis of the bone?

- Do bedclothes and other objects not impinge on the traction?

- Is the footplate positioned above, not resting against, the end of the bed?

- Is the spreader bar wide enough to prevent the traction tape from rubbing on bony prominences?

For skin traction applications, assess

- Presence of skin allergies.

- Skin for signs of infection or injury. Generally, skin traction is contraindicated if the client has hypersensitive skin, an infection, open wound, swelling, or neurovascular impairments.

RELATED DIAGNOSTIC CATEGORIES

- High risk for Disuse syndrome

- High risk for Infection (at pin site)

- Pain

- High risk for Impaired skin integrity

- Constipation

- Self-care deficit

- Social isolation

PLANNING

Client Goals
The client will

- Remain free of complications associated with immobility.

- Remain free of complications associated with the specific traction.

Outcome Criteria
The client

- *Maintains normal musculoskeletal function:*

  - Demonstrates usual range of motion in all unaffected body joints.

  - Is able to move all fingers or toes of the affected extremity.

  - Feels normal sensation in all fingers or toes of the affected extremity.

  - Performs isotonic (and/or isometric) exercises as taught every 4 hours to specified body joints.

  - Retains baseline muscle mass.

  - Participates actively in self-care activities without fatigue.

- *Has minimum cardiovascular alterations:*

  - Maintains baseline vital signs.

Nursing Process Guide *CONTINUED*

- Has normal skin color of toes and fingers in the affected extremity.

- Has skin temperature in the affected extremity equal to that of the opposite limb.

- Has normal capillary refill in the nail of the large thumb or toe of the affected limb.

- Has a peripheral pulse in the affected limb equal in rate and volume to that of the opposite limb.

- Indicates signs of adequate venous blood flow (absence of edema, calf pain, inflammation, venous distention, skin changes).

- *Maintains normal respiratory function:*

  - Takes five deep breaths and coughs every waking hour.

  - Has normal breath sounds on auscultation.

  - Retains normal chest expansion.

  - Experiences no chest pain, fever, or other respiratory signs indicative of pulmonary infection, emboli, or atelectasis.

- *Maintains appropriate nutritional and fluid pattern:*

  - Maintains baseline weight.

- Has normal serum protein values.

- Has adequate tissue turgor.

- Has a balanced fluid intake and output.

- *Maintains normal elimination pattern:*

  - Voids at least 1500 ml per day.

  - Has an acidic urine.

  - Is free of signs of urinary retention, infection, and renal calculi.

  - Passes a formed semisolid stool at least every 2 or 3 days.

  - Remains free of signs of fecal impaction.

- *Maintains intact integument:*

  - Has clean, intact, well-hydrated skin.

  - Is free of pressure signs (pallor, redness, increased warmth or tenderness) over pressure areas.

- *Maintains normal psychosocial function:*

  - Participates actively in decisions about care.

  - Develops ways to overcome boredom.

  - Verbalizes concerns and feelings.

  - Accepts help from others.

Traction

Traction, like a cast, is a means by which a part of the body is immobilized. But unlike a cast, traction involves a pulling force that is applied to a part of the body while a second force, called **countertraction**, pulls in the opposite direction. Too much force can cause damage to nerves and tissues; too little force can produce painful muscle spasms and impair healing.

The pulling force of traction is provided through a system of pulleys, ropes, and weights attached to the client; the countertraction is often achieved by elevating the foot or head of the bed and therefore is supplied by the client's body. In *balanced traction*, the amount of force in the traction is equal to the amount of force in the countertraction. A *suspension* is a mechanism that suspends a body part by using traction equipment, but it does not involve a pulling force. However, traction may be added to a suspension.

In *straight, or running, traction*, the traction force is pulled against the long axis of the body, and the countertraction is supplied by the client's body. In a suspension or in a balanced traction, the affected part is supported by a sling, hammock, or ring splint, and countertraction is supplied partly by the body and partly by a system of weights attached to an overhead frame with pulleys and ropes.

People who have traction are often confined to bed for weeks or even months. Nursing implementation therefore involves ADLs, maintenance of the traction, and the prevention of problems related to immobility such as pressure sores.

Purposes of Traction
Traction is applied for several purposes:

- To reduce and/or immobilize a bone fracture for healing

- To maintain proper bone alignment

- To prevent soft tissue injury

- To correct, reduce, or prevent deformities

- To decrease muscle spasm and pain

- To treat inflammatory conditions by immobilizing a joint, e.g., for arthritis or tuberculosis of a joint

Types of Traction

There are four types of traction: manual, skin, skeletal, and encircling.

1. *Manual traction* is applied by the hands; i.e., the nurse holds the limb while exerting pulling force. It is a temporary measure used while skin traction is being prepared (e.g., when a cast is being applied) or in an emergency (e.g., when a traction rope breaks).

2. *Skin traction* is a pulling force applied to the skin and soft tissues through the use of tape or traction straps and a system of ropes, pulleys, and weights. The **traction tape** or **strap** is often made of vented foam rubber or cloth, and it may have either an adhesive or nonadhesive backing. Adhesive skin traction is used only for continuous traction. Nonadhesive skin traction is used intermittently; it can easily be removed and reapplied. The tape is applied lengthwise along a limb and attached to a **spreader bar**, which is designed to spread the tape away from the bony prominences of the involved body part (Figure 44–11, later in this chapter). The bar must be wider than the involved part.

3. *Skeletal traction* is applied by inserting metal pins, wires, or tongs directly into or through a bone. The metal device is then attached to a system of ropes, pulleys, and weights by means of a metal frame attached to the bed.

4. *Encircling traction* is often considered a type of skin traction. A halter or sling is placed around a body part and attached by means of a rope and pulley to a weight that pulls in a straight line. Examples of encircling traction are cervical head halter traction and pelvic traction.

Traction can be either continuous or intermittent. Continuous traction (skeletal or skin) is applied and released by a physician, who is responsible for handling the affected part when it is not in traction. Intermittent traction (nonadhesive skin traction) can be applied and released by nursing personnel with the appropriate order. However, the amount of weight to be applied is prescribed by the physician.

Traction Equipment

The following equipment is required for all skin and skeletal tractions:

- *An overhead frame:* This frame is attached to the hospital bed and provides a means for attach-

ment of the traction apparatus (Figure 44–1). There are numerous kinds of overhead frames, which attach to the bed in different ways; each frame, however, has at least two upright bars (one at each end of the bed), and one overhead bar.

- *A trapeze:* Attached to the overhead frame, the trapeze can be used by the client for moving in bed, unless contraindicated by the client's health.

- *A firm mattress:* To maintain body alignment and the efficiency of the traction, a firm mattress is essential. Some beds are manufactured with a solid bottom instead of springs, to provide firm support. If a firm bed is not available, a bedboard can be used to provide the needed support.

- *Ropes, pulleys, weight hangers, and weights.* These are not used, however, for the halo-thoracic vest traction (Figure 44–16, later in this chapter).

Guidelines for Traction

- All traction should have countertraction to prevent the client from being pulled by the force of traction against the pulleys or the bed, thus negating the traction.

- To apply and maintain the correct amount of traction, all traction weights should be hanging freely and the ropes should not touch any part of the bed.

- The traction force should follow an established line of pull. The line of pull determines the position and alignment of the body as prescribed by the physician. All ropes should be on the center track of a pulley, and the line of pull should always be from (a) the point of attachment to the client to (b) the first pulley (Figure 44–1).

- Traction should always be applied while the client is in proper body alignment in a supine position.

- To be effective, traction should be maintained continuously unless ordered otherwise.

Skin Tractions

A discussion of selected tractions that nurses may see in a hospital follows.

Buck's extension (Figure 44–1) is a simple traction used to immobilize fractures of the hip and reduce muscle spasm before surgical repair. It can be applied to one leg (unilateral) or both legs (bilateral). Buck's extension is a skin traction and may use either adhesive or nonadhesive tape. Sometimes commercially made foam rubber boot-type splints with

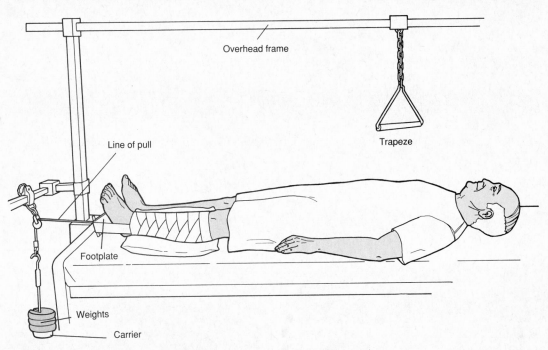

FIGURE 44–1 Unilateral Buck's extension traction.

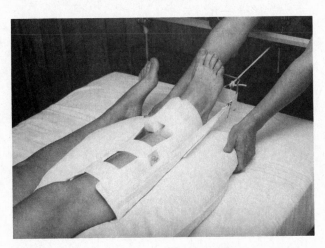

FIGURE 44–2 A commercially made Buck's boot.

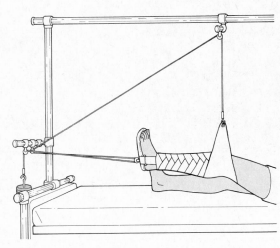

FIGURE 44–3 Russell traction.

self-adhering straps are used (Figure 44–2). Countertraction is applied by elevating the foot of the bed.

Russell traction (Figure 44–3) is a skin traction (adhesive or nonadhesive) applied to one or both legs. It is commonly used to immobilize fractures of the femur before surgical repair. A sling under the thigh is used to suspend the limb, and the knee is slightly flexed. The pull on the limb is both vertical (through the sling) and horizontal (through the footplate). The degree of flexion of the knee depends on the angle needed as determined by the physician. The placement of the overhead pulley and the pulley on the foot of the bed varies. The latter may be raised so that it is in line with the pulley on the footplate. The foot of the bed may or may not be elevated for countertraction. The head of the bed should remain flat. A pillow may or may not be ordered to support the lower leg.

Pelvic belts, or **girdles** (Figure 44–4), provide traction around the client's hips and relieve lower back, hip, and leg pain. The belts in common use today are disposable and adjustable, with self-adhering or Velcro straps. The belt is fitted directly on the skin over the iliac crests (i.e., the top margin is at the level of the umbilicus) and fastened over the abdomen. The straps, which attach to the pulley and

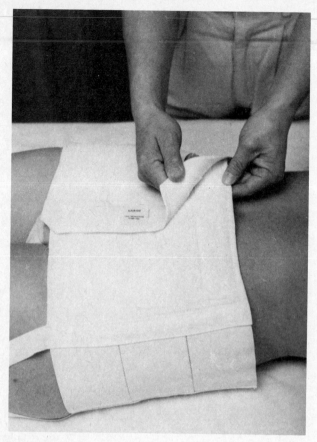

FIGURE 44–4 A pelvic belt.

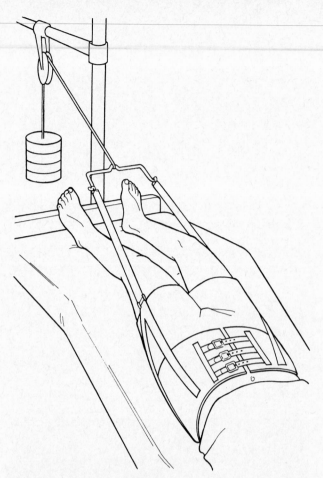

FIGURE 44–5 Pelvic girdle traction.

weight system, may be attached either at the client's sides, so that the pull of the traction is toward the foot of the bed, or at the back (under the client), so that the traction pull is downward and toward the foot of the bed (Figure 44–5). Countertraction is provided by elevating the foot of the bed or by placing the client in William's position, i.e., elevating the head of the bed and the knee gatch to approximately the same angle. This type of traction is frequently intermittent.

In **cervical head halter traction** (Figure 44–6), the cervical head halter provides skin (encircling) traction on the cervical spine. It relieves muscle spasms and nerve compression in the neck, upper arms, or shoulders that may be associated with cervical injuries, e.g., "whiplash." The head halter is attached to a spreader bar that is wide enough to prevent the halter from pressing on the client's ears, jaws, or sides of the head. Countertraction from the client's body weight is provided by elevating the head of the bed. Head halter traction may be applied intermittently or continuously. If traction is required for a long period of time, however, skeletal traction is applied.

Bryant's traction (Figure 44–7) is an adaptation of a bilateral Buck's extension. It is used to stabilize

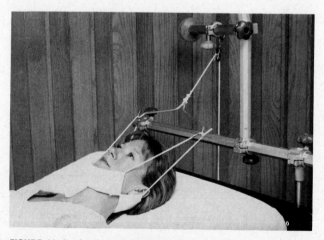

FIGURE 44–6 Cervical head halter traction.

fractured femurs or correct congenital hip dislocations in young children under 18 kg (40 lbs). In Bryant's traction, skin traction is applied to both the affected and the unaffected leg to maintain the position of the affected leg. A spreader bar attached to the strips maintains leg alignment. Unless otherwise ordered, the hips are flexed at right angles (90°) to the body, and the buttocks raised about 2.5 cm (1 in)

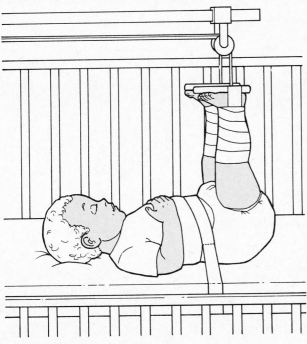

FIGURE 44–7   Bryant's traction.

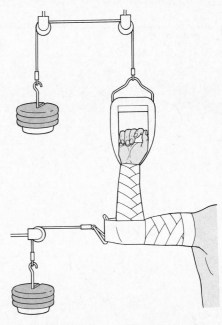

FIGURE 44–8   Side-arm (Dunlop's) traction.

off the mattress. The weight of the child's torso provides countertraction. A jacket or belt restraint may be necessary to prevent the child from turning and to supplement countertraction.

Side-arm, or Dunlop's, traction (Figure 44–8) is a combined horizontal and vertical adaptation of Buck's extension to the humerus and forearm. The traction pull outward from the upper arm is used to align fractures of the humerus, and the pull upward from the forearm maintains the forearm in the desired alignment relative to the humerus (e.g., a 45° or 90° angle). Countertraction is provided by the posi-

tioning of the body; e.g., a folded blanket placed under the mattress on the side of the traction frame augments countertraction.

A skeletal form of Dunlop's skin traction may be applied. Instead of the horizontal Buck's extension, a pin is drilled through the lower humerus and attached to a spreader, ropes, pulleys, and weights. The forearm is held in vertical Buck's extension, as it would be in the skin traction. Skeletal traction is indicated for severe fractures of the humerus that require a greater weight to overcome muscle spasms and produce effective bone alignment.

Technique 44–1 describes the steps involved in applying nonadhesive skin traction.

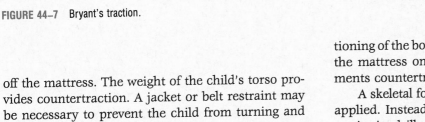

44-1   Applying Nonadhesive Skin Traction

Nonadhesive skin traction does not cause the skin irritations that are associated with adhesive tape. Furthermore, nurses with the appropriate order can release and apply it. Before applying this type of traction, verify the order to apply and/or remove the traction, including times and amount of weight. Manual traction should be applied when the traction apparatus is removed.

PURPOSES
- To promote and maintain alignment of a lower extremity
- To prevent neurovascular impairment
- To decrease muscle spasm and pain

► **Technique 44–1 Applying Nonadhesive Skin Traction** CONTINUED

ASSESSMENT FOCUS

Bruises and abrasions in the area where the traction is to be applied (report any open areas to the nurse in charge and/or physician before applying the traction); the neurovascular status of the extremity (i.e., the color, amount of movement, temperature, capillary filling, edema, numbness, sensation; see the Nursing Process Guide in Chapter 43, page 1001); any pain in the area (exact location, degree, duration, and description of the pain, and the identification or any movement or activity that initiates the pain); any history of circulatory problems and skin allergies; mental and emotional status and ability to understand activity restrictions.

EQUIPMENT

- Basin of water, soap, and towels
- Doughnut of stockinette
- Nonadhesive traction straps
- 2-inch or 3-inch elastic bandage, depending on the circumference of the extremity
- Adhesive tape
- Footplate or block or spreader bar wide enough to prevent the traction straps from irritating the skin over the sides of the foot and ankle (these come equipped with an attachment for the rope)
- Rope, weight hanger, and weights

INTERVENTION

1. Prepare the limb for traction.

- Wash and dry the extremity, e.g., the foot and leg.

- Apply a piece of rolled stockinette over the foot to a point just above the malleoli of the ankle. *This protects the skin over these bony prominences from abrasion and pressure from the traction tape.*

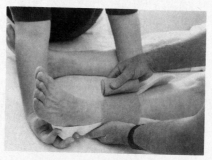

FIGURE 44–9 Securing a nonadhesive skin traction with an elastic bandage.

2. Apply the traction straps.

- Place the nonadhesive traction strap down the inner aspect of the leg, around the foot, and up the lateral aspect of the leg, leaving the tape slack around the foot. *The slack of the tape will be taken up by the spreader bar or footplate.*

- Secure an elastic bandage over the strap, starting just above the ankle, using spiral-reverse or modified figure-eight turns (Figure 44–9). *Starting just above the ankle avoids placing pressure on the Achilles tendon, and a spiral-reverse or modified figure-eight secures the bandage better than a simple spiral.*

- Secure the elastic bandage with adhesive tape.

3. Attach the spreader bar or footplate.

- Connect the spreader bar or footplate to the traction straps below the foot. *These prevent the traction straps from irritating the skin over the sides of the foot and ankle. A footplate will also help keep the foot in a normal position, i.e., neither acutely flexed nor extended* (Figures 44–10 and 44–11).

- Tie the rope to whatever footpiece or spreader is being used. Use a slip knot which can be untied easily and rapidly. Figure

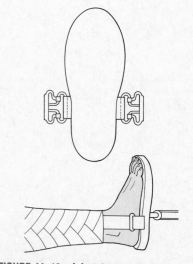

FIGURE 44–10 A footplate.

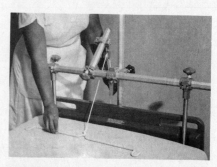

FIGURE 44–11 A spreader bar.

44–12 shows how to tie a slip knot.

4. Attach the weights.

▶ **Technique 44–1** CONTINUED

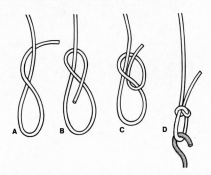

FIGURE 44–12 Tying a slip knot: *A,* make a figure eight; *B,* bring the free end of the rope through the lower loop; *C,* bring the free end of the rope under and through the upper loop; *D,* tighten the knot by pulling on the free end.

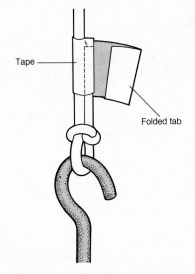

Tape

Folded tab

FIGURE 44–13 Taping traction rope ends using a folded tab.

- Thread the rope through a pulley over the foot of the bed.

- Using a slip knot, attach the end of the rope to a weight carrier.

- Fasten the short ends of the ropes with tape to prevent them from slipping. When taping the ends of the ropes, make a folded tab at the end of the tape to facilitate its removal (Figure 44–13).

- Determine the amount of weight to be used, and slowly place the weights on the carrier (Figure 44–1, earlier). *Sudden weight can jar the extremity and cause pain.*

5. Ensure appropriate traction.

- Elevate the foot of the bed to ensure appropriate countertraction.

- Ensure that the affected leg is immobilized in a straight plane with the line of traction.

- Ensure that the client's heel is supported off the bed and away from the foot of the bed.

6. Assess the neurovascular status and skin of the affected limb.

- Assess neurovascular signs every 2 to 4 hours. See the neurovascular assessment for Chapter 43, page 1001.

- Remove and reapply the skin traction every 8 hours or more frequently as required to assess and maintain skin integrity.

7. Assess the psychosocial responses of the client.

- Determine the client's perceptions of the consequences and effects of being in traction.

- Observe and validate nonverbal responses and cues.

8. Document all relevant information.

- Record the procedure and the amount of weight applied, as well as all nursing assessments.

EVALUATION FOCUS	Neurovascular status of the affected limb (see Chapter 43, page 1001); status of skin beneath traction and over other bony prominences; integrity of the traction apparatus; client response to traction; any discomfort.

SAMPLE RECORDING

Date	Time	Notes
12/22/93	1700	Buck's skin traction applied to R lower leg as ordered. Skin intact, equal in temperature and color to L leg. Able to move all toes, and plantar flex and dorsiflex ankle. Sensation felt in web between great and second toe, and medial and lateral surfaces of sole of foot. Resting comfortably. ——— Carrie A. Murphy, RN

KEY ELEMENTS OF APPLYING NONADHESIVE SKIN TRACTION

- Assess the neurovascular status of the affected limb before applying the traction, and then every 2 to 4 hours.
- Maintain proper body alignment.
- Remove and reapply the traction at least every 8 hours.
- Maintain skin integrity.
- Document and promptly report any neurovascular problems.

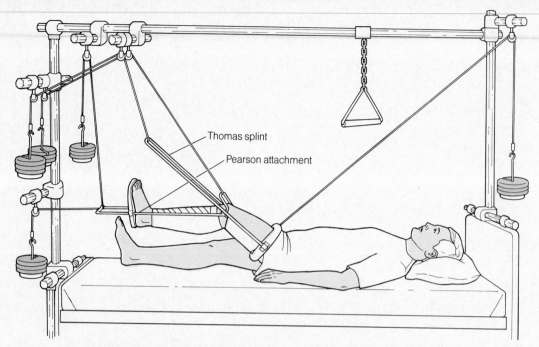

FIGURE 44-14 Balanced suspension with Thomas leg splint and Pearson attachment.

Skeletal Tractions

Skeletal traction can be applied to the skull, the proximal end of the ulna, the distal end of the femur, the proximal and distal ends of the tibia, and the calcaneus (heel bone). Because bone withstands greater stress than skin, heavier weights can be used (e.g., up to 35 pounds). Metal pins, wires, or tongs are inserted into the bone to which the traction is applied. Common examples are the Steinmann pin, the Kirschner wire, and the Cructhfield tongs.

A Thomas leg splint and Pearson attachment is a balanced suspension that allows the client some degree of movement when skeletal traction is applied to the femur to prevent muscle spasm and overriding of bone fragments before surgical fixation. The **Thomas leg splint** consists of a full ring or half ring around the thigh with two rods on either side of the legs. The distal end is attached to a weighted rope for suspension. The **Pearson attachment** is a sling appliance that joins the Thomas splint at knee level. It supports the lower leg off the bed and permits the knee to be flexed (Figure 44-14). The pin or wire drilled through the bone is attached to a spreader, which in turn, is attached to ropes, pulleys, and weights. Countertraction is supplied mostly by the body's weight. The suspension weight, however, is counterbalanced by a weighted rope attached to the proximal end of the Thomas splint. To prevent footdrop, a footplate is attached to the Pearson apparatus. To prevent skin breakdown, the ischial ring of the

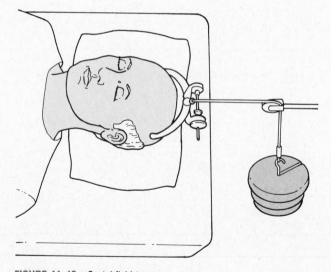

FIGURE 44-15 Crutchfield tongs.

Thomas splint is padded; sheepskin slings are positioned along the Pearson attachment.

Skull tongs (e.g., Crutchfield, Burton, Gardner-Wells, or Vinke) immobilize fractures of the cervical and upper thoracic vertebrae. The tongs are secured to each side of the skull. The center metal bar is attached to ropes, pulleys, and weights and creates a traction pull along the long axis of the spine (Figure 44-15).

An adaptation of the skull tong is the **halo ring** traction. This is a circular metal band secured by two anterior and two posterior pins that penetrate the skull only a fraction of an inch. The ring can be attached to a weighted rope, a plaster cast, or a molded plastic vest. The latter method is referred to as a **halo-thoracic vest traction** (Figure 44–16). The halo is attached to the plaster cast or plastic vest by metal rods. Some vests extend to the client's pelvic girdle. The vest, which is well padded with sheepskin, supports and suspends the weight of the entire apparatus around the chest.

The desired traction to the thoracic spine is achieved by adjusting the nuts and bolts that attach the metal bars to the halo apparatus. By increasing or decreasing the distance between the halo and the vest, traction is increased or decreased. The advantage of this traction over other types of head and neck traction is that it allows the client to sit, stand, and walk, thus decreasing the respiratory, circulatory, and muscular problems associated with prolonged immobility.

Care of a Client in Traction

The care of a client in traction involves understanding the principles of traction and its maintenance and preventing complications of the specific traction and complications associated with immobility. If skeletal traction has been applied in the operating room, postoperative care is usually needed as well. See Chapter 42.

Clients in traction generally require meticulous monitoring of the neurovascular status of the affected body part, and protective devices and measures to safeguard the skin. For clients in skeletal traction, pin site care may be ordered to prevent infection. According to a study by Jones-Walton (1991, p. 12) on pin site care, pin sites may or may not be treated. Some surgeons prefer no treatment. For agencies that do provide pin site care, this same study indicated the following findings:

* Two to three pin site treatments are provided per day.

* Clean or sterile technique is used.

* Hydrogen peroxide, povidone-iodine (Betadine) solutions, and normal saline are used for care.

* Application of Polysporin or Betadine ointments or alcohol is often applied after initial cleansing.

Technique 44–2 explains the steps involved in assisting a client in traction. Table 44–1 outlines the pressure areas associated with various kinds of traction.

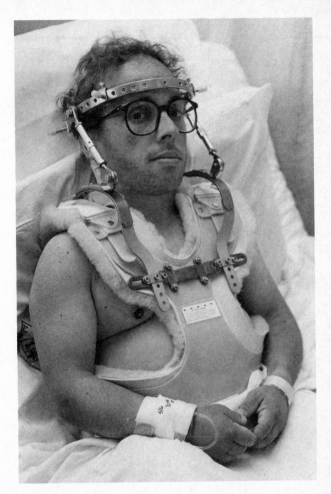

FIGURE 44–16   Halo-thoracic vest traction.

TABLE 44–1   TRACTION PRESSURE AREAS

Traction	Pressure Areas
Buck's extension	Skin over the tibia, if bandage slips; malleoli, hamstring tendon; heels; back
Russell traction	As above for Buck's extension; popliteal space due to sling; sole of foot due to footplate
Pelvic girdle	Iliac crests; back
Cervical head halter	Chin; occipit; ears; mandible
Bryant's traction	Skin over the tibia; malleoli; hamstrings tendon; sole of feet; upper back
Side arm	Soft tissues near shoulders; anterior surface of elbow joint due to bandages
Thomas leg splint and Pearson attachment	Groin, popliteal space; Achilles tendon; heel; peroneal nerve if splint misplaced
Halo-thoracic vest	Areas where jacket edges touch the skin; skin under vest

44-2 Assisting a Client in Traction

PURPOSES
- To support the client psychologically
- To maintain the traction
- To assist the client with ADLs, as required
- To prevent the occurrence of complications (e.g., pressure sores, pneumonia, muscle contractures, and constipation)

ASSESSMENT FOCUS

Clinical signs of embolism; pressure areas for skin irritation or breakdown; neurovascular status of affected extremity; clinical signs of complications of immobility (e.g., pressure sores, constipation, hypostatic pneumonia, and muscle atrophy); integrity of the traction apparatus and the client's body alignment; need for diversional activities; assistance required with ADLs. See the Nursing Process Guide on page 1016. For clients with *skeletal traction*, note also inflammation and amount and character of drainage at pin sites.

EQUIPMENT

- Trapeze, if needed
- Protective skin devices (e.g., heel protectors)
- Rubbing alcohol or lotion
- Supplies for pin care in skeleton traction (e.g., alcohol, hydrogen peroxide, povidone-iodine solution, or other agency-recommended antiseptic (optional)

INTERVENTION

1. Verify the physician's orders.
- Determine the degree of movement permitted and any special precautions, e.g., bed positions permitted.

2. Inspect the traction apparatus.
- Note the type of traction, and inspect the traction apparatus regularly, i.e., whenever you are at the bedside or at prescribed intervals, such as every 2 hours. See inspection of the traction apparatus in the Nursing Process Guide on page 1016. *Any articles that impinge on the traction can negate its effectiveness.*
- For *Russell traction*, check the sling position frequently and maintain hip flexion at the correct angle.
- For *Bryant's traction*, ensure that the sacrum is elevated sufficiently to allow the nurse to slip a hand between the child's buttocks and the bed.

3. Maintain the client in the appropriate traction position.
- Maintain the client in the supine position unless there are other orders. *Changing position can change the body alignment and the amount of force supplied by the traction.*
- Maintain body alignment when turning the client. In some cases, the person can turn to a lateral position if body alignment is maintained by a pillow placed between the legs. Refer to the client's record for information about permitted movement.
- Provide a trapeze to assist the client to move and lift the body for back care if the person is unable to turn, e.g., if the client has balanced suspension traction.
- Provide a fracture or slipper bedpan as required to minimize the client's movement.
- Restrain a child as needed to prevent slipping toward the foot of

the bed (Russell traction).
- For clients with skull tongs, a halo ring, or a cervical head halter, turn the client as a unit, using a special bed.
- If skull tongs or pins become dislodged, notify the physician immediately and place sandbags on either side of the head to maintain alignment.

4. Assess the neurovascular status of the affected extremity.
- For clients who have adhesive skin traction or skeletal traction, provide a neurovascular assessment every hour for the first 24 hours. If the client's status is "normal," then assess every 4 hours during the traction. If the client's status is not normal, continue hourly assessments.
- For clients who have nonadhesive skin traction, provide a neurovascular assessment 30 minutes following reapplication of the bandage, then every 2 hours for

▶ **Technique 44–2** *CONTINUED*

the first 24 hours, then every 4 hours if the client's status is normal.

- For details about neurovascular assessment, see Chapter 43, page 1001.

5. Provide protective devices and measures to safeguard the skin.

- Place heel protectors or sheepskins under the heels, sacrum, shoulders, and other pressure areas. See Table 44–1.

- Massage the skin with rubbing alcohol or lotion every 4 hours and, if redness and signs of pressure appear, every 2 hours. *Alcohol tends to toughen the skin and leave it less vulnerable to breakdown.* Because alcohol is drying to the skin, however, lotion may be preferred for those who have dry skin (e.g., elderly people).

- Make sure the spreader bar is wide enough to prevent the traction tape from rubbing on the client's bony prominences.

- For clients with a cervical head halter, keep the chin dry, using alcohol or cornstarch.

- For clients with a halo-thoracic vest, open or remove the vest daily to inspect the skin and provide skin care. Change or clean the sheepskin lining at least weekly.

6. Remove only intermittent nonadhesive skin traction in accordance with agency protocol or orders.

- Removal of skeletal and adhesive skin traction is a physician's responsibility. A reduced fracture can be malpositioned if skeletal or adhesive traction is removed.

- To remove a *nonadhesive* skin traction,

   a. Remove the weights first.

   b. Then unwrap the bandage

and provide skin care.

   c. Rewrap the limb and slowly reattach the weights.

7. Provide pin site care two or three times daily if indicated by the physician's orders and agency protocol.

- Carefully inspect the site. *Regular inspection of the pin site ensures early detection of minor infections, as manifested by signs of serosanguinous drainage, crusting, swelling, and erythema.*

- Use clean or sterile technique as agency protocol dictates. See Chapter 39 for information about sterile dressing supplies.

- Remove crusts with a rolling technique by using half-strength hydrogen peroxide, povidone-iodine solution, normal saline, or other agent recommended by the agency. Use a gentle rolling technique to reduce irritation to the tissue. *Removing all crusted secretions permits the pin site to drain freely. Initial crusts around pins do not create a problem and can be left, but accumulated crusts around external fixator pins may cause secondary infection.*

- Cover the pin site with a sterile barrier, i.e., sterile gauze or sterile ointment. One method is to soak 2 × 2 sterile gauze with povidone-iodine solution after the gauze has been applied around the pin (Celeste, Folcik, and Dumas 1984, p. 20). Procedures vary, so determine agency practices regarding pin site care.

- Adjust frequency of care according to the amount of drainage.

- If purulent drainage is present, notify the physician and obtain specimens for culture and sensitivity.

8. Teach the client ways to prevent problems associated with immobility.

- Teach the client deep-breathing and coughing exercises to prevent hypostatic pneumonia. See Chapter 30, page 743.

- Teach the client appropriate exercises to maintain and develop muscle tone, prevent muscle contracture and atrophy, and promote blood circulation:

   a Range-of-motion exercises are discussed in Chapter 21, page 512. For clients in a Thomas splint with a Pearson attachment, place the bed in a flat position for 20 to 30 minutes per shift to provide hip extension.

   b. Isometric exercises are discussed in Chapter 43, page 1012. Isometric exercises to strengthen the quadriceps muscles include tightening the knees; by pushing the knees down without moving them, the hamstring muscles are also strengthened. Tensing the buttocks and the inner thighs promotes stabilization of the hips; tensing the inner thighs also helps stabilize the knees.

   c. Circulation to the extremities can be promoted by encouraging the client to flex and extend the feet as well as to perform the isometric exercises.

   d. Specific exercises to strengthen the biceps and triceps muscles in preparation for using crutches can be taught as indicated. For example, raising the buttocks off the bed by pushing down with the arms develops the triceps, and pulling the body up with a trapeze develops the biceps. See Chapter 21, page 528.

9. Document all assessments and nursing interventions.

▶

▶ **Technique 44–2 Assisting a Client in Traction** *CONTINUED*

EVALUATION FOCUS

> Neurovascular status of affected extremity; comparison of vital signs to baseline data; skin integrity over skin pressure sites; status of pin site; breathing pattern and lung sounds; nutritional and fluid intake; elimination pattern; muscle size and strength; joint range of motion; participation in self-care activities; and psychosocial response to the traction.

KEY ELEMENTS OF ASSISTING A CLIENT IN TRACTION

- Assess and document neurovascular status at least every 4 hours.
- Maintain proper body alignment.
- Maintain skin integrity over skin pressure sites.

- Monitor the status of the pin site and provide care according to agency protocol.
- Prevent complications of immobility.

CRITICAL THINKING CHALLENGE

Margaret O'Hara, a 46-year-old female, has been placed in pelvic traction to treat low back pain. While assessing her response to treatment, she tells you she is "bored lying flat on her back all day" and wants you to remove the apparatus. What will you say? What will you do?

RELATED RESEARCH

Jones-Walton, P. March/April 1991. Clinical standards in skeletal traction pin site care. *Orthopaedic Nursing* 10:12–16.

Olson, B.; Ustanko, L.; and Warner, S. January/February 1991. The patient in a halo brace: Striving for normalcy in body image and self-concept. *Orthopaedic Nursing* 10:44–50.

REFERENCES

Celeste, S. M.; Folcik, M. A.; and Dumas, K. M. July/August 1984. Identifying a standard for pin site care using the quality assurance approach. *Orthopaedic Nursing* 3:17–24.

Jobes, R. D. July/August 1982. Cranial nerve assessment with halo traction. *Orthopaedic Nursing* 1:11–15.

Jones, I. H. June 6, 1990. Making sense of . . . traction. *Nursing Times* 86:39–41.

Jones-Walton, P. March/April 1991. Clinical standards in skeletal traction pin site care. *Orthopaedic Nursing* 10:12–16.

Morris, L.; Kraft, S.; Tessem, S.; and Reinisch, S. January 1988. Nursing the patient in traction. *RN* 51:26–31.

————. February 1988. Special care for skeletal traction. *RN* 51:24–29.

Osborne, L. J., and Digiacomo, I. July/August 1987. Traction: A review with nursing diagnoses and interventions. *Orthopaedic Nursing* 6:13–19.

Rutecki, B., and Seligson, D. October 1980. Caring for the client in a halo apparatus. *Nursing 80* 10:73–77 (Canadians ed. pp. 19–23).

Sproles, K. J. January/February 1985. Nursing care of skeletal pins: A closer look. *Orthopaedic Nursing* 4:11–12, 15–19.

York, N., and Cowan, D. January 1980. Halo traction. *Canadian Nurse* 76:28–31.

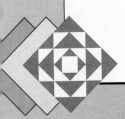

45

Therapeutic Beds

CONTENTS

NURSING PROCESS GUIDE
THERAPEUTIC BEDS

ASSESSMENT

Assess

- Specific complaints of discomfort.

- Neurologic status, e.g., feelings of numbness or tingling in the extremities, ability to move extremities, and motor strength of extremities. Most agencies have a checklist for neurologic assessments.

- Condition of the client's skin for irritation and pressure areas.

- Client's tolerance for specific positions. Some people tolerate the supine position for longer periods than the prone position.

- Other special needs required by the client, e.g., range-of-motion exercises.

RELATED DIAGNOSTIC CATEGORIES

- Anxiety

- Fear

- High risk for Disuse syndrome

- High risk for Infection

- High risk for Injury

- High risk for Impaired skin integrity

- Self-care deficit: Bathing/hygiene

- Potential Altered tissue perfusion (peripheral)

PLANNING

Client Goals
The client will

- Remain free of complications associated with immobility.

- Maintain adequate neurovascular status and tissue perfusion of affected extremities.

- Experience minimal anxiety.

Outcome Criteria
See Chapter 44, pages 1016–1017. Also see Chapter 21, page 499, for joint range of motion and Chapter 20, page 480, for pressure sores.

Therapeutic Beds

Therapeutic beds, also referred to as **specialty beds**, are bed units that provide a healing environment. They are used primarily to stabilize the spine, treat the complications of immobility (e.g., pulmonary congestion), and to relieve pressure and/or subsequent skin breakdown. Five major types of therapeutic beds are commonly used today. See Table 45–1.

Nurses should understand how to operate therapeutic beds before providing care. Operating instructions should be attached to the bed in a prominent place. They should be conveniently located for both the client and the nurse and have a lockout mechanism to prevent accidental activation. Beds that are operated electrically should have a backup source of power or be manually controlled. Before placing a client on a therapeutic bed, the nurse needs to test it to make sure it is in good working order. Clients and support persons usually require an explanation, and a demonstration can be reassuring. Mattress sections of therapeutic beds must be covered by sheets; special sheets are often available.

The Stryker Frame and Stryker Wedge Frame

The **Stryker frame** (Figure 45–1) consists of two removable rectangular metal frames (anterior and posterior) with canvas stretched across them. Thin, sponge-rubber mattresses, covered with special sheets with ties, are placed over the canvas. The frames are fastened by a knurled nut to a metal attachment at the head and the foot.

To allow use of the bedpan, the canvas and mattress on the posterior frame (used for the supine position) have a section that can be removed under the buttocks. An opening in the canvas and mattress of the anterior frame (used for the prone position) may be used to allow a male client to void. In the prone position, the canvas and mattress should extend from below the shoulders to the ankles. Narrow forehead and chin straps support the head. The bed is also equipped with armboard and footboard attachments. Three restraining straps (often fastened with Velcro) are placed around both frames when turning the client. Because the bed is so narrow, these restraints

TABLE 45–1   COMMONLY USED THERAPEUTIC BEDS

Type	Description	Brand Name	Indicated Use
Air-fluidized (AF) beds	Forced temperature-controlled air is circulated around millions of tiny silicone-coated beads.	Clinitron	Pressure relief
		Skytron	Treatment of pressure sores, burns
		FluidAir	As above for Skytron
Spinal stabilization	Permits frequent turning while maintaining spinal alignment.	Stryker Frame CircOlectric Bed Roto Rest	Spinal injury Immobilized clients
Static low-air-loss (LAL)	Consists of many air-filled cushions divided into 4 or 5 sections. Separate controls permit each section to be inflated to a different level of firmness.	Mediscus Flexicair	Pressure relief on bony prominences and/or compromised areas
		KenAir	Burns
Active or second generation low-air-loss	Like the static LAL but in addition gently pulsates or rotates from side to side, thus stimulating capillary blood flow and facilitating movement of pulmonary secretions.	Therapulse Rescue BioDyne	Immobilized clients who have pulmonary problems and compromised skin integrity
Special feature beds	*Obesity beds* permit care of obese clients. Some can assume sitting and Trendelenburg positions.	MegaBed Paragon	For clients over 300 lbs (some beds accommodate up to 800 lbs)
	Orthopedic beds can be used as a tilt table, recliner, or chair.	Nelson Bed	Immobilized clients

Adapted from C. M. Ceccio, Understanding therapeutic beds, *Orthopaedic Nursing*, May/June 1990, 9:57–70 and M. Martes, Put your patient on the right bed, *Orthopaedic Nursing*, July/August 1984, 3:51–54.

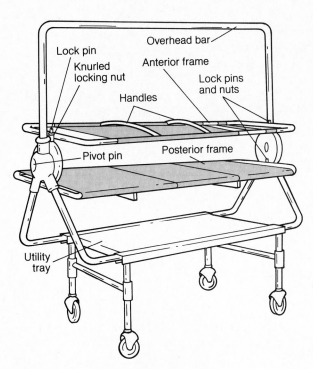

FIGURE 45–1   A standard Stryker turning frame.

 may also be fastened around the client as a safety precaution either continuously or at night.

An adaptation of the Stryker frame is the **Stryker wedge frame**, which by design requires only one nurse to turn the client (Figure 45–2). The upper frame is angled toward the lower frame at the side

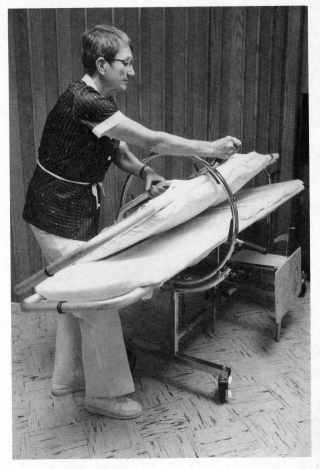

FIGURE 45–2   A Stryker wedge frame. Note the wedge shape formed by the anterior and posterior frames.

on which the frame will turn. This wedge prevents the client from sliding out between the frames during the turn. The frames are attached to a turning ring that the nurse can adjust to tighten the frame snugly over the client. The turning ring opens to form anterior and posterior rings, i.e., two half rings.

Clients on turning frames are generally turned every 2 hours, but the frequency of turning depends on the person's health status, care requirements, and tolerance. The nurse needs to establish the schedule for turning needs with the client and record it on the nursing care plan. The nurse usually schedules turns so that the client can sleep on the posterior frame and have meals on the anterior one.

Two nurses are essential to turn the client on standard frames; one nurse stands at the foot, the other at the head; on a signal, the nurses turn the client in unison. A third person may be required to ensure security of tubes and drains during turning. Only one nurse is required for the Stryker wedge frame unless agency protocol indicates that two nurses must be present. Technique 45–1 details the steps involved in turning a client on a Stryker wedge frame.

45-1 Turning a Client on a Stryker Wedge Frame

Before turning a client on a Stryker wedge frame, determine (a) skin care or other special needs, e.g., range-of-motion (ROM) exercises; (b) scheduled times for the turn; (c) whether restraining straps are applied continuously or only at night; (d) the client's record of tolerance for specific positions; and (e) which positioning supports are required. Footboards are generally attached to prevent footdrop when the client is in the supine position. When the client is prone, the feet should hang over the end of the canvas in a flexed position. To prevent external rotation of the hips, a sandbag or trochanter roll may be placed against the hips.

PURPOSES
- To maintain body alignment while changing the position
- To prevent skin, respiratory, and circulatory problems related to immobility

ASSESSMENT FOCUS
Body alignment; condition of the skin (i.e., any irritation or pressure areas); discomfort; neurologic status (e.g., numbness or tingling in the extremities, ability to move extremities, and motor strength of extremities). See also Table 43–1, page 1003.

EQUIPMENT
- Anterior or posterior frame, depending on the turn (these are usually kept at the bedside)
- Clean linen for the frame, as required
- Positioning devices (e.g., pillow supports, footboards)
- Restraining straps
- Protective devices for the skin (e.g., sheepskin)
- Incontinence pads, if required

INTERVENTION

1. Prepare the client.
- Before turning, ensure that all nursing care requirements are completed. For example, if the client is on the posterior frame, bathe all but the back, and place a clean gown on the person. *This eliminates the necessity of turning the client again for care.*

- Explain the direction in which the turn will take place, e.g., to the client's right or left. *This explanation provides reassurance.*

- If the client has suction or drainage tubes, place this equipment carefully at the head of the bed before the turn. Be sure that the tubing is long enough to accommodate the turn. *This will avoid pulling or tangling the tubing.* Place urinary drainage bags on the mattress beside the client; they must not pass above the client during the turn. *Drainage bags that pass above the client can cause backflow into the client.*

▶ **Technique 45–1** CONTINUED

Turning from Supine to Prone Position

2. Prepare the equipment.

- ⓢ Ensure that the wheels of the frame are locked. *The wheels are locked to prevent the frame from moving during the turn.*

- Remove the armboards and bed linen or bath blanket.

- Ensure that the anterior frame has clean linen on it.

3. Position the client.

- Make sure the client's arms are not extended beyond the turning radius. If the client is unconscious, do not remove the armboards until the arms are secured with straps.

- Place a pillow lengthwise over the lower legs. *The pillow provides security during the turn and maintains the alignment of the feet and legs.*

- Place the anterior frame over the client, and tighten the knurled nut at the head of the frame (Figure 45–3). The anterior frame will be angled with the posterior frame to form a wedge. If a standard Stryker frame, rather than the wedge frame, is used, fasten the knurled nuts at *both* the head and the foot of the frame, and do not angle the frames. *Tightening the knurled nut(s) keeps the frame securely in place during the turn.*

- Ensure that the forehead and chin bands are placed appropriately, i.e., that they do not obstruct the nose, mouth, and eyes. A pillow may be placed beside the head. *The pillow prevents lateral movement during the turn.*

- Close the turning ring over the anterior frame, making sure that it is locked securely and that the frame fits snugly over the client. The nuts on the anterior turning ring can be adjusted to tighten the frame against the client. Di-

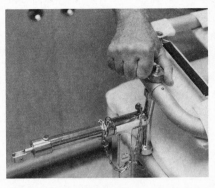

FIGURE 45–3　Tightening the knurled nut at the head of the frame.

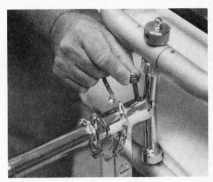

FIGURE 45–4　Pulling out the lock pin at the head of the frame.

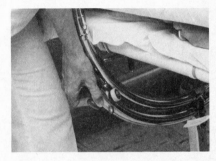

FIGURE 45–5　Pulling out the lock knob on the turning ring.

rections for doing this are written on the frame.

- Place the two restraining straps around both the frame and the client's legs and chest. Buckle the straps at the side of the client. If the standard Stryker frame is used, a third restraining strap is usually placed over the hips (on the wedge frame, the turning ring is positioned over the hips). *The straps prevent the client from slipping, especially the arms, if the client is unable to use them. Placing the strap buckle at the side makes it easier to open after the turn.*

4. Turn the client.

- Ask the client to wrap both arms around the anterior frame, if able. Otherwise, make sure that the arms are restrained. *This provides greater security when turning.*

- Pull out the positive lock pin at the head of the frame (Figure 45–4). *The frame can pivot when this pin is out.*

- Pull out the red turning lock knob on the turning ring (Figure 45–5). *This allows the frame to turn.*

- Grasp the handle on the turning ring, and inform the client that you will turn on the count of 3. When two nurses are present, the nurse at the head of the stan-

dard bed usually gives the directions for turning.

- Count to 3, and turn the frame toward you and toward the narrower side of the wedge, using a smooth, gradual motion. *People feel more secure when turned toward the nurse.*

5. Secure the frame.

- Replace the positive lock pin. *The pin stabilizes the frame and prevents it from pivoting.*

- Push in the circular silver lock knob (Figure 45–6). *This opens the turning ring.*

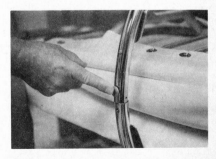

FIGURE 45–6　Pushing in the silver lock knob.

▶

▶ **Technique 45–1 Turning a Client on a Stryker Wedge Frame** *CONTINUED*

• Release the knurled nut, and remove the posterior frame.

6. Provide necessary care, and position the client.

Turning from Prone to Supine Position

7. Prepare the client as in step 1 above.

🅢 • Ensure that the wheels of the frame are locked.

• Remove the armboards and bed linen or bath blanket, and ensure that the posterior frame has clean linen on it.

• Make sure the client's arms are not extended beyond the turning radius. If the client is unconscious, do not remove the armboards until the arms are secured with straps.

• Place incontinence pads or sheepskins over the client's sacrum, if necessary, and put a small pillow under the lumber curvature, if required.

8. Secure the frame.

• Place the posterior frame over the person, and fasten it securely by tightening the knurled nut at the head of the frame.

• Close and lock the turning ring as in step 3.

• Place the two restraining straps around both the frame and the client's legs and chest as in step 3.

9. Turn the client as in steps 4 to 5, making necessary adjustments for the person moving from the prone to the supine position.

For Either Position

10. Provide care to the client.

• Provide skin care to pressure areas as required.

• Position the client in correct body alignment.

• Attach the armboards, and position the client's arms appropriately to prevent adduction contractures of the shoulders and flexion contractures of the

elbows. The armboards should be slightly below the level of the frame when the client is in the prone position and level with the frame when the client is in the supine position.

• Cover the client appropriately for warmth.

• Place restraining straps around the client as a protective measure if required. Generally, one restraining strap is placed around the hips for clients receiving narcotics or sedatives and for all people at bedtime.

• Instruct the client about foot or leg exercises, e.g., dorsiflexion and plantar flexion, inversion and eversion of the foot, if health indicates.

• Put clean linen and a pillow on the frame that was removed, in readiness for the next turn.

11. Document turning the client and all assessments and interventions according to agency practice.

EVALUATION FOCUS

Skin condition, joint range of motion; neurologic status; discomfort; tolerance of positions.

SAMPLE RECORDING

Date	Time	Notes
11/07/93	1700	Alternated prone and supine positions q3h. A 6 cm diameter area on sacrum remains reddened. No breaks in the skin. No discomfort or vertigo with turning but states does not like it. Left plantar reflex +1, Right plantar +2, Range-of-motion exercises performed. ——————— Ross Tom, SN

KEY ELEMENTS OF TURNING A CLIENT ON A STRYKER WEDGE FRAME

• Make sure the client understands the turning procedure.

• Before each turn, explain the direction in which the turn will occur and when it will take place.

• Provide skin care to bony prominences before and after the turn.

• Position the arms appropriately before the turn.

• Arrange tubing and containers appropriately before the turn.

• Lock the wheels of the bed before and after turns.

• Maintain the client's alignment during the turn.

• Make sure the frame is fastened securely before the turn.

• Apply restraining straps before the turn and around the client after turning as needed.

• Secure the frame after the turn.

The CircOlectric Bed

The **CircOlectric bed** (Figure 45–7) offers a greater variety of positions than the Stryker wedge frame. A CircOlectric bed can turn 210°, thus permitting a client to assume a variety of positions. For example, clients can be placed in standing position, Trendelenburg's position, and even sitting positions. Positions that tilt the client vertically toward the standing position are particularly useful for preventing postural hypotension and preparing the client for ambulation. From the standing position, a person can walk directly off the bed without changing the spinal alignment. Another advantage of the CircOlectric bed is that it can be operated independently by the client. Even very helpless people may be able to adjust their positions slightly and assume a greater degree of independence.

As Figure 45–8 shows, the CircOlectric bed consists of the following:

- An electrically operated circular framework and motor, which can be operated manually in case of a power failure.

- A posterior (basic) frame, for lying in the supine position, with a foam mattress, a mattress cover, and a headboard. A circular section of the mattress and a metal plate under the perineal area can be removed to insert a bedpan. The bedpan is held in place by special fasteners.

- An anterior frame, for lying in the prone position, with a foam mattress and cover.

- Special sheets that fasten to the mattresses with elastic bands.

- A footboard that attaches to the frame.

- A control switch to adjust the bed and a hand crank if it needs to be operated manually. The control switch has two labels, "Face" and "Back." The face switch turns the bed slowly to the prone position while the back switch turns it to supine position.

- Adjustable side rails.

- Forehead and chin supports for the anterior frame.

- Accessory equipment includes traction bars, an IV pole, exercise apparatus, and canvas arm slings to support the arms.

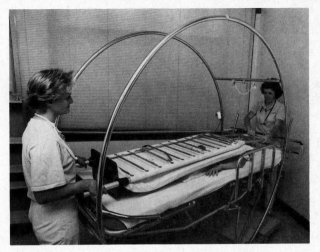

FIGURE 45–7 A CircOlectric bed with the anterior frame in place.

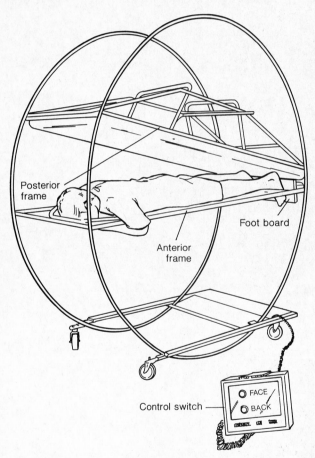

FIGURE 45–8 Some of the functional parts of a CircOlectric bed.

Technique 45–2 explains how to turn a client on a CircOlectric bed.

45-2 Turning a Client on a CircOlectric Bed

Before turning a client on a CircOlectric bed, determine (a) skin care requirements, (b) the position of pillows and other supports, (c) scheduled times for turning, and (d) tolerance of specific positions.

PURPOSES
- To maintain body alignment while changing position
- To permit the client to assume sitting, standing, and lying positions
- To prevent skin, respiratory, and circulatory problems related to immobility

ASSESSMENT FOCUS

Body alignment; condition of the skin; discomfort; neurologic status; vital signs.

EQUIPMENT

- Positioning devices (e.g., pillows, folded bath blankets, towels)
- Canvas arm slings and/or

- safety belt
- Restraining straps for the client in a prone position

- Skin care materials, including padding for bony prominences, if needed

INTERVENTION

1. Prepare the client.

- Describe the technique and the sensations the client may experience. People often need considerable reassurance the first few times they are turned, because they experience vertigo (dizziness) from the turning. They also feel helpless and sometimes imagine that they will fall. It is important to discuss these sensations and reassure them that the turning is carefully controlled and can be stopped at any time.

2. Prepare the equipment.

All Turns

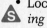 • Lock the wheels of the bed. *Locking the wheels prevents the bed from moving during turning.*

- Free any tubing, and arrange tubing and containers appropriately prior to the turn. *Tubing can become tangled during the turn if it is not arranged beforehand.*

- Maintain eye contact with the client during any turn. *Maintaining eye contact is reassuring to the client and allows you to become immediately aware of any problem.*

- Do not stop a turn until the client reaches the intended position unless it is absolutely necessary. *Stopping and then starting a turn can increase a client's nausea and vertigo.*

- Maintain traction (e.g., skull tongs) during the turn. *Lack of traction can result in nonalignment of the vertebral column.*

Turning from Supine to Upright or Prone Position

- Measure the distance from the client's shoulders to ankles, and adjust the canvas of the anterior frame to fit the body. *The anterior frame should support the body from the shoulders to the ankles.*

- Remove the restraining strap and top covers from the client.

- Place a pillow or folded bath blanket lengthwise over the lower legs. *This padding maintains their alignment and prevents movement during the turn.*

- Remove the pillow under the head.

- Place the anterior frame over the client and fasten the bolts at both ends.

- Adjust the head support, and pad

it if necessary.

3. Position the client.

• Make sure the client's feet are placed where they will not be injured by the footboard.

- Assist the client to place both arms around the anterior frame. If the client cannot grasp the frame, place the arms alongside the body and secure them with a restraining strap, or place the arms in the canvas slings (Figure 45–9).

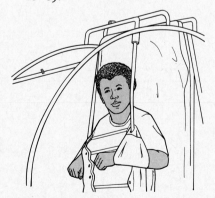

FIGURE 45–9 Supporting the arms in canvas slings.

4. Turn the client.

- Inform the client, then turn on the control marked "Face." The bed will move slowly, turning the client toward a prone position.

► **Technique 45–2** CONTINUED

(For an upright position, stop the bed when the client is vertical. The upright position is first established with the anterior frame in place. When the person tolerates standing between the frames for 5 to 10 minutes, the client then progresses to standing with only restraining straps at the waist and the knees.)

- Release the switch when the client is in position, e.g., when the client is horizontal.

- Release the locks on the posterior frame, and push the frame upward until it locks in its gatched (raised) position.

- Adjust the client's body to ensure correct alignment.

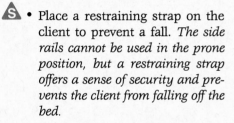 • Place a restraining strap on the client to prevent a fall. *The side rails cannot be used in the prone position, but a restraining strap offers a sense of security and prevents the client from falling off the bed.*

Turning from Prone to Supine Position

5. Prepare the equipment.

- Remove the restraining strap and top covers from the client.

- Make sure that the footboard is placed against the feet. *The footboard helps to stabilize the client during the turn.*

- Disengage the posterior frame from its raised position by releasing the lock and pushing the frame upward.

- Lower the frame so that it fits over the client, then fasten the bolts at both ends.

6. Turn the client.

- Secure the client's arms as in step 3.

- Inform the client, then turn on the control marked "Back." The bed will move slowly to turn the client toward a supine position.

- Release the switch when the bed is horizontal or in the desired position.

- Release the locks on the anterior frame, and remove the frame.

7. Assist the client to a comfortable position.

- Remove the pillow or bath blanket over the legs.

- Adjust the body for correct alignment. Provide supports, e.g., a head pillow, as required.

- Adjust the side rails, if necessary.

All Turns

8. Provide any nursing interventions as required.

- Provide skin care to bony prominences before and after the turn. *Skin care before a turn treats the pressure areas onto which the client will be moved; after a turn it will treat pressure areas the client has been lying on.*

9. Document relevant assessments and interventions.

- In many agencies, turns are recorded in a summary statement at the end of a shift.

EVALUATION FOCUS | Tolerance of the turns (i.e., discomfort, vertigo, syncope, nausea, pallor); condition of the skin; neurologic status; vital signs.

SAMPLE RECORDING

Date	Time	Notes
11/06/93	1600	Alternated supine, prone and sitting position q3h. Verbalized vertigo after supine to sitting position. B.P. 90/70 -P.96-R.30. Vertigo stopped in 5 minutes. Skin reddened over coccyx; no broken areas. Full range-of-motion exercises performed q3h. Left plantar, achilles reflexes +1. Right plantar achilles reflex +3. Right patellar +4, Left patellar +1. ———————— Rosanne L. Russel, RN

KEY ELEMENTS OF TURNING A CLIENT ON A CIRCOLECTRIC BED

- Make sure the client understands the turning procedure.
- Before each turn, explain the direction in which the turn will occur and when it will take place.
- Provide skin care to bony prominences before and after the turn.
- Apply alignment supports as required.

- Arrange tubing and containers appropriately before the turn.
- Lock the wheels of the bed before and after turns.
- Maintain the client's alignment during the turn.
- Make sure the bed is fastened securely before the turn.
- Apply restraining straps before the turn and after the turn as required.

The Nelson Bed

The **Nelson bed** is used in orthopedic practice. It can be tilted or used in the reclining position or as a chair (Figure 45–10). For clients who cannot flex their hip joints, the bed can be tipped to a vertical position so that the client can step from the bed without hip flexion. This bed is frequently used for clients who have bilateral spica casts, amputations, or fractured femurs. It does not have pressure-relieving properties.

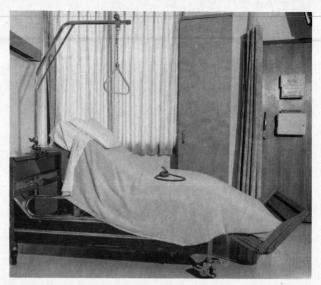

FIGURE 45–10   A Nelson bed in a sitting position.

CRITICAL THINKING CHALLENGE

Adam Graves, a 38-year-old male with a spinal cord injury, has been placed on a CircOlectric bed to facilitate care. When you prepare to turn him from the supine to the prone position, what signs would indicate that he is anxious? If he is anxious, how will you respond? What will you do?

RELATED RESEARCH

Pieper, B.; Mikols, C.; Adams, W.; and Mance, B. May/June 1990. Low and high air-loss beds in acute care hospitals. *Journal of Enterstomal Therapy* 17:131–36.

Walsh, M., and Brescia, F. J. February 1990. Clinitron therapy and pain management in advanced cancer patients. *Journal of Pain and Symptom Management* 5:46–50.

REFERENCES

Allan, D. August 15–21, 1984. Care of the patient in a wedge turning frame . . . Stryker frame. *Nursing Times* 80:40–41.

Ceccio, C. M. May/June 1990. Understanding therapeutic beds. *Orthopaedic Nursing* 9:57–70.

Lovell, H. W., and Anderson, C. L. May 1990. Put your patient on the right bed. *RN* 53:66–72.

Martes, M. July/August 1984. The Nelson bed on an orthopaedic unit. *Orthopaedic Nursing* 3:51–54.

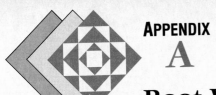

Root Words, Prefixes, and Suffixes

Word element	Meaning
ROOT WORDS	
Circulatory System	
cardio	heart
angio, vaso	vessel
hem, hema, hemato	blood
vena, phlebo	vein
arteria	artery
lympho	lymph
thrombo	clot (of blood)
embolus	moving clot
Digestive System	
bucca	cheek
os, stomato	mouth
gingiva	gum
glossa	tongue
pharyngo	pharynx
esophago	esophagus
gastro	stomach
hepato	liver
cholecyst	gallbladder
pancreas	pancreas
entero	intestines
duodeno	duodenum
jejuno	jejunum
ileo	ileum
caeco	cecum
appendeco	appendix
colo	colon
recto	rectum
ano, procto	anus
Skeletal System	
skeleto	skeleton
Respiratory System	
naso, rhino	nose
tonsillo	tonsil
laryngo	larynx
tracheo	trachea
bronchus, broncho	bronchus (pl. bronchi)
pulmo, pneuma, pneum	lung (sac with air)
Nervous System	
neuro	nerve

Word element	Meaning
cerebrum	brain
oculo, ophthalmo	eye
oto	ear
psych, psycho	mind
Urinary System	
urethro	urethra
cysto	bladder
uretero	ureter
reni, reno, nephro	kidney
pyelo	pelvis of kidney
uro	urine
Female Reproductive System	
vulvo	vulva
perineo	perineum
labio	labium (pl. labia)
vagino, colpo	vagina
cervico	cervix
utero	womb; uterus
tubo, salpingo	fallopian tube
ovario, oophoro	ovary
Male Reproduction System	
orchido	testes
Regions of the Body	
crani, cephalo	head
cervico, tracheo	neck
thoraco	chest
abdomino	abdomen
dorsum	back
Tissues	
cutis, dermato	skin
lipo	fat
musculo, myo	muscle
osteo	bone
myelo	marrow
chondro	cartilage
Miscellaneous	
cyto	cell
genetic	formation, origin
gram	tracing or mark

Word element	Meaning	Word element	Meaning
graph	writing, description	hepa, hepato	liver
kinesis	motion	histo	tissue
meter	measure	homo	same
oligo	small, few	hydro	water
phobia	fear	hygro	moisture
photo	light	hyper	too much, high
pyo	pus	hypo	under, decreased
scope	instrument for visual examination	hyster	uterus
		ileo	ileum
roentgen	x-ray	in	in, within, into
lapar	flank; through the abdominal wall	inter	between
		intra	within
		intro	in, within, into
PREFIXES		juxta	near, close to
a, an, ar	without or not	laryngo	larynx
ab	away from	latero	side
acro	extremities	lapar	abdomen
ad	toward, to	leuk	white
adeno	glandular	macro	large, big
aero	air	mal	bad, poor
ambi	around, on both sides	mast	breast
amyl	starch	medio	middle
ante	before, forward	mega, megalo	large, great
anti	against, counteracting	meno	menses
bi	double	mono	single
bili	bile	multi	many
bio	life	myelo	bone marrow, spinal cord
bis	two		
brachio	arm	myo	muscle
brady	slow	neo	new
broncho	bronchus (pl. bronchi)	nephro	kidney
cardio	heart	neuro	nerve
cervico	neck	nitro	nitrogen
chole	gall or bile	noct	night
cholecysto	gallbladder	non	not
circum	around	ob	against, in front of
co	together	oculo	eye
contra	against, opposite	odonto	tooth
costo	ribs	ophthalmo	eye
cyto	cell	ortho	straight, normal
cysto	bladder	os	mouth, bone
demi	half	osteo	bone
derma	skin	oto	ear
dis	from	pan	all
dorso	back	para	beside, accessory to
dys	abnormal, difficult	path	disease
electro	electric	ped	child, foot
en	into, in, within	per	by, through
encephal	brain	peri	around
entero	intestine	pharyngo	pharynx
equi	equal	phlebo	vein
eryth	red	photo	light
ex	out, out of, away from	phren	diaphragm, mind
extra	outside of, in addition to	pneumo	air, lungs
ferro	iron	pod	foot
fibro	fiber	poly	many, much
fore	before, in front of	post	after
gastro	stomach	pre	before
glosso	tongue	proct	rectum
glyco	sugar	pseudo	false
hemi	half	psych	mind
hemo	blood	pyel	pelvis of the kidney
		pyo	pus

Word element	Meaning	Word element	Meaning
pyro	fever, heat	emia	blood
quadri	four	esis	action
radio	radiation	form	shaped like
re	back, again	genesis, genetric	formation, origin
reno	kidney	gram	tracing, mark
retro	backward	graph	writing
rhin	nose	ism	condition
sacro	sacrum	itis	inflammation
salpingo	fallopian tube	ize	to treat
sarco	flesh	lith	stone, calculus
sclero	hard, hardening	lithiasis	presence of stones
semi	half	lysis	disintegration
sex	six	megaly	enlargement
skeleto	skeleton	meter	instrument that measures
steno	narrowing, constriction		
sub	under	oid	likeness, resemblance
super	above, excess	oma	tumor
supra	above	opathy	disease of
syn	together	orrhaphy	surgical repair
tachy	fast	osis	disease, condition of
thyro	thyroid, gland	ostomy	to form an opening or outlet
trache	trachea		
trans	across, over	otomy	to incise
tri	three	pexy	fixation
ultra	beyond	phage	ingesting
un	not, back, reversal	phobia	fear
uni	one	plasty	plastic surgery
uretero	ureter	plegia	paralysis
urethro	urethra	rhage	to burst forth
uro	urine, urinary organs	rhea	excessive discharge
vaso	vessel	rhexis	rupture
		scope	lighted instrument for visual examination

SUFFIXES

Word element	Meaning	Word element	Meaning
able	able to	scopy	to examine visually
algia	pain	stomy	to form an opening
cele	tumor, swelling	tomy	incision into
centesis	surgical puncture to remove fluid	uria	urine
cide	killing, destructive		
cule	little		
cyte	cell		
ectasia	dilating, stretching		
ectomy	excision, surgical removal of		

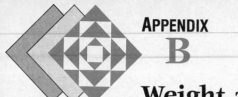

Weight and Volume Equivalents

Metric Equivalents

WEIGHTS

1 picogram	=	10^{-12} gram
1 nanogram	=	10^{-9} gram
1 microgram	=	10^{-3} milligram = 10^{-6} gram
1 milligram	=	1000 micrograms = 10^{-6} gram
1 centigram	=	10 milligrams = 10^{-1} decigram = 10^{-2} gram
1 decigram	=	100 milligrams = 10 centigrams = 10^{-1} gram
1 gram	=	1000 milligrams = 100 centigrams = 10 decigrams
1 kilogram	=	1000 grams

VOLUME

1 milliliter	=	1 gram
1 liter	=	1 kilogram = 1000 grams (milliliters)

Approximate Weight Equivalents: Metric and Apothecaries' Systems

METRIC	APOTHECARIES'	METRIC	APOTHECARIES'
0.1 mg	1/600 grain	30 mg	1/2 grain
1.12 mg	1/500 grain	40 mg	2/3 grain
0.15 mg	1/400 grain	50 mg	3/4 grain
0.2 mg	1/300 grain	60 mg	1 grain
0.25 mg	1/250 grain	100 mg (0.1 gm)	1-1/2 grains
0.3 mg	1/200 grain	150 mg (0.15 gm)	2-1/2 grains
0.4 mg	1/150 grain	200 mg (0.2 gm)	3 grains
0.5 mg	1/120 grain	300 mg (0.3 gm)	5 grains
0.6 mg	1/100 grain	400 mg (0.4 gm)	6 grains
0.8 mg	1/80 grain	500 mg (0.5 gm)	7-1/2 grains
1 mg	1/60 grain	600 mg (0.6 gm)	10 grains
1.2 mg	1/50 grain	1 gram	15 grains
1.5 mg	1/40 grain	1.5 gm	22 grains
2 mg	1/30 grain	2 gm	30 grains
3 mg	1/20 grain	3 gm	45 grains
4 mg	1/15 grain	4 gm	60 grains (1 dram)
5 mg	1/12 grain	5 gm	75 grains
6 mg	1/10 grain	6 gm	90 grains
8 mg	1/8 grain	7.5 gm	120 grains (2 drams)
10 mg	1/6 grain	10 gm	2-1/2 drams
12 mg	1/5 grain	30 gm	1 ounce (8 drams)
15 mg	1/4 grain	500 gm	1.1 pounds
20 mg	1/3 grain	1000 gm	2.2 pounds (1 kilogram)
25 mg	3/8 grain		

Approximate Volume Equivalents: Metric, Apothecaries', and Household Systems

METRIC	APOTHECARIES'	HOUSEHOLD
0.06 ml	1 minim (m)	1 drop (qt)
0.3 ml	5 minims	
0.6 ml	10 minims	
1 ml	15 minims	15 drops (gtt)
2 ml	30 minims	
3 ml	45 minims	
4 ml	60 minims (1 fluid dram [f$\mathfrak{Z}$])	60 drops (1 teaspoon [tsp])
8 ml	2 fluid drams	2 teaspoons
15 ml	4 fluid drams	4 teaspoons (1 tablespoon [Tbsp])
30 ml	8 fluid drams (1 fluid ounce f$\mathfrak{Z}$])	2 tablespoons
60 ml	2 fluid ounces	
90 ml	3 fluid ounces	
200 ml	6 fluid ounces	1 teacup
250 ml	8 fluid ounces	1 large glass
500 ml	16 fluid ounces (1 pint)	1 pint
750 ml	1½ pints	
1000 ml (1 liter)	2 pints (1 quart)	1 quart
4000 ml	4 quarts	1 gallon

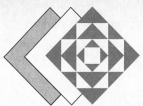

Glossary

abdominal paracentesis removal of fluids from the peritoneal cavity

abduction movement of a bone away from the midline of the body

abortion termination of a pregnancy before the fetus reaches the stage of viability; may be accidental or spontaneous, or induced

abruptio placenta premature partial or complete separation of a normally implanted placenta after the 20th week of gestation

accountability being responsible for one's actions and accepting the consequences of one's behavior

acholic clay colored and free from bile

acidemia (acidosis) a condition that occurs with increases in blood carbonic acid or with decreases in blood bicarbonate; blood pH below 7.35

acidosis (acidemia) a condition that occurs with increases in blood carbonic acid or with decreases in blood bicarbonate; blood pH below 7.35

acne an inflammatory condition of the sebaceous glands

acromegaly a disorder caused by excessive growth hormone secretion

active assistive range-of-motion (ROM) exercise the client—with the nurse's assistance—uses a stronger, opposite arm or leg to move each of the joints of a limb incapable of active motion

active range-of-motion (ROM) exercise isotonic exercise in which the client moves each joint in the body through its complete range of movement, maximally stretching all muscle groups within each plane, over the joint

actual health problem deviations from health that can be clinically validated by identifiable defining characteristics

adduction movement of a bone toward the midline of the body

ADL's, activities of daily living the tasks of daily life, e.g., eating, bathing, and dressing

adipose fat; of a fatty nature

adventitious breath sounds abnormal or acquired breath sounds

advocate an individual who pleads the cause of another or argues or pleads for a cause or proposal

aerobic requiring oxygen

affect feelings, emotions

afterbirth the placenta and membranes that are expelled during the third stage of labor after the birth of the infant

afterpains abdominal pains that are "cramp like", caused by uterine contractions that occur after childbirth

agglutinin a specific antibody formed in the blood

agglutinogen a substance that acts as an antigen and stimulates the production of agglutinins

albinism the complete or partial lack of melanin in the skin, hair, and eyes

albumin the main protein found in the blood, also found in breast milk

algor mortis the gradual decrease of the body's temperature after death

alignment (posture) the proper relationship of body segments to one another

alkalemia (alkalosis) a condition that occurs with increases in blood bicarbonate or decreases in blood carbonic acid; blood pH above 7.45

alkalosis (alkalemia) a condition that occurs with increases in blood bicarbonate or decreases in blood carbonic acid; blood pH above 7.45

alopecia the loss of scalp (baldness) or body hair

alternating pressure mattress (airbed) a specialized mattress attached to a motor that lowers or raises the air pressure inside the mattress, designed to decrease pressure on bony prominences

amblyopia reduced visual acuity in one eye

Ambu bag (resuscitation bag) a device used to provide oxygen to a client when they are unable to breathe for themselves

ambulation the act of walking

amino acid one of a group of organic acids containing nitrogen that are considered the components of protein

ammonia dermatitis diaper rash

amniocentesis removal of a specimen of amniotic fluid from the amniotic sac in the uterus

amniotic fluid the clear fluid inside the amnion surrounding the fetus that provides physical protection for and helps maintain temperature of the fetus and facilitates its movement

ampule a small glass container for individual doses of liquid medications

anabolism a process in which simple substances are converted by the body cells into more complex substances, e.g., building tissue, positive nitrogen balance

anaerobic not requiring oxygen to live

analysis the separation into components, breaking down the whole into its parts

anemia a condition in which the blood is deficient in red blood cells or hemoglobin

anesthesia loss of sensation or feeling; induced loss of the sense of pain

angiography a diagnostic procedure enabling X-ray visual examination of the vascular system after injection of a radiopaque dye

angle of Louis the junction between the body of the sternum and the manubrium

anions ions that carry a negative charge; chloride, bicarbonate, phosphate, sulfate

anisocoria unequal pupils

ankylosis permanent fixation of a joint

anorexia lack of appetite

anoscopy visual examination of the anal canal using an anoscope (a lighted instrument)

anoxia systemic absence or reduction of oxygen in the body tissues below physiologic levels

antecubital fossa or space the point on the arm located in front of the elbow

anthropometric measurements measurements of the size and composition of the body, e.g., height, weight, skinfold

antimicrobial destructive to or preventing the development of microorganisms

antiseptic an agent that inhibits the growth of specific microorganisms

anuria the failure of the kidneys to produce urine, resulting in a total lack of urination or output of less than 100 ml per day in an adult

apical pulse a central pulse located at the apex of the heart

APIE an acronym for a charting method that follows the sequence of assessment, planning, implementation, evaluation

apnea a complete absence of respirations

apothecary a system of medication measurement that derives from England

approximate (wound edges) to bring close together

aquathermia to treat with warm water

arm muscle circumference (AMC) considered an index of the body's protein reserves, calculated from the triceps skinfold and mid-upper arm circumference

arrector pili muscles the erector muscle attached to the hair follicle

arterial blood pressure the measure of the pressure exerted by the blood as it pulsates through the arteries

arteriosclerosis a condition in which the elastic and muscular tissues of the arteries are replaced with fibrous tissue

arrhythmia (dysrhythmia) a pulse that has an abnormal rhythm

ascites the accumulation of fluid in the abdominal cavity

aspirate to remove gases or fluids from a cavity by using suction

asepsis freedom from infection or infectious material

assault an attempt or threat to touch another person unjustifiably

assessing the process of collecting, verifying, and organizing data (information) about a client's health status

associative thinking thinking that involves random, unstructured thoughts (day dreaming)

astigmatism an uneven curvature of the cornea that prevents horizontal and vertical rays from focusing on the retina

atalectasis a condition that occurs when ventilation is decreased in which pooled secretions accumulate in a dependent area of a bronchiole and block it

ataxia abnormally altered muscular coordination

atelectasis collapse of lung tissue

athlete's foot a fungal infection of the foot caused by tinea pedis

atomizer a device that produces large droplets for inhalation

atony lack of normal muscle tone

atrioventricular (AV) node the neuromuscular tissue of the heart at the base of the atrial septum that conveys impulses to the ventricles

atrophy wasting away; decrease in size or organ or tissue, e.g., muscle

attitude a feeling or belief directed toward a person, object, or idea

audit (nursing) a process in which nursing interventions are monitored and measured against established standards

auricle the visible part of the ear

auscultation the process of listening to sounds produced within the body

auscultatory gap the temporary disappearance of sounds normally heard over the brachial artery when the sphygmomanometer cuff pressure is high and the sounds reappear at a lower level

autonomy the state of being independent and self-directed without outside control

autopsy (postmortem examination) an examination of the body after death to determine the cause of death and to learn more about a disease process

axilla armpit

bactericidal capable of killing bacteria

bag of waters the membranes (amnion and chorion) that contain the amniotic fluid and fetus

balance stability; steadiness; equilibrium

bandage a strip of cloth used to wrap a part of the body

barium enema an X-ray filming of the large intestine using a contrast medium; also called a lower gastrointestinal series or lower GI series

barium swallow an X-ray filming of the esophagus, stomach, and duodenum; also referred to as an upper gastrointestinal series or upper GI series

barrel chest a variation of shape in the chest where the ratio of the anteroposterior to lateral diameter is 1 to 1

basal metabolic rate (BMR) the rate of energy utilization in the body required to maintain essential activities such as breathing

base of support the area on which an object rests

battery the willful or negligent touching of a person (or the person's clothes or even something the person is carrying), which may or may not cause harm

Beau's lines transverse white lines or grooves in the nail resulting from severe injury or illness

bed cradle a device designed to keep the top bedclothes off the feet, legs, and abdomen

belief (opinion) something people judge to be true on the basis of probability rather than actuality, an attitude whose cognitive component is based more on faith than on fact

binder a type of bandage applied to large body areas (abdomen or chest) or for a specific body part (arm sling); used to provide support

binocular vision ability to focus on images with both eyes

bioethics ethical rules or principles that govern right conduct concerning life

biofeedback a stress management technique that brings under conscious control bodily processes normally thought to be beyond voluntary command

biopsy the removal and examination of tissue from the living body

blood volume expanders solutions used to increase the volume of blood following severe loss of blood

bloody show pink or blood-tinged vaginal mucous discharge caused by the rupture of small capillaries as the cervix dilates and effaces in early labor

body mass index (BMI) indicates whether weight is appropriate for height

body mechanics the efficient and coordinated use of the body to produce motion and maintain balance during activity

body temperature the balance between the heat produced by the body and the heat lost from the body

boggy uterus a soft and spongy feeling of the uterus upon palpation, reflecting an inadequately contracted uterus

bowel diversion the surgical creation of an ostomy to enable the excretion of fecal waste while at the same time rerouting the feces away from a specific segment of the intestine

bowel incontinence (fecal incontinence) refers to loss of voluntary ability to control fecal and gaseous discharges through the anal sphincter

bradycardia abnormally slow pulse rate, less than 60 per minute

bradypnea abnormally slow respiratory rate, usually less than 10 respirations per minute

Braxton Hicks contractions painless, periodic uterine contractions that occur during pregnancy and are often mistaken for true labor

breech presentation a common abnormality of delivery where the fetal buttocks or feet present rather than the head

bromhidrosis foul-smelling perspiration

bronchoscopy visual examination of the bronchi using a bronchoscope

bruit a blowing or swishing sound created by turbulence of blood flow

bruxism grinding of the teeth during sleep

Bryant's traction a type of traction used to stabilize fractured femurs or correct congenital hip dislocation in young children

buccal pertaining to the cheek

Buck's extension a type of simple traction used to immobilize fractures of the hip and reduce muscle spasm before surgical repair

buffer an agent or system that tends to maintain constancy or that prevents changes in the chemical concentration of a substance

bunion lateral deviation of the big toe with swelling or callus formation over the metatarsophalangeal joint

burn to undergo an alteration or destruction of the skin and/or other body tissues by fire, hot substance, chemical, or radiation

cafe-au-lait spots spots of patchy pigmentation of skin, usually light brown in color

callus (bone) early bone, formed following fracture of a bone, that is normally ultimately replaced by hard bone

callus (skin) a thickened portion of the skin

caloric value the amount of energy that nutrients or foods supply to the body

calorie a unit of heat energy

cannula a tube with a lumen (channel) that is inserted into a cavity or duct and is often fitted with a trocar during insertion

canthus the angular junction of the eyelids at each corner of the eyes

carbohydrate a nutrient composed of carbon, hydrogen, and oxygen, e.g., starches and sugars

cardiac monitor a machine used to enable continual observation or monitoring of the electrical function of the heart

cardiac output the amount of blood ejected by the heart with each ventricular contraction

caries (dental) tooth cavities

carrier a person or animal that harbors a specific infectious agent and serves as a potential source of infection, yet does not manifest any clinical signs of disease

cast a rigid cylindrical dressing or casing used to immobilize various parts of the body

catabolism a destructive process in which complex substances are broken down into simpler substances, e.g., breakdown of tissue

cataracts opacity of the lens or capsule of the eye

catheter a tube of rubber, plastic, metal, or other material used to remove or inject fluids into a cavity such as the bladder

cations ions that carry a positive charge; sodium, potassium, calcium, magnesium

CAT scan *see* tomography

cementum calcified tissue covering the root of a tooth

center of gravity the point at which the mass (weight) of the body is centered

centigrade (Celsius) a thermometer scale used to measure heat; the freezing point of water is 0 C and the boiling point is 100 C

central venous line a catheter inserted into a large vein located centrally in the body, e.g., the superior vena cava, right atrium

central venous pressure (CVP) the measurement of the pressure of the blood, in millimeters of water, within the vena cava or the right atrium of the heart

cephalic pertaining to the head

cephalic presentation fetal delivery in which the head is the presenting part

cerebral death the higher brain center or cerebral cortex is irreversibly destroyed

cerumen the wax-like substance secreted by glands in the external ear canal

cervical dilation the process in which there is a widening of the cervical os and canal allowing the passage of the infant

cervical head halter traction a device that provides skin-encircling traction on the cervical spine to relieve muscle spasm and nerve compression related to cervical injuries in the neck, upper arms, or shoulders

cervical os the opening of the uterus

Chadwick's sign violet, bluish color of vaginal mucosa seen at 8 to 11 weeks of gestation

change agent a person or group who initiates changes or who assists others in making modifications in themselves or in the system

charting by exception a documentation method in which only significant findings or exceptions to norms are recorded

chemical restraints medications used to control socially disruptive behavior

chemical thermogenesis the stimulation of heat production in the body through increased cellular metabolism caused by increases in thyroxine output

choanal atresia congenital occlusion of the opening between the nasal cavities and the nasopharynx

cholangiography (cholangiogram) an X-ray film of the biliary tract taken after the injection of a dye

cholecystogram (cholecystography, oral cholecystography) an X-ray film of the gallbladder after ingestion of a contrast dye

cholesterol a lipid that does not contain fatty acid but possesses many of the chemical and physical properties of other lipids

chronologic charting a written record of information in sequence as time moves forward

Chvostek's sign an indication of tetany; spasm of facial muscles in response to a tap over the facial nerve

cilia hairlike projections of the respiratory mucous membrane

CircOlectric bed a therapeutic bed that enables a variety of client positions

circumduction movement of the distal part of the bone in a circle while the proximal end remains fixed

clapping (percussion, cupping) the forceful striking of the skin with cupped hands to loosen secretions in the lungs

clean free of potentially infectious agents

client a person who engages the advice or services of another who is qualified to provide this service

client advocate an individual who advocates or pleads the cause of clients' rights

client goal a broad statement about the expected or desired change in the status of the client after the client receives nursing interventions

closed bed an unoccupied bed with the top covers drawn up to the top of the bed under the pillows

closed wound a tissue injury without a break in the skin

clubbing (of a nail) elevation of the proximal aspect of the nail and softening of the nail bed

coarctation (of the aorta) severe narrowing of the aorta

cochlea a seashell-shaped structure located in the inner ear; it has numerous apertures for passage of the cochlear division of the auditory nerve

code of ethics a means by which professional standards of practice are established, maintained, and improved

cognitive referring to intellectual processes such as remembering, thinking, perceiving, abstracting, and generalizing

cognitive appraisal (Lazarus) an evaluative process that determines why and to what extent a particular transaction or series of transactions between the person and the environment is stressful

collaborative nursing action those activities performed either jointly with another member of the health care team or as a result of a joint decision by the nurse and another health care team member

colonization the presence of organisms in body secretions or excretions in which strains of bacteria become resident flora but do not cause illness

colonoscopy visual examination of the interior of the colon with a colonoscope

colostomy an opening into the colon (large bowel)

colostrum breast secretions that may occur from the second trimester of pregnancy onward, more commonly noted in the first 2 to 3 days after birth and before the onset of lactation. The immune properties of colostrum cleanse mucus and meconium from the gastrointestinal tract of the newborn

comedo a blackhead, a plug of dried sebum in a sebaceous gland

communication an interactive process (verbal and/or nonverbal) between two or more people with the goal of exchanging ideas, thoughts, information, or feelings

compartment syndrome the condition in which increased pressure in a limited space compromises or reduces the circulation and function of the tissues within the space

compliance the individual's desire to learn and to act on the learning

compliance (of arteries) the distensibility of the arteries, i.e., their ability to contract and expand

compound fracture fracture in which there is an open wound over the broken bone, or where bone fragments protrude through the skin

compress a moist gauze dressing applied frequently to an open wound; sometimes medicated

compromised host any person at increased risk for an infection

computerized axial tomography (CAT) *see* tomography

concave hollowed or rounded inward

concept a mental image of reality

conceptualization the intellectual process of forming a concept

condom a sheath or cover, usually made of rubber or plastic, worn over the penis during coitus to prevent conception or infection; urinary condoms are used to catch urine

conduction the transfer of heat from one molecule in direct contact to another

congruence in communication, when words and behavior coincide or are unified

conjunctiva a membrane covering the eyelids and eyeball

conjunctivitis inflammation of the bulbar and palpebral conjunctiva

constant data data or information that does not change, e.g., birthdate

constipation passage of small, dry, hard stool or passage of no stool for an abnormally long time

consumer an individual, a group of people, or a community that uses a service or commodity

contraction an intermittent tightening and shortening of uterine muscle fibers that cause cervical dilation and effacement during labor

contracture permanent shortening of a muscle and subsequent shortening of tendons and ligaments

contraindicate not indicated or inappropriate

convection the dispersion of heat by air currents

convex curved or rounded like the external surface of a sphere

coping (Lazarus) the process through which the individual manages the demands of the person-environment relationship that are appraised as stressful, and the emotions it generates

core temperature the temperature of the deep tissues of the body, e.g., thorax, abdominal cavity; relatively constant at 98.6F

corn a conical, circular, painful, raised area on the toe or foot

coroner a public official, not necessarily a physician, appointed or elected to inquire into the causes of death

costal breathing (thoracic breathing) breathing involving the external intercostal muscles and other accessory muscles, such as the sternocleidomastoid muscles

counseling the process of helping a client to recognize and cope with stressful psychologic or social problems, to improve interpersonal relationships, and to promote personal growth

countertraction a force that counteracts the direct pull of traction

covert data (symptoms, subjective data) information (data) apparent only to the person affected and can be described or verified only by that person

crackles (rales) bubbling or rattling sounds, audible by ear or stethoscope on inhalation; they are a result of fluid in the lungs

cradle cap a yellowish, oily crusting of the scalp of infants

creative thinking a productive intellectual skill that creates original ideas by establishing relationships among thoughts and concepts

crepitation (1) a dry, crackling sound like that of crumpled cellophane, produced by air in the subcutaneous tissue or by air moving through fluid in the alveoli of the lungs; (2) a crackling, grating sound produced by bone rubbing against bone

critical thinking a pattern of thinking based on knowledge, experience, and the ability to conceptualize and analyze relationships

cross-contamination the transfer of microorganisms from one surface to another

cross-referencing method listing all problems separately, using consecutive numbers and matching them with major health problems

crown (of tooth) the exposed part of a tooth outside the gum

crowning the appearance of the presenting fetal part at the vaginal opening during the labor process

crutch palsy a weakness of the muscles of the forearm, wrist, and hand caused by prolonged pressure of the crutch on the axillary nerve

cryotherapy therapeutic use of cold

cue a piece of information or data acquired through one of the five senses that influences decision-making

Cushing's syndrome a disorder in which there is increased adrenal hormone production

cuticle the flat, thin rim of skin surrounding the nail

cyanosis bluish discoloration of the skin and mucous membranes caused by reduced oxygen in the blood

cystectomy removal of the bladder

cystoscopy visual examination of the urinary bladder with a cystoscope

dacryocystitis inflammation of the lacrimal sac

dandruff dry or greasy, scaly material shed from the scalp

debilitated having lost strength

debridement removal of infected and necrotic tissue

decidua the endometrial lining of the uterus that encases the impregnated ovum and sloughs off after delivery as a part of lochia

decision making the process of choosing the best action to meet a desired goal

decode to relate the message perceived to the receiver's storehouse of knowledge and experience and to sort out the meaning of the message

decubitus ulcer an ulcer of the skin and underlying tissues produced by prolonged pressure

defecation expulsion of feces from the rectum and anus

defervescence the stage of abatement of a fever

dehydration insufficient fluid in the body

demise death

dentifrice a paste or powder used to clean or polish the teeth

dentin the chief substance of teeth, forming the body, neck, and roots; it is covered by enamel

dentures a natural or artificial set of teeth; usually the term designates artificial teeth

dependent edema edema of the lowest or most dependent parts of the body

dependent nursing action those activities carried out on the order of the physician, under the physician's supervision, or according to specified routines

depilatory a cream used to remove body hair

depolarize (cardiac muscle) to reduce toward a nonpolarized state; to cause loss of charge

dermatologic related to the skin

descent the channeling of the presenting part of the fetus through the birth canal

diagnosing the process that results in a diagnostic statement or nursing diagnosis that provides the basis for the selection of nursing interventions for the client

diaphoresis profuse perspiration

diaphragm the muscle structure separating the abdominal and thoracic cavities

diaphragmatic breathing (abdominal breathing) breathing that involves the contraction and relaxation of the diaphragm

diarrhea defecation of liquid feces and increased frequency of defecation

diastole the period during which the ventricles relax

diastolic pressure the pressure of the blood against the arterial walls when the ventricles of the heart are at rest

directive interview a highly structured communication to elicit specific information

directed thinking thinking that is purposeful and goal-directed

dirty contaminated by potentially infectious agents

disinfectant agent that destroys microorganisms other than spores

distal farthest from the point of reference

diuresis (polyuria) the production of abnormally large amounts of urine by the kidneys without an increased fluid intake

diuretic an agent that increases urine secretion

dorsal (supine) position a back-lying position without a pillow

dorsal recumbent position a back-lying position with the head and shoulders slightly elevated

douche vaginal irrigation, washing of the vagina by a liquid at a low pressure

drain a substance or appliance that assists in the discharge of serosanguinous fluid and purulent material from a wound and promotes healing of underlying tissues

drawsheet (half sheet) a special sheet, made of cotton, plastic, or rubber, that is placed across the center of the foundation of the bed used to facilitate moving bed bound clients

drip factor (drop factor) the number of drops per milliliter of solution delivered for a particular drip chamber before calculating the drip rate

droplet nuclei residue of evaporated droplets that remain in the air for long periods of time

drug (medication) a substance administered for the diagnosis, cure, treatment, mitigation, or prevention of disease

Duchenne muscular dystrophy a genetically acquired disease that causes gradual progressive muscle wasting

dullness a thud-like sound produced during percussion by dense tissue of body organs, such as the liver, spleen, or heart

dumping syndrome a condition experienced by jejunostomy clients when hypertonic foods and liquids suddenly distend the jejunum

Dunlop's traction (side-arm traction) combined horizontal and vertical adaptation of Buck's extension traction to the humerus and forearm

duration (of sound) the length of time that a sound is heard

dynorphins compounds found in the pituitary gland, hypothalamus, and spinal cord that seem to have an analgesic effect

dysphagia difficulty or inability to swallow

dyspnea difficult or labored breathing

dysrhythmia (arrhythmia) a pulse with an irregular rhythm

dysuria painful or difficult voiding

ecchymosis a bruise that changes in color from blue-black to greenish brown or yellow

ectopic pregnancy a pregnancy characterized by implantation of the ovum in an abnormal position outside the uterus

ectropion eversion or outturning of the eyelid

edema the presence of excess interstitial fluid in the body

effacement the process of thinning and shortening of the cervix that occurs during labor

effleurage a stroking massage technique

egg crate mattress a specialized foam rubber mattress designed to provide support while relieving pressure on the body's bony prominences

electrocardiogram (ECG, EKG) a graph of the electrical activity of the heart

electrocardiograph a machine that measures and records the electrical impulses from the heart on an electrocardiogram

electroencephalogram (EEG) a graph of the electrical activity of the brain

electroencephalograph a machine that measures and records electrical impulses from the brain on an electroencephalogram

electrolyte a chemical substance that develops an electric charge and is able to conduct an electric current when placed in water; an ion

electromyogram (EMG) a record of the electrical potential created by the contraction of a muscle

electromyograph a machine that measures and records electrical impulses from the muscles on an electromyogram

emaciated excessively lean

embolus a clot that has moved from its place of origin, causing obstruction to circulation elsewhere

emmetropic normal refraction so that the eyes focus images on the retina

emollient an agent that soothes and softens skin or mucous membrane; often an oily substance

empathy the ability to discriminate what the other person's world is like and to communicate to the other this understanding in a way that shows the other that the helper understands the client's feelings and the behavior and experience underlying these feelings

emphysema a chronic pulmonary condition in which the alveoli are dilated and distended

enamel (of tooth) the covering over the crown of the tooth

encoding the selection of specific signs or symbols (codes) to transmit the message, such as which language and words to use, how to arrange the words, what tone of voice and gestures and/or other body language to use

endocervical referring to the lining of the uterine cervix or the cervical os

endogenous opiods chemical regulators in the body that may modify pain

endorphins a polypeptide found throughout the body that is thought to relieve pain

endoscope an instrument used for examining the interior of a hollow organ, e.g., the bladder, rectum, stomach, or bronchi

endotracheal tube a tube that is inserted through the mouth or nose into the trachea

enema a solution introduced into the rectum and sigmoid colon to remove feces and/or flatus

engagement (lightening) the entrance of the presenting fetal part at the upper entrance of the pelvis (pelvic inlet)

enkephalins a pentapeptide naturally occurring in the brain that has opiate-like effects

enteric referring to the intestines

entropion inversion or inturning of the lid

enuresis bedwetting, involuntary passing of urine in children after bladder control is achieved

environment the aggregate of surrounding things, conditions, or influences, with particular reference to those aspects that affect the existence or development of people and other living things

epistaxis nose bleed

Epstein's pearls white nodules found on the palate of newborns

equipoise a state of equilibrium or balance

eructation belching; the expulsion of swallowed gases through the mouth

erythema a redness associated with a variety of skin rashes

eschar thick necrotic tissue produced by burning, by a corrosive application, or by death of tissue associated with loss of vascular supply, bacterial invasion, and putrefaction

esophagoscopy visual examination of the interior of the esophagus with a lighted instrument

ethics the rules or principles that govern right conduct

evaluating determining the client's response to nursing interventions and comparing the response to predetermined standards

eversion turning the sole of the foot outward by moving the ankle joint

eupnea normal, quiet breathing

eustachian tube a channel lined with mucous membrane that connects the middle ear and the nasopharynx; it acts as an air pressure stabilizer

evaporation conversion of a liquid into a vapor

excoriation loss of the superficial layers of the skin

exhalation (expiration) the movement of gases from the lungs to the atmosphere

exophthalmus a protrusion of the eyeballs with elevation of the upper eyelids, resulting in a startled or staring expression

expectorate to cough and spit up mucus or other materials

extension increasing the angle of a joint

external respiration the interchange of oxygen and carbon dioxide between the alveoli of the lungs and the pulmonary blood

extracellular fluid (ECF) fluid found outside the body cells

exudate material, such as fluid and cells, that has escaped from blood vessels during the inflammatory process and is deposited in tissue or on tissue surfaces

face mask a mask covering the client's nose and mouth used to deliver oxygen and/or other gases

face tent a device that covers the face used to deliver oxygen to the client when a face mask is not tolerated

Fahrenheit a thermometer scale used to measure heat; the freezing point of water is 32F and the boiling point is 212F

false imprisonment the unjustifiable detention that deprives a person of personal liberty for any length of time

fasciculation an abnormal contraction or shortening of a bundle of muscle fibers

fast abstain from food

fat embolism fat globules that are released from the bone marrow and from local tissue trauma into the blood circulation

febrile pertaining to a fever; feverish

fecal impaction a mass or collection of hardened, putty-like feces in the folds of the rectum

fecal incontinence (bowel incontinence) refers to loss of voluntary ability to control fecal and gaseous discharges through the anal sphincter

feedback in the communication process, the response that the message receiver sends back to the sender; in teaching/learning, the response the learner gives when receiving new instruction, or the response the teacher gives to the learner relating to the learner's performance of desired objectives

femoral torsion abnormal medial or lateral rotation of the femur

fenestrated drape a drape with an opening in its center

fetomaternal pertaining to the fetus and the mother

fiber an indigestible carbohydrate derived from plants

FiO$_2$ fraction of inspired oxygen

fissure a cleft or groove

flatness an extremely dull sound produced during percussion by very dense tissue, such as muscle or bone

flatulence the presence of excessive amounts of gas in the stomach or intestines

flexion decreasing the angle of a joint (between two bones); the act of bending

flowmeter a device used to control the flow of oxygen delivery

flowsheet a record used to record the progress of specific or specialized data such as vital signs, fluid balance, or routine medications

fluoroscopy an examination using a device (fluoroscope) that views internal structures using X-rays

focus charting a method of charting that uses key words or foci to describe what is happening to the client

fomite an inanimate object other than food that can harbor disease producing microorganisms and transmit an infection

fontanels unossified membranous gaps in the bone structure of the skull

footboard a board placed at the foot of the client bed to support the feet and prevent foot drop; may also be used to keep bed covers of the client's feet

force an external influence, a push or a pull exerted on an object

Fowler's position a bed-sitting position with the head of the bed raised to 45°

fracture a break in the continuity of a bone

fremitus vibrations felt through the chest wall by palpation

frenulum a midline fold connecting the undersurface of the tongue to the floor of the mouth

frequency (of urination) voiding at more frequent intervals than usual

friction rubbing; the force that opposes motion

friction strokes a massage technique in which strong circular massage is followed by centripetal stroking

functional hemoglobin the ratio of oxygen bound to hemoglobin compared to the amount of hemoglobin that is available for binding

fundus the upper part of the uterus located between the fallopian tubes

funnel chest (pectus excavatum) a congenital defect of the chest where the sternum is depressed, narrowing the anteroposterior diameter

gait the way a person walks

gastric pertaining to the stomach

gastroscopy visual examination of the stomach with a lighted instrument (gastroscope)

gastrostomy an opening through the abdominal wall into the stomach

gastrostomy feeding the instillation of liquid nourishment through a tube that enters the stomach through a surgical opening through the abdominal wall

gatch bed a bed fitted with movable joints beneath the hips and knees of the client

gavage administration of nourishment to the stomach through a nasogastric or orogastric tube; tube feeding

general adaptation syndrome (GAS, stress syndrome) (Selye) a general arousal response of the body to a stressor that is characterized by certain physiologic events and that is dominated by the sympathetic nervous system

genupectoral kneeling position with torso at a 90° angle to hips

genu valgum knock-knee, a condition in which knees are very close to each other and the ankles are apart

genu varum bowleg, a condition of curving out of the legs

gestation referring to pregnancy; the point of conception to the point at which birth occurs, normally 38 to 42 weeks

gingiva the gum

gingivitis acute or chronic inflammation of the gums

glaucoma a disturbance in the circulation of aqueous fluid, which causes an increase in intraocular pressure

glossitis inflammation of the tongue

glucometer a device used to measure the amount of glucose in a blood sample

goal attainment the resolution of the client concern or health problem specified in the nursing diagnosis

Goodell's sign a softening of the cervix and vagina identified as a sign of pregnancy

goniometer a device used to measure the angle of a joint in degrees

granulation tissue young connective tissue with new capillaries formed in the wound healing process

gravity the force that pulls objects toward the earth

ground (electrical) to transmit electric current from an object or surface to the ground

guided imagery a relaxation technique using self-chosen positive images to achieve specific health-related goals, i.e., stress reduction, pain control

gynecomastia development of an abnormally large mammary gland in the male

hair follicle a pouch-like depression in the skin enclosing the root of a hair

hair shaft the visible part of the hair

halo ring a type of traction consisting of a circular metal band secured by two anterior and two posterior pins that penetrate the skull only a fraction of an inch, used to immobilize fractures of the cervical and upper thoracic vertebrae

halo-thoracic vest traction a device where a halo ring is attached to a plaster cast or plastic vest by metal rods, used to immobilize fractures of the cervical and upper thoracic vertebrae

hangnail a shred of epidermal tissue at either side of the nail

health care system the totality of services offered by all health disciplines

health care team health personnel from different disciplines who coordinate their skills to assist a client and/or support persons, commonly includes nurses, physicians, pharmacists, dietitians, physiotherapists, and so on

health problem any condition or situation in which a client requires help to promote, maintain, or regain a state of health or to achieve a peaceful death

heat balance when the amount of heat produced by the body exactly equals the amount of heat lost

heave an abnormal lateral movement of the chest related to enlargement of the left ventricle

hemangioma a large, persistent, bright red or dark purple vascular area of the skin

hematocrit the proportion of red blood cells (erythrocytes) to the total blood volume

hematoma a collection of blood in a tissue, organ, or space due to a break in the wall of a blood vessel

hemiplegia loss of movement on one side of the body

hemorrhage excessive loss of blood from the vascular system

hemostat a small pair of forceps used to constrict blood vessels

hemothorax a collection of blood in the pleural cavity

heparin lock the airtight cap covering the end of a client's intravenous or central venous tubing

hernia a protrusion of the organ or tissue through an abdominal or inguinal opening

hirsutism abnormal hairiness, particularly in women

hordeolum (sty) a redness, swelling, and tenderness of the hair follicle and glands that empty at the edge of the eyelids

horizontal recumbent a back-lying position with legs extended and a small pillow under the head

humidifier a device that adds water vapor to inspired air

hydatidiform mole degenerative process of chorionic villi of the uterus

hydrocephalus a condition in which there is excessive cerebrospinal fluid within the skull

hydrometer (urinometer) an instrument used to measure the specific gravity of urine

hygiene the science of health and its maintenance

hyperalimentation (total parenteral nutrition, TPN) the intravenous infusion of water, protein, carbohydrates, electrolytes, minerals, and vitamins through a central vein

hypercalcemia an excess of calcium in the blood plasma

hypercapnea (hypercarbia) accumulation of carbon dioxide in the blood

hyperchloremia an excess of chloride in the blood plasma

hyperesthesia greater than normal sensation

hyperextension further extension between two bones or stretching out of a joint

hyperglycemia an excessive concentration of sugar in the blood

hyperhidrosis excessive perspiration

hyperkalemia an excess of potassium in the blood plasma

hypermagnesia an excess of magnesium in the blood plasma

hypernatremia an excess of sodium in the blood plasma

hyperopia farsightedness; abnormal refraction in which light rays focus behind the retina

hyperphosphatemia an excess of phosphate in the blood plasma

hyperpyrexia (hyperthermia) an extremely elevated body temperature

hyperresonance an abnormal booming sound produced during percussion of the lungs

hypertelorism wide spacing between the eyes

hypertension an abnormally high blood pressure over 140 mm Hg systolic and/or 90 mm Hg diastolic

hyperthermia (hyperpyrexia) an extremely high fever, e.g., 105.8F (41C)

hypertonic solution a fluid possessing a greater concentration of solutes than plasma

hypertrophy enlargement of a muscle or organ

hyperventilation very deep, rapid respirations

hypervolemia an abnormal increase in the body's blood volume; circulatory overload

hypesthesia (hypoesthesia) less than normal sensation

hypocalcemia deficiency of calcium in the blood plasma

hypochloremia deficiency of chloride in the blood plasma

hypodermic (subcutaneous) under the skin

hypoesthesia (hypesthesia) less than normal sensation

hypoglycemia a reduced amount of glucose in the blood

hypokalemia deficiency of potassium in the blood plasma

hypomagnesia deficiency of magnesium in the blood plasma

hyponatremia deficiency of sodium in the blood plasma

hypophosphatemia deficiency in phosphate in the blood plasma

hypostatic pneumonia an infection of lung tissue resulting from poor circulation or stagnation of secretions

hypotension an abnormally low blood pressure with a systolic pressure less than 100 mm Hg in an adult

hypothalamic integrator the center that controls the core temperature, located in the preoptic area of the hypothalamus

hypothermia a core body temperature below the lower limit of normal

hypoventilation very shallow respirations

hypovolemia an abnormal reduction in blood volume

hypoxemia low partial pressure of oxygen or low saturation of oxyhemoglobin in the arterial blood

hypoxia insufficient oxygen anywhere in the body

ileostomy an opening into the ileum (small bowel)

implementing carrying out the planned nursing interventions to help the client attain the goals, putting the care plan into action

incentive spirometers (sustained maximal inspiration devices [SMIs]) instruments that measure the flow of air inhaled through the mouthpiece

incontinence involuntary urination

incurvated nail (ingrown toenails) penetration of the edges of the nail plate into the surrounding tissues

incus an anvil-shaped ossicle of the middle ear; it communicates sound waves from the malleus to the stapes

independent nursing action an activity that the nurse initiates as a result of the nurse's own knowledge and skills

inertia inactivity; inability to move spontaneously

infarct a localized area of necrosis (dead cells) usually owing to obstructed arterial blood flow to the part

informed consent a client's agreement to accept a course of treatment or a procedure after receiving complete information—including the risks of treatment and facts relating to it—from the physician

infusion controller a device used with intravenous infusions to control the infusion rate by using gravitational force

infusion pump a device used with intravenous fluids to deliver a desired infusion rate by exerting positive pressure on the tubing or on the fluid

inhalation (inspiration) refers to the intake of air into the lungs

inhalation therapy (aerosolization) deliverance of droplets of medication or moisture suspended in a gas, such as oxygen, by inhalation through the nose or mouth

inorganic substances substances not derived from hydrocarbons and not of organic origin

inquest a legal inquiry into the cause or manner of a death

in situ in place; localized

inspection visual examination to detect features detectable to the eye

instillation application of a medication into a body cavity or orifice

intensity (amplitude) the loudness or softness of a sound

intermittent positive pressure breathing (IPPB) delivery of oxygen into the lungs at positive pressure and release of the pressure passively during expiration

internal respiration the interchange of oxygen and carbon dioxide between the circulating blood and the cells of the body tissues

interstitial fluid fluid that surrounds the cells, includes lymph

interview a planned communication or a conversation with the purpose of obtaining information

intra-arterial into an artery

intra-cardiac into the heart muscle

intradermal under the epidermis; into the dermis

intracellular fluid (ICF) fluid found within the body cells, also called cellular fluid

intralipid therapy the infusion of essential fatty acids or fat emulsions through a central venous line

intramuscular into the muscle

intraoperative period the phase during surgery that begins when the client is transferred to the operating room bed and ends when the client is admitted to the recovery room

intraosseous into the bone

intrapartal the phase of childbirth from the onset of labor through the expulsion of the placenta

intraspinal (intrathecal) into the spinal canal

intrathecal (intraspinal) into the spinal canal

intravascular within a blood vessel

intravenous within a vein

intravenous push (IVP, bolus) the direct intravenous administration of a medication that cannot be diluted or that is needed in an emergency

intravenous pyelography (IVP); intravenous urography (IVU) an X-ray filming of the kidney and ureters after injection of a radiopaque material into the vein

intubation the insertion of a tube

involution a process of progressive reduction in the size of the uterus after delivery has occurred

iritis inflammation of the iris

irrigation (lavage) a flushing or washing-out of a body cavity, organ or wound with a specified solution

ischemia deficiency of blood supply caused by obstruction of circulation to the body part

isolation practices that prevent the spread of infection and communicable disease

isometric (static, setting) exercise tensing of a muscle against an immovable outer resistance, which does not change muscle length or produce joint motion

isotonic (dynamic) exercise exercise in which muscle tension is constant and the muscle shortens to produce muscle contraction and movement

IV filters devices attached to intravenous infusion tubing to filter or remove air, particulate matter, and microbes to prevent contamination

jaundice a yellowish color of the sclera, mucous membranes, and/or skin

jejunostomy an opening through the abdominal wall into the jejunum

jejunostomy feeding the instillation of liquid nourishment through a tube that enters the jejunum through a surgical opening into the abdominal wall

joint the place where two or more bones join

JVD jugular venous distention

Kardex a widely used, concise method of organizing and recording data about a client, making information quickly accessible to all members of the health team

Kelly clamp (forceps) a type of hemostat

keratin the type of protein found in epidermis, hair, and nails

keratotic spots horny growths, such as warts or calluses

ketone any compound containing the carbonyl group, CO, and having hydrocarbon groups attached to the carbonyl group

ketone bodies products of incomplete fat metabolism that appear in the urine

kinesthesia the ability to perceive extent, direction, or weight of movement

Koplick's spots red spots on the buccal mucosa associated with measles

Korotkoff's sounds a series of five sounds produced by blood within the artery with each ventricular contraction

kyphosis excessive convex curvature of the thoracic spine

lacrimal canaliculi (canals) a passageway from the inner-most corner of the eye to the lacrimal sac

lacrimal duct a small passageway from the lacrimal gland draining the tears onto the conjunctiva at the upper outer corner of the eye

lacrimal glands the organ that lies over the upper outer corner of the eye and secretes tears

lacrimal sac a pouch-like structure located in a groove in the lacrimal bone between the inner corner of the eye and the bridge of the nose

lacrimation tearing of the eyes

lactation milk production during the postpartum period

lanugo the fine, woolly hair or down on the shoulders, back, sacrum, and earlobes of the unborn child that may remain for a few weeks after birth

large calorie (calorie, kilocalorie [kcal]) the amount of heat required to raise the temperature of 1 kg of water 1 degree C

laryngoscopy visual examination of the larynx with a laryngoscope

lateral position a side-lying position

lavage an irrigation or washing of a body organ, such as the stomach

laxative a medication that stimulates bowel activity

learning a change in human disposition or capability that persists over a period of time and that cannot be solely accounted for by growth, is represented by a change in behavior

learning need a need to change behavior or "a gap between the information an individual knows and the information necessary to perform a function or care for self"

Leopold's maneuver a systematic way of palpating the obstetrical client's abdomen to determine the position of the fetus

leukoplakia white patches or spots on the mucous membrane of the tongue or cheek

lever a rigid bar that moves on a fixed axis called a fulcrum

leverage force applied with the use of a lever

lice parasitic insects that infest mammals

life processes normal life events

lift an abnormal anterior movement of the chest related to enlargement of the right ventricle

lightening (engagement) the descent of the fetus and uterus into the maternal pelvis

linea nigra the dark pigmented line extending from the umbilicus to the pubis during pregnancy

line of gravity an imaginary vertical line running through the center of gravity

lipid an organic substance that is greasy and insoluble in water

lithotomy position a back-lying position in which the feet are supported in stirrups

livor mortis discoloration of the skin caused by breakdown of the red blood cells that occurs after blood circulation has ceased, appears in the dependent areas of the body

local adaptation syndrome (LAS) the reaction of one organ or body part to stress

lochia the vaginal discharge of blood, white blood cells, mucus, and shreds of decidua that come from the uterus during the postpartal period

long board (smooth mover, Easyglide) a lacquered or smooth polyethylene board with handholds along its edges used to facilitate moving the client from bed to stretcher or stretcher to bed

lordosis an exaggerated concavity in the lumbar region of the vertebral column

low-Fowler's (semi-Fowler's) position a bed-sitting position in which the head of the bed is elevated between 15° and 45°, with or without knee flexion

lumbar puncture (LP, spinal tap) insertion of a needle into the subarachnoid space at the lumbar region

lumen a channel within a tube

lymph transparent, slightly yellow fluid found within the lymphatic vessels

macrocephaly abnormally large head circumference

macrognathia abnormally large jaw

malleus a hammer-shaped ossicle of the middle ear; it is connected to the tympanic membrane and transmits sound waves to the incus

malocclusion malposition and imperfect contact of the mandibular and maxillary teeth

mammography an X-ray study of breast tissue

management the use of delegated authority within the formal organization to organize, direct, or control responsible subordinates so that all service contributions are coordinated to attain a goal

manometer an instrument used to measure the pressure of fluids or gases

mastication the act of chewing

mastitis inflammation of the breast

mastoid breast-shaped; the bony prominence of the temporal bone behind the ear

mature milk breast milk that has a high percentage of water and 20 calories per ounce

mean blood pressure the midway point between the systolic and diastolic pressures

mediastinal shift a lateral movement of the organs in the mediastinum, i.e., the heart and major vessels

medical asepsis all practices intended to confine a specific microorganism to a specific area, limiting the number, growth, and spread of microorganisms

medical examiner a physician who usually has advanced education in pathology or forensic medicine who determines causes of death

medical record (chart) an account of the client's health history, current health status, treatment, and progress

medication (drug) a substance administered for the diagnosis, cure, treatment, mitigation, or prevention of disease

melanin the pigment that gives color to the skin

meniscus the crescent-shaped upper surface of a column of fluid

metabolism the sum of all the physical and chemical processes by which living substance is formed and maintained and by which energy is made available for use by the organism

microcephaly abnormally small head circumference

micrognathia abnormally small jaw

micromineral minerals that people require daily in amounts less than 100 mg

micronutrient nutrients, such as vitamins and minerals, required in small quantities by the body

micturition (voiding, urination) the process of emptying the bladder

milk, milking (a tube) the compression and movement of fingers along the length of a tube in order to move its contents toward an opening for removal

minitracheostomy (MT, cricotracheotomy) a technique in which a cannula with an internal diameter of 4 mm is inserted into the trachea, through the cricothyroid membrane

midwife a female who practices the art of aiding in the delivery of infants; may be a nurse who has received special training in obstetrics and is qualified to deliver infants

milia small, white nodules (whiteheads) usually found over the nose and face of newborns

miliaria rubra a prickly heat rash of the face, neck, trunk, or perineal area of infants

minim an apothecary unit of measurement, a volume of water equal in weight to a grain of wheat

miosis constricted pupils

miter a method of folding the bedclothes at the corners to secure them in place while the bed is occupied

Mongolian spots blue-gray areas of discoloration of the skin of the lower back, thighs, and sometimes shoulders of the infant and small children; more often seen in non-white children

motivation in learning, the desire to learn

mucous membrane epithelial tissue that forms mucus, concentrates bile, and secretes or excretes enzymes

mucus plug a pool of thick mucus that occludes the cervical os during pregnancy to protect the fetus from infection

multigravida a woman who has been pregnant more than once

multilumen catheter a catheter that has more than one channel, each channel or lumen has a separate port located along or at the catheter tip

multiparous a female who has more than one child

multiple pregnancy a pregnancy characterized by more than one fetus in the uterus

murmurs an adventitious or abnormal sound heard on auscultation of the heart during systole and diastole

mydriasis enlarged pupils

myelogram (myelography) an X-ray film of the spinal cord, nerve roots, and vertebrae after injection of a contrast medium into the subarachnoid space

myopia nearsightedness; abnormal refraction in which light rays focus in front of the retina

myxedema (hypothyroidism) underactivity of the thyroid

myxedema facies dry, puffy face with dry skin and coarse features caused by under activity of the thyroid

Nagele's rule a rule of measurement used to determine the onset of labor; seven days are added to the first date of the last menstrual period, then three months subtracted

nail atrophy abnormally decreased thickness of the nail

nail hypertrophy abnormally increased thickness of the nail

narrative charting a written description in the medical record of client responses to health problems and medical and nursing interventions

nasal cannula (nasal prongs) a device used to administer low-flow oxygen

nasogastric tube a plastic or rubber tube inserted through the nose into the stomach for the purpose of feeding or irrigating the stomach

nasolacrimal duct the channel between the lacrimal sac and the nose

nasopharyngeal tube a tube that is inserted through a nostril and terminates in the pharynx, below the upper edge of the epiglottis

nausea the urge to vomit

nebulization the conversion of a fine mist or spray from a liquid

nebulizer a device that produces a fine mist; atomizer or sprayer

necrotic death of tissue caused by inadequate blood supply

needle recapper a device that allows the nurse to uncap and recap a needle safely

negative reinforcement punishment for undesirable responses

Nelson bed a therapeutic bed used in the treatment of orthopedic client, it can be tilted, used in the reclining position, or as a chair

nerve conduction study a procedure to determine the excitability and conduction velocity of motor and sensory nerves and the presence of disease of the peripheral nerves

nociceptor a pain receptor

nocturia (nycturia) increased frequency of urination at night that is not a result of increased fluid intake

nondirective interview a communication in which the nurse allows the client to control the purpose, subject matter, and pacing

nonverbal communication an interaction between two or more people that uses gestures, facial expressions or body language; does not include the written or spoken word

normocephaly head size and shape that is considered normal

nose culture a specimen collected from the mucosa of the nasal passages using a culture swab

nulliparous a female who has never had a child

nursing care plan (client care plan) a written guide that organizes information about a client's health into a meaningful whole and focuses on the actions nurses must take to address the client's identified nursing diagnoses and meet the stated goals

nursing diagnosis the nurse's clinical judgment about individual, family, or community responses to actual and potential health problems/life processes to provide the basis for selecting nursing interventions to achieve outcomes for which the nurse is accountable

nursing health history a record compiled by nurses by a systematic method, containing data about a client's past and current health status

nursing leadership a process of interpersonal influence through which the nurse helps the client establish and achieve goals to improve well-being

nursing order the specific actions the nurse takes to help the client meet established health care goals

nursing process a systematic rational method of planning and providing nursing care

nursing strategy nursing actions or interventions that address a specific nursing diagnosis to achieve client goals

nutrients the organic and inorganic chemicals found in foods and required for proper body functioning

nutrition what a person eats and how the body uses it

obese to weigh greater than 20% of the ideal for height and frame

objective data (signs, overt data) information (data) that are detectable by an observer or can be tested against an accepted standard; information that can be seen, heard, felt, or smelled

obligatory loss the essential fluid loss required to maintain body functioning

observe gathering data by using the five senses

occlusive closed

occult hidden

occupied bed a bed currently being used by a client

oligohydramnios an inadequate or decreased amount of amniotic fluid in the uterus

oliguria production of abnormally small amounts of urine by the kidney

open bed a bed not presently being used by its occupant, with the top covers folded back

ophthalmic pertaining to the eye

oral referring to the mouth

organic substances substances containing carbon and derived from living organisms

orifice an external opening of a body cavity

oropharyngeal tube a tube that is inserted in the oropharynx (mouth and pharynx) to suction secretions

orthopnea ability to breathe only when in an upright position (sitting or standing)

orthopneic position a sitting position to relieve respiratory difficulty in which the client leans over and is supported by an overbed table across the lap

orthostatic hypotension decrease in blood pressure related to positional changes from lying to sitting or standing positions

ossicles the bones of sound transmission in the middle ear

osteitis deformans (Paget's disease) a disorder in which bony thickness increases, especially seen in the head

osteoporosis demineralization of the bone

ostomy a suffix denoting the formation of an opening or outlet

otic pertaining to the ear

otitis externa inflammation of the external auditory canal

otitis media inflammation of the middle ear

otoscope an instrument used to examine the ears

outcome criteria statements that describe specific, observable, and measurable responses of the client

overhydration similar to extracellular fluid excess; results in edema

overt data (signs, objective data) information (data) that are detectable by an observer or can be tested against an accepted standard; information that can be seen, heard, felt, or smelled

oxidation a chemical process by which a substance combines with oxygen; energy is released, and other substances are formed

oxygen analyzer a device used to measure the concentration of oxygen being received by the client

pace number of steps taken per minute or the distance taken in one step when walking

pack an unsterile hot or cold moist cloth applied to an area of the body

pain threshold the amount of pain stimulation a person requires before feeling pain

pain tolerance the maximum amount and duration of pain that an individual is willing to endure

palate the roof of the mouth

pallor the absence of underlying red tones in the skin; may be most readily seen in the buccal mucosa

palpation the examination of the body using the sense of touch

Pap (Papanicolaou) smear a method of taking a sample of cervical cells for microscopic examination to detect malignancy

papavirus hominis the virus that causes plantar warts

paraphrasing (restating) actively listening for the client's basic message and then repeating those thoughts and/or feelings in similar words

parasite a microorganism that lives in or on another from which it obtains nourishment

parenteral drug administration occurring outside the alimentary tract; injected into the body through some route other than the alimentary canal, e.g., intramuscularly

paresthesia an abnormal sensation of burning or prickling

Parkinson position a position used for the administration of nasal medications in which the client assumes a back-lying position with the head turned toward the side to be treated

paronychia infection of the tissue surrounding the nail

parotitis inflammation of the parotid salivary gland

passive range-of-motion (ROM) exercise exercise in which another person moves each of the client's joints through their complete range of movement, maximally stretching all muscle groups within each plane over each joint

patent open, unobstructed; not closed

patent ductus arteriosis congenital defect in which the ductus arteriosus fails to close at birth

patient a person who is waiting for or undergoing medical treatment and care

patient controlled analgesia (PCA) a pain management technique that allows the client to take an active role in managing pain

PCM protein-calorie malnutrition

Pearson attachment a sling appliance that joins the Thomas splint at knee level to support the lower leg off the bed and permit the knee to be flexed

pediculosis infestation with head lice

pelvic belt (girdle) a device that provides traction around the client's hips to relieve lower back, hip, and leg pain

Penrose drain a flexible rubber drain

perception checking (consensual validation) a method of clarifying or verifying the meaning of specific words rather than the overall meaning of a message

percussion an assessment method in which the body surface is struck to elicit sounds that can be heard or vibrations that can be felt

percussion (clapping, cupping) the forceful striking of the skin with cupped hands to loosen secretions in the lungs

perfusion passage of blood constituents through the vessels of the circulatory system

perioperative period the time before, during, and after an operation

peripheral at the edge or outward boundary

peripherally inserted central catheter (PIC catheter, PICC) a long venous catheter inserted into a distal vein and threaded so that the tip is located in the superior vena cava or right atrium

peripheral parenteral nutrition (PPN) intravenous parenteral nutrition administered through peripheral vein sites

perinatal period the period from the 28th week of gestation through 28 days following birth

perineum the area between the anus and the posterior (back) aspect of the genitals

periodontal disease (pyorrhea) disorder of the supporting structures of the teeth

peripheral pulse a pulse located in the periphery of the body, e.g., foot, wrist

peristomal around a stoma

peritoneal dialysis the instillation and drainage of a solution (dialysate) from the peritoneal cavity

personal space the distance people prefer to maintain when interacting with others; in North Americans usually 1½ to 4 feet

PES format the three essential components of nursing diagnostic statements, including the terms describing the problem, the etiology of the problem, and the defining characteristics or cluster of signs and symptoms

pes valgus (talipes valgus) clubfoot in which the toe turns outward

pes varus (talipes varus) clubfoot in which the sole turns inward

petechiae pinpoint red areas in the skin

petrissage a massage technique consisting of kneading or large, quick pinches of the skin, subcutaneous tissue, and muscle

pH a measure of the relative alkalinity or acidity of a solution; a measure of the concentration of hydrogen ions

phimosis a condition in which the opening of the foreskin of the penis is extremely narrow

phlebitis inflammation of the vein

photophobia sensitivity to light

physical examination (assessment) the means by which the nurse obtains the objective data needed to complete the assessment phase of the nursing process

physical restraint any manual method or physical or mechanical device, material, or equipment attached to the client's body that restricts the client's movement

physiotherapy (physical therapy) treatment with physical and mechanical means, such as massage and electricity

pigeon chest (pectus carinatum) a permanent deformity of the chest characterized by a narrow transverse diameter, an increased anteroposterior diameter, and a protruding sternum

pitch the frequency or number of the vibrations heard during auscultation

pitting edema edema in which firm finger pressure on the skin produces an indentation (pit) that remains for several seconds

placenta the oval-shaped body or structure in the uterus that provides fetal nourishment, oxygenation, eliminates fetal wastes, and serves as an organ of exchange between mother and fetus

placenta previa a condition of pregnancy in which the placenta is abnormally implanted in the lower uterine segment

planning the process in which the nurse and client set priorities, write goals or expected outcomes, and establish a written care plan designed to resolve or minimize the identified problems of the client and to coordinate the care provided by all health team members

plantar flexion movement of the ankle so that the toes point downward

plantar wart a wart on the sole of the foot

plaque an invisible soft film consisting of bacteria, molecules of saliva, and remnants of epithelial cells and leukocytes that adheres to the enamel surface of teeth

pleximeter in percussion, the middle finger of the non-dominant hand placed firmly on the client's skin

plexor in percussion, the middle finger of the dominant hand or a percussion hammer used to strike the pleximeter

pneumothorax accumulation of gas or fluid in the pleural cavity

point of maximal impulse (PMI) the point where the apex of the heart touches the anterior chest wall

poison any substance that injures or kills through its chemical action when inhaled, injected, applied, or absorbed in relatively small amounts

polarized (cardiac muscle) electrically charged

polyhydramnios excessive amniotic fluid

polyuria (diuresis) the production of abnormally large amounts of urine by the kidneys without an increased fluid intake

portal of entry in communicable disease, the opening through which infectious organisms invade the body, e.g., urinary tract, respiratory tract, open wound

possible nursing diagnosis clinical judgment statements used when evidence about a response is unclear or when the related factors are unknown

postoperative period the period following surgery that begins with the admission to the recovery room and ends when the client has completely recovered from the surgery

postpartal the period after birth of the placenta

postpartal hemorrhage a 500 ml or greater blood loss during the postpartal period following a vaginal delivery; greater than 1000 ml blood loss following a cesarean section

postural drainage the drainage, by gravity, of secretions from various lung segments

potential health problem risk factors that predispose persons and families to health problems

potential nursing diagnosis (high risk nursing diagnosis) a clinical judgment that an individual, family, or community is more vulnerable to develop a problem than others in the same or similar situation

precordium an area of the chest overlying the heart

preeclampsia an abnormal condition of pregnancy in which the client develops hypertension, albuminuria/proteinuria, and edema

preoperative period the period before an operation that begins when the decision for surgery has been made and ends when the client is transferred to the operating room bed

presbyopia loss of elasticity of the lens and thus loss of ability to see close objects

prescription the written direction for the preparation and administration of a drug

pressure (skin) the perpendicular force exerted on the skin by gravity

pressure sores (decubitus ulcers, bedsores, distortion sores) reddened areas, sores, or ulcers of the skin occurring over bony prominences

preterm labor labor taking place between the 20th and 38th week of pregnancy

primary data data or information that is obtained from the client

primary intention healing (primary union, first intention healing) healing that occurs in a wound in which the tissue surfaces are or have been approximated and there is minimal or no tissue loss; it is characterized by the formation of minimal granulation tissue and scarring

primigravida a female pregnant for the first time; gravida 1

priority setting the process of establishing a preferential order for nursing strategies

privileged communication information given to a professional who is forbidden by law from disclosing the information in a court without the consent of the person who provided it

PRN an order that enables the nurse to give a medication or treatment when, in the nurse's judgment, the client needs it

problem a need that the client is unable to meet without assistance from members of the health care team

problem-oriented medical record (POMR or POR) data about the client are recorded and arranged according to the client's problems, rather than according to the source of the information

proctoscopy visual examination of the interior of the rectum with a proctoscope

Proetz position a position used for the administration of nasal medications in which the client assumes a back-lying position with the head over the edge of the bed or pillow under the shoulders so that the head is tipped backward

progressive relaxation a formalized relaxation technique designed to reduce stress and chronic pain

pronation moving the bones of the forearm so that the palm of the hand faces downward when held in front of the body

prone position a face-lying position, with or without a small pillow

prosthesis an artificial part, e.g., a glass eye, an artificial limb, or dentures

protein an organic substance that is composed of carbon, hydrogen, oxygen, and nitrogen and that yields amino acids upon hydrolysis

protocol a written plan specifying the procedure to be followed in a particular situation

protraction moving a part of the body forward in the same plane parallel to the ground

proximal closest to the point of reference

pruritus itching

ptosis eyelids that lie at or below the pupil margin

puerperium the period extending from placental delivery through complete involution of the uterus, usually about 6 weeks

pull sheet (turn sheet) a sheet placed beneath the client from the shoulders—as in a draw sheet—to the buttocks, which facilitates turning the client and moving him up or down in bed

pulp cavity the cavity in the central part of the crown of a tooth that contains pulp

pulse the wave of blood within an artery that is created by contraction of the left ventricle of the heart

pulse deficit the difference between the apical pulse and the radial pulse

pulse oximeter a noninvasive device that measures the arterial blood oxygen saturation by means of a sensor attached to the finger

pulse pressure the difference between the systolic and the diastolic blood pressure

pulse rate the number of pulse beats per minute

pulse rhythm the pattern of the beats and intervals between the beats

pulse volume the strength or amplitude of the pulse, the force of blood exerted with each beat

Purkinje's fibers a network of modified cardiac muscle fibers concerned with the conduction of impulses in the heart; dense networks of these fibers form the sinoatrial and atrioventricular nodes

purulent containing pus

pyrexia (hyperthermia) a body temperature above the normal range; fever

quality (of sound) a subjective description of a sound, e.g., whistling, gurgling

quickening the first fetal movements felt by the pregnant female

radiation the transfer of heat from the surface of one object to the surface of another without contact between the two objects

rales (crackles) bubbling or rattling sounds, audible by ear or stethoscope on inhalation; they are a result of fluid in the lungs

range of motion the degree of movement possible for each joint

rationality thinking based on reasons, rather than prejudice, preferences, self-interest or fears

reactive hyperemia the increased presence of blood in an area after restoration of blood flow following a decreased supply

readiness in learning, the behavior that reflects motivation to learn at a specific time; includes emotional and experiential readiness

rebound phenomenon (thermal) the time when the maximum therapeutic effect of a hot or cold application is achieved and the opposite effect begins

recording (charting) the process of making entries on the client's medical record (chart)

rectal referring to the distal portion of the large intestine

reduction the realignment of fractured bone fragments to their normal position

reflex an automatic response of the body to a stimulus

reflux backward flow

regeneration (tissue) renewal, regrowth

regurgitation the spitting up or backward flow of undigested food

renal calculi calcium crystals or stones in the renal system

repolarized (cardiac muscle) reacquiring an electric charge

resistive exercise exercise in which the client contracts a muscle against an opposing force, e.g., a weight

resonance a hollow sound produced during percussion by lungs filled with air

respiration the act of breathing

respiratory excursion (chest expansion) the amount of chest expansion or movement from full expiration to full inspiration

respiratory quality (character) refers to those aspects of breathing that are different from normal, effortless breathing, includes the amount of effort exerted to breathe and the sounds produced by breathing

respiratory rhythm (pattern) refers to the regularity of the expirations and the inspirations

restraints protective devices used to limit physical activity of the client or a part of the client's body

resuscitation bag Ambu bag; a device used to provide oxygen to clients when they are unable to breathe for themselves

retention sutures (stay sutures) large sutures used in addition to skin sutures to attach underlying tissues of fat and muscle as well as skin; used to support incisions in obese individuals or when healing may be prolonged

retraction (mobility) moving a part of the body backward in same plane parallel to the ground

retrograde pyelography an X-ray film taken after a contrast medium is injected through ureteral catheters into the kidneys

Rh factor antigens present on the surface of some people's erythrocytes; persons who possess this factor are referred to as *Rh positive*, and those who do not are referred to as *Rh negative*

rhonchi (gurgles) coarse, dry, wheezy, or whistling sounds, more audible during exhalation, as the air moves through tenacious mucus or a constricted bronchus

rigor mortis the stiffening of the body that occurs about 2 to 4 hours after death

roller bar a metal frame covered with longitudinal rollers used to facilitate the transfer of the client from bed to stretcher or stretcher to bed

root (of tooth) the structure embedded in the jaw that supports and anchors the tooth

rotation movement of the bone around its central axis

rupture of membranes the spontaneous breaking of the amniotic sac membrane with the release of amniotic fluid before or during labor

Russell traction skin traction which is applied to one or both legs to immobilize fractures of the femur before surgical repair

S$_1$ the first heart sound that occurs when the atrioventricular valves (mitral and tricuspid) close

S$_2$ the second heart sound that occurs when the semilunar valves (aortic and pulmonic) close

saliva the clear liquid secreted by the salivary glands in the mouth

sanguinous containing blood

scabies a contagious skin infestation caused by an arachnid, the itch mite

scald a burn from a hot liquid or vapor, such as steam

scan a noninvasive type of X-ray procedure capable of distinguishing minor differences in the radiodensity of soft tissues

scientific method a logical, systematic approach to solving problems

scoliosis an abnormal lateral deviation of the spine

sebaceous glands glands that secrete sebum

sebum the oily, lubricating secretion of glands in the skin called sebaceous glands

secondary data data or information that is obtained from a source other than the client, e.g., family, friends, medical records

secondary intention healing (secondary union) healing that occurs in a wound in which the tissue surfaces are not approximated and there is extensive tissue loss; it is characterized by the formation of excessive granulation tissue and scarring

semicircular canals passages shaped like half circles in the inner ear that control the sense of balance by the effect of fluid moving against hairlike nerves

semi-Fowler's (low-Fowler's) position a bed-sitting position in which the head of the bed is elevated between 15° and 45°, with or without knee flexion

semiprone position (Sims' position) a side-lying position with lowermost arm behind the body and uppermost leg flexed

serosanguinous composed of serum and blood

serous consisting of serum

serous otitis inflammation of the eustachian tube

serum the clear liquid portion of the blood that does not contain fibrinogen

shearing force a combination of friction and pressure that, when applied to the skin, results in damage to the blood vessels and tissues

shock acute circulatory failure

side-arm traction (Dunlop's) combined horizontal and vertical adaptation of Buck's extension traction to the humerus and forearm

side rails (safety rails) movable rails attached to the sides of hospital beds and stretchers designed to decrease the risk of client falls

sigmoidoscopy visual examination of the interior of the sigmoid colon with a sigmoidoscope

signs (objective data, overt data) information (data) that are detectable by an observer or can be tested against an accepted standard; information that can be seen, heard, felt, or smelled

Sims' position (semiprone position) a side-lying position with lowermost arm behind the body and uppermost leg flexed

single order an order that is to carried out one time only at a specified time

sinoatrial (SA) node the pacemaker of the heart; the collection of the Purkinje's fibers in the right atrium of the heart where the rhythm of contraction is initiated

sitz bath (hip bath) used to soak a client's pelvic or perineal area

skin fold measurement the fold of skin that includes the subcutaneous tissue but not the underlying muscle, indicates the amount of body fat

skull tongs devices used to immobilize fractures of the cervical and upper thoracic vertebrae

small calorie the amount of heat required to raise the temperature of 1 g of water 1 degree C

smegma a thick, white, cheeselike secretion that tends to collect between the labia of females and under the foreskin of the penis of males

soak refers to immersing a body part in a solution or wrapping the part in gauze dressings and then saturating the dressing with a solution

SOAP an acronym for a charting method that follows a recording sequence of subjective data, objective data, assessment, and planning

social communication unplanned communication, often carried out in an informal setting and usually at a leisurely pace

solute a substance dissolved in a liquid

solvent the liquid in which a solute is dissolved

sordes accumulation of foul matter (food, microorganisms and epithelial elements) on the teeth and gums

source-oriented medical record a medical record in which the health care worker makes notations in a specific separate section or sections of the record specific to the health care worker's discipline, i.e., the nurse records on the Nurse's Notes, the physician records on the physician's Progress Notes

specific gravity the weight or degree of concentration of a substance compared with that of an equal volume of another, such as distilled water, taken as a standard

spectrophotometry a means of measuring the amount of red and infrared light absorbed by oxygenated and deoxygenated hemoglobin in arterial blood, used in the pulse oximetry

speculum a funnel-shaped instrument used to widen and examine canals of the body, e.g., the vagina or nasal canal

sphygmomanometer an instrument used to measure blood pressure

splint a rigid bar or appliance used to stabilize or immobilize a body part

splinter hemorrhages (nails) red or brown longitudinal streaks in the nail

spoon-shaped nail a thin nail with a concave profile

spore a round or oval structure enclosed in a tough capsule

spreader bar a bar designed to spread traction tape away from the bony prominences of the involved body part

sputum the mucus secretion from the lungs, bronchi, and trachea

standing order a written document about policies, rules, regulations, or orders regarding client care that gives the nurse authority to carry out specific actions under certain circumstances, often when a physician is not available; an order that may be carried out indefinitely until another order is written to cancel it

stapes a stirrup-shaped ossicle of the middle ear, it communicates sound waves from the incus to the internal ear

stasis dermatitis inflammation of the skin in the lower extremities caused by poor venous circulation

STAT indicates an order that is to be carried out immediately and only once

station (in pregnancy) the estimated relationship of the fetal presenting part to the ischial spines of the pelvis; based on a numerical scale of −5 to +5 cm, depending upon height above or below the ischial spines

station (mobility) the way a person stands

stereognosis the ability to recognize objects by touching and manipulating them

sterile free from microorganisms, including spores

sterile field a specified area considered free of microorganisms

sterilization a process that destroys all microorganisms, including spores

stoma an artificial opening in the abdominal wall; it may be permanent or temporary

stomatitis inflammation of the oral mucosa

stopcock a valve that controls the flow of fluid or air through a tube

strabismus squinting or crossing of the eyes; uncoordinated eye movements

stress (as a response) the disruption caused by a noxious stimulus or stressor;
(as a stimulus) an event or set of circumstances causing a disrupted response

stressor any factor that produces stress or alters the body's equilibrium

striae skin streaked with reddish or whitish lines on various parts of the body (e.g., breasts, abdomen, thighs, upper arms) as a result of skin stretching from pregnancy, obesity, tumor, or edema

stridor a harsh, crowing sound made on inhalation caused by constriction of the upper airway

stroke volume the amount of blood ejected from the heart with each ventricular contraction

structured communication an interaction between two or more people with a definite planned content

Stryker frame a device consisting of two removable rectangular metal frames (anterior and posterior) with canvas stretched across them

Stryker wedge frame an adaptation of the Stryker frame that is designed so that only one nurse is required to turn the client

stump distal portion of a limb that remains after an amputation

stylet a metal or plastic probe inserted into a needle or cannula to render it stiff and to prevent occlusion of the needle by particles of tissue

subarachnoid space the area between the arachnoid membrane and the pia mater

subcutaneous (hypodermic) under the skin

subjective data (symptoms, covert data) information (data) apparent only to the person affected and can be described or verified only by that person

sublingual under the tongue

substance P a neurotransmitter that acts to enhance transmission of pain impulses across a synapse to other neurons

suctioning the aspiration of secretions by a catheter connected to a suction machine or wall outlet

sudoriferous glands a gland of the dermis that secretes sweat

sulcular technique a technique of brushing the teeth under the gingival margins; it is also referred to as the Bass method

sulcus the groove between the surface of the tooth and the gum

supination moving the bones of the forearm so that the palm of the hand faces upward when held in front of the body

supine hypotensive syndrome a condition characterized by low blood pressure and bradycardia secondary to the uterus compressing the inferior vena cava as the uterus enlarges

supine position a back-lying position

suppository a solid, cone-shaped, medicated substance inserted into the rectum, vagina, or urethra

suprapubic above the pubic arch

surface temperature the temperature of the skin, the subcutaneous tissue, and fat; variable in response to environmental temperature changes

surfactant a lipoprotein mixture secreted in the alveoli that reduces surface tension of the fluid lining the alveoli

surgical asepsis (sterile technique) those practices that keep an area or object free of all microorganisms

surgical bed (anesthetic, recovery, or postoperative bed) a bed with the top covers fanfolded to one side or to the end of the bed

susceptible host any person who is at risk for infection

sutures (of the skull) junction lines of the skull bones

sutures (wound) the surgical stitches used to close accidental or surgical wounds, can also refer to the material used to sew the wound

symmetry correspondence in shape, size, and relative position of parts on opposite sides of a body

symptoms (covert data, subjective data) information (data) apparent only to the person affected and can be described or verified only by that person

syncope faintness

synthesis putting together the parts into the whole

syringe an instrument used to inject or withdraw liquids

systole the period during which the ventricles contract

systolic pressure the pressure of the blood against the arterial walls when the ventricles of the heart contract

tachycardia an abnormally rapid pulse rate, greater than 100 beats per minute

tachypnea abnormally fast respirations, usually more than 24 respirations per minute

talipes (clubfoot) a number of deformities of the foot, especially those occurring congenitally

tartar a visible, hard deposit of plaque and dead bacteria that forms at the gum lines

teaching refers to activities by which one person helps another to learn, the goal of which is to achieve specific learning objectives or behavior changes, a system of activities intended to produce learning

technical skills "hands-on" skills, such as skills required to manipulate equipment, administer injections, and move or reposition clients

tactile related to touch

tension the elasticity of the arteries

terminal hair long, coarse, pigmented body hair

territoriality a concept of the space and things that individuals consider their own

tetany a syndrome manifested by muscle twitching, cramps, convulsions, and sharp flexion of the wrist and ankle joints

thecal whitlow acute inflammation of the tissue surrounding the nail

therapeutic (specialty) bed a bed unit designed to provide a healing environment

therapeutic communication an interactive process between nurse and client that helps the client overcome temporary stress, to get along with other people, to adjust to the unalterable, and to overcome psychological blocks which stand in the way of self-realization

therapeutic touch (TT) a process by which energy is transmitted or transferred from one person to another with the intent of potentiating the healing process of one who is ill or injured

thermography the use of an infrared camera to photograph the surface of the body, thus indicating surface temperatures

thermometer an instrument used to determine body temperature

Thomas leg splint a device which consists of a full ring or half ring around the thigh with two rods on either side of the legs for the purpose of immobilizing and stabilizing a fractured femur

thoracentesis (thoracocentesis) insertion of a needle into the pleural cavity for diagnostic or therapeutic purposes

thrill a vibrating sensation over a blood vessel which indicates turbulent blood flow

throat culture a specimen collected from the mucosa of the oropharynx and tonsillar regions using a culture swab

thrombophlebitis inflammation of a vein followed by formation of a blood clot

ticks parasites that bite into tissue and suck blood

tinea pedis (athlete's foot) a fungal infection of the foot

toe pleat a fold made in the top bedclothes to provide additional space for the client's toes and feet

tomogram an image acquired from a CAT scan

tomography a scanning procedure during which a narrow X-ray beam passes through the body part from different angles; *see also* scan

tonus the slight, continual contraction or tension of muscles

tonic neck reflex (Fencer's position) a reflex in which, when the head is forcibly turned to one side, the arm and leg on that side are extended while the opposite limbs are flexed

topical applied externally, e.g., to the skin or mucous membranes

torsion twisting

total nutrient admixture (TNA) a mixture of dextrose, amino acids, lipids, vitamins and minerals in a single container administered over a 24-hour period

total parenteral nutrition (TPN, hyperalimentation) is the intravenous infusion of water, protein, carbohydrates, electrolytes, minerals, and vitamins through a central vein

tourniquet a device, e.g., a rubber strip, that is wrapped around a body extremity to compress the blood vessels

tracheal lavage the insertion of sterile normal saline through a tracheostomy tube into the trachea

tracheostomy a surgical incision in the trachea below the first or second tracheal cartilage

tracheostomy tube a tube inserted into the trachea through a surgical incision

traction exertion of a pulling force either manually or by a device in order to stabilize and immobilize a fracture

traction tape (strap) adhesive or nonadhesive tape, made of various materials (e.g., elastic, porous) that is applied lengthwise along a limb and attached to a spreader bar

tragus a cartilaginous protrusion at the entrance to the ear canal

transabdominal through or across the abdomen or abdominal wall

transactional stress theory (Lazarus) a set of cognitive, affective, and adaptive responses that arise out of person–environment transactions

transcutaneous electric nerve stimulation (TENS) a non-invasive, nonanalgesic pain control technique that allows the client to assist in the management of acute and chronic pain

transdermal a method of medication administration in which medication is applied to the skin in a gel and is then absorbed

transferrin a blood protein that binds with iron and transports it throughout the body

transfusion (blood) the introduction of whole blood or its components into the venous circulation

transitional milk breast milk produced from 2 to 4 days after delivery until approximately 2 weeks postpartum

transverse lie a lateral or crosswise positioning of the fetus in the uterus

trapeze bar a triangular handgrip suspended from an overbed frame, used by the client

tremor an involuntary trembling of a limb or body part

trimester a three month period during pregnancy

trochanter roll a rolled towel support placed against the hips to prevent external rotation of the legs

trocar a sharp, pointed instrument that fits inside a cannula and is used to pierce body tissues

Trousseau's sign an indicator of tetany; muscular spasm that results when pressure is applied to nerves and vessels of the upper arm

turgor normal fullness and elasticity

turn sheet (pull sheet) a sheet placed beneath the client from the shoulders, as in a draw sheet, to the buttocks which facilitates turning the client and moving him up or down in bed

tympanic membrane the eardrum

tympanites when the presence of excessive flatus leads to stretching and inflation or distention of the intestines

tympany a musical or drum-like sound produced during percussion over an air-filled stomach and abdomen

ultrasonography the use of ultrasound to produce an image of an organ or tissue

ultrasound a noninvasive diagnostic technique that uses sound waves to measure the acoustic density of tissues

unoccupied bed a bed not currently being used by a client

ureterostomy an opening into the ureter

urgency (of urination) the feeling that one must urinate

urinary diversion the surgical rerouting of the urine produced in the kidneys to a site other than the bladder

urinary incontinence a temporary or permanent inability of the external sphincter muscles to control the flow of urine from the bladder

urinary pH the measurement of the concentration of hydrogen ions in the urine that indicates its acidity or alkalinity

urinary reflux backward flow of urine

urinary retention the accumulation of urine in the bladder and inability of the bladder to empty itself

urinary stasis stagnation of urinary flow

urinary suppression the sudden stoppage of urine secretion or excretion

urination (micturition, voiding) the process of emptying the bladder

urinometer (hydrometer) an instrument used to measure the specific gravity of urine

urography an X-ray of any part of the urinary tract after the introduction of a radiopaque dye

uterine prolapse a displacing of the uterus as it pulls downward through the vaginal orifice

uvula a fleshy mass suspended at the midline and back of the palate

vacutainer a device used in the collection of blood specimens that allows the collection of multiple specimens with one needle stick

value something of worth, or a belief held dear by a person

Valsalva maneuver forceful exhalation against a closed glottis, which increases intrathoracic pressure and thus interferes with venous return to the heart

vaporization continuous evaporation of moisture from the respiratory tract and from the mucosa of the mouth and from the skin

variable data data or information that changes over time, e.g., blood pressure, temperature

varicose veins (varicosities) enlarged, twisted, superficial veins, most commonly seen in the lower extremities

vasoconstriction a decrease in the caliber (lumen) of blood vessels

vasodilation an increase in the caliber (lumen) of blood vessels

vasovagal syncope a sudden fainting caused by hypotension induced by the response of the nervous system to abrupt vagal stimulation

vellus fine, nonpigmented body hair

venipuncture puncture of a vein for collection of a blood specimen or for infusion of therapeutic solutions

ventilation the movement of air in and out of the lungs; the process of inhalation and exhalation

verbal communication an interaction between two or more people that uses the spoken or written word

vernix caseosa the whitish, cheesy, greasy protective material found on the skin at birth

vertex the top of the head; crown of the head

vertigo dizziness

vesicostomy an artificial opening into the bladder in which the anterior wall of the bladder is sutured to the abdominal wall and a stoma is formed from the bladder wall

vestibule (ear) a cavity at the entrance to the ear

vial a glass medication container with a sealed rubber cap, for single or multiple doses

vibration a series of vigorous quiverings produced by hands that are placed flat against the chest wall to loosen thick secretions

Virchow's triad three factors that predispose a client to the formation of a thrombophlebitis include impaired venous return to the heart, hypercoagulability of the blood, and injury to a vessel wall

viscosity the physical property that results from friction of molecules in a fluid; the greater the viscosity, the "thicker" the fluid

visual acuity the degree of detail the eye can discern in an image

visual fields the area an individual can see when looking straight ahead

vital capacity the maximum amount of air that can be exhaled after a maximum inhalation

vital signs (cardinal signs) measurements of physiologic functioning, specifically temperature, pulse, respiration, and blood pressure

vitiligo patches of hypopigmented skin, caused by the destruction of melanocytes in the area

voiding (urination, micturition) the process of emptying the bladder

volume-control set a small fluid container attached below the primary infusion container used to administer intermittent intravenous medications

walker a metal, rectangular frame used as an aid to ambulation

water mattress a plastic hollow mattress filled with water designed to reduce pressure on bony prominences

wheezing a rasping or whistling sound in breathing caused by constriction in the upper airway

wound a break in the continuity of a body tissue

xerography (xeromammography) type of X-ray procedure used in examining different body tissues (breast tissue)

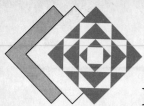

Photographic Credits

Chapter 3 Figure 3–2: Richard Tauber.

Chapter 4 Figure 4–1: William Thompson. Figure 4–3: Richard Tauber.

Chapter 5 Figure 5–1: Richard Tauber.

Chapter 6 Figures 6–1, 6–3, 6–10, 6–11, 6–15: Richard Tauber. Figures 6–4 through 6–8: Ambularm Co.

Chapter 9 Figures 9–2 through 9–6, 9–11, 9–16, 9–17, 9–20, 9–29 through 9–33: William Thompson. Figures 9–18, 9–19: Richard Tauber.

Chapter 10 Figures 10–7, 10–26: Richard Tauber. Figure 10–17: Suzanne Arms Wimberley.

Chapter 11 Figures 11–7, 11–8, 11–31: William Thompson. Figures 11–11, 11–21 through 11–25, 11–27, 11–34 through 11–37, 11–42 through 11–45, 11–49 through 11–53, 11–70, 11–90, 11–92 through 11–99, 11–101 through 11–104: Richard Tauber. Figures 11–62, 11–66, 11–87 through 11–89, 11–100: Tom Ferentz.

Chapter 12 Figures 12–3 through 12–5: Richard Tauber.

Chapter 13 Figure 13–2: Amy H. Snyder.

Chapter 14 Figures 14–3, 14–5: William Thompson.

Chapter 15 Figures 15–8, 15–9: Richard Tauber.

Chapter 16 Figure 16–10: Richard Tauber. Figures 16–18, 16–19: William Thompson.

Chapter 17 Figure 17–2: Tom Ferentz. Figures 17–5, 17–6: Richard Tauber. Figure 17–12: William Thompson.

Chapter 18 Figures 18–3, 18–11: Tom Ferentz. Figure 18–10: George B. Fry III.

Chapter 19 Figures 19–8, 19–14, 19–15, 19–19: William Thompson. Figures 19–21, 19–24: George B. Fry III. Figure 19–22: Richard Tauber.

Chapter 21 Figures 21–7 through 21–36, 21–40, 21–59, 21–60: Tom Ferentz. Figure 21–37: Danninger Medical Technology, Inc. Figures 21–41, 21–42, 21–46: Richard Tauber. Figure 21–40: George B. Fry III. Figures 21–39, 21–43, 21–58: William Thompson.

Chapter 22 Figures 22–1 through 22–3: Tom Ferentz. Figures 22–5, 22–6, 22–12 through 22–15: Richard Tauber. Figure 22–7: Judy Braginsky.

Chapter 23 Figure 23–1: Tom Ferentz. Figures 23–2, 23–5, 23–7: William Thompson.

Chapter 25 Figures 25–3, 25–10, 25–14, 25–17, 25–25 through 25–27: William Thompson. Figures 25–12, 25–13, 25–20, 25–21, 25–24: Tom Ferentz. Figures 25–22, 25–31: Richard Tauber.

Chapter 26 Figure 26–5: William Thompson. Figures 26–7, 26–8: Richard Tauber.

Chapter 28 Figures 28–4, 28–11 through 28–13: William Thompson. Figure 28–25: George B. Fry III.

Chapter 29 Figure 29–3: Judy Braginsky. Figures 29–5 through 29–7, 29–9, 29–10, 29–12, 29–14: William Thompson.

Chapter 30 Figures 30–1, 30–7, Table 30–2: Richard Tauber. Figures 30–3 through 30–5, 30–10 through 30–14: William Thompson. Figure 30–6: Tom Ferentz.

Chapter 31 Figure 31–2: William Thompson. Figure 31–6: Elizabeth D. Elkin. Figure 31–7: Suzanne Arms Wimberley.

Chapter 32 Figures 32–2, 32–3, 32–5, 32–8, 32–9, 32–12: William Thompson. Figures 32–6, 32–7, 32–10, 32–14, 32–15: Richard Tauber.

Chapter 33 Figures 33–7, 33–13, 33–17: William Thompson. Figures 33–11, 33–12: Tom Ferentz. Figures 33–14, 33–15, 33–18: Richard Tauber.

Chapter 34 Figures 34–4 through 34–6, 34–8, 34–10: Richard Tauber. Figure 34–9: William Thompson.

Chapter 35 Figure 35–6: Tom Ferentz. Figures 35–7 through 35–9: Richard Tauber. Figure 35–11: William Thompson. Figure 35–15: George B. Fry III.

Chapter 36 Figures 36–3, 36–4: George B. Fry III. Figures 36–27, 36–29: Richard Tauber. Figures 36–8 through 36–11, 36–16, 36–34, 36–36, 36–39 through 36–42: William Thompson.

Chapter 38 Figures 38–4, 38–5: Richard Tauber.

Chapter 39 Figure 39–13: Tom Ferentz. Figures 39–14, 39–15: George B. Fry III.

Chapter 40 Figures 40–1, 40–2, 40–6, 40–8, 40–15: William Thompson.

Chapter 41 Figure 41–1: Tom Ferentz. Figures 41–2, 41–4: William Thompson. Figures 41–3, 41–5 through 41–7: Richard Tauber.

Chapter 42 Figures 42–3 through 42–5, 42–9: William Thompson.

Chapter 43 Figures 43–2, 43–4, 43–6 through 43–11: William Thompson.

Chapter 44 Figures 44–2, 44–4, 44–6, 44–9, 44–16: William Thompson.

Chapter 45 Figure 45–10: Richard Tauber. Figures 45–3, 45–4, 45–6: George B. Fry III. Figures 45–2, 45–5, 45–7: William Thompson.

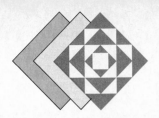

Index

Abbreviations, commonly used, 58, 59
  in medication orders, 828
Abdomen, 262–263
  See also Gastrointestinal tract
  assessing, 263–268
  in pediatric client, 316
  in pregnant client, 329
  changes in pregnancy, 328–329
  divisions and landmarks, 262–263
Abdominal (ABD) pads, 922
  with binders, 951, 953, 954
Abdominal binder, 951, 954, 955
Abdominal breathing exercises, 738, 743
  teaching, 744
Abdominal distention, assessing for, 264
Abdominal paracentesis, 347, 351
  assisting with, 351–353
Abdominal sounds, assessing, 265
  in pregnant client, 329
Abducens nerve, assessing, 274
Abduction, defined, 500
Abrasions, 209
Abruptio placentae, indications of, 330, 334
Absorption powders, as wound dressings, 921
Abuse, assessing child for, 303
Accessory nerve, assessing, 274
Accidents, incident reports on, 60, 61
Accountability, 7
Accuracy concerns, in record keeping, 57
Achilles reflex, assessing, 276
Acid-base balance, 582–583
  wound healing and, 915
Acidemia, 583
Acid-fast bacillus (AFB) test, sputum specimen for, 739
Acidifying IV solutions, 589
Acidosis, 583
  metabolic (base bicarbonate deficit), 583
  respiratory (carbonic acid excess), 583
Acne/Acne vulgaris, 209, 379
  assessing for, 209
Acquired immune deficiency syndrome. *See* AIDS
Acrochordons (cutaneous tags), in elderly, 211
Acromegaly, 214
Actinic keratoses, 211
Active-assistive ROM exercises, 514
Active involvement, as learning factor, 78
Active listening, 68, 70–73
  for pain relief, 906
Active ROM exercises, as isotonic, 512
Activities of daily living (ADLs)
  active ROM exercises vs., 512
  assessing for discharge, 118
  as isotonic exercise, 512
  in traction care, 1017
Activity
  fecal elimination and, 658
  pulse rate and, 169, 171

Activity deficit, nursing diagnosis, 26
Activity-exercise pattern, assessing, 24, 28
Activity intolerance, nursing strategies and, 35. *See also* Immobility
Activity tolerance
  assessing for, 498
  defined, 500
Acupressure (shiatsu massage), 896
Adaptability, in verbal communication, 65
Adduction, defined, 500
ADD-Vantage IV delivery system, 878
Adenosine triphosphate (ATP), body heat production and, 159
Adhesive skin traction, 1018
ADLs. *See* Activities of daily living
Administration sets
  for blood transfusion, 617
  for IV infusion, 591
  preparing, 594–595
  selecting, 594
Admission, 104–116
  discharge planning at, 107
  nursing process guide, 105–106
  practices and trends, 106–109
  techniques for adult client, 109–112
  techniques for pediatric client, 113–115
Admission sheet, 45
Adolescents
  breast assessment in, 315, 316
  breast development in, 258
  dietary needs, 539, 540
  female, genitals assessment in, 283
  hair development in, 425
  nutritional needs, 539, 540
  preadmission procedures for, 108
  preoperative preparation for, 985
Adrenal glands
  in Cushing's syndrome, 214
  locating, 263
Adult, competent, defined, 8
Advocate, defined, 6
Aerobic culture, wound drainage specimen for, 918
Aerosolization (inhalation therapy), 847
Aerosol spray or foam, defined, 824
AF (air-fluidized) beds, 1031
AFB. *See* Acid-fast bacillus
Affect, assessing, 205, 206
African-American clients, hair care for, 426, 428–429
Afternoon care, 378
Afterpains, postpartal, 340
Against medical authority (AMA) form, 8, 121, 122
Age
  See also specific age groups
  adjusting for prematurity, 297
  arterial compliance and, 186
  as barrier to learning, 80

blood pressure and, 161, 186, 187
body temperature and, 160–161
chest shape changes with, 243
eyelid abnormalities and, 217
fecal elimination and, 658, 660
fluid and electrolyte balance and, 578
fluid proportions and, 575–576
fluid requirements and, 577
glaucoma and, 216
informed consent and, 8
male secondary sex characteristics and, 286
medication administration and, 857
pain tolerance and, 904
presbyopia and, 215–216
pulse rate and, 161, 169
pulse rate assessment site and, 171
respiratory rate and, 161
skin atrophy with, 209
teaching goals and, 81
vital signs and, 161. *See also specific signs*
Agglutinins (antibodies), 617
Agglutinogens, blood transfusions and, 617
AIDS, wound care precautions, 920. *See also specific procedures*
Air, as contrast agent, 368
Air (alternating pressure) mattress, 443
Airborne transmission of microorganisms, 133–134
Air conduction of sound, 224
Air detector, in infusion pumps or controllers, 612
Air-fluidized (AF) beds, 1031
Airway, artificial. *See* Artificial airways
Alarms, on infusion pumps or controllers, 611–612
Albinism, 209
Alcohol, in cooling sponge bath, 976
Alcohol use, communication process and, 67
Algor mortis, 125
Alignment of body. *See* Body alignment
Alkalemia, 583
Alkalinity of body fluids, 582–583
Alkalizing IV solutions, 589
Alkalosis, 583
  metabolic (base bicarbonate excess), 583
  respiratory (carbonic acid deficit), 583
Allergies
  diets for, 539
  heat or cold therapy and, 957
  infant formulas and, 551
  recording at admission, 111–112
  skin sensitivity and, 379–380
  tube feedings and, 561
Alopecia (hair loss), 211, 425
  assessing for, 212
  in pediatric client, 304
Altered health maintenance, as nursing diagnosis, 26, 27

Altered nutrition, as nursing diagnosis, 26
Alternating pressure (air) mattress, 443
AMA (against medical authority) form, 8, 121, 122
Amblyopia (lazy eye), 307
Ambu bag, in tracheostomy or endotracheal suctioning, 799–780
Ambularm safety monitoring device, 91–93
Ambulation, 520–533
  assisting with, 521–524
    with cane, 524–526
    with crutches, 527, 529–533
    with walker, 526
  common problems, 520
  nursing process guide, 498–499
  postoperative, 994
  preambulatory exercises, 520–521
AMC (arm muscle circumference), 541, 543
American Hospital Association, Patient's Bill of Rights, 12, 13
American Nurses' Association (ANA)
  on assessment focus, 18
  code of ethics, 11–12
  nursing practice defined by, 2, 7
Amino acid urine test, 686
Ammonia dermatitis. *See* Diaper rash
Amniocentesis, 347, 360
  assisting with, 360–362
Amniotic fluid, assessing, 334
Ampules, for parenteral medications, 859
  mixing medications from vial and, 862–863
  preparing medications from, 860–861
Amputation, stump bandage for, 949–951
Amylase urine test, 686
Anabolism/catabolism, immobility and, 509–510
Anaerobic culture, wound drainage specimen for, 918–919
Analgesia
  administering, 906–907
    narcotics caution, 906–907
    patient-controlled analgesia (PCA) pumps, 907–910
  endogenous, 904–905
Analysis, in diagnosis, 16
ANA. *See* American Nurses' Association
Anderson frame (bed cradle), 444
Anemia
  nail atrophy and, 435
  pressure sores and, 482
Aneroid sphygmomanometers, 187, 188
Anesthesia
  fecal elimination and, 660
  as flatulence cause, 661
  reports on, as part of record, 46
Anesthesia (loss of touch sensation), 279
Anesthetic bed. *See* Surgical bed

Anger
allowing expression of, 69
mediating, 894
as response to fear, 905–906
Angina pectoris, nitroglycerine
patch for, 827
Angiocatheter, for IV therapy, 591
starting an infusion with,
596–600
Angiography, 368, 371
contrast agent for, 372
Angle of Louis, 242
Anions/cations, 576
Anisocoria (unequal pupils), 217
Ankle, hinge joint in, 505
Ankle muscles, assessing, 270,
498
Ankle restraints, 96
applying, 98, 100
Ankylosed collagen tissue, 507
Anorexia, immobility as cause
of, 510
Anoscopy, 364, 366
Antepartal period, 326. See also
Pregnancy
Anterior axillary lines, 241
Anterior cervical nodes, 236
assessing, 238
Anterior chamber of eye, assess-
ing, 220
Anterior superior iliac spines, as
abdominal landmark, 263
Anthelix of ear, 224
Anthelmintics, 662
Anthropometric measurements,
541
techniques for taking, 542–543
Antibiotic solutions, for irrigating
a wound, 936
Anticipatory grieving, as nursing
diagnosis, 26, 30, 31
Antiemboli stockings, 990
applying, 990–992
Antiemetic, transdermal administration of, 827
Antimicrobial solutions, for irrigating a wound, 936
Antiseptics, role of, 134
Anuria, 685
Anus, assessing, 290–291
in pediatric client, 321
in pregnant client, 327, 331
Anxiety
at admission, 106
assessing for, in intrapartal
period, 333
body temperature and, 161
bruxism (teeth grinding) as
sign of, 311
communication process and,
68, 75
as learning barrier, 78, 82
minimizing, 893–894
guided imagery for, 898–900
for pain relief, 905–906
progressive relaxation for,
896–898
nonverbal communication of,
66
preoperative, 984
special studies and, 346
Aorta
in abdominal assessment, 266
locating, 262, 263
Aortic area of precordium, locating, 253
in children, 314
Apex of heart, 251
Aphasia, 271–272
Apical lung expansion exercises,
738, 743
teaching, 744–745
Apical (mitral) area of precordium. See Point of maximal
impulse (PMI)

Apical pulse, 168
assessing, 174–176
reasons for using, 169
Apical-radial pulse, assessing,
176–177
APIE format, 54–55
Apnea, 184, 739
Apocrine glands, developmental
changes in, 378
Apothecaries' system of mea-
sures, 829, 830
Appearance, assessing, 205–206
Appendix, locating, 263
Appropriateness, in record keep-
ing, 57–58
Approximation, in wound heal-
ing, 916
Aquathermia or aquamatic pads,
961
applying, 961–964
Aqueous solution, defined, 824
Aqueous suspension, defined, 824
Arcus senilis, in eye, 223
Argyle chest drainage system,
814, 815
setting up, 816
Arm amputation, stump bandage
for, 949
Arm casts, 1006
pressure areas with, 1007
Arm muscle circumference
(AMC), 541, 543
Arm slings, 951, 952–953, 955
Arm traction, 1021
Arrector pili muscles, 424
Arterial blood flow, assessing, 257
Arterial blood pressure, 186
Arterial wall elasticity
assessing, 173
pulse rate and, 170
Arteriography, 371
Arteriosclerosis, blood pressure
and, 186, 187
Arthritis
heat therapy for, 958
pain relief measures, 907
Artificial airways, 791–811
endotracheal, 793
suctioning, 798–801
nursing process guide, 792
oropharyngeal/nasopharygeal,
792–793
inserting and maintaining,
795–797
tracheostomy, 793–795
types of, 792–795
Artificial dentures
assessing, 233
cleaning, 406–407
Artificial eyes, care of, 416–418
Ascending colon, locating, 262,
263
Ascites, 351
Asepsis, 134–135
surgical, 134–135, 136–137,
138–139
Aspirin, 907
Assault, implications for nurses,
8
Assessing, 198–292
See also Physical examination;
specific areas of body; specific systems
at admission, 105, 109, 112
artificial airway, 792
for bandage or binder, 944, 945
bathing as opportunity for, 380
blood pressure
equipment for, 187–189
in infants, 194–195
methods, 189–190
sites for, 189
techniques, 191–195
body temperature, sites for,
162–163

in cast care, 1001, 1007–1009,
1010
for central venous line, 629
of chest drainage, 813
for cold therapy, 957
cultural behaviors relevant to,
199
with pediatric client, 295,
296, 297, 306
data collection methods, 20–24
data evaluation, 40
data sources, 19–20
data structure or framework,
24
data types, 19
at discharge, 118
for ear care, 401
for exercise and ambulation,
498
for eye care, 400–401
for fecal elimination, 656
fetal heart rate (FHR), 177–181
for fluid and electrolyte balance, 57
for foot care, 424
for gastric or jejunal feeding,
559
for hair care, 423
for heat and cold therapy, 957
for infection risk, 132
for intravenous therapy, 588
medications, 823
for mouth care, 400
for moving clients, 453
for nail care, 423
nursing health history, 199
in nursing process, 16, 19–24
reassessing, 38
for nutrition needs, 536
in ostomy care, 722
for oxygen therapy, 775
pain, 903
perioperative, 981–982
pictorial guide to, 240a
for positioning client, 479
in postoperative period,
982–983
for postural drainage, 737
pulse rate
apical pulse, 174–176
apical-radial pulse, 176–177
fetal heart rate (FHR),
177–181
peripheral pulse, 169–173
for respiratory assistive
devices, 737
respiratory rate, 183–186
in antepartal period, 328
in intrapartal period, 333
for safety problems, 87
for skin hygiene care, 377
in SOAP/SOAPIER/APIE for-
mats, 54, 55
for special studies, 346
stress and coping, 891
in therapeutic touch, 900
in traction care, 1016,
1026–1027
urinary elimination, 681
vital signs, 158–196. See also
specific signs
for wound care, 915
Associative thinking, 18
Astigmatism, 216
Ataxia, 276
Atelectasis
immobility as cause of, 509
in pediatric client, 313
as postoperative complication,
983
Athlete's foot (tinea pedis), 438
fissures as sign of, 209
Athletics, pulse rate and, 171
Atony, fecal elimination and, 660
ATP. See Adenosine triphosphate

Atrioventricular (AV) node, 366
Atrophy
assessing muscles for, 269
disuse, 507
of nails, 435
of skin
described, 209
immobility and, 511
Attention span, assessing, 272
Attentive listening, 68, 70–73
Attitudes
assessing, 205, 206
communication process and,
68
defined, 11
ethical aspects of nursing and,
11
Audiometric evaluation, 224–225
Audiotape reports, 60, 61
Audio-visual aids, as teaching
strategy, 81, 82
Audit, record as tool for, 45
Auditory aphasia, 272
Auditory meatus, external, 224
Auditory nerve, assessing, 274
Auricles, 224
assessing, 225–226
in pediatric client, 309
Auscultation, 204
in blood pressure assessment,
189–190, 192, 193
for infants, 194, 195
in pulse rate assessment, 170
Auscultatory gap, 190
Automated client care plan,
48–49
Autonomy, as environmental fac-
tor, 87–88
Autopsy, 126
AV (atrioventricular) node, 366
Axillae
assessing, 258–260
in pregnant client, 329
temperature assessment in,
162–163, 165, 166
temperature variations in,
162
Axillary crutch, 527
Axillary lymph nodes, assessing,
260
in pediatric client, 316
Axillary muscles, 260
Axillary tail of Spence, 258

Babinski (plantar) reflex, assessing, 276, 320
Back-lying position. See Dorsal
recumbent position
Back pain, heat therapy for, 958
Back rubs
for pressure sore prevention,
387–389
for stress reduction, 894,
895–896
Bacteria
fecal elimination and, 658, 660
on normal skin, 378
hygienic care and, 379
Bactericidal action of skin, 378
Bagging contaminated material,
145–146
Balance
body mechanics and, 454–455,
456
defined, 454
tests of, 277
Ball-and-socket joints
in hip, 504–505
in shoulder, 501–502
Ballard Trach Care Suction System, 798
Bandages, 946
basic techniques, 945, 946–948
binder, 951–955
clinical guidelines, 945

(continued)

Suprarenal gland, locating, 263
Suprasternal retraction, defined, 184
Surface temperature, core temperature vs., 159
Surfactants, immobility and, 509
Surgery
See also Perioperative period; Postoperative period; Preoperative period
central venous line insertion by, 630, 631
consent for, 984
fecal elimination and, 660
as flatulence cause, 661
fluid and electrolyte balance and, 578
intentional wounds in, 916
drains for, 932
dry dressings for, 922–926
postoperative complications, 983, 994
sutures, 937–941
medication orders and, 827
reports on, as part of record, 46
Surgical asepsis, 134–135
maintaining, 136–137, 138–139
sterile field, 148–152
sterile gloves, 153–156
sterile gown, 155–156
surgical hand scrub, 146–148
Surgical bed, 445
making, 992–993
Surgical drains, 932–936
Surgipads, 922
Susceptible host, 134
Sustained maximal inspiration (SMI) devices, 738, 746
assisting client with, 747–748
Sutures, 937–938
common types, 938
removing, 939–941
Sutures (skull), assessing, 305
Suture scissors, 938
Sweating (diaphoresis)
body heat lowered by, 160
fluid loss through, 577
Sweat (sudoriferous) glands, 378
Swelling, with cast
See also Edema
assessing for, 1001
preventing, 1008
Swing carry, 89–90
Symbols, commonly used, 58, 59, 828
Sympathetic stimulation, body heat production and, 160
Symptoms
in PES format, 26–27, 30
as subjective data, 19
Synthesis, in diagnosis, 16
Synthetic casts, 1005
care of, 1007, 1011–1012
preventing irritation by, 1010–1011
Synthetic dressings, 921
moist transparent wound barriers, 928–930
Syringes
oral, for administering medication, 833
for parenteral medication, 857–858
for wound irrigation, 936
Syrup, defined, 824
Systole, 252, 254
Systolic pressure, 186
changes in pregnancy, 328

Tablets, 834
administering, 833–836
sublingually, 825
defined, 824
Tachycardia, 169

Tachypnea, 184, 739
Tactile discrimination, 279, 282. *See also* Sensory function
Tactile fremitus, assessing, 246–247, 249
in pediatric client, 313
Tail of Spence, 258
Talipes, 318
Tandem intravenous alignment, 592–593
medication delivery with, 882–883
Tape-recorded reports, 60, 61
Tapeworms, 662
Tartar, on teeth, 232
Taste, changes in elderly, 235
T-binder, 951, 954, 955
TB. *See* Tubercle bacillus
Teaching, 76–85
See also specific procedures
active ROM exercises, 512
biofeedback, 900
breathing exercises, 743–745
before surgery, 984–986
cast care, 1012–1013
crutch use, 527, 529–533
defined, 5, 79
at discharge, 123
exercises with cast, 1012
flatulence prevention, 676
guided imagery, 898–900
implementing plan for, 82–84
learning factors, 78–79
learning vs., 78
nursing process guide, 77
as nursing role, 5
ostomy care, 722
irrigation, 730–731
urinary diversion ostomy, 735
peritoneal dialysis methods, 716
planning for, 77, 80–82
poisoning prevention, 94
preadmission, 106–107
preoperative, 984–988
principles of, 80
progressive relaxation, 897–898
as structured communication, 64
technique, 83–84
tooth decay prevention, 403
walker use, 526
Teaching role of nurse, 5
See also Teaching; *specific procedures*
learning factors, 78–79
nursing process guide, 77
Technical skills requirements, 4–5
Teeth, 231, 402
anatomy of, 402
assessing, 233
in pediatric client, 311
brushing and flossing, 403–406
developmental changes in, 235, 311, 402
diagrams, 232, 311
Tegaderm, 928
Telangiectasias, 209
in elderly, 211
Telepaque tablets, 372
Telephone orders, for medication, 827. *See also* Verbal orders
Telfa gauze, 921–922
Temperature, body. *See* Body temperature
Temperature, environmental
as comfort factor, 88
communication and, 68
fluid and electrolyte balance and, 578
Temperature sensation, 279, 281. *See also* Sensory function
Temperature-sensitive tape, 164

Temporal pulse, 168
reasons for using, 169
Temporary carriers, 133
Temporomandibular joint (TMJ), 501
TENS (transcutaneous electric nerve stimulation), 910–912
Tents
face, 781
administering oxygen by, 783–785
humidity, 781
administering oxygen by, 785–786
Tepid sponge bath, 976
Tepid water, defined, 960
Terminal hair, 424
Terminology, standard, 58, 59
in medication orders, 828
Territoriality, as environmental factor, 88
Testes
assessing, in pediatric client, 320, 321
development of, 286
palpating, 288
Tetany, hypocalcemia and, 581
Thecal whitlow, 435
Therapeutic baths, 380
Therapeutic beds, 1029–1038
CircOlectric, 1031, 1035
turning client on, 1036–1037
Nelson bed, 1031, 1038
Stryker frame/Stryker wedge frame, 1030–1032
turning client on, 1032–1034
Therapeutic communication, 64
nontherapeutic responses, 71, 73–74
techniques for, 70–73
Therapeutic environment, 87
Therapeutic touch (TT), 900–901
Therapulse bed, 1031
Thermal receptor adaptation, heat or cold therapy and, 959
Thermography, 372
Thermometers, 163–164, 165
Thermoplastic casts, 1005
Thigh blood pressure, 189
techniques, 193
Thinking/Thinking skills
creative, 4, 18
critical, 4, 17–18, 19
directed vs. associative, 18
Thomas leg splint, 1024
pressure areas in, 1025
Thoracentesis, 347, 353
assisting with, 354–355
Thoracic expansion, assessing, 246
Thora-Drain chest drainage system, 815
Thorax, 241–244
assessing, 241, 245–251
in pediatric client, 313
in pregnant client, 326, 328
changes in elderly, 243, 251
changes in pregnancy, 328
chest shape and size, 243–244
chest wall landmarks, 241–243
Thought processes, assessing, 206
Thready pulse, 170
"3 in 1" TPN preparation, 651
Thrill, assessing carotid artery for, 255
Throat culture, specimen collection for, 739, 741–743
Thromboembolism, as cast complication, 1001, 1003
Thrombophlebitis
formation of, 508
as postoperative complication, 983

Thrombus (blood clot)
as immobility danger, 508–509
massage caution, 387
as postoperative complication, 983
as traction complication, 1016
Thumb, saddle joint in, 504
Thumb spica, 945, 947–948
Thyroid disorders, 214
Thyroid cartilage, 236
assessing, 239
Thyroid gland, 236
assessing, 239–240
in pediatric client, 313
Thyroxine
body heat production and, 160
body temperature and, 161
Ticks, 425
Tie tapes (Montgomery straps), 922, 923
Time, recording, 56–57
Timed urine specimens, 685, 686
collecting, 690–692
Timing
communication process and, 65, 68
as learning factor, 79
of vital sign assessment, 159
Tincture, defined, 824
Tinea pedis. *See* Athlete's foot
Tissue damage. *See* Pressure sores
Tissue forceps, 151
Tissue perfusion, postoperative assessment, 982
Tissue removal procedures. *See* Body fluid or tissue removal procedures
Titles, using on records, 57
TMJ (temporomandibular joint), 501
TNA (total nutrient admixture), 651
Toenails, ingrown (incurvated), 435. *See also* Nails
Toes, joints in, 505–506
Toilet training, assisting with, 660
Tomogram, 374
Tongue
assessing, 234
in pediatric client, 311
inflammation of (glossitis), 232
role of, 402
special cleaning techniques, 409
Tonic neck reflex (Fencer's position), 312
assessing, 319
Tonsils, 231
assessing, 235
in pediatric client, 311, 312
Tonus, 454
Tooth care. *See* Teeth
Topical enzymes, as wound dressings, 921
Topical medication, 825, 826, 837
administering, 837–838
assessing client for, 823
types of, 824, 825, 837. *See also specific types*
Total nutrient admixture (TNA), 651
Total parenteral nutrition (TPN), 647–649
See also Nutrient solutions
catheter type for, 630
central venous line used for, 629
complications of, 648
components of, 647
initiating and monitoring, 649–650
intralipid therapy and, 647, 651–653